DISEASES OF THE LIVER
AND BILIARY SYSTEM

Diseases of the Liver and Biliary System

SHEILA SHERLOCK
DBE, MD (Edin.), Hon. DSc (Edin., New York, Yale),
Hon. MD (Cambridge, Dublin, Leuven, Lisbon,
Mainz, Oslo, Padua, Toronto), Hon. LLD (Aberd.),
FRCP, FRCPE, FRACP, Hon. FRCCP,
Hon. FRCPI, Hon. FACP

Professor of Medicine,
Royal Free Hospital School of Medicine,
University of London

JAMES DOOLEY
BSc, MD, FRCP

Senior Lecturer and Honorary Consultant in Medicine,
Royal Free Hospital School of Medicine,
University of London

TENTH EDITION

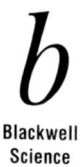

Blackwell
Science

© 1963, 1968, 1975, 1981,
1985, 1989, 1993, 1997 by
Blackwell Science Ltd
Editorial Offices:
Osney Mead, Oxford OX2 0EL
25 John Street, London WC1N 2BL
23 Ainslie Place, Edinburgh EH3 6AJ
350 Main Street, Malden
    Massachusetts 02148-5018, USA
54 University Street, Carlton
    Victoria 3053, Australia

Other Editorial Offices:
Arnette Blackwell SA
    224, Boulevard Saint Germain
    75007 Paris, France

Blackwell Wissenschafts-Verlag GmbH
    Kurfürstendamm 57
    10707 Berlin, Germany

    Zehetnergasse 6
    A-1140 Wien
    Austria

Set by Excel Typesetters Co., Hong Kong
Printed and bound in Italy
by Rotolito Lombarda, Milan

The Blackwell Science Logo is a
trade mark of Blackwell Science Ltd,
registered at the United Kingdom
Trade Marks Registry

First published 1955
Reprinted 1956
Second edition 1958
Reprinted 1959, 1961
Third edition 1963
Reprinted 1965, 1966
Fourth edition 1968
Reprinted 1969, 1971
Fifth edition 1975
Sixth edition 1981
Reprinted 1982, 1983
Seventh edition 1985
Reprinted 1986, 1987
Eighth edition 1989
Reprinted 1991
Ninth edition 1993
Reprinted 1993
Tenth edition 1997

German third edition 1965
Greek fourth edition 1972
Japanese fourth edition 1973
    fifth edition 1980
Spanish first edition 1956
    third edition 1966
    fifth edition 1976
    eighth edition 1991
Portuguese fourth edition 1970
    fifth edition 1978
    seventh edition 1988
    eighth edition 1991
Turkish fifth edition 1981
Italian eighth edition 1991
Italian ninth edition 1994
Spanish ninth edition 1996

DISTRIBUTORS

Marston Book Services Ltd
PO Box 269
Abingdon
Oxon OX14 4YN
(*Orders*: Tel: 01235 465500
            Fax: 01235 465555)
USA
Blackwell Science, Inc.
Commerce Place
350 Main Street
Malden, MA 02148-5018
(*Orders*: Tel: 800 215-1000
            617 876-7000
            Fax: 617 492-5263)
Canada
Copp Clark Professional
200 Adelaide St, West, 3rd Floor
Toronto, Ontario M5H 1W7
(*Orders*: Tel: 800 759-6102
            617 388-8250
            Fax: 617 388-8255)
Australia
Blackwell Science Pty Ltd
54 University Street
Carlton, Victoria 3053
(*Orders*: Tel: 3 9347 0300
            Fax: 3 9347 5001)

A catalogue record for this title
is available from the British Library

ISBN 0-86542-906-5

Library of Congress
Cataloging-in-publication Data

Sherlock, Sheila, Dame.
    Diseases of the liver and
    biliary system/Sheila Sherlock,
    James Dooley.—10th ed.
    p. cm.
    Includes bibliographical references
    and index.
    ISBN 0-86542-906-5
    1. Liver—Diseases.
    2. Biliary tract—Diseases.
    I. Dooley, James. II. Title.
    [DNLM: 1. Liver Diseases.
    2. Biliary Tract Diseases.
    WI 700 S552d 1996]
    RC845.S52   1997
    616.3'6—dc20
    DNLM/DLC
    for Library of Congress   96-23961
                                            CIP

Contents

20   Alcohol and the Liver, 385

21   Iron Overload States, 405

22   Wilson's Disease, 417

23   Nutritional and Metabolic Liver Diseases, 427

xiv   *Contents*

Preface to the Tenth Edition

Since the ninth edition was published in 1993, over 20,000 papers focusing on the liver and its diseases have been published. Included in this massive literature are a remarkable number of discoveries and new treatments. These have made revision of of this tenth edition an exciting and challenging project.

Molecular genetics has identified the gene for several hepatic diseases including Wilson's disease, and a candidate gene for haemochromatosis. These findings should help patients in diagnosis and management and scientists in explaining mechanisms and clinical variations. Molecular virology has advanced the understanding of hepatitis C and given us hepatitis G. Banding of oesophageal varices and experience with TIPS have influenced the treatment of portal hypertension. Magnetic resonance cholangiography and endoscopic ultrasonography have added considerable momentum to imaging of the biliary tract. Liver transplantation has become part of today's routine for the failing liver, both acute and chronic.

The tenth edition reflects these wide-ranging advances in hepatobiliary disease. There are more than 1000 new references and 100 new figures. We have endeavoured to distil the new and often complex concepts and findings to make them accessible to students, interns, postgraduate trainees as well as generalists. In a subject of increasing complexity we hope that specialists will find our approach to the new concepts and discoveries appealing.

We owe a great debt to our colleagues, especially Professor P.J. Scheuer and Dr A.P. Dhillon for histological material and Dr R. Dick, who has generously provided many of the figures. We would also like to express our indebtedness to Dr Leslie Berger, Dr Andrew Burroughs, Professor Geoffrey Dusheiko, Dr David Harry, Professor Kenneth Hobbs, Professor Neil McIntyre, Professor John Summerfield, Dr Tony Watkinson and Professor Roger Williams.

Miss Aileen Duggan and Miss Catherine Purcell have made light of the secretarial burden. Miss Anne Fletcher and her staff in the Royal Free Hospital Library have been meticulous with the bibliography. The clarity and style of the figures, both new and those preserved from previous editions, owes much to the artistry of Miss Janice Cox over many years.

We are particularly grateful to Rebecca Huxley and her colleagues at Blackwell Science for help with both manuscript and proofs. We would also like to thank Jane Fallows, who has worked on reformatting all the line drawings for the computer and drawn several new figures for this tenth edition.

In the course of nine editions and 40 years, many readers have followed the senior author's steps through marriage and motherhood as though prefaces were some form of soap opera. Encouraged by the many letters of friendship, she and her husband, Dr D. Geraint James, are delighted to announce that their grandchild, Alice, born on 28 October 1991, has been joined by a sister, Emily, on 30 August 1994. As Alice and Emily grow into the 21st century, they will see from these ten editions that hepatology has succeeded as a discipline in its own right, moulded by a close teamwork of clinicians, radiologists, pathologists and molecular biologists.

SHEILA SHERLOCK
JAMES DOOLEY
November 1996

Preface to the First Edition

My aim in writing this book has been to present a comprehensive and up-to-date account of diseases of the liver and biliary system, which I hope will be of value to physicians, surgeons and pathologists and also a reference book for the clinical student. The modern literature has been reviewed with special reference to articles of general interest. Many older more specialized classical contributions have therefore inevitably been excluded.

Disorders of the liver and biliary system may be classified under the traditional concept of individual diseases. Alternatively, as I have endeavoured in this book, they may be described by the functional and morphological changes which they produce. In the clinical management of a patient with liver disease, it is important to assess the degree of disturbance of four functional and morphological components of the liver—hepatic cells, vascular system (portal vein, hepatic artery and hepatic veins), bile ducts and reticulo-endothelial system. The typical reaction pattern is thus sought and recognized before attempting to diagnose the causative insult. Clinical and laboratory methods of assessing each of these components are therefore considered early in the book. Descriptions of individual diseases follow as illustrative examples. It will be seen that the features of hepatocellular failure and portal hypertension are described in general terms as a foundation for subsequent discussion of virus hepatitis, nutrition liver disease and the cirrhoses. Similarly blood diseases and infections of the liver are included with the reticulo-endothelial system, and disorders of the biliary tract follow descriptions of acute and chronic bile duct obstruction.

I would like to acknowledge my indebtedness to my teachers, the late Professor J. Henry Dible, the late Professor Sir James Learmonth and Professor Sir John McMichael, who stimulated my interest in hepatic disease, and to my colleagues at the Postgraduate Medical School and elsewhere who have generously invited me to see patients under their care. I am grateful to Dr A. G. Bearn for criticizing part of the typescript and to Dr A. Paton for his criticisms and careful proof reading. Miss D. F. Atkins gave much assistance with proof reading and with the bibliography. Mr Per Saugman and Mrs J. M. Green of Blackwell Scientific Publications have co-operated enthusiastically in the production of this book.

The photomicrographs were taken by Mr E. V. Willmott, FRPS, and Mr C. A. P. Graham from sections prepared by Mr J. G. Griffin and the histology staff of the Postgraduate Medical School. Clinical photographs are the work of Mr C. R. Brecknell and his assistants. The black and white drawings were made by Mrs H. M. G. Wilson and Mr D. Simmonds. I am indebted to them all for their patience and skill.

The text includes part of unpublished material included in a thesis submitted in 1944 to the University of Edinburgh for the degree of MD, and part of an essay awarded the Buckston–Browne prize of the Harveian Society of London in 1953. Colleagues have allowed me to include published work of which they are jointly responsible. Dr Patricia P. Franklyn and Dr R. E. Steiner have kindly loaned me radiographs. Many authors have given me permission to reproduce illustrations and detailed acknowledgments are given in the text. I wish also to thank the editors of the following journals for permission to include illustrations: *American Journal of Medicine, Archives of Pathology, British Heart Journal, Circulation, Clinical Science, Edinburgh Medical Journal, Journal of Clinical Investigation, Journal of Laboratory and Clinical Investigation, Journal of Pathology and Bacteriology, Lancet, Postgraduate Medical Journal, Proceedings of the Staff Meetings of the Mayo Clinic, Quarterly Journal of Medicine, Thorax* and also the following publishers: Butterworth's Medical Publications, J. & A. Churchill Ltd, The Josiah Macy Junior Foundation and G. D. Searle & Co.

Finally I must thank my husband, Dr D. Geraint James, who, at considerable personal inconvenience, encouraged me to undertake the writing of this book and also criticized and rewrote most of it. He will not allow me to dedicate it to him.

SHEILA SHERLOCK

Chapter 1
Anatomy and Function

The liver, the largest organ in the body, weighs 1200–1500 g and comprises one-fiftieth of the total adult body weight. It is relatively larger in infancy, comprising one-eighteenth of the birth weight. This is mainly due to a large left lobe.

Sheltered by the ribs in the right upper quadrant, the upper border lies approximately at the level of the nipples. There are two anatomical lobes, the right being about six times the size of the left (figs 1.1, 1.2, 1.3). Lesser segments of the right lobe are the *caudate lobe* on the posterior surface and the *quadrate lobe* on the inferior surface. The right and left lobes are separated anteriorly by a fold of peritoneum called the falciform ligament, posteriorly by the fissure for the ligamentum venosum and inferiorly by the fissure for the ligamentum teres.

The liver has a double blood supply. The *portal vein* brings venous blood from the intestines and spleen and the *hepatic artery*, coming from the coeliac axis, supplies the liver with arterial blood. These vessels enter the liver through a fissure, the *porta hepatis*, which lies far back on the inferior surface of the right lobe. Inside the porta, the portal vein and hepatic artery divide into branches to the right and left lobes, and the right and left hepatic bile ducts join to form the common hepatic duct. The *hepatic nerve plexus* contains fibres from the sympathetic ganglia T7 to T10, which synapse in the coeliac plexus, the right

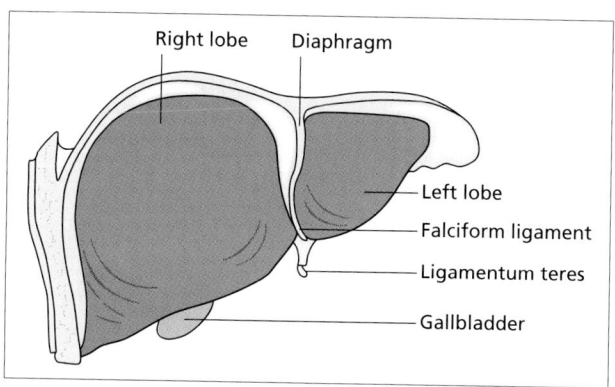

Fig. 1.1. Anterior view of the liver.

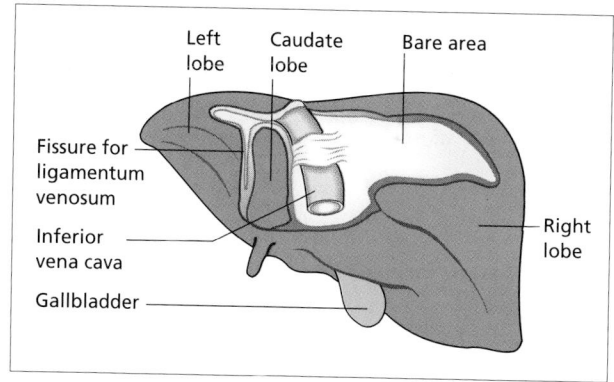

Fig. 1.2. Posterior view of the liver.

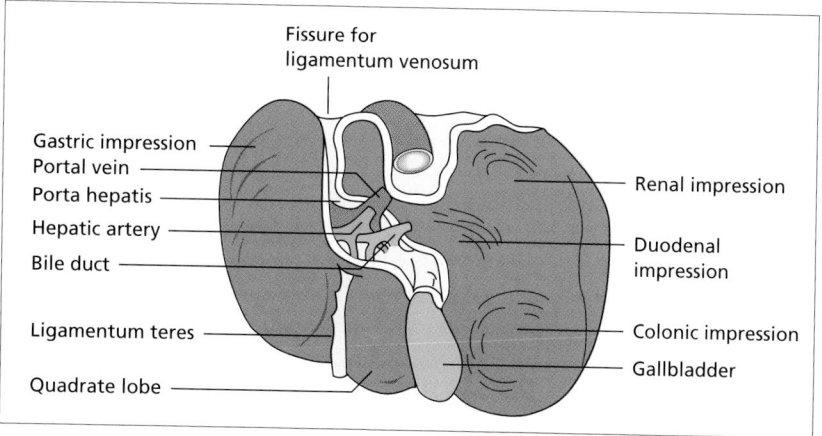

Fig. 1.3. Inferior view of the liver.

and left vagi and the right phrenic nerve. It accompanies the hepatic artery and bile ducts into their finest ramifications, even to the portal tracts and hepatic parenchyma [7].

The *ligamentum venosum*, a slender remnant of the ductus venosus of the fetus, arises from the left branch of the portal vein and fuses with the inferior vena cava at the entrance of the left hepatic vein. The *ligamentum teres*, a remnant of the umbilical vein of the fetus, runs in the free edge of the falciform ligament from the umbilicus to the inferior border of the liver and joins the left branch of the portal vein. Small veins accompanying it connect the portal vein with veins around the umbilicus. These become prominent when the portal venous system is obstructed inside the liver.

The venous drainage from the liver is into the *right* and *left hepatic veins* which emerge from the back of the liver and at once enter the inferior vena cava very near its point of entry into the right atrium.

Lymphatic vessels terminate in small groups of glands around the porta hepatis. Efferent vessels drain into glands around the coeliac axis. Some superficial hepatic lymphatics pass through the diaphragm in the falciform ligament and finally reach the mediastinal glands. Another group accompanies the inferior vena cava into the thorax and ends in a few small glands around the intrathoracic portion of the inferior vena cava.

The *inferior vena cava* makes a deep groove to the right of the caudate lobe about 2 cm from the mid-line.

The *gallbladder* lies in a fossa extending from the inferior border of the liver to the right end of the porta hepatis.

The liver is completely covered with peritoneum except in three places. It comes into direct contact with the diaphragm through the bare area which lies to the right of the fossa for the inferior vena cava. The other areas without peritoneal covering are the fossae for the inferior vena cava and gallbladder.

The liver is kept in position by peritoneal ligaments and by the intra-abdominal pressure transmitted by the tone of the muscles of the abdominal wall.

Functional anatomy: sectors and segments

Based on the external appearances described above, the liver has a right and left lobe separated along the line of insertion of the falciform ligament. This separation, however, does not correlate with blood supply or biliary drainage. A *functional anatomy* is now recognized based upon studies of vascular and biliary casts made by injecting vinyl into the vessels and bile ducts. This classification correlates with that seen by imaging techniques.

The main portal vein divides into right and left

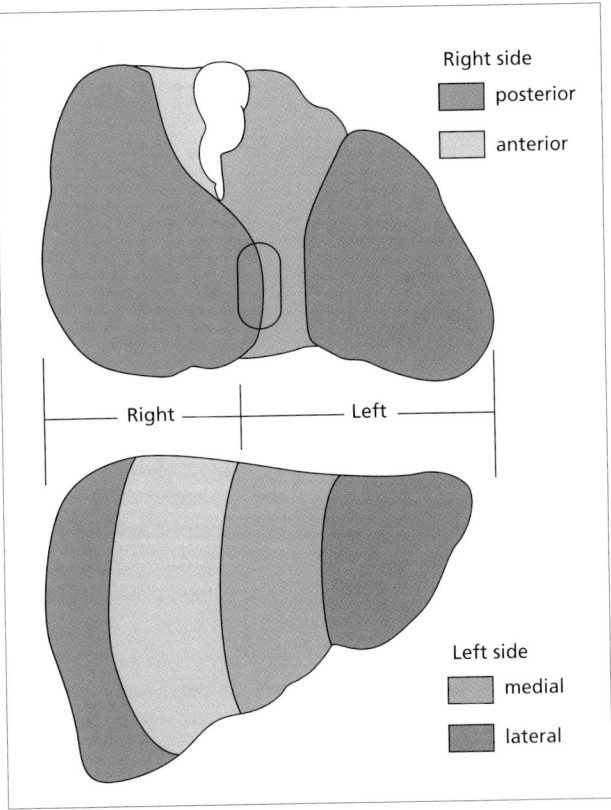

Fig. 1.4. The sectors of the human liver.

branches and each of these supplies two further subunits (variously called sectors). The sectors on the right side are anterior and posterior and, in the left lobe, medial and lateral—giving a total of four sectors (fig. 1.4). Using this definition, the right and left side of the liver are divided not along the line of the falciform ligament, but along a slightly oblique line to the right of this, drawn from the inferior vena cava above to the gallbladder bed below. The right and left side are independent with regard to portal and arterial blood supply, and bile drainage. Three plains separate the four sectors and contain the three major hepatic vein branches.

Closer analysis of these four hepatic sectors produces a further subdivision into segments (fig. 1.5). The right anterior sector contains segments V and VIII; right posterior sector, VI and VII; left medial, IV; left lateral sector, segments II and III. There is no vascular anastomosis between macroscopic vessels of the segments but communications exist at sinusoidal level. Segment I, the equivalent of the caudate lobe, is separate from the other segments and does not derive blood directly from the major portal branches or drain by any of the three major hepatic veins.

This functional anatomical classification allows interpretation of radiological data and is of importance to the surgeon planning a liver resection. There are wide variations in portal and hepatic vessel anatomy which can

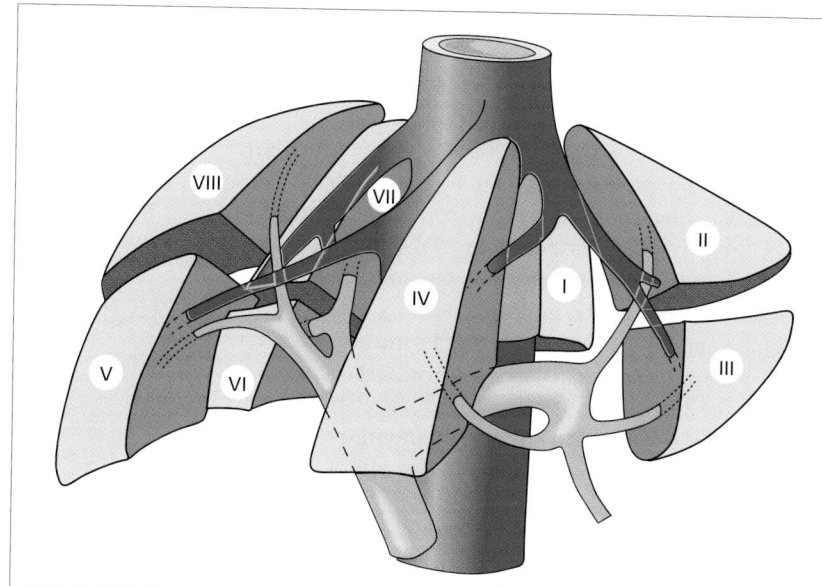

Fig. 1.5. Schematic representation of the functional anatomy of the liver. Three main hepatic veins (dark blue) divide the liver into four sectors, each of them receiving a portal pedicle; hepatic veins and portal veins are intertwined as the fingers of two hands [8].

be demonstrated by spiral CT and MRI reconstruction [44, 45].

Anatomy of the biliary tract (fig. 1.6)

The *right* and *left hepatic ducts* emerge from the liver and unite in the porta hepatis to form the *common hepatic duct*. This is soon joined by the *cystic duct* from the gallbladder to form the common bile duct.

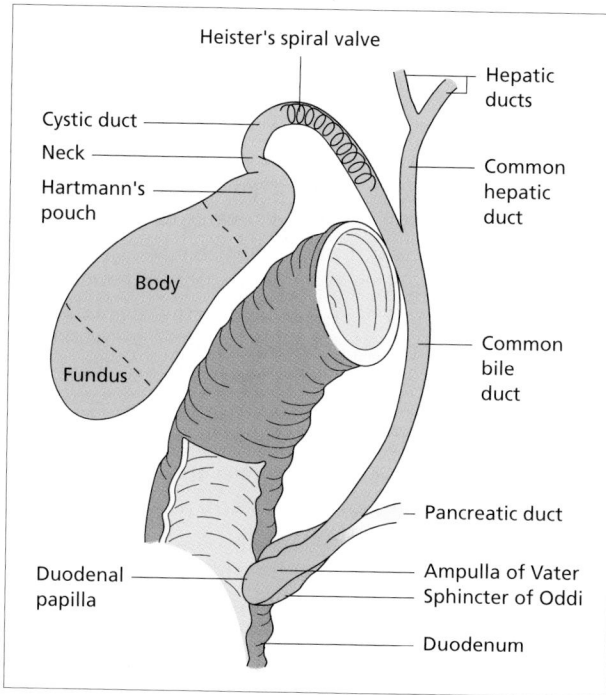

Fig. 1.6. Gallbladder and biliary tract.

The *common bile duct* runs between the layers of the lesser omentum, lying anterior to the portal vein and to the right of the hepatic artery. Passing behind the first part of the duodenum in a groove on the back of the head of the pancreas, it enters the second part of the duodenum. The duct runs obliquely through the posteromedial wall, usually joining the main pancreatic duct to form the *ampulla of Vater* (1720). The ampulla makes the mucous membrane bulge inwards to form an eminence: the *duodenal papilla*. In about 10–15% of subjects the bile and pancreatic ducts open separately into the duodenum.

The dimensions of the common bile duct depend on the technique used. At operation it is about 0.5–1.5 cm in diameter. Using endoscopic cholangiography it is usually less than 11 mm and values greater than 18 mm are pathological [28]. By ultrasound the values are less, the common bile duct being 2–7 mm and values greater than this are abnormal.

The duodenal portion of the common bile duct is surrounded by a thickening of both longitudinal and circular muscle fibres derived from the intestine. This is called the *sphincter of Oddi* (1887).

The *gallbladder* is a pear-shaped bag 9 cm long with a capacity of about 50 ml. It always lies above the transverse colon, and is usually next to the duodenal cap overlying, but well anterior to, the right renal shadow.

Any decrease in concentrating power is accompanied by reduced distensibility. The fundus is the wider end and is directed anteriorly; this is the part palpated when the abdomen is examined. The body extends into a narrow neck which continues into the cystic duct. The *valves of Heister* are spiral folds of mucous membrane in the wall of the cystic duct and neck of the gallbladder.

Hartmann's pouch is a sacculation at the neck of the gallbladder; this is a common site for a gallstone to lodge.

The wall consists of a musculo-elastic network without definite layers, the muscle being particularly well developed in the neck and fundus. The mucous membrane is in delicate closely woven folds; instead of glands there are deep indentations of mucosa, the *crypts of Luschka*, which penetrate into the muscular layer. There is no submucosa or muscularis mucosae.

The *Rokitansky–Aschoff sinuses* are branching evaginations from the lumen into the mucosa and muscularis of the gallbladder. They play an important part in acute cholecystitis and gangrene of the gallbladder wall.

Blood supply. The gallbladder receives blood from the *cystic artery*. This branch of the hepatic artery is large, tortuous and variable in its anatomical relationships. Smaller blood vessels enter from the liver through the gallbladder fossa. The venous drainage is into the *cystic vein* and thence into the portal venous system.

The arterial blood supply to the supra-duodenal bile duct is generally by two main (axial) vessels which run beside the bile duct. These are supplied predominantly by the retro-duodenal artery from below, and the right hepatic artery from above, although many other vessels contribute. This pattern of arterial supply would explain why vascular damage results in bile duct stricturing [29].

Lymphatics. There are many lymphatic vessels in the submucous and subperitoneal layers. These drain through the cystic gland at the neck of the gallbladder to glands along the common bile duct, where they anastomose with lymphatics from the head of the pancreas.

Nerve supply. The gallbladder and bile ducts are liberally supplied with nerves, from both the parasympathetic and the sympathetic system.

Development of the liver and bile ducts

The liver begins as a hollow endodermal bud from the foregut (duodenum) during the third week of gestation. The bud separates into two parts—hepatic and biliary. The *hepatic* part contains bipotential progenitor cells that differentiate into hepatocytes or ductal cells, which form the early primitive bile duct structures (ductal plates). Differentiation is accompanied by changes in cytokeratin type within the cell [42]. Experimental deletion of *c-jun*, a component of the AP1 gene activation complex, specifically prevents liver development [21]. Normally, this collection of rapidly proliferating cells penetrates adjacent mesodermal tissue (the septum transversum) and is met by ingrowing capillary plexuses from the vitelline and umbilical veins which will form the sinusoids. The connection between this proliferating mass of cells and the foregut, the *biliary* part of the endodermal bud, will form the gallbladder and extra-hepatic bile ducts. Bile begins to flow at about the twelfth week. Haemopoietic cells, Kupffer cells and connective tissue cells are derived from the mesoderm of the septum transversum. The fetal liver has a major haemopoietic function which subsides during the last 2 months of intra-uterine life so that only a few haemopoietic cells remain at birth.

Anatomical abnormalities of the liver

These are being increasingly diagnosed with more widespread use of CT and ultrasound scanning.

Accessory lobes. The liver of the pig, dog and camel is divided into distinct and separate lobes by strands of connective tissue. Occasionally, the human liver may show this reversion and up to 16 lobes have been reported. This abnormality is rare and without clinical significance. The lobes are small and usually on the under surface of the liver so that they are not detected clinically but noted incidentally at scanning, operation or necropsy. Rarely they are intra-thoracic. An accessory lobe may have its own mesentery containing hepatic artery, portal vein, bile duct and hepatic vein [32]. This may twist and demand surgical intervention.

Riedel's lobe [35] is fairly common and is a downward tongue-like projection of the right lobe of the liver. It is a simple anatomical variation; it is not a true accessory lobe. The condition is more frequent in women. It is detected as a mobile tumour on the right side of the abdomen which descends with the diaphragm and on inspiration. It may come down as low as the right iliac region. It is easily mistaken for other tumours in this area, especially a visceroptotic right kidney. It does not cause symptoms and treatment is not required. Scanning may be used to identify Riedel's lobe and other anatomical abnormalities.

Cough furrows on the liver are parallel grooves on the convexity of the right lobe. They are one to six in number and run antero-posteriorly, being deeper posteriorly. They are said to be associated with a chronic cough.

Corset liver [31]. This is a fibrotic furrow or pedicle on the anterior surface of both lobes of the liver just below the costal margin. The mechanism is unknown, but it affects elderly women who have worn corsets for many years. It presents as an abdominal mass in front of and below the liver and is isodense with the liver. It may be confused with a hepatic tumour.

Lobar atrophy. Interference with the portal supply or biliary drainage of a lobe may cause atrophy. There is usually hypertrophy of the opposite lobe. Left lobe atrophy found at post-mortem or during scanning is not uncommon and is probably related to reduced blood supply via the left branch of the portal vein. The lobe is decreased in size with thickening of the capsule, fibrosis and prominent biliary and vascular markings. The vascular problem may date from the time of birth [13].

Obstruction to the right or left hepatic bile duct by benign stricture or cholangiocarcinoma is now the most common cause of lobar atrophy [20]. The alkaline phosphatase is usually elevated. The bile duct may not be dilated within the atrophied lobe. Relief of obstruction may reverse the changes if cirrhosis has not developed. Distinction between a biliary and portal venous aetiology may be made using technetium labelled iminodiacetic acid (IDA) and colloid scintiscans. A small lobe with normal uptake of IDA and colloid is compatible with a portal aetiology. Reduced or absent uptake of both isotopes favours biliary disease.

Agenesis of the right lobe [33]. This rare lesion may be an incidental finding associated, probably coincidentally, with biliary tract disease and also with other congenital abnormalities. It can cause pre-sinusoidal portal hypertension. The other liver segments undergo compensatory hypertrophy. It must be distinguished from lobar atrophy due to cirrhosis or hilar cholangiocarcinoma.

Anatomical abnormalities of gallbladder and biliary tract (see Chapter 30).

Surface marking (figs 1.7, 1.8)

Liver. The upper border of the right lobe is on a level with the 5th rib at a point 2 cm medial to the right mid-clavicular line (1 cm below the right nipple). The upper border of the left lobe corresponds to the upper border of the 6th rib at a point in the left mid-clavicular line (2 cm below the left nipple). Here only the diaphragm separates the liver from the apex of the heart.

The lower border passes obliquely upwards from the 9th right to the 8th left costal cartilage. In the right nipple line it lies between a point just under to 2 cm below the costal margin. It crosses the mid-line about mid-way between the base of the xiphoid and the umbilicus and the left lobe extends only 5 cm to the left of the sternum.

Gallbladder. Usually the fundus lies at the outer border

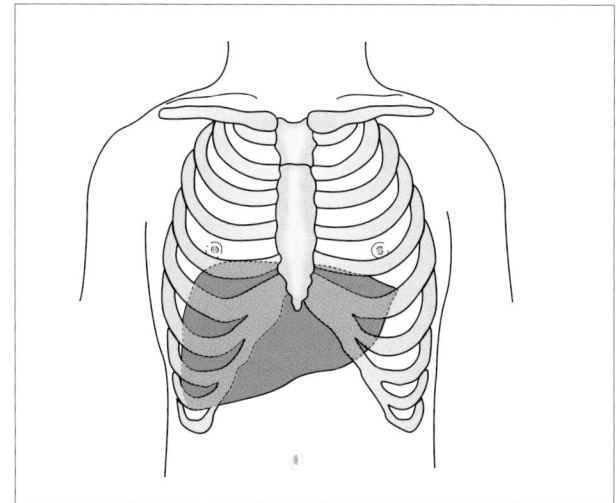

Fig. 1.7. The surface marking of the liver.

of the right rectus abdominis muscle at its junction with the right costal margin (9th costal cartilage) (fig. 1.8). In an obese subject it may be difficult to identify the outer border of the rectus sheath and the gallbladder may then be located by the Grey–Turner method. A line is drawn from the left anterior superior iliac spine through the umbilicus; its intersection with the right costal margin indicates the position of the gallbladder. These guidelines depend upon the individual's somatotype. The fundus may occasionally be found below the iliac crest.

Methods of examination

Liver. The lower edge should be determined by palpation just lateral to the right rectus muscle. This avoids mistaking the upper intersection of the rectus sheath for the liver edge.

The liver edge moves 1–3 cm downwards with deep inspiration. It is usually palpable in normal subjects inspiring deeply. The edge may be tender, regular or irregular, firm or soft, thickened or sharp. The lower

Fig. 1.8. Surface markings of the gallbladder. Method I: the gallbladder is found where the outer border of the right rectus abdominis muscle intersects the 9th costal cartilage. Method II: a line drawn from the left anterior superior iliac spine through the umbilicus intersects the costal margin at the site of the gallbladder.

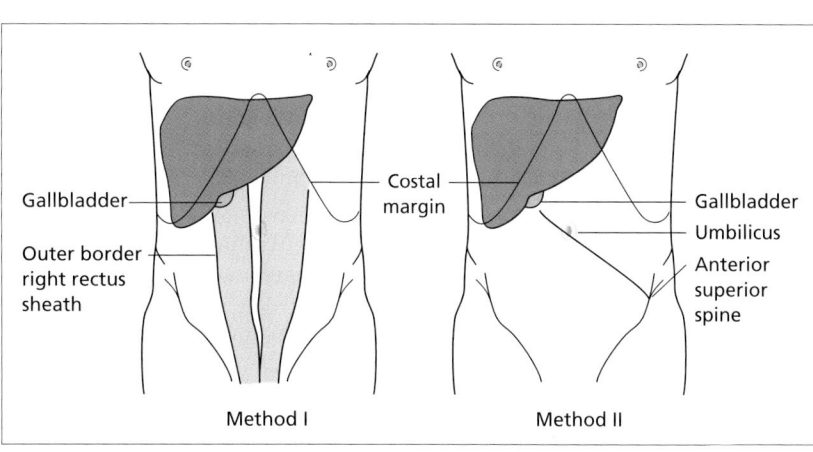

Gallbladder

Outer border right rectus sheath

Costal margin

Gallbladder

Umbilicus

Anterior superior spine

Method I   Method II

edge may be displaced downwards by a low diaphragm, for instance in emphysema. Movements may be particularly great in athletes or singers. Some patients with practice become very efficient at 'pushing down' the liver. The normal spleen can become palpable in similar fashion. Common causes of a liver palpable below the umbilicus are malignant deposits, polycystic or Hodgkin's disease, amyloidosis, congestive cardiac failure, and gross fatty change. Rapid change in liver size may occur when congestive cardiac failure is corrected, cholestatic jaundice relieved, severe diabetes controlled, or when fat is dispersed. The surface can be palpated in the epigastrium and any irregularity or tenderness noted. An enlarged caudate lobe, as in the Budd–Chiari syndrome or with some cases of cirrhosis, may be palpated as an epigastric mass.

Pulsation of the liver, usually associated with tricuspid valvular incompetence, is felt by manual palpation with one hand behind the right lower ribs posteriorly and the other anteriorly on the abdominal wall.

The upper edge is determined by fairly heavy percussion passing downwards from the nipple-line. The lower edge is recognized by very light percussion passing upwards from the umbilicus towards the costal margin. Percussion is a valuable method of determining liver size and is the only clinical method of determining a small liver.

The anterior liver span is obtained by measuring the vertical distance between uppermost and lowermost points of hepatic dullness by percussion in the right midclavicular line. This is usually 12–15 cm. Direct percussion is as accurate as ultrasound in estimating liver span [38].

Friction may be palpable and audible, usually due to recent biopsy, tumour or peri-hepatitis [17]. The venous hum of portal hypertension is audible between the umbilicus and the xiphisternum. An arterial murmur over the liver may indicate a primary liver cancer or acute alcoholic hepatitis.

The *gallbladder* is palpable only when it is distended. It is felt as a pear-shaped cystic mass usually about 7 cm long. In a thin person, the swelling can sometimes be seen through the anterior abdominal wall. It moves downwards on inspiration and is mobile laterally but not downwards. The swelling is dull to percussion and directly impinges on the parietal peritoneum, so that the colon is rarely in front of it. Gallbladder dullness is continuous with that of the liver.

Abdominal tenderness should be noted. Inflammation of the gallbladder causes a positive *Murphy's sign*. This is the inability to take a deep breath when the examining fingers are hooked up below the liver edge. The inflamed gallbladder is then driven against the fingers and the pain causes the patient to catch his breath.

The enlarged gallbladder must be distinguished from a *visceroptotic right kidney*. This, however, is more mobile, can be displaced towards the pelvis and has the resonant colon anteriorly. A *regenerative* or *malignant nodule* feels much firmer.

Imaging. A plain film of the abdomen, including the diaphragms, may be used to assess liver size and in particular to decide whether a palpable liver is due to actual enlargement or to downward displacement. On moderate inspiration the normal level of the diaphragm, on the right side, is opposite the 11th rib posteriorly and the 6th rib anteriorly.

Ultrasound, CT or MRI can also be used to study liver size, shape and consistence.

Hepatic morphology

Kiernan (1833) introduced the concept of hepatic lobules as the basic architecture. He described circumscribed pyramidal lobules consisting of a central tributary of the hepatic vein and at the periphery a portal tract containing bile duct, portal vein radicle and hepatic artery branch. Columns of liver cells and blood-containing sinusoids extended between these two systems.

Stereoscopic reconstructions and scanning electron microscopy have shown the human liver as columns of liver cells radiating from a central vein, and interlaced in orderly fashion by sinusoids (fig. 1.9).

The liver tissue is pervaded by two systems of tunnels, the portal tracts and the hepatic central canals which dovetail in such a way that they never touch each other; the terminal tunnels of the two systems are separated by about 0.5 mm (fig. 1.10). As far as possible the two systems of tunnels run in planes perpendicular to each other. The sinusoids are irregularly disposed, normally in a direction perpendicular to the lines connecting the central veins. The terminal branches of the portal vein discharge their blood into the sinusoids and the direction of flow is determined by the higher pressure in the portal vein than in the central vein.

The *central hepatic canals* contain radicles of the hepatic vein and their adventitia. They are surrounded by a limiting plate of liver cells.

The *portal triads* (syn. portal tracts, Glisson's capsule) contain the portal vein radicle, the hepatic arteriole and bile duct with a few round cells and a little connective tissue (fig. 1.11). They are surrounded by a limiting plate of liver cells.

The liver has to be divided *functionally*. Traditionally, the unit is based on a central hepatic vein and its surrounding liver cells. However, Rappaport [34] envisages a series of functional acini, each centred on the portal triad with its terminal branch of portal vein, hepatic artery and bile duct (zone 1) (figs 1.12, 1.13). These interdigitate, mainly perpendicularly, with terminal hepatic veins of adjacent acini. The circulatory peripheries of

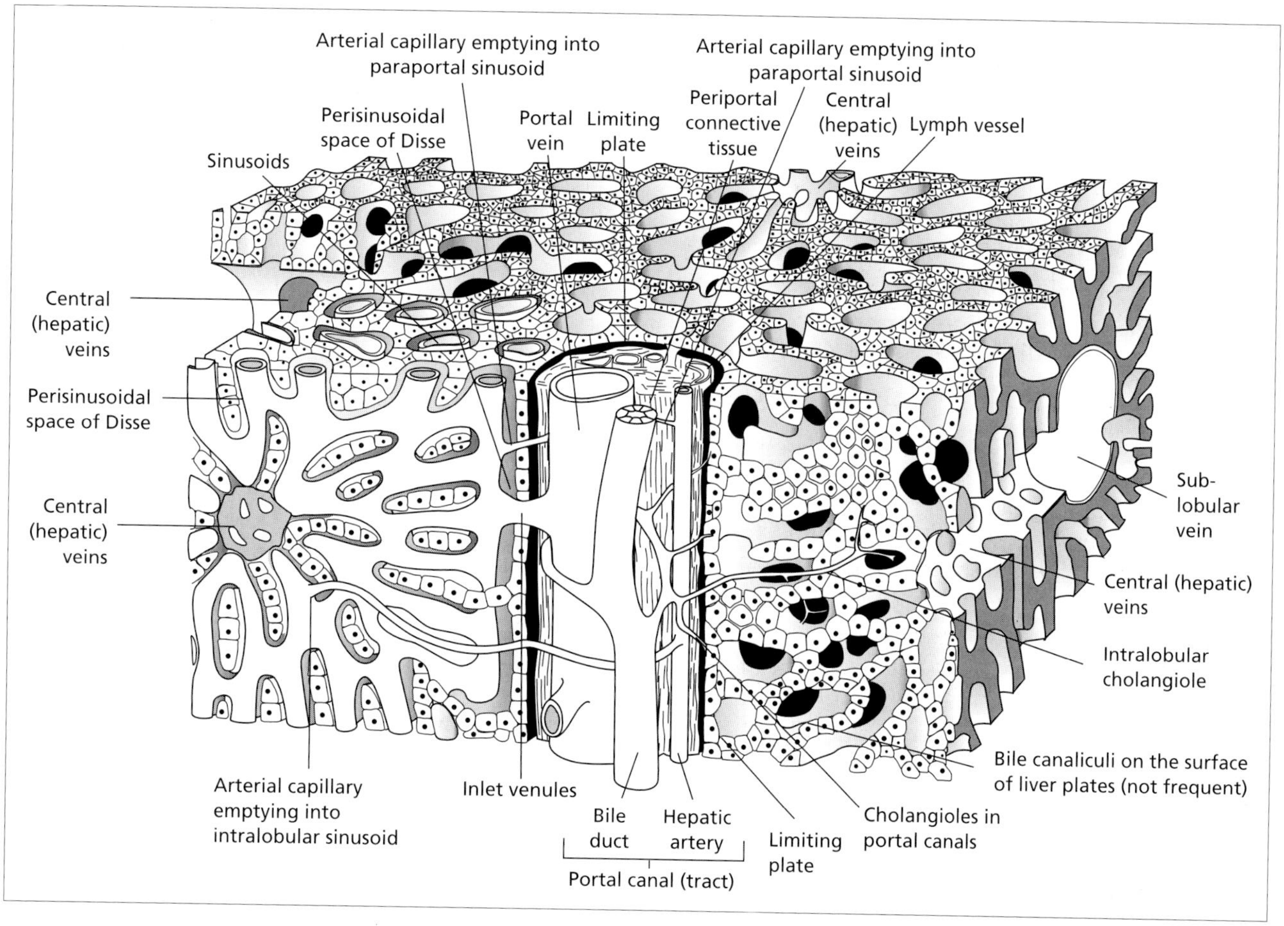

Arterial capillary emptying into
paraportal sinusoid

Arterial capillary emptying into
paraportal sinusoid

Perisinusoidal
space of Disse

Portal
vein

Limiting
plate

Periportal
connective
tissue

Central
(hepatic)
veins

Lymph vessel

Sinusoids

Central
(hepatic)
veins

Perisinusoidal
space of Disse

Central
(hepatic)
veins

Sub-
lobular
vein

Central (hepatic)
veins

Intralobular
cholangiole

Arterial capillary
emptying into
intralobular sinusoid

Inlet venules

Bile
duct

Hepatic
artery

Limiting
plate

Cholangioles in
portal canals

Bile canaliculi on the surface
of liver plates (not frequent)

Portal canal (tract)

Fig. 1.9. The structure of the normal human liver.

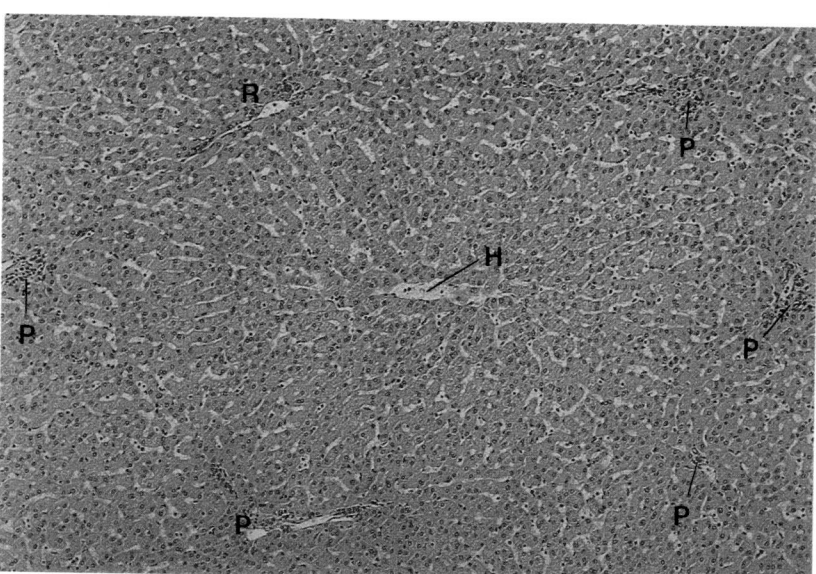

Fig. 1.10. Normal hepatic histology. H =
terminal hepatic vein; P = portal tract.
(Stained H & E, ×60.)

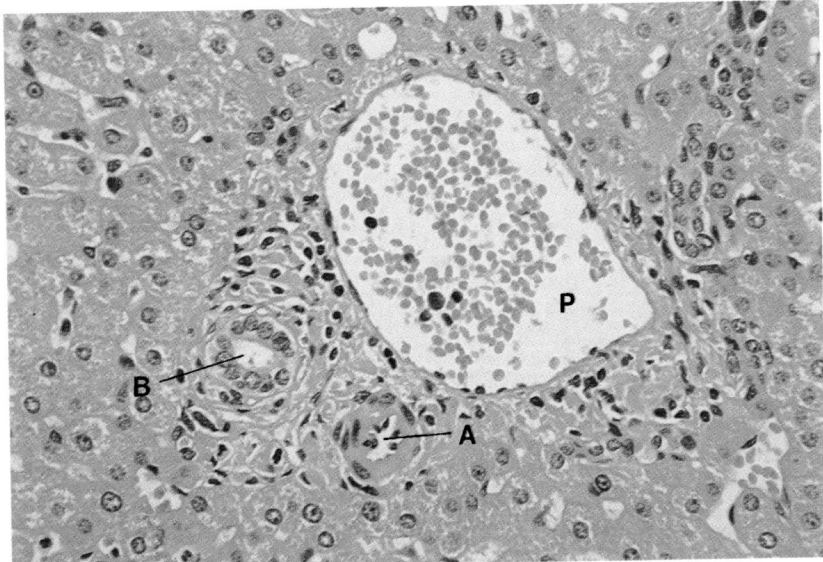

Fig. 1.11. Normal portal tract. A = hepatic artery; B = bile duct; P = portal vein. (Stained H & E.)

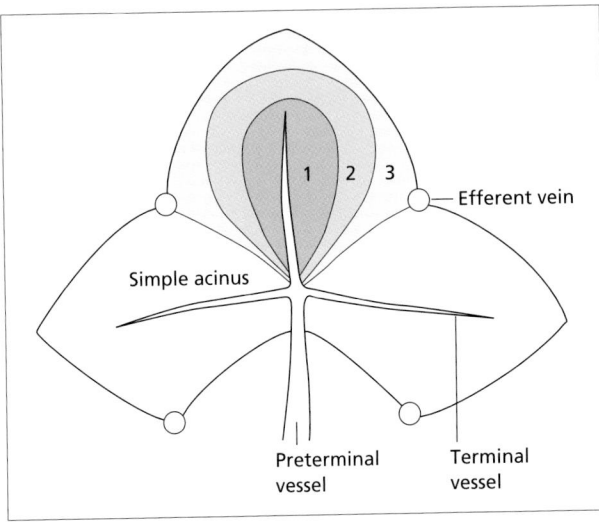

Fig. 1.12. The complex acinus according to Rappaport. Zone 1 is adjacent to the entry (portal venous) system. Zone 3 is adjacent to the exit (hepatic venous) system.

acini (adjacent to terminal hepatic veins) (zone 3) suffer most from injury whether viral, toxic or anoxic. Bridging necrosis is located in this area. The regions closer to the axis formed by afferent vessels and bile ducts survive longer and may later form the core from which regeneration will proceed. The contribution of each acinar zone to liver cell regeneration depends on the acinar location of damage [30, 34].

The liver cells (*hepatocytes*) comprise about 60% of the liver. They are polygonal and approximately 30 μm in diameter. The nucleus is single or, less often, multiple and divides by mitosis. The lifespan of liver cells is about 150 days in experimental animals. The hepatocyte has three surfaces: one facing the sinusoid and space of Disse, the second facing the canaliculus and the third facing neighbouring hepatocytes. There is no basement membrane.

The sinusoids are lined by endothelial cells. Associated with the sinusoids are the phagocytic cells of the reticulo-endothelial system (Kupffer cells), and the hepatic stellate cells, which have also been called fat-storing cells, Ito cells and lipocytes.

There are approximately 202×10^3 cells in each milligram of normal human liver, of which 171×10^3 are parenchymatous and 31×10^3 littoral (sinusoidal, including Kupffer cells).

The *space of Disse* is a tissue space between hepatocytes and sinusoidal endothelial cells. The *hepatic lymphatics* are found in the peri-portal connective tissue and are lined throughout by endothelium. Tissue fluid seeps through the endothelium into the lymph vessels.

The branch of the *hepatic arteriole* forms a plexus around the bile ducts and supplies the structures in the portal tracts. It empties into the sinusoidal network at different levels. There are no direct hepatic arteriolar–portal venous anastomoses.

The excretory system of the liver begins with the *bile canaliculi* (see figs 13.2, 13.3). These have no walls but are simply grooves on the contact surfaces of liver cells (see fig. 13.1). Their surfaces are covered by microvilli. The plasma membrane is reinforced by microfilaments forming a supportive cytoskeleton (see fig. 13.2). The canalicular surface is sealed from the rest of the intercellular surface by junctional complexes including tight junctions, gap junctions and desmosomes. The intralobular canalicular network drains into thin-walled terminal bile ducts or ductules (cholangioles, canals of Hering) lined with cuboidal epithelium. These terminate in larger (interlobular) bile ducts in the portal canals.

Fig. 1.13. Blood supply of the simple liver acinus, zonal arrangements of cells and the microcirculatory periphery. The acinus occupies adjacent sectors of neighbouring hexagonal fields. Zones 1, 2 and 3 respectively represent areas supplied with blood of first, second and third quality with regard to oxygen and nutrient content. These zones centre on the terminal afferent vascular branches, bile ductules, lymph vessels and nerves (PS) and extend into the triangular portal field from which these branches crop out. Zone 3 is the microcirculatory periphery of the acinus since its cells are as remote from their own afferent vessels as from those of adjacent acini. The *perivenular* area is formed by the most peripheral portions of zone 3 of several adjacent acini. In injury progressing along this zone, the damaged area assumes the shape of a seastar (darker tint around a terminal hepatic venule, THV, in the centre). 1, 2, 3 = microcirculatory zones; 1', 2', 3' = zones of neighbouring acinus [34].

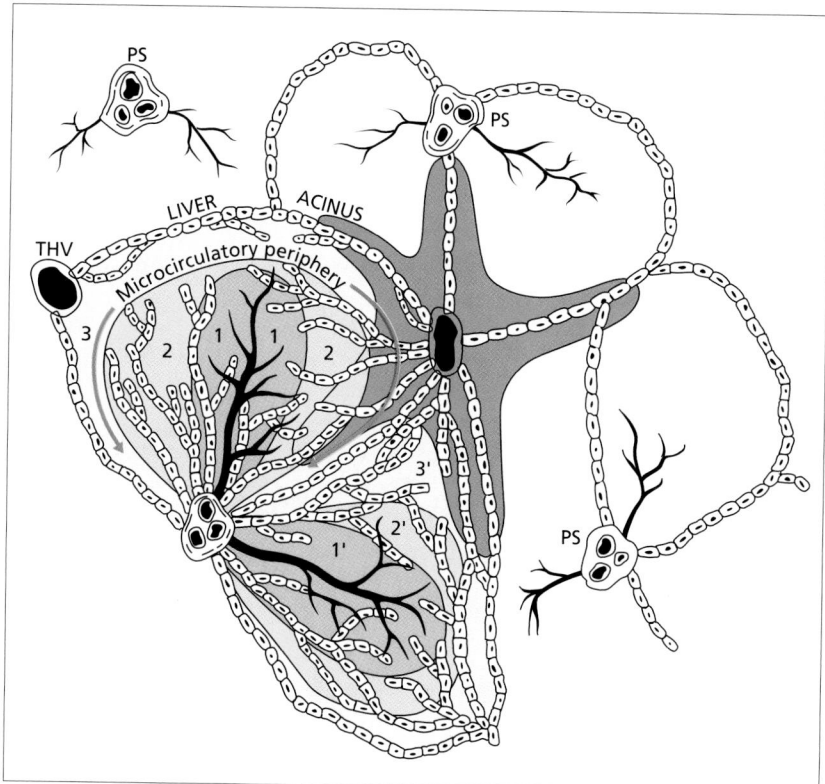

They are classified into small (less than 100 μm in diameter), medium (±100 μm), and large (more than 100 μm).

Electron microscopy and hepato-cellular function (figs 1.14, 1.15)

The liver cell margin is straight except for a few anchoring pegs (desmosomes). From it, equally sized and spaced microvilli project into the lumen of the bile canaliculi. Along the sinusoidal border, irregularly sized and spaced microvilli project into the peri-sinusoidal tissue space. The microvillous structure indicates active secretion or absorption, mainly of fluid.

The *nucleus* contains deoxyribonucleo-protein. Human liver after puberty contains tetraploid nuclei and, at about age 20, in addition, octoploid nuclei are found. Increased polyploidy has been regarded as pre-cancerous. In the chromatin network one or more nucleoli are embedded. The nucleus has a double contour with pores allowing interchange with the surrounding cytoplasm.

The *mitochondria* also have a double membrane, the inner being invaginated to form grooves or cristae. An enormous number of energy-providing processes take place within them, particularly those involving oxidative phosphorylation. They contain many enzymes, particularly those of the citric acid cycle and those involved in β-oxidation of fatty acids. They can transform energy so released into adenosine diphosphate (ADP). Haem synthesis occurs here.

The *rough endoplasmic reticulum* (RER) is seen as lamellar profiles lined by ribosomes. These are responsible for basophilia under light microscopy. They synthesize specific proteins, particularly albumin, those used in blood coagulation and enzymes. They may adopt a helix arrangement, as polysomes, for coordination of this function. Glucose-6-phosphatase is synthesized. Triglycerides are synthesized from free fatty acids and complexed with protein to be secreted by exocytosis as lipoprotein. The RER may participate in glycogenesis.

The *smooth endoplasmic reticulum* (SER) forms tubules and vesicles. It contains the microsomes. It is the site of bilirubin conjugation and the detoxification of many drugs and other foreign compounds (P450 systems). Steroids are synthesized, including cholesterol and the primary bile acids which are conjugated with the amino acids glycine and taurine. The SER is increased by enzyme inducers such as phenobarbital.

Peroxisomes are distributed near the SER and glycogen granules. Their function is unknown.

The *lysosomes* are dense bodies adjacent to the bile canaliculi. They contain many hydrolytic enzymes which, if released, could destroy the cell. They are probably intracellular scavengers which destroy organelles with shortened lifespans. They are the site of deposition

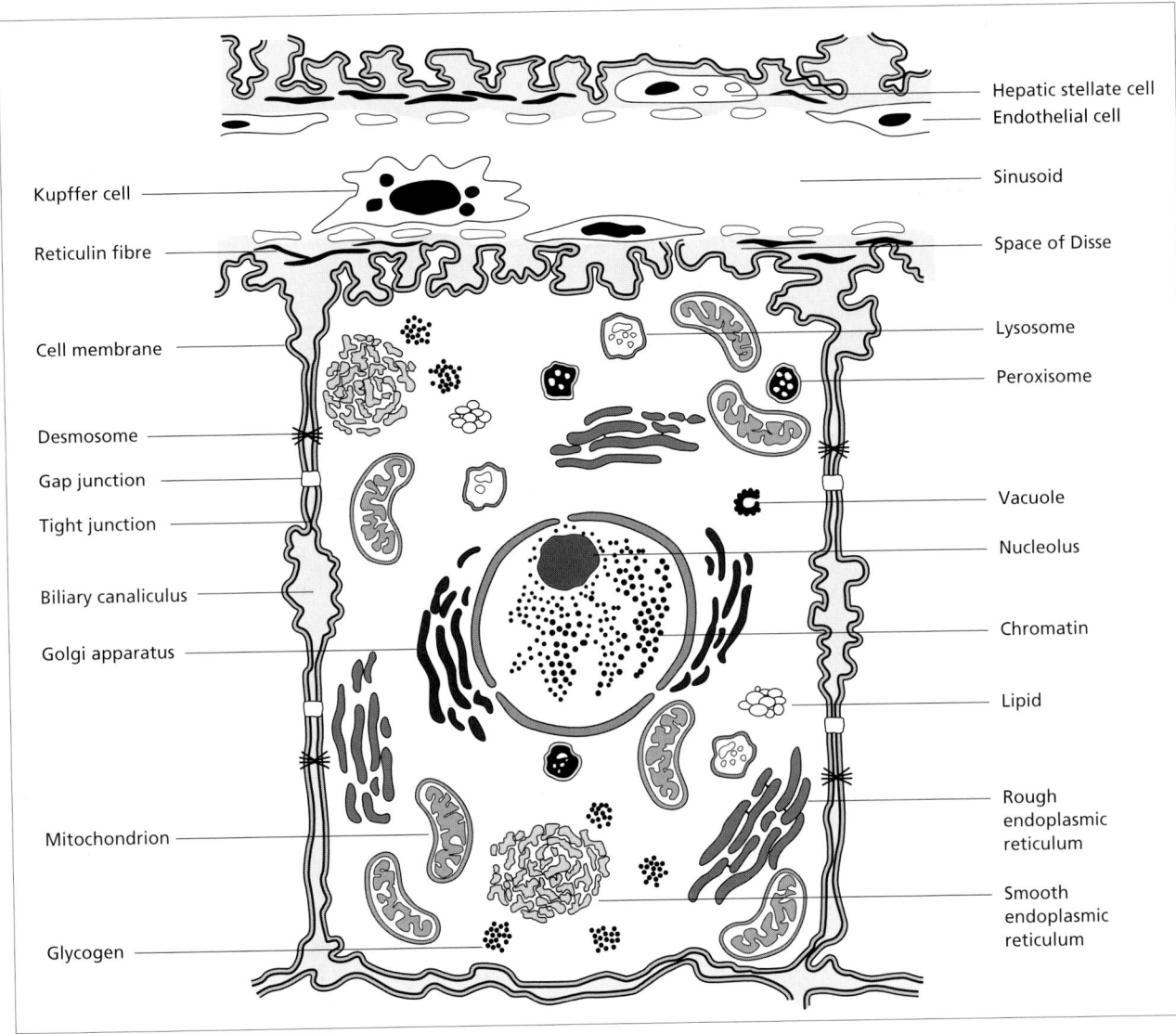

Fig. 1.14. The organelles of the liver cell.

of ferritin, lipofuscin, bile pigment and copper. Pinocytic vacuoles may be observed in them. Some pericanalicular dense bodies are termed *microbodies*.

The *Golgi apparatus* consists of a system of particles and vesicles again lying near the canaliculus. It may be regarded as a 'packaging' site before excretion into the bile. This entire group of lysosomes, microbodies and Golgi apparatus is a means of sequestering any material which is ingested and has to be excreted, secreted or stored for metabolic processes in the cytoplasm. The Golgi apparatus, lysosomes and canaliculi are concerned in cholestasis (Chapter 13).

The intervening cytoplasm contains granules of glycogen, lipid and fine fibrils.

The *cytoskeleton* supporting the hepatocyte consists of microtubules, microfilaments and intermediate filaments [15]. Microtubules contain tubulin and control subcellular mobility, vesicle movement and plasma protein secretion. Microfilaments are made up of actin, are contractile and are important for the integrity and motility of the canaliculus, and for bile flow. Intermediate filaments are elongated branched filaments comprising cytokeratins [42]. They extend from the plasma membrane to the peri-nuclear area and are fundamental for the stability and spatial organization of the hepatocyte.

Sinusoidal cells

The sinusoidal cells (endothelial cells, Kupffer cells, hepatic stellate cells and pit cells) form a functional and histological unit together with the sinusoidal aspect of the hepatocyte [39].

Endothelial cells line the sinusoids and have fenestrae

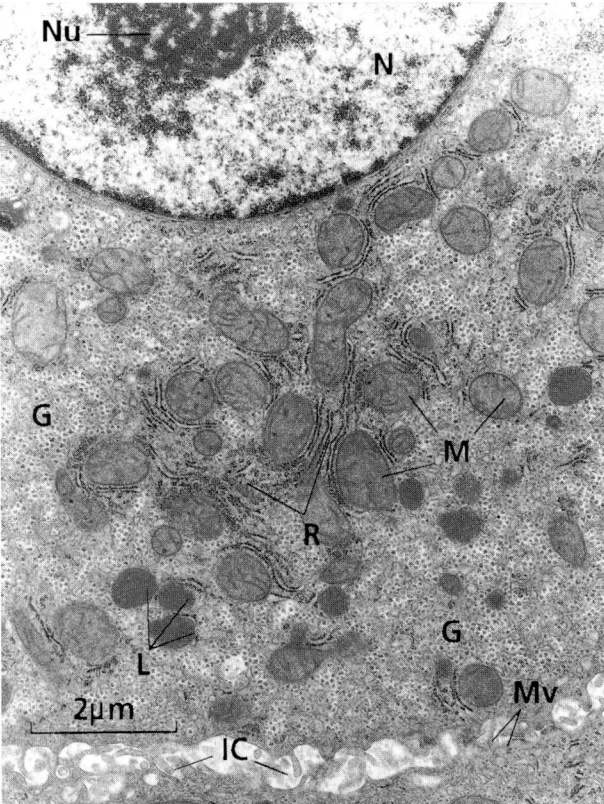

Fig. 1.15. Electron microscopic appearances of part of a normal human liver cell. N = nucleus; Nu = nucleolus; M = mitochondria; R = rough endoplasmic reticulum; G = glycogen granules; Mv = microvilli in intracellular space; L = lysosomes; IC = intercellular space (courtesy Ms J. Lewin).

which provide a graded barrier between sinusoid and space of Disse (fig. 1.16). The Kupffer cells are attached to the endothelium.

The hepatic stellate cells lie in the space of Disse between the hepatocytes and the endothelial cells (fig. 1.17). *Disse's space* contains tissue fluid which flows outwards into lymphatics in the portal zones. When sinusoidal pressure rises, lymph production in Disse's space increases and this plays a part in ascites formation where there is hepatic venous outflow obstruction.

Kupffer cells. These are highly mobile macrophages attached to the endothelium. They are peroxidase staining and have a nuclear envelope. They phagocytose large particles and contain vacuoles and lysosomes. They are derived from blood monocytes and have only limited capabilities of division. They phagocytose by endocytosis (pinocytosis or phagocytosis) which may be absorptive (receptor-mediated) or fluid phase (non-receptor-mediated) [41]. Kupffer cells endocytose old cells, foreign particles, tumour cells, bacteria, yeast, viruses and parasites. They take up and process oxidized low-density lipoproteins (thought to be atherogenic) [14], and remove denatured proteins and fibrin in disseminated intravascular coagulation.

The Kupffer cell has specific membrane receptors for ligands including the Fc portion of immunoglobulin and C3b component of complement, which are important for antigen presentation.

With generalized infections or trauma, Kupffer cells become activated. They specifically endocytose endotoxin and, in response, secrete a series of factors such as tumour necrosing factor (TNF), interleukins, collagenase and lysosomal hydrolases. These increase discomfort and sickness. The toxicity of endotoxin is caused

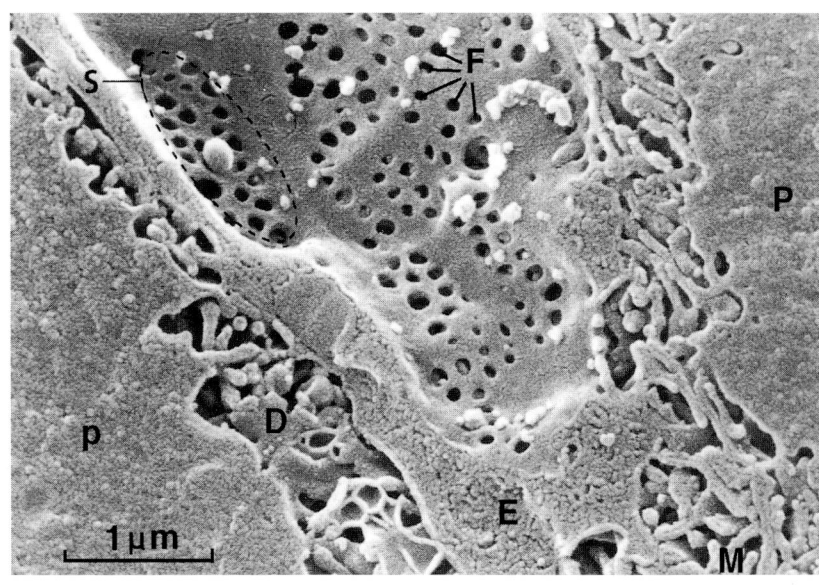

Fig. 1.16. Scanning electron micrograph of sinusoid showing fenestrae (F) grouped into sieve plates (S). P = parenchymal cell; D = space of Disse; M = microvilli; E = endothelial cell (courtesy Prof. E. Wisse).

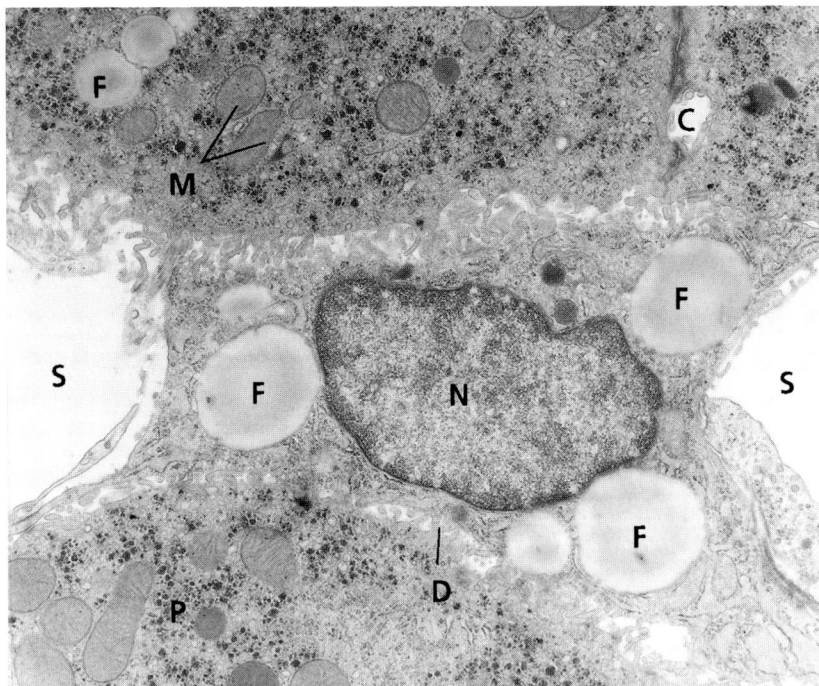

Fig. 1.17. Transmission electron micrograph of hepatic stellate cell. Note characteristic fat droplets (F). S = lumen of sinusoid; D = space of Disse; P = parenchymal cell; C = bile canaliculus; N = nucleus; M = mitochondria (magnification ×12 000) (courtesy Prof. E. Wisse).

by the secretory products of Kupffer cells since endotoxin itself is not toxic.

The Kupffer cell secretes arachidonic acid metabolites including prostaglandins [39].

The Kupffer cell has specific membrane receptors for insulin, glucagon and lipoproteins. The carbohydrate receptor, which recognizes *N*-acetyl glucosamine, mannose and galactose may mediate the pinocytic uptake of certain glycoproteins, particularly lysosomal hydrolases. It also mediates the uptake of IgM-containing immune complexes.

Kupffer cells have erythroblastoid function in fetal liver.

Opsonins, plasma fibronectin, immunoglobulins and tuftsin, a natural immunomodulatory peptide [25], promote recognition and speed of endocytosis by Kupffer cells.

Endothelial cells. These sessile cells form a continuous wall to the lumen of the sinusoid. Fenestrae (0.1 µm in diameter) in the endothelial cells (see fig. 1.16), clustered in sieve plates, function as a biofilter between the sinusoidal blood and the plasma within the space of Disse. They have a dynamic cytoskeleton which maintains and regulates their size [11]. This 'liver sieve' filters macromolecules of differing size. Large triglyceride-rich parent chylomicrons cannot pass, while smaller triglyceride-depleted, cholesterol- and retinol-rich remnants can enter the space of Disse [16]. Endothelial cells have lobular gradients. Scanning electron microscopy has shown, particularly in zone 3 in alcoholic patients, a

striking reduction in the number of fenestrae with formation of a basal lamina [22].

Sinusoidal endothelial cells are active in clearing macromolecules and small particles from the circulation by receptor-mediated endocytosis [40]. They carry surface receptors for hyaluronan (major polysaccharide from connective tissue), chondroitin sulphate, and mannose-terminated glycoprotein, as well as receptors II and III for the Fc fragment of IgG and a receptor for the lipopolysaccharide-binding protein [37]. The endothelial cells act as scavenger cells removing harmful enzymes and pathogens. They also clear denatured collagen from blood, and bind and take up lipoprotein.

Hepatic stellate cells (fat-storing cells, lipocytes, Ito cells). These cells lie within the subendothelial space of Disse. They have long cytoplasmic extensions some giving close contact with parenchymal cells, and others reaching several sinusoids, where they may regulate blood flow and hence influence portal hypertension [6]. In normal liver they are the major storage site of retinoids, giving the morphological characteristic of cytoplasmic lipid droplets. When empty of these droplets, they resemble fibroblasts. They contain actin and myosin and contract in response to endothelin-1 and substance P [36]. With hepatocyte injury, hepatic stellate cells lose their lipid droplets, proliferate, migrate to zone 3 of the acinus, change to a myofibroblast-like phenotype, and produce collagen type I, III and IV and laminin. Stellate cells also release matrix proteinases and inhibitory molecules of matrix proteinases (tissue inhibitor of metalloproteinases, TIMP) [4, 23] (see Chapter 19). Collagenization of the space of Disse results in decreased access of protein-bound substrates to the hepatocyte [46].

Pit cells. These are highly mobile natural killer lymphocytes attached to the sinusoidal surface of the endothelium [10]. Microvilli or pseudopods penetrate the endothelial lining, making contact with the microvilli of the parenchymal cells in the space of Disse. They are short-lived cells and are renewed from circulating lymphocytes which differentiate within the sinusoids [43]. They show characteristic granules and rod-cored vesicles. Pit cells show spontaneous cytotoxicity against tumour and virus infected hepatocytes.

Sinusoidal cell interactions

There are complex interactions between Kupffer and endothelial cells, as well as sinusoidal cells and hepatocytes. Kupffer cell activation by lipopolysaccharide suppresses hyaluronan uptake by endothelial cells, an effect probably mediated by leukotrienes [12]. Cytokines produced by sinusoidal cells can both stimulate and inhibit hepatocyte proliferation [26].

Extra-cellular matrix

This is obvious when there is liver disease, but also exists in a subtle form even in normal liver. In or around the space of Disse, all major constituents of a basement membrane can be found including type IV collagen, laminin, heparan sulphate, protoglycan and fibronectin [9]. All cells impinging on the sinusoid can contribute to this matrix. The matrix within Disse's space influences hepato-cellular function, affecting expression of tissue-specific genes such as albumin as well as the number and porosity of sinusoidal fenestrations [27]. It may be important in liver regeneration.

Altered hepatic microcirculation and disease [46]

In liver disease, particularly in the alcoholic, the liver microcirculation may be altered by collagenization of the space of Disse, formation of a basal lamina beneath the endothelium and modification of the endothelial fenestrations [22]. All these processes are maximal in zone 3. They contribute to deprivation of nutrients intended for the hepatocyte and to the development of portal hypertension.

Adhesion molecules

In hepatic inflammation lymphocytes are often the cells infiltrating the liver. There is an interaction between the receptor on the leucocyte surface, lymphocyte function

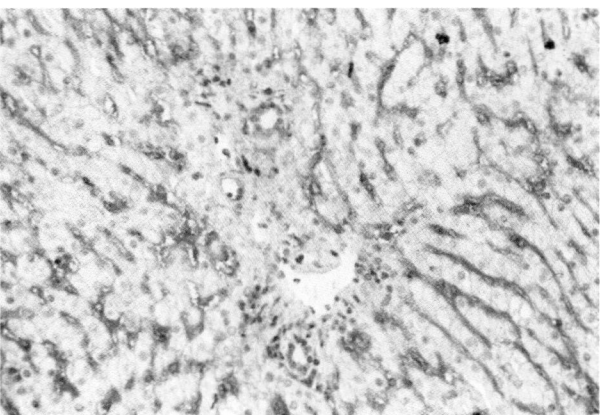

Fig. 1.18. Normal liver tissue stained for ICAM-1. Note: diffuse staining of sinusoidal lining cells; faint membranous staining of occasional hepatocytes; bile ducts are negative. (Courtesy Dr S.G. Hubscher.)

associated antigen (LFA-1) and an intercellular adhesion molecule (ICAM-1 or -2). ICAM-1 is expressed strongly on sinusoidal lining cells and weakly on portal and hepatic endothelium in normal liver [1] (fig. 1.18). Induction of ICAM-1 on biliary epithelium, vascular endothelium and peri-venular hepatocytes is found in post-transplant rejection. Expression of this adhesion molecule on bile ducts has been found in primary biliary cirrhosis and primary sclerosing cholangitis [2].

Functional heterogeneity [18]

The relative functions of cells in the circulation periphery of acini (zone 3) adjacent to terminal hepatic veins are different from those in the circulatory area adjacent to terminal hepatic arteries and portal veins (zone 1) (see figs 1.12, 1.13) (table 1.1) [19].

Krebs' cycle enzymes (urea synthesis and glutaminase) are found in highest concentration in zone 1 whereas glutamine synthetase is peri-venous.

Oxygen supply is an obvious difference; cells in zone 3 receive their oxygen supply last and are particularly prone to anoxic liver injury.

The drug-metabolizing P450 enzymes are present in greater amounts in zone 3. This is particularly so after enzyme induction, for instance with phenobarbital. Hepatocytes in zone 3 receive a higher concentration of any toxic product of drug metabolism. They also have a reduced glutathione concentration. This makes them particularly susceptible to hepatic drug reactions.

Hepatocytes in zone 1 receive blood with a high bile salt concentration and therefore are particularly important in bile-salt-dependent bile formation. Hepatocytes in zone 3 are important in non-bile-salt-dependent bile formation. There are also zonal differences in the hepatic transport rate of substances from sinusoid to canaliculus.

Table 1.1. Metabolism related to the zonal location of the hepatocyte whether acinar zone 3 ('central') or zone 1 ('peri-portal') [19]

	Zone 1	Zone 3
Carbohydrates	Gluconeogenesis	Glycolysis
Proteins	Albumin ⎫ synthesis Fibrinogen ⎭	Albumin ⎫ synthesis Fibrinogen ⎭
Cytochrome P450	+	++
after phenobarbital	+	++++++++
Glutathione	++	–
Oxygen supply	+++	+
Bile formation		
Bile-salt-dependent	++	–
Non-bile-salt-dependent	–	++
Sinusoids	Small	Straight
	Highly anastomotic	Radial

The cause of the metabolic difference between the zones varies. For some functions (gluconeogenesis, glycolysis, ketogenesis) it appears to be dependent upon the direction of blood flow along the sinusoid. For others (cytochrome P450) the gene transcription rate differs between peri-venous and peri-portal hepatocytes [18]. The differential expression of glutamine synthetase across the acinus is already established in fetal liver.

Sinusoidal membrane traffic [5]

The sinusoidal plasma membrane is a receptor-rich and metabolically dynamic domain which is separated from the bile canaliculus by a lateral domain which participates in cell–cell interactions (see fig. 1.14). Receptor-mediated endocytosis (RME) is responsible for transfer of large molecules such as glycoproteins, growth factors and carrier proteins (transferrin). These ligands bind to receptors on the sinusoidal membrane, the occupied receptors cluster into a coated (clatharin) pit and endocytosis proceeds. The fate of the ligand within the cell varies according to the molecule involved and the pathways are complex (fig. 1.19). Many ligands terminate in lysosomes where they are broken down while the recep-

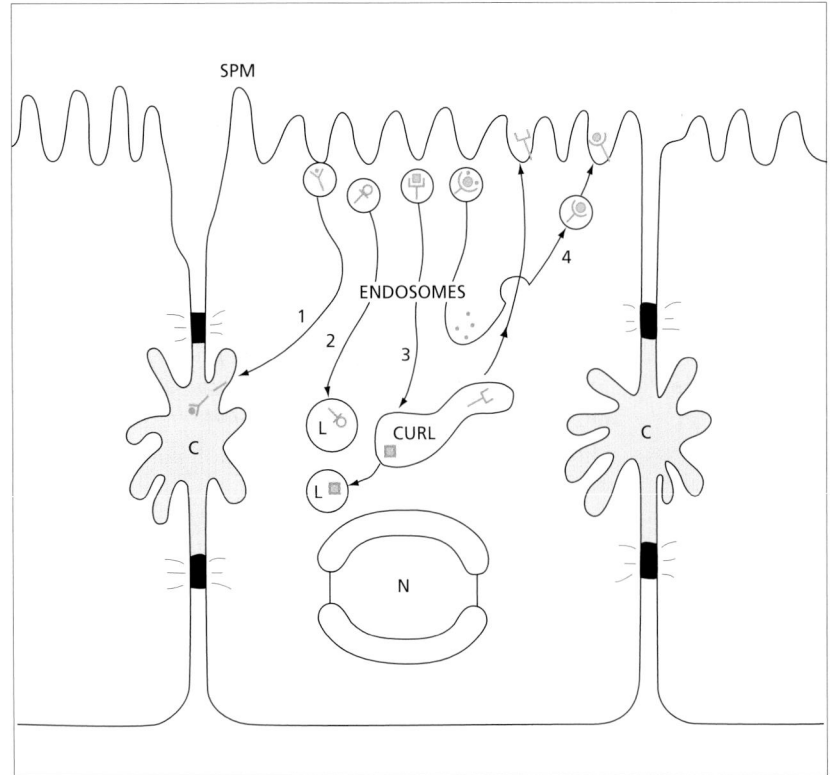

Fig. 1.19. Pathways of endocytosis from the sinusoidal membrane (SPM = sinusoidal plasma membrane; C = bile canaliculus; L = lysosome; N = nucleus; CURL = compartment of uncoupling of receptor and ligand). Receptors bound to ligand group together in coated pit. There is endocytosis resulting in a coated vesicle which then loses its clatharin coat and fuses with other vesicles to form early endosomes (the site of sorting). Subsequent pathways include:
1 vesicular transport to bile canaliculus where ligand and receptor are released (transcytosis) (e.g. polymeric IgA);
2 transfer of ligand and receptor to lysosome where they are degraded;
3 receptor and ligand are transferred to CURL. Receptor and ligand separate. The receptor returns to sinusoidal plasma membrane. Ligand enters lysosome and is degraded (e.g. LDL, asialoglycoprotein, insulin);
4 ligand and receptor return to plasma membrane (e.g. transferrin and its receptor after release of iron).

tor returns to the sinusoidal plasma membrane to perform again. Some ligands pass by vesicular transport across the cell to be discharged into the bile canaliculi.

Bile duct epithelial cells

These can be isolated from rat liver [3] and grown in short-term culture. Studies show receptor-mediated endocytosis of epidermal growth factor by the cells [24] and exocytosis under the control of secretin.

References

1 Adams DH, Hubscher SG, Shaw J *et al*. Intercellular adhesion molecule 1 on liver allografts during rejection. *Lancet* 1989; **ii**: 1122.

2 Adams DH, Hubscher SG, Shaw J *et al*. Increased expression of intercellular adhesion molecule 1 on bile ducts in primary biliary cirrhosis and primary sclerosing cholangitis. *Hepatology* 1991; **14**: 426.

3 Alpini G, Phillips JO, Vroman B *et al*. Recent advances in the isolation of liver cells. *Hepatology* 1994; **20**: 494.

4 Arthur MJP, Iredale JP. Hepatic lipocytes, TIMP-1 and liver fibrosis. *J. Royal Coll. Phys. Lond.* 1994; **28**: 200.

5 Austen BM, Westwood OMR. *Protein Targeting and Secretion*. IRL Press at Oxford University Press, Oxford, 1991, pp. 54–59.

6 Bhathal PS, Grossman HJ. Reduction of the increased portal vascular resistance of the isolated perfused cirrhotic rat liver by vasodilators. *J. Hepatol.* 1985; **1**: 325.

7 Bioulac-Sage P, Lafon ME, Saric J *et al*. Nerves and perisinusoidal cells in human liver. *J. Hepatol.* 1990; **10**: 105.

8 Bismuth H. Surgical anatomy and anatomical surgery of the liver. *World J. Surg.* 1982; **6**: 3.

9 Bissell DM, Choun MO. The role of extracellular matrix in normal liver. *Scand. J. Gastroenterol.* 1988, **23** (suppl 151): 1.

10 Bouwens L, Wisse E. Pit cells in the liver. *Liver* 1992; **12**: 3.

11 Braet F, De Zanger R, Baekeland M *et al*. Structure and dynamics of the fenestrae-associated cytoskeleton of rat liver sinusoidal endothelial cells. *Hepatology* 1995; **21**: 180.

12 Deaciuc IV, Bagby GJ, Niesman MR *et al*. Modulation of hepatic sinusoidal endothelial cell function by Kupffer cells: an example of intercellular communication in the liver. *Hepatology* 1994; **19**: 464.

13 Emery JL. Degenerative changes in the left lobe of the liver in the newborn. *Arch. Dis. Child.* 1952; **27**: 558.

14 Esbach S, Pieters MN, Van Der Boom J *et al*. Visualisation of the uptake and processing of oxidized low-density lipoproteins in human and rat liver. *Hepatology* 1993; **18**: 537.

15 Feldmann G. The cytoskeleton of the hepatocyte. *J. Hepatol.* 1989; **8**: 380.

16 Fraser R, Dobbs BR, Rogers GWT. Lipoproteins and the liver sieve: the role of the fenestrated sinusoidal endothelium in lipoprotein metabolism, atherosclerosis, and cirrhosis. *Hepatology* 1995; **21**: 863.

17 Fred HL, Brown GR. The hepatic friction rub. *N. Engl. J. Med.* 1962; **266**: 554.

18 Gumucio JJ. Hepatocyte heterogeneity: the coming of age from the description of a biological curiosity to a partial understanding of its physiological meaning and regulation. *Hepatology* 1989; **9**: 154.

19 Gumucio JJ, Miller DL. Functional implications of liver cell heterogeneity. *Gastroenterology* 1981; **80**: 393.

20 Hadjis NS, Blumgart LH. Clinical aspects of liver atrophy. *J. Clin. Gastroenterol.* 1989; **11**: 3.

21 Hilberg F, Aguzzi A, Howells N *et al*. c-Jun is essential for normal mouse development and hepatogenesis. *Nature* 1993; **365**: 179.

22 Horn T, Christoffersen P, Henriksen JH. Alcoholic liver injury: defenestration in non-cirrhotic livers. A scanning microscopic study. *Hepatology* 1987; **7**: 77.

23 Iredale JP, Murphy G, Hembry RM *et al*. Human hepatic lipocytes synthesize tissue inhibitor of metalloproteinase-1. Implication for regulation of matrix degradation in liver. *J. Clin. Invest.* 1992; **90**: 282.

24 Ishii M, Vroman B, LaRusso NF. Morphologic demonstration of receptor-mediated endocytosis of epidermal growth factor by isolated bile duct epithelial cells. *Gastroenterology* 1990; **98**: 1284.

25 Kubo S, Rodriguez Jr T, Roh MS *et al*. Stimulation of phagocytic activity of murine Kupffer cells by Tuftsin. *Hepatology* 1994; **19**: 1044.

26 Maher JJ, Friedman SL. Parenchymal and nonparenchymal cell interactions in the liver. *Semin. Liver Dis.* 1993; **13**: 13.

27 McGuire RF, Bissell DM, Boyles J *et al*. Role of extracellular matrix in regulating fenestrations of sinusoidal endothelial cells isolated from normal rat liver. *Hepatology* 1992; **15**: 989.

28 Niederau C, Sonnenberg A, Mueller J. Comparison of the extrahepatic bile duct size measured by ultrasound and by different radiographic methods. *Gastroenterology* 1984; **87**: 615.

29 Northover JMA, Terblanche J. A new look at the arterial supply of the bile duct in man and its surgical implications. *Br. J. Surg.* 1979; **66**: 379.

30 Nostrant TT, Miller DL, Appelman HD *et al*. Acinar distribution of liver cell regeneration after selective zonal injury in the rat. *Gastroenterology* 1978; **75**: 181.

31 Philips DM, La Brecque DR, Shirazi SS. Corset liver. *J. Clin. Gastroenterol.* 1985; **7**: 361.

32 Pujari BD, Deodhare SG. Symptomatic accessory lobe of liver with a review of the literature. *Postgrad. Med. J.* 1976; **52**: 234.

33 Radin DR, Colletti PM, Ralls PW *et al*. Agenesis of the right lobe of the liver. *Radiology* 1987; **164**: 639.

34 Rappaport AM. The microcirculatory acinar concept of normal and pathological hepatic structure. *Beitr. Path.* 1976; **157**: 215.

35 Reitemeier RJ, Butt HR, Baggenstoss AH. Riedel's lobe of the liver. *Gastroenterology* 1958; **34**: 1090.

36 Sakamoto M, Ueno T, Kin M *et al*. Ito cell contraction in response to endothelin-1 and substance P. *Hepatology* 1993; **18**: 978.

37 Scoazec J-Y, Feldmann G. *In situ* immunophenotyping study of endothelial cells of the human hepatic sinusoid: results and functional implications. *Hepatology* 1991; **14**: 789.

38 Skrainka B, Stahlhut J, Fullbeck CL *et al*. Measuring liver span. Bedside examination versus ultrasound and scintiscan. *J. Clin. Gastroenterol.* 1986; **8**: 267.

39 Smedsrod B, De Bleser PJ, Braet F *et al*. Cell biology of liver endothelial and Kupffer cells. *Gut* 1994; **35**: 1509.

40 Smedsrod B, Pertoft H, Gustafson S *et al*. Scavenger functions of the liver endothelial cell. *Biochem. J.* 1990; **266**: 313.

41 Toth CA, Thomas P. Liver endocytosis and Kupffer cells. *Hepatology* 1992; **16**: 255.

42 Van Eyken P, Desmet VJ. Cytokeratins and the liver. *Liver* 1993; **13**: 113.

43 Vanderkerken K, Bouwens L, De Neve W *et al.* Origin and differentiation of hepatic natural killer cells (Pit cells). *Hepatology* 1993; **18**: 919.

44 van Leeuwen MS, Fernandez MA, van ES HW *et al.* Variation in venous and segmental anatomy of the liver: two- and three-dimensional MR imaging in health volunteers. *Am. J.* *Roentgenol.* 1994; **162**: 1337.

45 van Leeuwen MS, Noordzij J, Fernandez MA *et al.* Portal venous and segmental anatomy of the right hemiliver: observations based on three-dimensional spiral CT renderings. *Am. J. Roentgenol.* 1994; **163**: 1395.

46 Villeneuve J-P, Huet P-M. Microcirculatory abnormalities in liver diseases. *Hepatology* 1987; **7**: 186.

Chapter 2
Assessment of Liver Function

Selection of biochemical tests

Tests are needed to detect disease, to direct the diagnostic work-up, to estimate the severity, to assess prognosis and to evaluate therapy (table 2.1). There is no 'magic' test and it is unnecessary to use a large number of methods. The more investigations are multiplied, the greater chance there is of a biochemical deficiency being demonstrated. This type of 'shotgun' investigation adds to the confusion. A few simple tests of established value should be used.

If an abnormality is found it may need to be confirmed by a repeat estimation to show that it is real and not a laboratory error.

Tests most useful in the *diagnostic work-up of jaundice* (Chapter 12) are the serum alkaline phosphatase level, and serum transaminase values. An isolated rise in serum unconjugated bilirubin suggests Gilbert's syndrome or haemolysis.

The *severity of liver cell damage* is assessed by serial measurement of serum total bilirubin, albumin, transaminase and prothrombin time after vitamin K.

The diagnosis of *minimal hepato-cellular damage* may be suspected by noting minimally elevated serum transaminase values and sometimes serum bilirubin. Causes will include alcoholic liver damage, where serum gamma glutamyl transpeptidase (γ-GT) is of particular value, and well-compensated cirrhosis — although similar changes may be seen in heart failure and fever.

Hepatic infiltrations such as primary or secondary cancer, amyloid disease or the reticuloses are suggested by an elevated serum alkaline phosphatase value without jaundice.

Fibrosis may be estimated by the serum procollagen type III peptide (Chapter 19).

The pattern of *conventional tests* (bilirubin, enzymes) indicate which more-specialist tests are likely to be valuable. These more specific methods include viral hepatitis markers and immunological tests such as the mitochondrial antibody for primary biliary cirrhosis. Imaging by ultrasonography and CT are important links in the diagnostic pathway as is liver biopsy.

The liver is central to the metabolism of protein, carbohydrate and fat (fig. 2.1) as well as being important in

Table 2.1. Essential serum methods in hepato-biliary disease

Test	Normal range	Value
Bilirubin		
Total	5–17 µmol/litre*	Diagnosis jaundice. Assess severity
Conjugated	<5 µmol/litre	Gilbert's disease, haemolysis
Alkaline phosphatase	35–130 iu/litre	Diagnosis cholestasis, hepatic infiltrations
Aspartate transaminase (AST/SGOT)	5–40 iu/litre	Early diagnosis of hepato-cellular disease, follow progress
Alanine transaminase (ALT/SGPT)	5–35 iu/litre	ALT relatively lower than AST in alcoholism
γ-glutamyl transpeptidase (γ-GT)	10–48 iu/litre	Diagnosis alcohol abuse, marker biliary cholestasis
Albumin	35–50 g/litre	Assess severity
γ-globulin	5–15 g/litre	Diagnosis chronic hepatitis and cirrhosis—follow course
Prothrombin time (PT) (after vitamin K)	12–16 seconds	Assess severity

* 0.3–1.0 mg/dl.

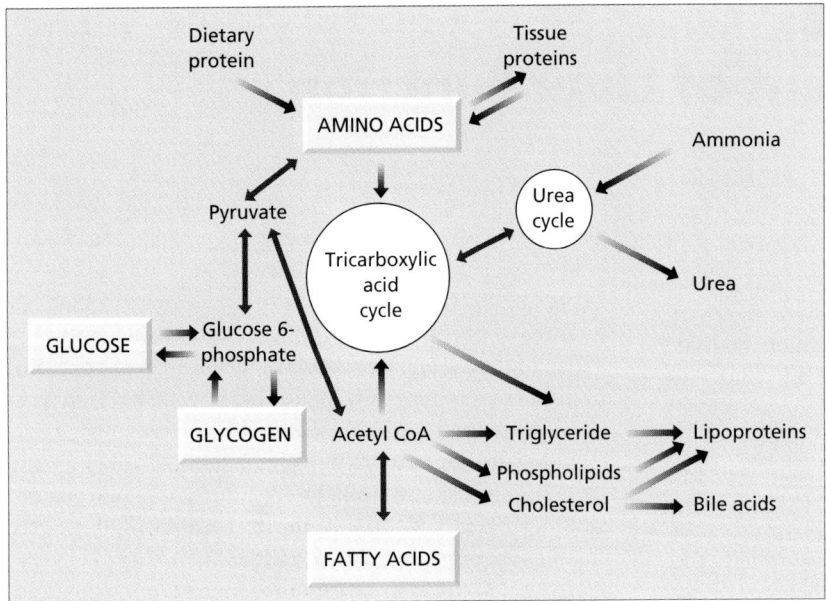

Fig. 2.1. The important metabolic pathways of protein, carbohydrate and fat in the liver.

drug metabolism. Quantitative methods of assessment of liver function using substrates for a specific hepatic pathway, including galactose, caffeine and lignocaine give a better measure of hepatic *function* rather than *damage* (see p. 21). Quantitation of the asialoglycoprotein receptor also provides a measure of the 'functional mass' of the liver.

Bile pigments

Bilirubin

Bilirubin metabolism is described in detail in Chapter 12.

The serum bilirubin may be increased in both cholestatic and hepato-cellular disease with an associated rise in liver enzymes. In these cases the bilirubin is predominantly conjugated. An isolated rise in serum bilirubin (without enzyme elevation) may be familial, or due to haemolysis (fig. 2.2).

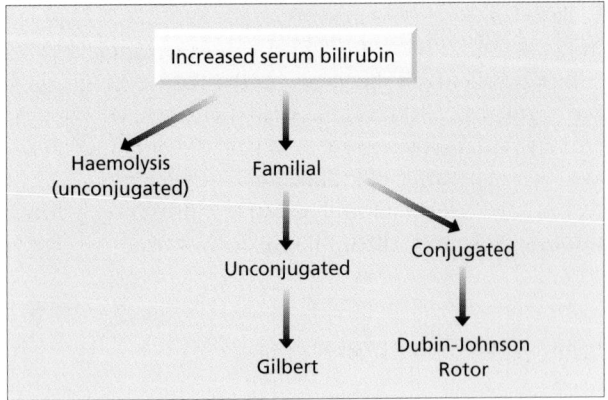

Fig. 2.2. Algorithm for managing a patient with an isolated increase in serum total bilirubin.

Serum bilirubin estimations are based on the van den Bergh diazo reaction. A direct reaction at 10 minutes gives an estimate of the conjugated bilirubin present. The total bilirubin is determined in the presence of an accelerator such as caffeine-benzoate or methanol. An approximate value for the unconjugated (indirect) bilirubin is obtained by subtracting the value for conjugated from that for the total bilirubin.

These diazo reactions are subject to error and diagnosis should not be based solely upon them [5]. Other more accurate methods for estimation such as thin layer chromatography, high performance gas liquid chromatography and alkaline methanolysis are available but are too elaborate to be clinically useful [3].

Inspection of *faeces* is an important investigation in jaundice. Clay-coloured stools indicate cholestatic jaundice but may also occur in hepato-cellular jaundice. The colour will be normal in haemolytic jaundice. Rarely pale stools occur in very severe bilirubin glucuronyl-transferase deficiency.

Bilirubin cannot be detected in the *urine* of normal subjects or patients with unconjugated hyperbilirubinaemia. In cholestatic patients a small fraction of the conjugated bilirubin in plasma is dialysable and filtered by the glomerulus, some is re-absorbed by the tubules, and the remainder gives the dark colour to the urine.

'Dipsticks' are commercially available, easy to use and give satisfactory results for the detection of conjugated bilirubin in urine.

Uses. In acute virus hepatitis bilirubin appears in the urine before urobilinogen or before jaundice. In an undiagnosed febrile illness, bilirubinuria favours the diagnosis of hepatitis.

As a screening test urinary bilirubin has some value in general practice detecting the pre-icteric patient. It is, however, an insensitive test for patients with enzyme elevation alone [1].

Urobilinogen

Bacterial action converts bilirubin in the colon to a series of colourless tetrapyrroles collectively called urobilinogen. Approximately 20% is absorbed and undergoes an enteric circulation with re-excretion into bile by the liver. A small proportion is excreted in the urine. Urinary urobilinogen has been used in the evaluation of liver problems. In complete bile duct obstruction where no bilirubin enters the intestine, urinary urobilinogen may be absent. However, measurement of this substance in the urine has been superseded by more sensitive serum tests as well as imaging, which give a more direct path to diagnosis. As with urinary bilirubin measurements, spot urinary urobilinogen is a poor predictor of hepatic disease with a high proportion of false negative results [1].

Bromsulphalein

The dye bromsulphalein (BSP) is rapidly removed by the liver and excreted in the bile. The intravenous test was used to assess liver dysfunction in the absence of jaundice. However, in view of the cost, the occasional side-effects (which may be fatal) and the inconvenience, it is rarely performed nowadays.

In patients suspected of Dubin–Johnson hyperbilirubinaemia a blood sample is taken not only at 45 minutes after injection but also at 2 hours. A higher level of BSP at 2 hours than at 45 minutes is diagnostic and reflects release of conjugated BSP back into the blood-stream after a normal initial uptake [4].

Indocyanine green

This dye is removed from the circulation by the liver. It is not conjugated and there is no extra-hepatic removal or entero-hepatic circulation. It is safer, more expensive and more specific than BSP. It is used for liver blood flow studies [2].

References

1 Binder L, Smith D, Kupka T *et al*. Failure of prediction of liver function test abnormalities with the urine urobilinogen and urine bilirubin assays. *Arch. Pathol. Lab. Med.* 1989; **113**: 73.

2 Caesar J, Shaldon S, Chiandussi L *et al*. The use of indocyanine green in the measurement of hepatic blood flow and as a test of hepatic function. *Clin. Sci.* 1961; **21**: 43.

3 Fevery J, Blanckaert N. What can we learn from analysis of the serum bilirubin? *J. Hepatol.* 1986; **2**: 113.

4 Mandema E, DeFraiture WH, Nieweg HO *et al*. Familial chronic idiopathic jaundice (Dubin–Sprinz disease) with a note on bromsulphalein metabolism in this disease. *Am. J. Med.* 1960; **28**: 42.

5 Rosenthal P. The laboratory method as a variable in the diagnosis of hyperbilirubinemia. *Am. J. Dis. Child.* 1987; **141**: 1066.

Serum enzyme tests

These tests will usually indicate the type of liver injury, whether hepato-cellular or cholestatic, but cannot be expected to differentiate one form of hepatitis from another or to determine whether cholestasis is intra- or extra-hepatic. They are valuable in directing the choice of specific serological tests, imaging or liver biopsy to reach the diagnosis. Only a few tests are necessary and the combination of a serum aspartate transaminase (AST formerly SGOT) and alkaline phosphatase, with occasionally serum alanine transaminase (ALT formerly SGPT) is adequate. The degree of elevation of some biochemical tests in patients with liver disease may be effected by dietary intake, for example of fats [2].

Alkaline phosphatase

The level of alkaline phosphatase rises in cholestasis and to a lesser extent when liver cells are damaged (fig. 2.3). The mechanisms of the increase are complex [6]. Synthesis of the alkaline phosphatase by the hepatocyte is increased and this depends on intact protein and RNA synthesis. Secretion into the serum may arise through leakage from canaliculus into the sinusoid because of leaky tight junctions. Increased release of alkaline phosphatase into sinusoids from the hepatocyte plasma membranes may contribute.

Serum hepatic alkaline phosphatase may be distinguished from bony phosphatase by fractionation into iso-enzymes, but this is not routinely carried out. An isolated rise in alkaline phosphatase may be of intestinal origin [7]. A rise in γ-GT confirms the likely source of alkaline phosphatase as being hepato-biliary. Raised levels are sometimes observed with primary or secondary hepatic tumours, even without jaundice or involvement of bone. Increased values without a rise in serum bilirubin are also found with other space-occupying lesions or infiltration, such as amyloid, abscess, leukaemia or granulomas. Non-specific mild elevations are seen in a variety of conditions including Hodgkin's disease and heart failure. The cause is presumably focal, intra-hepatic bile duct obstruction caused by these lesions.

Gamma glutamyl transpeptidase

Serum values are increased in cholestasis and hepato-cellular disease. Levels parallel serum alkaline phosphatase in cholestasis and may be used to confirm that a

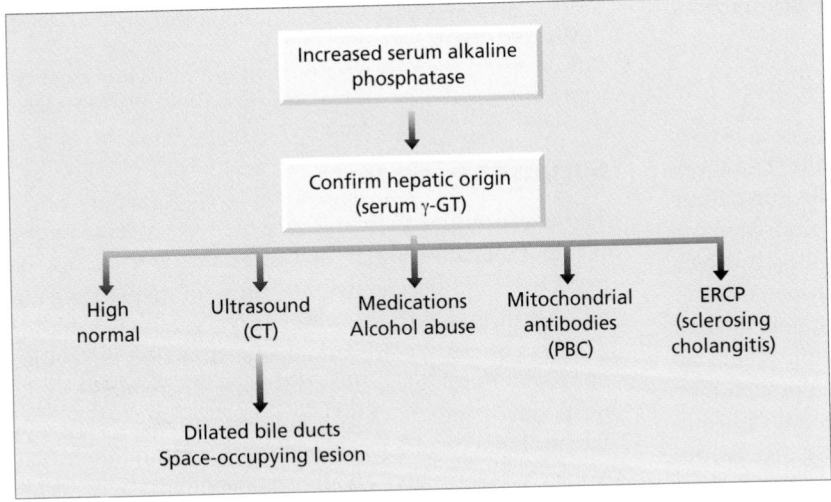

Fig. 2.3. Algorithm for managing a patient with an isolated increase in serum alkaline phosphatase or serum gamma glutamyl transpeptidase (γ-GT). PBC = primary biliary cirrhosis; ERCP = endoscopic retrograde cholangiopancreatography.

raised serum phosphatase is of hepato-biliary origin (see above). Levels are increased with hepatic metastases, not consistently but more so than for alkaline phosphatase.

An isolated rise in serum γ-GT is seen in patients with alcohol abuse, even without liver disease, perhaps because of microsomal enzyme induction. More often there is steatosis. In fibrosis, cirrhosis and hepatitis due to alcohol, other liver enzymes are elevated in conjunction with γ-GT [5].

Unfortunately many factors influence the level so that increases are non-disease-specific. Disorders include hepato-biliary disease, alcoholism, and concomitant drug administration for instance with barbiturates or phenytoin. Screening with serum γ-GT may have led to more alcohol abusers being identified although in a third of such individuals the serum γ-GT does not rise. The finding of increased levels, however, often leads to over-investigation of an elevated level in an innocent person who has never taken alcohol or a social drinker who has never abused alcohol.

Aminotransferases

Glutamic oxaloacetic transaminase (GOT, aspartate transaminase) is a mitochondrial enzyme present in large quantities in heart, liver, skeletal muscle and kidney and the serum level increases whenever these tissues are acutely destroyed, presumably due to release from damaged cells.

Glutamic pyruvic transaminase (GPT, alanine transaminase) is a cytosolic enzyme also present in liver [8]. Although the absolute amount is less than SGOT, a greater proportion is present in liver compared with heart and skeletal muscles. A serum increase is therefore more specific for liver damage than SGOT.

Transaminase determinations are useful in the early diagnosis of virus hepatitis. Measurements must be made early, for normal values may be reached within a week of the onset. The patient may develop fatal acute hepatic necrosis in spite of falling transaminase values. Serial estimations are essential.

Very high levels may be seen in the early stages of acute cholestasis particularly choledocholithiasis [3], and with circulatory failure.

Routine screening may show unexpectedly raised amino transferase levels (fig. 2.4). These are often due to obesity, diabetes mellitus, alcohol abuse, hepatic drug reaction or circulatory failure. Chronic viral and autoimmune hepatitis must be considered, as must haemochromatosis. Rarer causes include α₁-antitrypsin deficiency.

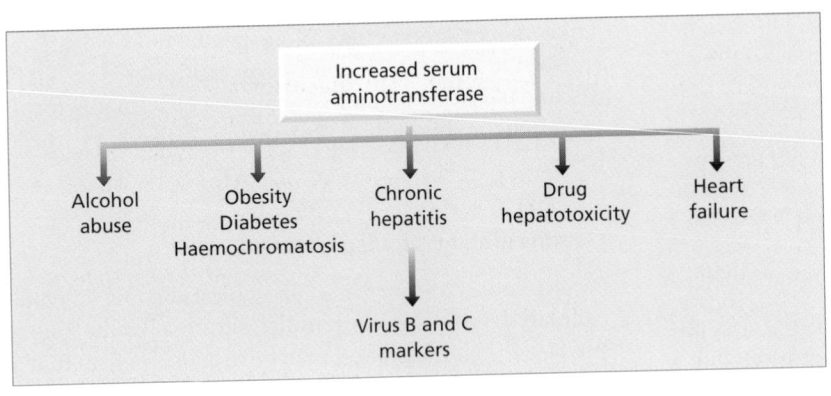

Fig. 2.4. Algorithm for managing a patient with an isolated increase in serum aminotransferase on routine screening.

Liver biopsy is usually necessary to make the diagnosis [4]. However, this should be delayed if the patient is asymptomatic and the increase in transaminase is modest. The value should be monitored.

Results vary in cirrhosis, and are particularly high in chronic hepatitis with active inflammation. Very high levels are unusual in alcoholic liver disease. A high ratio of SGOT to SGPT (greater than two) may be useful in diagnosing alcoholic hepatitis and cirrhosis [1]. This is due not only to hepatocyte damage but to pyridoxal 5-phosphate (vitamin B_6) deficiency.

Other serum enzymes

Lactic dehydrogenase (LDH) is a relatively insensitive index of hepato-cellular injury and is not routinely used. Marked increases are found in patients with neoplasms, especially with hepatic involvement.

References

1 Cohen JA, Kaplan MM. The SGOT : SGPT ratio—an indicator of alcoholic liver disease. *Dig. Dis. Sci.* 1979; **24**: 835.

2 Deems RO, Friedman LS, Friedman MI *et al*. Relationship between liver biochemical tests and dietary intake in patients with liver disease. *J. Clin. Gastroenterol.* 1994; **18**: 304.

3 Fortson WC, Tedesco FJ, Starnes EC *et al*. Marked elevation of serum transaminase activity associated with extrahepatic biliary tract disease. *J. Clin. Gastroenterol.* 1985; **7**: 502.

4 Hultcrantz R, Glaumann H, Lindberg G *et al*. Liver investigation in 149 asymptomatic patients with moderately elevated activities of serum aminotransferases. *Scand. J. Gastroenterol.* 1986; **21**: 109.

5 Ireland A, Hartley L, Ryley N *et al*. Raised γ-glutamyl-transferase activity and the need for liver biopsy. *Br. Med. J.* 1991; **302**: 388.

6 Kaplan MM. Serum alkaline phosphatase—another piece is added to the puzzle. *Hepatology* 1986; **6**: 526.

7 Rosalki SB, Foo AY, Dooley JS. Benign familial hyperphosphatasaemia as a cause of unexplained increase in plasma alkaline phosphatase activity. *J. Clin. Pathol.* 1993; **46**: 738.

8 Sherman KE. Alanine aminotransferase in clinical practice: a review. *Arch. Intern. Med.* 1991; **151**: 260.

Quantitative assessment of hepatic function (table 2.2)

Chronic liver diseases pass through a long period of minimum non-specific symptoms ('compensated') until the final stage of ascites, jaundice, encephalopathy and pre-coma ('decompensated'). Serum albumin and prothrombin time give some indication of the synthetic function of the liver, but this is usually maintained until late disease. Serial estimates of *quantitative liver function* in the early stages would be helpful both in monitoring treatment and in prognosis but are of no value in diagnosis.

In the rat model of biliary cirrhosis, serial breath tests

Table 2.2. Quantitative hepatic function tests

Site	Substrate	Function
Cytosol	Galactose*	Galactokinase (phosphorylation)
Microsome (cytochrome P450 system)	Aminopyrine	N-demethylation
	Caffeine	N-demethylation
	Lignocaine	N-deethylation
	Antipyrine	Hydroxylation/ demethylation
Plasma membrane	Galactose terminated glycoprotein	Asialoglycoprotein receptor

* Low dose assesses hepatic perfusion.

allow prediction of the time of death from cirrhosis. In 78 patients with cirrhosis, galactose elimination capacity, aminopyrine breath test and indocyanine green clearance predicted survival (fig. 2.5) but were not significantly better than the Child (Pugh) score [7]. In 190 alcoholic cirrhotics, the aminopyrine breath test had added prognostic value in Child grade A and B, but not grade C patients [11].

Such tests suffer from the drawback of their complexity. The lack of a major impact above routine laboratory tests and Child grading is reflected in their present role in clinical research rather than the routine management of patients.

Galactose elimination capacity

Galactose is pharmacologically safe and can be injected intravenously in a dose sufficient to saturate the enzyme system responsible for its elimination. The rate-limiting step is the initial phosphorylation by galactokinase. Account must be taken of the substantial fraction of the dose eliminated extrahepatically. This test seems to reflect hepato-cellular function fairly accurately but requires multiple determinations over a 2-hour period.

Breath tests

Aminopyrine is metabolized (*N*-demethylated) by the cytochrome P450 (microsomal) system to carbon dioxide. It has many of the characteristics of an ideal breath test substance for the measurement of hepatic function [2]. The aminopyrine is labelled with ^{14}C and given by mouth. Samples of breath are collected at intervals over 2 hours for analysis. The expired $^{14}CO_2$ correlates with the rate of disappearance of radioactivity from the plasma. The test reflects the residual functional microsomal mass and viable hepatic tissue. Results in cirrhotic rats suggest that reduced *N*-demethylation is

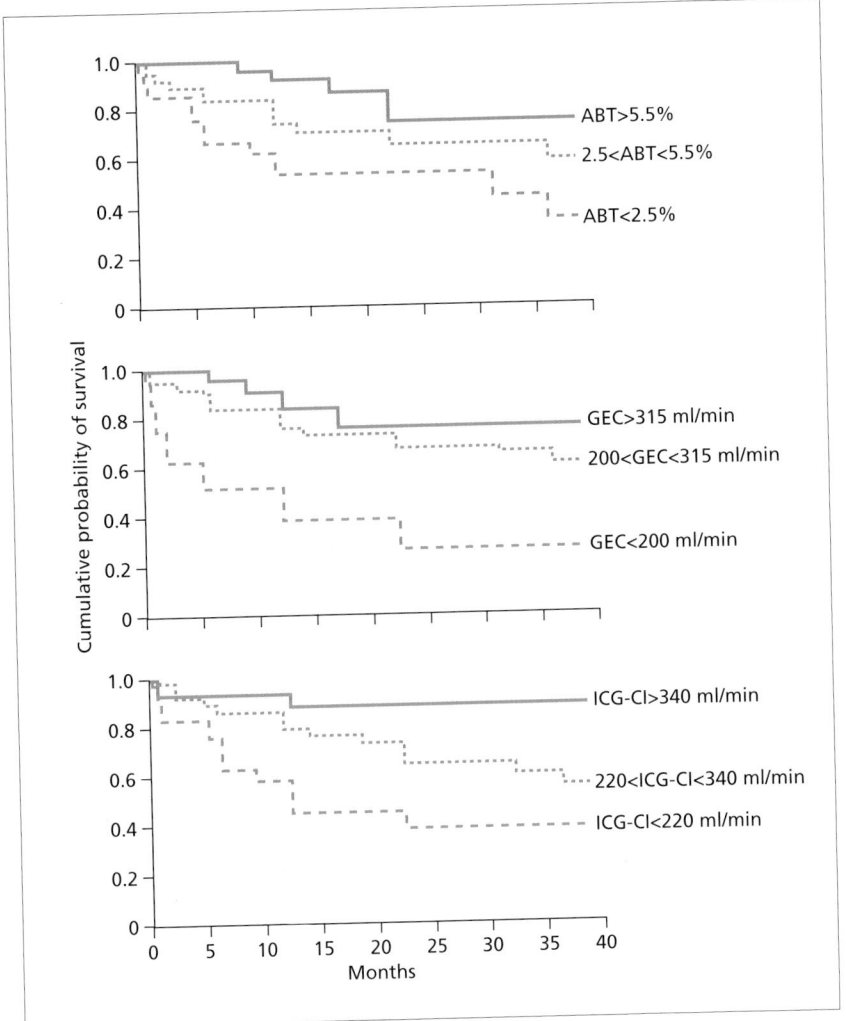

Fig. 2.5. Kaplan–Meier survival curves in 78 patients with cirrhosis stratified according to the results of an aminopyrine breath test (ABT), galactose elimination capacity (GEC) and ICG clearance (ICG-Cl) [7].

due to loss of liver cell volume. The function per hepatocyte remains constant. It is of value in prognosis [7] and to assess therapy rather than for screening or diagnosis. It may be useful to assess the effect of drugs on hepatic microsomal enzyme function.

^{14}C-caffeine and phenacetin have been used as breath test substances. The ^{14}C-galactose breath test measures cytosolic function. All breath tests are complex and costly. They are unlikely to achieve general popularity.

Salivary caffeine clearance

Caffeine (1,3,7-trimethylxanthine) is metabolized almost exclusively by N-demethylation in the hepatic microsomal enzyme system (cytochrome P448). The methylxanthines are excreted in the urine. Serum and salivary caffeine levels can be assayed simply using an enzyme multiplied immuno-assay technique [6, 13]. Overnight caffeine clearance in saliva correlates well with serum clearance and also with the aminopyrine breath test [13]. Salivary caffeine clearance is a simple

method to measure hepatic functional impairment. There is, however, reduced caffeine clearance with increasing age, induction of metabolism by cigarette smoking and interference with metabolism by certain drugs such as cimetidine. Serial caffeine clearance testing in the same patient should be done with a standardized dose of caffeine since clearance is dose dependent [3].

Lignocaine metabolite formation

Lignocaine is metabolized by oxidative N-deethylation by the cytochrome P450 system. Monoethylglycinexylidide (MEGX) is formed and correlates with the rate of lignocaine clearance. Serum MEGX concentration after intravenous injection of lignocaine gives a quantitative assessment of liver function. MEGX concentrations vary widely both in patients without liver disease as well as those with only mild abnormalities [8, 10]. They are significantly lower in cirrhotics and correlate with a worse prognosis [1]. Galactose elimination and aminopyrine breath test may discriminate mild disease from cirrhosis better than MEGX formation [8].

Antipyrine

Antipyrine has a long half-life, which in patients with severe liver disease may increase to 30 hours or more. Sampling of blood or saliva has to be over an extended period which limits the practicability of this agent.

Asialoglycoprotein receptor

Hepatocytes clear asialoglycoproteins (galactose terminated) from the circulation by a specific receptor on the sinusoidal plasma membrane. The number of receptors falls with hepato-cellular damage. Receptor number is quantified by computer analysis of the hepatic uptake of ^{99m}Tc-labelled galactosyl-neoglycalbumin (an asialoglycoprotein analogue) using a standard scintillation camera and a single blood test. Results correlate with severity of liver disease (Child score), aminopyrine breath test and indocyanine green clearance. Mean receptor concentration in end-stage cirrhosis (0.35 ± 0.07 µmol/l) compares with 0.83 ± 0.06 µmol/l in controls [9]. There are similar results with Tc-diethylanetriamine-pentaacetic acid-galactosyl human serum albumin [5]. Receptor number is reduced in acute hepatitis, increasing with recovery [12]. Despite promising results, application of this functional test remains experimental.

Excretory capacity (bromsulphalein)

The old intravenous bromsulphalein disappearance technique allowed an estimate of the storage capacity of the hepatocyte (S) and its excretory function (Tm). It was abandoned because of its complexity, its cost and the untoward reactions to BSP [4].

References

1 Arrigoni A, Gindro T, Aimo G *et al.* Monoethylglycinexylidide test: a prognostic indicator of survival in cirrhosis. *Hepatology* 1994; **20**: 383.
2 Baker AL, Kotake AN, Schoeller DA. Clinical utility of breath tests for the assessment of hepatic function. *Semin. Liv. Dis.* 1983; **3**: 318.
3 Cheng WSC, Murphy TL, Smith MT *et al.* Dose-dependent pharmacokinetics of caffeine in humans: relevance as a test of quantitative liver function. *Clin. Pharmacol. Ther.* 1990; **47**: 516.
4 Hacki W, Bircher J, Preisig R. A new look at the plasma disappearance of sulfobromophthalein (BSP): correlation with the BSP transport maximum and the hepatic plasma flow in man. *J. Lab. Clin. Med.* 1976; **88**: 1019.
5 Kudo M, Todo A, Ikekubo K *et al.* Quantitative assessment

of hepatocellular function through *in vivo* radioreceptor imaging with technetium-99m galactosyl human serum albumin. *Hepatology* 1993; **17**: 814.
6 McDonagh JE, Nathan VV, Bonavia IC *et al.* Caffeine clearance by enzyme multiplied immunoassay technique: a simple, inexpensive, and useful indicator of liver function. *Gut* 1991; **32**: 681.
7 Merkel C, Gatta A, Zoli M *et al.* Prognostic value of galactose elimination capacity, aminopyrine breath test, and ICG clearance in patients with cirrhosis: comparison with the Pugh score. *Dig. Dis. Sci.* 1991; **36**: 1197.
8 Meyer-Wyss B, Renner E, Luo H *et al.* Assessment of lidocaine metabolite formation in comparison with other quantitative liver function tests. *J. Hepatol.* 1993; **19**: 133.
9 Pimstone NR, Stadalnik RC, Vera DR *et al.* Evaluation of hepatocellular function by way of receptor-mediated uptake of a technetium-99m labeled asialoglycoprotein analog. *Hepatology* 1994; **20**: 917.
10 Shiffman ML, Luketic VA, Sanyal AJ *et al.* Hepatic lidocaine metabolism and liver histology in patients with chronic hepatitis and cirrhosis. *Hepatology* 1994; **19**: 933.
11 Urbain D, Muls V, Thys O *et al.* Aminopyrine breath test improves long-term prognostic evaluation in patients with alcoholic cirrhosis in Child classes A and B. *J. Hepatol.* 1995; **22**: 179.
12 Virgolini I, Müller C, Höbart J *et al.* Liver function in acute viral hepatitis as determined by a hepatocyte-specific ligand: ^{99m}Tc-galactosyl-neoglycoalbumin. *Hepatology* 1992; **15**: 593.
13 Wahllander A, Mohr S, Paumgartner G. Assessment of hepatic function: comparison of caffeine clearance in serum and saliva during the day and at night. *J. Hepatol.* 1990; **10**: 129.

Lipid and lipoprotein metabolism

Lipids

The liver is central to lipid (cholesterol, phospholipid, triglyceride) and lipoprotein metabolism. Lipids are insoluble in water. Lipoproteins, hydrophobic within and hydrophilic on the outside, allow their transport in the plasma.

Cholesterol is found in cell membranes and is a precursor of bile acids and steroid hormones. It is synthesized in the liver, small intestine and in other tissues. Some is derived from intestinal absorption, reaching the liver in chylomicron remnants. Cholesterol synthesis takes place mainly from acetyl CoA in the microsomal fraction and in cytosol (fig. 2.6). Hepatic synthesis is inhibited by cholesterol feeding and by fasting, and is increased by a biliary fistula or bile duct ligation and also by an intestinal lymph fistula. The rate-limiting step is the conversion of 3-hydroxy-3-methylglutaryl-CoA (HMG-CoA) to mevalonate by the enzyme HMG-CoA reductase. The mechanism controlling this process is uncertain. Cholesterol in membranes and in bile is present almost exclusively as free cholesterol. Bile provides the only significant route for cholesterol excretion. In plasma and

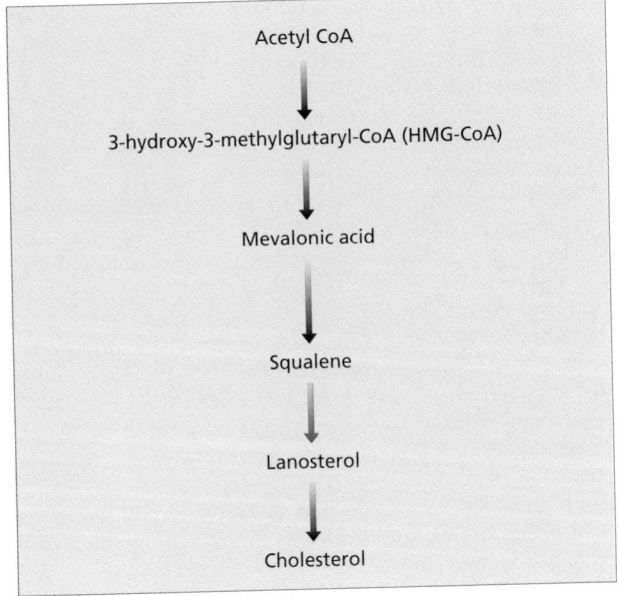

Fig. 2.6. Cholesterol biosynthesis.

in certain tissues such as liver, adrenal and skin, cholesterol esters (cholesterol esterified with long-chain fatty acids) are also found. Cholesterol esters are more non-polar than free cholesterol and therefore are even less soluble in water. Esterification is carried out in plasma by the enzyme lecithin cholesterol acyl transferase (LCAT) which is synthesized in the liver.

Phospholipids are a heterogeneous group of compounds. They contain one or more phosphoric acid groups and another polar group. This may be a heterogeneous base such as choline or ethanolamine. In addition there are one or more long-chain fatty acid residues. The phospholipids are much more complex in terms of chemical reactivity than cholesterol and cholesterol esters. They are important constituents of cell membranes and take part in a large number of chemical reactions. The most abundant phospholipid in plasma and most cellular membranes is phosphatidyl choline (lecithin).

Triglycerides are simpler compounds than the phospholipids. They have a backbone of glycerol, the hydroxy groups of which have been esterified with fatty acids. Naturally occurring triglycerides contain a variety of fatty acids; they act as a store of energy and also a method of transport of energy from the gut and liver to peripheral tissues.

Lipoproteins

These are essential for the circulation and metabolism of lipids. They are particles and are separated by their differing density on ultracentrifugation. This explains their nomenclature. Their surface comprises apolipoprotein, of several different types (table 2.3), free cholesterol and phospholipids. Inside there is cholesterol ester, triglycerides and fat-soluble vitamins.

There are several metabolic cycles for lipoprotein, of which two are prominent: one is involved in fat absorbed from the intestine, and the other is responsible for the handling of endogenously synthesized lipid (fig. 2.7). There is overlap between the two.

Dietary fat is absorbed from the small intestine, and incorporated into chylomicrons. These enter the circulation (via the thoracic duct) where the triglyceride is removed by the action of lipoprotein lipases. The triglyceride is utilized or stored in tissue. The chylomicron remnant is taken up by the liver and the cholesterol enters metabolic pathways or plasma membranes, or is excreted in bile.

In the endogenous pathway, triglyceride leaves the liver in VLDL. In the circulation the triglyceride is removed by the action of lipoprotein lipases. As a result VLDL particles become smaller, forming intermediate density lipoprotein (IDL), and then LDL, the major carrier for cholesterol. The predominant route for removal of LDL is by LDL receptors on the liver surface, but there are receptors on other cells which become important in the formation of atheromatous plaques.

HDL is the particle facilitating cholesterol removal from peripheral tissues. The HDL cholesterol is either taken up by the liver, or is incorporated into IDL resulting in the mature LDL. This removal of peripheral cholesterol is an important pathway, as reflected in the protective effect of a high HDL–cholesterol level against

Table 2.3. Properties of lipoprotein

Lipoproteins	Apolipoprotein	Source	Carries
Chylomicrons	B48, AI, C-II, E	Intestine	Dietary fat
Very low density lipoprotein (VLDL)	B100, C-II, E	Liver	Hepatic triglyceride and cholesterol
Low density lipoprotein (LDL)	B100	From VLDL	Cholesterol
High density lipoprotein (HDL)	A-I, A-II	Peripheral tissue	Cholesterol ester

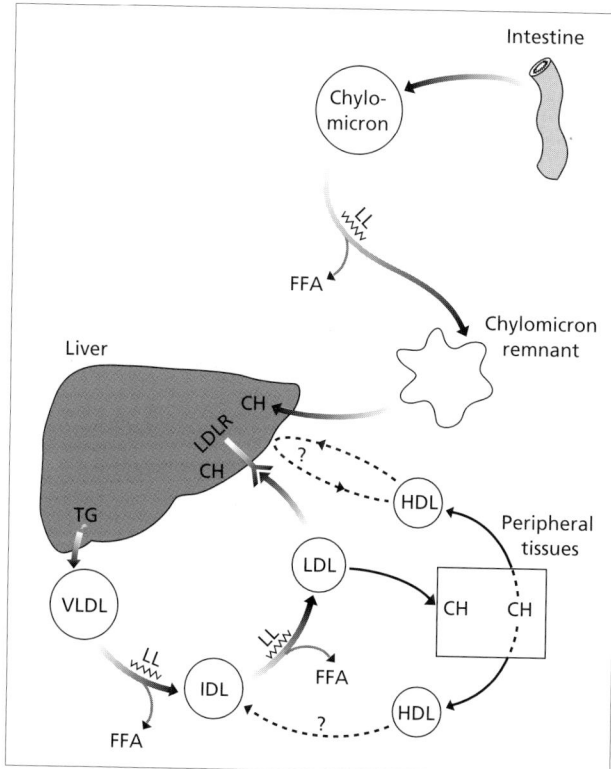

Fig. 2.7. The role of the liver in lipoprotein metabolism. LL = lipoprotein lipase; FFA = free fatty acid; CH = cholesterol; TG = triglyceride; LDLR = LDL receptor. (For lipoproteins see table 2.3.)

coronary artery disease. The metabolism of the HDL particle is still unclear.

Most apolipoproteins are made by the liver, some by the intestines. Apart from being components of lipoproteins, some have other functions; Apo A-1 activates plasma LCAT; C-11 activates lipoprotein lipase.

Changes in liver disease [1]

Cholestasis. Total and free cholesterol are increased. This is not due simply to the retention of cholesterol normally excreted in the bile. The mechanism is uncertain. Four factors have been implicated: regurgitation of biliary cholesterol into the circulation; increased hepatic synthesis of cholesterol; reduced plasma LCAT activity; and regurgitation of biliary lecithin, which produces a shift of cholesterol from pre-existing tissue cholesterol into the plasma. Whereas slight increases to 1.5–2 times normal are sometimes seen in acute cholestasis, very high values are found in chronic conditions, especially post-operative stricture and primary biliary cirrhosis. Values of over five times the upper limit of normal are associated with skin xanthomas. Malnutrition lowers the serum cholesterol so that values may be normal in carcinomatous biliary obstruction.

The level of cholesterol ester is decreased due to LCAT deficiency. Triglycerides tend to be increased. An abnormal lipoprotein, lipoprotein X, very rich in free cholesterol and lethicin is found which appears on electron microscopy as bilamellar discs. The red cell changes in cholestasis are related to abnormalities in cholesterol and lipoprotein.

Parenchymal injury. Triglyerides tend to be increased related to an accumulation of triglyceride-rich LDL. Cholesterol ester is reduced due to a low LCAT. In cirrhosis total serum cholesterol values are usually normal. Low results indicate malnutrition or decompensation. In the fatty liver due to alcohol, VLDL is increased, together with triglycerides. With drug toxicity, failure of apolipoprotein synthesis leads to difficulty in export of triglycerides as VLDL, and hence fatty liver.

Serum cholesterol esters, lipoproteins, LCAT and lipoprotein X are not estimated routinely. They are not of any established value in the diagnosis or assessment of liver function, although low plasma LCAT levels early following liver transplantation may indicate allograft malfunction [2].

References

1 Harry DS, McIntyre N. Plasma lipoproteins and the liver. In *Wright's Liver and Biliary Disease*, 3rd edn, Millward-Sadler GH, Wright R, Arthur MJP, eds. WB Saunders, 1992: 61.

2 Shimada M, Yanaga K, Makowka L *et al.* Significance of lecithin: cholesterol acyltransferase activity as a prognostic indicator of early allograft function in clinical liver transplantation. *Transplantation* 1989; **48**: 600.

Bile acids

Bile acids are synthesized only in the liver, 250–500 mg being produced and lost in the faeces daily. Synthesis is under negative feedback control. The primary bile acids, cholic acid and chenodeoxycholic acid, are formed from cholesterol (fig. 2.8). Synthesis is controlled by the amount of bile acid returning to the liver in the enterohepatic circulation. When exposed to colonic bacteria the primary bile acids undergo 7α-dehydroxylation with the production of the secondary bile acids, deoxycholic and a very little lithocholic acid. Tertiary bile acids, largely ursodeoxycholic acid, are formed in the liver by epimerization of secondary bile acids. In human bile the amount of the trihydroxy acid (cholic acid) roughly equals the sum of the two dihydroxy acids (chenodeoxycholic and deoxycholic).

The bile acids are conjugated in the liver with the amino acids glycine or taurine. This prevents absorption in the biliary tree and small intestine but permits conservation by absorption in the terminal ileum. Sulphation and glucuronidation (as a detoxifying mechanism) may be increased with cirrhosis or cholestasis when these

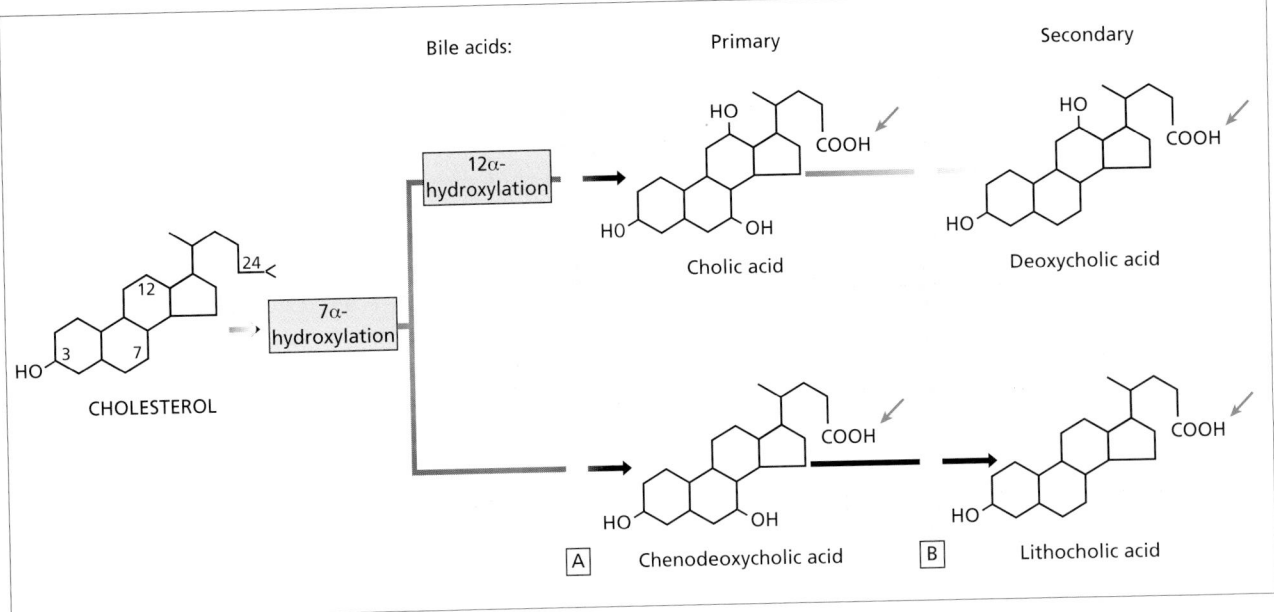

Fig. 2.8. Production of primary and secondary bile acids from cholesterol. A = oxidation cleavage of side chain, from C27 steroid to C24 carboxylic acid; B = 7α-dehydroxylation by intestinal bacteria; arrows = site of conjugation with glycine and taurine.

conjugates are found in excess in the urine and also in bile [11]. Bacteria can hydrolyse bile salts to bile acid and glycine or taurine.

Bile salts are excreted into the biliary canaliculus against an enormous concentration gradient between liver and bile. This depends in part on the intracellular negative potential of approximately –35 mV, which provides potential-dependent facilitated diffusion, and also on a carrier mediated process involving a 100 kDa glycoprotein [7, 9]. The bile salts enter into micellar and vesicular association with cholesterol and phospholipids. In the upper small intestine the bile salt micelles are too large and too polar (hydrophilic) to be absorbed. They are intimately concerned with the digestion and absorption of lipids. When the terminal ileum and proximal colon are reached, absorption of bile acid takes place by an active transport process found only in the ileum. Non-ionic passive diffusion occurs throughout the whole intestine and is most efficient for unconjugated, dihydroxy bile acid. Oral administration of ursodeoxycholic acid interferes with the small intestinal absorption of both chenodeoxycholic and cholic acid [10].

The absorbed bile salts enter the portal venous system and reach the liver where they are taken up with great avidity by the hepatocytes. This depends upon a sodium coupled co-transport system using the sodium gradient across the sinusoidal membrane as a driving force. Chloride ions may also be involved. The most hydro-

phobic bile acids (unconjugated mono and dihydroxy bile acids) probably enter the hepatocyte by simple diffusion ('flip-flop') across the lipid membrane. The mechanism of bile acid passage across the liver cell from sinusoid to bile canaliculus is controversial. Cytosolic bile acid binding proteins, for example 3α-hydroxysteroid dehydrogenase, are involved [12]. The role of microtubules is uncertain. Vesicles seem to play a role but only at higher bile acid concentrations [2]. The bile acids are reconjugated and re-excreted into bile. Lithocholic acid is not re-excreted.

This entero-hepatic circulation of bile salts takes place 2–15 times daily (fig. 2.9). Because absorption efficiency varies among the individual bile acids they have different synthesis and fractional turnover rates.

In cholestasis bile acids are excreted in the urine by active transport and passive diffusion. They tend to be sulphated and these conjugates are actively secreted by the renal tubule [13].

Changes in disease

Bile salts increase the biliary excretion of water, lecithin, cholesterol and conjugated bilirubin. Ursodeoxycholic acid produces a much greater choleresis than chenodeoxycholic or cholic acid [8].

Altered biliary excretion with defective biliary micelle formation is important in the pathogenesis of gallstones (Chapter 31). It also leads to the steatorrhoea of cholestasis.

Bile salts form a micellar solution with cholesterol and phospholipid, and in this way help to emulsify dietary fat and also play a part in the mucosal phase of absorption. Diminished secretion leads to steatorrhoea

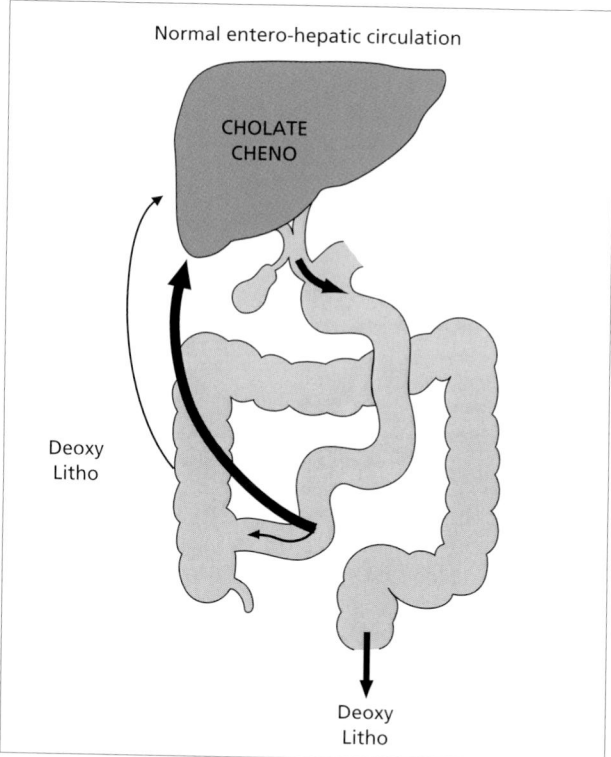

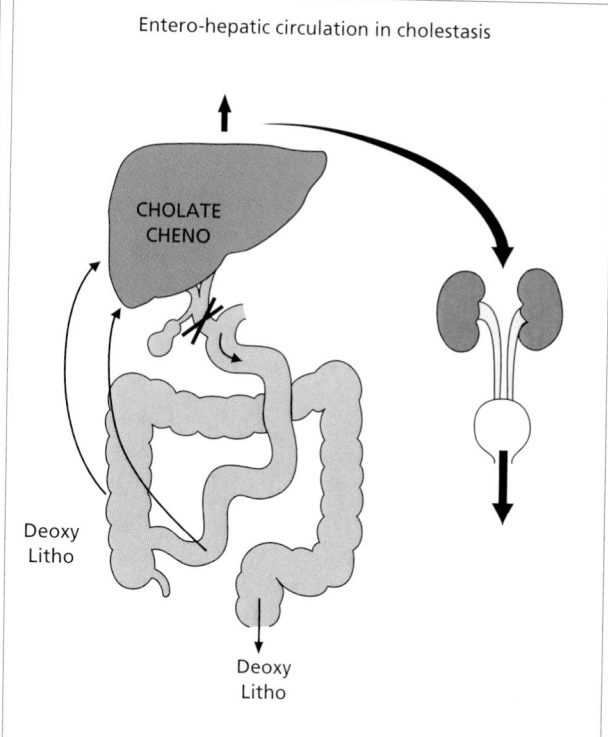

Fig. 2.9. The entero-hepatic circulation of bile acids in normal subjects and in cholestasis.

(fig. 2.10). They assist pancreatic lipolysis. They release gastrointestinal hormones.

Disordered intra-hepatic metabolism of bile salts may be important in the pathogenesis of cholestasis (Chapter 13). They used to be thought to have a role in the pruritus of cholestasis but data now suggest that other substances are responsible (Chapter 35).

They may be responsible for target cells in the peripheral blood of jaundiced patients (Chapter 4) and for the secretion of conjugated bilirubin in urine. If bile acids are deconjugated by small intestinal bacteria, the resulting free bile acids are absorbed. Micelle formation and absorption of fat are then impaired. This may partly explain the malabsorption complicating diseases with stasis and bacterial overgrowth in the small intestine.

Removal of the terminal ileum interrupts the entero-hepatic circulation and allows large amounts of primary bile acids to reach the colon and to be dehydroxylated by bacteria, thus reducing the body's bile salt pool. The altered bile salts in the colon excite a profound electrolyte and water loss with diarrhoea.

Lithocholic acid is mostly excreted in the faeces and only slightly absorbed. It is cirrhotogenic to experimental animals and can be used to produce experimental gallstones. Taurolithocholic acid can also cause intra-hepatic cholestasis perhaps by interfering with the bile-salt independent fraction of bile flow.

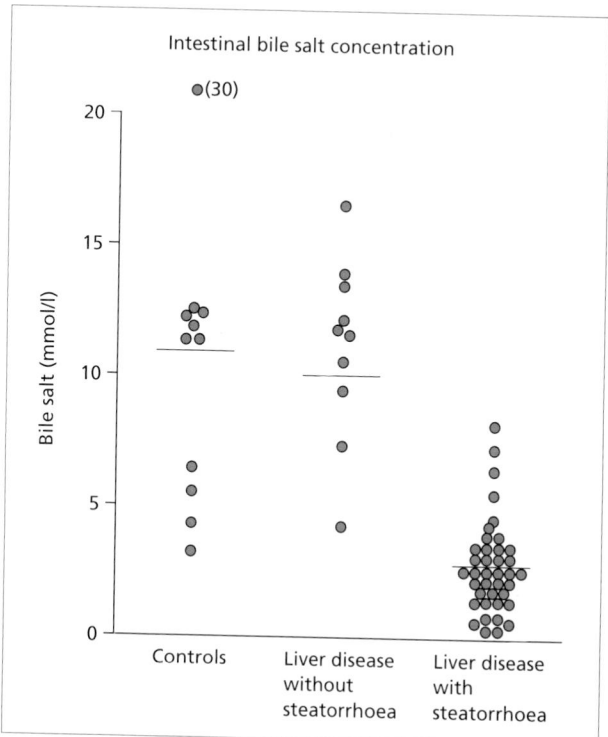

Fig. 2.10. Patients with chronic, non-alcoholic liver disease and steatorrhoea show a reduced bile salt concentration in their aspirated intestinal contents compared with control subjects and patients with chronic liver disease without steatorrhoea.

Serum bile acids

Gas–liquid chromatography allows individual bile acids to be distinguished, but the method is time consuming and the equipment expensive.

Enzymatic assays are based on the use of bacterial 3-hydroxysteroid dehydrogenase. The use of a bioluminescence assay, capable of detecting bile salts in the picomolar range, has improved the sensitivity of this enzymatic technique up to that of radio-immunoassay. The method is simple and inexpensive if the equipment is available. Radio-immunoassay techniques can also measure individual bile acids. Commercial kits are available.

The serum concentration of total bile acids reflects the extent to which bile acids re-absorbed from the intestine have escaped extraction on first passage through the liver. The value reflects the instantaneous balance between intestinal absorption and hepatic uptake. Intestinal load is more important than hepatic extraction in regulating peripheral serum bile acid levels.

Raised levels of serum bile acids are specific for hepato-biliary disease [3]. Sensitivity of serum bile acid estimations is less than originally thought for detecting hepato-cellular damage in viral hepatitis or chronic liver disease. It is, however, better than the serum albumin or the prothrombin time because the value depends not only on hepatic injury, but also on excretory function and portal systemic shunting [6]. It may be useful in determining prognosis. Normal serum bile acids are found in Gilbert's syndrome [14].

The addition to the fasting serum bile acid value of a 2-hour post-prandial level adds little in sensitivity [5].

Estimations of individual bile acids are not diagnostic. In cholestasis the ratio of serum trihydroxy to dihydroxy acid increases. Patients with hepato-cellular failure usually have a low ratio, the main bile acid being chenodeoxycholic acid. This is due to a reduction in the activity of the 12α-hydroxylase enzyme in the hepatocyte.

Amino acid conjugation is preserved even with severe hepato-cellular damage [1].

Serum conjugated cholic acid, measured by radio-immunoassay, may be the best screening method for liver disease [4].

In cholestasis bile acids are excreted in the *urine*. The pattern is similar to that in the serum, but sulphate esters account for a larger proportion of the total bile acids [13].

References

1 Arisaka M, Arisaka O, Nittono H *et al.* Conjugating ability of bile acids in hepatic failure. *Acta Paediatr. Scand.* 1986; **75**: 875.
2 Crawford JM, Gollan JL. Transcellular transport of organic anions in hepatocytes: still a long way to go. *Hepatology* 1991; **14**: 192.
3 Ferraris R, Colombatti G, Florentini MT *et al.* Diagnostic value of serum bile acids and routine liver function tests in hepatobiliary diseases: sensitivity, specificity, and predictive value. *Dig. Dis. Sci.* 1983; **28**: 129.
4 Ferraris R, Florentini T, Galatola G *et al.* Diagnostic value of serum immunoreactive conjugated cholic or chenodeoxycholic acids in detecting hepatobiliary diseases. Comparison with levels of 3 alpha-hydroxy bile acids determined enzymatically and with routine liver tests. *Dig. Dis. Sci.* 1987; **32**: 817.
5 Greenfield SM, Soloway RD, Carithers RL Jr. *et al.* Evaluation of postprandial serum bile acid response as a test of hepatic function. *Dig. Dis. Sci.* 1986; **31**: 785.
6 Hofmann AF. The aminopyrine demethylation breath test and the serum bile acid level: nominated but not yet elected to join the common liver tests. *Hepatology* 1982; **2**: 512.
7 Hofmann AF. Bile acid secretion, bile flow and biliary lipid secretion in humans. *Hepatology* 1990; **12**: 17S.
8 Loria P, Carulli N, Medici G *et al.* Determinants of bile secretion: effect of bile salt structure on bile flow and biliary cation secretion. *Gastroenterology* 1989; **96**: 1142.
9 Meier PJ. The bile salt secretory polarity of hepatocytes. *J. Hepatol.* 1989; **9**: 124.
10 Stiehl A, Raedsch R, Rudolph G. Acute effects of ursodeoxycholic and chenodeoxycholic acid on the small intestinal absorption of bile acids. *Gastroenterology* 1990; **98**: 424.
11 Stiehl A, Raedsch R, Rudolph G *et al.* Biliary and urinary excretion of sulfated, glucuronidated and tetrahydroxylated bile acids in cirrhotic patients. *Hepatology* 1985; **5**: 492.
12 Stolz A, Takikawa H, Ookhtens M *et al.* The role of cytoplasmic proteins in hepatic bile acid transport. *Ann. Rev. Physiol.* 1989; **51**: 161.
13 Summerfield JA, Cullen J, Barnes S *et al.* Evidence for renal control of urinary excretion of bile acids and bile acid sulphates in the cholestatic syndrome. *Clin. Sci. Mol. Med.* 1977; **52**: 51.
14 Vierling JM, Berk PD, Hofmann AF *et al.* Normal fasting-state levels of serum cholyl-conjugated bile acids in Gilbert's syndrome: an aid to diagnosis. *Hepatology* 1982; **2**: 340.

Amino acid metabolism

Amino acids derived from the diet and from tissue breakdown reach the liver for metabolism. Some are transaminated or deaminated to keto-acids which are then metabolized by many pathways including the tricarboxylic acid cycle (Krebs–citric acid cycle). Others are metabolized to ammonia and urea (Krebs–Henseleit urea cycle). The maximal rate of urea synthesis in chronic liver disease is markedly reduced [7]. However, experimentally, at least 85% of liver must be removed before this mechanism fails significantly and before blood and urinary amino acid levels increase. A low blood urea concentration is a rare accompaniment of fulminant liver failure. A rise in blood ammonia level also represents a failure of the Krebs–Henseleit cycle and this increase has been related to hepatic encephalopathy.

Clinical significance

A generalized or selective amino aciduria is a feature of hepato-cellular disease. In patients with severe liver disease the usual picture is an increase in the plasma concentration of one or both of the aromatic amino acids tyrosine and phenylalanine, together with methionine, and a reduction in the branched-chain amino acids valine, leucine and isoleucine (fig. 2.11) [5]. The changes are explained by impaired hepatic function, portosystemic shunting of blood and hyperinsulinaemia and hyperglucagonaemia. Patients with minimal liver disease also show changes, particularly a reduction in plasma proline, perhaps reflecting increased collagen production. There is no difference in the ratio between branched-chain and aromatic amino acids whether or not the patients show hepatic encephalopathy.

In fulminant hepatitis there is marked generalized aminoaciduria involving particularly cystine and tyrosine and this carries a bad prognosis.

Plasma proteins

The plasma proteins produced by the hepatocyte are synthesized on polyribosomes bound to the rough endoplasmic reticulum, from which they are discharged into the plasma [10]. Falls in concentration usually reflect decreased hepatic synthesis although changes in plasma volume and losses, for instance into gut or urine, may contribute.

The hepatocyte makes albumin, fibrinogen, α_1-antitrypsin, haptoglobin, caeruloplasmin, transferrin and prothrombin (table 2.4). Some liver-produced proteins are acute phase reactors and rise in response to tissue injury such as inflammation (table 2.4). These include fibrinogen, haptoglobin, α_1-antitrypsin, C_3 component of complement and caeruloplasmin. An acute phase response may contribute to well-maintained or increased serum concentrations of these proteins, even with hepato-cellular disease.

The mechanism is complex but cytokines (IL1, IL6, TNF-α) play a role [1, 9]. IL6 binds to the cell-surface receptor and this stimulates a message from the hepatocyte membrane to the nucleus where there is induction of specific nuclear factors with responsive promoter elements at the 5' end of several acute phase genes. There are also post-transcriptional as well as transcriptional mechanisms. Cytokines not only stimulate production of acute phase proteins but also inhibit the synthesis of albumin, transferrin and a range of other proteins.

The *immunoglobulins* IgG, IgM and IgA are synthesized by the B cells of the lymphoid system.

Some 10 g *albumin* is synthesized by the normal liver daily, whereas those with cirrhosis can only synthesize about 4 g. In liver disease, the fall in serum albumin concentration is slow, for the half-life of albumin is about 22 days. Thus a patient with fulminant liver failure may die with a virtually normal serum albumin value. A patient with decompensated cirrhosis would be expected to have a low level (figs 2.12, 2.13).

α_1-*antitrypsin* deficiency is genetically determined.

Haptoglobin is a glycoprotein composed of two types of polypeptide chains, α and β, which are covalently associated by disulphide bonds. Haptoglobin is largely synthesized by the hepatocyte. Hereditary deficiencies are frequent in American Blacks. Low values are found in severe chronic hepato-cellular disease and in haemolytic crises.

Caeruloplasmin is the major copper-containing protein in plasma and is responsible for the oxidase activity. A

Table 2.4. Serum (plasma) proteins synthesized by the liver

	Normal concentration
Albumin	40–50 g/litre
α_1-antitrypsin*	2–4 g/litre
α-fetoprotein	<10 Ku/litre
α_2-macroglobulin	2.2–3.8 g/litre
Caeruloplasmin*	0.2–0.4 g/litre
Complement components (C_3, C_6 and C_1)	
Fibrinogen*	2–6 g/litre
Haemopexin	0.8–1.0 g/litre
Prothrombin (factor II)†	
Transferrin	2–3 g/litre

* Acute phase proteins.
† Vitamin K dependent; also factors VII and X.

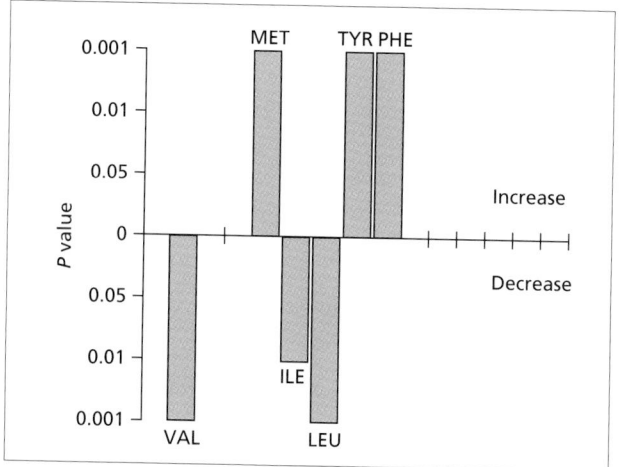

Fig. 2.11. The plasma amino acid pattern in cryptogenic cirrhosis (mean of 11 patients) compared with normal individuals. The aromatic amino acids and methionine are increased while the branched-chain amino acids are decreased. MET = methionine; TYR = tyrosine; PHE = phenylalanine; VAL = valine; ILE = isoleucine; LEU = leucine [5].

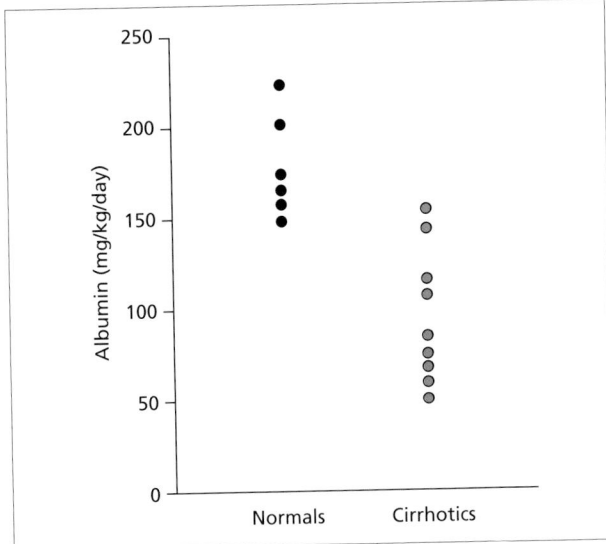

Fig. 2.12. The absolute synthesis of serum albumin (^{14}C carbonate method) in cirrhosis is reduced [11].

low concentration is found in 95% of those who are homozygous and about 10% of those heterozygous for Wilson's disease [8]. Caeruloplasmin increases to normal if a patient with Wilson's disease has a hepatic transplant. One must estimate caeruloplasmin in all patients with chronic hepatitis so that Wilson's disease, with its

mandatory penicillamine therapy, may be diagnosed. However, low values are also found in very severe decompensated cirrhosis which is not due to Wilson's disease. High values are found in pregnancy, following oestrogen therapy and with large bile duct obstruction.

Transferrin is the iron transport protein. The plasma transferrin is more than 90% saturated with iron in patients with untreated idiopathic haemochromatosis. Reduced values may be found with cirrhosis.

The C_3 *component of complement* tends to be reduced in cirrhosis, normal in chronic hepatitis and increased in compensated primary biliary cirrhosis. Low values in fulminant hepatic failure and alcoholic cirrhosis with or without hepatitis reflect reduced hepatic synthesis and there is a correlation with prolonged prothrombin time and depression of serum albumin concentration [2]. There is also a contribution from increased consumption due to activation of the complement system. Transient reductions are found in the early 'immune complex' stage of acute hepatitis B.

Alpha-fetoprotein is a normal component of plasma protein in human fetuses older than 6 weeks, and reaches maximum concentration at between 12 and 16 weeks of fetal life. A few weeks after birth it disappears from the circulation but reappears in the blood of patients with primary liver cancer and can be shown in the tumour by indirect immunofluorescence. Raised values are also found with embryonic tumours of ovary

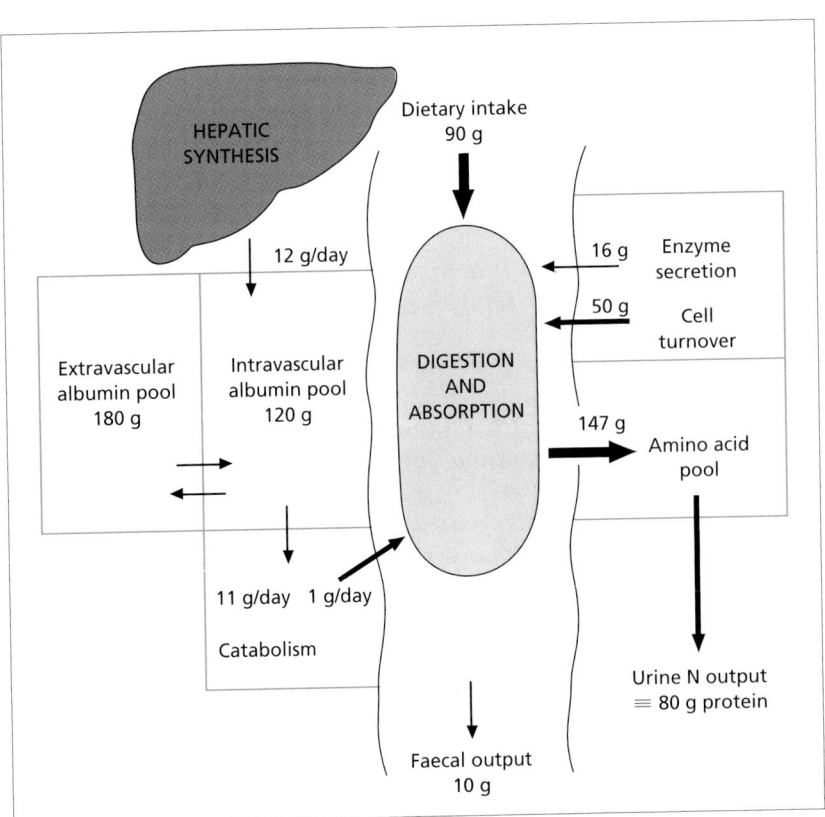

Fig. 2.13. The turnover of plasma albumin in a 70 kg adult seen in the context of the daily protein economy of the gastrointestinal tract and overall nitrogen balance. The total exchangeable albumin pool of about 300 g is distributed between the intravascular and extravascular compartments in a ratio of approximately 2 : 3. In this simplified schema the balance sheet is expressed in terms of grams of protein ($\equiv 6.25 \times$ g of N). Losses do not include relatively minor routes, e.g. 2 g per day from the skin [10].

and testis and in embryonic hepatoblastoma. It may also be present with carcinomas of the gastrointestinal tract with hepatic secondaries. Raised values are also found in hepatitis B surface antigen negative chronic hepatitis and during acute viral hepatitis where they may indicate hepato-cellular regeneration. However, very high values are virtually confined to primary liver cancer. In a hepatitis-B-positive patient, rising values are of particular significance as an indicator of the development of hepato-cellular carcinoma (see Chapter 28).

Electrophoretic pattern of the serum proteins

Electrophoresis is used to determine the proportions of the various serum proteins [12].

In cirrhosis, albumin is reduced. In acute hepatitis these changes are much less conspicuous. Plasma pre-albumin may be a very sensitive index of hepatic functional capacity [6].

The α_1-globulins contain glycoproteins and hormone-binding globulins. They tend to be low in hepato-cellular disease, falling in parallel with the serum albumin. An increase accompanies acute febrile illnesses and malignant disease. Ninety per cent of α_1-globulin consists of α_1-antitrypsin and an absent α_1-globulin may indicate α_1-antitrypsin deficiency.

The α_2- and β-globulins include lipoproteins. In cholestasis the increase in α_2- and β-globulin components correlates with the height of serum lipids. This pattern may be useful in distinguishing biliary from non-biliary cirrhosis. High lipoprotein components strongly support a biliary aetiology.

The γ-globulins rise in hepatic cirrhosis due to increased production. The increased numbers of plasma cells in marrow, and even in the liver itself, may be the source. The γ-globulin peak in hepato-cellular disease shows a wide base (*polyclonal gammopathy*). *Monoclonal gammopathy* is rare and may be age- rather than chronic liver disease-related. The dip between β- and γ-globulins tends to be bridged.

Immunoglobulins. IgG is markedly increased in chronic hepatitis and cryptogenic cirrhosis. In autoimmune hepatitis the raised level of IgG falls during treatment with corticosteroids. There is a slow and sustained increase in viral hepatitis and it is also increased in alcoholic cirrhosis [3].

IgM is markedly increased in primary biliary cirrhosis and to a lesser extent in viral hepatitis and cirrhosis.

IgA is markedly increased in cirrhosis of the alcoholic but also in primary biliary and cryptogenic cirrhosis.

The increase in serum secretory IgA, the predominant immunoglobulin in bile, may be related to communication of the bile canaliculus with the space of Disse and/or through the bile duct into the portal blood vessels [4].

In chronic hepatitis with active inflammation and cryptogenic cirrhosis the pattern is surprisingly similar, with increases in IgG, IgM and to a lesser extent IgA [3].

About 10% of patients with chronic cholestasis due to large bile duct obstruction show increases in all three main immunoglobulins.

Patterns are not diagnostic of any one disease but together with other data add support to considering a particular diagnosis.

References

1 Andus T, Bauer J, Gerok W. Effects of cytokines on the liver. *Hepatology* 1991; **13**: 364.
2 Ellison RT, Horsburgh CR Jr, Curd J. Complement levels in patients with hepatic dysfunction. *Dig. Dis. Sci.* 1990; **35**: 231.
3 Feizi T. Serum immunoglobulins in liver disease. *Gut* 1968; **9**: 193.
4 Fukuda Y, Nagura H, Asai J *et al.* Possible mechanisms of elevation of serum secretory immunoglobulin A in liver disease. *Am. J. Gastroenterol.* 1986; **81**: 315.
5 Morgan MY, Marshall AW, Milsom JP *et al.* Plasma amino-acid patterns in liver disease. *Gut* 1982; **23**: 362.
6 Rondana M, Milani L, Merkel C *et al.* Value of prealbumin plasma levels as a liver test. *Digestion* 1987; **37**: 72.
7 Rudman D, Difulco TJ, Galambos JT *et al.* Maximal rates of excretion and synthesis of urea in normal and cirrhotic subjects. *J. Clin. Invest.* 1973; **52**: 2241.
8 Scheinberg IH, Sternlieb I. *Wilson's Disease.* WB Saunders, Philadelphia, 1984.
9 Sehgal PB. Interleukin-6: a regulator of plasma protein gene expression in hepatic and non-hepatic tissues. *Mol. Biol. Med.* 1990; **7**: 117.
10 Tavill AS. The synthesis and degradation of liver-produced proteins. *Gut* 1972; **13**: 225.
11 Tavill AS, Craigie A, Rosenoer VM. The measurement of the synthetic rate of albumin in man. *Clin. Sci.* 1968; **34**: 1.
12 Wolf PL. Interpretation of electrophoretic patterns of serum proteins. *Clin. Lab. Med.* 1986; **6**: 441.

Carbohydrate metabolism

The liver occupies a key position in carbohydrate metabolism (see fig. 2.1) [2, 4]. The changes in cirrhosis are complex and not fully understood.

In fulminant acute hepatic necrosis the blood glucose level may be low. This is rare in chronic liver disease.

In fasted patients with cirrhosis the contribution of carbohydrates to energy production is reduced (2 vs. 38% in normal controls) with the contribution from fat increasing (86 vs. 45%) [3]. This may be caused by impaired release of hepatic glucose or reduced reserve of glycogen in the liver. After eating a meal, however, cirrhotics like controls make immediate use of dietary carbohydrate, indeed perhaps to a greater degree, because of a reduced ability to store and then mobilize energy as triglyceride [1].

The oral and intravenous glucose tolerance tests may show impairment in cirrhosis and there is relative insulin resistance (Chapter 23).

Galactose tolerance is also impaired in hepato-cellular disease and oral and intravenous tests have been devised. Results are independent of insulin secretion. Galactose removal by the liver has been used to measure hepatic blood flow.

References

1 Avgerinos A, Harry D, Bousboulas S *et al*. The effect of an eucaloric high carbohydrate diet on circulating levels of glucose, fructose and non-esterified fatty acids in patients with cirrhosis. *J. Hepatol.* 1992; **14**: 78.
2 Kruszynska YT, McIntyre N. Carbohydrate metabolism. In *Oxford Textbook of Clinical Hepatology*. McIntyre N, Benhamou P-J, Bircher J, Rizzetto M, Rodes J, eds. Oxford University Press, Oxford, 1991: 129.
3 Schneeweiss B, Graninger W, Ferenci P *et al*. Energy metabolism in patients with acute and chronic liver disease. *Hepatology* 1990; **11**: 387.
4 Sherlock S. Carbohydrate changes in liver disease. *Am. J. Clin. Nutr.* 1970; **23**: 462.

Effects of ageing on the liver [3, 4]

The liver weight and volume decreases with ageing [8]. Liver blood flow is reduced and there is compensatory hypertrophy of hepatocytes [5]. Routine biochemical tests are similar to those of the general population.

In animals, protein synthesis by the liver falls with age. Since the total protein content of cells remains relatively constant it is thought that protein turnover is also reduced [6].

First-pass metabolism of drugs is reduced and drugs handled in this way have a greater effect. Hepatic microsomal mono-oxygenase enzyme activity does not appear to decline with age [1, 7]. There is, however, a reduction in metabolism of drugs handled by oxidation but not by acetylation. More fatal reactions to halothane and drugs such as benoxyprofen are found in the elderly. The elderly are also liable to have adverse reactions related to the multiplicity of drugs they are taking.

Cholesterol saturation of bile increases with age due to enhanced hepatic secretion of cholesterol and decreased bile acid synthesis [2]. This may explain age as a risk factor for cholesterol gallstones.

References

1 Arora S, Kassarjian Z, Krasinski SD *et al*. Effect of age on tests of intestinal and hepatic function in healthy humans. *Gastroenterology* 1989; **96**: 1560.
2 Einarsson K, Nilsell K, Leijd B *et al*. Influence of age on secretion of cholesterol and synthesis of bile acids by the liver. *N. Engl. J. Med.* 1985; **313**: 277.
3 Mooney H, Roberts R, Cooksley WGE *et al*. Alterations in the liver with ageing. *Clin. Gastroenterol.* 1985; **14**: 757.
4 Popper H. Aging and the liver. In *Progress in Liver Diseases VIII*, Popper H, Schaffner F, eds. Grune & Stratton, Orlando, 1986: 659.
5 Rawlins MD, James OFW, Williams FM *et al*. Age and the metabolism of drugs. *Q. J. Med.* 1987; **64**: 545.
6 Ward W, Richardson A. Effect of age on liver protein synthesis and degradation. *Hepatology* 1991; **14**: 935.
7 Woodhouse KW, Mutch E, Williams FM *et al*. The effect of age on pathways of drug metabolism in human liver ageing. *Age Ageing* 1984; **13**: 328.
8 Wynne HA, Cope LH, Mutch E *et al*. The effect of age upon liver volume and apparent liver blood flow in healthy man. *Hepatology* 1989; **9**: 297.

Chapter 3
Biopsy of the Liver

A needle biopsy of the liver was said to have been first performed by Paul Ehrlich in 1883 (table 3.1) [14] in a study of the glycogen content of the diabetic liver, and later in 1895 by Lucatello in Italy, for the diagnosis of tropical liver abscess. The first published series was by Schüpfer (1907) [42] in France, where the technique was used for the diagnosis of cirrhosis and hepatic tumours. The method, however, never achieved early popularity until the 1930s when it was used for general purposes by Huard and co-workers [22] in France, and by Baron [3] in the USA. The Second World War saw a rapid increase in the use of liver biopsy, largely to investigate the many cases of non-fatal viral hepatitis which were affecting the armed forces of both sides [23, 43].

Now, in the course of training, almost every junior doctor will have learnt to perform needle liver biopsy, under supervision. The indications and techniques have changed, the complications are better recognized and the risks have decreased. Interpretation of the biopsy is an important part of a histopathologist's training.

Selection and preparation of the patient

The patient is usually admitted to hospital. Outpatients selected must not be jaundiced or show any sign of decompensation such as ascites or encephalopathy. Outpatient biopsy should be avoided in cirrhotic patients or in those with tumours [38]. Outpatient biopsies are usually indicated because of patient preference and reduction of cost. The American Gastroenterological Association recommends that clinicians should be allowed to decide whether the biopsy is done as an in-patient or outpatient, and this should not be dictated by insurance coverage [24].

The one-stage prothrombin time should not be more than 3 seconds prolonged over control values after 10 mg vitamin K is given intramuscularly. The platelet count should exceed 80 000.

In thrombocytopenic patients the risk of haemorrhage depends on the function of the platelets rather than on their numbers. A patient with 'hypersplenism' and a platelet count of less than 60 000 is much less likely to bleed than one with leukaemia who has a similar platelet count. This distinction particularly arises in patients with haematological problems or after organ transplants where the effects on the liver of cytotoxic therapy, viruses and other infective agents and of the graft-versus-host reaction have to be resolved. In such patients, if the platelet count can be raised to greater than 60 000 by platelet infusion, biopsy seems to be safe. Care should also be taken in recently imbibing alcoholic patients who may have reduced platelet counts and platelet dysfunction, especially if acetyl salicylic acid has been consumed. In such patients the platelet count may be 100 000 and the prothrombin time only 3 seconds prolonged over control values, yet the bleeding time may be 25 minutes.

The patient's blood group should be known and facilities for blood transfusion must always be available.

Biopsy should not be done with tense ascites as a specimen will not be obtained.

Clinically significant haemorrhage complicated 12.5% of 155 liver biopsies in haemophiliacs [1]. Liver biopsy should not be performed in haemophilia A unless there are very definite indications when the factor VIII level should be raised, and maintained, to about 50% for at least 48 hours.

Anatomical abnormalities are common and liver size varies. A small liver may not be penetrated by the needle and distortion may result in puncture of the gallbladder or large blood vessels in the hilum. If possible, before any biopsy, ultrasound should be done and attention paid to liver size, the site of the gallbladder and any anatomical abnormality [11].

Table 3.1. History of liver biopsies [44]

Author	Date	Country	Purpose
Ehrlich	1883	Germany	Glycogen
Lucatello	1895	Italy	Tropical
Schüpfer	1907	France	Cirrhosis
Huard et al.	1935	France	General
Baron	1939	USA	General
Iversen & Roholm	1939	Denmark	Hepatitis
Axenfeld & Brass	1942	Germany	Hepatitis
Dible et al.	1943	UK	Hepatitis

Techniques

The Menghini needle obtains a specimen by aspiration (fig. 3.1) [33]. The sheathed 'Trucut' is a modification of the old Vim–Silverman needle. It is of particular value in cirrhotic patients [9]. Fragmentation of the biopsy is greater with the Menghini technique but the procedure is quicker, easier and the costs of the needle less. Complications are less than with the Trucut procedure [38].

Menghini 'one second' needle biopsy (fig. 3.1). The 1.4 mm diameter needle is used routinely. A short needle is available for paediatric use. The tip of the needle is oblique and slightly convex towards the outside. The needle is fitted within its shaft with a blunt nail. This internal block prevents the biopsy from being fragmented or distorted by violent aspiration into the syringe.

Sterile solution (3 ml) is drawn into the syringe which is inserted through the anaesthetized track down to but not through the intercostal space. Two millilitres of solution are injected to clear the needle of any skin fragments. Aspiration is now commenced and maintained. This is the slow part of the procedure. With the patient holding his breath in expiration, the needle is rapidly introduced perpendicularly to the skin into the liver substance and extracted. This is the quick part of the procedure. The tip of the needle is now placed on sterile filter paper and some of the remaining saline flushed through the needle to deposit the biopsy gently onto the paper. The piece of tissue is transferred into fixative.

Sedation is not given routinely before biopsy as it may interfere with the patient's co-operation. However, analgesia is sometimes needed after the procedure.

The *intercostal technique* is the most frequently used method [44]. It rarely fails, provided care is taken to assess liver size carefully by light percussion. A preliminary ultrasound or CT scan is useful. A small fibrotic liver is a contraindication. After adequate local anaesthesia, the needle is inserted in the 8th or 9th intercostal space in the mid-axillary line at the end of expiration with the patient breathing quietly. The direction is slightly posterior and cranial which helps to avoid

the gallbladder. If an epigastric mass is present or imaging indicates left lobe disease an anterior approach is made.

Transjugular liver biopsy. A special Trucut needle is inserted through a catheter placed in the hepatic vein via the jugular vein. The needle is then introduced into the liver tissue by transfixing the hepatic venous wall (fig. 3.2).

This technique is indicated in those who have a coagulation disorder, massive ascites, a small liver or who are unco-operative. It is useful in fulminant liver failure to determine prognosis and the need for liver transplantation [12, 30]. An advantage is that wedged and free hepatic venous pressure may be measured at the same time. The procedure may be attempted after percutaneous biopsy has failed (table 3.2).

Adequate tissue is obtained in 81–97% of those with fibrosis or cirrhosis [28, 30]. Complications are reported between 0 and 20%. The mortality is very low, but perforation of the liver capsule can be fatal [28]. The disadvantage is the greater complexity and cost compared

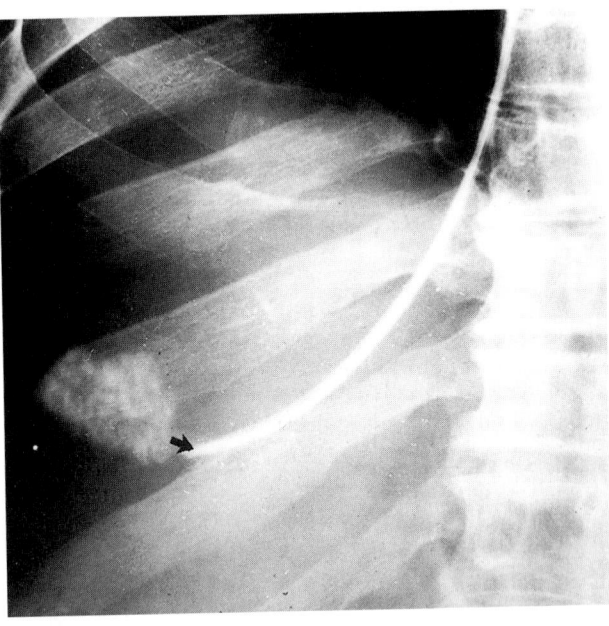

Fig. 3.2. Transjugular liver biopsy. The catheter is in the hepatic vein and contrast has been injected to show the wedged position. The Trucut needle is taking the liver biopsy (arrow).

Table 3.2. Indications for transjugular liver biopsy

Coagulation defects
Fulminant liver failure pre-transplant
Massive ascites
Small liver
Measurement wedged hepatic venous pressure
Unco-operative patient

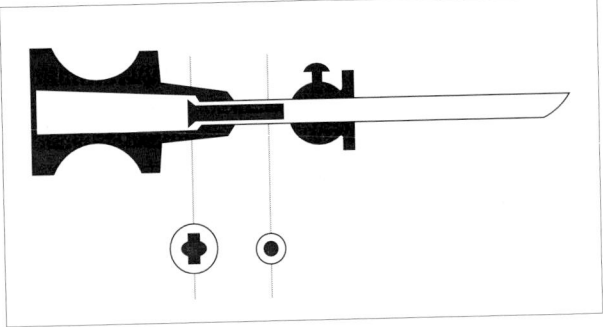

Fig. 3.1. Longitudinal section of the Menghini liver biopsy needle. Note the nail in the shaft of the needle [33].

with the percutaneous approach. Although usually successful, the liver fragments are sometimes very small.

Directed (guided) biopsy. A lesion is recognized under imaging and, assuming coagulation and other conditions are satisfactory, a Trucut biopsy needle is advanced into it. The method of imaging includes ultrasound, CT and hepatic angiography (fig. 3.3). In patients with poor coagulation, a gel foam plug may be injected through the outer cannula of the Trucut needle after the inner cutting needle, with its contained specimen, has been removed [50]. This is effective in preventing major bleeding after image-guided biopsies. Directed liver biopsy gives a higher percentage of positives than the blind percutaneous technique. The overall accuracy for chronic liver disease using the blind technique is approximately 81%, but this can be raised to 95% if a directed form of liver biopsy is used [37].

The *Biopty gun* uses a modified 18- or 14-gauge Trucut needle and is operated with one hand (figs 3.4, 3.5). It is fired by a fast and powerful spring mechanism. It allows precise positioning of the needle and is less painful than the manual procedure. It is particularly useful for focal lesions [48].

Fine-needle-guided biopsy. Using a 22 swg (0.7 mm) needle adds to the safety. It is particularly useful for the diagnosis of focal lesions although diagnostic accuracy is variable [5, 7]. Because of the size, fine-needle biopsy cannot be expected to be so useful in generalized disease such as chronic hepatitis or cirrhosis.

A Surecut (0.66 mm) liver biopsy needle can be used when the Menghini is contraindicated. Risk of complications even following puncture of a hydatid cyst or haemangioma is minimal [27].

Cytological examination of the aspirate is useful for tumour typing [17].

After-care. Bleeding is most likely within the first 3–4 hours after biopsy [25]. Pulse rate and blood pressure are charted every 15 minutes for the first hour and every 30 minutes for the next 2 hours.

Inpatients continue to have pulse rate charted for 24

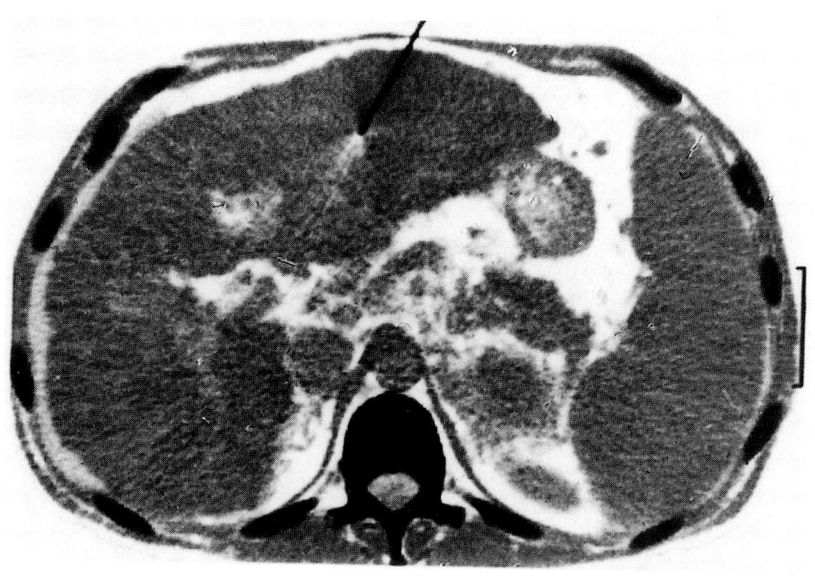

Fig. 3.3. CT of a 45-year-old male with hepatitis-B-positive cirrhosis. An irregular liver outline and splenomegaly are clearly seen. Directed biopsy of suspected neoplasm of the left lobe of liver diagnosed hepato-cellular carcinoma.

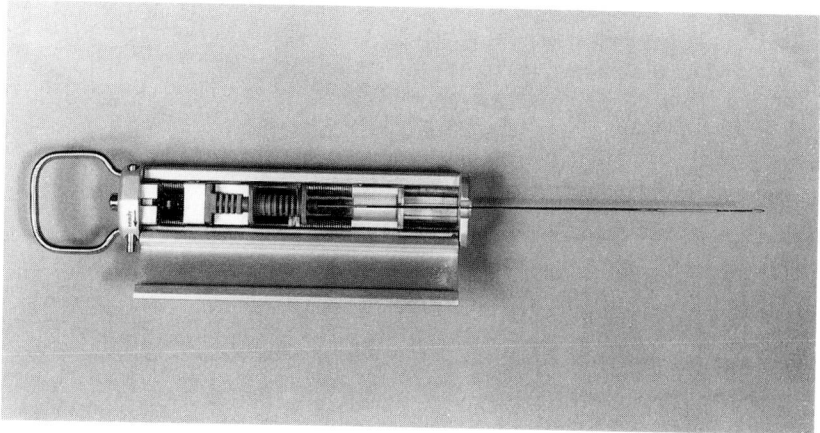

Fig. 3.4. The Biopty (TM) gun (Biopter).

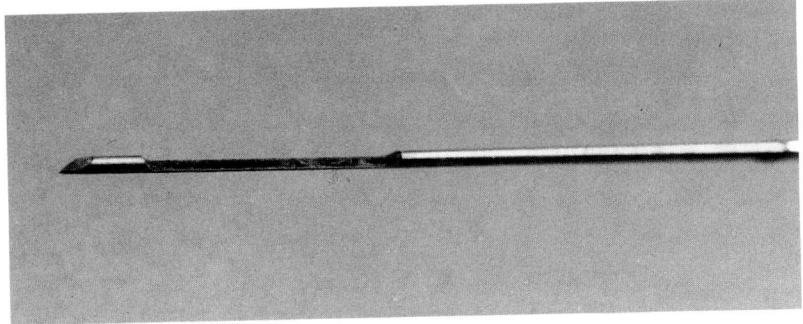

Fig. 3.5. The Trucut needle tip has an outer cannula and inner cutting needle. The inner needle is advanced and a liver biopsy is cored out.

hours and routine visits are paid 4 and 8 hours post-biopsy. A very careful watch must be kept on the patient. Rest in bed is essential for 24 hours.

Outpatients are admitted to a supervised day ward at 9.00 a.m. The biopsy is never done later than 11.00 a.m. Pulse and blood pressure are monitored as for inpatients. The patient remains recumbent until 4.00 p.m., is seen at 4.30 p.m., by the physician and is allowed to go home at 5.00 p.m., accompanied and being driven. The patient stays not more than 30 minutes drive from the hospital. The patient should not be alone and must have a telephone available. The usual indication for outpatient biopsy is the diagnosis and management of chronic hepatitis, cirrhosis or alcoholic liver disease.

During the puncture the patient may complain of a drawing feeling across the epigastrium. Afterwards some patients have a slight ache in the right side for about 24 hours and some complain of pain referred from the diaphragm to the right shoulder.

Difficulties

Failures arise in patients with cirrhosis, especially with ascites, for the tough liver is difficult to pierce and a few liver cells may be extracted, leaving the fibrous framework behind. Another difficulty may be pulmonary emphysema; the liver is then pushed downwards by the low diaphragm so that the trocar passes above it.

Failure is often due to the needle not being sharp enough to penetrate the capsule. Disposable needles are an advantage for they are sharp.

The percentage of successes increases with diameter of the needle used but so does the complication rate and one must be weighed against the other. The 1 mm Menghini needle, for instance, which is extremely safe, often fails to procure adequate hepatic tissue for diagnosis. The Trucut needle causes more haemorrhages.

Liver biopsy in paediatrics

The Menghini technique may be employed. In infants a local anaesthetic, with 15–60 mg pentobarbital 30 minutes before the biopsy, is adequate. The child is restrained by adhesive strapping across the upper thighs and chest and the subcostal approach used. If the liver is small then the intercostal route is employed, the assistant compressing the chest at the end of expiration to arrest respiration.

Complications (4.5%) are more frequent in children than in adults and bleeding is particularly likely in those with cancer or having bone marrow transplants [8]. In older children, general anaesthesia is usually preferred, depending on the co-operation of the child.

Transjugular biopsy can be used in children [15].

Risks and complications

The mortality from various large combined series is about 0.01% (table 3.3). Complications are reported in 0.06–0.32% of patients [45].

In 17 years, some 8000 needle biopsies of the liver have been performed at the Royal Free Hospital with only two deaths, one in a haemophiliac and one in a patient with acute viral hepatitis [44]. In spite of the low mortality and complication rate, liver biopsy must only be performed when the patient can be expected to benefit from the information and where it cannot be obtained by less invasive means.

Table 3.3. Fatalities from needle liver biopsy

Source	Date	Reference	Biopsies	Mortality (%)
USA	1953	[1, 2]	20 016	0.17
Europe combined	1964	[3]	23 382	0.01
Germany	1967	[4]	80 000	0.015
Italy	1986	[5]	68 276	0.009
USA	1990	[6]	9 212	0.11

1 Zamcheck. *N. Engl. J. Med.* 1953; **249**: 1020.
2 Zamcheck. *N. Engl. J. Med.* 1953; **249**: 1062.
3 Thaler. *Wien. Klin. Wchschr.* 1964; **29**: 533.
4 Lindner. *Dtsch. Med. Wschr.* 1967; **92**: 1751.
5 Piccinino. *J. Hepatol.* 1986; **2**: 165.
6 McGill. *Gastroenterology* 1990; **99**: 1396.

Pleurisy and peri-hepatitis

A friction rub caused by fibrinous peri-hepatitis or pleurisy may be heard on the next day. It is of little consequence and pain subsides with analgesics. A chest X-ray may show a small pneumothorax.

Haemorrhage

In a recent series of 9212 biopsies, there were 10 (0.11%) fatal and 22 (0.24%) non-fatal haemorrhages [31]. Malignancy, age, female sex and number of passes were the only predictable factors for bleeding. The complication rate is higher when referrals are from a haematological department than when predominantly hepatological problems are being investigated. Haemorrhage usually develops when least expected and when, at the time of biopsy, the risk seemed small. It might be related to factors other than peripheral clotting, for instance, the concentration of clotting factors in hepatic parenchyma, and the failure of mechanical compression of the needle tract by elastic tissue [13].

Bleeding from the puncture wound usually consists of a thin trickle lasting 10–60 seconds and the total blood loss is only 5–10 ml. Serious haemorrhage is usually intra-peritoneal but may be intra-thoracic from an intercostal artery. The bleeding results from perforation of distended portal or hepatic veins or aberrant arteries. The occasional laceration of a major intra-hepatic vessel cannot be avoided. In some cases, a tear of the liver follows deep breathing during the intercostal procedure.

Perforation of the capsule with intra-peritoneal haemorrhage may follow transvenous biopsy.

Spontaneous recovery may ensue, otherwise angiography followed by transcatheter embolization is usually successful (figs 3.6, 3.7).

Severe haemothorax usually responds to blood transfusion and chest aspiration.

Haemorrhage is rare in the non-jaundiced.

Intra-hepatic haematomas

At 2–4 hours post-biopsy, intra-hepatic haematomas are detected by ultrasound in only about 2% [20]. This is probably an underestimate as the haematomas remain isoechoic for the first 24–48 hours and are not detected by ultrasound. The day after biopsy, haematomas, usually asymptomatic, are detected in 23% [34]. They can cause fever, rises in serum transaminases, a fall in haematocrit and, if large, right upper-quadrant tenderness and an enlarging liver. They may be seen in the arterial phase of a dynamic CT scan as triangular hyperdense segments. Sometimes a distal portal vein branch may be noted during the arterial phase. Occasionally, haematomas are followed by delayed haemorrhage.

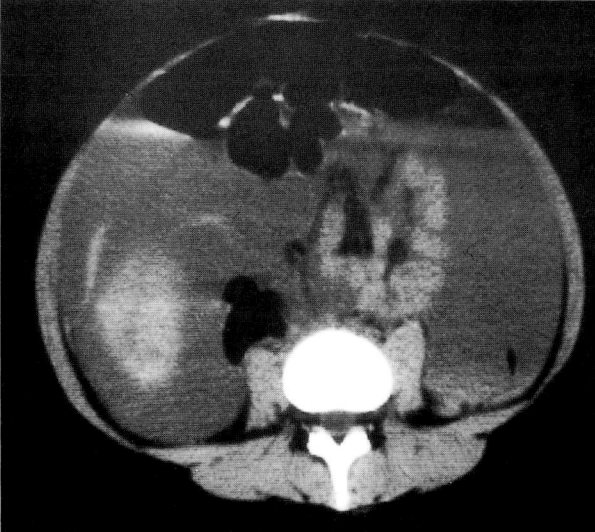

Fig. 3.6. CT scan taken 4 hours post-biopsy in a patient with hepatic metastases and jaundice showing haemorrhage around and into the liver.

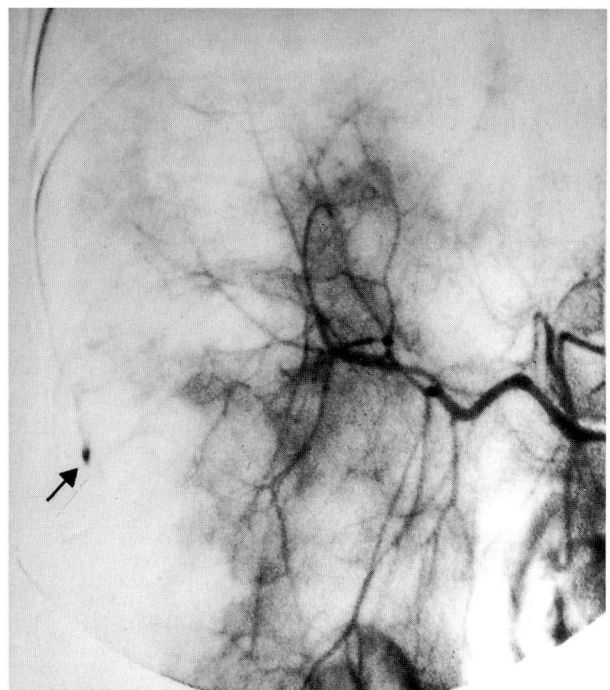

Fig. 3.7. Same patient as in fig. 3.6. Hepatic arteriography (DSA technique) shows blood beside the liver (arrow). The bleeding point was later successfully embolized via the hepatic artery.

Haemobilia

Haemobilia follows bleeding from a damaged hepatic vessel, artery or vein, into bile duct (fig. 3.8). It is marked by biliary colic with enlargement and tenderness of the

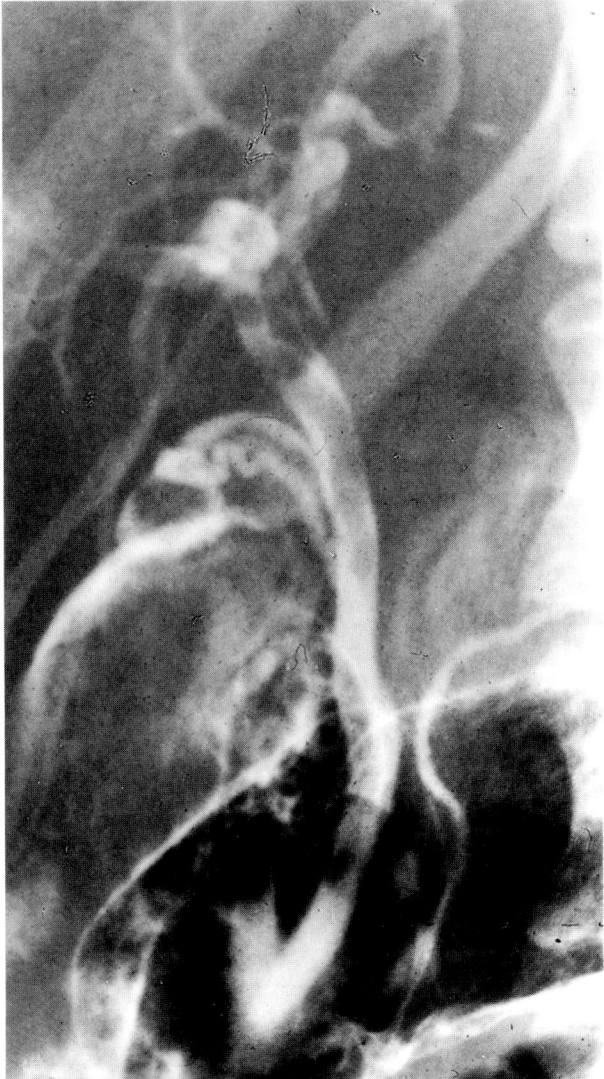

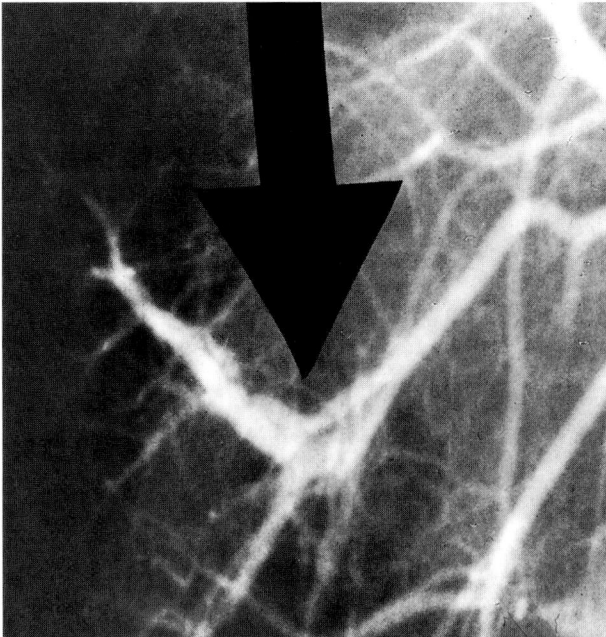

Fig. 3.9. Hepatic arteriography taken post-liver biopsy shows an arteriovenous fistula (arrow).

Fig. 3.8. Haemobilia following needle liver biopsy. ERCP shows linear filling defects in the common bile duct.

liver and sometimes the gallbladder [49]. The diagnosis is confirmed by ultrasound or ERCP. It may be treated by hepatic arterial embolization; however, spontaneous recovery is usual.

Arteriovenous fistula

An arteriovenous fistula, shown by hepatic arteriography, follows 5.4% of liver biopsies (figs 3.9, 3.10) [35].

Histology shows marked phlebosclerosis of the portal vein tributaries [18]. The fistula may close spontaneously, otherwise it can be treated by direct hepatic arterial catheterization and embolization of the feeding artery.

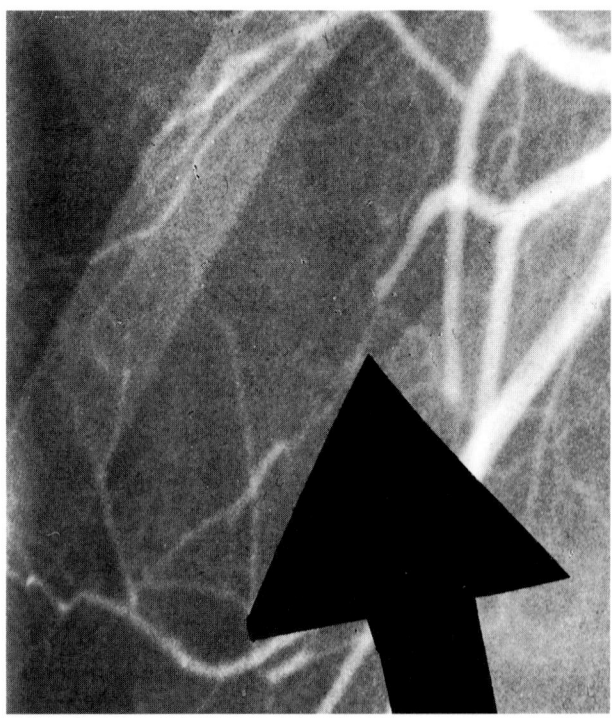

Fig. 3.10. Same patient. The arteriovenous fistula has been successfully embolized (arrow).

Biliary peritonitis

This is the second commonest complication after haemorrhage. It was seen 49 times in 123000 biopsies with 12 deaths [49]. The bile usually comes from the gallbladder, which may be in an unusual position, or from dilated bile ducts. Biliary scintigraphy demonstrates the leak [47]. Surgical management is usually necessary although conservative measures with intravenous fluids, antibiotics and intensive care monitoring may be successful [40].

Puncture of other organs

Puncture of organs such as the kidney or colon is rarely clinically significant.

Infection

Transient bacteraemia is relatively common, particularly in patients with cholangitis. Septicaemia is rarer; blood cultures are usually positive for *Escherichia coli*. Septic complications are not more common in transplant patients with Roux-en-Y than with choledochocholedochostomy anastomoses [16].

Carcinoid crisis

This can follow percutaneous biopsy [4].

Sampling variability

It is surprising that such a small biopsy should so often be representative of changes in the whole liver. Cholestasis, steatosis, viral hepatitis and the reticuloses are fortunately diffuse. This is also true of most cirrhoses, although in macronodular cirrhosis it is possible to aspirate a large nodule and find normal architecture. There is sampling variability in the diagnosis of cirrhosis in the presence of acute hepatitis or chronic hepatitis. The focal granulomatous diseases such as sarcoidosis, tumour deposits and abscesses may be missed; this is infrequent if serial sections are cut.

Misdiagnosis is often due to smallness of sample, especially failure to obtain portal zones, to the focal nature of the disease process and particularly to the inexperience of the interpreter.

The diagnostic yield may be improved if three consecutive samples are obtained by redirecting the biopsy needle through a single entry site [32].

Fibrous tissue is increased under the capsule in operative biopsies and this may give a false impression of the liver as a whole.

Operative biopsies may also show artefactual changes such as patchy loss of glycogen, haemorrhages, polymorph infiltration and even focal necrosis. These are presumably related to the effects of trauma, circulatory changes and hypoxia accompanying surgery.

Naked eye appearances

A satisfactory biopsy is 1–4 cm long and weighs 10–50 mg.

The cirrhotic liver tends to crumble into fragments of irregular contour. The fatty liver has a pale greasy look and floats in the formol–saline fixative. The liver containing malignant deposits is dull white in colour. The liver from a patient with Dubin–Johnson hyperbilirubinaemia is diffusely chocolate coloured (see fig. 12.10).

In cholestatic jaundice, the greenish central areas contrast with the less green periphery. The vascular centres of lobules in hepatic congestion may be obvious.

Preparation of the specimen

The biopsy is usually fixed in 10% formol–saline. The time taken to fix such a small piece is less than for a larger specimen. Routine stains include haematoxylin and eosin and a good stain for connective tissue. All specimens are stained for iron and by the diastase/PAS method. Orcein staining is also useful. This shows hepatitis B surface antigen in the hepatocyte as a uniform, finely granular, brown material. It also stains copper-associated protein in lysosomes as black–brown granules, usually in the peri-portal area (zone 1). This is a useful indicator of cholestasis and is also sometimes found in Wilson's disease.

Adequate biopsies (3 mm in length) excised from paraffin blocks can be analysed retrospectively for iron and copper by atomic absorption spectrophotometry [36]. If iron overload is suspected, the specimen must not be fixed in saline as this leads to rapid loss of iron.

Specimens for electron microscopy are fixed within seconds in glutaraldehyde and preserved at 4°C until processed. Electron microscopy is particularly valuable for diagnosis of tumours of uncertain origin and storage disorders, including Wilson's disease, Niemann–Pick disease and the Dubin–Johnson syndrome.

Serial sections are important for the diagnosis of lesions such as granulomas which may be scattered through the liver.

Cytological preparations are made by smearing the aspirated tissue core on a slide.

Interpretation

The specimen should preferably be at least 2 cm in length with four portal zones if a reliable opinion is to be given. In the normal liver zone 1 (portal) bears a regular relation to zone 3 (central). This may be difficult to establish in small biopsies especially if no portal zones have been obtained, but this orientation is an essential first step. Each portal zone consists of one or two bile ductules, a branch of the hepatic artery and of the portal vein, a few mononuclears and an occasional fibroblast. The liver cell plates are one cell thick and contain abundant glycogen. Mitoses are not seen in the liver cells which are usually mononucleate and of regular size. The sinusoids are lined by Kupffer cells and can be seen converging upon the central hepatic vein.

Isolated sinusoidal dilatation prompts a search for a tumour or a disease associated with granulomas.

Liver biopsy appearances are described in individual chapters, and detailed histology can be found in the monographs of Klatskin and Conn [26] and Scheuer and Lefkowitch [41].

Indications (table 3.4) [29, 44]

The numbers of liver biopsies performed in any liver unit are tending to fall due to the increasing diagnostic use of trans-hepatic and endoscopic cholangiography, imaging procedures, virological markers and immunological diagnosis, particularly of primary biliary cirrhosis and autoimmune chronic hepatitis. Numbers are maintained by biopsies for the management of patients with chronic hepatitis and for hepatic transplantation.

Drug-related acute liver disease can be difficult to identify and the history is essential. Sometimes the distinction from acute viral hepatitis is impossible.

Chronic hepatitis remains the most important indication. Biopsy is needed to establish the diagnosis, follow the progress and in particular, the effects of therapy. A semi-quantitative assessment can be made of inflammation (grading) and fibrosis (progression) (Knodell score) [10] (Chapter 17).

Anatomical diagnosis of a cirrhosis demands connective tissue stains.

Alcohol-related disease liver biopsy is used for diagnosis and for prognosis but also as a deterrent to further consumption.

Cholestasis. Extra-hepatic cholestasis can usually be diagnosed by trans-hepatic and endoscopic cholangio-graphy with ultrasound and CT scans and without recourse to liver biopsy. Liver biopsy is particularly useful in small duct disease (ductopenia) including primary biliary cirrhosis, small duct sclerosing cholangitis, chronic drug cholestasis, cholestatic sarcoidosis and graft-versus-host disease [29].

Infections. These include tuberculosis, brucellosis, syphilis, histoplasmosis, coccidioidomycosis, pyogenic infection, leptospirosis, amoebiasis and opportunistic infections such as herpes, cytomegala and cryptosporidosis. When indicated, the appropriate stains for the causative organism should be applied and a portion of the biopsy cultured.

Liver biopsy is useful in elucidating the cause of *fever* of unknown origin [21].

Storage diseases. These include amyloidosis and glycogen disease (Chapter 23). Haemochromatosis and Wilson's disease can be diagnosed and the effect of therapy is assessed by serial biopsies.

Orthotopic liver transplant. Liver biopsy is useful in the pre-transplant work-up. Post-transplant pathology includes rejection, infection and bile leaks. Liver biopsy is essential to unravel these complications. The protocol 5-day biopsy is particularly useful in diagnosing episodes of rejection [6].

Renal transplants. Liver biopsy is useful in evaluating the chronic liver disease in kidney recipients [39].

Space-occupying lesions are diagnosed by direct biopsy under imaging.

Other indications include obscure hepatomegaly or splenomegaly, and abnormal biochemical tests of uncertain cause particularly where fatty liver is suspected [46].

Special methods [41]

Histochemical techniques have been widely applied. Bile canaliculi may be shown by staining for adenosine triphosphatase (ATPase), and staining for glucose-6-phosphatase may be used. Electron microscopy may be combined with histochemistry. ATPase is localized to the microvilli of the canaliculi and 5-nucleotidase to the microvilli of the sinusoidal border. Acid phosphatase is found in Kupffer cells, degenerating foci and regenerating nodules; alkaline phosphatase defines cholangioles.

Immunohistochemical stains may be used to demonstrate antigens of viral hepatitis A, C, D and E, and of hepatitis B, also herpes and adenovirus. Immunohistochemistry is also used to diagnose amyloid disease and α_1-antitrypsin deficiency.

Immunohistochemistry is used to investigate neoplastic conditions and to demonstrate α-fetoprotein in hepatocellular carcinoma and high molecular weight cytokeratin in cholangiocaricinoma. Factor VIII-related antigen is used to diagnose angiosarcoma and epithelioid haemangioendothelioma.

Table 3.4. Indications for liver biopsy

Acute hepatitis
Drug-related hepatitis
Chronic hepatitis
Cirrhosis and portal hypertension
Liver disease in the alcoholic
Intra-hepatic (ductopenia) cholestasis
Infective conditions
Storage diseases
Post-hepatic transplantation
Liver complications of renal transplantation
Space-occupying lesions
Unexplained hepatomegaly or enzyme elevations

In situ hybridization using complementary DNA or RNA sequences is done on formal fixed paraffin embedded material and with light microscopy. It is useful in demonstrating viral antigens (e.g. cytomegala, herpes and hepatitis B).

PCR is useful in HIV and HCV RNA infections but the whole biopsy is required for the analysis.

Mononuclear cells derived from liver biopsies may be studied by immunohistochemical methods using monoclonal antibodies specific for various surface antigens [19].

Quantitative analysis of liver biopsy specimens is plagued by sampling difficulties and by failure to find a suitable standard of reference. In the liver with normal structure, results are reasonably reliable. Difficulties arise particularly in biopsies from cirrhotic livers where the proportion of fibrous tissue is uncertain. DNA, which is confined to the nucleus, is probably the best reference base although this may be valueless where the proportion of cells of different types is variable. Alternatively, the substance being investigated may be referred to dry weight or to total nitrogen content of the biopsy.

References

1 Aledort LM, Levine PH, Hilgartner M *et al.* A study of liver biopsies and liver disease among hemophiliacs. *Blood* 1985; **66**: 367.

2 Axenfeld H, Brass K. Klinische und bioptische Untersuchungen über den sogenannten Icterus catarrhalis. *Frankfurt. Z. Pathol.* 1942; **57**: 147.

3 Baron E. Aspiration for removal of biopsy material from the liver. *Arch. Intern. Med.* 1939; **63**: 276.

4 Bissonnette RT, Gibney RG, Berry BR *et al.* Fatal carcinoid crisis after percutaneous fine-needle biopsy of hepatic metastasis: case report and literature review. *Radiology* 1990; **174**: 751.

5 Bru C, Maroto A, Bruix J *et al.* Diagnostic accuracy of fine-needle aspiration biopsy in patients with hepatocellular carcinoma. *Dig. Dis. Sci.* 1989; **34**: 1765.

6 Brunt EM, Peters MG, Flye MW *et al.* Day-5 protocol liver allograft biopsies document early rejection episodes and are predictive of recurrent rejection. *Surgery* 1992; **111**: 511.

7 Buscarini L, Fornari F, Bolondi L *et al.* Ultrasound-guided fine-needle biopsy of focal liver lesions: techniques, diagnostic accuracy and complications. *J. Hepatol.* 1990; **11**: 344.

8 Cohen MB, A-Kader HH, Lambers D *et al.* Complications of percutaneous liver biopsy in children. *Gastroenterology* 1992; **102**: 629.

9 Colombo M, del Ninno E, de Franchis R *et al.* Ultrasound assisted percutaneous liver biopsy: superiority of the Tru-Cut over the Menghini needle for diagnosis of cirrhosis. *Gastroenterology* 1988; **95**: 487.

10 Desmet VJ, Gerber M, Hoofnagle JH *et al.* Classification of chronic hepatitis: diagnosis, grading and staging. *Hepatology* 1994; **19**: 1513.

11 Dixon AK, Nunez DK, Bradley JR *et al.* Failure of percutaneous liver biopsy: anatomical variation. *Lancet* 1987; **2**: 437.

12 Donaldson BW, Gopinath R, Wanless IR *et al.* The role of transjugular liver biopsy in fulminant liver failure: relation to other prognostic indicators. *Hepatology* 1993; **18**: 1370.

13 Ewe K. Bleeding after liver biopsy does not correlate with indices of peripheral coagulation. *Dig. Dis. Sci.* 1981; **26**: 388.

14 Frerichs FT von. *Über den Diabetes.* Hirschwald, Berlin, 1884.

15 Furuya KN, Burrows PE, Phillips MJ *et al.* Transjugular liver biopsy in children. *Hepatology* 1992; **15**: 1036.

16 Galati JS, Monsour HP, Donovan JP *et al.* The nature of complications following liver biopsy in transplant patients with Roux-en-Y choledochojejunostomy. *Hepatology* 1994; **20**: 651.

17 Glenthoj A, Sehested M, Torp-Pedersen S. Diagnostic reliability of histological and cytological fine needle biopsies from focal liver lesions. *Histopathology* 1989; **15**: 375.

18 Hashimoto E, Ludwig J, MacCarty RL *et al.* Hepatoportal arteriovenous fistula: morphologic features studied after orthotopic liver transplantation. *Hum. Pathol.* 1989; **20**: 707.

19 Hata K, Van Thiel DH, Herberman RB *et al.* Phenotypic and functional characteristics of lymphocytes isolated from liver biopsy specimens from patients with active liver disease. *Hepatology* 1992; **15**: 816.

20 Hederstrom E, Forsberg L, Floren C-H *et al.* Liver biopsy complications monitored by ultrasound. *J. Hepatol.* 1989; **8**: 94.

21 Holtz T, Moseley RH, Scheiman JM. Liver biopsy in fever of unknown origin: a reappraisal. *J. Clin. Gastroenterol.* 1993; **17**: 29.

22 Huard P, May JM, Joyeux B. La ponction biopsie du foie et son utilté dans le diagnostique des affections hépatiques. *Ann. Anat. Path. Anat. Norm. Méd-chir* 1935; **12**: 1118.

23 Iversen P, Roholm K. On aspiration biopsy of the liver, with remarks on its diagnostic significance. *Acta. Med. Scand.* 1939; **102**: 1.

24 Jacobs WH, Goldberg SB and The Patient Care Committee of the American Gastroenterological Association. Statement on outpatient percutaneous liver biopsy. *Dig. Dis. Sci.* 1989; **34**: 322.

25 Janes CH, Lindor KD. Outcome of patients hospitalized for complications after outpatient liver biopsy. *Ann. Intern. Med.* 1993; **118**: 96.

26 Klatskin G, Conn HO. *Histopathology of the Liver*, vols 1 and 2. Oxford University Press, New York, 1993.

27 Langlois S le P. Fine-needle biopsy of hepatic hydatids and haemangiomas: an overstated hazard. *Australas. Radiol.* 1989; **33**: 144.

28 Lebrec D, Goldfarb G, Degott C *et al.* Transvenous liver biopsy—an experience based on 1000 hepatic tissue samplings with this procedure. *Gastroenterology* 1982; **82**: 338.

29 Ludwig J, Batts KP, Moyer TP *et al.* Advances in liver biopsy diagnosis. *Mayo Clin. Proc.* 1994; **69**: 677.

30 McAfee JH, Keeffe EB, Lee RG *et al.* Transjugular liver biopsy. *Hepatology* 1992; **15**: 726.

31 McGill DB, Rakela J, Zinsmeister AR *et al.* A 21-year experience with major hemorrhage after percutaneous liver biopsy. *Gastroenterology* 1990; **99**: 1396.

32 Maharaj B, Maharaj RJ, Leary WP *et al.* Sampling variability and its influence on the diagnostic yield of percutaneous needle biopsy of the liver. *Lancet* 1986; **i**: 523.

33 Menghini G. One-second needle biopsy of the liver. *Gastroenterology* 1958; **35**: 190.

34 Minuk GY, Sutherland LR, Wiseman DA *et al.* Prospective study of the incidence of ultrasound-detected intrahepatic and subcapsular hematomas in patients randomized to 6 or

24 hours of bed rest after percutaneous liver biopsy. *Gastroenterology* 1987; **92**: 290.

35 Okuda K, Musha H, Nakajima Y *et al.* Frequency of intra-hepatic arteriovenous fistula as a sequela to percutaneous needle puncture of the liver. *Gastroenterology* 1978; **74**: 1204.

36 Olynyk JK, O'Neill R, Britton RS *et al.* Determination of hepatic iron concentration in fresh and paraffin-embedded tissue: diagnostic implications. *Gastroenterology* 1994; **106**: 674.

37 Pagliaro L, Rinaldi F, Craxi A *et al.* Percutaneous blind biopsy versus laparoscopy with guided biopsy in diagnosis of cirrhosis: a prospective, randomised trial. *Dig. Dis. Sci.* 1983; **28**: 39.

38 Piccinino F, Sagnelli E, Pasquale G *et al.* Complications following percutaneous liver biopsy. A multicentre retrospective study on 68 276 biopsies. *J. Hepatol.* 1986; **2**: 165.

39 Rao KV, Anderson WR, Kasiske BL *et al.* Value of liver biopsy in the evaluation and management of chronic liver disease in renal transplant recipients. *Am. J. Med.* 1993; **94**: 241.

40 Ruben RA, Chopra S. Bile peritonitis after liver biopsy: non-surgical management of a patient with an acute abdomen: a case report with review of the literature. *Am. J. Gastroenterol.* 1987; **82**: 265.

41 Scheuer PJ, Lefkowitch JH. *Liver Biopsy Interpretation*, 5th edn. WB Saunders, Philadelphia, 1994.

42 Schüpfer F. De la possibilité de faire 'intra vitam' un diagnostic histo-pathologique précis des maladies du foie et de la rate. *Sem. Méd.* 1907; **27**: 229.

43 Sherlock S. Aspiration liver biopsy, technique and diagnostic application. *Lancet* 1945; **ii**: 397.

44 Sherlock S, Dick R, van Leeuwen DJ. Liver biopsy today. The Royal Free Hospital experience. *J. Hepatol.* 1984; **1**: 75.

45 Tobkes AI, Nord HJ. Liver biopsy: review of methodology and complications. *Digestion* 1995; **13**: 267.

46 Van Ness MM, Diehl AM. Is liver biopsy useful in the evaluation of patients with chronically elevated liver enzymes? *Ann. Intern. Med.* 1989; **111**: 473.

47 Veneri RJ, Gordon SC, Fink-Bennett D. Scintigraphic and culdoscopic diagnosis of bile peritonitis complicating liver biopsy. *J. Clin. Gastroenterol.* 1989; **11**: 571.

48 Whitmire LF, Galambos JT, Phillips VM *et al.* Imaging guided percutaneous hepatic biopsy: diagnostic accuracy and safety. *J. Clin. Gastroenterol.* 1985; **7**: 511.

49 Yoshida J, Donahue P, Nyhus LM. Hemobilia: review of recent experience with a worldwide problem. *Am. J. Gastroenterol.* 1987; **82**: 448.

50 Zins M, Vilgrain V, Gayno S *et al.* US-guided percutaneous liver biopsy with plugging of the needle track: a prospective study in 72 high-risk patients. *Radiology* 1992; **184**: 841.

Chapter 4
The Haematology of Liver Disease

General features

Hepato-cellular failure, portal hypertension and jaundice may affect the blood picture. Chronic liver disease is usually accompanied by 'hypersplenism'. Diminished erythrocyte survival is frequent. In addition both parenchymal hepatic disease and cholestatic jaundice may produce blood coagulation defects. Dietary deficiencies, alcoholism, bleeding and difficulties in hepatic synthesis of proteins used in blood formation or coagulation add to the complexity of the problem.

Spontaneous bleeding, bruising and purpura, together with a history of bleeding after minimal trauma such as venepuncture, are more important indications of a bleeding tendency in patients with liver disease than are laboratory tests.

Blood volume

Plasma volume is frequently increased in patients with cirrhosis, especially with ascites and also with long-standing obstructive jaundice or with hepatitis. This hypervolaemia may partially, and sometimes totally, account for a low peripheral haemoglobin or erythrocyte level. Total circulating haemoglobin is reduced in only about half the patients.

Erythrocyte changes

The red cells may be *hypochromic*. This is often due to gastrointestinal bleeding leading to iron deficiency. In portal hypertension anaemia follows gastro-oesophageal bleeding and is enhanced by thrombocytopenia and disturbed blood coagulation. In cholestasis or cirrhosis of the alcoholic, haemorrhage may be from an ulcer or gastritis. Epistaxis, bruising and bleeding gums add to the anaemia.

The erythrocytes are usually *normocytic*. This is a combination of the microcytosis of chronic blood loss and the macrocytosis inherent in patients with liver disease. Thus the red cell membrane cholesterol and phospholipid content and/or ratio is changed and this results in various morphological abnormalities including thin macrocytes and target cells.

Thin macrocytes are frequent and are associated with a macronormoblastic marrow. These resolve when liver function improves.

Target cells are also thin macrocytes. They are found in both hepato-cellular and cholestatic jaundice. They are flat, macrocytic and have an increased surface area and increased resistance to osmotic lysis. They are particularly prominent in cholestasis where a rise in bile acids may contribute by inhibiting lecithin cholesterol acyl transferase (LCAT) activity [10]. The red cell membrane LCAT is decreased, resulting in loading of the membrane with both cholesterol and lecithin. Membrane fluidity is unchanged.

Spur cells are cells with unusual thorny projections. They are also termed *acanthocytes* (fig. 4.1). They are associated with far advanced liver disease usually in alcoholics. Severe anaemia and haemolysis are also found [13, 14]. Their appearance is a bad prognostic sign. The mechanism of their formation is unclear but they may be derived from *echinocytes*, also called burr cells [22]. These spiculated cells are not usually seen on dry blood films but are present on wet films or scanning electron microscopy in many patients with liver disease. They form because of an interaction with the abnormal HDL found in liver disease [22]. There is excess accumulation of unesterified cholesterol compared with phospholipid, with resultant reduced membrane fluidity and the formation of thorny projections. Reticulo-endothelial cells in the spleen modify these rigid cells with removal of membrane.

Alcoholics show genuine *thick macrocytes* probably related to the toxic effect of alcohol on the bone marrow. Folic acid and B_{12} deficiency may contribute.

Erythrocytosis may complicate hepato-cellular carcinoma due to production of erythropoietin by the tumour cells [30].

Bone marrow of chronic hepato-cellular failure is hyperplastic and macronormoblastic. In spite of this, erythrocyte volume is depressed and the marrow therefore does not seem able to compensate completely for the anaemia (*relative marrow failure*).

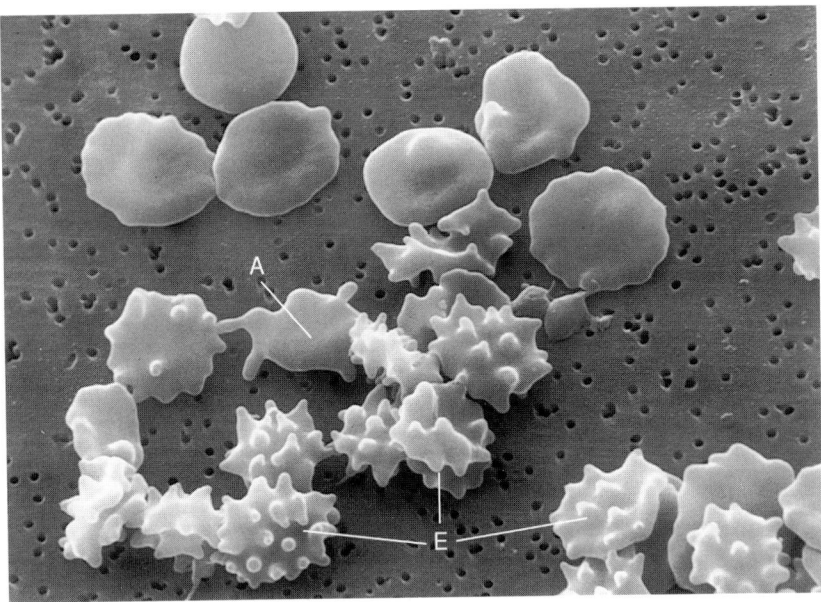

Fig. 4.1. Scanning electron micrograph of abnormal red cells from a patient with alcoholic hepatitis, showing echinocytes (E) at various stages of development, and an acanthocyte (A) (courtesy Dr J. Owen and Ms J. Lewin).

Folate and B_{12} metabolism

The liver stores folate and converts it to its active storage form, tetrahydrofolate [9]. Folate deficiency may accompany chronic liver disease, usually in the alcoholic. This is largely due to dietary deficiency. Serum folate levels are low. Folate therapy is useful. The liver also stores vitamin B_{12}. Hepatic levels are reduced in liver disease. When hepatocytes become necrotic the vitamin is released into the blood and high serum B_{12} levels are recorded. This is shown in hepatitis, active cirrhosis and with primary liver cancer. Values in cholestatic jaundice are normal.

Megaloblastic anaemia is rare with chronic liver disease and vitamin B_{12} therapy is rarely needed.

Erythrocyte survival and haemolytic anaemia

Increased red cell destruction is almost constant in hepato-cellular failure and jaundice of all types [27]. This is reflected in erythrocyte polychromasia and reticulocytosis.

The mechanism is extremely complex. The major factor is hypersplenism with destruction of red blood cells in the spleen. Also, spur cells have membrane defects, particularly decreased fluidity, and this with altered architecture exacerbates splenic destruction. In some instances, however, the spleen is not the site of erythrocyte destruction. Splenectomy or corticosteroid therapy have little effect [27].

Haemolysis may occur in Wilson's disease (Chapter 22), and this diagnosis is likely in the young patient presenting with haemolysis and liver dysfunction.

Haemolysis may be acute in patients with alcoholic

hepatitis who also have hypercholesterolaemia (*Zieve's syndrome*) [39].

Very rarely an autoimmune haemolytic anaemia with a positive Coombs' test is seen in chronic hepatitis, primary biliary cirrhosis and primary sclerosing cholangitis [7]. Haemolytic anaemia may also follow liver transplantation due to 'passenger lymphocytes' in a mismatch donor organ [11] or a delayed transfusion reaction.

Aplastic anaemia is a rare complication of acute viral hepatitis, usually type non-A non-B non-C [28]. It carries a very bad prognosis and has been treated by bone marrow transplantation [37]. It may follow liver transplantation for fulminant non-A non-B hepatitis.

Hepatitis B virus positive serum inhibits a normal human marrow cell [38].

Changes in the leucocytes and platelets

Leucopenia and thrombocytopenia are commonly found in patients with cirrhosis, usually with a mild anaemia ('*hypersplenism*').

Leucocytes

The leucopenia is of the order of $1.5–3.0 \times 10^9/l$, the depression mainly affecting polymorphs. Occasionally it may be more severe.

Leucocytosis accompanies cholangitis, fulminant hepatitis, alcoholic hepatitis, hepatic abscess and malignant disease. It is also found with extra-hepatic tumours producing colony-stimulating factor, which may be associated with hepatic damage [32]. Atypical lymphocytes are found in the peripheral blood in viral infections such as infectious mononucleosis and virus hepatitis.

Platelets

Abnormalities in platelet count, structure and function are common in patients with all forms of liver disease.

In patients with portal hypertension a reduced platelet count, rarely severe, is due to increased splenic sequestration. This is related to a greatly increased splenic platelet pool. Increased destruction of platelets is minimal. Platelet half-life is normal. Platelet volume is low [15]. Similar haematological changes occur with thrombosis of the portal vein and other diseases with splenomegaly.

In some patients there may be increased destruction of platelets. Platelet-associated IgG antibodies are found in patients with chronic hepatitis, particularly due to hepatitis C (88% of patients) and hepatitis B (47%) [21]. The antibody level correlates with the degree of thrombocytopenia.

Platelet function, in particular aggregation, is impaired in patients with cirrhosis, particularly Child's grade C. There is a reduced availability of arachidonic acid for prostaglandin production [23], and also a reduction in platelet adenosine triphosphate and 5-hydoxytryptamine [17].

Abnormal platelet aggregation due to disseminated intravascular coagulation may be important in severe liver failure.

Decreased production of platelets from the bone marrow follows alcohol excess, folic acid deficiency and viral hepatitis.

The thrombocytopenia (usually $60–90 \times 10^9/l$) of chronic liver disease is extremely frequent and is largely due to hypersplenism. It is very rarely of clinical significance. Unless the patient is actually *suffering* from the leucopenia or thrombocytopenia the spleen should *not* be removed; mere demonstration of a low platelet or leucocyte count is not sufficient. The circulating platelets and leucocytes, although in short supply, are, in contrast to those of leukaemia, functioning well. Splenectomy is contraindicated. The mortality in patients with liver disease is high and the operation is liable to be followed by splenic and portal vein thrombosis which preclude later operations on the portal vein and may make hepatic transplantation more difficult.

The liver and blood coagulation

[20, 25, 36]

Disturbed blood coagulation in patients with hepatobiliary disease is particularly complex. This is due to the many often conflicting changes in the pathways which lead to fibrin production at the same time as changes in

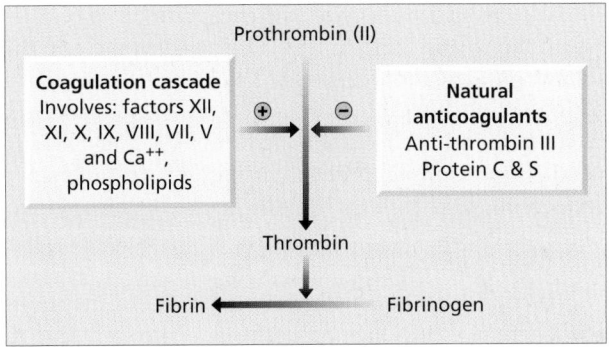

(a)

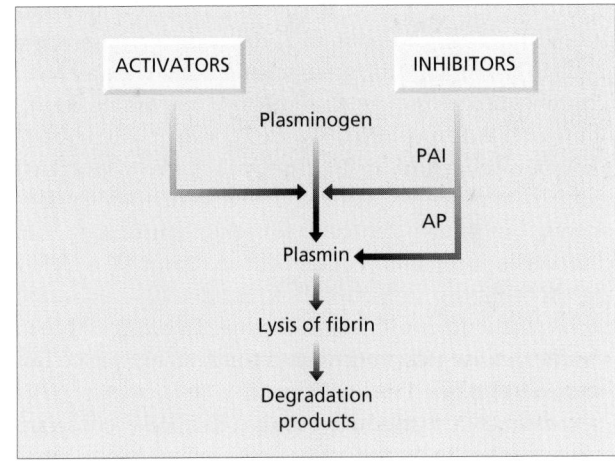

(b)

Fig. 4.2. Normal pathways of (a) coagulation and (b) fibrinolysis. Liver disease effects virtually all components. PAI = plasminogen activator inhibitor; AP = antiplasmin.

Table 4.1. Effect of liver disease on haemostasis

Reduced synthesis of clotting factors
hepatic dysfunction *per se*
vitamin K deficiency/malabsorption
Reduced synthesis of inhibitors of coagulation
Production of abnormal/dysfunctional proteins
Enhanced fibrolytic activity
reduced clearance of activators of fibrinolysis
reduced production of inhibitors of fibrinolysis
Reduced hepatic clearance of activated clotting factors
Disseminated intravascular coagulation
multifactorial including endotoxaemia
Platelet abnormalities
number
function

the fibrinolytic process (fig. 4.2; table 4.1). Changes in platelet number and function are discussed in the previous section. Despite the complexity of the changes, the end result is reduced coagulation which needs therapeutic intervention if there is bleeding or if a procedure is planned that risks haemorrhage.

The hepatocyte is the principal site of *synthesis* of all

the *coagulation proteins* with the exception of von Willebrand factor and factor VIIIC. The proteins include the vitamin K-dependent factors II, VII, IX and X, also labile factor V, factor VIII, contact factors XI and XII, fibrinogen and fibrin-stabilizing factor XIII. The half-life of all these clotting proteins is very short and hence reductions can rapidly follow acute hepato-cellular necrosis. Factor VII is particularly affected with a half-life of 100–300 minutes.

Vitamin K is a fat-soluble vitamin produced by intestinal bacteria. Deficiency occurs most commonly due to cholestasis, intra- and extra-hepatic, but may also follow treatment with bile acid chelators (cholestyramine) or oral antibiotics. The vitamin K-dependent proteins are made in the rough endoplasmic reticulum. They all have a number of glutamic acid residues in their amino-terminal region that must be converted, post-ribosomally, to gamma-carboxyglutamic acid by a carboxylase that requires vitamin K [12]. The function of these blood-clotting proteins depends on this conversion. In cholestasis parenteral replacement of vitamin K corrects the prothrombin time rapidly to normal (24–48 hours) and is useful diagnostically. If the coagulopathy is due to hepatic disease the prothrombin time may improve but not to normal.

Inhibitors which modulate the coagulation cascade are also synthesized by the liver. These include antithrombin III (ATIII), protein C and S, and heparin co-factor II. Protein C and S are vitamin K-dependent. In fulminant hepatic failure [18] and cirrhosis [2] these inhibitors are reduced but their deficiency is not associated with thrombotic events, probably because of the other changes in coagulation. Homozygous protein C deficiency has been cured by hepatic transplantation [8].

In liver disease, structurally and functionally *inadequate clotting factors and proteins* may be produced. *Dysfibrinogenaemia* is particularly frequent in cirrhosis, chronic hepatitis and acute liver failure. The fibrinogen may contain an excessive number of sialic acid residues. These are thought to lead to abnormal polymerization of fibrin monomers. There may also be a low molecular weight fibrinogen. Abnormalities of fibrinogen account for the prolongation of thrombin time in many patients with liver disease. This should be suspected if the partial thromboplastin time is increased but fibrinogen levels are normal and fibrinogen degradation products not increased.

There is evidence for *enhanced fibrinolytic activity* in patients with liver disease. Goodpasture first described the accelerated lysis of incubated clotted blood taken from cirrhotic patients in 1914. Hepatocytes synthesize plasminogen, and plasmin inhibitors such as α_2-antiplasmin, as well as inhibitors of tissue plasminogen activator (PAI-1). In patients with cirrhosis, plasminogen activator inhibitor antigen is reduced even without features of clotting activation (increased fibrin/fibrinogen degradation products; D-dimer) [35]. Increased tissue plasminogen activator activity relative to plasminogen activator *inhibitor* activity and α_2-antiplasmin are thought to lead to increased fibrinolysis [19]. Patients with severe liver disease and markers of hyperfibrinolysis are at higher risk of bleeding [34].

Whether there is background *disseminated intravascular coagulation* (DIC) in patients with cirrhosis, chronic hepatitis and acute hepatitis has been debated for some time. The complex changes in coagulation proteins, inhibitors and protein fragments usually associated with DIC could have been due to liver disease. Studies of thrombin–antithrombin (TAT) complexes, soluble fibrin, fibrin and fibrinogen degradation products (D-dimer, D-monomer) suggest that low grade DIC is a component of the coagulopathy in some patients with severe liver disease [1, 16, 24]. The mechanisms stimulating this are thought to include impaired clearance of activated clotting factors, and endotoxaemia [33].

Whatever the background state, cirrhotic patients are, however, at greater risk of overt DIC than patients with normal liver function, particularly in the presence of sepsis and hypotension [6].

Ascitic fluid contains fibrin monomers, fibrin degradation products and low levels of fibrinogen. This indicates active intra-peritoneal coagulation. Fibrinolysis, induced by infusion of plasminogen activators, accounts for the coagulopathy [31] which complicates intravenous infusion of ascitic fluid as in the LeVeen shunt.

Thrombotic complications can occur in cirrhotic patients. The relationship between antiphospholipid antibodies (lupus anticoagulant, anticardiolipin antibodies) reported in cirrhotics [29], the reduction in physiological anticoagulants (antithrombin III, protein C and S) and thrombotic events remains to be established.

Tests of coagulation

The prothrombin time (PT) before and after 10 mg vitamin K intramuscularly is the most satisfactory test for a coagulation defect in patients with hepato-biliary disease. It is also a most sensitive indication of hepato-cellular necrosis and/or prognosis. The partial thromboplastin time (PTT) is sometimes performed and is slightly more sensitive than the PT. Prolongation indicates not only deficiency of the prothrombin complex but also factors XI and XII.

Estimation of individual clotting factors is rarely necessary although in patients with fulminant hepatic failure the level of factor V is related to outcome. Thus, in patients with paracetamol-induced hepatic failure a factor V concentration of <10% on admission predicts a poor outcome [26]. The ratio of factor VIII (increased in liver disease) to factor V on admission is also valuable.

The platelet count is done. Measurement of the bleeding time assesses the contribution of platelet number and function to haemostasis.

Fibrinolysis and disseminated intravascular coagulation are diagnosed by marked prolongation of the PT, fibrinogen levels below 1.0 g/l, FDPs greater than 100 µg/l and thrombocytopenia less than 100×10^9/l.

Management of coagulation defect

Vitamin K_1 should be given to all patients with a prolonged prothrombin time. The usual course is 10 mg vitamin K_1 by intramuscular injection for 3 days. This is effective in about 3 hours and will correct hypoprothrombinaemia related to malabsorption of vitamin K secondary to bile salt deficiency. Defects predominantly due to hepato-cellular disease will not be restored by the vitamin K_1 treatment. Nevertheless, even in patients with predominantly hepato-cellular jaundice there may be a component of bile salt secretory failure and the prothrombin time often improves by a few seconds. A prolongation of the prothrombin time of more than 3 seconds (INR 1.2) after intramuscular vitamin K_1 contraindicates such procedures as liver biopsy, splenic venography, percutaneous cholangiography or laparotomy. If such procedures are essential, the clotting defect may be improved by fresh-frozen plasma which is effective for a few hours (table 4.2). However, even patients with prothrombin times and platelet counts regarded as acceptable for invasive procedures (PT < 17 seconds; platelets > 80×10^9/l) may have prolonged bleeding times [3]. Multiple linear regression analysis shows bleeding time to correlate independently with serum bilirubin concentration and platelet count.

In general, apart from vitamin K_1 therapy, it is not necessary to restore blood coagulation to normal in patients with liver disease unless there is active bleeding. Stored blood transfusion will supply prothrombin, VII, VIII and X. Fresh blood also supplies factor V and platelets. Fresh-frozen plasma is a good source of clotting factors, especially V.

Desmopressin (DDAVP), a vasopressin analogue, causes transient shortening of the bleeding time and PTT (but not PT) with increases in factor VIII and von Willebrand factor. Infusions may be helpful for the control of bleeding in patients with chronic liver disease [5].

DIC is treated by control of trigger factors such as infection, shock and dehydration. Fresh blood is most useful but, if unavailable, fresh-frozen plasma and packed red blood cells may be used. DIC is never severe enough to merit heparin therapy.

Platelet-rich plasma concentrates are used if thrombocytopenia is a problem and may be given to cover a procedure such as transjugular liver biopsy in a severely thrombocytopenic patient.

Hepatic transplantation

Pre-operative coagulation defects are due to the diseased liver. This and operative blood loss lead to replacement usually with about 20 units red blood cells and 15 units platelets. Prognosis is related to the amount of blood and blood products required [4]. During surgery, coagulation and fibrolysis are activated. In the anhepatic phase there is reduced clearance of activated proteins and inhibitors. The state of preservation of the donor liver determines post-operative coagulation problems. Revascularization of a compromised liver may lead to extensive defibrination and uncontrolled bleeding.

References

1 Bakker CM, Knot EAR, Stibbe J *et al.* Disseminated intravascular coagulation in liver cirrhosis. *J. Hepatol.* 1992; **15**: 330.
2 Bell H, Odegaard OR, Andersson T *et al.* Protein C in patients with alcoholic cirrhosis and other liver diseases. *J. Hepatol.* 1992; **14**: 163.
3 Blake JC, Sprengers D, Grech P *et al.* Bleeding time in patients with hepatic cirrhosis. *Br. Med. J.* 1990; **301**: 12.
4 Bontempo FA, Lewis JH, Van Thiel DH *et al.* The relation of preoperative coagulation findings to diagnosis, blood usage, and survival in adult liver transplantation. *Transplantation* 1985; **39**: 532.
5 Burroughs AK, Matthews K, Qadiri M *et al.* Desmopressin and bleeding time in patients with cirrhosis. *Br. Med. J.* 1985; **291**: 1377.
6 Carr JM. Disseminated intravascular coagulation in cirrhosis. *Hepatology* 1989; **10**: 103.
7 Case Records of the Massachusetts General Hospital. Case 3–1991. *N. Engl. J. Med.* 1991; **324**: 180.
8 Casella JF, Lewis JH, Bontempo FA *et al.* Successful treatment of homozygous protein C deficiency by hepatic transplantation. *Lancet* 1988; **i**: 435.
9 Chanarin I, Hutchinson M, McLean A *et al.* Hepatic folate in man. *Br. Med. J.* 1966; **1**: 396.
10 Cooper RA, Arner EC, Wiley JS *et al.* Modification of red cell membrane structure by cholesterol-rich lipid dispersions: a model for the primary spur cell defect. *J. Clin. Invest.* 1975; **55**: 115.
11 Dzik WH, Jenkins RL. Renal failure from ABO hemolysis due to anti-A of graft origin following liver transplantation. *Transfusion* 1987; **27**: 550.

Table 4.2. Routine before invasive techniques (including surgery)

Measure	Prothrombin time Partial thromboplastin time Platelet count
Routine	Abstain from alcohol for one week Vitamin K_1 10 mg intramuscularly
If necessary	Fresh-frozen plasma Platelet infusion

12 Furie B, Furie BC. Molecular basis of vitamin K-dependent γ-carboxylation. *Blood* 1990; **75**: 1753.

13 Gisselbrecht C, Metreau J-M, Dhumeaux D *et al.* L'acanthocytose au cours des cirrhoses. *Gastroenterol. Clin. Biol.* 1977; **1**: 621.

14 Grahn EP, Dietz AA, Stefani SS *et al.* Burr cells, hemolytic anemia and cirrhosis. *Am. J. Med.* 1968; **45**: 78.

15 Jørgensen B, Fischer E, Ingeberg S *et al.* Decreased blood platelet volume and count in patients with liver disease. *Scand. J. Gastroenterol.* 1984; **19**: 492.

16 Kruskal JB, Robson SC, Franks JJ *et al.* Elevated fibrin-related and fibrinogen-related antigens in patients with liver disease. *Hepatology* 1992; **16**: 920.

17 Laffi G, Marra F, Gresele P *et al.* Evidence for a storage pool defect in platelets from cirrhotic patients with defective aggregation. *Gastroenterology* 1992; **103**: 641.

18 Langley PG, Williams R. Physiological inhibitors of coagulation in fulminant hepatic failure. *Blood Coag. Fibrinol.* 1992; **3**: 243.

19 Leebeek FWG, Kluft C, Knot EAR *et al.* A shift in balance between profibrinolytic and antifibrinolytic factors causes enhanced fibrinolysis in cirrhosis. *Gastroenterology* 1991; **101**: 1382.

20 Mammen EF. Coagulation defects in liver disease. *Med. Clin. North Am.* 1994; **78**: 545.

21 Nagamine T, Ohtuka T, Takenhara K *et al.* Thrombocytopenia associated with hepatitis C viral infection. *J. Hepatol.* 1996; **24**: 135.

22 Owen JS, Brown DJC, Harry DS *et al.* Erythrocyte echinocytosis in liver disease. Role of abnormal plasma high density lipoproteins. *J. Clin. Invest.* 1985; **76**: 2275.

23 Owen JS, Hutton RA, Day RC *et al.* Platelet lipid composition and platelet aggregation in human liver disease. *J. Lipid Res.* 1981; **22**: 423.

24 Paramo JA, Rifon J, Fernandez J *et al.* Thrombin activation and increased fibrinolysis in patients with chronic liver disease. *Blood Coag. Fibrinol.* 1991; **2**: 227.

25 Paramo JA, Rocha E. Hemostasis in advanced liver disease. *Semin. Thromb. Hemostasis* 1993; **19**: 184.

26 Pereira LMMB, Langley PG, Hayllar KM *et al.* Coagulation factor V and VIII/V ratio as predictors of outcome in paracetamol induced fulminant hepatic failure: relation to other prognostic indicators. *Gut* 1992; **33**: 98.

27 Pitcher CS, Williams R. Reduced red cell survival in jaundice and its relation to abnormal glutathione metabolism. *Clin. Sci.* 1963; **24**: 239.

28 Pol S, Driss F, Devergie A *et al.* Is hepatitis C virus involved in hepatitis-associated aplastic anemia? *Ann. Intern. Med.* 1990; **113**: 435.

29 Quintarelli C, Ferro D, Valesini G *et al.* Prevalence of lupus anticoagulant in patients with cirrhosis: relationship with beta-2-glycoprotein 1 plasma levels. *J. Hepatol.* 1994; **21**: 1086.

30 Sakisara S, Watanabe M, Tateishi H *et al.* Erythropoietin production in hepatocellular carcinoma cells associated with polycythemia: immunohistochemical evidence. *Hepatology* 1993; **18**: 1357.

31 Schölmerich J, Zimmerman U, Köttgen E *et al.* Proteases and antiproteases released to the coagulation system in plasma and ascites. Prediction of coagulation disorder in ascites retransfusion. *J. Hepatol.* 1988; **6**: 359.

32 Suzuki A, Takahasi T, Okuno Y *et al.* Liver damage in patients with colony-stimulating-factor producing tumors.

Am. J. Med. 1993; **94**: 125.

33 Violi F, Ferro D, Basili S *et al.* Assocation between low-grade disseminated intravascular coagulation and endotoxaemia in patients with liver cirrhosis. *Gastroenterology* 1995; **109**: 531.

34 Violi F, Ferro D, Basili S *et al.* Hyperfibrinolysis increases the risk of gastrointestinal hemorrhage in patients with advanced cirrhosis. *Hepatology* 1992; **15**: 672.

35 Violi F, Ferro D, Basili S *et al.* Hyperfibrinolysis resulting from clotting activation in patients with different degrees of cirrhosis. *Hepatology* 1993; **17**: 78.

36 Violi F, Ferro D, Quintarelli C *et al.* Clotting abnormalities in chronic liver disease. *Dig. Dis.* 1992; **10**: 162.

37 Witherspoon RP, Storb R, Shulman H *et al.* Marrow transplantation in hepatitis-associated aplastic anemia. *Am. J. Hematol.* 1984; **17**: 269.

38 Zeldis J, Mugishima H, Steinberg H *et al.* In vitro hepatitis B virus infection of human bone marrow cells. *J. Clin. Invest.* 1986; **78**: 411.

39 Zieve L. Hemolytic anemia in liver disease. *Medicine (Baltimore)* 1966; **45**: 497.

Haemolytic jaundice

Haemoglobin is released in excessive amounts, increasing from the normal of 6.25 g to as much as 45 g daily. Consequently there is an increase in the serum bilirubin, 85% of which is unconjugated. The rise in conjugated bilirubin is probably due to retention.

Even if bile pigment production reaches its maximum of 1500 mg daily (six times normal), serum bilirubin rises only to about 2–3 mg/100 ml (35–50 µmol/l). This is because of the great capacity of the liver to handle pigment. If patients with haemolytic jaundice show serum bilirubin values greater than 70–85 µmol/l there is probably the additional factor of hepato-cellular dysfunction or kidney failure. Anaemia itself will, of course, depress liver function.

Unconjugated bilirubin is not water soluble and does not pass into the urine. A little bilirubin may be detected in the urine by sensitive tests if the conjugated level in the blood rises to values that are unusually high for haemolysis.

Bile pigment excretion is greatly increased and large quantities of stercobilinogen are found in the stools. Each milligram of stercobilinogen corresponds to the breakdown of 24 mg haemoglobin. This estimate can only be approximate, for a significant proportion of the faecal haem pigment is derived from sources other than haemoglobin of mature erythrocytes.

PATHOLOGICAL CHANGES

The breakdown of haemoglobin yields iron. *Tissue siderosis* is a feature of most types of haemolytic anaemia.

The *liver* is normal sized and is reddish-brown due to increased amounts of iron. Histology shows iron in

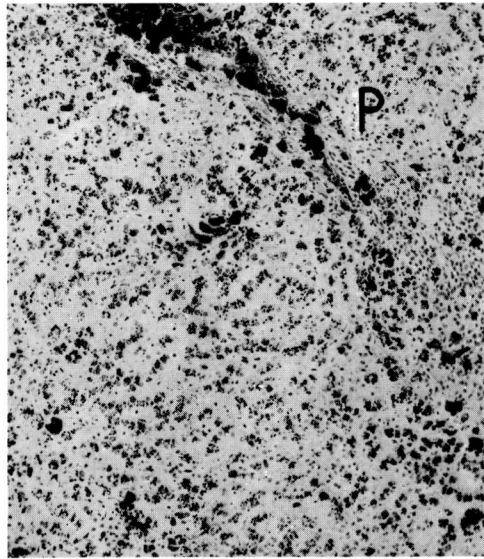

Fig. 4.3. Haemolytic jaundice. The hepatic architecture is normal. Increased amounts of iron are seen in the liver cells, Kupffer cells and especially the large macrophages of the portal tracts (P). (Stained ferro-cyanide, ×90.)

Kupffer cells, large macrophages of the portal tracts, and to a lesser extent in hepatic parenchyma (fig. 4.3). In the severely anaemic, there is centrizonal sinusoidal distention with fatty change. Focal areas of liver cell necrosis are attributed to vascular obstruction of sinusoids by impacted cells undergoing lysis or to the direct effect of haemolysis on the liver cells. The Kupffer cells are generally swollen and hyperplastic foci of erythropoiesis are uncommon. The *gallbladder* and *bile passages* contain dark viscid bile. Calcium bilirubinate pigment calculi are found in one-half to two-thirds of patients. Secondary cholecystitis may be followed by crops of multiple, faceted, mixed gallstones.

The *spleen* is enlarged, fleshy and packed with erythrocytes. The *red bone marrow* is hyperplastic.

CLINICAL FEATURES

The picture varies with the cause, but certain symptoms and signs are common to all forms of haemolysis.

Anaemia depends on the rate of destruction compared with regeneration of red blood cells. It increases rapidly with crises where the patient becomes ill with aching pains in the abdomen and limbs, fever, headache and sometimes even a fall in blood pressure and collapse.

Jaundice is usually mild and lemon yellow. It increases rapidly with haemolytic crises or if there is a coincidental difficulty in biliary excretion such as virus hepatitis or choledocholithiasis or if the kidney fails.

Pigment *gallstones* may be associated with the features of chronic cholecystitis. Stones in the common bile duct

may cause obstructive jaundice, and the coexistence of two types of jaundice provides a confusing clinical picture. Gallstones in children always suggest a haemolytic aetiology.

Splenomegaly is present in the chronic forms.

Ulcers or pigmentation from healed ulcers, usually over the internal or external malleoli, occur in some types.

HAEMATOLOGICAL CHANGES

Anaemia is variable and the peripheral blood shows active regeneration. Reticulocytes are increased to 20%. Leucocytes are usually increased.

The bone marrow is hyperplastic and the proportion of erythroid to leucopoietic cells rises.

The survival of labelled erythrocytes is reduced and increased uptake can be shown in the spleen.

In some hereditary anaemias iron overload may occur without transfusion. This is particularly when there is a high degree of ineffective erythropoiesis — for example, congenital dyserythropoietic anaemias, congenital sideroblastic anaemia and thalassaemia intermedia. It may also occur in pyruvate kinase deficiency [15]. The role of hetero- or homozygosity for the genetic haemochromatosis gene remains unclear.

FAECES AND URINE

The faeces are dark and stercobilinogen is increased. Urobilinogen is increased in the urine. Bilirubin is detected in the urine only rarely, when jaundice is deep. When blood destruction is rapid, free haemoglobin may be found in the urine and microscopy reveals pigmented casts.

SERUM BIOCHEMISTRY

Serum unconjugated bilirubin levels are raised but conjugated bilirubin is only slightly increased.

The serum alkaline phosphatase, albumin and globulin concentrations are normal. Serum haptoglobins are diminished. The serum cholesterol level is low.

If haemolysis is particularly acute, methaemalbumin can be detected in the serum. Serum ferritin is increased. Free haemoglobin may be detected.

DIFFERENTIAL DIAGNOSIS

The diagnosis of haemolytic from other forms of jaundice is usually easy. The absence of pain, pruritus, the dark colour of the stools and normal alkaline phosphatase are points of difference from cholestatic jaundice. The absence of stigmas of hepato-cellular disease, the normal serum alanine transaminase and protein values distinguish it from virus hepatitis and cirrhosis.

Distinction from the congenital unconjugated hyper-bilirubinaemias may be difficult, particularly as many patients with Gilbert's disease show a decreased erythrocyte survival.

The liver in haemolytic anaemias

Hereditary spherocytosis [4]

The main signs are jaundice, anaemia, splenomegaly and gallstones, but the spectrum of disease is wide from no clinical expression to death *in utero*. Inheritance is dominant or recessive. In 70% of cases the molecular defect is a mutation in ankyrin, one of the components of the red cell skeleton [5].

Jaundice is rarely noticed before school age or adolescence. The mean serum bilirubin level is 35 μmol/l (2 mg/dl) (range 10–100 μmol/l). Deep jaundice is rare. This may develop in the neonatal period and be associated with incipient kernicterus.

Gallstones are related to age and are rare at less than 10 years old. They are symptomatic in about half the patients. The stones are usually removed at the time of splenectomy.

Hereditary elliptocytosis, another genetic defect due to a mutation in a protein within the red cell membrane skeleton, is usually a harmless trait, the haemolysis being compensated. It may occasionally develop into active decompensated haemolytic anaemia.

Various enzyme defects

Many of the hereditary non-spherocytic anaemias are now known to be due to various defects in the metabolism of the red cells. They include deficiency of pyruvate kinase or triose phosphate isomerase, or deficiency in the pentose phosphate pathway such as glucose-6-phosphate dehydrogenase (G6PD). These conditions may be of particular importance in the aetiology of neonatal jaundice. The gene responsible for G6PD deficiency has now been cloned and a wide range of mutations recognized. These are beginning to explain the wide spectrum of clinical pictures seen in this condition ranging from haemolysis during the neonatal period, after infection or after the ingestion of certain drugs, to chronic anaemia irrespective of any of these factors. Variants of the gene are now recognized where there is no significant reduction in enzyme activity in red cells [1].

Viral hepatitis can precipitate destruction of G6PD-deficient cells and so cause acute haemolytic anaemia and very high serum bilirubin concentrations.

Sickle-cell disease

The abnormal haemoglobin crystallizes in the erythrocytes when the oxygen tension is reduced. There are crises of blood destruction with acute attacks of pain. The liver may be affected acutely by sickling crises. There is right upper quadrant pain, fever and increased jaundice, associated with systemic and haematological features of sickling. This should help differentiate the clinical picture from a common bile duct stone. Fulminant liver failure is rare [13]. A distinct clinical picture of intra-hepatic cholestasis is also recognized but is unusual [10]. Histologically there is intracanalicular cholestasis, sinusoidal dilatation, Kupffer cell hyperplasia and erythrophagocytosis.

There may be chronic elevation of transaminases and/or alkaline phosphatase with hepatic scarring. Several factors have been implicated including microvascular stasis, with recurrent ischaemic episodes, and trans-fusion-related disease (haemosiderosis and viral hepatitis) [3].

Jaundice accompanying sickle-cell disease is always particularly deep, the high serum bilirubin levels being related to the combination of haemolysis and impaired hepato-cellular function. Depth of jaundice *per se* should not be regarded as an indication of severity. Concomitant viral hepatitis or obstructed bile ducts lead to exceptionally high serum bilirubin values.

Gallstones are found in 25% of children and 50–70% of adults with homozygous sickle cell disease. They are usually in the gallbladder; duct calculi are rare. In two-thirds of adults the stones are asymptomatic [2]. About 55% of stones are radio-opaque. The high frequency of gallbladder stones may be due in part to changes in gallbladder volume and motility [6].

HEPATIC HISTOLOGY

Active and healed areas of necrosis may have followed anoxia due to vascular obstruction by impacted sickle cells or by Kupffer cells swollen with phagocytosed erythrocytes following intra-hepatic sickling. The widened sinusoids show a foam-like fibrin reticulum within their lumen. This intra-sinusoidal fibrin may later result in fibre deposition in the space of Disse and narrowed sinusoids. Bile plugs are prominent. Fatty change is related to anaemia and haemosiderosis to multiple transfusions.

The classic findings are of intra-sinusoidal sickling, Kupffer cell erythrophagocytosis and ischaemic necrosis. It is difficult to explain the severe liver dysfunction on these histological findings [8]. These changes have been reported largely on autopsy specimens. In biopsies, the histological picture is more likely to be that of a complicating disease such as septicaemia or concurrent viral hepatitis [11].

ELECTRON MICROSCOPY

The changes are those of hypoxia. There are sinusoidal aggregates of sickled erythrocytes, fibrin and platelets, with increased collagen and occasional basement membranes in the space of Disse.

CLINICAL FEATURES

Asymptomatic patients commonly have raised serum transaminases and hepatomegaly [12]. Hepatitis B and C, and iron overload may have complicated transfusions.

In about 10% the crisis selectively affects the liver. It lasts 2–3 weeks. It is marked by abdominal pain, fever, jaundice, an enlarged tender liver and a rise in serum transaminases. In some patients the crisis is precipitated by salmonella infection or by folic acid deficiency.

Acute liver failure, usually with cholestasis, is rare. Jaundice is very deep with a markedly increased prothrombin time and encephalopathy but with only modestly increased serum transaminases. Liver biopsy shows the changes of sickle-cell disease with marked zone 2 necrosis and cholestasis. The diagnosis of hepatic sickle crisis from viral hepatitis is difficult. In general, in viral hepatitis pain is less, jaundice deeper and transaminase elevations more prolonged. Liver biopsy and hepatitis viral markers usually help to make the distinction. Exchange transfusion has been successful [13].

Prolonged intra-hepatic cholestasis associated with sickle cell anaemia has also responded to exchange transfusion [10].

Acute cholecystitis and choledocholithiasis may simulate hepatic crisis or viral hepatitis. Endoscopic or percutaneous cholangiography are important investigations in excluding biliary obstruction. Complications after cholecystectomy are common, and this is indicated only if there is great difficulty in making a distinction from abdominal crisis or where symptoms are clearly related to gallbladder disease. Pre-operative exchange transfusion may lessen later complications [2].

General features include leg ulcers, which are frequent. The upper jaw is protuberant and hypertrophied. The fingers are clubbed. Bone deformities seen radiologically include rarefaction and narrowing of the cortex of the long bones and a 'hair-on-end' appearance in the skull.

Thalassaemia

Crises of blood destruction and fever and the reactionary changes in bone are similar to those seen in sickle-cell disease. The liver shows siderosis and sometimes fibrosis. The haemosiderosis may progress to an actual haemochromatosis and indicate treatment by continuous desferrioxamine therapy (see Chapter 21). The stainable iron in the liver cells may be greater in those who have lost the spleen as a storage organ for iron.

Transfusion-acquired hepatitis B and C may lead to chronic liver disease.

Episodes of intra-hepatic cholestasis of uncertain nature can also develop. Gallstones may be a complication.

Previously the commonest cause of death in thalassaemia major was heart failure but the clinical course of the disease is changing with improved therapy including, in particular, iron chelation.

TREATMENT

This may include folic acid, blood transfusion, iron chelation therapy, antiviral treatment, pneumococcal vaccination and occasionally splenectomy. Bone marrow transplantation may be considered but the survival is worse in those with liver disease [9].

Paroxysmal nocturnal haemoglobinuria

In this rare acquired disease, there is intravascular, complement-mediated haemolysis. The defect is due to mutation of the PIG-A gene on chromosome X [14] which results in deficient biosynthesis of the glycosylphosphatidylinositol (GPI) anchor. This leads to an absence of certain proteins on the red cell surface. The cells are sensitive to lysis when the pH of the blood becomes more acid during sleep. During an episode of haemolysis the urine passed in the morning may be brown or reddish brown due to haemoglobinuria.

Acutely the patients show a dusky, reddish jaundice and the liver enlarges. Aspartate transaminase may be increased (due to haemolysis) and serum studies show iron deficiency (due to urinary loss of haemoglobin). Liver histology shows some centrizonal necrosis and siderosis.

Hepatic vein thrombosis may be a complication. Bile duct changes similar to primary sclerosing cholangitis, perhaps due to ischaemia, have been reported [7].

Acquired haemolytic anaemia

The haemolysis is due to extra-corpuscular causes. Spherocytosis is slight and osmotic fragility only mildly impaired.

The patient is moderately jaundiced. The increased pigment is unconjugated, but in severe cases conjugated bilirubin increases and appears in the urine. This may be related to bilirubin overload in the presence of liver damage. Blood transfusion accentuates the jaundice, for transfused cells survive poorly.

The haemolysis may be *idiopathic*. The increased haemolysis is then due to autoimmunization. Coombs' test is positive.

The *acquired* type may complicate other diseases, especially those involving the reticuloendothelial system. These include Hodgkin's disease, the leukaemias, reticulosarcoma, carcinomatosis and uraemia. The anaemia of hepato-cellular jaundice is also partially haemolytic. Coombs' test is usually negative.

Autoimmune haemolytic anaemia is a rare complication of autoimmune chronic hepatitis and primary biliary cirrhosis.

Wilson's disease may present as a haemolytic crisis (Chapter 22).

Haemolytic disease of the newborn

See Chapter 24.

Incompatible blood transfusion

Chills, fever and backache are followed by jaundice. Urobilinogen is present in the urine. Liver function tests give normal results. In severe cases free haemoglobin is detected in blood and urine. Diagnostic difficulties arise when a patient suffering from a disease that may be complicated by hepato-cellular failure or biliary obstruction becomes jaundiced soon after a blood transfusion.

References

1 Beutler E. Glucose-6-phosphate dehydrogenase deficiency. *N. Engl. J. Med.* 1991; **324**: 169.
2 Bond LR, Hatty SR, Horn MEC *et al.* Gallstones in sickle cell disease in the United Kingdom. *Br. Med. J.* 1987; **295**: 234.
3 Comer GM, Ozick LA, Sachdev RK *et al.* Transfusion-related chronic liver disease in sickle cell anemia. *Am. J. Gastroenterol.* 1991; **86**: 1232.
4 Croom RD III, McMillan CW, Sheldon GF *et al.* Hereditary spherocytosis. Recent experience and current concepts of pathophysiology. *Ann. Surg.* 1986; **203**: 34.
5 Delaunay J. Genetic disorders of the red cell membranes. *FEBS Letters* 1995; **369**: 34.
6 Everson GT, Nemeth A, Kourourian S *et al.* Gallbladder function is altered in sickle hemoglobinopathy. *Gastroenterology* 1989; **96**: 1307.
7 Huong DLT, Valla D, Franco D *et al.* Cholangitis associated with paroxysmal nocturnal hemoglobinuria: another instance of ischemic cholangiopathy? *Gastroenterology* 1995; **109**: 1338.
8 Johnson CS, Omata M, Tong MJ *et al.* Liver involvement in sickle cell disease. *Medicine* 1985; **64**: 349.
9 Lucarelli G, Galimberti M, Polchi P *et al.* Marrow transplantation in patients with thalassemia responsive to iron chelation therapy. *N. Engl. J. Med.* 1993; **329**: 840.
10 O'Callaghan A, O'Brien SG, Ninkovic M *et al.* Chronic intrahepatic cholestasis in sickle cell disease requiring exchange transfusion. *Gut* 1995; **37**: 144.
11 Omata M, Johnson CS, Tong M *et al.* Pathological spectrum of liver diseases in sickle cell disease. *Dig. Dis. Sci.* 1986; **31**: 247.
12 Schubert TT. Hepatobiliary system in sickle cell disease. *Gastroenterology* 1986; **90**: 2013.
13 Stephan JL, Merpit-Gonon E, Richard O *et al.* Fulminant liver failure in a 12-year-old girl with sickle cell anaemia: favourable outcome after exchange transfusion. *Eur. J. Pediatr.* 1995; **154**: 469.
14 Takeda J, Miyata T, Kawagoe K *et al.* Deficiency of the GPI anchor caused by mutation of the PIG-A gene in paroxysmal nocturnal hemoglobinuria. *Cell* 1993; **73**: 703.
15 Zanella A, Berzuini A, Colombo MB *et al.* Iron status in red cell pyruvate kinase deficiency: study of Italian cases. *Br. J. Haematol.* 1993; **83**: 485.

The liver in myelo- and lymphoproliferative disease

The liver contains multipotential cells that can differentiate into reticulo-endothelial, myeloid and lymphoid cells. These can be affected by malignant disease (leukaemia, lymphoma), usually in association with systemic disease, rarely as a primary hepatic disease. Reduced haemopoietic activity in marrow is followed by extramedullary haemopoiesis in the liver. Reticulo-endothelial storage diseases affect the liver as well as other organs. This section outlines the involvement of the liver in this broad group of diseases.

The liver is involved to a variable extent, usually with no functional effect, but mildly abnormal liver function tests. However, liver biopsies are helpful for diagnosis. Staining of sections with monoclonal antibodies may be necessary to define the cell type or disease. Involvement may be focal, so that serial sections should be cut. If scanning shows a focal lesion, guided biopsy is worthwhile.

Rarely fulminant liver failure complicates the primary disease, due to replacement of hepatocytes with malignant cells. This is reported in acute lymphoblastic leukaemia [10], non-Hodgkin's lymphoma [51], monoblastic transformation in chronic myeloid leukaemia [36] and malignant histiocytosis [5]. It is important to differentiate these from liver failure due to viral or drug hepatitis, since liver transplantation is contraindicated when there is underlying haematological malignancy [51].

Acute and chronic abnormalities of liver function tests may be due to treatment. Drugs given should be reviewed. More aggressive chemotherapy has increased hepato-toxic drug reactions. Multiple blood transfusions are a frequent cause of viral hepatitis, particularly hepatitis C and non-A, non-B, non-C, and to a lesser extent B. This is usually mild in the immunocompromised host. Hepatitis B may be reactivated during cytotoxic or immunosuppressive therapy, and there may be a fulminant hepatitis-like episode following withdrawal of treatment. This is thought to be due to a rebound effect with the return of immunity, and clearance of a large number of hepatocytes containing the virus [7, 27].

Gastrointestinal haemorrhage may complicate myeloproliferative diseases, leukaemia or lymphoma. In some this is caused by peptic ulceration or erosions. There may be portal hypertension due to hepatic, portal or splenic vein thrombosis related to a hypercoagulable state. Evidence for a myeloproliferative disorder was found in 14 of 33 patients with non-tumour-related portal vein thrombosis [47].

Occasionally the portal hypertension is pre-sinusoidal and seems to be secondary to infiltrative lesions in the portal zones and sinusoids. In others, increased blood flow due to splenomegaly may be important. If the wedged hepatic venous pressure is increased and the gradient with the intra-splenic pressure is normal, splenectomy may be indicated [29]. In systemic mastocytosis [9] and myeloid metaplasia [38] new fibre formation in the sinusoids may contribute. Portal and central zone fibrosis can be related to cytotoxic therapy.

Leukaemia

Myeloid

The enlarged liver is smooth and firm, and the cut section shows small, pale nodules.

Microscopically (figs 4.4, 4.5) both portal tracts and sinusoids are infiltrated with immature and mature cells

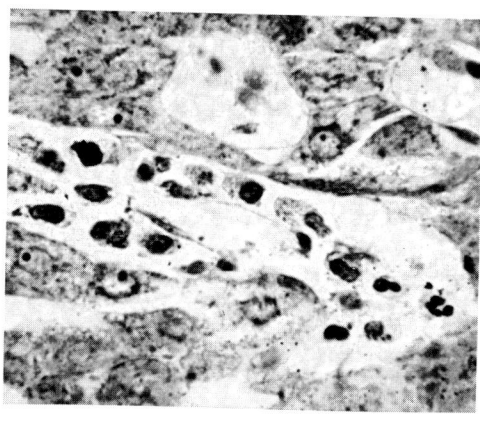

Fig. 4.5. Myeloid leukaemia. Cells of the myeloid and lymphocytic series can be seen in the sinusoidal wall, but outside the endothelial lining. (Stained Leishman, ×350.)

of the myeloid series. The immature cells lie outside the sinusoidal wall.

The portal tracts are enlarged with myelocytes and polymorphs, both neutrophil and eosinophil; round cells are also conspicuous. The liver cell cords are compressed by the leukaemic deposits.

Lymphoid

Macroscopically, the liver is moderately enlarged, with pale areas on section.

Microscopically (fig. 4.6) the leukaemic infiltration

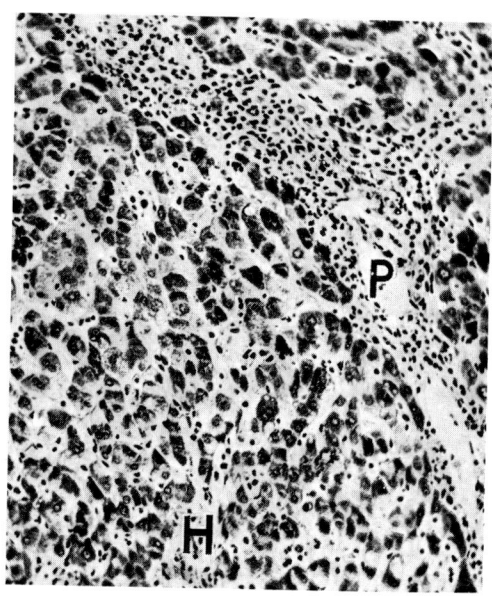

Fig. 4.4. Myelogenous leukaemia. Hepatic architecture is normal, but the sinusoids and a portal tract (P) contain increased numbers of cells of the myeloid series. H = hepatic venule. (Stained Best's carmine, ×70.)

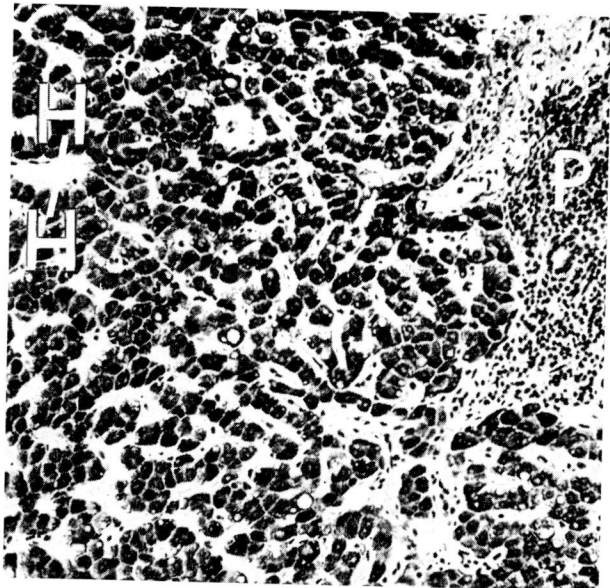

Fig. 4.6. Lymphoid leukaemia. Essential hepatic architecture is normal, but a portal tract (P) contains many cells of the lymphocyte series. The sinusoids are not affected. H = hepatic venule. (Stained Best's carmine, ×70.)

involves only the portal tracts—the normal sites of lymphoid tissue in the liver. The portal areas are enlarged and contain both mature and immature cells of the lymphatic series. The sinusoids are not affected. The liver cells are normal.

Hairy cell leukaemia

The liver is usually involved although specific clinical and biochemical features are rare. Sinusoidal and portal infiltration with mononuclear 'clear' cells is seen with sinusoidal congestion and beading [52]. Angiomatous lesions, usually periportal, consist of blood spaces lined by hairy cells. Methacrylate embedded liver biopsy sections show tartrate-resistant acid phosphatase activity in the hairy cells [52].

Bone marrow transplantation

Liver abnormalities occur at some time in the majority of patients within 12 months of bone marrow transplantation [15]. The changes range from abnormal liver function tests alone, to coagulation abnormalities, ascites and hepato-renal failure. There are many possible causes (table 4.3); more than one may be responsible at any one time. Pre-existing liver disease increases the risk.

Table 4.3. Hepato-biliary disease and bone marrow transplantation

Problem	Related to
Pre-existing	
Fungal	Granulocytopenia
Viral (type B, C)	Blood products
Drug	Medication
Biliary	Stones
Post-transplantation	
Early neutropenic phase (to 4 weeks)	
Acute graft-versus-host	Donor marrow
Veno-occlusive disease	Cytoreductive therapy
Nodular regenerative hyperplasia	
Drug induced	Including TPN
Extra-hepatic bacterial sepsis	Bacteria/endotoxin
Fungal	
Biliary disease	Sludge
Intermediate (4–15 weeks)*	
Viral	CMV
	Hepatitis B/C
Late (>15 weeks)	
Chronic graft-versus-host	Multiorgan disease
Chronic viral infection	
Fungal	Immunosuppression
Tumour recurrence	

* As well as continuing early problems.

In the first 15 weeks, the most common causes of liver abnormality are acute graft-versus-host (GVH) disease, intra-hepatic veno-occlusive disease, drug-induced reactions and infection [44].

Jaundice and abnormal liver enzyme tests accompany the systemic manifestations of *acute GVH disease*—rash and diarrhoea. This usually begins 3–8 weeks post-transplant. The hepatic changes may persist to give cholestatic chronic GVH disease with intra-hepatic bile duct damage. Chronic GVH may also develop *de novo*.

The development of jaundice, painful hepatomegaly, weight gain and ascites in the first weeks after bone marrow transplantation suggests a diagnosis of *veno-occlusive disease*. This is due to high-dose cytoreductive therapy given 5–10 days before the marrow infusion. The incidence varies from one report to another, ranging from less than 5% to over 60%, probably reflecting different patient groups, conditioning regimens and diagnostic criteria. Mortality in severely affected individuals is high, around 50%. There is controversy whether histological evidence of venular occlusion is needed for diagnosis. Routine percutaneous liver biopsy is often contraindicated by a low platelet count, prolonged coagulation tests and ascites. Transvenous liver biopsy overcomes these problems, although bleeding complications may still occur [42]. This route also allows the wedged hepatic venous pressure to be measured [42]. Trials of treatment (e.g. thrombolytic therapy) are likely to need biopsy data to substantiate the diagnosis of veno-occlusive disease made on clinical grounds. Four histological abnormalities correlate with the clinical severity of disease: occluded hepatic venules, eccentric luminal narrowing/phlebosclerosis, hepatocyte necrosis and sinusoidal fibrosis [41]. These findings suggest that there is extensive injury to zone three structures by the cytoreductive therapy.

Opportunistic *fungal and bacterial infections* occur during neutropenic periods and may cause abnormal liver function; *viral infections* occur later.

Helpful data to identify the cause of the hepatic abnormality include: (i) timing of the changes related to drugs, chemotherapy, radiation, and bone marrow infusion; (ii) the dose of cytoreductive (conditioning) therapy; (iii) the source of donor marrow; (iv) pretreatment viral serology; (v) the degree of immunosuppression; and (vi) evidence of systemic disease. Bacteriological and virological data are important. Often more than one process is involved. In one series transvenous liver biopsy provided useful data for patient management in over 80% of cases [42].

After bone marrow transplantation, hepato-biliary scintiscanning and ultrasound commonly show abnormalities of questionable clinical significance [21]. Doppler ultrasonography is not reliable for the diagnosis of veno-occlusive disease [45].

Lymphoma

Hepatic involvement occurs in about 70% of cases and immediately puts the patient into stage IV [22]. It may be seen as diffuse infiltrates, as focal tumour-like masses, as portal zone cellularity, as an epithelioid cell reaction or as lymphoid aggregates [22]. Rarely lymphomatous infiltration presents as acute liver failure [51].

In *Hodgkin's disease*, typical tissue is seen spreading out from the portal tracts, with lymphocytes, large pale epithelioid cells, eosinophils, plasma cells and giant Reed–Sternberg cells (fig. 4.7). Later, fibroblasts are found in a supporting connective tissue reticulum.

In patients with known extra-hepatic Hodgkin's disease, but without obvious Reed–Sternberg cells in sections of the liver, hepatic involvement is suggested by portal infiltrates larger than 1 mm in diameter, changes of acute cholangitis, portal oedema and portal infiltrates with a predominance of atypical lymphocytes. These changes should stimulate a wider search for the diagnostic Reed–Sternberg cell in further sections [12].

In *non-Hodgkin's lymphoma*, the portal zones are usually involved. In small cell lymphocytic lymphoma, a dense, monotonous proliferation of normal appearing lymphocytes is seen. The more aggressive lymphomas also involve portal zones and form tumour nodules. Large cell lymphoma may infiltrate sinusoids [46].

In *histiocytic medullary reticulosis*, large numbers of reticulum cells fill the sinusoids and portal tracts. Occasionally, the deposits may be single and large.

Liver granulomas with or without hepatic involvement are found with most lymphomas. Caseation without evidence of tuberculosis has been reported [25].

Paraproteinaemia and amyloidosis may be complications.

DIAGNOSIS OF HEPATIC INVOLVEMENT

Detection of hepatic involvement can be extremely difficult. It is unlikely if hepatomegaly is not found. Fever, jaundice and splenomegaly increase the likelihood. Increases in serum γ-GT and transaminase values are suggestive, although often non-specific [3].

Focal defects may be shown by ultrasound, CT and MRI scanning. Enlarged abdominal lymph nodes may also be seen. Hodgkin's disease may present with sterile liver abscesses [54].

Needle liver biopsy rarely reveals Hodgkin's tissue if the CT scan is normal. Laparotomy, peritoneoscopy, or directed ultrasound or CT liver biopsy add to the chances of obtaining Hodgkin's tissue. Needle biopsy does not exclude hepatic involvement if only an epithelioid histiocyte reaction is seen. Sinusoidal dilatation in zone 2 and 3 is found in 50% and may give a clue to the diagnosis [8].

Presentation as jaundice may provide great diagnostic difficulties (table 4.4). Lymphoma should always be considered in patients with jaundice, fever and weight loss.

JAUNDICE IN THE LYMPHOMAS (table 4.4)

Hepatic infiltrates may be massive or present as space-occupying lesions. Large intra-hepatic deposits are the commonest cause of deep jaundice. Histological evidence is essential for diagnosis.

Biliary obstruction is more frequent with non-Hodgkin's lymphoma than with Hodgkin's disease [13]. It is usually due to hilar glands which are less mobile than those along the common bile duct which can be pushed aside. Occasionally the obstructing glands are peri-ampullary. Investigations include endoscopic or percutaneous cholangiography, and brush cytology. Known lymphoma elsewhere draws attention to this as a possible cause of bile duct obstruction. Differentiation from other causes of extra-hepatic biliary obstruction is difficult, and depends on the appearances on scanning and at cholangiography, and the results of cytology and biopsy.

Rarely, an idiopathic intra-hepatic usually cholestatic jaundice may be seen in Hodgkin's [19] and non-Hodgkin's lymphoma [49]. It is unrelated to deposits in the liver or bile duct compression. Hepatic histology shows canalicular cholestasis. These changes are unre-

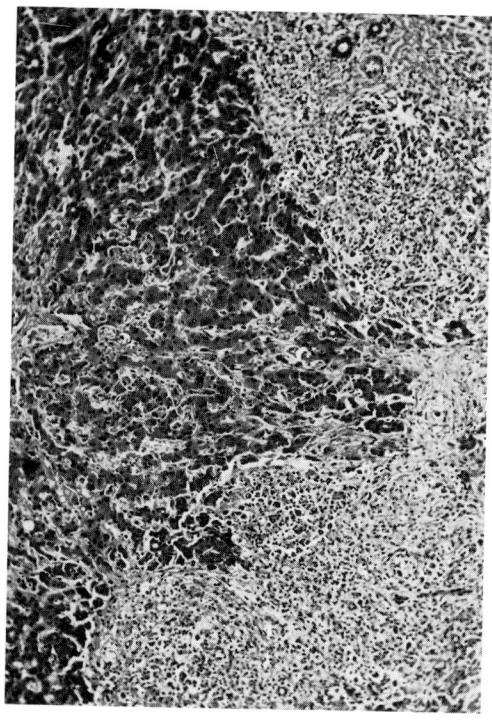

Fig. 4.7. Hodgkin's disease. The portal zones are infiltrated by Hodgkin's tissue. (Stained H & E, ×70.)

Table 4.4. Jaundice in lymphoma—features

Related to lymphoma	

Hepatic infiltrates
    Massive
    Tumour mass
	Scans. Liver biopsy

Biliary obstruction	Usually hilar Investigate endoscopic or percutaneous cholangiography Non-Hodgkin's usually

Intra-hepatic cholestasis	Rare
	Liver biopsy
	    'pure' cholestasis
	    loss of bile ducts
	Usually Hodgkin's

Haemolysis	Autoimmune haemolytic anaemia Positive Coombs' test
Related to therapy	
Chemotherapy	High dose can cause fulminant liver failure (see Chapter 18)
Hepatic irradiation	More than 3000 rads (see Chapter 18)
Post-transfusion (hepatitis C)	(See Chapter 16)
Hepatitis B reactivation	(See Chapter 16)
Opportunist infections	(See Chapter 27)

lated to therapy. The diagnosis is difficult and is made after full investigation. Liver histology may show loss of intra-hepatic bile ducts [19].

Rarely haemolysis causes deep jaundice. It may be due to Coombs' positive autoimmune haemolytic anaemia. Jaundice is exacerbated by bilirubin overload following blood transfusion.

Chemotherapy may cause jaundice. Almost all the cytotoxic drugs can be incriminated if given in sufficient dose. Common culprits include methotrexate, 6-mercaptopurine, cytosine arabinoside, procarbazine and vincristine. A death has been reported in a patient given ABVD [24]. Hepatic irradiation in a dose usually exceeding 3500 rads may cause jaundice.

Post-transfusion viral hepatitis B, C, or non-A, non-B, non-C, may affect the immunocompromised patient. Opportunist infections are also encountered.

PRIMARY HEPATIC LYMPHOMA [2, 53]

This rare lymphoma by definition affects only the liver. There is a solitary mass in 60%, multiple masses in 35% and diffuse disease in 5% [35]. Histologically it is a non-Hodgkin's large cell B- or less often T-cell lymphoma. Presentation is mainly with pain, hepatomegaly, a palpable mass, and elevated alkaline phosphatase and bilirubin. Fever, night sweats and weight loss occur in 50% of

cases. There is no lymphadenopathy. Ultrasound and CT show a non-specific space-occupying lesion in the liver in the majority but there may be diffuse hepatomegaly without tumour. Diagnosis is by liver biopsy. Sometimes histology may initially be confusing suggesting carcinoma or chronic hepatitis, or showing extensive haemorrhagic necrosis suggesting Budd–Chiari syndrome. The destructiveness of the infiltrate is a helpful diagnostic feature.

Primary lymphoma of the liver may be found incidentally or complicating AIDS [39]. Patients with pre-existing cirrhosis have a poor prognosis. Negative alpha-fetoprotein and CEA with a high LDH level in a patient with a liver mass should raise the possibility of lymphoma.

TREATMENT OF HEPATIC INVOLVEMENT

More aggressive combination chemotherapy has considerably improved the prognosis of intra-hepatic Hodgkin's deposits causing jaundice. Treatment is the same as for other stage IV patients regardless of the jaundice. Similarly, those with 'idiopathic' cholestasis should receive the therapy appropriate for their lymphoma. If MOPP has failed ABVD should be tried. If jaundice is persistent, some palliation may be achieved by moderate local irradiation.

Extra-hepatic biliary obstruction is treated by external radiation and, if necessary, the insertion of internal stents by the endoscopic or percutaneous route.

If drug toxicity is the cause, treatment may have to be changed or doses reduced.

Treatment for non-Hodgkin's lymphoma causing jaundice is the same as that for Hodgkin's disease.

Primary hepatic lymphoma is treated by chemotherapy or occasionally by lobectomy [2].

Lymphosarcoma

Nodules of lymphosarcomatous tissue may be found in the liver, especially in the portal tracts. Macroscopically they resemble metastatic carcinoma. The liver may also be involved in giant follicular lymphoma.

Multiple myeloma

The liver may be involved in plasma cell myeloma, the portal tracts and sinusoids being filled with plasma cells. Associated amyloidosis may involve the hepatic arterioles.

Angio-immunoblastic lymphadenopathy

This resembles Hodgkin's disease. The liver shows a pleomorphic portal zone infiltrate (lymphocytes, plasma cells and blast cells) without histiocytes or Reed–Sternberg cells [16].

Extramedullary haemopoiesis

The primitive reticulum cells of hepatic sinusoids and portal tracts possess the capacity to mature into adult erythrocytes, leucocytes or platelets. If the stimulus to blood regeneration is sufficiently strong, this function can be resumed. This is rare in the adult although myeloid metaplasia in the liver of the anaemic infant is not unusual. In the adult, it occurs with bone marrow replacement or infiltration, and especially in association with secondary carcinoma of bone, myelofibrosis, myelosclerosis, multiple myeloma, and the marble bone disease of Albers–Schoenberg. It complicates all conditions associated with a leucoerythroblastic anaemia.

The condition is well exemplified by myelofibrosis and myelosclerosis, where the liver is enlarged, with a smooth firm edge. The spleen is enormous, and its removal results in even greater enlargement of the liver and an increase in bilirubin, alkaline phosphatase and gamma-glutamyl transpeptidase, rather than transaminases [31]. The mortality after splenectomy is 10–20%, some caused by hepatic dysfunction due to the increase in extramedullary haemopoiesis.

Ascites occurs in a low percentage of patients with extramedullary haemopoiesis, and may be due to portal hypertension, or, after splenectomy, peritoneal deposits of extramedullary haemopoiesis [26].

MICROSCOPIC FEATURES

The conspicuous abnormality is a great increase in the cellular content, both in the portal tracts and in the distended sinusoids (fig. 4.8). The cells are of all types and varying maturity. Myeloblasts and myelocytes are prominent. There are many reticulum cells and these may be converted into giant cells. The haemopoietic tissue may form discrete foci in the sinusoids.

Peri-sinusoidal fibrosis may be a feature with collagen bundles in Disse's space [38].

Electron microscopy shows haematological cells in the sinusoids with transformation of peri-sinusoidal cells into fibroblasts and myofibroblast-like cells.

Portal hypertension. This may be due to portal vein thrombosis or sinusoidal infiltration with haemopoietic cells. Disse's space fibrosis contributes [11]. Nodular regenerative hyperplasia may also cause portal hypertension [11].

Systemic mastocytosis

This is a disease of mast cell hyperplasia that may effect several organ systems. It can present with hepatomegaly [9] as well as lymphadenopathy and skin lesions. Liver biopsy, stained with haematoxylin and eosin, shows polygonal cells with eosinophilic granules predominantly in portal tracts, with fewer in the sinusoids [18]. On staining with Giemsa and toluidine blue, the typical metachromatic cytoplasmic granules may be identified. Mast cell infiltration is a common finding, but severe liver disease is unusual except in those with haematological involvement or aggressive mastocytosis. Nodular regenerative hyperplasia, portal venopathy and veno-occlusive disease are reported [32] and may be responsible for portal hypertension and ascites. The latter carries a poor prognosis. Cirrhosis occurs in up to 5% of patients [18].

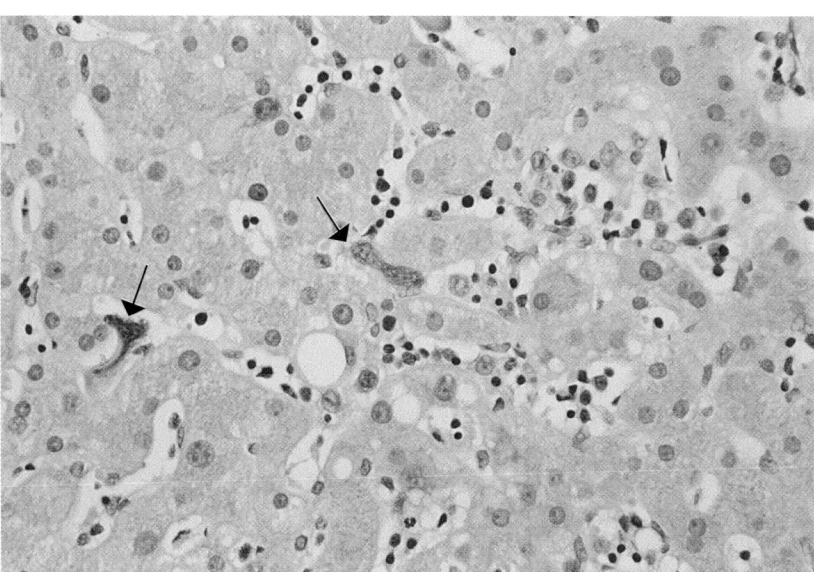

Fig. 4.8. Extramedullary haemopoiesis— megakaryocytes (arrows), erythroblasts, normoblasts and polymorphs are seen in the hepatic sinusoids. (Stained H & E.)

Langerhans' cell histiocytosis (histiocytosis X)

The underlying pathology of this rare condition is proliferation and aggregation of Langerhans' cells in the reticulo-endothelial system. Electron microscopy shows trilamellar rod-shaped structures (Birbeck granules) within the cells which also contain the neural-specific protein S-100. Langerhans' cell histiocytosis comprises several entities (which overlap) including eosinophilic granuloma (bone lesions), Hand–Schüller–Christian disease (endocrine lesions; skin) and Letterer–Siwe disease (disseminated type; lungs, bone marrow, skin, lymph nodes, spleen, liver). The mechanism of liver injury is not known. Cholestasis is due to sclerosing cholangitis affecting intra-hepatic ducts [28] or proliferating histiocytic cells in peri-portal areas [20]. Liver disease is present in one-third of patients. Portal hypertension and variceal haemorrhage may develop. Liver failure due to biliary cirrhosis is unusual. Transplantation has been successful with no evidence of recurrent disease up to 7 years [55].

Lipid storage diseases

The lipidoses are disorders in which abnormal amounts of lipids are stored in the cells of the reticulo-endothelial system. They may be classified according to the lipid stored: xanthomatosis, cholesterol; Gaucher's disease, cerebroside; Niemann–Pick disease, sphingomyelin.

Primary and secondary xanthomatosis

Cholesterol is stored mainly in the skin, tendon sheaths, bone and blood vessels. The liver is rarely involved but there may be isolated nests of cholesterol-containing foamy histiocytes in the liver. Investigation of the liver is of little diagnostic value.

Cholesteryl ester storage disease [4]

This rare, recessive, relatively benign disease is associated with acid cholesteryl ester hydrolase deficiency. It presents with symptomless hepato-splenomegaly. The liver is orange in colour and hepatocytes contain excess cholesteryl ester and neutral fat. A septate fibrosis is also present.

Gaucher's disease

This rare, autosomal recessive disease first described in 1882 [17] affects mainly Askenazi Jews. It is the commonest lysosomal storage disorder. It is due to a deficiency of lysosomal β-glucocerebrosidase so that the substrate β-glucocerebroside accumulates in the reticulo-endothelial system throughout the body, particularly liver, bone marrow and spleen.

Three types are recognized:
• Type 1 (adult, chronic, non-neuronopathic) is the mildest and most common (1 in 500–2000 among Askenazi Jews). The central nervous system is spared.
• Type 2 (infantile, acute, neuronopathic) is rare. In addition to the visceral involvement there is massive fatal neurological involvement, with death in infancy.
• Type 3 (juvenile, subacute, neuronopathic) is also rare. There is gradual and heterogeneous neurological involvement.

The various forms represent different mutations in the structural gene for glucocerebrosidase on chromosome 1, although there is a variability in severity of disease within a specific genotype [33]. The key to the degree of damage appears to be the macrophage response to glucocerebroside accumulation, but the mechanisms are unknown. Overall, however, analysis of the gene for specific mutations allows prediction of the clinical course for particular genotypes [56].

The characteristic Gaucher cell is approximately 70–80 μm in diameter, oval or polygonal in shape and with pale cytoplasm. It contains two or more peripherally placed hyperchromatic nuclei between which fibrils pass parallel to each other (fig. 4.9). It is quite different from the foamy cell of xanthomatosis or Niemann–Pick disease.

Electron microscopy. The accumulated β-glucocerebroside formed from degraded cell membranes precipitates within the lysosomes and forms long

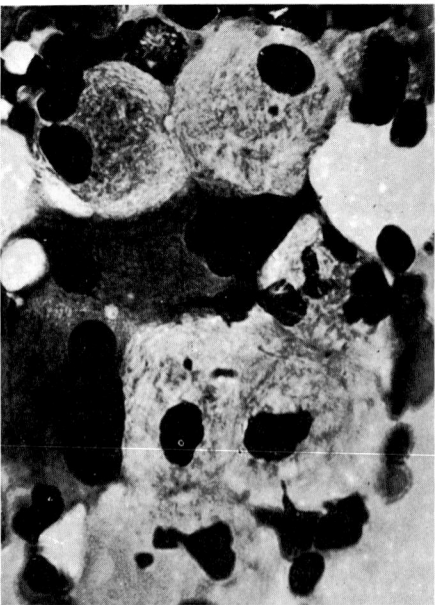

Fig. 4.9. Gaucher's disease. Smears of sternal marrow show large pale Gaucher cells with fibrillary cytoplasm and eccentric hyperchromatic nuclei. (Stained Leishman, ×600.)

(20–40 nm) rod-like tubules. These are seen by light microscopy. A somewhat similar cell is seen in chronic myeloid leukaemia and in multiple myeloma due to increased turnover of β-glucocerebroside.

Chronic adult form (type 1)

This is the most common type. It is of variable severity and age of onset but usually commences insidiously before the age of 30 years. It is chronic and may be recognized in quite old people.

The mode of presentation is variable, with unexplained hepato-splenomegaly (especially in children), spontaneous bone fractures, or bone pain with fever. Alternatively there may be a bleeding diathesis, with non-specific anaemia.

The clinical features include pigmentation which may be generalized or a patchy, brownish tan. The lower legs may have a symmetrical pigmentation, leaden grey in colour and containing melanin. The eyes show yellow pingueculae (fig. 4.10).

The spleen is enormous and the liver is moderately enlarged, smooth and firm. Superficial lymph glands are not usually involved.

Hepatic involvement is often associated with fibrosis and abnormal liver function tests. Serum alkaline phosphatase is usually increased, sometimes with a rise in transaminase [23]. Cirrhosis may develop [43] with ascites. Portal hypertension may lead to bleeding oesophageal varices [1].

Bone X-rays. The long bones, especially the lower ends of the femora, are expanded, so that the waist normally seen above the condyles disappears. The appearance has been likened to that of an Erlenmeyer flask or hock bottle.

Sternal marrow shows the diagnostic Gaucher cells (fig. 4.9).

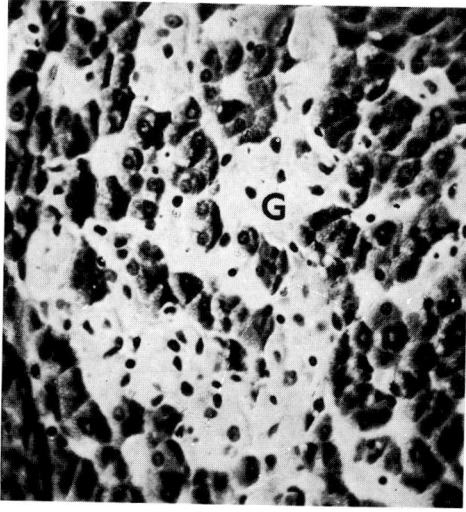

Fig. 4.11. Gaucher's disease. Liver sections show areas between the liver cell cords filled with large pale cells (G) with small dark nuclei. (Stained Best's carmine, × 250.)

Aspiration liver biopsy should be performed if sternal puncture has yielded negative results. The liver is diffusely involved (fig. 4.11).

Peripheral blood changes. With diffuse bone marrow involvement, a leucoerythroblastic picture may be seen. Alternatively leucopenia and thrombocytopenia with prolonged bleeding time may be associated with only a moderate hypochromic microcytic anaemia [40].

Diagnosis may be made by measuring β-glucocerebrosidase in mixed mononuclear cells obtained from venous blood.

Blood biochemical changes. Serum alkaline phosphatase is usually increased, sometimes with a rise in transaminase [23]. Serum cholesterol is normal.

TREATMENT

Previously there was no specific therapy. Recently, however, intravenous infusions of a modified placental glucocerebrosidase, deglycosylated so as to be preferentially taken up by the mannose lectin on macrophages, has had clinical success. Spleen and liver size reduced and there was haematological improvement. Smaller doses than initially used have been found to produce a clinical improvement [6, 34]. This will reduce the cost of treatment.

Splenectomy, partial or total, has been done for the very large spleen causing abdominal discomfort, and occasionally for thrombocytopenia or an acquired haemolytic anaemia. Total splenectomy is followed by more aggressive bone disease and a pre-disposition to malignancy [14]. In the future successful enzyme replacement therapy should obviate the need for surgical intervention.

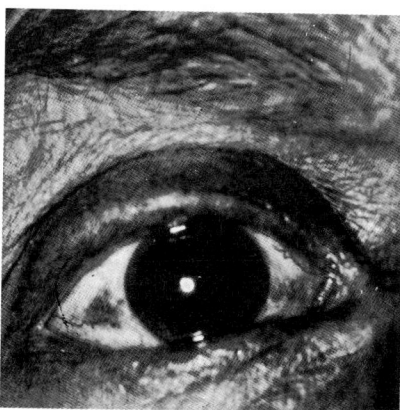

Fig. 4.10. Gaucher's disease. On either side of the pupil are wedge-shaped pingueculae consisting of yellow thickenings, fatty in appearance.

Liver transplantation for decompensated cirrhosis has been done [43]. This does not correct the metabolic defect, and longer follow-up is needed to evaluate the extent of lipid reaccumulation in the liver. Bone marrow transplantation has been done, but the risks are considered prohibitive in comparison with enzyme replacement therapy.

Acute infantile Gaucher's disease (type 2)

This acute form of the disease presents within the first 6 months of life and is usually fatal before 2 years. The child appears normal at birth. There is cerebral involvement, progressive cachexia and mental deterioration. The liver and spleen are enlarged and superficial lymph nodes may also be palpable.

Autopsy shows Gaucher cells throughout the reticulo-endothelial system. They are, however, not found in the brain and the pathogenesis of the cerebral disease is not understood.

Niemann–Pick disease

This rare, familial disease, inherited as autosomal recessive, mainly affects the Jewish race. The deficiency is in the enzyme, sphingo-myelinase, in the lysosomes of the reticulo-endothelial system. This results in the lysosomal storage of sphingomyelin. The liver and spleen are predominantly involved.

The characteristic cell is pale, ovoid or round, $20–40\,\mu m$ in diameter. In the unfixed state it is loaded with granules; when fixed in fat solvents the granules are dissolved, giving a vacuolated and foamy appearance. There are usually only one or two nuclei. Electron microscopy shows lysosomes as laminated myelin-like figures. These contain the abnormal lipid.

Niemann–Pick disease *type A* (acute neuronopathic form) occurs in infants, who die before the age of 2 years. The condition starts in the first 3 months, with anorexia, weight loss and retardation of growth. The liver and spleen enlarge, the skin becomes waxy and acquires a yellowish-brown coloration on exposed parts. The superficial lymph nodes are enlarged. There are pulmonary infiltrates. The patient is blind, deaf and mentally retarded.

The fundus may show a cherry-red spot due to retinal degeneration at the macula.

The peripheral blood shows a microcytic anaemia and in the later stages the foamy Niemann–Pick cell may be found.

The disease may present as *neonatal cholestatic jaundice* which remits. Progressive neurological deterioration appears in late childhood [50].

A further *type B* (chronic, non-neuronopathic form) is associated with neonatal cholestasis which resolves.

Cirrhosis develops slowly and may lead to portal hypertension, ascites and liver failure [37]. Liver transplantation for hepatic failure has been successful [43]. Although hepatic lipid accumulation was not seen at 10 months, longer follow-up is needed to assess the metabolic outcome.

Diagnosis is made by marrow puncture, which reveals characteristic Niemann–Pick cells or by finding a low level of sphingomyelinase in leucocytes.

Bone marrow transplant has been done for patients with early severe liver disease [48]. Preliminary reports were promising with reduction of sphingomyelin from liver, spleen and bone marrow, but longer follow-up is needed.

Sea-blue histiocyte syndrome

This rare condition is characterized by histiocytes staining a sea-blue colour with Wright or Giemsa stain in bone marrow and in reticulo-endothelial cells of the liver. The cells contain deposits of phosphosphingolipid and glucosphingolipid. Clinically the liver and spleen are enlarged. The prognosis is usually good although thrombocytopenia and hepatic cirrhosis have been reported. It probably represents adult Niemann–Pick disease [30].

References

1 Aderka D, Garfinkel D, Rothem A *et al.* Fatal bleeding from esophageal varices in a patient with Gaucher's disease. *Am. J. Gastroenterol.* 1982; **77**: 838.

2 Anthony PP, Sarsfield P, Clarke T. Primary lymphoma of the liver: clinical and pathological features of 10 patients. *J. Clin. Pathol.* 1990; **43**: 1007.

3 Bagleyk CM Jr, Roth JA, Thomas LB *et al.* Liver biopsy in Hodgkin's disease. Clinicopathologic correlations in 127 patients. *Ann. Intern. Med.* 1972; **76**: 219.

4 Beaudet AL, Ferry GD, Nichols BL Jr *et al.* Cholesterol storage disease: clinical, biochemical and pathological studies. *J. Paediatr.* 1977; **90**: 910.

5 Beaugrand M, Trinchet JC, Callard P *et al.* Malignant histiocytosis presenting as a fulminant hepatic disease. *Gastroenterology* 1983; **84**: 447.

6 Bembi B, Zanatta M, Carrozzi M *et al.* Enzyme replacement treatment in type 1 and 3 Gaucher's disease. *Lancet* 1994; **344**: 1679.

7 Bird GLA, Smith H, Portmann B *et al.* Acute liver decompensation on withdrawal of cytotoxic chemotherapy and immunosuppressive therapy in hepatitis B carriers. *Q. J. Med.* 1989; **73**: 895.

8 Bruguera M, Caballero T, Carreras E *et al.* Hepatic sinusoidal dilatation in Hodgkin's disease. *Liver* 1987; **7**: 76.

9 Capron J-P, Lebrec C, Degott C *et al.* Portal hypertension in systemic mastocytosis. *Gastroenterology* 1978; **74**: 595.

10 Conway EE, Santorineou M, Mitsudo S. Fulminant hepatic failure in a child with acute lymphoblastic leukaemia. *J. Pediatr. Gastroenterol. Nutr.* 1992; **15**: 194.

11 Degott C, Capron J-P, Bettan L *et al.* Myeloid metaplasia, perisinusoidal fibrosis, and nodular regenerative hyperplasia of the liver. *Liver* 1985; **5**: 276.

12 Dich NH, Goodman ZD, Klein MA. Hepatic involvement in Hodgkin's disease: clues to histologic diagnosis. *Cancer* 1989; **64**: 2121.

13 Feller E, Schiffman FJ. Extrahepatic biliary obstruction by lymphoma. *Arch. Surg.* 1990; **125**: 1507.

14 Fleshner PR, Aufses AH, Grabowski GA *et al.* A 27 year experience with splenectomy for Gaucher's disease. *Am. J. Surg.* 1991; **161**: 69.

15 Forbes GM, Davies JM, Herrmann RP *et al.* Liver disease complicating bone marrow transplantation: a clinical audit. *J. Gastroenterol. Hepatol.* 1995; **10**: 1.

16 Frizzera G, Moran EM, Rappaport H. Angio-immunoblastic lymphadenopathy: diagnosis and clinical course. *Am. J. Med.* 1975; **59**: 803.

17 Gaucher E. De l'epithéliome primitif de la rate. *Thèse de Paris* 1882.

18 Horny H-P, Kaiserling E, Campbell M *et al.* Liver findings in generalized mastocytosis: a clinicopathologic study. *Cancer* 1989; **63**: 532.

19 Hubscher SG, Lumley MA, Elias E. Vanishing bile duct syndrome: a possible mechanism for intrahepatic cholestasis in Hodgkin's lymphoma. *Hepatology* 1993; **17**: 70.

20 Iwai M, Kashiwadani M, Okuno T *et al.* Cholestatic liver disease in a 20 yr old woman with histiocytosis X. *Am. J. Gastroenterol.* 1988; **83**: 164.

21 Jacobson AF, Teefey SA, Lee SP *et al.* Frequent occurrence of new hepatobiliary abnormalities after bone marrow transplantation: results of a prospective study using scintigraphy and sonography. *Am. J. Gastroenterol.* 1993; **88**: 1044.

22 Jaffe ES. Malignant lymphomas: pathology of hepatic involvement. *Semin. Liv. Dis.* 1987; **7**: 257.

23 James SP, Stromeyer FW, Chang C *et al.* Liver abnormalities in patients with Gaucher's disease. *Gastroenterology* 1981; **80**: 126.

24 Joensuu H, Söderström K-O, Nikkaen V. Fatal necrosis of the liver during ABVD chemotherapy for Hodgkin's disease. *Cancer* 1986; **58**: 1437.

25 Johnson LN, Iseri O, Knodell RG. Caseating hepatic granulomas in Hodgkin's lymphoma. *Gastroenterology* 1990; **99**: 1837.

26 Knobel B, Melamud E, Virag I *et al.* Ectopic medullary hematopoiesis as a cause of ascites in agnogenic myeloid metaplasia. *Acta Haematol.* 1993; **89**: 104.

27 Lau JYN, Lai CL, Lin HJ *et al.* Fatal reactivation of chronic hepatitis B virus infection following withdrawal of chemotherapy in lymphoma patients. *Q. J. Med.* 1989; **73**: 911.

28 Leblanc A, Hadchouel M, Jehan P *et al.* Obstructive jaundice in children with histiocytosis X. *Gastroenterology* 1981; **80**: 134.

29 Lindor K, Rakela J, Perrault J *et al.* Non-cirrhotic portal hypertension due to lymphoma. Reversal following splenectomy. *Dig. Dis. Sci.* 1987; **32**: 1056.

30 Long RG, Lake BD, Pettit JE *et al.* Adult Niemann–Pick disease: its relationship to the syndrome of the sea-blue histiocyte. *Am. J. Med.* 1977; **62**: 627.

31 Lopez-Guillermo A, Cervantes F, Bruguera M *et al.* Liver dysfunction following splenectomy in idiopathic myelofibrosis: a study of 10 patients. *Acta Haematol.* 1991; **85**: 184.

32 Mican JM, Di Bisceglie AM, Fong T-L *et al.* Hepatic involve-

ment in mastocytosis: clinicopathologic correlations in 41 cases. *Hepatology* 1995; **22**: 1163.

33 Mistry PK. Genotype/phenotype correlations in Gaucher's disease. *Lancet* 1995; **346**: 982.

34 Niederau C, Holderer A, Heintges T *et al.* Glucocerebrosidase for treatment of Gaucher's disease: first German long-term results. *J. Hepatol.* 1994; **21**: 610.

35 Ohsawa M, Aozasa K, Horiuchi K *et al.* Malignant lymphoma of the liver: report of five cases and review of the literature. *Dig. Dis. Sci.* 1992; **37**: 1105.

36 Ondreyco SM, Kjeldsberg CR, Fineman RM *et al.* Monoblastic transformation in chronic myelogenous leukemia: presentation with massive hepatic involvement. *Cancer* 1981; **48**: 957.

37 Putterman C, Zelingher J, Shouval D. Liver failure and the sea-blue/adult Niemann–Pick disease. Case report and review of the literature. *J. Clin. Gastroenterol.* 1992; **15**: 146.

38 Roux D, Merlio JP, Quinton A *et al.* Agnogenic myeloid metaplasia, portal hypertension and sinusoidal abnormalities. *Gastroenterology* 1987; **92**: 1067.

39 Scoazec J-Y, Degott C, Brousse N *et al.* Non-Hodgkin's lymphoma presenting as a primary tumor of the liver: presentation, diagnosis and outcome in eight patients. *Hepatology* 1991; **13**: 870.

40 Sherlock SPV, Learmonth JR. Aneurysm of the splenic artery; with an account of an example complicating Gaucher's disease. *Br. J. Surg.* 1942; **30**: 151.

41 Shulman HM, Fisher LB, Schoch LG *et al.* Veno-occlusive disease of the liver after marrow transplantation: histologic correlates of clinical signs and symptoms. *Hepatology* 1994; **19**: 1171.

42 Shulman HM, Gooley T, Dudley MD *et al.* Utility of transvenous liver biopsies and wedged hepatic venous pressure measurements in 60 marrow transplant recipients. *Transplantation* 1995; **59**: 1015.

43 Smanik EJ, Tavill AS, Jacobs GH *et al.* Orthotopic liver transplantation in two adults with Niemann–Pick and Gaucher's diseases: implications for the treatment of inherited metabolic disease. *Hepatology* 1993; **17**: 42.

44 Storek J, Gale RP, Goldstein L. Analysing early liver dysfunction after bone marrow transplantation. *Transplant Immunol.* 1993; **1**: 163.

45 Teefey SA, Brink JA, Borson RA *et al.* Diagnosis of veno-occlusive disease of the liver after bone marrow transplantation: value of duplex sonography. *AJR* 1995; **164**: 1397.

46 Trudel M, Aramendi T, Caplan S. Large-cell lymphoma presenting with hepatic sinusoidal infiltration. *Arch. Pathol. Lab. Med.* 1991; **115**: 821.

47 Valla D, Casadevall N, Huisse MG *et al.* Etiology of portal vein thrombosis in adults. *Gastroenterology* 1988; **94**: 1063.

48 Vellodi A, Hobbs JR, O'Donnell NM *et al.* Treatment of Niemann–Pick disease type B by allogeneic bone marrow transplantation. *Br. Med. J.* 1987; **295**: 1375.

49 Watterson J, Priest JR. Jaundice as a paraneoplastic phenomenon in a T-cell lymphoma. *Gastroenterology* 1989; **97**: 1319.

50 Wenger DA, Barth G, Githens JH. Nine cases of sphingomyelin lipidosis, a new variant in Spanish-American children. Juvenile variant of Niemann–Pick disease with foamy and sea-blue histiocytes. *Am. J. Dis. Child.* 1977; **131**: 955.

51 Woolf GM, Petrovic LM, Rojter SE *et al.* Acute liver failure due to lymphoma: a diagnostic concern when considering liver transplantation. *Dig. Dis. Sci.* 1994; **39**: 1351.

52 Yam LT, Janckila AJ, Chan CH *et al.* Hepatic involvement in

hairy cell leukemia. *Cancer* 1983; **51**: 1497.

53 Zafrani ES, Gaulard P. Primary lymphoma of the liver. *Liver* 1993; **13**: 57.

54 Zaman A, Bramley PN, Wyatt J *et al*. Hodgkin's disease presenting as liver abscesses. *Gut* 1991; **32**: 959.

55 Zandi P, Panis Y, Debray D *et al*. Pediatric liver transplantation for Langerhans' cell histiocytosis. *Hepatology* 1995; **21**: 129.

56 Zimran A, Sorge J, Gross E *et al*. Prediction of severity of Gaucher's disease by identification of mutations at DNA level. *Lancet* 1989; **ii**: 349.

Chapter 5
Ultrasound, Computed Tomography and Magnetic Resonance Imaging

Hepato-biliary scanning can detect and characterize tumours in the liver, and demonstrate obstruction of blood vessels and bile ducts (see Chapter 29). It is an essential step in the diagnostic work-up of most hepatic problems. It may show some types of diffuse disease. Ultrasound (US) and computed tomography (CT) are most often used; magnetic resonance imaging (MRI) is increasingly available and experience is growing rapidly. Radio-isotope scanning for space-occupying lesions and diffuse disease has been superseded generally by the above techniques; it retains a role for biliary tract disease (see Chapter 29).

US, CT and MRI all perform well with the optimal equipment, technique and operator. Selection of the method used will depend to an extent on the availability and cost. The clinician plays a major role in maintaining the quality of the report by specifying clearly the clinical problem.

Radio-isotope scanning

99mTc-labelled tin colloid and colloids of human albumin are taken up by reticulo-endothelial cells. Introduced in the 1960s they were used to detect hepatic tumours, but could not differentiate cystic from solid ones. Lesions 4 cm in diameter are usually demonstrated, but sensitivity falls below this size. Reduced patchy hepatic uptake with increased activity from bone marrow and spleen denoted chronic liver disease. US has replaced isotope scanning for the detection of space-occupying lesions, and can show the irregular liver outline and change in echogenicity in cirrhosis. Isotope scanning has also been replaced in other situations such as Budd–Chiari syndrome where the characteristic findings (preferential uptake by the caudate lobe) are not reliable enough to be of routine clinical value.

67Gallium citrate is taken up by liver tumours and by inflammatory processes, for example abscess, but again the newer techniques, US and CT, are more appropriate for the majority of patients and centres. Gallium scanning retains a role in the complex patient with chronic sepsis of unknown origin when a focus of increased radioactivity may suggest an inflammatory collection.

99mTc IDA derivatives have a role in the imaging of the biliary tract [14] (see Chapter 29).

99mTc-labelled red blood cells can be used to establish the diagnosis of cavernous haemangioma. A dynamic scan after intravenous injection will show an area of low activity initially. The lesion will then fill in as pooling of the red cells occurs. The delayed film will show an area of higher activity than the surrounding liver. Such a dynamic scan is equivalent to the appearances with CT following enhancement.

99mTc-neoglycalbumin binds to the asialoglycoprotein receptor. Using computer analysis, hepatic blood flow, receptor concentration and binding data can be derived. Such modelling can be applied to several labelled compounds to give a quantitative measure of liver function (see Chapter 2). Different components of liver perfusion can be calculated. The technique is not routinely used.

Positron emission tomography (PET)

This requires a cyclotron as it is based upon the principle that a positron emitted from a radioactive substance combines with an electron to form two photons travelling in opposite directions and that these can be localized by confidence detection. Positron-emitting radio elements include ^{15}O, ^{13}N, ^{11}C and ^{18}F, and these can be used to study regional blood flow and metabolism. This technique has been used to study hepatic blood flow [5]. Because of increased glucose utilization in malignant tissue, PET scanning with 2[^{18}F]-fluoro-2-deoxy-D-glucose can detect carcinomas. This method shows promise in pancreatic carcinoma, with a sensitivity and specificity of about 90% [10]. Further evaluation is awaited.

Ultrasound

Most imaging units use real-time high resolution US scanners. These are inexpensive compared with CT and MRI. US takes only a few minutes to perform. Dilated bile ducts, gallbladder disease, hepatic tumours and some diffuse hepatic abnormalities are shown. Residents who are not specialists in US can master the basic technique [23] and apply it in the outpatient department or on the ward, for example to image liver and gallbladder before liver biopsy or to detect dilated bile ducts.

US has problems with hepato-biliary examination in the fat or gaseous patient, those with a high liver lying entirely covered by the rib margin and postoperative patients with dressings and painful scars.

A normal US shows the liver to have mixed echogenicity (fig. 5.1). Portal and hepatic veins, inferior vena cava and aorta are shown. The normal intra-hepatic bile ducts are thin and run parallel to large portal vein branches. The right and left hepatic ducts are 1–3 mm in diameter and the common duct 2–7 mm in diameter. US is the screening investigation of choice for patients with cholestasis (Chapter 29). The gallbladder is an ideal organ for sonography (Chapter 31).

The portal vein originates at the junction of the superior mesenteric and splenic veins. US can show a dilated portal vein and collaterals in portal hypertension, an obstructed or scarred portal vein due to tumour or thrombus, and the bunch of vessels of cavernomatous transformation in chronic portal vein thrombosis [25]. Assessment of portal vein patency by real-time US, however, is not always accurate, particularly in patients with previous portal or biliary surgery. Doppler US has a greater sensitivity and specificity [1]. In the absence of Doppler US, real-time US remains a useful first investigation in patients who have bled from oesophageal varices, to assess patency of the portal vein. The patency of portal systemic shunts can also be confirmed.

In heart failure, US shows dilated hepatic veins and inferior vena cava (IVC). In Budd–Chiari syndrome, hepatic veins may not be seen. Doppler US again adds diagnostic information over and above real-time US [4].

Focal hepatic lesions are better detected by US than diffuse disease. Lesions down to 1 cm in diameter can be seen [20]. Simple cysts have smooth walls and echo-free contents with through transmission of the sound waves (fig. 5.2). The appearance is diagnostic and with small cysts more accurate than CT. Hydatid cysts produce a characteristic appearance with the contained daughter cysts. Cavernous haemangioma, the commonest liver neoplasm, is usually hyper-echoic often with through transmission (fig. 5.3). Such a lesion less than 3 cm in diameter detected incidentally in a patient with normal liver function tests and defined by an experienced ultrasonographer generally needs no further investigation. Lesions more than 3 cm or where the appearances are not classic, or where metastases (especially hyper-vascular) are suspected, would need further confirma-

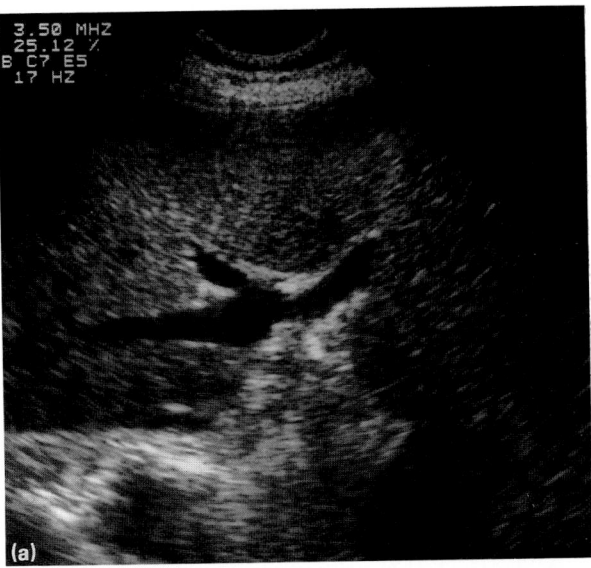

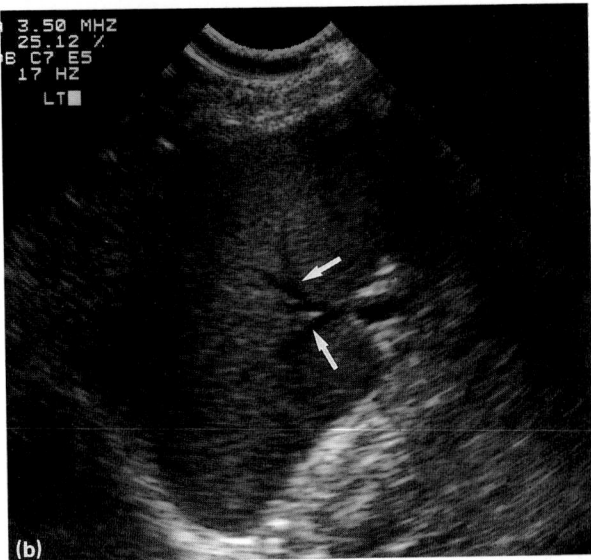

Fig. 5.1. Ultrasound appearance of normal liver. (a) Normal homogeneous echo pattern and the echo-free portal vein and its intra-hepatic branches. (b) Hepatic veins (arrowed) converge to enter the inferior vena cava.

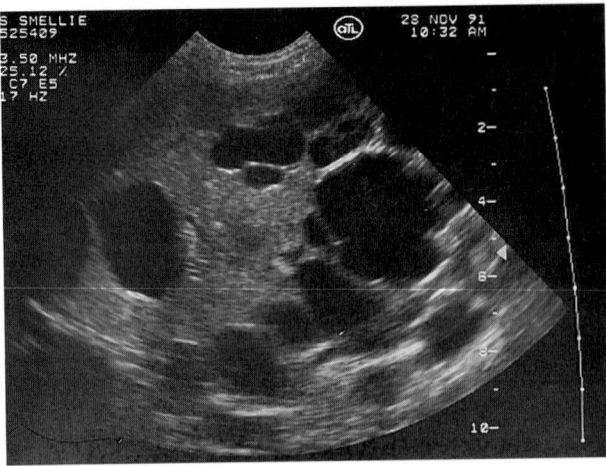

Fig. 5.2. Ultrasonography in polycystic liver disease shows multiple echo-free spaces with through transmission signals.

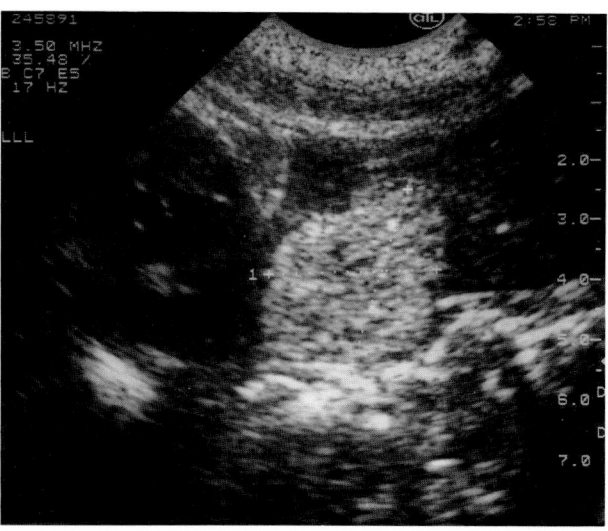

Fig. 5.3. Ultrasonography showing a 3 cm hyper-echoic mass in the liver. This is characteristic of a cavernous haemangioma.

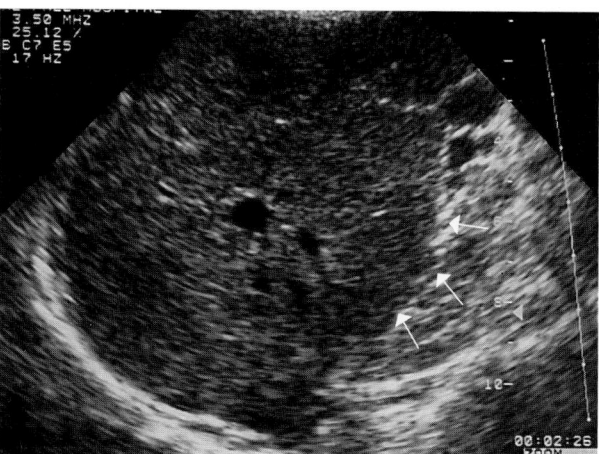

Fig. 5.5. Ultrasound scan in cirrhosis showing irregular edge of liver (arrowed) together with coarse echo pattern.

tion by dynamic enhanced CT, red blood cell scintiscan or MRI.

Malignant masses (primary or secondary carcinoma) produce a range of appearances on US including a hyper- or hypo-echoic pattern (fig. 5.4), well circumscribed or infiltrative. Appearances highly suggestive of metastases include the bull's eye appearance (a hyper-echoic rim surrounding a hypo-echoic centre). Necrotic tumours may mimic abscess or cyst. Clinical data are paramount — underlying cirrhosis, a proven primary tumour or raised tumour markers in the serum being

important. Guided biopsy or aspiration will usually follow to establish the actual pathology.

Diffuse hepatic disease may be detected by US as may anatomical anomalies. In cirrhosis the edge of the liver may be irregular (fig. 5.5), the hepatic echo pattern coarse (i.e. increased irregular echogenicity) and there may be ascites. A fatty liver may show bright echoes. Accurate quantitation of fat, however, is not possible, partly because of the normal variation in echo pattern between normal individuals.

US is the current first choice (together with alpha-fetoprotein) to screen for the development of hepato-cellular carcinoma in patients with cirrhosis.

US is the first choice examination when a hepatic abscess is suspected. There is an area of reduced echogenicity with or without a surrounding capsule. Sometimes the pus has a similar echogenicity to liver and the abscess is not detected. Clinical features should draw attention to the possibility of a false negative result and CT ordered as a second option. US-guided aspiration for microbiology is necessary. Therapeutic aspiration or catheter drainage may follow.

Doppler ultrasound [19]

Doppler US depends upon the principle that the velocity and direction of flow in a vessel can be derived from the difference between the frequency of the US signal emitted from the transducer and that reflected back (echo) from the vessel. The technique is difficult and needs an experienced sonographer. Hepatic veins (fig. 5.6), hepatic artery and portal vein (see fig. 10.23) each have unique Doppler signals (Chapter 10). This technique may aid diagnosis in suspected hepatic vein block [4], hepatic artery thrombosis (after liver transplantation) and portal vein thrombosis [1]. In portal hyperten-

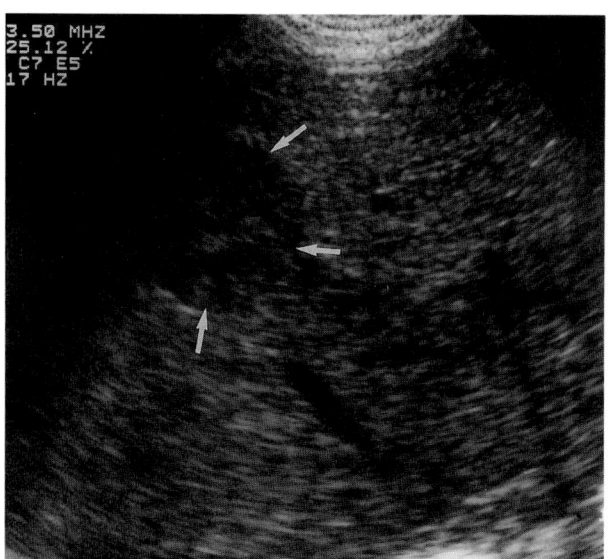

Fig. 5.4. Ultrasound of liver showing round hypo-echoic mass (arrowed) with altered echo pattern. Hepato-cellular carcinoma within a cirrhotic liver.

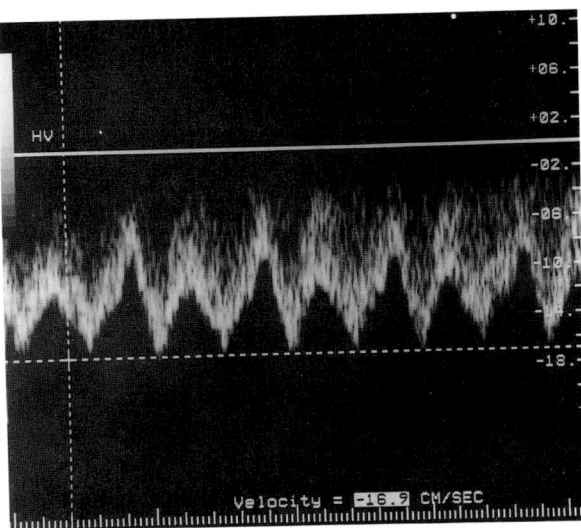

Fig. 5.6. Duplex doppler ultrasound of hepatic vein flow showing normal variation in flow with right atrial systole.

sion the direction of portal flow and the patency of portosystemic shunts can be seen. Flattening of the Doppler waveform of the hepatic veins suggests the presence of cirrhosis [7].

Monitoring of flow through transjugular intra-hepatic porto-systemic shunts (TIPS) by 2–3 monthly Doppler US is useful in detecting shunt dysfunction before clinical signs occur [15].

Endoscopic ultrasound

This technique can detect small periampullary carcinomas and demonstrate the bile duct and gallbladder better than transcutaneous US [2]. Its use is restricted, however, by the availability of the equipment, and endoscopic and ultrasonic expertise.

Computed tomography [3, 9]

The liver is displayed as a series of adjacent cross-sectional slices. The hard copy scan is depicted as if seen from below. Typically 10–12 images are needed to examine the whole liver. Conventional CT is being replaced by spiral CT. In the conventional method, individual exposures are taken at 7–10 mm intervals through the area of interest. The breath must be held for each slice.

Spiral CT, where a continuous spiral exposure is made, can be completed during a single breath-hold, and thus more quickly (15–30 seconds). Images are still reconstructed as individual cross-sections. The great advantage of this method is that the scan can be completed while there is peak concentration of contrast medium in the blood vessels of interest [3]. The detail is superior to

conventional CT particularly for small blood vessels. Tumour detection is improved. Computer reconstruction allows three-dimensional pictures which show the relationship of blood vessels to tumours, and, with intravenous cholangiographic medium, the biliary tree.

The CT scan demonstrates detailed anatomy across the whole abdomen at the level of the slice (fig. 5.7). Oral contrast is usually given to help identify stomach and duodenum. Enhancement by intravenous contrast medium, given as a bolus, an infusion or by arterioportography, demonstrates blood vessels, followed by the hepatic parenchyma. There is renal excretion of contrast. Intravenous cholangiography as a source of contrast is very occasionally used to delineate the biliary system but is restricted to patients with normal liver function tests. CT gives good visualization of adjacent organs, particularly kidneys, pancreas, spleen and retroperitoneal lymph nodes.

CT demonstrates focal hepatic lesions and some diffuse conditions. Advantages over US are that it is less operator dependent and hard copy films can be more readily understood by the clinician. It is more reproducible and obese patients are well suited for CT. Gas-filled bowel may rarely produce some artefact—solved by altering the patient's position. Pain, post-operative scars and dressings are no hindrance. CT-guided biopsy and aspiration are accurate.

Disadvantages are cost, the exposure to radiation and lack of portability—the patient must be brought to the scanner.

The liver appears homogeneous with an attenuation value (in Hounsfield units) similar to kidney and spleen. Portal vein branches are seen at the hilum. Intravenous enhancement is necessary to confidently differentiate these from dilated bile ducts. Hepatic veins are usually seen. Enhanced CT shows the portal vein and can be

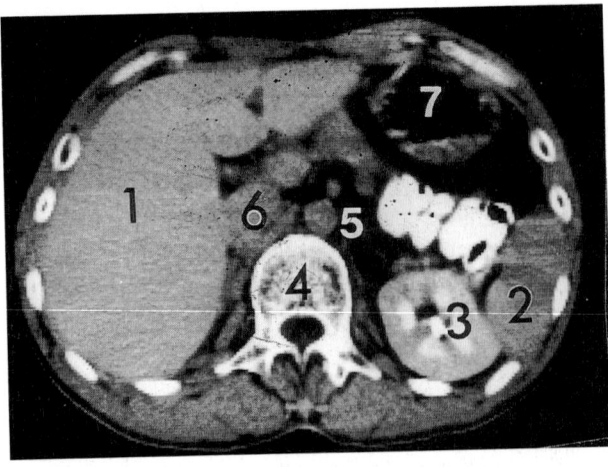

Fig. 5.7. CT scan (enhanced by contrast) showing liver (1), spleen (2), kidney (3), vertebral body (4), aorta (5), pancreas (6) and stomach (7).

used to check patency. Invading tumour or obstructing thrombus may be seen. Cavernomatous transformation can be recognized with two or more enhancing vessels in place of the obstructed portal vein. Doppler US, however, remains the better technique to demonstrate abnormalities of the portal vein.

In Budd–Chiari syndrome there may be a patchy pattern of hepatic enhancement ('pseudotumour' appearance) (fig. 5.8) which may wrongly be interpreted as tumour within the liver. The caudate lobe is enlarged.

An enhanced CT demonstrates the splenic vein and in portal hypertension the collaterals around spleen and retroperitoneum (fig. 5.9). Spontaneous and surgical shunts can be demonstrated.

Normal bile ducts, both intra-hepatic and extra-hepatic, are difficult to see. In the gallbladder calcified stones are demonstrated and CT is used in the evalu-ation of patients for non-surgical therapy of gallbladder stones. US rather than CT, however, is the technique of choice to search for gallbladder stones *per se*.

The shape of the liver, any anatomical abnormalities or lobe atrophy are seen. Liver volume can be calculated from the slices taken but is a research tool.

CT demonstrates diffuse liver disease due to cirrhosis (fig. 5.10), fat (fig. 5.11) and iron (fig. 5.12). A nodular, uneven edge to the liver which may be shrunken suggests cirrhosis. Ascites and splenomegaly support this diagnosis. CT is of particular value in suspected cirrhosis when clotting deficiencies preclude routine percutaneous liver biopsy. Fatty liver shows a lower attenuation value than normal. Even in an unenhanced scan the blood vessels stand out with a higher attenuation value than liver parenchyma. Mono-energetic CT scanning

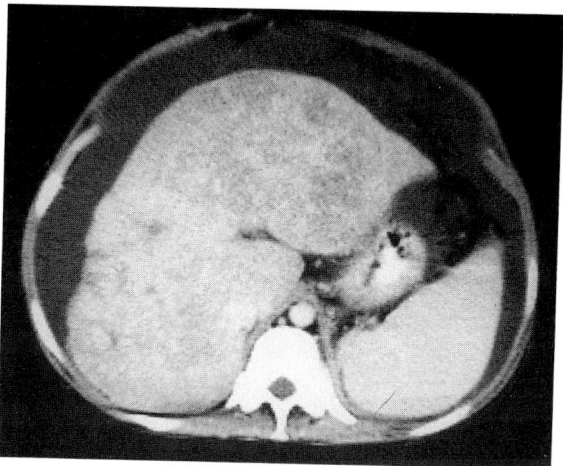

Fig. 5.8. Enhanced CT scan showing patchy areas of low attenuation in the liver (pseudotumour appearance) and ascites in a patient with Budd–Chiari syndrome.

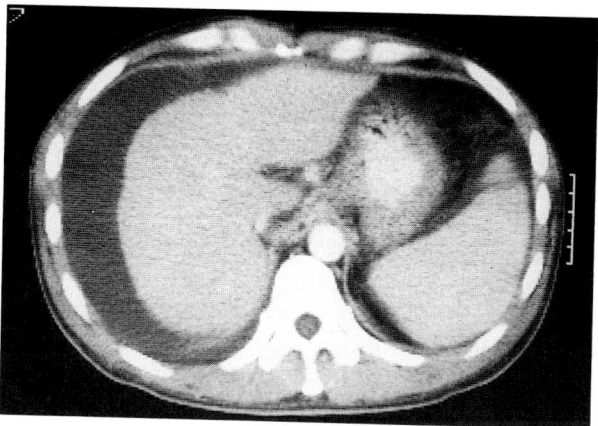

Fig. 5.10. Enhanced CT scan showing shrunken liver with a nodular margin and ascites due to cirrhosis.

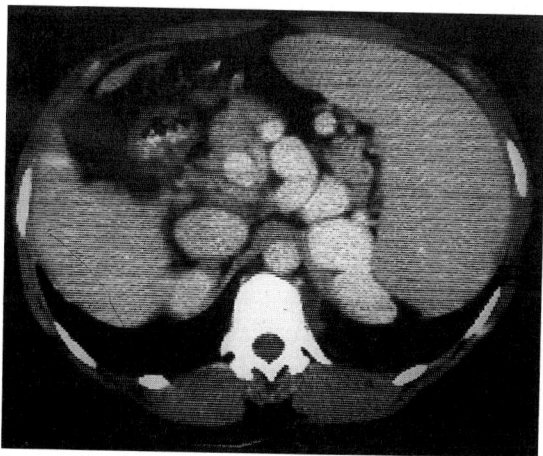

Fig. 5.9. Enhanced CT scan showing massive collaterals (white) around the large spleen due to portal hypertension.

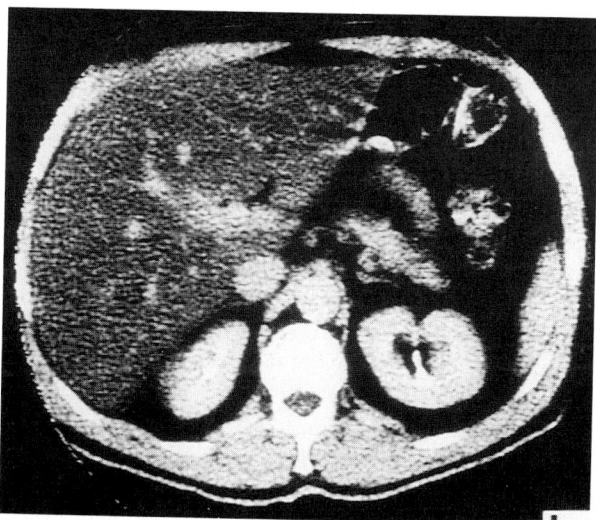

Fig. 5.11. Enhanced CT scan in a patient with a fatty liver showing blood vessels outlined within the hepatic parenchyma which has a very low attenuation value.

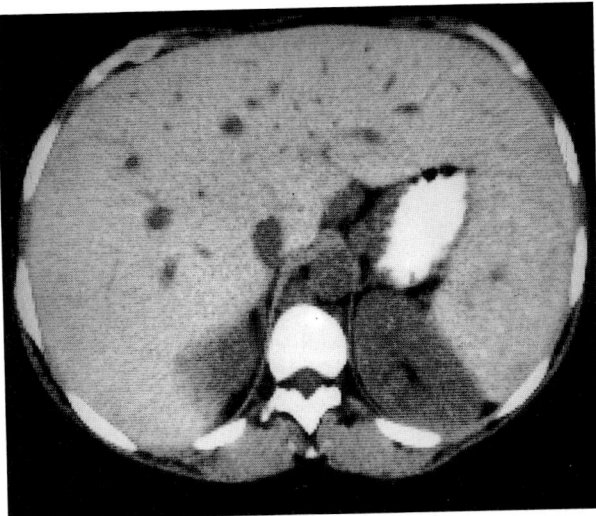

Fig. 5.12. Unenhanced CT scan of secondary iron over load in thalassaemia major. The liver shows increased density, greater than that of the kidney. Portal vein radicles are very prominent.

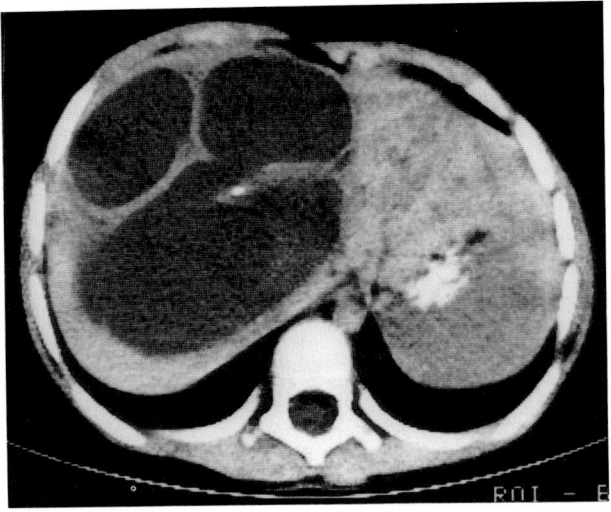

Fig. 5.13. CT scan (enhanced by contrast) showing simple cysts in the liver.

may be used to assess liver fat content in alcoholic patients. Results agree with chemical and hepatic histological assessment. Fatty liver thus may be diagnosed without the need for liver biopsy.

In iron overload, hepatic density is increased on CT and the unenhanced liver is brighter than the spleen or kidney (fig. 5.12). Using dual energy CT there is a correlation with liver iron but this is insufficient with moderate siderosis to make the method of practical value in the management of patients with haemochromatosis.

Liver with a high copper content usually has a normal attenuation value.

Space-occupying lesions of 1 cm and more in diameter can be detected by CT. Both unenhanced and enhanced scans should be done. Thus a filling defect on an unenhanced scan may be rendered isodense by intravenous contrast injection and missed. Conversely, an area isodense with normal liver on the unenhanced scan may only be seen after enhancement.

Benign lesions (often detected by chance) include simple cysts and cavernous haemangioma. Simple cysts can usually be confidently identified because of the low attenuation value of the centre, equivalent to water (fig. 5.13). Smaller cysts, however, may suffer from a partial volume effect (i.e. an artificially high attenuation value because of averaging with the surrounding block of normal tissue). US is useful to confirm the small cyst.

Cavernous haemangioma appears as a low attenuation area on an enhanced scan which subsequently fills in with contrast from the periphery (fig. 5.14). In only 55% of cases is this unequivocal and in the disputed case confirmation by radio active labelled red cell scan, MRI or angiography may be necessary.

CT scan can detect solid lesions greater than 1 cm in

diameter due to primary or secondary malignant tumour (figs 28.9, 28.28). They usually have a lower attenuation value than normal liver which remains on enhancement. Calcification is present in some metastases such as from colon. Highly vascular metastases (kidney, choriocarcinoma, carcinoid) may fill in with enhancement. Most primary tumours do not. Whether confirmation by image guided biopsy is necessary will depend upon the clinical situation and the results of tumour markers, alpha-fetoprotein and CEA. The sensitivity of CT in showing hepato-cellular carcinoma is 87%, compared with 80% for US and 90% for hepatic angiography [18]. The sensitivity for satellite lesions is lower at 59% for CT and angiography, and 17% for US. Injection of iodized oil (Lipiodol) into the hepatic artery followed by CT 2 weeks later (see fig. 28.11) may be used to detect small lesions, but many still escape detection—the sensitivity in a study of lesions 9–40 mm in diameter being only 53% [24].

CT scanning after injection of contrast into the splenic or superior mesenteric artery (CT arterioportography) is the most sensitive method for detecting hepatic metastases (fig. 5.15) and also shows benign and malignant primary hepatic tumours [22]. Because it is invasive it is generally reserved for candidates for surgical resection. CT portography detects 75% of hepato-cellular carcinomas less than 2 cm in diameter [11] and 88% of primary and secondary hepatic malignant lesions [12].

Adenomas and focal nodular hyperplasia usually give negative defects but can be missed both by CT and US because they have characteristics close to that of normal liver tissue. Focal nodular hyperplasia classically has a central scar but this is not specific enough to be of guaranteed diagnostic value.

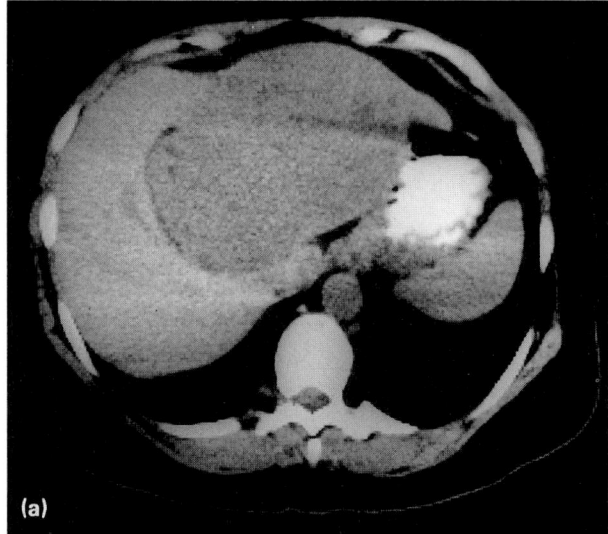

(a)

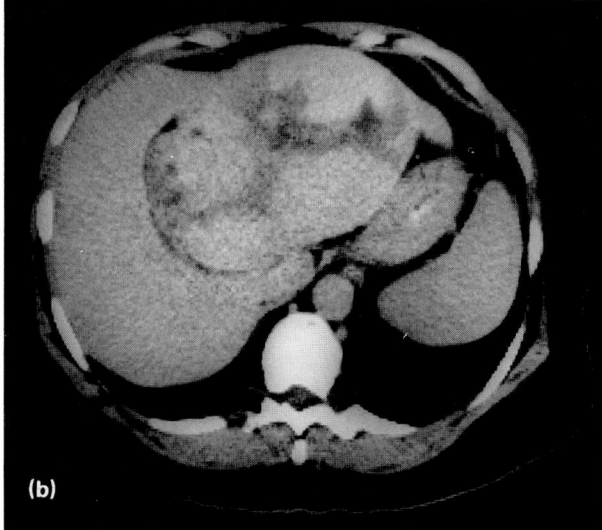

(b)

Fig. 5.14. CT scan shows a large, low attenuation lesion in the left lobe of the liver (a). Following enhancement (b), dynamic scanning shows gradual infilling of the lesion which eventually became isodense with the remainder of the liver. These are the characteristic appearances of a cavernous haemangioma.

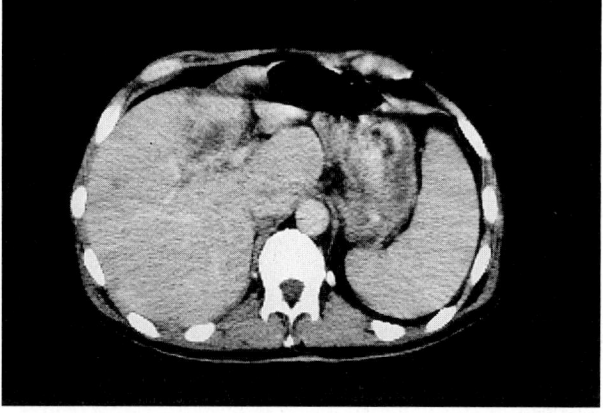

(a)

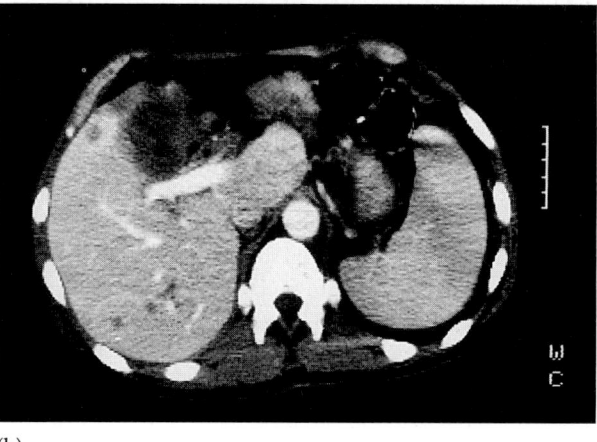

(b)

Fig. 5.15. Value of CT portography. (a) Conventional enhanced CT scan of liver in patient with cholangiocarcinoma in left lobe. There was a suspicion of metastases in the right lobe. (b) CT portography clearly showing multiple small metastases in the right lobe. The portal vein is well seen as is the lesion in the left lobe.

Abscesses usually show a lower attenuation than normal liver (fig. 5.16). Aspiration under guidance is possible as with US. An enhanced rim around the abscess on CT is said to be more characteristic of amoebic abscess. Hydatid cysts, particularly those that are old and inactive, may have a calcified rim. Daughter cysts can be seen in active disease.

Enhanced CT is a valuable aid in abdominal trauma, the size of any laceration or contusion being noted, and the extent of any haemoperitoneum [17]. False aneurysms of the hepatic artery should be searched for.

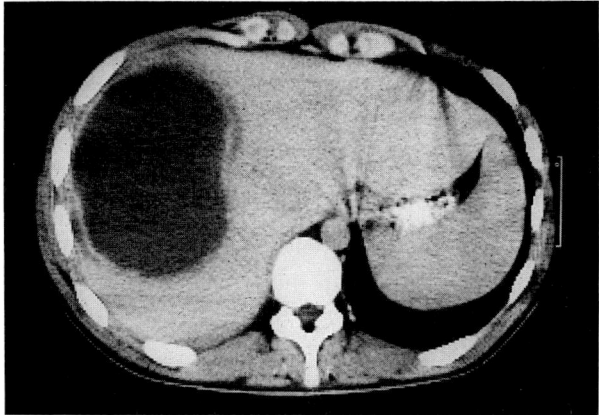

Fig. 5.16. CT scan of liver in a 21-year-old man with fever and right upper quadrant pain. CT shows a large space-occupying lesion from which 1 litre of pus was drained. This was an infected amoebic abscess.

An important function of CT, more so than US, is to define the anatomy for the surgeon considering hepatic resection. The segmental position of the lesion can be identified. CT portography will show whether more lesions exist than seen on the conventionally enhanced scan (fig. 5.15).

Magnetic resonance imaging [9, 13]

This is the most expensive scanning technique, at approximately six times the cost of US and twice that of CT. The detection of lesions with MRI is comparable to that with CT, although most protocols for MRI at present have lower spatial resolution than that available for CT. The detection and characterization of lesions less than 1 cm in diameter is difficult. Although there are advances in fast scanning techniques, respiratory artefacts may be a problem. Some hepatic lesions have specific MRI signal characteristics, but others do not. Tissue-specific contrast agents may refine this in the future. CT has the benefit over MRI of demonstrating structures around the liver.

MRI depends upon detection of energy released from hydrogen protons after forcible alignment in a strong magnetic field. The technique is safe with certain provisos. Patients with cardiac pacemakers and internal magnetic material (clips, metallic foreign bodies) are excluded as are pregnant patients; it is difficult to scan and monitor the ventilated patient from intensive care.

Several measurements of tissue can be made but those most commonly employed are the relaxation times T_1 and T_2, and proton density. Tissues appear greatly different according to the mode used. Blood vessels and bile ducts are visualized without the need for contrast material. There is excellent contrast resolution (better than CT) and good spatial resolution (not as good as CT). As scanning times (currently 5–10 minutes for each sequence) shorten with technological advances, artefact from respiratory movement particularly in the breathless patient will decrease and spatial resolution will improve. Multiple planes (axial, coronal, sagittal) can be reconstructed according to need. Reproducibility is good. Tissue characterization is possible.

T_1 relaxation time is the time taken for hydrogen protons to re-align within the external magnetic field after a radio-wave pulse. T_2 relaxation time describes the rate at which the axes of the protons move out of phase with each other because of the differing electromagnetic influence of adjacent protons. Protein density simply depicts the number of protons per unit area. Tissues respond differently to the MRI process and scans can therefore characterize cyst fluid, sub-acute and chronic haematoma, fat, neoplasm, fibrotic tissue and vessels.

On T_1 weighted (T_1W) scans the liver usually appears grey and homogeneous, with a signal greater than spleen. On T_2W the hepatic signal is less than that from spleen (fig. 5.17). Dilated bile ducts are easily seen.

Normal blood vessels usually appear black with T_1W and T_2W scans because the energy donated during the radiopulse has passed out of the slice with blood flow by the time the return signal is recorded. With gradient echo sequence, used only in selected cases, recording is less delayed after excitation, and blood vessels may appear bright.

Which ever technique is used, portal vein, hepatic veins, IVC, aorta and biliary tract are seen. Note that no contrast injection is needed for blood vessel or bile duct visualization.

MRI can show cysts, haemangioma, primary and secondary tumour (fig. 5.18). Malignant tumour usually appears dark (low signal) on T_1W scan and bright (high signal) on T_2W. Differentiation between hepato-cellular carcinoma and metastases is not possible. Preliminary reports suggest that adenomatous hyperplastic nodules without dysplasia are hypointense on T_2W scans, differentiating them from hepato-cellular carcinoma [16]. Cavernous haemangioma is particularly bright on T_2W scans and can be distinguished from carcinoma using a spin–echo sequence of 2000/150 [6].

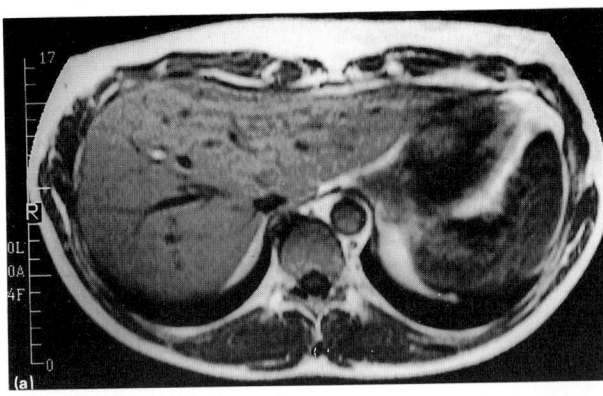

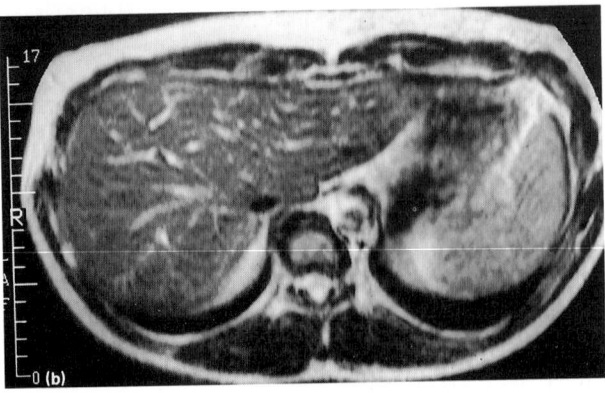

Fig. 5.17. MRI scan in a normal adult volunteer. (a) T_1W scan (spin echo 300/12). (b) T_2W scan (spin echo 1500/80). Blood vessels within the homogenous liver (left) are easily seen without intravenous contrast.

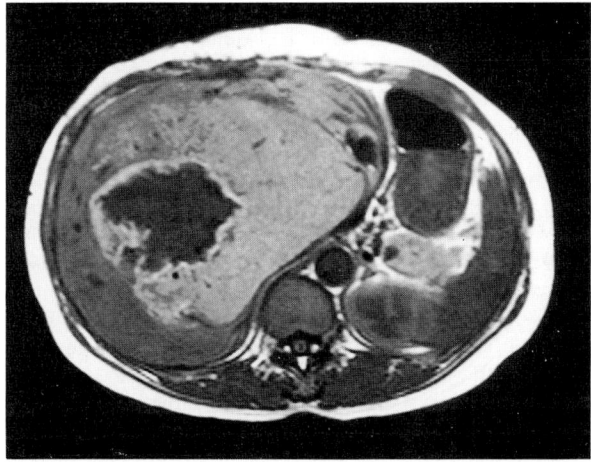

(a)

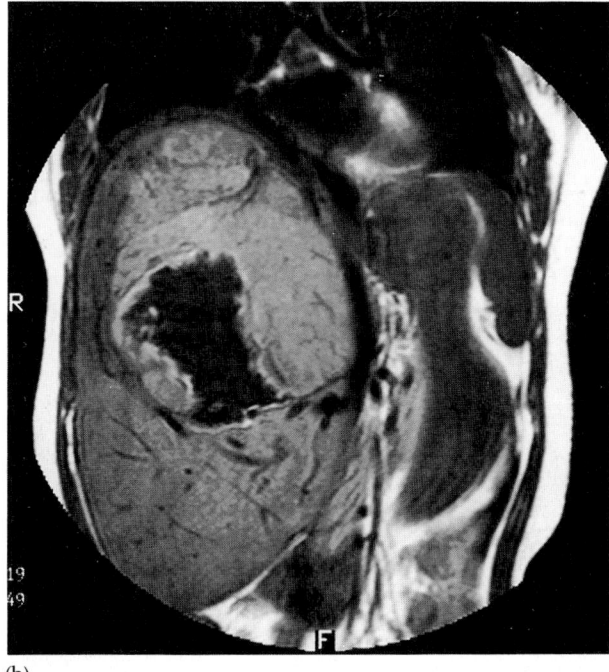

(b)

Fig. 5.18. MRI scan (T_1W): (a) axial and (b) coronal sequences. There is a large mass within the anterior/superior part of the liver with an abnormal vascular pattern. A low signal area within this is necrotic tissue. Normal liver is seen behind and below the tumour (courtesy Dr W. Curati).

MRI detects an increase in hepatic iron but is not yet quantitatively accurate enough to help in the management of patients with haemochromatosis. The liver appears black on T_1W and T_2W scans.

MR cholangiography (see fig 29.7) is a relatively new technique limited to only a few centres. It can show bile duct strictures and stones non-invasively [21]. It remains to be seen whether this technique will find a role compared with the conventional approach for biliary tract disease of US followed by diagnostic and, if necessary, therapeutic ERCP.

Many data are accumulating on MRI. Developments will include optimizing the spin–echo sequence, using fast imaging sequences and applying new contrast media such as gadolinium derivatives and ferrite. At present the results for MRI of the liver are comparable to CT. MRI promises much for the future but its use may well be limited by cost, availability and expertise. At present, the clinical hepatologist need not feel deprived if he does not have access to abdominal MRI.

CT remains the better choice if scanning of the chest or pelvis as well as liver is needed to investigate malignant disease, or if guided biopsy is necessary.

MR spectroscopy

MR spectroscopy allows non-invasive evaluation of bio-chemical changes in tissue *in vivo*. Changes in molecules involved in selected areas of cellular metabolism can be detected. This technique has been applied to patients with liver disease. Phosphorus-31 spectroscopy of the liver shows changes in tumours and 40% of patients with diffuse liver disease [8]. These are not specific, and the technique currently remains experimental.

Conclusions and choice

The choice of technique for hepato-biliary imaging depends upon the availability of the appropriate apparatus, operator and interpreter, and the problem that has to be solved (table 5.1). Strict diagnostic algorithms cannot be formulated that will service *all units*. Radio-isotope scanning has been superseded by US and CT which are better in detecting lesions and characterizing them. With an experienced ultrasonographer, this technique is the initial examination of choice for the majority of problems. Equivocal results can be further studied by CT if necessary.

CT and MRI characterize most lesions better than US but are more costly and less widely available. In some centres CT replaces US as the primary procedure, often more out of availability and convenience (for the clinician) than need. MRI is at present the most costly method of scanning and is likely to be used in most units only for difficult problems which cannot be solved by US or CT.

For the diagnosis of jaundice, US is the preferred screening investigation. If necessary this may be followed by CT scanning to help in the diagnosis and to show the extent of disease.

For the diagnosis of gallbladder stones, US is the primary method of choice.

Tc-IDA scanning provides an alternative non-invasive method to US for determining bile duct obstruction, in the diagnosis of acute cholecystitis, and in demonstrating post-operative biliary patency and leaks.

Table 5.1. Non-invasive imaging for hepato-biliary disease

	Choice		
Question	First	Second	Third
Mass in liver	US	CT	MRI
Hepatic metastases	US/CT	MRI	
Screen cirrhotic for HCC	US	CT	
Tumour resectable	CT*	MRI	
Haemangioma	US	CT	RBC scan/MRI
Abscess	US/CT		
Hydatid cyst	US	CT	
Portal vein patent	USDop	US/CT	MRI
Portal hypertension	USDop	US	CT
Budd–Chiari	USDop	US	CT
Shunt patent	USDop	US/CT	
Assessment of trauma	US/CT		
Cirrhosis	US/CT		
Fatty liver	CT	US	MRI
Iron	CT	MRI	
Gallbladder stone	US		
Acute cholecystitis	US/IDA		
Dilated bile ducts	US		
Duct stone	US†		
Bile leak	IDA		
Pancreatic tumour	US/CT		

* CT portography.
† Only of value if positive.
HCC = hepato-cellular carcinoma; RBC = red blood cell;
USDop = Doppler ultrasound; IDA = scintiscan with
iminodiacetic acid derivative.

References

1 Alpern MB, Rubin JM, Williams DM *et al*. Porta hepatis: duplex Doppler US with angiographic correlation. *Radiology* 1987; **162**: 53.

2 Amouyal P, Amouyal G, Levy P *et al*. Diagnosis of choledocholithiasis by endoscopic ultrasonography. *Gastroenterology* 1994; **106**: 1062.

3 Bluemke DA, Urban B, Fishman EK. Spiral CT of the liver: current applications. *Semin. Ultrasound CT MRI* 1994; **15**: 107.

4 Bolondi L, Gaiani S, Li Bassi S *et al*. Diagnosis of Budd–Chiari syndrome by pulsed Doppler ultrasound. *Gastroenterology* 1991; **100**: 1324.

5 Chen BC, Huang S-C, Germano G *et al*. Noninvasive quantification of hepatic arterial blood flow with nitrogen-13-ammonia and dynamic positron emission tomography. *J. Nucl. Med.* 1991; **32**: 2199.

6 Choi BI, Han MC, Kim C-W. Small hepatocellular carcinoma versus small cavernous hemangioma: differentiation with MR imaging at 2.0T. *Radiology* 1990; **76**: 103.

7 Colli A, Cocciolo M, Riva C *et al*. Abnormalities of Doppler waveform of hepatic veins in patients with chronic liver disease: correlation with histologic findings. *AJR* 1994; **162**: 833.

8 Cox IJ, Menon DK, Sargentoni J *et al*. Phosphorus-31 magnetic resonance spectroscopy of the human liver using chemical shift imaging techniques. *J. Hepatol.* 1992; **14**: 265.

9 de Lange EE. Cross-sectional imaging of the liver. *Baillière's Clin. Gastroenterol.* 1995; **9**: 97.

10 Friess H, Langhans J, Ebert M *et al*. Diagnosis of pancreatic cancer by 2[^{18}F]-fluoro-2-deoxy-D-glucose positron emission tomography. *Gut* 1995; **36**: 771.

11 Ikeda K, Saitoh S, Koida I *et al*. Imaging diagnosis of small hepatocellular carcinoma. *Hepatology* 1994; **20**: 82.

12 Irie T, Takeshita K, Wada Y *et al*. CT evaluation of hepatic tumors: comparison of CT with arterial portography, CT with infusion hepatic arteriography, and simultaneous use of both techniques. *AJR* 1995; **164**: 1407.

13 Johnson CD. Magnetic resonance imaging of the liver: current clinical applications. *Mayo Clin. Proc.* 1993; **68**: 147.

14 Krishnamurthy S, Krishnamurthy GT. Technetium-99m-iminodiacetic acid organic anions: review of biokinetics and clinical application in hepatology. *Hepatology* 1989; **9**: 139.

15 Lafortune M, Martinet J-P, Denys A *et al*. Short- and long-term hemodynamic effects of transjugular intrahepatic portosystemic shunts: a Doppler/manometric correlative study. *AJR* 1995; **164**: 997.

16 Matsui O, Kadoya M, Kameyama T *et al*. Adenomatous hyperplastic nodules in the cirrhotic liver: differentiation from hepatocellular carcinoma with MR imaging. *Radiology* 1989; **173**: 123.

17 Moon KL, Federle MP. Computed tomography in hepatic trauma. *Am. J. Roentgenol.* 1983; **141**: 309.

18 Rizzi PM, Kane PA, Ryder SD *et al*. Accuracy of radiology in detection of hepatocellular carcinoma before liver transplantation. *Gastroenterology* 1994; **107**: 1425.

19 Scoutt LM, Zawin ML, Taylor KJW *et al*. Doppler US. Part II: clinical applications. *Radiology* 1990; **174**: 309.

20 Shinagawa T, Ohto M, Kimura K *et al*. Diagnosis and clinical features of small hepatocellular carcinoma with emphasis on the utility of real-time ultrasonography: a study in 51 patients. *Gastroenterology* 1984; **86**: 495.

21 Soto JA, Barish MA, Yucel EK *et al*. Magnetic resonance cholangiography: comparison with endoscopic retrograde cholangiopancreatography. *Gastroenterology* 1996; **110**: 589.

22 Soyer P, Bluemke DA, Fishman EK. CT during arterial portography for the preoperative evaluation of hepatic tumors: how, when, and why? *AJR* 1994; **163**: 1325.

23 Tandon BN, Rana S, Acharya SK. Bedside ultrasonography: a low-cost definitive diagnostic procedure in obstructive jaundice. *J. Clin. Gastroenterol.* 1987; **9**: 353.

24 Taourel PG, Pageaux GP, Coste V *et al*. Small hepatocellular carcinoma in patients undergoing liver transplantation: detection with CT after injection of iodized oil. *Radiology* 1995; **197**: 377.

25 Webb LJ, Berger LA, Sherlock S. Grey-scale ultrasonography of portal vein. *Lancet* 1977; **ii**: 675.

Chapter 6
Hepato-cellular Failure

Hepato-cellular failure can complicate almost all forms of liver disease. It may follow virus hepatitis, or the cirrhoses, fatty liver of pregnancy, hepatitis due to drugs, overdose with drugs such as acetaminophen (paracetamol), ligation of the hepatic artery near the liver, or occlusion of the hepatic veins. The syndrome does not complicate portal venous occlusion alone. Circulatory failure, with hypotension, may precipitate liver failure, especially in the cirrhotic.

It may be terminal in chronic cholestasis, such as primary biliary cirrhosis or surgical cholestatic jaundice associated with malignant replacement of liver tissue or acute cholangitis. It should be diagnosed cautiously in a patient suffering from acute biliary obstruction.

Although the clinical features may differ, the overall picture and treatment are similar, irrespective of the aetiology. Acute fulminant hepato-cellular failure poses special problems (Chapter 8).

There is no constant hepatic pathology and in particular necrosis is not always seen. The syndrome is therefore functional rather than anatomical. It comprises some or all of the following features.
• General failure of health.
• Jaundice.
• Hyperdynamic circulation and cyanosis.
• Fever and septicaemias.
• Neurological changes (hepatic encephalopathy) (Chapters 7, 8).
• Ascites (Chapter 9).
• Changes in nitrogen metabolism.
• Skin and endocrine changes.
• Disordered blood coagulation (Chapter 4).

General failure of health

The most conspicuous feature is weakness and easy fatiguability. Wasting can be related to difficulty in synthesizing tissue proteins. Anorexia and poor dietary habits add to the malnutrition.

Jaundice

Jaundice is largely due to failure of the liver cells to metabolize bilirubin, so it is some guide to the severity of liver cell failure.

In acute failure, due to such causes as virus hepatitis, jaundice parallels the extent of liver cell damage. This is not so evident in cirrhosis, where jaundice may be absent or mild. This is due to the balance achieved between hepatic necrosis and regeneration. When present it represents active hepato-cellular disease and indicates a bad prognosis. Diminished erythrocyte survival adds a haemolytic component to the jaundice.

Vasodilatation and hyperdynamic circulation

This is associated with all forms of hepato-cellular failure, but especially with decompensated cirrhosis [35]. It is shown by flushed extremities, bounding pulses and capillary pulsations. Peripheral blood flow is increased and this is due mainly to increased skin blood flow [24]. Arterial blood flow is increased in the lower limbs [6]. Portal blood flow is increased. Renal blood flow, and particularly cortical perfusion, is reduced. Cardiac output is raised [13, 29] and evidenced by tachycardia, an active precordial impulse and frequently an ejection systolic murmur (figs 6.1, 6.2). These circulatory changes only rarely result in heart failure.

The blood pressure is low and, in the terminal phase, further reduces kidney function. At this stage the

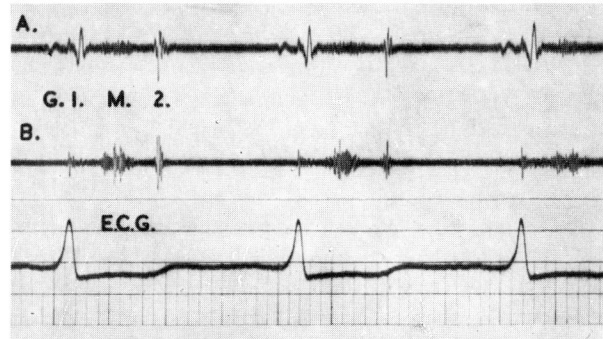

Fig. 6.1. Cirrhosis. Phonocardiogram at apex (A) and base (B) shows ejection-type systolic murmur (M) and an auricular sound (presystolic gallop) (G) [23].

73

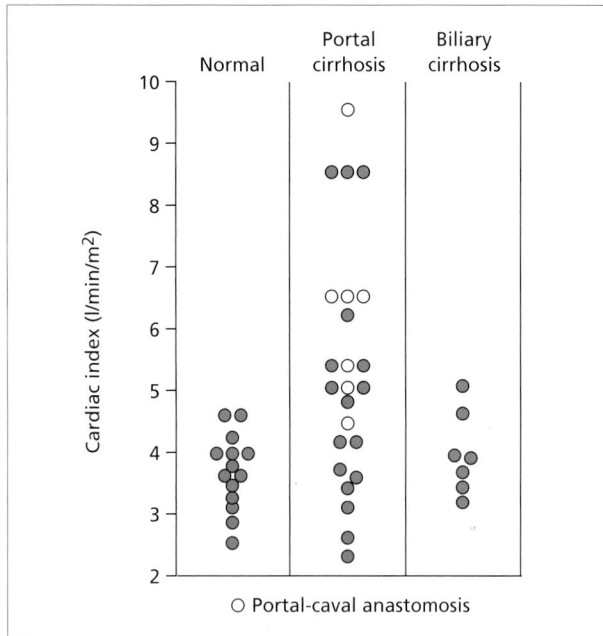

Fig. 6.2. The cardiac output is raised in many patients with hepatic cirrhosis but within normal limits in biliary cirrhosis. Mean normal cardiac index is $3.68 \pm 0.60\,l/min/m^2$. Mean in hepatic cirrhosis is $5.36 \pm 1.98\,l/min/m^2$ [29].

impaired liver blood flow contributes to hepatic failure and the fall in cerebral blood flow adds to the mental changes [10]. Such hypotension is ominous and attempts at elevation by raising circulatory volume by blood transfusion or by such drugs as dopamine are of only temporary benefit (see fig. 9.13).

Systemic vascular peripheral resistance is reduced as is the arteriovenous oxygen difference. In patients with cirrhosis, whole body oxygen consumption is decreased and tissue oxidation is abnormal [28]. This has been related to the hyperdynamic circulation and to arteriovenous shunting. Thus, the vasodilator state of liver failure may contribute to general tissue hypoxia.

Vasomotor tone is decreased as shown by reduced vasoconstriction in response to mental exercise, the Valsalva manoeuvre and tilting from horizontal to vertical [23, 24]. Autonomic neuropathy is a poor prognostic indicator [7]. It seems possible that large numbers of normally present, but functionally inactive, arteriovenous anastomoses have opened under the influence of a vasodilator substance. The effective arterial blood volume falls as a consequence of the enlargement of the arterial vascular compartment induced by arterial vasodilatation. This activates the sympathetic and renin–angiotensin systems and is important in sodium and water retention and ascites formation (Chapter 9). The hyperdynamic splanchnic circulation is related to portal hypertension (Chapter 10).

The nature of the vasodilators concerned remains speculative. They are likely to be multiple. Whatever the nature, the substances might be formed by the sick hepatocyte, fail to be inactivated by it or bypass it through intra- or extra-hepatic porto-systemic shunts. The vasodilators are likely to be of intestinal origin. In cirrhosis, increased permeability of the intestinal mucosa and porto-systemic shunting allow endotoxin and cytokines to reach the systemic circulation and these could be responsible (see fig. 6.9) [21, 22].

Nitric oxide (NO), a potent vasodilator, may be related to the hyperdynamic circulation hence to ascites development and to the hepato-renal syndrome (Chapter 9) and portal hypertension (Chapter 10) (fig. 6.3) [38]. NO is released in endothelial cells from L-arginine and acts by inactivation of guanylate cyclase. NO synthase is the responsible enzyme and L-arginine analogues such as NG-monomethyl-L-arginine (L-NMMA) inhibit this conversion and have been shown to reverse many of the vasodilator effects of NO. Inhibitors have been shown to reverse the hyperdynamic circulation in portal hypertensive rats [19]. Cirrhotic rats show increased sensitivity to the pressor effect of NO inhibition and portal pressure rises [30]. NO synthase is inducible after stimulation with bacterial endotoxin or cytokines [26].

Various gastrointestinal peptides such as vasoactive intestinal polypeptide (VIP), substance P and CGRP (II) [2] have little effect on the portal circulation. Glucagon is a vasodilator and increases azygous flow in patients with cirrhosis but has little effect on cardiac index or haemodynamics so implying little effect on systemic vascular resistance [20]. It is unlikely to be the sole vasodilator responsible.

Prostaglandins (E_1, E_2 and E_{12}) have vasodilatory actions and prostanoids are released into the portal vein in patients with chronic liver disease [40]. They may play a part in vasodilatation.

The cirrhotic shows arterial hyporeactivity to endogenous vasoconstrictors [27].

After hepatic transplantation, portal pressure becomes normal, cardiac index and splanchnic flow remain high due to the persistence of porto-systemic collateral flow [9, 11].

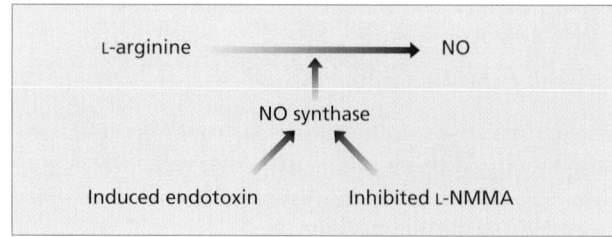

Fig. 6.3. Nitric oxide (NO) is a general vasodilator. It is produced from L-arginine, NO synthase being the responsible enzyme. This is induced by endotoxin and inhibited by L-NMMA.

Hepato-pulmonary syndrome [18]

About a third of patients with decompensated cirrhosis have reduced arterial oxygen saturation and are sometimes cyanosed [32] (table 6.1, fig. 6.4). This is probably due to intrapulmonary shunting through microscopic arteriovenous fistulae [12, 34]. Injection studies of the pulmonary artery in cirrhotic patients have shown a marked arterial dilatation in fine peripheral branches of the pulmonary artery both within the respiratory parts of the lung and on the pleura where spider naevi are sometimes seen (fig. 6.5) [3]. Rarely, actual pulmonary arteriovenous shunts have been demonstrated by pulmonary angiography (fig. 6.6). Cardiac catheterization studies in one cyanosed patient with cirrhosis showed a right-to-left shunt with an arterial oxygen saturation of 91% falling to 68% on exercise. Such shunts may be confirmed by infusions of micropaque gelatin into the pulmonary vascular tree at autopsy [3].

The pulmonary vascular dilatation and arteriovenous shunting may be shown by contrast-enhanced echocardiography [16]. ^{99m}Tc macro-aggregated albumin lung scanning or pulmonary angiography shows the spongy appearance of the basal pulmonary vessels corresponding to the infiltrates seen on the chest X-ray.

Table 6.1. Pulmonary changes complicating chronic hepato-cellular disease

Hypoxia	Raised diaphragms
Intra-pulmonary shunting	Basal atelectasis
Ventilation–perfusion mismatch	Primary pulmonary hypertension
	Porto-pulmonary shunting
Reduced transfer factor	Chest X-ray mottling
Pleural effusion	

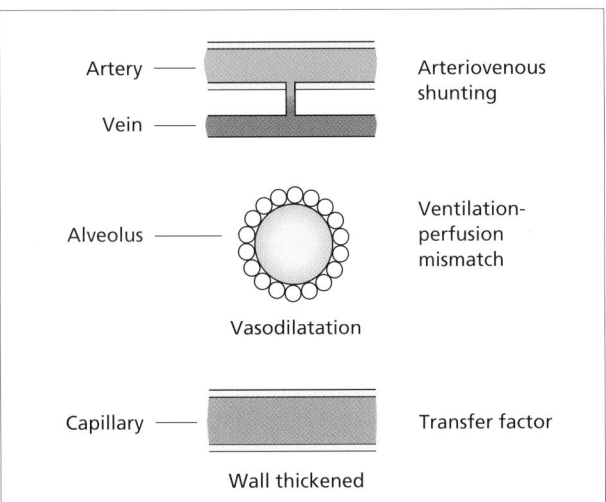

Fig. 6.4. Pulmonary changes in liver failure.

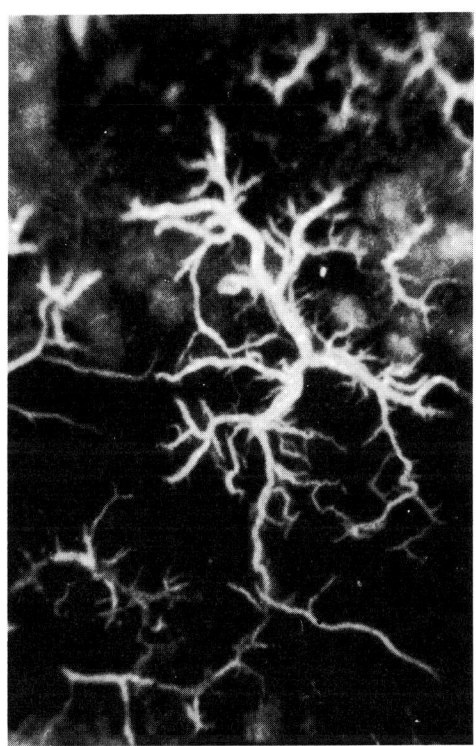

Fig. 6.5. Cirrhosis. Macroscopic appearances of the pleura showing dilated pleural vessels resembling a spider naevus [3].

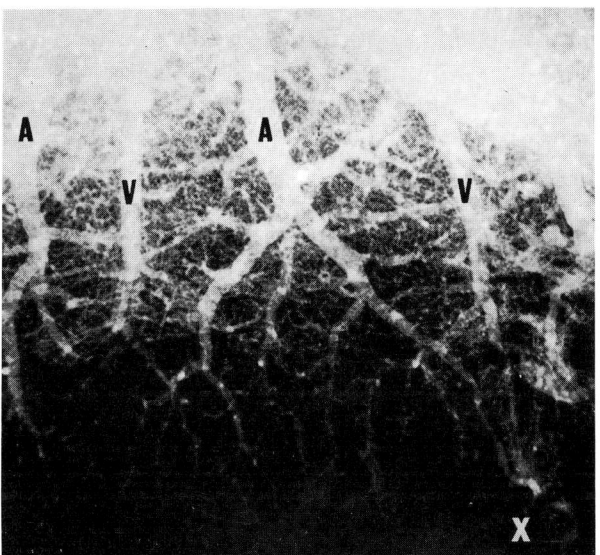

Fig. 6.6. Arteriogram from a patient with cirrhosis showing a slice of the basal region of the left lung. Arteries (A) and veins (V) alternate: X is the site of the arteriovenous shunting, into which a large arterial branch can be directly traced. The injection medium was barium suspension [3].

Reduction of diffusing capacity is present without a restrictive ventilatory defect [37]. This is likely to be due to dilatation of small pulmonary blood vessels, a complication both of advanced cirrhosis and fulminant hepatic failure [3, 36, 42]. A reduction in transfer factor is a consistent finding, perhaps related to thickening of the walls of the small veins and capillaries by a layer of collagen [36].

The pulmonary vasodilatation is associated with a low pulmonary vascular resistance which fails to respond to hypoxia or exercise [1]. This also leads to failure of the lung to match perfusion with ventilation [33]. Even in those who retain hypoxic pulmonary vasoconstriction, the pulmonary artery pressure is low in the face of hypoxia and a raised carbon dioxide. Porto-pulmonary anastomoses have been demonstrated but are unlikely to contribute to arterial oxygen desaturation as the portal vein has a high oxygen content. Moreover, the flow from them is probably small.

Finally, pulmonary function in cirrhotics may be reduced by a high diaphragm (secondary to hepatomegaly or massive ascites), a pleural effusion or the chronic lung disease of the heavy smoking alcoholic.

Finger clubbing is a frequent but not constant association of the cyanosis and increased cardiac index. Platypnoea and also orthodeoxia are usual [15].

The most profound cyanosis and clubbing are associated with chronic active hepatitis and long-standing cirrhosis. Improvement in liver function is associated with both lessening of the cyanosis and the nodularity seen on the chest radiograph.

The mechanisms remain uncertain. A pulmonary dilator is probably responsible, but whether this is related to failure of production by the diseased liver or failure of hepatic metabolism is unknown [14].

Relation to liver transplantation

Pulmonary assessment is essential in any candidate for liver transplant [14]. A chest X-ray is necessary. Pa_{O_2} should be measured erect and supine to allow diagnosis of orthodeoxia, a good indication of pulmonary vascular dilatation. This is confirmed by contrast echocardiography [15]. Technetium-labelled macro-aggregated albumin can also be used to demonstrate the pulmonary dilatations [15].

Resolution of intra-pulmonary shunting follows liver transplant, especially with diffuse precapillary dilatations (fig. 6.7) [39]. In paediatrics, pulmonary shunting reversed within weeks of the operation [17]. Reversal is not always the case with large pulmonary arteriovenous shunts and these may require coil embolotherapy which should precede transplant [31].

Pulmonary hypertension

This affects 2% of patients with portal hypertension both intra- and extra-hepatic [8]. Histometric study of the muscular pulmonary arteries shows dilatation and thickening of the wall and, rarely, thrombi [25]. Plexogenic pulmonary arteriopathy, involving arteries 10–200 mm in diameter and once thought to be diagnostic of pulmonary hypertension has been found at autopsy [25].

The pulmonary hypertension may be part of the general hyperdynamic circulatory state of cirrhosis. Porto-systemic and porto-pulmonary collaterals could deliver vasomotor factors of intestinal origin into the pulmonary circulation (fig. 6.8). The factors responsible are not known, but endothelin-1, a potent pulmonary constrictor related to endotoxaemia, is a possibility.

Pulmonary hypertension should be suspected in hypoxaemic patients without pulmonary vascular dilatation. It is confirmed by echocardiography with Doppler assessment of pulmonary artery pressures [15]. If positive, measurements of the pulmonary circulation should be made by right heart catheterization.

Significant pulmonary hypertension (exceeding 40 mmHg) and pulmonary vascular resistance more than 250 dynes/second/cm or reduced cardiac output

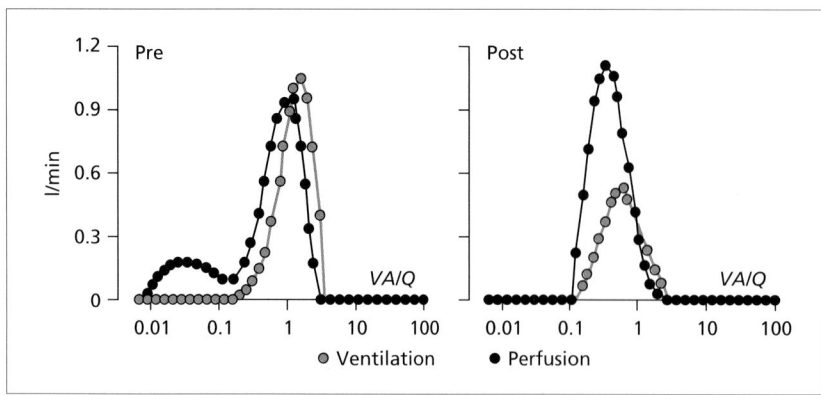

Fig. 6.7. Using the multiple inert gas elimination technique, intra-pulmonary shunting and ventilation–perfusion mismatch disappeared after liver transplant [5].

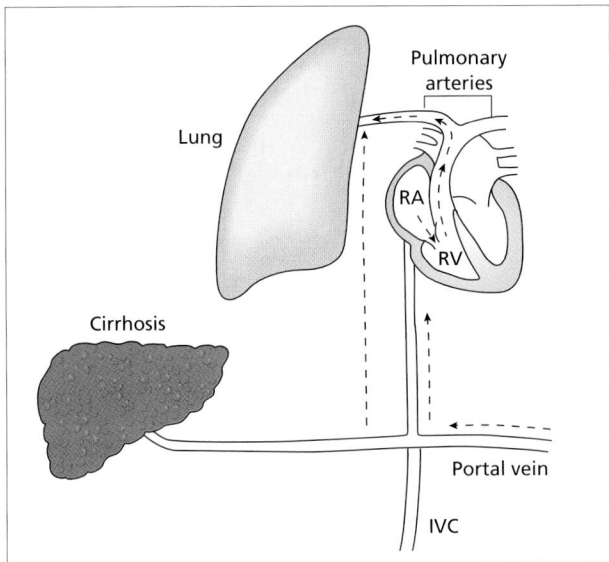

Fig. 6.8. Pulmonary hypertension in cirrhosis might be related to portal-systemic and porto-pulmonary shunting of vasoconstrictor substances.

increases the risk of liver transplantation resulting in peri-operative deaths from acute right ventricular failure [4].

Pulmonary hypertension can also follow multiple tumour emboli to the pulmonary microvasculature in patients with hepato-cellular carcinoma [41].

References

1 Agusti AGN, Roca J, Bosch J *et al*. The lung in patients with cirrhosis. *J. Hepatol*. 1990; **10**: 251.

2 Bendtsen F, Schifter S, Henriksen JH. Increased circulating calcitonin gene-related peptide (CGRP) in cirrhosis. *J. Hepatol*. 1991; **12**: 118.

3 Berthelot P, Walker JG, Sherlock S *et al*. Arterial changes in the lungs in cirrhosis of the liver—lung spider nevi. *N. Engl. J. Med*. 1966; **274**: 291.

4 Cheng EY, Woehlck HJ. Pulmonary artery hypertension complicating anesthesia for liver transplantation. *Anesthesiology* 1992; **77**: 389.

5 Eriksson LS, Söderman C, Ericzon B-G *et al*. Normalization of ventilation/perfusion relationships after liver transplantation in patients with decompensated cirrhosis: evidence for a hepatopulmonary syndrome. *Hepatology* 1990; **12**: 1350.

6 Fernández-Rodriguez CM, Prieto J, Zozaya JM *et al*. Arteriovenous shunting, hemodynamic changes, and renal sodium retention in liver cirrhosis. *Gastroenterology* 1993; **104**: 1139.

7 Fleckenstein JF, Frank SM, Thuluvath PJ. Presence of autonomic neuropathy is a poor prognostic indicator in patients with advanced liver disease. *Hepatology* 1996; **23**: 471.

8 Hadengue A, Benhayoun MK, Lebrec D *et al*. Pulmonary hypertension complicating portal hypertension: prevalence and relation to splanchnic hemodynamics. *Gastroenterology* 1991; **100**: 520.

9 Hadengue A, Lebrec D, Moreau R *et al*. Persistence of systemic and splanchnic hyperkinetic circulation in liver transplant patients. *Hepatology* 1993; **17**: 175.

10 Hecker R, Sherlock S. Electrolyte and circulatory changes in terminal liver failure. *Lancet* 1956; **ii**: 1121.

11 Henderson JM. Abnormal splanchnic and systemic hemodynamics of end-stage liver disease: what happens after liver transplantation? *Hepatology* 1993; **17**: 514.

12 Hutchison DCS, Sapru RP, Sumerling MD *et al*. Cirrhosis, cyanosis and polycythaemia: multiple pulmonary arteriovenous anastomoses. *Am. J. Med*. 1968; **45**: 139.

13 Kowalski HJ, Abelman WH. The cardiac output at rest in Laennec's cirrhosis. *J. Clin. Invest*. 1953; **32**: 1025.

14 Krowka MJ, Cortese DA. Hepatopulmonary syndrome: an evolving perspective in the era of liver transplantation. *Hepatology* 1990; **11**: 138.

15 Krowka MJ, Dickson ER, Cortese DA. Hepatopulmonary syndrome: clinical observations and lack of therapeutic response to somatostatin analogue. *Chest* 1993; **104**: 515.

16 Krowka MJ, Tajik AJ, Dickson ER *et al*. Intrapulmonary vascular dilatations (IPVD) in liver transplant candidates. Screening by two-dimensional contrast-enhanced echocardiography. *Chest* 1990; **97**: 1165.

17 Laberge J-M, Brandt ML, Lebecque P *et al*. Reversal of cirrhosis-related pulmonary shunting in two children by orthotopic liver transplantation. *Transplantation* 1992; **53**: 1135.

18 Lange PA, Stoller JK. The hepatopulmonary syndrome. *Ann. Intern. Med*. 1995; **122**: 521.

19 Lee F-Y, Colombato LA, Albillos A *et al*. N-ω-nitro-L-arginine administration corrects peripheral vasodilation and systemic capillary hypotension and ameliorates plasma volume expansion and sodium retention in portal hypertensive rats. *Hepatology* 1993; **17**: 84.

20 Lee SS, Moreau R, Hadengue A *et al*. Glucagon selectively increases splanchnic blood flow in patients with well-compensated cirrhosis. *Hepatology* 1988; **8**: 1501.

21 Lin R-S, Lee F-Y, Lee S-D *et al*. Endotoxemia in patients with chronic liver disease: relationship to severity of liver diseases, presence of esophageal varices, and hyperdynamic circulation. *J. Hepatol*. 1995; **22**: 165.

22 Lopez-Talavera JC, Merrill WW, Groszmann RJ. Tumor necrosis factor alpha: a major contributor to the hyperdynamic circulation in prehepatic portal-hypertensive rats. *Gastroenterology* 1995; **108**: 761.

23 Lunzer MR, Manghani KK, Newman SP *et al*. Impaired cardiovascular responsiveness in liver disease. *Lancet* 1975; **ii**: 382.

24 Lunzer MR, Newman SP, Sherlock S. Skeletal muscle blood flow and neurovascular reactivity in liver disease. *Gut* 1973; **14**: 354.

25 Matsubara O, Nakamura T, Uehara T *et al*. Histometrical investigation of the pulmonary artery in severe hepatic disease. *J. Pathol*. 1984; **143**: 31.

26 Moncada S, Palmer RM, Higgs EA. Nitric oxide: physiology, pathophysiology, and pharmacology. *Pharmacol. Rev*. 1991; **43**: 109.

27 Moreau R, Lebrec D. Endogenous factors involved in the control of arterial tone in cirrhosis. *J. Hepatol*. 1995; **22**: 370.

28 Moreau R, Lee SS, Hadengue A *et al*. Relationship between oxygen transport and oxygen uptake in patients with cirrhosis: effects of vasoactive drugs. *Hepatology* 1989; **9**: 427.

29 Murray JF, Dawson AM, Sherlock S. Circulatory changes in

chronic liver disease. *Am. J. Med.* 1958; **24**: 358.

30 Niederberger M, Gines P, Tsai P *et al.* Increased aortic cyclic guanosine monophosphate concentration in experimental cirrhosis in rats: evidence for a role of nitric oxide in the pathogenesis of arterial vasodilation in cirrhosis. *Hepatology* 1995; **21**: 1625.

31 Poterucha JJ, Krowka MJ, Dickson ER *et al.* Failure of hepatopulmonary syndrome to resolve after liver transplantation and successful treatment with embolotherapy. *Hepatology* 1995; **21**: 96.

32 Rodman T, Sobel M, Close HP. Arterial oxygen unsaturation and the ventilation perfusion defect of Laennec's cirrhosis. *N. Engl. J. Med.* 1960; **263**: 73.

33 Ruff F, Hughes JMB, Stanley N *et al.* Regional lung function in patients with hepatic cirrhosis. *J. Clin. Invest.* 1971; **50**: 2403.

34 Sherlock S. The liver–lung interface. *Semin. Resp. Med.* 1988; **9**: 247.

35 Sherlock S. Vasodilatation associated with hepatocellular disease: relation to functional organ failure. *Gut* 1990; **31**: 365.

36 Stanley NN, Williams AJ, Dewar CA *et al.* Hypoxia and hydrothoraces in a case of liver cirrhosis: correlation of physiological, radiographic, scintigraphic and pathological findings. *Thorax* 1977; **32**: 457.

37 Stanley NN, Woodgate DJ. Mottled chest radiograph and gas transfer defect in chronic liver disease. *Thorax* 1972; **27**: 315.

38 Stark ME, Szurszewski JH. Role of nitric oxide in gastrointestinal and hepatic function and disease. *Gastroenterology* 1992; **103**: 1928.

39 Stoller JK, Moodie D, Schiavone WA *et al.* Reduction of intrapulmonary shunt and resolution of digital clubbing associated with primary biliary cirrhosis after liver transplantation. *Hepatology* 1990; **11**: 54.

40 Wernze H, Tittor W, Goerig M. Release of prostanoids into the portal and hepatic vein in patients with chronic liver disease. *Hepatology* 1986; **6**: 911.

41 Willett IR, Sutherland RC, O'Rourke MF *et al.* Pulmonary hypertension complicating hepato-cellular carcinoma. *Gastroenterology* 1984; **87**: 1180.

42 Williams A, Trewby P, Williams R *et al.* Structural alterations to the pulmonary circulation in fulminant hepatic failure. *Thorax* 1979; **34**: 447.

Fever and septicaemia

About one-third of patients with decompensated cirrhosis show a continuous low-grade fever which rarely exceeds 38°C. This is unaffected by antibiotics or by altering dietary protein. It seems to be related to the liver disease alone. Cytokines such as tumour necrosis factor may be responsible at least in alcoholics [8] (fig. 6.9). Cytokines released as part of the inflammatory response have undesirable effects particularly vasodilatation, endothelial activation and multi-organ failure.

The human liver is bacteriologically sterile and the portal venous blood only rarely contains organisms. However, in the cirrhotic, bacteria, particularly intesti-

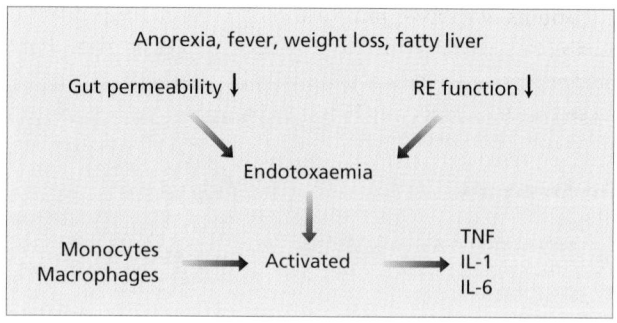

Fig. 6.9. Anorexia, fever, weight loss and a fatty liver in patients with hepato-cellular failure may be related to endotoxaemia with production of cytokines: tumour necrosis factor (TNF), interleukin 1 (IL1) and interleukin 6 (IL6).

nal, could reach the general circulation either by passing through a faulty hepatic filter or through porto-systemic collaterals [2].

Septicaemia is frequent in terminal hepato-cellular failure. Multiple factors contribute. Kupffer cell and polymorphonuclear function are impaired [3, 5]. Serum shows a reduction in factors such as fibronectin, opsonins and chemo-attractants, including members of the complement cascade. Systemic toxaemia of intestinal origin results in deterioration of the scavenger functions of the reticulo-endothelial system and also to renal damage [6] (fig. 6.9). These factors contribute to blood culture positive episodes. They are particularly important in spontaneous bacterial peritonitis which affects 75% of cirrhotic patients with ascites (Chapter 9).

Urinary tract infections are particularly common in cirrhotic patients and are usually Gram-negative. Indwelling urinary catheters play a part.

Pneumonia especially affects alcoholics. Community-acquired infection usually responds to erythromycin plus cefotaxine and septrin. Hospital-acquired infections are more serious and indicate a third-generation cephalosporin such as ceftaxidine. Other infections include lymphangitis and endocarditis [4]. Of patients with acute liver failure 50% show infections, often arising from soft tissues, the respiratory or urinary tract or central venous cannulas [7]. Clinical features may be atypical with inconspicuous fever, no rigors and only slight leucocytosis.

In both acute and chronic liver failure, about two-thirds of the infections are Gram-positive, often staphylococcal and Gram-negative in one-third [1, 7]. Grade C cirrhotics are usually affected. The hospital mortality is 38%. Bad prognostic features are an absence of fever, elevated serum creatinine and marked leucocytosis [1]. Recurrent infections are ominous and sufferers should be considered for liver transplant.

Patients with liver failure should receive prophylactic antibiotics during invasive practical procedures. Parenteral broad-spectrum antibiotics should be commenced when infection is suspected.

References

1 Barnes PF, Arevalo C, Chan LS *et al.* A prospective evaluation of bacteremic patients with chronic liver disease. *Hepatology* 1988; **8**: 1099.

2 Caroli J, Platteborse R. Septicémie porto-cave. Cirrhosis du foie et septicémie à colibacille. *Sem. Hôp. Paris* 1958; **34**: 472.

3 Imawari M, Hughes RD, Gove CD *et al.* Fibronectin and Kupffer cell function in fulminant hepatic failure. *Dig. Dis. Sci.* 1985; **30**: 1028.

4 McCashland TM, Sorrell MF, Zetterman RK. Bacterial endocarditis in patients with chronic liver disease. *Am. J. Gastroenterol.* 1994; **89**: 924.

5 Rajkovic IA, Williams R. Abnormalities of neutrophil phagocytosis, intracellular killing, and metabolic activity in alcoholic cirrhosis and hepatitis. *Hepatology* 1986; **6**: 252.

6 Rimola A, Soto R, Bory F *et al.* Reticuloendothelial system phagocytic activity in cirrhosis and its relation to bacterial infections and prognosis. *Hepatology* 1984; **4**: 53.

7 Rolando N, Harvey F, Brahm J *et al.* Prospective study of bacterial infection in acute liver failure: an analysis of fifty patients. *Hepatology* 1990; **11**: 49.

8 Yoshioka K, Kakumu S, Arao M *et al.* Tumor necrosis factor α production by peripheral blood mononuclear cells of patients with chronic liver disease. *Hepatology* 1989; **10**: 769.

Fetor hepaticus

This is a sweetish, slightly faecal smell of the breath which has been likened to that of a freshly opened corpse, or mice. It complicates severe hepato-cellular disease especially with an extensive collateral circulation. It is presumably of intestinal origin, for it becomes less intense after defaecation or when the gut flora is changed by wide-spectrum antibiotics. Methyl mercaptan has been found in the urine of a patient with hepatic coma who exhibited fetor hepaticus [1]. This substance can be exhaled in the breath and might be derived from methionine, the normal demethylating processes being inhibited by liver damage.

In patients with acute liver disease, fetor hepaticus, particularly if so extreme that it pervades the room, is a bad omen and often precedes coma. It is very frequent in patients with an extensive portal-collateral circulation, when it is not such a grave sign. Fetor may be a useful diagnostic sign in patients seen for the first time in coma.

Reference

1 Challenger F, Walshe JM. Fœtor hepaticus. *Lancet* 1995; **i**: 1239.

Changes in nitrogen metabolism

Ammonia metabolism (Chapter 9). The failing liver is unable to convert ammonia to urea.

Urea production is impaired, but the reserve powers of synthesis are so great that the blood urea concentration in hepato-cellular failure is usually normal. Low values may be found in fulminant hepatitis. Maximal rate of urea synthesis is a good measure of hepato-cellular function, but is too complicated for routine use [2].

Amino acid metabolism. An almost constant excess of amino acid is present in the urine [3]. In both acute and chronic liver disease a common pattern of plasma amino acids is found. The aromatic amino acids, tyrosine and phenylalanine, are raised together with methionine. The concentration of the three branched-chain amino acids, valine, isoleucine and leucine, is reduced [1]. This results in a lowering of the ratio of branched-chain to aromatic amino acids and this is irrespective of the presence or absence of hepatic encephalopathy.

Serum albumin level falls in proportion to the degree of hepato-cellular failure and its duration. Protein is absorbed and retained, but is not used for serum protein manufacture. The low serum protein values may also reflect an increased plasma volume.

Plasma prothrombin falls with the serum protein levels. The consequent prolonged prothrombin time is not restored to normal by vitamin K therapy. Other proteins concerned in blood clotting may be deficient. In terminal liver failure the bleeding diathesis may be so profound that the patient is exsanguinated by such simple procedures as a paracentesis abdominis (see Chapter 4).

References

1 Morgan MY, Milsom JP, Sherlock S. Plasma amino acid patterns in liver disease. *Gut* 1982; **23**: 362.

2 Rudman D, Di Fulco TJ, Galambos JT *et al.* Maximal rates of excretion and synthesis of urea in normal and cirrhotic subjects. *J. Clin. Invest.* 1973; **52**: 2241.

3 Walshe JM. Disturbances of amino-acid metabolism following liver injury. *Q. J. Med.* 1953; **22**: 483.

Skin changes

An older Miss Muffett
Decided to rough it
And lived upon whisky and gin.
Red hands and a spider
Developed outside her—
Such are the wages of sin. [1]

Vascular spiders [1, 3, 5]

Synonyms: *arterial spider, spider telangiectasis, spider angioma.*

Arterial spiders are found in the vascular territory of the superior vena cava and very rarely below a line joining the nipples. Common sites are the necklace area, the face, forearms and dorsum of the hand (fig. 6.10). They are rarely found in the mucous membrane of the nose, mouth and pharynx. They fade after death.

An arterial spider consists of a central arteriole, radiating from which are numerous small vessels resembling a spider's legs (fig. 6.11). It ranges in size from a pinhead to 0.5 cm in diameter. When sufficiently large it can be seen or felt to pulsate, and this effect is enhanced by pressing on it with a glass slide. Pressure on the central prominence with a pinhead causes blanching of the whole lesion, as would be expected from an arterial lesion.

Arterial spiders may disappear with improving hepatic function, whereas the appearance of fresh spiders is suggestive of progression. The spider may also disappear if the blood pressure falls due to shock or haemorrhage. Spiders can bleed profusely.

In association with vascular spiders, and having a similar distribution, numerous small vessels may be scattered in random fashion through the skin, usually on the upper arms. These resemble the silk threads in American dollar bills and the condition is called *paper money skin*.

A further association is the appearance of *white spots* on arms and buttocks on cooling the skin [3]. Examination with a lens shows that the centre of each spot represents the beginnings of a spider.

Vascular spiders are most frequently associated with cirrhosis, especially of the alcoholic. They may appear transiently with viral hepatitis. Rarely they are found in normal persons, especially children. During pregnancy,

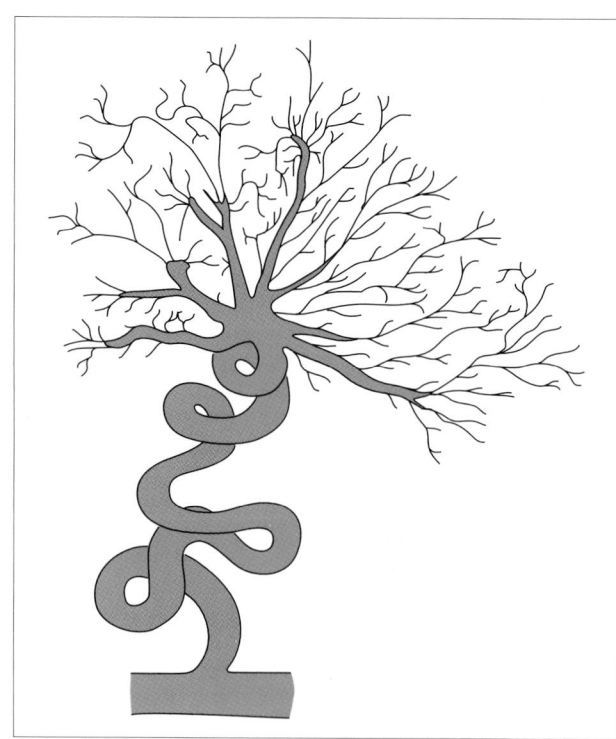

Fig. 6.11. Schematic diagram of an arterial spider [3].

they appear between the second and fifth months, disappearing within 2 months of delivery. A few spiders should not be sufficient to diagnose liver disease, but many new ones, with increasing size of old ones, arouse suspicion.

Differential diagnosis

Hereditary haemorrhagic telangiectasis. The lesions are usually on the upper body. Mucosal ones are common inside the nose, on the tongue, lips, palate, in the pharynx, oesophagus and stomach. The nail beds, palmar surfaces and fingers are frequently involved. Visceral angiography usually shows lesions elsewhere.

The telangiectasis is punctiform, flat or a little elevated, with sharp margins. It is connected with a single vessel, or with several, which makes it resemble the vascular spider. Pulsation is difficult to demonstrate.

The lesion is a thinning of the telangiectatic vessel but the veins show muscular hypertrophy [4].

Telangiectasia may be associated with cirrhosis. Calcinosis, Raynaud's phenomenon, sclerodactyly and telangiectasia (*CRST syndrome*) may be found in patients with primary biliary cirrhosis.

Campbell de Morgan's spots are very common, increasing in size and number with age. They are bright red, flat or slightly elevated and occur especially on the front of the chest and the abdomen.

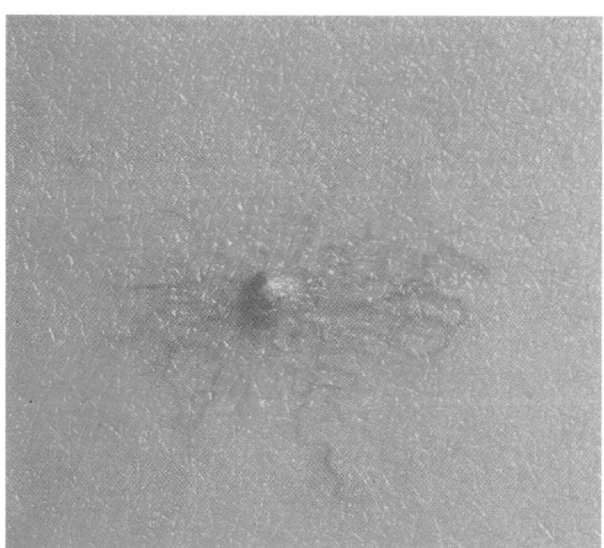

Fig. 6.10. A vascular spider. Note the elevated centre and radiating branches.

The venous star is found with elevation of venous pressure. It usually overlies the main tributary to a vein of large size. It is 2–3 cm in diameter and is not obliterated by pressure; the blood flow is from the periphery to the central collecting vein (opposite to that of the vascular spider). Venous stars are seen on the dorsum of the foot, legs, back and on the lower border of the ribs.

Palmar erythema (liver palms)

The hands are warm and the palms bright red in colour, especially the hypothenar and thenar eminences and pulps of the fingers (fig. 6.12). Islets of erythema may be found at the bases of the fingers. The soles of the feet may be similarly affected. The mottling blanches on pressure and the colour rapidly returns. When a glass slide is pressed on the palm it flushes synchronously with the pulse rate. The patient may complain of throbbing, tingling palms.

Palmar erythema is not so frequently seen in cirrhosis as are vascular spiders. Although both may be present, they may appear independently, making it difficult to define a common aetiology.

Many normal people have *familial* palmar flushing, unassociated with liver disease. A similar appearance may be seen in prolonged rheumatoid arthritis, in pregnancy, with chronic febrile diseases, leukaemia and thyrotoxicosis.

White nails

White nails, due to opacity of the nail bed, were found in 82 of 100 patients with cirrhosis and occasionally in certain other conditions (fig. 6.13) [2]. A pink zone is seen at the tip of the nail and in a severe example the lunula

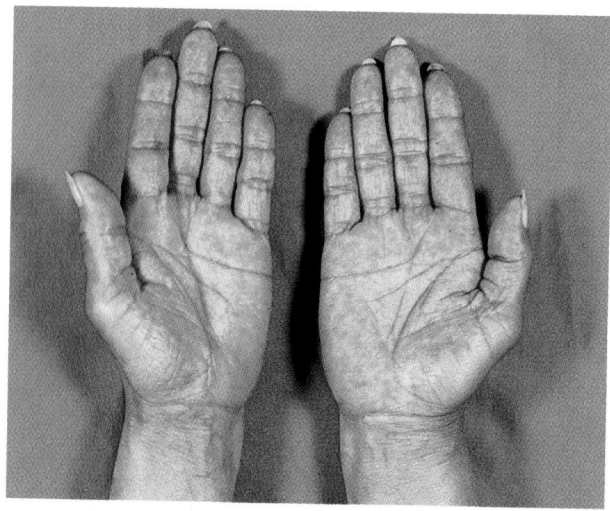

Fig. 6.12. Palmar erythema ('liver palms') in a patient with hepatic cirrhosis.

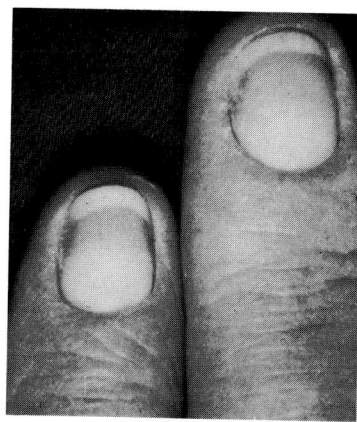

Fig. 6.13. White nails in a patient with hepatic cirrhosis.

cannot be distinguished. The lesions are bilateral, thumb and index being especially involved.

Mechanism of skin changes

The selective distribution of vascular spiders is not understood. Exposure of upper parts of the body to the elements may damage the skin so that it becomes susceptible to the development of spiders when the appropriate internal stimulus exists. Children may develop spiders on the knees and one nudist with cirrhosis was said to be covered with vascular spiders. The number of spiders does not correlate with the hyperdynamic circulation, although when the cardiac output is very high the spiders pulsate particularly vigorously.

The vascular spiders and palmar erythema have been traditionally attributed to oestrogen excess. They are also seen in pregnancy when circulating oestrogens are increased. Oestrogens have an enlarging, dilating effect on the spiral arterioles of the endometrium, and such a mechanism may explain the closely similar cutaneous spiders [1]. Oestrogens have induced cutaneous spiders in man [1] although this is not usual when such therapy is given for prostatic carcinoma. The liver certainly inactivates oestrogens although oestradiol levels in cirrhosis are often normal. The ratio between oestrogens and androgens may be more important. In male cirrhotics, although the serum oestradiol was normal, free serum testosterone was reduced. The oestradiol/free testosterone ratio was highest in male cirrhotics with spiders [5].

The aetiology of the other skin lesions remains unknown.

References

1 Bean WB. *Vascular Spiders and Related Lesions of the Skin.* Blackwell Scientific Publications, Oxford, 1959.

2 Lloyd CW, Williams RH. Endocrine changes associated with Laennec's cirrhosis of the liver. *Am. J. Med.* 1948; **4**: 315.

3 Martini GA. Über Gefässveränderungen der Haut bei Leberkranken. *Z. Klin. Med.* 1955; **150**: 470.

4 Martini GA, Straubesand J. Zur Morphologie der Gefässspinnen ('vascular spiders') in der Haut Leberkranker. *Virchows Arch.* 1953; **324**: 147.

5 Pirovino M, Linder R, Boss C *et al.* Cutaneous spider nevi in liver cirrhosis: capillary microscopical and hormonal investigations. *Klin. Wochenschr.* 1988; **66**: 298.

Endocrine changes

Endocrine changes may be found in association with cirrhosis. They are more common in cirrhosis of the alcoholic and if the patient is in the active, reproductive phase of life. In the male, the changes are towards feminization. In the female the changes are less and are towards gonadal atrophy.

Hypogonadism

Diminished libido and potency are frequent in men with active cirrhosis and a large number are sterile. The impotence and its severity are greater if the cirrhotic patient is alcoholic [7]. Patients with well-compensated disease may have large families.

The testes are soft and small. Seminal fluid is abnormal in some.

Secondary sexual hair is lost and men shave less often. Prostatic hypertrophy has a lower incidence in men with cirrhosis [5].

Other signs include female body habitus and a female escutcheon. Gynaecomastia is particularly common in alcoholics.

The female has ovulatory failure. The pre-menopausal patient loses feminine characteristics particularly breast and pelvic fat. She is usually infertile; menstruation is erratic, diminished or absent, but rarely excessive. Any breast or uterine atrophy is of little significance in the post-menopausal woman.

In women with non-alcoholic liver disease, sexual behaviour, desire, frequency and performance are not impaired [1].

Gynaecomastia, sometimes unilateral, is rare, and the incidence in cirrhotics may not differ from that of controls [6] (fig. 6.14). Total oestrogen/free testosterone and oestrodial/free testosterone ratios are higher in cirrhotic patients, but cannot be correlated with the presence of gynaecomastia.

The breasts may be tender. Enlargement is caused by hyperplasia of the glandular elements [5]. Young men with chronic active hepatitis may develop gynaecomastia but alcoholic liver disease is the commonest association.

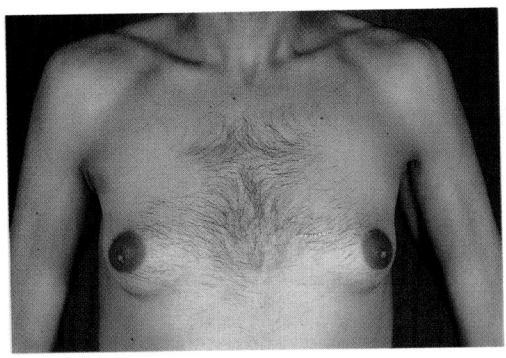

Fig. 6.14. Gynaecomastia in a patient with cirrhosis.

Spironolactone therapy is the commonest cause of gynaecomastia in cirrhotic patients. This decreases serum testosterone levels and reduces hepatic androgen-receptor activity [10].

Relation to alcohol

It is difficult to disentangle the hypothalamic–pituitary–gonadal dysfunction in patients with chronic liver disease from the aetiology of the liver disease and particularly from the effects of alcohol.

Feminization is more frequent with alcoholic cirrhosis than with other types. Acute administration of alcohol to normal men increases the hepatic metabolism of testosterone.

The hepatic uptake of sex steroids depends on liver function. Chronic administration of alcohol raises sex hormone binding globulin (SHBG) so reducing the free fraction of plasma testosterone and the amount presented to the liver [11]. However, low dehydroepiandosterone with raised oestradiol and androstenedione are found in patients with non-alcoholic liver disease [3]. The direct effect of alcohol on the testes may add to the general effects of liver disease. Acutely, alcohol also raises plasma gonadotrophins. Impotence is greater if the cirrhotic patient is alcoholic [7].

Mechanism

The three principal unconjugated oestrogens (oestrone, oestradiol and oestriol) are found in the plasma of normal men. They are produced by the testes and adrenals and also from peripheral conversion of major circulating androgens. Oestradiol is the most biologically potent oestrogen. It is bound to SHBG and to albumin. The biologically active unbound form is marginally raised in patients with cirrhosis and the total only minimally increased. The changes in plasma oestrogens are insufficient to account for the degree of feminization.

The human liver has both androgen and oestrogen

receptors which render it sensitive to androgens and oestrogens [9, 15]. Reduced oestrogen receptor concentrations in patients with chronic liver disease reflect the degree of liver dysfunction and not the specific type of liver disease [4]. In cirrhosis, the end organ sensitivities to sex hormones may be changed. Hepatic androgen receptors fall and hepatic oestrogen receptor concentrations increase [15].

Feminization may be related to hepatic regeneration [16]. Partial hepatic resection or liver transplantation are associated with increases in serum oestrogens and reductions in testosterone while oestrogen receptors increase [13].

Primary liver cancer occasionally presents with feminization [14]. Serum oestrone levels are high and can return to normal when the tumour is removed. The tumour can be shown to function as trophoblastic tissue.

Hypothalamic–pituitary function

Plasma gonadotrophins are usually normal although a minority of cirrhotic patients have high values. These normal levels, in spite of testicular failure, suggest either a primary testicular defect or a failure of the pituitary–hypothalamus. Impaired release of luteinizing hormone suggests a possible hypothalamic defect, at least in those with alcoholic liver disease [2].

Hypothalamic–pituitary dysfunction in some women with non-alcoholic liver disease may lead to amenorrhoea and oestrogen deficiency and also to osteoporosis [8].

Metabolism of hormones [12]

A reduced rate of hormonal metabolism might be related to a decrease in hepatic blood flow, to shunting of blood

through or around the liver or to an increase in SHBG which would reduce the free diffusible fraction of circulating hormone [11].

Steroid hormones are conjugated in the liver. Derivatives of oestrogens, cortisol and testosterone are conjugated as a glucuronide or sulphate and so excreted in the bile or urine. There seems to be little difficulty in the process even in the presence of hepato-cellular disease. The conjugated hormones excreted in the bile undergo an entero-hepatic circulation. In cholestasis the biliary excretion of oestrogens and especially of polar conjugates is greatly reduced. There are changes in the urinary pattern of excretion. Any failure of hormone metabolism results in a rise in blood hormone levels. This alters the normal homeostatic balance between secretion rates of hormones and their utilization. These feedback mechanisms between plasma hormone levels and hormone secretion prevent any but temporary rises in circulating levels. This may explain some of the difficulty in relating plasma hormone levels to clinical features.

Testosterone is converted to a more potent metabolite — dihydrotestosterone. It is degraded in the liver and conjugated for urinary excretion as 17-oxysteroids.

Oestrogens are metabolized and conjugated for excretion in urine or bile.

Cortisol is degraded primarily in the liver by a ring reduction to tetrahydrocortisone and subsequently conjugated with glucuronic acid (fig. 6.15).

Prednisone is converted to prednisolone.

References

1 Bach N, Schaffner F, Kapelman B. Sexual behavior in women with nonalcoholic liver disease. *Hepatology* 1989; **9**: 698.
2 Bannister P, Handley T, Chapman C *et al*. Hypogonadism in chronic liver disease: impaired release of luteinising hormone. *Br. Med. J.* 1986; **293**: 1191.
3 Bannister P, Oakes J, Sheridan P *et al*. Sex hormone changes in chronic liver disease: a matched study of alcoholic versus non-alcoholic liver disease. *Q. J. Med.* 1987; **63**: 305.
4 Becker U, Andersen J, Poulsen HS *et al*. Variation in hepatic estrogen receptor concentrations in patients with liver

Fig. 6.15. The metabolism of cortisol by the liver. In hepato-cellular disease there is difficulty in reducing the 4–3 ketonic group but not in conjugation. Urinary 17-ketosteroids and 17-hydroxycorticoids are therefore reduced.

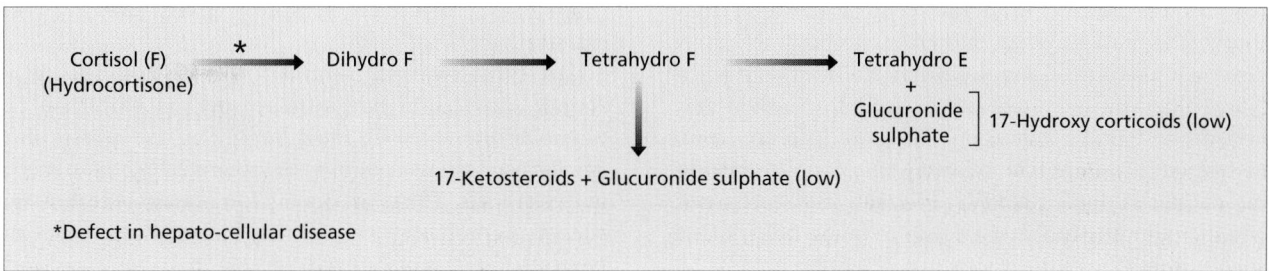

disease. A multivariate analysis. *Scand. J. Gastroenterol.* 1992; **27**: 355.

5 Bennett HS, Baggenstoss AH, Butt HR. The testis, breast and prostate of men who die of cirrhosis of the liver. *Am. J. Clin. Pathol.* 1950; **20**: 814.

6 Cavanaugh J, Niewoehner CB, Nuttall FQ. Gynecomastia and cirrhosis of the liver. *Arch. Intern. Med.* 1990; **150**: 563.

7 Cornely CM, Schade RR, Van Thiel DH *et al.* Chronic advanced liver disease and impotence: cause and effect? *Hepatology* 1984; **4**: 1227.

8 Cundy TF, Butler J, Pope RM *et al.* Amenorrhoea in women with non-alcoholic chronic liver disease. *Gut* 1991; **32**: 202.

9 Eagon PK, Elm MS, Stafford EA *et al.* Androgen receptor in human liver: characterization and quantitation in normal and diseased liver. *Hepatology* 1994; **19**: 92.

10 Francavilla A, Di Leo A, Eagon PK *et al.* Effect of spironolactone and potassium canrenoate on cytosolic and nuclear androgen and estrogen receptors of rat liver. *Gastroenterology* 1987; **93**: 681.

11 Guechot J, Vaubourdolle M, Ballet F *et al.* Hepatic uptake of sex steroids in men with alcoholic cirrhosis. *Gastroenterology* 1987; **92**: 203.

12 Johnson PJ. Sex hormones and the liver. *Clin. Sci.* 1984; **66**: 369.

13 Kahn D, Makowka L, Zeng P *et al.* Estrogen and androgen receptors in the liver after orthotopic liver transplantation. *Transplant Proc.* 1989; **21**: 409.

14 Kew MC, Kirschner MA, Abrahams GE *et al.* Mechanism of feminization in primary liver cancer. *N. Engl. J. Med.* 1977; **296**: 1084.

15 Porter LE, Elm MS, Van Thiel DH *et al.* Hepatic estrogen receptor in human liver disease. *Gastroenterology* 1987; **92**: 735.

16 Van Thiel DH, Stauber RE, Gavaler JS *et al.* Evidence for modulation of hepatic mass by estrogens and hepatic 'feminization'. *Hepatology* 1990; **12**: 547.

General treatment

Results are at the same time depressing and encouraging. Once the liver is disorganized, as in cirrhosis, it will never regain normal structure. Much can be achieved by symptomatic measures. The liver cells retain such an enormous regenerative capacity that, even though liver structure may not return to normal, functional compensation may be achieved.

Precipitating factors

Any factor depressing hepato-cellular function may throw the patient with hitherto compensated liver disease into failure. Gastrointestinal haemorrhage or the fall in blood pressure following surgical operation may necessitate blood transfusion. An acute infection must be treated. If failure has followed an alcoholic episode, the patient is denied alcohol. Electrolyte disturbances, whether diuretic-induced or due to some other factor such as vomiting or diarrhoea, must be corrected.

General measures

Bed rest reduces the functional demands on the liver. In the acute case, it is advisable; in the subacute and chronic case, bed rest is continued while improvement is maintained. If, after 4 weeks' bed rest, the condition remains static, the patient should be allowed moderate activity.

Diet. A high-protein diet may be of particular value in the alcoholic. In most cirrhotic patients 80–100 g protein and 2500 calories suffice. Fat need not be restricted within the calorie total. Folic acid may be deficient. Meals must be attractively presented — the patient with hepato-cellular failure has a fickle appetite, but if he can be persuaded to eat well clinical improvement will follow.

Diet is more important in the alcoholic who has been depriving himself of food than in the non-alcoholic who has usually been eating well.

Dietary supplements. Methionine, choline and amino acid supplements do not increase the rate of recovery. Very high methionine and cystine levels are found in the plasma in severe hepatitis and cirrhosis. There is no deficiency but rather difficulty in utilization.

Alcohol. Patients with acute hepato-cellular failure should abstain from all alcohol for between 6 months and 1 year after recovery. If alcoholism can be incriminated the patient should, if possible, become a total and life-long abstainer. If the chronic liver disease is non-alcoholic, one glass of wine or of beer daily will not be harmful.

Anaemia. The haemoglobin level must be kept above 10 g/100 ml. The anaemia may remit only when liver function improves.

Corticoid hormones. Prednisolone and ACTH do not affect the basic cirrhotic process. They have complications including an increased risk of serious infection.

Sex hormones. Hormone therapy to impotent men suffering from alcoholic cirrhosis may lead to the plasma hormone levels returning to normal but normal sexual potency is not restored. Cessation of alcohol and attention to social problems are more important than hormone therapy.

Oral testosterone has no beneficial effect in alcoholic cirrhosis other than to cause a slight decrease in gynaecomastia [1]. Mortality is increased.

Sedatives (Chapter 18). Morphine is very likely to precipitate coma.

Barbiturates vary in their mode of excretion. The long-acting, short-chain barbiturates such as barbitone or phenobarbitone are excreted largely by the kidney and small doses are reasonably well tolerated by the patient with cirrhosis. The short-acting, long-chain barbiturates such as pentobarbitone and the thiobarbitones such as pentothal are metabolized largely by the liver and should be avoided. If a barbiturate is used, the initial dose must be small.

Chlordiazepoxide (Librium) may lead to over-sedation in patients with liver disease [2]. The disposition of oxazepam is normal and this may be the drug of choice in cirrhosis [3].

References

1 Copenhagen Study Group for Liver Diseases. Testosterone treatment of men with alcoholic cirrhosis: a double blind study. *Hepatology* 1986; **6**: 807.

2 Roberts RK, Wilkinson GR, Branch RA *et al*. Effect of age and parenchymal liver disease on the disposition and elimination of chlordiazepoxide (Librium). *Gastroenterology* 1978; **75**: 479.

3 Shull HJ, Wilkinson GR, Johnson R *et al*. Normal disposition of oxazepam in acute viral hepatitis and cirrhosis. *Ann. Intern. Med.* 1976; **84**: 420.

Chapter 7
Hepatic Encephalopathy

Hepatic encephalopathy is a reversible neuropsychiatric state that complicates liver disease. The pathogenetic mechanism is not fully understood. Studies show derangement of several neurotransmitter systems. The changes are complex and no one defect provides a unifying explanation. The brain is exposed to increased levels of ammonia, neurotransmitters and their precursors because of failed hepatic clearance or the abnormal peripheral metabolism of the cirrhotic.

A spectrum of syndromes exists (table 7.1). In acute (fulminant) hepatic failure, encephalopathy accompanies the features of a virtual hepatectomy (Chapter 8). The encephalopathy of cirrhosis has portal-systemic shunting as a component but hepato-cellular dysfunction is also important; various precipitating factors play a part. Chronic neuropsychiatric states exist, usually in those with chronic portal–systemic shunting, and may be associated with irreversible brain damage. In these cases the hepato-cellular disease is relatively mild.

The different syndromes of hepatic encephalopathy also probably reflect the amount and range of 'toxic' metabolites/transmitters produced. The coma of acute liver failure, often with manic features and cerebral oedema, contrasting with the hypomanic lethargic picture of chronic encephalopathy, where astrocyte changes may occur.

Historical perspective

The relationship of the liver to mental function has been recognized from earliest times. The Babylonians (*circa* 2000 BC) attributed powers of augury and divination to the liver, designating it by the term also used for 'soul' or 'mood'. In the medicine of ancient China (Neiching 1000 BC) the liver was regarded as the storer of blood containing the soul. Hippocrates (460–370 BC) described a patient with hepatitis who 'barked like a dog, could not be held and said things which could not be comprehended'. Frerichs, the father of modern hepatology, described the terminal mental changes in patients with liver disease [23].

> Cases have occurred to me in which individuals who for a long period have suffered from cirrhosis of the liver have suddenly presented a series of morbid symptoms which are foreign to that disease. They have become unconscious, and have been afterwards seized with noisy delirium, from which they passed into deep coma and in this state have died.

It is now recognized that a neuropsychiatric syndrome of the same basic pattern may complicate liver disease of almost all types. It can culminate in coma and death.

Clinical features [1, 19, 65]

The picture is complex and affects all parts of the brain. There are neurological and psychiatric components. Variability between patients is a marked feature. The diagnosis may be easy — for example in the known cirrhotic admitted with gastrointestinal haemorrhage or sepsis, who is confused and on examination has a 'flapping' tremor. Without the clinical background data and obvious precipitating event, however, the slide into early hepatic encephalopathy may go unrecognized unless subtle changes of the syndrome are appreciated. A history obtained from a family member who has noticed a change may be valuable.

However, in cirrhotics with neuropsychiatric deterio-

Table 7.1. Factors in hepatic encephalopathy

Type of encephalopathy	% survival	Aetiological factors
Acute liver failure	20*	Viral hepatitis Alcoholic hepatitis Drug reactions and overdose
Cirrhosis with precipitant	70–80	Diuresis Haemorrhage Paracentesis Diarrhoea and vomiting Surgery Alcoholic excess Sedatives Infections Constipation
Chronic portal-systemic encephalopathy	100	Portal-systemic shunting Dietary protein intake Intestinal bacteria

* Without transplantation.

ration, particularly when sudden, the clinician should be on guard for the occasional patient with intracranial haemorrhage, trauma, infection or tumour with the associated neurological signs, as well as a drug-induced or other metabolic cause.

With hepatic encephalopathy, differences in clinical history and examination are usual, particularly in the more chronic cases. The picture depends on the nature and severity of aetiological and precipitating factors. Children may show a particularly acute reaction, often with mania.

For descriptive purposes, features of encephalopathy can be separated into changes in consciousness, personality, intellect and speech.

Disturbed consciousness with disorder of sleep is usual. Hypersomnia appears early and progresses to reversal of the normal sleep pattern. Reduction of spontaneous movement, a fixed stare, apathy and slowness and brevity of response are early signs. Further deterioration results in reaction only to intense or noxious stimuli. Coma at first resembles normal sleep, but progresses to complete unresponsiveness. Deterioration may be arrested at any level. Rapid changes in the level of consciousness are accompanied by delirium.

Personality changes are most conspicuous with chronic liver disease. These include childishness, irritability and loss of concern for family. Even in remission the patient may present similar personality features suggesting frontal lobe involvement. They are usually co-operative, pleasant people with an ease in social relationships and frequently a jocular, euphoric mood.

Intellectual deterioration varies from slight impairment of organic mental function to gross confusion. Isolated abnormalities appearing in a setting of clear consciousness relate to disturbances in visual spatial gnosis. These are most easily elicited as constructional apraxia, shown by inability to reproduce simple designs with blocks or matches (fig. 7.1). The *Reitan trail-making test* (fig. 7.2) may be used serially to assess progress [17]. Writing is oblivious of ruled lines and a daily writing chart is a good check of progress (fig. 7.1). Failure to distinguish objects of similar size, shape, function and position leads to symptoms such as micturating and defaecating in inappropriate places. Insight into such anomalies of behaviour is frequently preserved.

Speech is slow and slurred and the voice is monotonous. In deep stupor, dysphasia becomes marked and is always combined with perseveration.

Some patients have *fetor hepaticus*. This is a sour, faecal smell in the breath, due to volatile substances normally formed in the stool by bacteria. These mercaptans if not removed by the liver are excreted through the lungs and appear in the breath. Fetor hepaticus does not correlate with the degree or duration of encephalopathy and its absence does not exclude hepatic encephalopathy.

The most characteristic neurological abnormality is the 'flapping' tremor ('*asterixis*'). This is due to impaired inflow of joint and other afferent information to the brain-stem reticular formation resulting in lapses in posture. It is demonstrated with the patient's arms outstretched and fingers separated or by hyperextending the wrists with the forearm fixed (fig. 7.3). The rapid flexion–extension movements at the metacarpophalangeal and wrist joints are often accompanied by lateral movements of the digits. Sometimes arms, neck, jaw, protruded tongue, retracted mouth and tightly closed eyelids are involved and the gait is ataxic. Absent at rest, less marked on movement and maximum on sustained posture, the tremor is usually bilateral, although not bilaterally synchronous, and one side may be affected

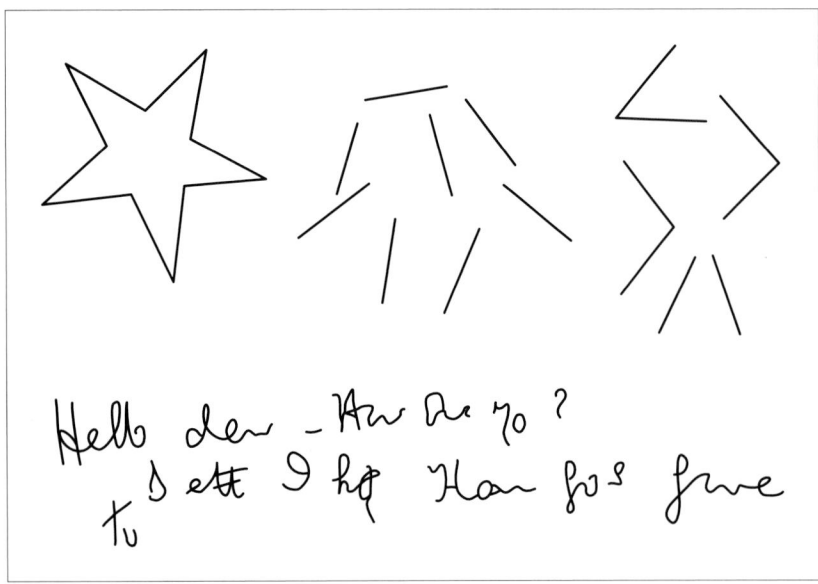

Fig. 7.1. Focal disorders in chronic portal-systemic encephalopathy elicited in patients with full consciousness and minimal intellectual defect, in the absence of gross tremor or visual disorder. (*Above*) Constructional apraxia. (*Below*) Writing difficulty. 'Hello dear. How are you? Better I hope. That goes for me too' [19].

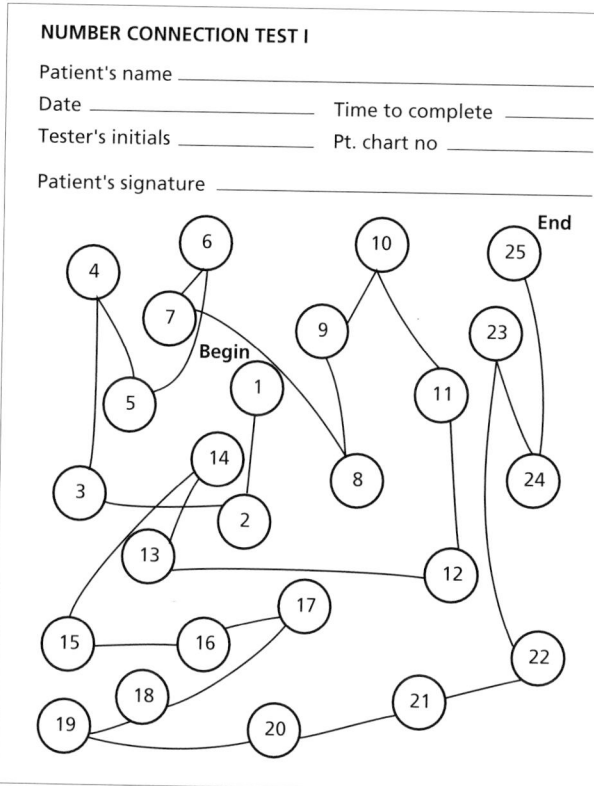

NUMBER CONNECTION TEST I

Patient's name _____

Date _____ Time to complete _____

Tester's initials _____ Pt. chart no _____

Patient's signature _____

Fig. 7.2. The Reitan number connection test.

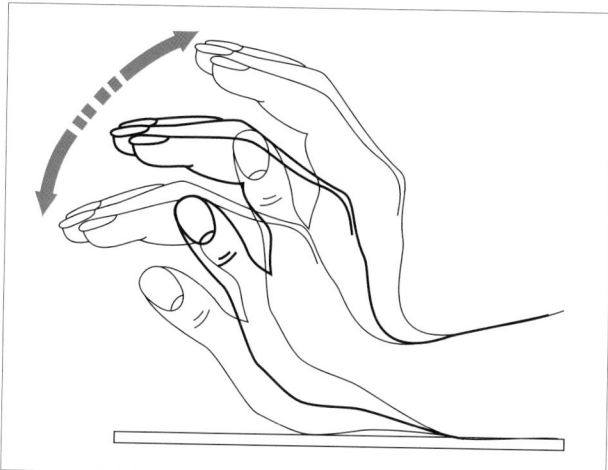

Fig. 7.3. 'Flapping' tremor elicited by attempted dorsiflexion of the wrist with the forearm fixed.

more than the other. It may be appreciated by gentle elevation of a limb or by the patient gripping the physician's hand. In coma the tremor disappears. A 'flapping' tremor is not specific for hepatic pre-coma. It can also be observed in uraemia, in respiratory failure and in severe heart failure.

Deep tendon reflexes are usually exaggerated. Increased muscle tone is present at some stage and sus-

tained ankle clonus is often associated with rigidity. During coma patients become flaccid and lose their reflexes.

The plantar responses are usually flexor becoming extensor in deep stupor or coma. Hyperventilation and hyperpyrexia may be terminal. The diffuse nature of the cerebral disturbance is further shown by excessive appetite, muscle twitchings, grasping and sucking reflexes. Disorders of vision include reversible cortical blindness [39].

The clinical course fluctuates, and frequent observation of the patient is necessary. Clinical grading should be used as a part of the clinical record of neuropsychiatric signs:

Grade 1. Confused. Altered mood or behaviour. Psychometric defects.

Grade 2. Drowsy. Inappropriate behaviour.

Grade 3. Stuporous but speaking and obeying simple commands. Inarticulate speech. Marked confusion.

Grade 4. Coma. Cannot be roused.

Investigations

Cerebrospinal fluid

This is usually clear and under normal pressure. Patients in hepatic coma may show an increased CSF protein concentration, but the cell count is normal. Glutamic acid and also glutamine may be increased.

Electroencephalogram [52]

There is a bilateral synchronous slowing of the wave frequency (with an increase in wave amplitude) from the normal α rhythm of 8–13 cycles per second (Hz) down to the δ range of below 4 cycles per second (fig. 7.4). This is best graded using frequency analysis. Alerting stimuli, such as opening the eyes, fail to reduce the background rhythmic activity. The change starts in the frontal or central region and progresses posteriorly.

This technique is useful for diagnosis and to assess treatment.

In very chronic cases with permanent neuronal damage, the tracing may be slow or rapid and flat. Such changes may be 'fixed' and unaltered by diet.

EEG changes occur very early even before psychological or biochemical disturbances. They are non-specific, being found also in conditions such as uraemia, CO_2 retention, vitamin B_{12} deficiency or hypoglycaemia. These changes, however, in a conscious patient with liver disease are virtually diagnostic.

Evoked potentials

These are electrical potentials from the sub-cortical and

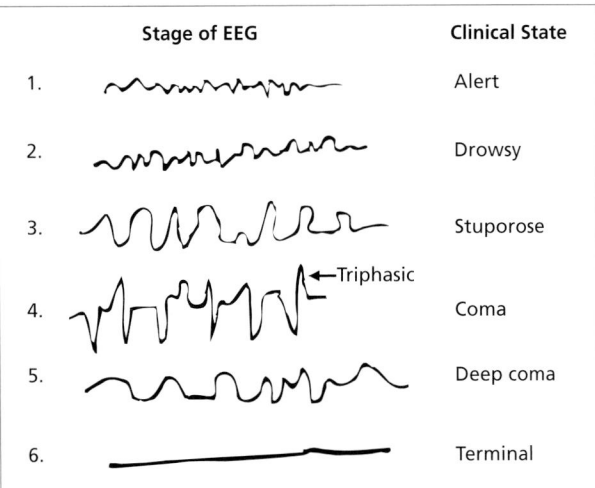

Stage of EEG	Clinical State
1.	Alert
2.	Drowsy
3.	Stuporose
4. ←Triphasic	Coma
5.	Deep coma
6.	Terminal

Fig. 7.4. Changes in EEG during phases of encephalopathy. There is a slowing in frequency with increasing amplitude until in stage 4 triphasic waves appear. The amplitude then decreases. Finally there is absence of rhythmic activity.

cortical neurones triggered by visual or auditory stimuli, or stimulation of somatosensory nerves. They test the conduction and function of afferent pathways between the stimulated peripheral tissue and the cortex. Abnormalities of visual (VEPs), brain-stem auditory (BAEPs) and somatosensory (SEPs) evoked potentials have been found in clinical and sub-clinical encephalopathy. They remain a research rather than clinical tool. Because the sensitivity has varied from one study to another, VEPs and BAEPs have little place in the evaluation of sub-clinical encephalopathy particularly compared with psychometric testing. The value of SEPs awaits further study [32].

A newer method recording event-related *endogenous* potentials is under study. The patient's co-operation is needed, limiting it to encephalopathy grade 0–2. Such visual P300 potentials have been found to be more sensitive than psychometric tests in cirrhotics with sub-clinical encephalopathy [31].

Brain scans

CT and MRI show cerebral atrophy even with apparently well-compensated cirrhosis and results are related to the severity of the liver dysfunction. Atrophy is particularly marked in those with chronic persistent encephalopathy and may be potentiated by alcoholism [71]. The CT scan can be quantitated to show cerebral oedema and cortical atrophy even in those with sub-clinical portal-systemic encephalopathy [7].

Increased signal in the basal ganglia on T_1-weighted MRI scanning in cirrhotic patients does not seem to relate to hepatic encephalopathy, but correlates with serum bilirubin [71] and blood manganese concentration [30].

Neuropathological changes [1, 74]

Grossly the brain may be normal, but cerebral oedema (fig. 8.3) is seen in about half of the patients, particularly the younger cases dying with prolonged deep coma.

Microscopically, the characteristic changes in patients with cirrhosis who die in hepatic coma are in astrocytes rather than neurones. The astrocytes proliferate and develop enlarged nuclei, prominent nucleoli, margination of chromatin and accumulation of glycogen — changes referred to as Alzheimer type 2 astrocytosis. These changes are found particularly in the cerebral cortex and basal ganglia and are related to hyperammonaemia [12]. Neurones show minor alterations. Early astrocyte changes are probably reversible.

In very long-standing cases, the structural changes may be irreversible and the patient unresponsive to treatment (chronic hepato-cerebral degeneration) [74]. Apart from the astrocytic changes there is cortical thinning with loss of neurones in cortex, basal ganglia and cerebellum.

Demyelination in the pyramidal tracts is associated with spastic paraplegia.

Experimental hepatic coma

In acute hepatic failure the blood–brain barrier shows increased permeability with specific alterations in transport systems [78]. However, in the precomatosed rat with galactosamine-induced hepatic failure there is no generalized increased permeability of the blood–brain barrier [35]. There are obvious difficulties in equating animal models with humans.

Clinical variants in cirrhotics

PRE-CLINICAL

Clinically inapparent impairment in mental functions, sufficient to cause disruption in the routine of everyday living, is frequent in patients with cirrhosis [70]. The picture is similar to that associated with lesions of the fronto-parietal regions of the brain. About three-quarters of patients with cirrhosis, and seemingly normal neurological and mental status, fail psychometric tests, impairment of performance being more marked than for verbal skills [24]. Only 18% of 71 cirrhotic patients attending an outpatient clinic gave normal psychometric tests, 48% had sub-clinical and 34% overt encephalopathy [45].

In Germany only 15% of patients with chronic liver disease and portal hypertension, clinically not encephalopathic, were judged fit to drive a car [64]. This contrasts with a study from Chicago [67] in a small selected group of cirrhotic patients some of whom had sub-clinical encephalopathy. Patients with previous episodes of overt encephalopathy and those on treatment were excluded. The simulated and real driving performance of the cirrhotic group did not differ from the matched control group.

ACUTE TYPE

The syndrome may appear spontaneously, without a precipitant, usually in a deeply jaundiced patient with ascites and in the terminal stages. Most cases are related to a precipitating factor. These act by depressing liver cell or cerebral function, increasing nitrogenous material in the intestine, or raising the portal–collateral flow (table 7.2).

The commonest precipitant is a brisk response to a potent *diuretic*. Large *paracenteses* may also precipitate coma; the mechanism is uncertain. Electrolyte imbalance following removal of large quantities of electrolytes and water, changes in hepatic circulation and hypotension may contribute. Other causes of fluid and electrolyte depletion, such as *diarrhoea* or *vomiting*, may be precipitants.

Gastrointestinal haemorrhage, usually from oesophageal varices, is another common precipitant. Coma is precipitated by the large protein meal (as blood) in addition to depression of hepato-cellular function due to anaemia and reduction in liver blood flow.

Surgical procedures are tolerated extremely poorly. Hepatic function is depressed by the blood loss, anaesthesia and 'shock'.

Table 7.2. Precipitants of acute hepatic encephalopathy in the cirrhotic patient

Electrolyte imbalance
Diuretics
Vomiting
Diarrhoea
Bleeding
Oesophageal and gastric varices
Gastro-duodenal erosions
Mallory–Weiss tear
Drugs
Alcohol withdrawal
Infection
Spontaneous bacterial peritonitis
Urinary
Chest
Constipation
Large protein meal

Acute alcoholism precipitates coma both by depressing cerebral function and by the associated acute alcoholic hepatitis. *Opiates* [33], *benzodiazepines* and *barbiturates* depress cerebral function and have a prolonged action when hepatic detoxication is delayed.

Infections, especially with bacteraemia and including 'spontaneous' bacterial peritonitis, may be the precipitant.

Coma may occasionally be initiated by a large *protein meal* or *severe constipation*.

Transjugular intra-hepatic portal-systemic shunts (TIPS) precipitate or worsen hepatic encephalopathy in about 20–30% of cases. This incidence varies depending on the patient population and selection [27, 62, 66]. As with surgical shunts, the wider the diameter of TIPS inserted, the more likely is encephalopathy.

CHRONIC TYPE

This relates to extensive portal-systemic shunting, which may consist simply of the myriad of small anastomotic vessels developing in the cirrhotic patient or, more often, one major collateral channel, such as the spleno-renal, gastro-renal, umbilical or inferior mesenteric vein.

Fluctuations in encephalopathy are related to dietary protein and diagnosis can be confirmed by noting the effect clinically and on the EEG of a precipitant such as a high-protein diet or by demonstrating improvement by protein withdrawal. Clinical and biochemical evidence of liver disease may be equivocal or absent, and the neuropsychiatric disorder may dominate the picture.

The intermittent neuropsychiatric disturbance may continue for many years [68] and the diagnosis is very likely to fall between various specialist interests. The psychiatrist is interested in the non-specific organic reaction and may not consider underlying liver disease. The neurologist focuses attention on the neurological features, while the hepatologist, recognizing the cirrhosis, fails to elicit the neurological signs or assumes that the patient is just 'odd' or an alcoholic. The patient may be seen for the first time in coma or in remission, adding to the diagnostic difficulty.

The *acute psychiatric states* often present shortly (2 weeks to 8 months) after porta-caval anastomosis as a paranoid-schizophrenic picture or as hypomania [60]. 'Classical' portal-systemic encephalopathy, with EEG slowing, is usually present in addition. Formal psychiatric treatment may be required as well as treatment of the hepatic encephalopathy.

HEPATO-CEREBRAL DEGENERATION: MYELOPATHY

More persistent neuropsychiatric syndromes are probably related to organic changes in the central nervous system, not only in the brain but also in the spinal cord

[74]. Progressive *paraplegia* may commence insidiously in those with a large portal-systemic collateral circulation. The encephalopathy is not severe. The spinal cord shows demyelination. The paraplegia is progressive and the usual treatment for portal-systemic encephalopathy is ineffective.

Chronic cerebellar and *basal ganglia* signs with parkinsonism, the tremor being unaffected by intention, may develop after some years of chronic hepatic encephalopathy [60, 74]. Permanent cerebral damage is probably present, for treatment has little effect on the tremor. *Focal cerebral symptoms*, epileptic attacks and dementia have also been noted [60].

Differential diagnosis

A *low sodium state* can develop in cirrhotic patients on a restricted sodium diet and having diuretics and abdominal paracenteses. This is shown by apathy, headache, nausea and hypotension. The diagnosis is confirmed by finding low serum sodium levels with a rise in blood urea concentration. The condition may be combined with impending hepatic coma.

Acute alcoholism [19] provides a particularly difficult problem especially as the two syndromes may coexist (see Chapter 20). Many symptoms attributed to alcoholism may be due to portal-systemic encephalopathy. Delirium tremens is distinguished by the continuous motor and autonomic over-activity, total insomnia, terrifying hallucinations and a finer, more rapid tremor. The patient is flushed, agitated, inattentive and perfunctory in his replies. Tremor, absent at rest, becomes coarse and irregular on activity. Profound anorexia, often with retching and vomiting, is common.

Portal-systemic encephalopathy in an alcoholic has similar features to that in the non-alcoholic except for the frequent absence of rigidity, hyperreflexia and ankle clonus due to concomitant peripheral neuritis. An EEG is helpful, as is the observation of a favourable response to dietary protein withdrawal, lactulose and neomycin.

Wernicke's encephalopathy is common with profound malnutrition and with alcoholism.

Hepato-lenticular degeneration (*Wilson's disease*) is found in young people, often with a family history. The symptoms do not fluctuate, the tremor is choreo-athetoid rather than 'flapping', the Kayser–Fleischer corneal ring is seen and disturbances in copper metabolism can usually be demonstrated.

Latent *functional psychoses*, such as depression or paranoia, are frequently released by impending hepatic coma. The type of reaction is related to the previous personality, and to intensification of personality traits. The psychiatric importance of the syndrome is emphasized by such patients often being admitted to mental hospitals. Conversely, a chronic psychiatric state in patients with known liver disease may not be related to the liver dysfunction. In such patients investigations are designed to demonstrate the chronic syndrome and in particular a large collateral circulation by venography or by CT scanning after intravenous contrast enhancement. Clinical and EEG changes induced by high and low protein feeding may also be useful.

Prognosis

Prognosis depends on the extent of liver cell failure. The chronic group with relatively good liver function but with an extensive collateral circulation combined with increased intestinal nitrogen have the best prognosis and the acute hepatitis group the worst. In cirrhosis, the outlook is poor if the patient has ascites, jaundice and a low serum-albumin level—all indicative of liver failure. If treatment is begun early in the precomatose state, the chances of success are increased. The prognosis is better if the precipitant can be treated, for instance infection, diuretic overdose or haemorrhage.

Assessment of therapy is made difficult by fluctuations in the clinical course. The value of any new method can only be assessed after large numbers of patients have been treated by controlled regimes. Results in patients with chronic encephalopathy (largely related to porto-systemic shunting) with recovery as the rule, must be separated from acute hepato-cellular failure in which recovery is rare.

Older patients have the added disadvantage of cerebral vascular disease. Children with portal vein obstruction having a portal-systemic shunt develop no intellectual or psychological side-effects [2].

Pathogenetic mechanisms

The essentially reversible nature of the syndrome with such widespread cerebral changes suggests a metabolic mechanism. However, no single metabolic derangement accounts for hepatic encephalopathy. The basic processes are failure of hepatic clearance of gut-derived substances, either through hepato-cellular failure or shunting (fig. 7.5), and altered amino acid metabolism, both of which result in changes in cerebral neurotransmission. Several neuroactive toxins, in particular ammonia, and neurotransmitter systems (table 7.3) are thought to be involved and interconnect. Reduced cerebral metabolic rates for oxygen and glucose found in hepatic encephalopathy are thought to be due to the reduced neuronal activity.

PORTAL-SYSTEMIC ENCEPHALOPATHY

Every patient with hepatic pre-coma or coma has a circulatory pathway through which portal blood may enter

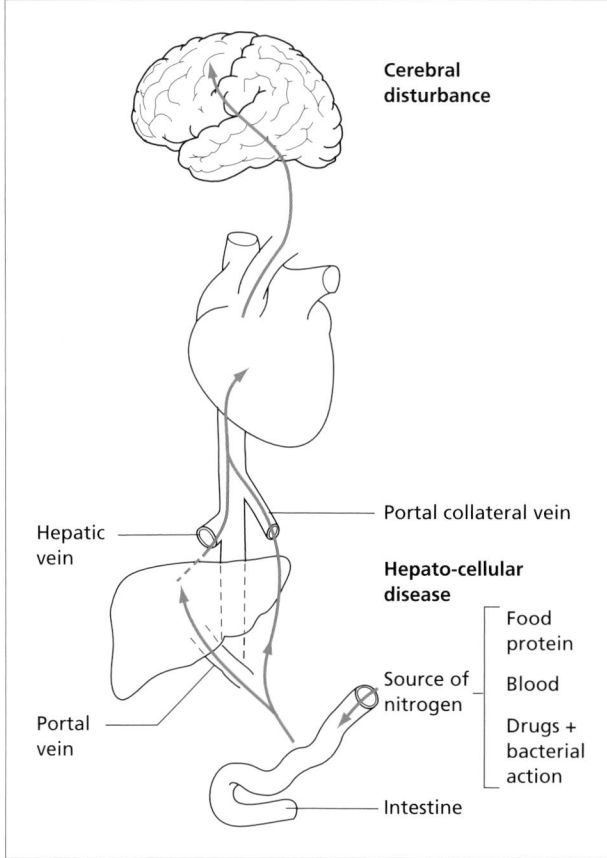

Fig. 7.5. The mechanism of portal-systemic encephalopathy [68].

the systemic veins and reach the brain without being metabolized by the liver [55].

In patients with poor hepato-cellular function, such as acute hepatitis, the shunt is through the liver itself. The damaged cells are unable to metabolize the contents of the portal venous blood completely so that they pass unaltered into the hepatic veins (fig. 7.5).

In patients with more chronic forms of liver disease, such as cirrhosis, the portal blood bypasses the liver through large natural 'collaterals'. The portal-hepatic vein anastomoses, developing around the nodules in a cirrhotic liver, may also act as internal shunts. The picture is a common complication of porta-caval anastomosis and TIPS. The condition is analogous to the neuropsychiatric disturbance developing in the dog with an Eck fistula (porta-caval shunt) if it is fed meat.

Encephalopathy is unusual if liver function is adequate. In hepatic schistosomiasis, where the collateral circulation is great and liver function good, coma is rare. If shunting is sufficiently great, however, encephalopathy may develop in the absence of obvious liver disease, for instance in extra-hepatic portal hypertension.

Patients going into hepatic coma are suffering from cerebral intoxication by intestinal contents which have not been metabolized by the liver (*portal-systemic encephalopathy*) [65]. The nature of the cerebral intoxicant is nitrogenous. A picture indistinguishable from impending hepatic coma can be induced in some patients with cirrhosis by the oral administration of a high-protein diet, ammonium chloride, urea, or methionine [54, 55, 65].

INTESTINAL BACTERIA

Symptoms can often be relieved by oral antibiotics. The intoxicants therefore seem to be produced by intestinal bacteria. Other measures which diminish the colonic flora, for instance colonic exclusion or purgation, may also be effective. Moreover, urea-splitting bacteria and the small intestinal flora generally are increased in patients with liver disease.

Table 7.3. Neurotransmitters implicated in hepatic encephalopathy

Neurotransmitter system	Normal action	Hepatic encephalopathy
Glutamate	Neuro-excitation	Dysfunction $\bullet$ $\downarrow$ receptors interference by NH_4^+
GABA/BZ	Neuro-inhibition	Increased endogenous BZs ??GABA
Dopamine Noradrenaline	Motor/cognitive	Inhibition false neurotransmitters (aromatic amino acids)
Serotonin	Arousal	?Dysfunction synaptic deficit? $\uparrow$ serotonin turnover

BZ, benzodiazepine.

Neurotransmission

Although there are many studies in experimental and human encephalopathy, the overall picture remains complex and in many areas conflicting and controversial. Definitive data are difficult to collect (table 7.4). Ammonia is thought to play an important role; other neurotransmitter systems are strongly implicated.

AMMONIA AND GLUTAMINE

Ammonia has been the most widely studied factor in the pathogenesis of hepatic encephalopathy. There is a considerable bank of data implicating it in the neuronal dysfunction that occurs (fig. 7.6) [48].

Ammonia is produced from the breakdown of proteins, amino acids, purines and pyrimidines. About half of the ammonia arising from the intestine is synthesized by bacteria, the remainder coming from dietary protein and glutamine. The liver normally converts ammonia to urea and glutamine. Disorders of the urea cycle (congenital defects, Reye's syndrome) lead to an encephalopathy.

In hepatic encephalopathy blood ammonia levels are elevated in 90% of patients. Brain levels are also increased. Encephalopathy can be reproduced in some patients by oral ammonium salts. Studies suggest that the permeability of the blood–brain barrier to ammonia is increased in cirrhotic patients [36].

Hyperammonaemia *per se* is associated with decreased excitatory neurotransmission. Ammonia intoxication leads to a hyperkinetic preconvulsive state which cannot be equated with hepatic coma.

The primary mechanisms proposed for ammonia in hepatic encephalopathy are a *direct* effect on neural membranes or on post-synaptic inhibition [69], and an *indirect* neuronal dysfunction due to disturbance of glutamate neurotransmission.

There is no urea cycle in the brain, and ammonia removal involves a different pathway. In astrocytes, glutamine synthetase converts glutamate plus ammonia to glutamine (fig. 7.7). With excess ammonia, glutamate (an important excitatory neurotransmitter) is depleted, and glutamine accumulates. CSF levels of glutamine and α-ketoglutarate correlate with the degree of encephalopa-

Table 7.4. Problem of investigating neurotransmitters in hepatic encephalopathy

---
Access to cerebral tissue
Lability of factors, e.g. NH3
Complexity of neurotransmitters
Applicability of animal models
Spectrum of human disease
Difficulty of interpreting ligand data which depend on:
   release
   metabolism (enzymes)
   removal/reuptake
   receptor binding

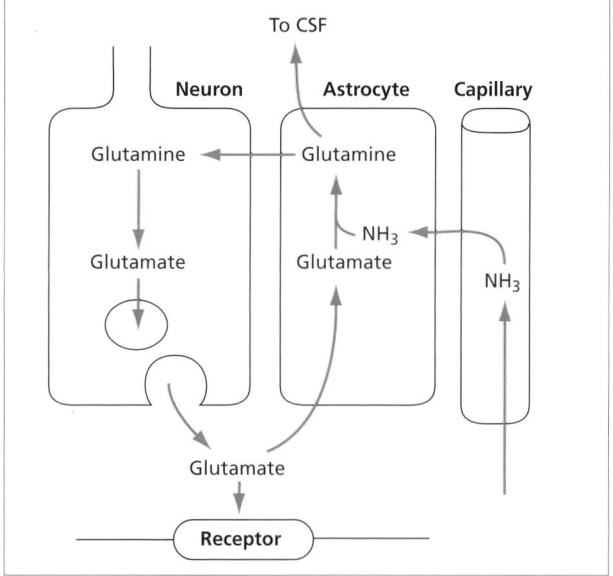

Fig. 7.7. Key steps in glutamatergic synaptic regulation and removal of ammonia by the brain. In the neuron, glutamate is synthesized from its precursor glutamine, stored in synaptic vesicles and ultimately released via a calcium-dependent mechanism. Once released glutamate can act upon any of the types of glutamate receptors found in the synaptic cleft. In the astrocyte, glutamate is taken up and converted to glutamine by glutamine synthetase using NH_3. In hepatic encephalopathy changes include increased cerebral NH_3, astrocyte damage, and a reduced number of glutamine receptors. (Reproduced with permission from [48].)

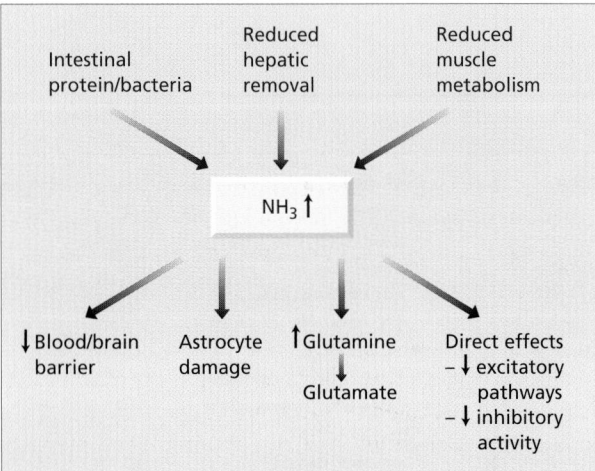

Fig. 7.6. Ammonia: source and potential role in hepatic encephalopathy.

thy. This description is, however, a simplification of the complex changes in glutamine/glutamate that have been found [48, 50]. A reduction in glutamate binding sites and in glutamate reuptake by astrocytes have been suggested.

The overall contribution of ammonia to the development of hepatic encephalopathy is difficult to quantitate, particularly since there are also changes in other neurotransmitter systems. That other mechanisms are involved is underlined by the finding that in 10% of patients with hepatic encephalopathy, blood ammonia values are within the normal range regardless of the depth of coma.

Methionine derivatives, mainly mercaptans, induce hepatic encephalopathy. This has led to the view that certain toxins, particularly ammonia, mercaptans, fatty acids and phenols act synergistically [79]. These observations need extension with the better techniques now available. However, in a recent study of experimental encephalopathy, methanephiol, an extremely toxic mercaptan, was not implicated in the pathogenesis of hepatic encephalopathy [11].

FALSE NEUROTRANSMITTERS

It has been proposed that dopamine and catecholamine-mediated cerebral neurotransmission is inhibited by amines generated either by bacterial action in the colon or by altered cerebral metabolism of precursors. The original hypothesis [22] suggested that decarboxylation of some amino acids in the colon leads to the formation of β-phenylethylamine, tyramine and octopamine—so-called false neurotransmitters. These might replace the true transmitter (fig. 7.8).

An alternative approach to interference with normal neurotransmission is based on a change in the availability of precursors. Thus plasma aromatic amino acids, tyrosine, phenylalanine and tryptophan, are increased in patients with liver disease probably due to failure of hepatic deamination. The branched-chain amino acids, valine, leucine and isoleucine, are decreased, perhaps due to increased metabolism by skeletal muscle and kidneys, secondary to the hyperinsulinaemia of chronic liver disease. The two groups of amino acids compete for uptake into the brain. The imbalance in plasma levels allows more aromatic amino acids to pass an abnormal blood–brain barrier. There may also be reduced efflux of aromatic amino acids from the brain [29]. An increase in phenylalanine level in the brain leads to inhibition of dopa production and the formation of false neurotransmitters such as phenylethanolamine and octopamine.

A change in this neurotransmitter system in hepatic encephalopathy has some support from the improve-

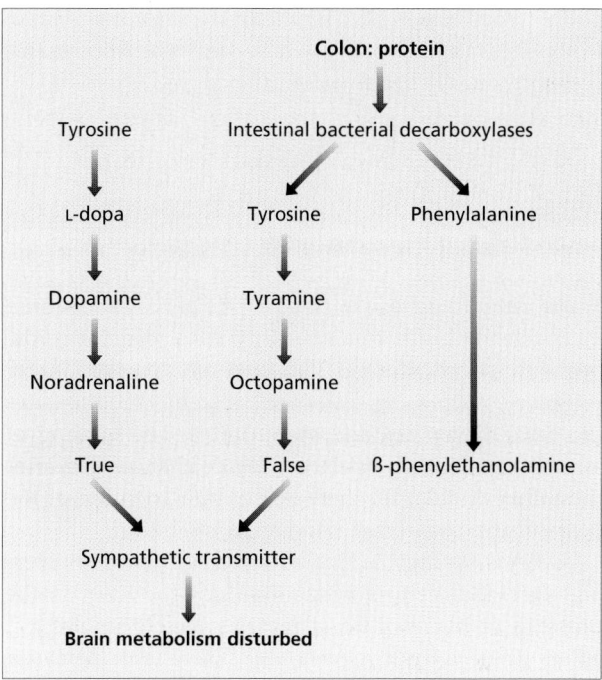

Fig. 7.8. The possible role of false sympathetic neurotransmitters in the disturbed cerebral metabolism in liver disease.

ment after L-dopa and bromocriptine treatment, but the number of patients who improve is limited and the results equivocal. Serum and urinary octopamine levels are increased in hepatic encephalopathy [38]. However, intraventricular infusion of enormous quantities of octopamine, with resulting depression of brain dopamine and adrenaline, failed to cause coma in normal rats [79]. Moreover, when brain catecholamines were measured post-mortem in cirrhotic patients with encephalopathy, no reduction was found compared with cirrhotics who were not encephalopathic at the time of death [18].

SEROTONIN

The neurotransmitter serotonin (5-hydroxytryptamine) is involved in the control of cortical arousal and thus the conscious state and the sleep/wake cycle. The precursor tryptophan is one of the aromatic amino acids increased in the plasma in liver disease. It is also increased in the CSF and brain of patients with hepatic coma and therefore has the potential to increase brain serotonin synthesis. In hepatic encephalopathy there are also other changes in serotonin metabolism including related enzymes (mono-amine oxidase), receptors and metabolites (5-HIAA). These changes, together with the appearance of encephalopathy in patients with chronic liver disease treated with ketanserin (a 5-HT blocker) for portal hypertension [75], implicate the serotonin system in hepatic encephalopathy. Where the dysfunction in this system primarily lies awaits further study.

GAMMA-AMINOBUTYRIC ACID (GABA) AND ENDOGENOUS BENZODIAZEPINES

GABA is the principal inhibitory neurotransmitter in the brain. It is usually synthesized from glutamate by glutamate dehydrogenase in presynaptic nerves and stored in vesicles. It binds to a specific GABA receptor in the post-synaptic membrane. This receptor is part of a larger receptor complex (fig. 7.9) which also has binding sites for benzodiazepines and barbiturates. The binding of any of these ligands opens a chloride channel and after the influx of chloride there is hyperpolarization of the post-synaptic membrane, and neuroinhibition.

GABA is synthesized by gut bacteria, and that entering the portal vein is metabolized by the liver. In the presence of liver failure or portal systemic shunting it enters the systemic circulation. There are increased GABA levels in the plasma of patients with liver disease and hepatic encephalopathy [34]. Suggestions that GABA might be involved in hepatic encephalopathy came mainly from experimental models of acute liver failure, but in subsequent studies in autopsied brain tissue from cirrhotic patients with encephalopathy, GABA *per se* does not seem to be involved.

However, the focus on the GABA–benzodiazepine receptor complex led to data suggesting that endogenous benzodiazepines are present in patients with hepatic encephalopathy and that these may interact with the receptor complex and cause neuroinhibition. Although benzodiazepine receptors are not altered in experimental or clinical hepatic encephalopathy, benzodiazepine-like compounds have been detected in the plasma and CSF of patients with hepatic encephalopathy due to cirrhosis [49] and in the plasma

in fulminant hepatic failure [5]. Cirrhotics with hepatic encephalopathy who had taken no synthetic benzodiazepines for at least 3 months showed significantly higher values for benzodiazepine activity than controls without liver disease, using a radioreceptor assay [49]. Severity of encephalopathy correlated with benzodiazepine activity in urine and plasma. Stool from cirrhotic patients contains five times the benzodiazepine-like activity as stool from controls [3].

However, it remains unclear whether the changes in the benzodiazepine receptor or endogenous ligands are significant pathogenetically or are simply associated phenomena. The endogenous benzodiazepine-receptor ligands require characterization and must be demonstrated in the central nervous system in sufficient quantities to induce encephalopathy [13]. Nevertheless involvement of this neurotransmitter system is consistent with the increased sensitivity to benzodiazepines of cirrhotic patients [6]. Moreover the benzodiazepine antagonist flumazemil reverses encephalopathy temporarily (the drug has a short half-life) in some patients.

OTHER METABOLIC ABNORMALITIES

These patients are often alkalotic. This may result from toxic stimulation of the respiratory centre by ammonium, from administration of alkalis such as citrate in transfusions or with potassium supplements, or from hypokalaemia.

Urea synthesis consumes bicarbonate. Progressive loss of urea cycle capacity is associated with increased plasma bicarbonate levels (and metabolic alkalosis) and ammonia excretion by the kidney increases [26].

Hypoxia increases cerebral sensitivity to ammonia. The stimulation of the respiratory centre results in increase in depth and rate of respiration. Hypocapnia follows and this reduces cerebral blood flow. The in-

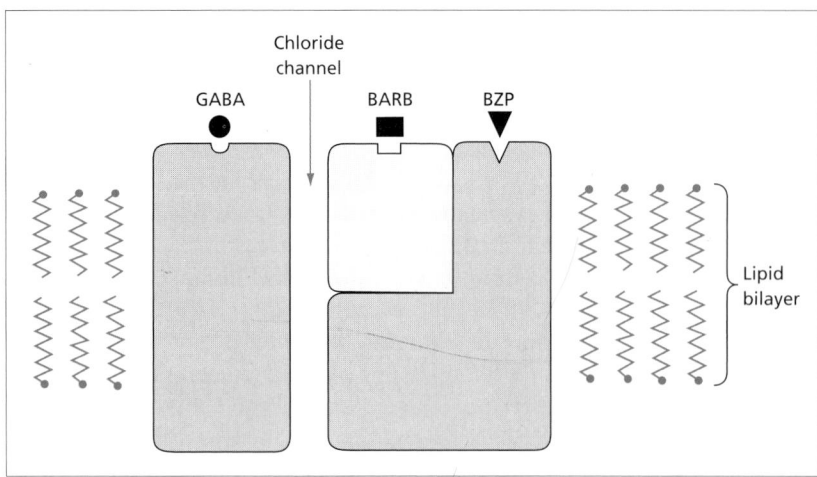

Fig. 7.9. Simplified model of the GABA-receptor/ionophore complex embedded in a post-synaptic neural membrane. Binding of any of the depicted ligands, GABA, barbiturates (BARB) or benzodiazepines (BZP), to its specific binding site increases chloride-ion conductance through the membrane with resultant hyperpolarization and neuroinhibition [63].

crease in the blood organic acids (lactate and pyruvate) is correlated with the reduction in CO_2 tension.

Any potent diuretic can precipitate hepatic coma. This may be related to hypokalaemia [16] and to readier penetration of ammonium ions through the blood–brain barrier in the presence of alkalosis. In addition to hypokalaemia, other electrolyte disturbances or a profound diuresis seem to initiate encephalopathy.

There are similarities between manganese neurotoxicity and chronic hepatic encephalopathy. Blood and brain manganese levels are increased in patients with cirrhosis and hepatic encephalopathy, and the signal from the globus pallidus on MRI scan is increased [30]. Such MRI changes are, however, also seen in cirrhotic patients without encephalopathy [71] leaving the link between manganese and hepatic encephalopathy unproven.

CHANGES IN CARBOHYDRATE METABOLISM

The hepatectomized dog dies in hypoglycaemic coma. Hypoglycaemic episodes are rare in chronic liver disease but may complicate fulminant hepatitis (Chapter 8).

Alpha-ketoglutaric and pyruvic acids are transported from the periphery to the metabolic pool in the liver, and blood levels increase as the neurological state deteriorates. These levels probably reflect severe liver damage. The fall in blood ketones also reflects severity of hepatic dysfunction. There is progressive impairment of intermediate carbohydrate metabolism as the liver fails.

Conclusion

No unifying mechanism explains hepatic encephalopathy. The brain controls neuropsychiatric behaviour through multiple inhibitory and stimulatory receptor-mediated pathways. Although neurotransmitters are produced locally they depend upon substrates and influences from further afield (fig. 7.10). When the liver fails or there is portal-systemic shunting there is a complex pattern of changes which influence multiple neurotransmitter systems.

Of the systems discussed, the effects of ammonia appear central to hepatic encephalopathy, with changes in glutamate, serotonin and endogenous benzodiazepine-mediated neurotransmission awaiting further study. The place of false neurotransmitters and GABA appears less persuasive than initially thought.

Cerebral metabolism is undoubtedly abnormal in liver disease. This is thought to be an effect rather than the cause of neurotransmitter-mediated changes. In the chronic case, actual structural changes in the brain can be demonstrated. The end result is a brain with abnormal neurotransmitter function, which is unduly sensitive to insults (opiates, electrolyte imbalance, sepsis, hypotension, hypoxia) that would be without effect in the normal patient.

Treatment of hepatic encephalopathy [41]

Treatment (table 7.5) broadly divides into three areas.

1 Identification and treatment of the precipitating cause.

2 Intervention to reduce the production and absorption of gut-derived ammonia and other toxins. This involves reduction and modification of dietary protein, alteration of enteric bacteria and the colonic environment (antibiotics, lactulose/lactilol), and stimulation of colonic emptying (enemas, lactulose/lactilol).

3 Prescription of agents to modify neurotransmitter balance directly (bromocriptine, flumazemil), or indirectly (branched-chain amino acids). These are of limited clinical value at present.

The choice of treatment depends on the clinical picture: sub-clinical, acute, or persistent chronic encephalopathy.

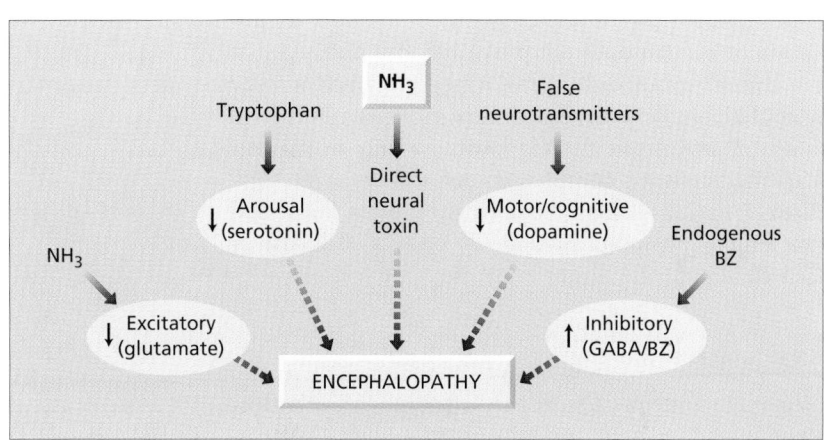

Fig. 7.10. Multifactorial mechanism of hepatic encephalopathy. The altered neurotransmitter state leaves the brain more sensitive to other insults including narcotics, sepsis, hypoxia and hypotension.

Table 7.5. Treatment of hepatic pre-coma and coma

Acute
1 Identify precipitating factor
2 Empty bowels of nitrogen-containing materials
   (a) stop haemorrhage
   (b) phosphate enema
3 Protein-free diet
   Raise dietary protein slowly with recovery
4 Lactulose or lactilol
5 Neomycin 1 g four times a day by mouth for 1 week
6 Maintain calorie, fluid and electrolyte balance
7 Stop diuretics, check serum electrolyte levels

Chronic
1 Avoid nitrogen-containing drugs
2 Protein, largely vegetarian intake, at limit of tolerance
   (about 50 g daily)
3 Ensure at least two free bowel movements daily
4 Lactulose or lactilol
5 If symptoms worsen adopt the regime for acute coma

DIET

In the acute attack dietary protein is reduced to 20 g/day. Calorie intake is maintained at 2000 calories/day or above, orally or intravenously.

During recovery, protein is added in 10 g increments on alternate days. Any relapse is treated by a return to the previous level. In patients after an acute episode of coma, a normal protein intake is soon achieved. In the chronic group, permanent protein restriction is needed to control mental symptoms [68]: the limits of tolerance are usually 40–60 g/day.

Vegetable protein is tolerated better than animal protein [72]. It is less ammoniagenic and contains small amounts of methionine and aromatic amino acids. It is also more laxative and increases the intake of dietary fibre so that there is increased incorporation and elimination of nitrogen contained in faecal bacteria [77]. It may be difficult to take because of flatulence, diarrhoea and bulk.

In the acute case, a few days' to a few weeks' deprivation of protein does not prove harmful and, even in the chronic group in whom dietary protein has to be restricted for many months, clinical protein malnutrition is rare. Protein restriction is indicated only in patients showing signs of encephalopathy. Others with liver disease may benefit from a high protein diet, and this may be achieved in combination with lactulose or lactitol.

ANTIBIOTICS

Neomycin, given orally, is very effective in decreasing gastrointestinal ammonium formation [20]. Little is absorbed from the gut although blood levels have been detected and impaired hearing or deafness may follow its long-term use. Thus it should only be used for the acute case for 5–7 days (4–6 g/day in divided doses). Clinical improvement is difficult to correlate with the changes in faecal flora [20].

Metronidazole (200 mg four times per day orally) seems to be as effective as neomycin [40]. Because of dose-related central nervous system toxicity, it should not be used long-term. In acute hepatic coma, lactulose is given, and neomycin added if the response is slow or partial. Surprisingly the two drugs seem to act synergistically [76], perhaps because of action on different bacterial populations.

LACTULOSE (fig. 7.11) [8] AND LACTILOL (table 7.6)

The human intestinal mucosa does not have an enzyme to split these synthetic disaccharides. When given by mouth *lactulose* reaches the caecum where it is broken down by bacteria predominantly to lactic acid. The faecal pH drops. The growth of lactose-fermenting organisms is favoured and organisms such as bacteroides, which are ammonia formers, are suppressed. It may 'detoxify' short-chain fatty acids produced in the presence of blood and proteins. The colonic fermentative bacteria prefer lactulose to blood when both are present [47]. It may be of particular value in hepatic encephalopathy induced by bleeding. The osmotic volume of the colon is increased.

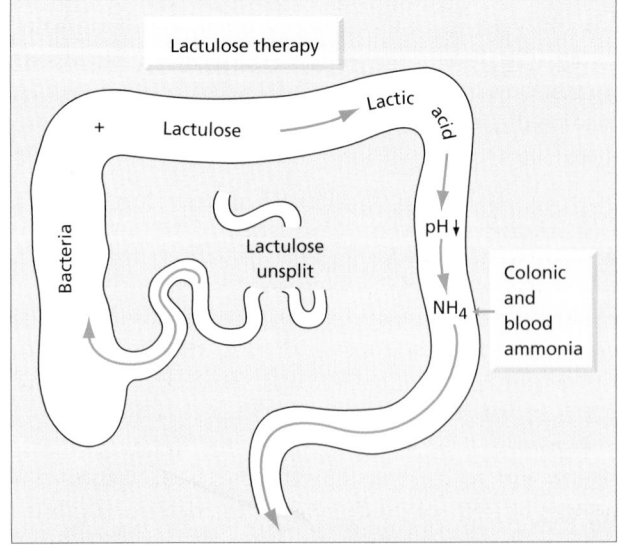

Fig. 7.11. Lactulose reaches the colon unsplit. It is then converted by bacteria to organic acids and an acid stool results. This may also affect the ionization of ammonia in the colon and reduce its absorption.

Table 7.6. The effects of lactilol compared with lactulose

Colonic effects similar
As effective in encephalopathy
Quicker action
More convenient (powder)
Less sweet
Less diarrhoea and flatulence

The mode of action is uncertain. Faecal acidity would reduce the ionization of ammonia and hence absorption of ammonia (also amines and other toxic nitrogenous compounds); faecal ammonia is not increased. Lactulose more than doubles the colonic output of bacterial mass and 'soluble' nitrogen [77]. This is no longer available for absorption as ammonia and a reduced urea production results [77].

The aim is to produce acid stools without diarrhoea. The dose is 10–30 ml three times a day and is adjusted to produce two semi-soft stools daily.

Side-effects include flatulence, diarrhoea and intestinal pain. Diarrhoea can be so profound that serum sodium increases to over 145 mmol/l, serum potassium falls and alkalosis develops. The blood volume falls so impairing renal function. These side-effects are particularly likely if the daily dose exceeds 100 ml. Some of the side-effects may be related to contamination of lactulose syrup with other sugars. Crystalline lactulose may be less toxic.

Lactilol (β-galactoside sorbitol) is a second-generation disaccharide easily produced in chemically pure, crystalline form which can be dispensed as a powder. It is not broken down or absorbed in the small intestine, but is metabolized by colonic bacteria [53]. As a powder, it is more convenient than the liquid lactulose and can be used as a sweetening agent. It is more palatable (tasting less sugary). The dose is approximately 30 g daily.

Lactilol seems to be as effective as lactulose in chronic [44] and acute portal-systemic encephalopathy. Patients respond more quickly to lactilol than lactulose, and there is less diarrhoea and flatulence [10, 44].

Lactilol and lactulose have been used for the treatment of sub-clinical hepatic encephalopathy [46]. Psychometric performance improved. A dose of lactitol of 0.3–0.5 g/kg per day is well tolerated and effective [61].

Purgation. Hepatic encephalopathy follows constipation and remissions are associated with return to a normal bowel action. The value of enemas and purgation with magnesium sulphate in patients with hepatic coma must be emphasized. Lactulose or lactose enemas may be used and are superior to water [73]. All enemas must be neutral or acid to reduce ammonium absorption. Magnesium sulphate enemas can cause dangerous hypermagnesaemia [15]. Phosphate enemas are safe.

OTHER PRECIPITATING FACTORS

Patients are extremely sensitive to sedatives and whenever possible these are avoided. If an overdose is suspected, the appropriate antagonist should be given. If the patient is uncontrollable and some sedation is necessary, a small dose of temazepam or oxazepam is given; morphine and paraldehyde are absolutely contraindicated. Chlordiazepoxide and heminevrin are valuable in the alcoholic with impending hepatic coma. Drugs known to induce hepatic coma such as oral amino acids and diuretics are disallowed.

Potassium deficiency can be treated by fruit juices or by effervescent or slow-release potassium chloride. If it is urgent, potassium chloride may be added to an intravenous infusion.

LEVODOPA AND BROMOCRIPTINE

If portal-systemic encephalopathy is related to a defect in dopaminergic neurotransmission then replenishment of cerebral dopamines should be beneficial. Dopamine does not pass the blood–brain barrier, but its precursor, levodopa, does and can cause temporary arousal in acute hepatic encephalopathy [37]. However, only a few patients benefit.

Bromocriptine is a specific dopamine receptor agonist with a prolonged action. As an adjunct to protein restriction and lactulose it has given clinical, psychometric and electro-encephalographic improvement in chronic portal-systemic encephalopathy [42]. It should be considered in the rare patient with intractable chronic portal-systemic encephalopathy and good, stable liver function resistant to dietary protein restriction and lactulose.

FLUMAZENIL

This is a benzodiazepine-receptor antagonist which can induce transient, variable but distinct improvement in about 70% of patients with hepatic encephalopathy associated with fulminant liver failure or cirrhosis [4, 25]. A randomized trial has confirmed the effect, and suggested that it may be blocking the effect of benzodiazepine-receptor agonist ligands synthesized *in situ* in the brain in liver failure [57]. The place of this group of compounds in the clinical situation has yet to be established.

BRANCHED-CHAIN AMINO ACIDS

A reduced ratio of branched-chain to aromatic amino acids has been related to the development of hepatic encephalopathy. Infusions of solutions containing a high concentration of branched-chain amino acids have been used to treat acute and chronic hepatic encephalopathy. Results have been extremely conflicting, perhaps related to differences in the nature of amino acid solutions, the ways of administration and the patients studied. Analysis of controlled trials shows that there is no consensus that intravenous branched-chain amino acids control hepatic encephalopathy [43].

Considering the high cost of intravenous amino acid mixtures, it is difficult to justify their use in hepatic encephalopathy where branched-chain amino acid blood levels are high anyway.

Despite individual studies showing benefit of oral branched-chain amino acid treatment [56] the benefit of this expensive treatment remains controversial [21, 41].

SHUNT OCCLUSION

Surgical shunt occlusion can reverse the severe portal-systemic encephalopathy following a porta-caval anastomosis. This may be preceded by an oesophageal transection to avoid the risk of re-bleeding [9]. Alternatively the shunt may be occluded by invasive radiology with the insertion of a balloon [58] or a steel coil [14]. This may also be done for a spontaneous spleno-renal shunt [28].

TEMPORARY HEPATIC SUPPORT

Complicated methods of temporary hepatic support are not applicable to hepatic coma in the cirrhotic. Such a patient is either terminal or can be expected to come out of coma without them. They are discussed under acute hepatic failure (Chapter 8).

HEPATIC TRANSPLANTATION

This may be the ultimate answer to the problem of chronic hepatic encephalopathy. One patient with a history of 3 years showed marked improvement lasting 9 months following transplantation [51]. Another patient with chronic hepatocerebral degeneration and spastic paraparesis showed remarkable improvement after orthotopic liver transplantation [59]. (See also Chapter 35.)

References

1 Adams RD, Foley JM. The neurological disorder associated with liver disease. *Res. Publ. Assn. Res. Nerv. Ment. Dis.* 1953; **32**: 198.

2 Alagille D, Carlier J-C, Chiva M *et al.* Long-term neuropsychological outcome in children undergoing portal-systemic shunts for portal vein obstruction without liver disease. *J. Pediat. Gastroenterol. Nutr.* 1986; **5**: 861.

3 Aronson L, Gacad RC, Kaminsky-Russ K *et al.* Evidence of gut production of 'endogenous' benzodiazepines: implications for hepatic encephalopathy. *Gastroenterology* 1996; **110**: A1144.

4 Bansky G, Meier PJ, Riederer E *et al.* Effects of the benzodiazepine receptor antagonist flumazenil in hepatic encephalopathy in humans. *Gastroenterology* 1989; **97**: 744.

5 Basile AS, Harrison PM, Hughes RD *et al.* Relationship between plasma benzodiazepine receptor ligand concentrations and severity of hepatic encephalopathy. *Hepatology* 1994; **19**: 112.

6 Batki G, Fisch HU, Karlaganis G *et al.* Mechanism of the excessive sedative response of cirrhotics to benzodiazepines. Model experiments with triazolam. *Hepatology* 1987; **7**: 629.

7 Bernthal P, Hays A, Tarter RE *et al.* Cerebral CT scan abnormalities in cholestatic and hepato-cellular disease and their relationship to neuro-psychologic test performance. *Hepatology* 1987; **7**: 107.

8 Bircher J, Haemmerli UP, Scollo-Lavizzari G *et al.* Treatment of chronic portal–systemic encephalopathy with lactulose. *Am. J. Med.* 1971; **51**: 148.

9 Bismuth H, Houssin D, Grange D. Suppression of the shunt and esophageal transection: a new technique for the treatment of disabling postshunt encephalopathy. *Am. J. Surg.* 1983; **146**: 392.

10 Blanc P, Daures J-P, Rouillon J-M *et al.* Lactitol or lactulose in the treatment of chronic hepatic encephalopathy: results of a meta-analysis. *Hepatology* 1992; **15**: 222.

11 Blom HJ, Chamuneau RAFM, Rothuizen J *et al.* Methanethiol metabolism and its role in the pathogenesis of hepatic encephalopathy in rats and dogs. *Hepatology* 1990; **11**: 682.

12 Butterworth RF. Portal-systemic encephalopathy: a disorder of neuron-astrocytic metabolic trafficking. *Dev. Neurosci.* 1993; **15**: 313.

13 Butterworth RF, Layrargues GP. Benzodiazepine receptors and hepatic encephalopathy. *Hepatology* 1990; **11**: 499.

14 Clarke B, Ellis MJC, Leung V *et al.* Reversal of hepatic encephalopathy and alteration in amino acid profiles after blocking a surgical splenorenal shunt by interventional radiological techniques. *J. Hepatol.* 1989; **8**: 325.

15 Collinson PO, Burroughs AK. Severe hypermagnesaemia due to magnesium sulphate enemas in patients with hepatic coma. *Br. Med. J.* 1986; **293**: 1013.

16 Conn HO. Effects of high–normal and low–normal serum potassium levels on hepatic encephalopathy: facts, half-facts or artifacts? *Hepatology* 1994; **20**: 1637.

17 Conn HO. Trailmaking and number-connection tests in the assessment of mental state in portal systemic encephalopathy. *Am. J. Dig. Dis.* 1977; **22**: 541.

18 Cuilleret G, Pomier-Layrargues G, Pons F *et al.* Changes in brain catecholamine levels in human cirrhotic hepatic encephalopathy. *Gut* 1981; **21**: 565.

19 Davidson EA, Summerskill WHJ. Psychiatric aspects of liver disease. *Postgrad. Med. J.* 1956; **32**: 487.

20 Dawson AM, McLaren J, Sherlock S. Neomycin in the treatment of hepatic coma. *Lancet* 1957; **ii**: 1263.

21 Fabbri A, Magrini N, Bianchi G *et al.* Overview of randomized clinical trials of oral branched-chain amino acid treatment in chronic hepatic encephalopathy. *J. Parent. Ent. Nutr.* 1996; **20**: 159.

22 Fischer JE, Baldessarini RJ. False neurotransmitters and

hepatic failure. *Lancet* 1971; **2**: 75.

23 Frerichs FT. *A Clinical Treatise on Diseases of the Liver*, Vol. I, p. 241. Translated by C Murchison. New Sydenham Society, London, 1960.

24 Gitlin N, Lewis DC, Hinkley L. The diagnosis and prevalence of subclinical hepatic encephalopathy in apparently healthy, ambulant non-shunted patients with cirrhosis. *J. Hepatol.* 1986; **3**: 75.

25 Grimm G, Ferenci P, Katzenschlager R *et al.* Improvement of hepatic encephalopathy with flumazenil. *Lancet* 1988; **ii**: 1392.

26 Haussinger D, Steeb R, Gerok W. Ammonium and bicarbonate homeostasis in chronic liver disease. *Klin. Wochenschr.* 1990; **68**: 75.

27 Jalan R, Gooday R, O'Carroll RE *et al.* A prospective evaluation of changes in neuropsychological and liver function tests following transjugular intrahepatic portosystemic stent-shunt. *J. Hepatol.* 1995; **23**: 697.

28 Kawanaka H, Ohta M, Hashizume M *et al.* Portosystemic encephalopathy treated with balloon-occluded retrograde transvenous obliteration. *Am. J. Gastroenterol.* 1995; **90**: 508.

29 Knudsen GM, Schmidt J, Almdal T *et al.* Passage of amino acids and glucose across the blood–brain barrier in patients with hepatic encephalopathy. *Hepatology* 1993; **17**: 987.

30 Krieger D, Krieger S, Jansen O *et al.* Manganese and chronic hepatic encephalopathy. *Lancet* 1995; **346**: 270.

31 Kügler CFA, Lotterer E, Petter J *et al.* Visual event-related P300 potentials in early portosystemic encephalopathy. *Gastroenterology* 1992; **103**: 302.

32 Kullmann F, Hollerbach S, Holstege A *et al.* Subclinical hepatic encephalopathy: the diagnostic value of evoked potentials. *J. Hepatol.* 1995; **22**: 101.

33 Laidlaw J, Read AE, Sherlock S. Morphine tolerance in hepatic cirrhosis. *Gastroenterology* 1961; **40**: 389.

34 Levy LJ, Leek J, Losowsky MS. Evidence for gamma aminobutyric acid as the inhibitor of gamma aminobutyric acid binding in the plasma of humans with liver disease and hepatic encephalopathy. *Clin. Sci.* 1987; **73**: 531.

35 Lo WD, Ennis SR, Goldstein GW *et al.* The effects of galactosamine-induced hepatic failure upon blood–brain barrier permeability. *Hepatology* 1987; **7**: 452.

36 Lockwood AH, Yap EWH, Wong WH. Cerebral ammonia metabolism in patients with severe liver disease and minimal hepatic encephalopathy. *J. Cereb. Blood Flow Metab.* 1991; **11**: 337.

37 Lunzer M, James IM, Weinman J *et al.* Treatment of chronic hepatic encephalopathy with levodopa. *Gut* 1974; **15**: 555.

38 Manghani KK, Lunzer MR, Billing BH *et al.* Urinary and serum octopamine in patients with portal systemic encephalopathy. *Lancet* 1975; **ii**: 943.

39 Miyata Y, Motomura S, Tsuji Y *et al.* Hepatic encephalopathy and reversible cortical blindness. *Am. J. Gastroenterol.* 1988; **83**: 780.

40 Morgan MH, Read AE, Speller DCE. Treatment of hepatic encephalopathy with metronidazole. *Gut* 1982; **23**: 1.

41 Morgan MY. The treatment of chronic hepatic encephalopathy. *Hepatogastroenterology* 1995; **38**: 377.

42 Morgan MY, Jakobovits AW, James IM *et al.* Successful use of bromocriptine in the treatment of chronic hepatic encephalopathy. *Gastroenterology* 1980; **78**: 663.

43 Morgan MY. Branched-chain amino acids in the management of chronic liver disease. Facts and fantasies. *J. Hepatol.* 1990; **11**: 133.

44 Morgan MY, Hawley KM. Lactilol versus lactulose in the treatment of acute hepatic encephalopathy in cirrhotic patients: a double-blind, randomized trial. *Hepatology* 1987; **7**: 1278.

45 Morgan MY, Stranger LC. The incidence of subclinical and overt hepatic encephalopathy in an unselected group of patients with cirrhosis. *Hepatogastroenterology* 1992; (submitted for publication).

46 Morgan MY, Alonso M, Stranger LC. Lactilol and lactulose for the treatment of subclinical hepatic encephalopathy in cirrhotic patients. A randomized, cross-over study. *J. Hepatol.* 1989; **8**: 208.

47 Mortensen PB, Rasmussen HS, Holtug K. Lactulose detoxifies *in vitro* short-chain fatty acid production in colonic contents induced by blood: implications for hepatic coma. *Gastroenterology* 1988; **94**: 750.

48 Mousseau DD, Butterworth RF. Current theories on the pathogenesis of hepatic encephalopathy. *PSEBM* 1994; **206**: 329.

49 Mullen KD, Szauter KM, Kaminsky-Russ K. 'Endogenous' benzodiazepine activity in body fluids of patients with hepatic encephalopathy. *Lancet* 1990; **336**: 81.

50 Oppong KNW, Bartlett K, Record CO *et al.* Synaptosomal glutamate transport in thioacetamide-induced hepatic encephalopathy in the rat. *Hepatology* 1995; **22**: 553.

51 Parkes JD, Murray-Lyon IM, Williams R. Neuropsychiatric and electroencephalographic changes after transplantation of the liver. *Q. J. Med.* 1970; **39**: 515.

52 Parsons-Smith BG, Summerskill WHJ, Dawson AM *et al.* The electroencephalograph in liver disease. *Lancet* 1957; **ii**: 867.

53 Patil DH, Westaby D, Mahida YR *et al.* Comparative modes of action of lactilol and lactulose in the treatment of hepatic encephalopathy. *Gut* 1987; **28**: 255.

54 Phear EA, Ruebner B, Sherlock S *et al.* Methionine toxicity in liver disease and its prevention by chlortetracycline. *Clin. Sci.* 1955; **15**: 93.

55 Phillips GB, Schwartz R, Gabuzda GJ Jr *et al.* The syndrome of impending hepatic coma in patients with cirrhosis of the liver given certain nitrogenous substances. *N. Engl. J. Med.* 1952; **247**: 239.

56 Plauth M, Egberts E-H, Hamster W *et al.* Long-term treatment of latent portosystemic encephalopathy with branched-chain amino acids. *J. Hepatol.* 1993; **17**: 308.

57 Pomier-Layrargues G, Giguère JF, Lavoie J *et al.* Flumazenil in cirrhotic patients in hepatic coma: a randomised double-blind placebo-controlled crossover trial. *Hepatology* 1994; **19**: 32.

58 Potts JR III, Henderson JM, Millikan WJ Jr *et al.* Restoration of portal venous perfusion and reversal of encephalopathy by balloon occlusion of portal systemic shunt. *Gastroenterology* 1984; **87**: 208.

59 Powell EE, Pender MP, Chalk JB *et al.* Improvement in chronic hepatocerebral degeneration following liver transplantation. *Gastroenterology* 1990; **98**: 1079.

60 Read AE, Sherlock S, Laidlaw J *et al.* The neuro-psychiatric syndromes associated with chronic liver disease and an extensive portal–systemic collateral circulation. *Q. J. Med.* 1967; **36**: 135.

61 Salerno F, Moser P, Maggi A *et al.* Effects of long-term administration of low-dose lactilol in patients with cirrhosis but without overt encephalopathy. *J. Hepatol.* 1994; **21**: 1092.

62 Sanyal AJ, Freedman AM, Shiffman ML *et al.* Portosystemic

encephalopathy after transjugular portosystemic shunt: results of a prospective controlled study. *Hepatology* 1994; **20**: 46.

63 Schafer DF, Jones EA. Hepatic encephalopathy and the γ-aminobutyric-acid neurotransmitter system. *Lancet* 1982; **i**: 18.

64 Schömerus H, Hamster W, Blunck H *et al.* Latent portal systemic encephalopathy, I. Nature of cerebral functional defects and their effect on fitness to drive. *Dig. Dis. Sci.* 1981; **26**: 622.

65 Sherlock S, Summerskill WHJ, White LP *et al.* Portal–systemic encephalopathy: neurological complications of liver disease. *Lancet* 1954; **ii**: 453.

66 Somberg KA, Riegler JL, LaBerge JM *et al.* Hepatic encephalopathy after transjugular intrahepatic portosystemic shunts: incidence and risk factors. *Am. J. Gastroenterol.* 1995; **90**: 549.

67 Srivastava A, Mehta R, Rothke SP *et al.* Fitness to drive in patients with cirrhosis and portal–systemic shunting: a pilot study evaluating driving performance. *J. Hepatol.* 1994; **21**: 1023.

68 Summerskill WHJ, Davidson EA, Sherlock S *et al.* The neuropsychiatric syndrome associated with hepatic cirrhosis and an extensive portal collateral circulation. *Q. J. Med.* 1956; **25**: 245.

69 Szerb JC, Butterworth RF. Effect of ammonium ions on synaptic transmission in the mammalian central nervous system. *Prog. Neurobiol.* 1992; **39**: 135.

70 Tarter RE, Hegedus AM, van Thiel DH *et al.* Non-alcoholic cirrhosis associated with neuropsychological dysfunction in the absence of overt evidence of hepatic encephalopathy. *Gastroenterology* 1984; **86**: 1421.

71 Thuluvath PJ, Edwin D, Yue CN *et al.* Increased signals seen in globus pallidus in T_1-weighted magnetic resonance imaging in cirrhotics are not suggestive of chronic hepatic encephalopathy. *Hepatology* 1995; **21**: 440.

72 Uribe M, Marquez A, Garcia Ramos G *et al.* Treatment of chronic portal–systemic encephalopathy with vegetable and animal protein diets: a controlled crossover study. *Dig. Dis. Sci.* 1982; **27**: 1109.

73 Uribe M, Campoll O, Vargas F *et al.* Acidifying enemas (lactilol and lactulose) versus nonacidifying enemas (tapwater) to treat acute portal–systemic encephalopathy: a double-blind, randomised clinical trial. *Hepatology* 1987; **7**: 639.

74 Victor M, Adams RD, Cole M. The acquired (non-Wilsonian) type of chronic hepatocerebral degeneration. *Medicine (Baltimore)* 1965; **44**: 345.

75 Vorobioff J, Garcia-Tsao G, Groszmann R *et al.* Long-term hemodynamic effects of ketanserin, a 5-hydroxytryptamine blocker, in portal hypertensive patients. *Hepatology* 1988; **9**: 88.

76 Weber FL, Fresard KM, Lally BR. Effects of lactulose and neomycin on urea metabolism in cirrhotic subjects. *Gastroenterology* 1982; **82**: 213.

77 Weber FL, Banwell JG, Fresard KM *et al.* Nitrogen in fecal bacterial fiber, and soluble fractions of patients with cirrhosis: effects of lactulose and lactulose plus neomycin. *J. Lab. Clin. Med.* 1987; **110**: 259.

78 Zaki AEO, Ede RJ, Davis M *et al.* Experimental studies of blood brain barrier permeability in acute hepatic failure. *Hepatology* 1984; **4**: 359.

79 Zieve L, Olsen RL. Can hepatic coma be caused by a reduction of brain noradrenaline or dopamine? *Gut* 1977; **18**: 688.

Chapter 8
Fulminant Hepatic Failure

Fulminant hepatic failure is the clinical syndrome of sudden and severe impairment of liver function in a previously healthy person. Encephalopathy is usually present. There is a severe coagulopathy, as well as other metabolic abnormalities. Cardiac, respiratory and renal failure may develop. Although usually due to an acute insult (virus or drug), fulminant hepatic failure may be the presentation of Wilson's disease, autoimmune chronic hepatitis or delta superinfection in a patient with chronic hepatitis B.

The original and generally accepted definition of fulminant hepatic failure includes a time framework of developing within 8 weeks of the first symptoms or jaundice. Within this time period, however, patterns have been recognized which relate to prognosis and aetiology. Patients progressing rapidly (time from jaundice to encephalopathy 7 days or less) are more likely to survive than those progressing more slowly [68], a clinical pattern seen more in hepatitis A and B than non-A non-B [68]. Such patterns have led to proposals of different time-based classifications, but agreement over these has not been reached [6, 7, 68].

However, the pattern of liver failure is important for management decisions and should be recognized whether classified as fulminant or subfulminant (jaundice to encephalopathy less or more than 2 weeks) [7], fulminant or late onset (less or more than 8 weeks) [37], or hyperacute (0–7 days), acute (8–28 days) or subacute (29 days to 12 weeks) [68]. The key to optimizing treatment is the *recognition* of acute liver failure and *transfer* of the patient to a liver unit with facilities for liver transplantation. The decision for liver transplantation needs to be made more rapidly in the patient with the fulminant, hyperacute and acute types. Strict classifications also have an important role in the interpretation of data from different units and countries, and in the planning of trials.

The prognosis for fulminant hepatic failure is much worse than that for chronic liver failure, but in fulminant failure the hepatic lesion is potentially reversible, and survivors usually recover completely. Complications that may lead to death include bacterial and fungal infections, circulatory instability, cerebral oedema, renal and pulmonary failure, acid–base and electrolyte disturbances and coagulopathy. These make intensive care, referral to a specialist unit, the availability of liver transplantation and temporary hepatic support vitally important. The survival of patients has improved with such facilities rising from about 20% in the early 1970s to 50% in the 1990s [94].

Causes (table 8.1)

In the USA and worldwide, the most frequent cause is viral hepatitis A, B and non-A non-B, accounting for 60–70% of cases [44, 57, 74]. In the UK the picture is different, paracetamol (acetaminophen) self-poisoning being the most common cause of fulminant hepatic failure [63, 94].

Of *identified* viral causes, hepatitis A and B are the most frequent, but in most series have been outnumbered by

Table 8.1. Causes of fulminant liver failure

Infective
Hepatitis virus A, B, C, D, E, ?G
Herpes simplex

Drug reactions and toxins
Acetaminophen (paracetamol) overdose
Halothane
Isoniazid–rifampicin
Antidepressants
Non-steroidal anti-inflammatory drugs
Valproic acid
Mushroom poisoning
Herbal remedies

Ischaemic
Ischaemic hepatitis
Surgical 'shock'
Acute Budd–Chiari syndrome

Metabolic
Wilson's disease
Fatty liver of pregnancy
Reye's syndrome

Miscellaneous (rare)
Massive malignant infiltration
Severe bacterial infection
Heat stroke

'hepatitis of unknown aetiology' also called sporadic non-A non-B hepatitis [32, 98]. These patients have typical prodromal symptoms and biochemical profiles, but no viral agent can be identified. HCV-RNA testing has shown that hepatitis C may be responsible for some of these cases, but the contribution varies geographically, being low (0–10%) [33, 64] in the USA and Europe and higher (40–60%) in Asia [16]. Local exceptions are reported. Serum HCV-DNA was detected in nine of 15 patients (60%) with fulminant hepatic failure of unknown cause in a series from Los Angeles [91] and was significantly associated with transmission risk factors.

Differences in the proportion of fulminant cases due to hepatitis A and B similarly vary with location, being about equal in areas such as the UK [94] compared with a high proportion of hepatitis B in countries such as Greece where the carriage of hepatitis B is higher [69]. In about 50% of hepatitis-B-positive patients, the fulminant course is precipitated by another factor, usually acute infection or superinfection with delta virus [82]. Sometimes a presumptive non-A non-B non-C infection may be responsible. However, if appropriate testing is not done hepatitis B may not be diagnosed since one-third to one-half of patients with fulminant hepatitis B become seronegative for hepatitis B surface antigen in a few days [82]. This may be due to a massive immunological assault on infected hepatocytes. Mutant hepatitis B virus types may complicate the picture further because of defective production of the normal viral antigens. Precore mutants have been associated with fulminant hepatitis B [59] but predisposition by this mutant to a more serious course has not been proven.

Reactivation of viral replication in carriers of hepatitis B may lead to fulminant hepatitis. This has been reported after anti-tumour chemotherapy and following cessation of immunosuppressive therapy. Withdrawal of even low doses of methotrexate (7.5–10 mg orally per week) has been followed by reactivation of hepatitis B and a fulminant course [35]. Withdrawal of chemotherapy in carriers of hepatitis C has also been associated with fulminant hepatitis [89].

Hepatitis E causes epidemics of acute hepatitis in India, central Asia, Mexico and China, where it is responsible for fulminant hepatic failure especially in pregnant women. In Western countries fulminant hepatitis due to hepatitis E has been reported in individuals with links to endemic areas [56]. Studies of sporadic non-A non-B fulminant hepatitis in England and the USA have not found hepatitis E [64, 98].

The overall fatality of an attack of acute hepatitis is about 1%, with the risk for non-A non-B (1.5–2.5%) being greater than that for hepatitis B (1%) or A (0.2–0.4%) [44].

Other viruses can cause a fatal hepatic necrosis especially in an immunocompromised individual. These include herpes simplex, cytomegalovirus, adenoviruses, Epstein–Barr [70] and varicella. Parvovirus B19 has been found in the liver of six of 10 paediatric patients with fulminant non-A non-B hepatic failure, some (four of six) with an associated aplastic anaemia [54].

Acetaminophen (paracetamol) is predictably hepatotoxic in overdosage and is the most common suicidal agent taken in the UK (Chapter 18). It can also be hepatotoxic in alcoholic patients even when taken in therapeutic doses. The classic picture is of very high serum aspartate transaminase levels (reported up to 48 000 iu/l) usually accompanied by a lower level of alanine transaminase [99]. The outcome is fatal in 20%.

Idiosyncratic drug reactions may cause fulminant hepatic failure. The most frequent culprits are anaesthetic agents, non-steroidal anti-inflammatory drugs [2], antidepressants and isoniazid given with rifampicin. Fatal hepatic injury is also reported with the 'recreational' drug ecstasy (3,4-methylenedioxymetamphetamine) [43].

Mushroom poisoning is common in France and in areas where unusual fungi are gathered and eaten. Hepatic failure is preceded by muscarinic effects, such as profuse sweating, vomiting and diarrhoea. Early recognition is important to optimize supportive measures and to be alerted to the possibility of liver failure [50].

Carbon tetrachloride poisoning usually causes more kidney than hepatic damage. This is true of most industrial poisons although fulminant hepatic failure can follow occupational exposure to the solvent 2-nitropropane [41].

At full term, pregnant women may develop fulminant hepatic necrosis due to eclampsia or fatty liver (Chapter 25).

Vascular causes of ischaemic hepatitis include an episode of low cardiac output in a patient with underlying cardiac disease, acute Budd–Chiari syndrome, and surgical shock with or without Gram-negative septicaemia.

Massive infiltration of the liver with tumour cells such as in lymphoma [97] can lead to fulminant hepatic failure. Such a cause should be considered in the differential diagnosis since liver transplantation is contraindicated, and specific therapy may be life saving. Disseminated tuberculosis very rarely may cause fulminant hepatic failure due to replacement of liver tissue [45].

Acute Wilson's disease must always be excluded in any patient who is less than 35 years old, particularly if haemolysis is associated. Fulminant hepatic failure may result in these patients from a superimposed acute viral hepatitis [80].

Clinical picture

The patient, previously having been well, typically develops non-specific symptoms — nausea and malaise. Jaundice follows and then features of hepatic encephalopathy. Coma may develop rapidly within a few days. Transfer of the patient to a specialist liver centre with a transplantation service needs to be done earlier rather than later. It has to be realized that a patient with acute liver disease and a prolonged coagulation can deteriorate and die. Advice from a liver centre should be sought. If on admission there is encephalopathy, immediate transfer should be discussed.

In the early stages jaundice bears little relation to the neuropsychiatric changes which may even develop before jaundice. Later, jaundice is deep. Liver size is usually small.

Vomiting is common but abdominal pain rare. Tachycardia, hypotension, hyperventilation and fever are later features. The clinician must be alert to the delay in liver damage following acetaminophen overdose which may present after a period of 2–3 days or apparent clinical recovery.

Focal neurological signs, high fever or a slow response to conventional treatment should prompt a search for alternative causes for encephalopathy.

In patients with a more gradual onset of hepatic insufficiency (over weeks rather than days, and variously called subfulminant, subacute or late onset) infrequently develop cerebral oedema. Ascites and renal failure appear, and the prognosis is worse than in those patients with a more rapid course.

Common complications of fulminant hepatic failure include infections, haemodynamic disturbances and cerebral oedema. These, hepatic encephalopathy, and other problems are discussed later.

Late onset hepatic failure. This term refers to a group of patients in whom encephalopathy develops after an illness of more than 8 weeks, but less than 24 weeks, from the first symptoms, in the absence of pre-existing liver disease. In most the cause cannot be found [30]. Nausea, malaise and abdominal discomfort are followed by ascites, encephalopathy and renal impairment. Survival was about 20% without transplantion. A 55% 1-year survival has been reported after transplant [30].

DISTINCTION FROM CHRONIC LIVER DISEASE

A note should be made of any history of liver disease, duration of symptoms, the presence of a hard liver, marked splenomegaly and vascular spiders on the skin (table 8.2). A problem arises in the alcoholic where recent heavy drinking adds acute hepatitis to underlying chronic liver disease. In these circumstances the liver is

Table 8.2. Fulminant hepatic failure: distinction between acute and acute-on-chronic types

	Acute	Acute-on-chronic
History	Short	Long
Nutrition	Good	Poor
Liver	±	+Hard
Spleen	±	+
Spiders	0	++

large. Potential reversibility of acute alcoholic hepatitis merits more supportive effort in these patients than could be given to the usual end-stage cirrhosis where the liver would not be expected to regenerate.

Investigations (table 8.3)

Blood is taken to identify problems needing immediate attention, to establish a baseline for hepatic and renal function, to establish the cause and to check criteria for survival/transplantation.

HAEMATOLOGY

The prothrombin time (together with the degree of encephalopathy) is central to assessment of the severity

Table 8.3. Investigations of acute hepato-cellular failure

Haematology
Haemoglobin, platelets, WBC, prothrombin, blood group

Biochemical
Blood glucose (urgent), serum bilirubin, aspartate transaminase, albumin, globulin, immunoglobulins
Serum urea, sodium, potassium, bicarbonate, chloride, calcium, phosphate, alkaline phosphatase
Serum amylase
Store 8 ml serum for later use

Microbiology, Virology
Hepatitis B antigen and IgM anticore
Hepatitis A (IgM) antibody
Hepatitis C antibody
Serum anti-delta
Blood culture aerobic and anaerobic
Sputum, urine, stool (culture and microscopy)
Store serum for virological studies

Other essential
Electro-encephalogram, electrocardiogram, X-ray of chest, fluid intake and output, blood gases

Additional (not always necessary)
Blood alcohol or other drug level
Urine electrolyte concentration
Plasma fibrin split products
Hepatic scan

of the clinical situation, and its progress. Haemoglobin and white count are obtained. A falling platelet count may reflect disseminated intravascular coagulation.

BIOCHEMISTRY

Blood glucose, blood urea, electrolytes and creatinine are measured. Bilirubin, albumin, transaminase, alkaline phosphatase and amylase are routinely done. Serum bilirubin is important prognostically for non-acetaminophen patients. Serum albumin is usually initially normal, but later a low albumin reflects a poor prognosis. The transaminases are of little prognostic value. Levels tend to fall as the patient's condition worsens. Blood gas analysis is important in the prognostic evaluation of acetaminophen liver failure.

VIROLOGICAL MARKERS

Acute hepatitis A should be diagnosed by a serum IgM anti-A. Serum hepatitis B surface antigen is checked, but the IgM core antibody is necessary for certain diagnosis. HBsAg may have been cleared and HBsAb will not have appeared. Serum HBV DNA is usually negative. Such rapid viral clearance indicates a favourable prognosis, perhaps because it implies a good immune response to the hepatitis B virus. In those positive for hepatitis B, serum anti-delta should be sought. Anti-HCV should

be performed, but is likely to be negative this early in the disease (Chapter 16).

ELECTRO-ENCEPHALOGRAM (EEG)

This has been used to assess the clinical state and determine prognosis (fig. 8.1). However, the guidelines used for decisions on clinical management, and in particular liver transplantation, no longer depend on the EEG. Repeated measurement may, however, be necessary when clinical and laboratory features do not move in the same direction.

Recently, it has been recognized that there may be epileptiform activity which is not clinically detected because the patient is paralysed and ventilated. Such fitting needs treatment and this argues for EEG monitoring [94].

SCANNING AND LIVER BIOPSY

CT scan will show a reduction in liver size. Some base the decision to transplant on the extent of this reduction on CT scanning at the time a donor liver becomes available [88] but correlation of liver size with survival is imprecise [52]. Most use clinical and laboratory data, because of concern with the feasibility and safety of moving a potentially unstable patient often with cerebral oedema from intensive care to radiology and back.

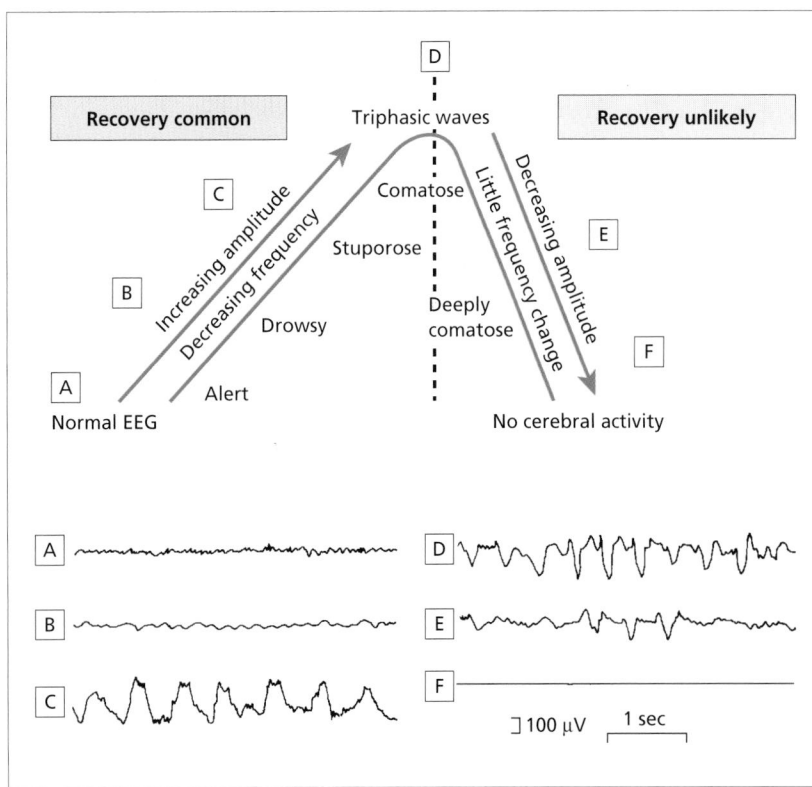

Fig. 8.1. Evolution of the EEG in liver failure. The progression from grade A to D is marked by increasing amplitude, decreasing frequency and increasing drowsiness. At D, triphasic waves appear and the interrupted line indicates the limit beyond which recovery is unlikely. From E to F amplitude decreases with little frequency change and at F there is no cerebral activity [49].

CT of the brain is unreliable in detecting early cerebral oedema, and the movement of the patient to the radiology unit carries the risk of deterioration.

Liver histology has been used in the decision making process for transplantation, based on whether or not submassive necrosis of 50% or more is present [88]. However, there is considerable variability of necrosis from area to area which may be prognostically misleading [40]. Moreover, most would prefer to avoid this procedure in the late stage fulminant patient.

Associations

HEPATIC ENCEPHALOPATHY

The neurological sequelae of fulminant hepatic failure are hepatic encephalopathy and cerebral oedema with raised intracranial pressure (ICP). Clinically they overlap (fig. 8.2). Early in the clinical course encephalopathy usually develops without evidence of increased ICP. Once stupor to deep coma with or without decerebrate posturing (grade 3–4 encephalopathy) develops, the patient is at high risk of developing cerebral oedema.

The pathogenesis of hepatic encephalopathy is multifactorial (Chapter 7) and centres on failure of the liver to remove toxic, mainly nitrogenous, substances from the circulation. In contrast to the coma of cirrhotic patients, portal-systemic encephalopathy due to shunting of blood past the liver is of minor importance. Blood ammonia (and presumably amine) levels are increased but do not correlate with the depth of coma or the prognosis. Such estimates are not necessary for management.

The onset of encephalopathy is often sudden. It may precede jaundice. The features are unlike those seen in chronic liver disease, with agitation, changes in personality, delusions and restlessness. The patient may show anti-social behaviour or character disturbance. Nightmares, headaches and dizziness are other inaugural, non-specific symptoms. Delirium, mania and fits indicate stimulation of the reticular system. Unco-operative behaviour often continues while consciousness is clouded. The delirium is of the noisy, restless variety and attacks of screaming are spontaneous or induced by minor stimuli. Violent behaviour is common. 'Flapping' tremor may be transient and overlooked. Fetor hepaticus is usually present.

The prognosis for patients with grade 1 or 2 encephalopathy (confused or drowsy) is good. For grade 3 or 4 it is much poorer.

CEREBRAL OEDEMA (INTRACRANIAL HYPERTENSION)

Fulminant hepatic failure is associated with cerebral oedema, which can lead to an increase in intracerebral pressure. This is uncommon in patients with grade 1 or 2 encephalopathy, but develops in the majority with grade 4. Raised intracerebral pressure can lead to brain stem herniation (fig. 8.3) and is the most common cause of death, being found in 81% of fatal cases [28]. There is a generalized or focal increase in brain volume due to an increase in water content. The cause is probably multifactorial [34], but two mechanisms have been proposed: vasogenic and cytotoxic. The vasogenic mechanism is based on disruption of the blood–brain barrier with leakage of plasma into the cerebrospinal fluid. The cytotoxic mechanism depends on cellular changes resulting

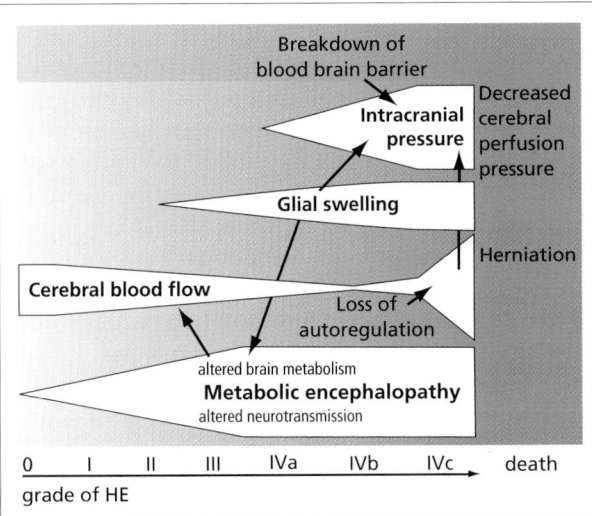

Fig. 8.2. Brain dysfunction in fulminant hepatic failure. Proposed interrelation of metabolic encephalopathy, intracranial pressure and changes in cerebral blood flow during the progression of the disease. HE = hepatic encephalopathy (reproduced with permission from [34]).

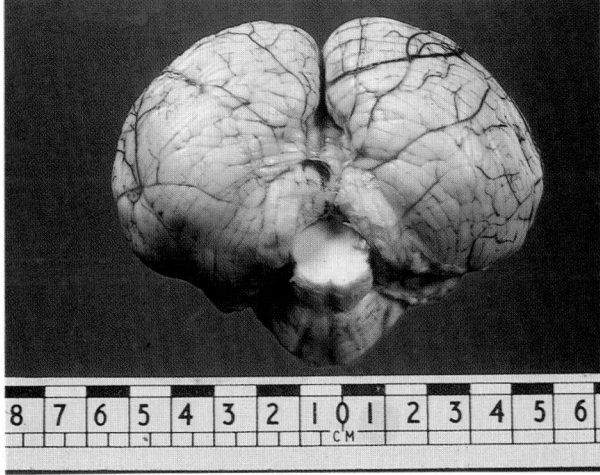

Fig. 8.3. Cerebral oedema in a patient who died in hepatic coma. Note the indented cerebellum.

in increased osmotic uptake of water into brain cells. Experimental data tend to favour the cytotoxic mechanism [74].

The net blood supply to the brain depends on the balance between carotid arterial pressure and intracerebral pressure. Cerebral blood flow appears to be inadequate in most patients with grade 4 encephalopathy resulting in cerebral hypoxia [92], and these changes may be related to the development of cerebral oedema. Moreover, a study has shown that cerebral blood flow autoregulation (maintained flow despite falling systemic blood pressure) is lost in an animal model of acute hepatic failure [55]. This would make systemic hypotension even more damaging in patients with fulminant hepatic failure.

Clinically, raised intracerebral pressure is suggested by systolic hypertension (sustained or intermittent) and increased muscle tone and myoclonus which progress to extension and hyperpronation of the arms and extension of the legs (decerebrate posturing). Dysconjugate eye movements and skewed positions of the eyes may be seen. If not controlled by treatment, this clinical picture progresses to loss of pupillary reflexes and respiratory arrest from brain-stem herniation.

COAGULOPATHY

The liver synthesizes all the coagulation factors (except factor VIII), inhibitors of coagulation and proteins involved in the fibrinolytic system (Chapter 4). It is also involved in the clearance of activated clotting factors. The coagulopathy of fulminant hepatic failure is thus complex and due not only to factor deficiency, but also enhanced fibrinolytic activity most likely caused by intravascular coagulation [72]. The platelet count may fall due to increased consumption or reduced production, and platelet function is also abnormal in fulminant hepatic failure.

The resulting coagulopathy predisposes to bleeding. This is a frequent cause of death; it may be spontaneous, from the mucous membranes, from the gastrointestinal tract or into the brain.

The prothrombin time is the most widely used test to assess coagulation. It is a guide to prognosis and is one of the criteria used in deciding whether transplantation should be done (see table 8.5) [66].

HYPOGLYCAEMIA, HYPOKALAEMIA, METABOLIC CHANGES

Hypoglycaemia is found in 40% of patients with fulminant hepatic failure [62]. It may be persistent and intractable. Plasma insulin levels are high due to reduced hepatic uptake; gluconeogenesis is reduced in the failing liver. Hypoglycaemia can cause rapid neurological deterioration and death in these patients and is one aspect

of the condition which can be treated satisfactorily.

Hypokalaemia is common and due in part to urinary losses with inadequate replacement, and high glucose feeding. Serum sodium levels tend to be low, falling markedly in the terminal stages. Other electrolyte changes include hypophosphataemia, hypocalcaemia and hypomagnesaemia.

Acid–base changes are common. Respiratory alkalosis is due to overbreathing, probably related to direct stimulation of the respiratory centre by unknown toxic substances. Respiratory acidosis can be caused by elevated intracranial pressure and respiratory depression, or pulmonary complications. Lactic acidosis develops in about half the patients reaching grade 3 coma. It is related to inadequate tissue perfusion due to hypotension and hypoxaemia. A metabolic acidosis is more frequent in acetaminophen-induced fulminant hepatic failure; the fall in pH is one of the criteria used in transplant decisions (see table 8.5).

INFECTION

Ninety per cent of patients with acute liver failure and grade 2 or more encephalopathy have clinical or bacteriological evidence of infection (fig. 8.4) [77]. Twenty-five per cent have associated bacteraemia. The majority of infections are respiratory. The high rate of infection can be related to poor host defences with impaired Kupffer cell and polymorph function and to the reduction of factors such as fibronectin, opsonins and chemoattractants, including components of the complement system [46]. Neutrophil superoxide and hydrogen peroxide production is reduced in patients with acute liver falure due to acetaminophen [17]. Poor respiratory effort and cough reflex, and the presence of endotracheal tubes, venous lines and urinary catheters place the patient at increased risk. Spontaneous bacterial peritonitis is also seen [15].

Infections in blood, respiratory tract and urine are usually detected within 3 days of admission. In some cases the source of infection may never be found, but distal tips of intravenous catheters should be cultured after removal, and are often incriminated. The typical manifestations of sepsis such as fever and leucocytosis may be absent (fig. 8.4). More than two-thirds of infections are due to Gram-positive organisms, usually staphylococci, but streptococci and Gram-negative bacilli are also found. Fungal infections are found in about one-third of patients, often unrecognized and ominous [78]. These patients share particular clinical features (table 8.4).

Overall, infections make a major contribution to clinical deterioration and death.

RENAL

Due to decreased urea synthesis by the liver, the blood

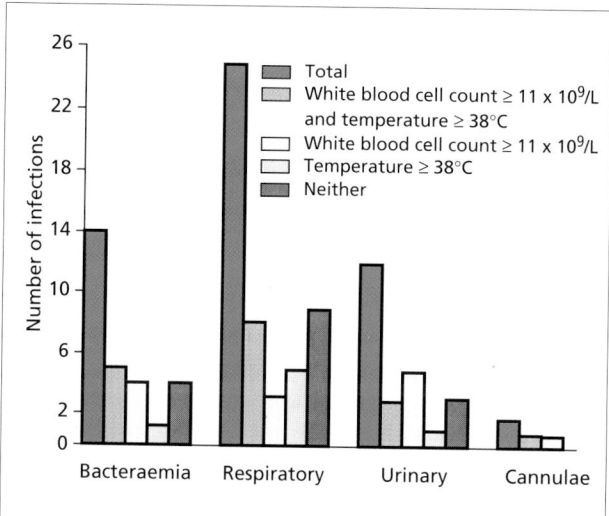

Fig. 8.4. Clinical signs of bacterial infection related to significant microbiological cultures in 50 patients with acute liver failure. Raised temperature and white cell count were poor indicators of bacterial infection.(Reproduced with permission from [77].)

Table 8.4. Features of systemic fungal infection [78]

Deterioration in coma grade after initial improvement
Pyrexia unresponsive to antibiotics
Established renal failure
Markedly elevated white cell count

urea concentration may not be a good indicator of kidney function, and the serum creatinine is preferred. Functional renal failure (hepato-renal syndrome) develops in about 55% with or without acute tubular necrosis [75]. There is marked renal vasoconstriction and reduced renal prostaglandin excretion [39]. Sepsis, endotoxaemia, bleeding and hypotension contribute to the acute tubular necrosis.

HAEMODYNAMIC CHANGES: SYSTEMIC HYPOTENSION

Hypotension is a feature of liver failure [84]. It is associated with a low peripheral vascular resistance and increased cardiac output which relate to the degree of hepatic damage. Apart from sepsis and endotoxaemia, the cause is unclear but possible mediators include prostaglandins and nitric oxide. There is covert tissue hypoxia at the microcirculatory level with consequent lactic acidosis. Oxygen extraction by tissues is reduced [9]. The circulatory changes are associated with decreased cerebral perfusion and renal vasoconstriction. Infusion of *N*-acetylcysteine improves oxygen delivery and extraction by tissues, perhaps through an effect on nitric oxide [42].

Cardiac arrhythmias of most types are noted in the late stages [9] and relate to electrolyte abnormalities, acidosis, hypoxia and the insertion of catheters into the pulmonary artery.

Depression of brain-stem function eventually leads to circulatory failure.

PULMONARY COMPLICATIONS

These include aspiration of gastric contents or blood, atelectasis, infection and respiratory depression due to brain-stem compression. Intrapulmonary arteriovenous shunting adds to the hypoxia. There may be pulmonary oedema. Adult respiratory distress syndome (ARDS) is usually refractory to treatment and fatal.

Chest X-rays show abnormalities in over half of patients [87]. These include lobar collapse, patchy consolidation, aspiration pneumonia and in one-quarter non-cardiogenic pulmonary oedema.

ACUTE PANCREATITIS

Acute haemorrhagic and necrotizing pancreatitis is frequent in patients dying with fulminant hepatic failure. It is difficult to recognize in the comatose patient but, rarely, it may be the cause of death. Serum amylase levels are raised in about one-third of patients and should be monitored.

Aetiological factors include 'duodenitis' found with fulminant hepatitis, haemorrhage into and around the pancreas, the causative virus, corticosteroid therapy and shock.

Prognosis

The overall survival for those reaching grade III or IV encephalopathy is 20% without transplantation. If only grade I or II coma is reached, survival is around 65%. Those who survive do not develop cirrhosis.

The advent of successful liver transplantation for acute hepatic failure has made prediction of survival particularly important. Indications, whether clinical or laboratory, that spontaneous recovery is unlikely are therefore of vital importance. Prognosis is worse in the older patients [73], although others have also found patients under 10 years old at particular risk [66]. Coexistence of other disease worsens the prognosis.

Aetiology is important. In one series, 12.5% of halothane-related patients survived compared with 66% for hepatitis A, 38.9% for hepatitis B and 50% for acetaminophen overdose [67].

If any precipitant of encephalopathy can be identified, particularly the administration of sedatives, the prognosis is better. The patient improves as the drug is eliminated.

Unfavourable clinical signs include a small liver [51] and ascites. Decerebrate rigidity, with loss of the oculo-vestibular reflex and respiratory failure are particularly ominous. Such patients, if they survive, may rarely be left with residual brain-stem and cerebral cortical injury [65].

Prothrombin time is the best indicator of survival [66]. The association of a clotting factor V concentration less than 15% with coma is also ominous [8]. At this level survival is only 10% for all aetiologies except hepatitis A and paracetamol overdose where the outlook is better. Hypoglycaemia is another bad sign.

Liver biopsy is rarely indicated but, if necessary, can be performed by the transjugular route. The extent of hepato-cellular necrosis and interlobular confluent necrosis is related to outcome [22]. Hepatocytes normally comprise about 85% of the total volume. If this falls below 35%, the survival rate is markedly reduced [93].

An important univariate and multivariate analysis was made of predictive factors in 586 patients with acute liver failure managed medically [66]. In patients with viral hepatitis and drug reactions, three static variables, aetiology (non-A non-B or drug), age (less than 11 years and more than 40 years) and duration of jaundice before encephalopathy (greater than 7 days) and two dynamic variables (a serum bilirubin exceeding 18 mg (300 µmol/l) and a prothrombin time exceeding 50 seconds) indicated a poor prognosis (table 8.5). In paracetamol overdose, survival correlated with arterial blood pH, peak prothrombin time and serum creatinine.

These criteria use clinical and laboratory data that are straightforward to collect. They have been validated by other studies [26, 58, 71], and are the current guide with which other prognostic schemes are compared [53]. The

Table 8.5. King's College Hospital criteria for liver transplantation in fulminant hepatic failure [66]

Acetaminophen
pH < 7.30 (irrespective of grade of encephalopathy)
or
Prothrombin time > 100 seconds and serum creatinine > 300 µmol/l
in patients with grade III or IV encephalopathy

Non-acetaminophen patients
Prothrombin time > 100 seconds (irrespective of grade of encephalopathy)
or
Any three of the following variables (irrespective of grade of encephalopathy):
Age < 10 or > 40 years
Aetiology: non-A, non-B hepatitis, halothane hepatitis, idiosyncratic drug reactions
Duration of jaundice before onset of encephalopathy > 7 days
Prothrombin time > 50 seconds
Serum bilirubin > 300 µmol/l

plasma unbound Gc protein concentration (an actin scavenger) is a good discriminant [58], but is not available for routine use. A complicated index based on laboratory and clinical data in another study was valuable, but data were analysed only for fulminant hepatitis B and non-A non-B [86]. Assessment of hepatocyte necrosis on liver biopsy, or reduced liver volume on CT scanning are used in some centres [88], and in the case of biopsy may alter the diagnosis in 17% of cases [26], but debate as to their discriminant value and practical problems in arranging them safely, at the appropriate time, have limited their use.

The causes of death are: bleeding, respiratory and circulatory failure, cerebral oedema, renal failure, infection, hypoglycaemia and pancreatitis.

Survival depends on the capacity of the liver to regenerate and this is almost impossible to predict. It is probably under humoral control and a hepatocyte growth factor has been identified. Human hepatocyte growth factor is increased in the blood in patients with fulminant hepatic failure, but this is not a useful prognostic measure.

No criteria are ever likely to predict the outcome of fulminant hepatic failure with certainty. However, predictions of a low chance of survival, for example 20%, are clinically useful in directing a decision to transplant with a 60–80% chance of survival.

Treatment [13]

Over the years survival of patients with fulminant hepatitis in deep coma has improved due to meticulous attention to the details of good supportive care combined with better knowledge of the most important functions lost when the liver cell fails. These patients are mercifully rare, and should be treated in a special unit with experience in their management, and, preferably, where facilities for liver transplantation are available. The complex problems associated with multiple organ failure require close monitoring and prompt treatment (table 8.6).

The measures described below apply to patients in grade III and IV coma and must be modified for those in the lower grades.

The usual measures for the unconscious patient are adopted. The patient is barrier nursed. Attendants should wear gloves, gowns and masks and should have been vaccinated against hepatitis B. The grade of coma (Chapter 7) must be charted hourly.

Liver size is determined daily by percussion and the lower margin marked on the abdominal wall. It may be confirmed by bedside ultrasound.

Temperature, pulse and blood pressure should be recorded at least hourly and preferably continuously. A strict fluid balance chart recording input and output is

Table 8.6. Management of acute hepato-cellular failure with coma

Problem	Treatment
Portal systemic encephalopathy	No protein by mouth Phosphate enema twice daily No sedation Lactulose 30 ml dose
Cerebral oedema	i.v. mannitol
Hypoglycaemia	100 ml 50% glucose if blood glucose falls below 60 mg/dl Up to 3 litres 10% glucose per 24 hours Correct hypokalaemia Check blood glucose hourly
Hypocalcaemia	10 ml 10% calcium gluconate i.v. daily
Renal failure	Haemofiltration Dialysis
Respiratory failure	Intubation (not tracheostomy) Ventilator Oxygen Maintain normal blood gases
Hypotension	Dopamine
Infection	Frequent cultures Antibiotic prophylaxis
Bleeding	Cimetidine or ranitidine i.v. Fresh frozen plasma and platelets

imperative. Pulmonary oedema is frequent, and care should be taken to avoid fluid overload.

A nasogastric tube is passed. An H_2-antagonist or omeprazole is given to prevent gastroduodenal erosions and bleeding.

To detect early evidence of complications, such as renal and respiratory failure, monitoring using invasive methods is necessary so that preventative measures can be taken. A urinary catheter, central venous catheter and arterial line should be placed, the last two after clotting factor and if necessary platelet infusion.

Hypoglycaemia is frequent, and on arrival the blood sugar is estimated. 100 ml of 50% glucose is given intravenously if the blood glucose is less than 60 mg/dl (3.5 mmol/l). A continuous infusion of dextrose 5 or 10% is given, the volume according to fluid needs. The blood sugar is checked every hour and further 50% glucose given if hypoglycaemia recurs. If it is necessary to move a patient from one centre to another, a 20% dextrose infusion should be given during the journey.

Respiratory status is monitored using pulse oximetry. Oxygen by mask is given. Endotracheal intubation is necessary for the comatose patient to prevent aspiration. Mechanical ventilation is necessary if respiratory failure

is shown by a rise in arterial $P\text{CO}_2$ (>6.5 kPa) or fall in $P\text{O}_2$ (<10 kPa).

To pre-empt *septic complications*, sputum and urine should be sent for culture daily. Venous and arterial line sites should be inspected regularly; cannulas should be replaced if inflamed, or if fever develops, or otherwise routinely every 3–5 days. The tip of the catheter is sent for culture.

Hypotension is extremely difficult, if not impossible to control. When crystalloid or albumin infusions do not correct the fall in blood pressure, dopamine can be given. If peripheral vascular resistance is particularly low, dopamine with noradrenaline or adrenaline can be tried.

When *renal failure* develops, monitoring of fluid balance becomes even more critical. Dopamine infusion may slow or reverse the change in renal function. Haemodialysis, or preferably arteriovenous haemofiltration [19] are indicated when the serum creatinine rises above about 400 µmol/l (4.5 mg/dl), and to correct fluid overload, acidosis and hyperkalaemia.

Coagulopathy is managed by routine intravenous vitamin K. Fresh frozen plasma and platelets are given if there is bleeding or for invasive procedures such as insertion of an arterial line or extradural pressure transducer.

Hepatic encephalopathy is treated by the usual routine (Chapter 7) with no protein by mouth, and phosphate enemas. Lactulose is given via the nasogastric tube in doses (initially 15–30 ml) sufficient to achieve two loose bowel motions daily. Exacerbating factors, such as sepsis, electrolyte imbalance and haemorrhage should be treated. Sedation must be avoided if at all possible. If absolutely necessary, if the patient is violent, a small dose of a short-acting benzodiazepine (e.g. midazolam) may be given. Neomycin is avoided because of possible nephrotoxicity. Antibiotics given to prevent or treat infection will also serve to treat the encephalopathy. Flumazemil is a benzodiazepine-receptor antagonist which can produce variable, short-lived but distinct improvement in about 70% of patients with hepatic encephalopathy [3, 38]. This drug at present has no formal role in the management of encephalopathy.

Cerebral oedema is an important cause of death. Intracranial pressure monitoring with an extradural pressure transducer is used in specialist units [12, 47, 60] allowing detection of subclinical episodes of intracranial hypertension. Control of cerebral oedema may prolong survival giving a greater chance of the patient reaching transplantation [47]. Complications of transducer insertion, including intracranial bleeding and sepsis, occur in about 4%, with fatal haemorrhage in 1% [12]. The type of transducer chosen depends on local expertise. A platelet count of less than 50×10^9/l is regarded as a contraindication because of the risk of bleeding [47]. Increases of intracranial pressure to 25–30 mmHg sustained for more than 5 minutes are treated with mannitol 1 g/kg body weight (up to 100 g given in a 20% solution as an intravenous bolus). Urine output must be monitored to confirm a diuresis. In patients with renal failure, mannitol should only be used in combination with ultrafiltration, to avoid hyperosmolarity and fluid overload.

It is important to nurse the patient with the upper trunk and head elevated between 20 and 30° above the horizontal since this lowers intracranial pressure. Further elevation may raise intracranial pressure and lower mean arterial pressure [18]. Corticosteroids are not effective, and hyperventilation has an effect which is not sustained [27]. Thiopental infusion is effective in some patients where mannitol and haemofiltration have failed [36] but because of possible haemodynamic effects should be done with intracranial pressure monitoring.

When intracranial pressure monitoring cannot be done, the clinical team should be alert for signs of raised intracranial pressure (see above), and administer mannitol if this is suspected.

Epileptiform activity detected by EEG should be treated with diazepam and/or phenytoin, to reduce the increase in cerebral oxygen consumption that occurs [94].

Infections occur in 90% of patients with fulminant hepatic failure [77]. A retrospective study showed a significantly lower rate of infection in patients who received selective intestinal decontamination (neomycin, colistin and nystatin or norfloxacin and nystatin) prophylactically compared with those who did not [81]. The reduction was predominantly in Gram-negative infection. A randomized controlled study has shown that selective parenteral (cefuroxime) and enteral (colistin, tobramycin, amphotericin B) antibiotic given before evidence of sepsis in patients reaching grade II encephalopathy, approximately halved the rate of infection (fig. 8.5) [76]. The majority of micro-organisms isolated in this study were Gram-positive. A subsequent randomized trial has shown that enteral decontamination gives no benefit over prophylactic parenteral antibiotic alone (ceftazidime, flucloxacillin) [79]. In this study, however, some multiresistant bacteria were encountered, thought related to the third-generation cephalosporin used. Thus the data show that prophylactic antibiotics are valuable in reducing infection in patients with fulminant hepatic failure. The most appropriate regimen will depend on the incidence, type and sensitivity of bacteria on the individual liver unit. Regular microbiological surveillance is essential. Without prophylaxis fungal infections are found in about 30% of patients [78]. Trials in which oral amphotericin B have been used have reduced the rate of fungal infection below 5% (fig. 8.5) [79]. Treatment of systemic fungal infection is with amphotericin B and flucytosine.

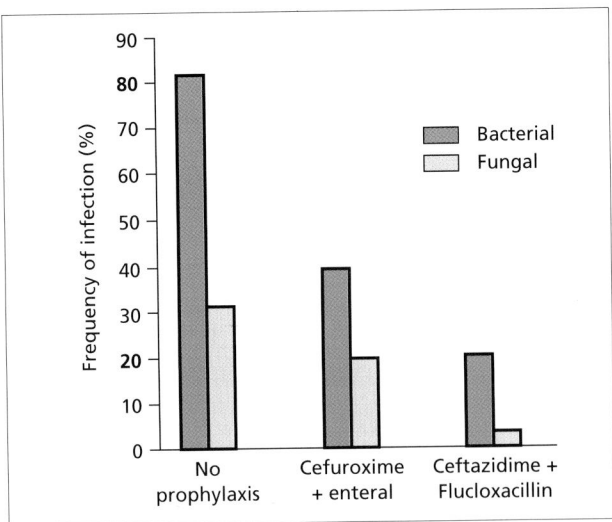

Fig. 8.5. Prevention of sepsis in fulminant hepatic failure: comparison of results from studies at King's College Hospital. Prophylactic parenteral antibiotics reduced infections. Enteral decontamination had no additional benefit. Oral amphotericin B (anti-fungal) was given with both antimicrobial regimes. (Data from [76, 77, 79] courtesy of Dr N. Rolando.)

N-acetylcysteine, initially introduced and validated for the acute treatment (12–15 hours) of acetaminophen self-poisoning, has been shown to improve blood flow, and oxygen delivery and extraction by both peripheral and cerebral tissue [42]. In a controlled trial clinical value has been demonstrated if acetylcysteine is continued (100 mg/kg in 16 hours) for longer than the first 16 hours in patients with fulminant hepatic failure due to acetaminophen [48]. Survival is increased, and cerebral oedema, hypotension and renal failure reduced. Although haemodynamic parameters are improved in non-acetaminophen-induced fulminant failure, studies are awaited to test clinical benefit in this group.

Prostaglandins. Although these may protect against hepatic injury experimentally, randomized clinical trials have not shown benefit in fulminant hepatic failure [5, 83].

Corticosteroids. Large doses of corticosteroids are of no benefit in fulminant hepatic failure. They may even be of negative value. The complications include infections and gastric erosions.

Artificial liver support

The aim is to provide support until the native liver recovers its function spontaneously, or until a donor liver is available. Much research has focused on the use of columns or membranes that would allow removal of toxic metabolites. Charcoal haemoperfusion, despite early promise, has not shown benefit in controlled trials

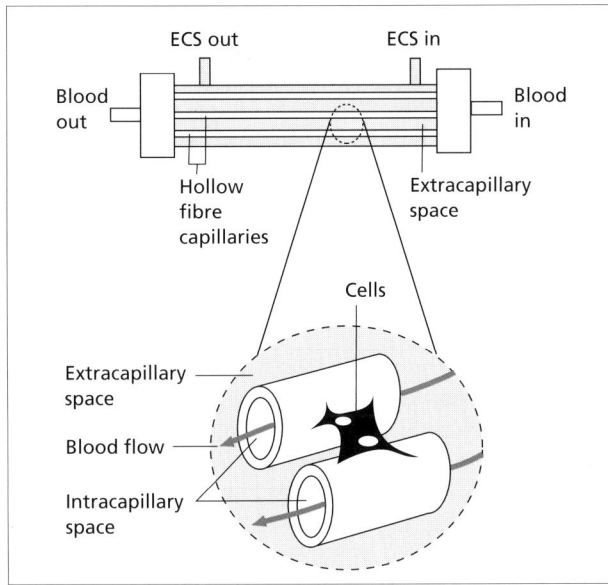

Fig. 8.6. Artificial liver support. Diagram of hollow fibre cartridge device. Cells are cultured on the extracapillary side of the semi-permeable fibres while blood or medium flows through the lumen. (Reproduced with permission from [85].)

[67]. Current studies are focusing on the use of cell-based extracorporeal devices. Plasma or blood is pumped through a network of fine, permeable capillary tubes housed in a chamber containing cultured hepatocytes (fig. 8.6) [85]. The capillary membrane is permeable to plasma components with a molecular weight cut off of about 70 000; cells and immunoglobulins cannot pass. Many types of liver cell have been used, human and non-human. Function of such bioartificial liver devices has been shown experimentally. Preliminary results in patients with fulminant hepatic failure are encouraging with a reduction in encephalopathy, serum ammonia and intracranial pressure, an increase in cerebral perfusion [21] and an improvement in prothrombin time, factor V level and galactose elimination capacity [29]. The technique holds promise for the future, but whether the results will ever regularly lead to recovery of the native liver rather than bridge the gap to successful transplantation remains to be seen. As with hepatocyte transplantation there are many problems to overcome [20].

Liver transplantation

Hepatic transplantation has to be considered for patients reaching grade III and IV coma due to fulminant hepatic failure. The survival rate for these patients without transplantation is usually less than 20%. Survival rates with transplantation are 60–80%. However, it is frequently difficult to judge both the right time and the necessity for transplant. If too early, the operation may be unnecessary and the patient will be committed to life-time immunosuppression; if too late, the chances of successful transplantation are reduced.

Indications [88, 96]

The decision to select ('list') an individual for potential transplant is based on many factors predicting severity. These include age, aetiology, time between onset of jaundice and encephalopathy, prothrombin time and serum bilirubin level [66], or plasma factor V level of less than 20% of normal [8]. In the original studies, use of these criteria identified about 95% of fatal cases. The lower predictive accuracy of these criteria (around 80%) in a subsequent study [71] does not detract from their value in assessing the patient admitted with fulminant hepatic failure. However, there is a delay in obtaining an acceptable donor liver, after putting out the request, of an average of about 2 days [1, 11]. Although the majority will have survived and still require a transplant, and some will have improved and not need a transplant, some will have died (tables 8.7, 8.8) or developed problems that make them inappropriate to transplant. The lower predictive value (0.50) of the prognostic criteria to identify which patients will *not* need a transplant has led to the suggestion that all patients with fulminant and subfulminant hepatic failure should be listed for transplantation on admission to hospital [23, 88] or when they

Table 8.7. Hepatic transplantation for fulminant liver failure (Paris experience) [4]

Number	112
Died waiting	18%
Transplanted	92
Alive	71%

Table 8.8. Transplant for fulminant liver failure (Paris experience) [4]

	Viral hepatitis	Drug-related	Wilson's	Uncertain
Number	53	20	4	33
Died waiting	21%	10%	25%	15%
Transplanted	42	18	3	28
Alive	78%	78%	100%	53%

Table 8.9. Checklist of information when referring patient with fulminant hepatic failure to liver unit

Patient details
Probable cause of liver failure
Risk factors
Drug overdose: when taken, blood levels, treatment
Past medical history
Previous surgery
Previous psychiatric history
Cardiorespiratory status
Current grade of encephalopathy
Assessment of renal and septic status
Obvious Kayser–Fleischer rings
Weight and height

Investigations
Full blood count, platelets
Prothrombin time (fibrin degradation products)
Urea, sodium, potassium, bicarbonate, creatinine, blood glucose, amylase
Bilirubin, transaminase, alkaline phosphatase, albumin
Blood gases, oximetry
Urine output
Positive bacteriological culture
Viral serology (HAV IgM, HBsAg, HBcore IgM)
Chest X-ray
Central venous pressure
Current medication/fluid regime
Scanning data: liver, brain
EEG

reach grade III encephalopathy [71], and that the decison as to whether or not transplantation is necessary should be reviewed when the donor liver becomes available.

These prognostic uncertainties emphasize the need for the early dialogue with (table 8.9), and transfer of patients with fulminant hepatic failure to, a specialist liver unit with the facilities for transplantation. Children in particular should be transferred before the development of hepatic encephalopathy [24].

Contraindications

Absolute contraindications are active ongoing infection;

adult respiratory distress syndrome and inspired oxygen of greater than 60%; fixed dilated pupils for prolonged periods of time (1 hour or more); and cerebral perfusion pressure <40 mmHg for longer than 1 hour or intracranial pressure >35 mmHg [96]. Relative contraindications are a rapidly increasing requirement for vasopressor support, infection under treatment and a history of psychiatric problems [63].

Results

Technically the operation is less difficult than that for chronic liver disease as portal venous collaterals and adhesions are not present. Coagulation defects can be controlled with plasma derivatives and platelets.

Published results worldwide show a survival between 40 and 90% (table 8.10), the variation probably reflecting the severity of illness at the time of transplantation and the criteria for proceeding with transplantation. These results compare with an estimated 20% survival of patients with fulminant hepatic failure reaching this stage of disease who are not transplanted. Donor livers are hard to find at short notice, and livers that are not ideal, for example with an incompatible blood group or steatosis, may be used. This worsens the results [10].

Analysis of the influence of pretransplantation status on outcome in fulminant hepatic failure has shown that in non-acetaminophen-induced liver failure, survival is related to aetiology and serum creatinine [23]. At the time of transplant indices of the severity of systemic illness (organ system failure and Apache III score) and serum creatinine discriminated survivors from non-survivors. In the acetaminophen group, time from ingestion to transplantation was significantly shorter in the survivors than non-survivors (4 ± 1 versus 6 ± 1 days). At the time of transplantation serum bilirubin and Apache III score correlated with survival [23].

Liver transplantation has been performed in patients with fulminant hepatitis A, B and presumed non-A non-B. Results in patients with hepatitis B are particularly satisfactory as the disease does not usually recur in the transplanted liver. Fulminant hepatitis developing in

Table 8.10. Transplantation for fulminant hepatic failure

Centre	References	Date	Number	Survival (%)
Birmingham, UK	Vickers *et al.* [90]	1988	16	56
Chicago	Emond *et al.* [31]	1989	19	58
London/Cambridge	Williams & O'Grady [95]	1990	56	58
Paris	Devictor *et al.* [24]	1992	19	68
San Francisco	Ascher *et al.* [1]	1993	35	92
Madrid	Moreno Gonzalez *et al.* [61]	1994	35	47
Pittsburgh	Dodson *et al.* [25]	1994	115	60
Paris	Bismuth *et al.* [10]	1995	116	68

hepatitis B carriers after withdrawal of immunosuppressive therapy has also been treated. Several patients transplanted for putative non-A non-B hepatitis have suffered acute fulminant hepatitis 5–8 days after the transplant. Togavirus-like particles have been demonstrated in the explanted as well as grafted liver [32]. Aplastic anaemia has occurred in 33% of children transplanted for fulminant non-A non-B hepatitis [14].

Auxiliary liver transplantation

The native liver is left in place, and the donor liver graft either placed in the right upper quadrant alongside the native liver (heterotopic), or part of the native liver is resected and replaced with a reduced size graft (orthotopic). The intention is to provide viable liver function from the graft, giving the native hepatitic liver time to recover and regenerate. The advantage is the temporary need for immunosuppression. Experience is limited, with survival of about 60% [44].

Conclusion

Liver transplantation cannot be accepted as the perfect and ideal treatment for fulminant hepatic failure, but it gives survival to many patients who otherwise would have died. Early referral of patients to a specialist centre must be emphasized. This will increase the chance of the patient being fit enough for transfer. Delayed action loses the window of opportunity for safe transfer and greater success of transplantation. There are still considerable selection difficulties. Some patients will clearly be candidates for transplant, some will obviously be unsuitable. The doubt lies in the intermediate cases and how many in this category will recover with conservative treatment alone. The initial selection of potential candidates for transplantation is separate from the final decision to proceed [23]. The success and role of artificial liver support systems and of auxiliary liver transplantation await further evaluation.

References

1 Ascher NL, Lake JR, Emond JC *et al*. Liver transplantation for fulminant hepatic failure. *Arch. Surg.* 1995; **128**: 677.

2 Banks AT, Zimmerman HJ, Ishak KG *et al*. Diclofenac-associated hepatotoxicity: analysis of 180 cases reported to the food and drug administration as adverse reactions. *Hepatology* 1995; **22**: 820.

3 Bansky G, Meier PJ, Riederer E *et al*. Effects of the benzodiazepine receptor antagonist flumazenil in hepatic encephalopathy in humans. *Gastroenterology* 1989; **97**: 744.

4 Benhamou JP. Fulminant hepatic failure. American Association for the Study of the Liver Disease Course Syllabus, 1990.

5 Bernuau J, Babany G, Pauwels A *et al*. Prostaglandin E_1 (PGE$_1$) has no beneficial effect in patients with either severe or fulminant hepatitis due to drugs or of undetermined etiology. *Hepatology* 1990; **12**: 373A.

6 Bernuau J, Benhamou JP. Classifying acute liver failure. *Lancet* 1993; **342**: 252.

7 Bernuau J, Rueff B, Benhamou JP. Fulminant and subfulminant liver failure: definitions and causes. *Semin. Liver Dis.* 1986; **6**: 97.

8 Bernuau J, Goudeau A, Poynard T *et al*. Multivariate analysis of prognostic factors in fulminant hepatitis B. *Hepatology* 1986; **6**: 648.

9 Bihari DJ, Gimson AES, Williams R. Cardiovascular, pulmonary and renal complications of fulminant hepatic failure. *Semin. Liver Dis.* 1986; **6**: 119.

10 Bismuth H, Samuel D, Castaing D *et al*. Orthotopic liver transplantation in fulminant and subfulminant hepatitis. The Paul Brousse experience. *Ann. Surg.* 1995; **222**: 109.

11 Bismuth H, Samuel D, Guggenheim J *et al*. Emergency liver transplantation for fulminant hepatitis. *Ann. Intern. Med.* 1987; **107**: 337.

12 Blei AT, Olafsson S, Webster S *et al*. Complications of intracranial pressure monitoring in fulminant hepatic failure. *Lancet* 1993; **341**: 157.

13 Caraceni P, Van Thiel DH. Acute liver failure. *Lancet* 1995; **345**: 163.

14 Cattral MS, Langnas AN, Markin RS *et al*. Aplastic anemia after liver transplantation for fulminant liver failure. *Hepatology* 1994; **20**: 813.

15 Chu C-M, Chiu K-W, Liaw Y-F. The prevalence and prognostic significance of spontaneous bacterial peritonitis in severe acute hepatitis with ascites. *Hepatology* 1992; **15**: 799.

16 Chu C-M, Sheen I-S, Liaw Y-F. The role of hepatitis C virus in fulminant viral hepatitis in an area with endemic hepatitis A and B. *Gastroenterology* 1994; **107**: 189.

17 Clapperton M, Rolando N, Sandoval L *et al*. Neutrophil superoxide (O^{-2}) and hydrogen peroxide (H_2O_2) production in patients with acute liver failure. *Eur. J. Invest.* (in press).

18 Davenport A, Will EJ, Davison AM. Effect of posture on intracranial pressure and cerebral perfusion pressure in patients with fulminant hepatic and renal failure after acetaminophen self-poisoning. *Crit. Care Med.* 1990; **18**: 286.

19 Davenport A, Will EJ, Losowsky MS *et al*. Continuous arteriovenous haemofiltration in patients with hepatic encephalopathy and renal failure. *Br. Med. J.* 1987; **295**: 1028.

20 Davies E, Hodgson HJF. Artificial livers — what's keeping them? *Gut* 1995; **36**: 168.

21 Demetriou AA, Rozga J, Podesta L *et al*. Early clinical experience with a hybrid bioartificial liver. *Scand. J. Gastroenterol.* 1995; **30** (Suppl. 208): 111.

22 Desmet VJ, De Groote J, Van Damme B. Hepato-cellular failure: a study of 17 patients with exchange transfusion. *Hum. Pathol.* 1972; **3**: 167.

23 Devlin J, Wendon J, Heaton N *et al*. Pretransplantation clinical status and outcome of emergency transplantation for acute liver failure. *Hepatology* 1995; **21**: 1018.

24 Devictor D, Desplanques L, Debray D *et al*. Emergency liver transplantation for fulminant liver failure in infants and children. *Hepatology* 1992; **16**: 1156.

25 Dodson SF, Dehara K, Iwatsuki S. Liver transplantation for fulminant hepatic failure. *ASAIO J.* 1994; **40**: 86.

26 Donaldson BW, Gopinath R, Wanless IR *et al*. The role of transjugular liver biopsy in fulminant liver failure: relation to other prognostic indicators. *Hepatology* 1993; **18**: 1370.

27 Ede RJ, Gimson AES, Bihari D *et al.* Controlled hyperventilation in the prevention of cerebral oedema in fulminant hepatic failure. *J. Hepatol.* 1986; **2**: 43.

28 Ede RJ, Williams RW. Hepatic encephalopathy and cerebral edema. *Semin. Liver Dis.* 1986; **6**: 107.

29 Ellis AJ, Wendon J, Hughes R *et al.* A controlled trial of the Hepatix Extracorporeal Liver Assist Device (ELAD) in acute liver failure. *Hepatology* 1994; **20**: 140A (Abstr.).

30 Ellis AJ, Saleh M, Smith H *et al.* Late-onset hepatic failure: clinical features, serology and outcome following transplantation. *J. Hepatol.* 1995; **23**: 363.

31 Emond JC, Aran PP, Whitington PF *et al.* Liver transplantation in the management of fulminant hepatic failure. *Gastroenterology* 1989; **96**: 1583.

32 Fagan EA. Acute liver failure of unknown pathogenesis: the hidden agenda. *Hepatology* 1994; **19**: 1307.

33 Feray C, Gigou M, Samuel D *et al.* Hepatitis C virus RNA and hepatitis B virus DNA in serum and liver of patients with fulminant hepatitis. *Gastroenterology* 1993; **104**: 549.

34 Ferenci P. Brain dysfunction in fulminant hepatic failure. *J. Hepatol.* 1994; **21**: 487.

35 Flowers MA, Heathcote J, Wanless IR *et al.* Fulminant hepatitis as a consequence of reactivation of hepatitis B virus infection after discontinuation of low-dose methotrexate therapy. *Ann. Intern. Med.* 1990; **112**: 381.

36 Forbes A, Alexander GJM, O'Grady JG *et al.* Thiopental infusion in the treatment of intracranial hypertension complicating fulminant hepatic failure. *Hepatology* 1989; **10**: 306.

37 Gimson AES, O'Grady JG, Ede RJ *et al.* Late-onset hepatic failure: clinical, serological and histological features. *Hepatology* 1986; **6**: 288.

38 Grimm G, Ferenci P, Katzenschlager R *et al.* Improvement of hepatic encephalopathy treated with flumazenil. *Lancet* 1988; **1**: 1392.

39 Guarner F, Hughes RD, Gimson AES *et al.* Renal function in fulminant hepatic failure: haemodynamics and renal prostaglandins. *Gut* 1987; **28**: 1643.

40 Hanau C, Munoz SJ, Rubin R. Histopathological heterogeneity in fulminant hepatic failure. *Hepatology* 1995; **21**: 345.

41 Harrison R, Letz G, Pasternak G *et al.* Fulminant hepatic failure after occupational exposure to 2-nitropropane. *Ann. Intern. Med.* 1987; **107**: 466.

42 Harrison PM, Wendon JA, Gimson AES *et al.* Improvement by acetylcysteine of hemodynamics and oxygen transport in fulminant hepatic failure. *N. Engl. J. Med.* 1991; **324**: 1852.

43 Henry JA, Jeffreys KJ, Dawling S. Toxicity and deaths from 3,4-methylenedioxymetamphetamine ('ecstasy'). *Lancet* 1992; **340**: 384.

44 Hoofnagle JH, Carithers RL, Shapiro C *et al.* Fulminant hepatic failure: summary of a workshop. *Hepatology* 1995; **21**: 240.

45 Hussain W, Mutimer D, Harrison R *et al.* Fulminant hepatic failure caused by tuberculosis. *Gut* 1995; **36**: 792.

46 Imawari M, Hughes RD, Gove CD *et al.* Fibronectin and Kupffer cell function in fulminant hepatic failure. *Dig. Dis. Sci.* 1985; **30**: 1028.

47 Keays RT, Alexander GJM, Williams R. The safety and value of extradural intracranial pressure monitors in fulminant hepatic failure. *J. Hepatol.* 1993; **18**: 205.

48 Keays R, Harrison PM, Wendon JA *et al.* Intravenous acetylcysteine in paracetamol induced fulminant hepatic failure: a prospective controlled trial. *Br. Med. J.* 1991; **303**: 1026.

49 Kennedy J, Parbhoo SP, MacGillivray B *et al.* Effect of extracorporeal liver perfusion on the electroencephalogram of patients in coma due to acute liver failure. *Q. J. Med.* 1973; **42**: 549.

50 Klein AS, Hart J, Brems JJ *et al.* Amanita poisoning: treatment and the role of liver transplantation. *Am. J. Med.* 1989; **86**: 187.

51 Komori H, Hirasa M, Takakuwa H *et al.* Concept of the clinical stages of acute hepatic failure. *Am. J. Gastroenterol.* 1986; **81**: 544.

52 Kumahara T, Muto Y, Moriwaki H *et al.* Determination of an integrated CT number of the whole liver in patients with severe hepatitis: an indicator of the functional reserve of the liver. *Gastroenterol. Jpn.* 1989; **24**: 290.

53 Lake JR, Sussman NL. Determining prognosis in patients with fulminant hepatic failure: when you absolutely, positively have to know the answer. *Hepatology* 1995; **21**: 879.

54 Langnas AN, Markin RS, Cattral MS *et al.* Parvovirus B19 as a possible causative agent of fulminant liver failure and associated aplastic anaemia. *Hepatology* 1995; **22**: 1661.

55 Larsen FS, Knudsen GM, Paulson OB *et al.* Cerebral blood flow autoregulation is absent in rats with thioacetamide-induced hepatic failure. *J. Hepatol.* 1994; **21**: 491.

56 Lau JYN, Sallie R, Fang JWS *et al.* Detection of hepatitis E virus genome and gene products in two patients with fulminant hepatitis E. *J. Hepatol.* 1995; **22**: 605.

57 Lee WM. Acute liver failure. *N. Engl. J. Med.* 1993; **329**: 1862.

58 Lee WM, Galbraith RM, Watt GH *et al.* Predicting survival in fulminant hepatic failure using serum Gc protein concentrations. *Hepatology* 1995; **21**: 101.

59 Liang TJ, Hasegawa K, Rimon N *et al.* A hepatitis B virus mutant associated with an epidemic of fulminant hepatitis. *N. Engl. J. Med.* 1991; **324**: 1705.

60 Lidofsky SD, Bass NM, Prager MC *et al.* Intracranial pressure monitoring and liver transplantation for fulminant liver failure. *Hepatology* 1992; **16**: 1.

61 Moreno Gonzalez E, Loinaz C, Garcia I *et al.* Orthotopic liver transplantation in 35 patients with fulminant hepatic failure. *Transplant Proc.* 1994; **26**: 3640.

62 Munoz SJ, Maddrey WC. Major complications of acute and chronic liver disease. *Gastroenterol. Clin. North Am.* 1988; **17**: 265.

63 Mutimer DJ, Ayres RCS, Neuberger JM *et al.* Serious paracetamol poisoning and the results of liver transplantation. *Gut* 1994; **35**: 809.

64 Mutimer D, Shaw J, Neuberger J *et al.* Failure to incriminate hepatitis B, hepatitis C, and hepatitis E viruses in the aetiology of fulminant non-A non-B hepatitis. *Gut* 1995; **36**: 433.

65 O'Brien CJ, Wise RJS, O'Grady JG *et al.* Neurological sequelae in patients recovered from fulminant hepatic failure. *Gut* 1987; **28**: 93.

66 O'Grady JG, Alexander GJM, Hayllar KM *et al.* Early indicators of prognosis in fulminant hepatic failure. *Gastroenterology* 1989; **97**: 439.

67 O'Grady JG, Gimson AES, O'Brien CJ *et al.* Controlled trials of charcoal hemoperfusion and prognostic factors in fulminant hepatic failure. *Gastroenterology* 1988; **94**: 1186.

68 O'Grady JG, Schalm SW, Williams R. Acute liver failure: redefining the syndromes. *Lancet* 1993; **342**: 273.

69 Papaevangelou G, Tassopoulos N, Roumeliotou-Karayannis A *et al.* Etiology of fulminant viral hepatitis in Greece. *Hepatology* 1984; **4**: 369.

70 Papatheodoridis GV, Delladetsima JK, Kavallierou L *et al.* Fulminant hepatitis due to Epstein–Barr virus infection. *J. Hepatol.* 1995; **23**: 348.

71 Pauwels A, Mostefa-Kara N, Florent C *et al.* Emergency liver transplantation for acute liver failure: evaluation of London and Clichy criteria. *J. Hepatol.* 1993; **17**: 124.

72 Pernambuco JR, Langley PG, Hughes RD *et al.* Activation of the fibrinolytic system in patients with fulminant liver failure. *Hepatology* 1993; **18**: 1350.

73 Redeker AG, Yamahiro HS. Controlled trial of exchange-transfusion therapy in fulminant hepatitis. *Lancet* 1973; **1**: 3.

74 Riegler JL, Lake JR. Fulminant hepatic failure. *Med. Clin. North Am.* 1993; **77**: 1057.

75 Ring-Larsen H, Palazzo U. Renal failure in fulminant hepatic failure and terminal cirrhosis: a comparison between incidence, types and prognosis. *Gut* 1981; **22**: 585.

76 Rolando N, Gimson A, Wade J *et al.* Prospective controlled trial of selective parenteral and enteral antimicrobial regimen in fulminant hepatic failure. *Hepatology* 1993; **17**: 196.

77 Rolando N, Harvey F, Brahm J *et al.* Prospective study of bacterial infection in acute liver failure: an analysis of fifty patients. *Hepatology* 1990; **11**: 49.

78 Rolando N, Harvey F, Brahm J *et al.* Fungal infection: a common, unrecognised complication of acute liver failure. *J. Hepatol.* 1991; **12**: 1.

79 Rolando N, Wade JJ, Stangou A *et al.* Prospective study comparing the efficacy of prophylactic parenteral antimicrobials, with or without enteral decontamination, in patients with acute liver failure. *Liver Transplant Surg.* 1996; **2**: 8.

80 Sallie R, Chiyende J, Tan KC *et al.* Fulminant hepatic failure resulting from coexistent Wilson's disease and hepatitis E. *Gut* 1994; **35**: 849.

81 Salmeron JM, Tito L, Rimola A *et al.* Selective intestinal decontamination in the prevention of bacterial infection in patients with acute liver failure. *J. Hepatol.* 1992; **14**: 280.

82 Saracco G, Macagno S, Rosina F *et al.* Serologic markers with fulminant hepatitis in persons positive for hepatitis B surface antigen. A worldwide epidemiologic and clinical survey. *Ann. Intern. Med.* 1988; **108**: 380.

83 Sheiner SB, Sinclair S, Greig P *et al.* A randomised control trial of prostaglandin E$_2$ (PGE$_2$) in the treatment of fulminant hepatic failure. *Hepatology* 1992; **16**: 88A.

84 Sherlock S. Vasodilatation associated with hepatocellular disease: relation to functional organ failure. *Gut* 1990; **31**: 365.

85 Sussman NL, Chong MG, Koussayer T *et al.* Reversal of fulminant hepatic failure using an extracorporeal liver assist device. *Hepatology* 1992; **16**: 60.

86 Takahashi Y, Kumada H, Shimizu M *et al.* A multicenter study on the prognosis of fulminant viral hepatitis: early prediction for liver transplantation. *Hepatology* 1994; **19**: 1065.

87 Trewby PN, Warren R, Contini S *et al.* Incidence and pathophysiology of pulmonary edema in fulminant hepatic failure. *Gastroenterology* 1978; **74**: 859.

88 Van Thiel DH. When should a decision to procede with transplantation actually be made in cases of fulminant or subfulminant hepatic failure: at admission to hospital or when a donor organ is made available? *J. Hepatol.* 1993; **17**: 1.

89 Vento S, Cainelli F, Mirandola F *et al.* Fulminant hepatitis on withdrawal of chemotherapy in carriers of hepatitis C virus. *Lancet* 1996; **347**: 92.

90 Vickers C, Neuberger J, Buckels J *et al.* Transplantation of the liver in adults and children with fulminant hepatic failure. *J. Hepatol.* 1988; **7**: 143.

91 Villamil FG, Hu K-Q, Yu C-H *et al.* Detection of hepatitis C virus with RNA polymerase chain reaction in fulminant hepatic failure. *Hepatology* 1995; **22**: 1379.

92 Wendon JA, Harrison PM, Keays R *et al.* Cerebral blood flow and metabolism in fulminant liver failure. *Hepatology* 1994; **19**: 1407.

93 Whelan J, Makk L, Tamburro CH. Early determination for liver transplantation in acute and subacute massive necrosis by use of the transvenous liver biopsy (TVLB). *Hepatology* 1988; **8**: 1446 (abstract).

94 Williams R. New directions in acute liver failure. *J. Roy. Coll. Phys. Ldn.* 1994; **28**: 552.

95 Williams R, O'Grady JG. Liver transplantation: results, advances and problems. *J. Gastroenterol. Hepatol.* 1990; suppl. **1**: 110.

96 Williams R, Wendon J. Indications for orthotopic liver transplantation in fulminant liver failure. *Hepatology* 1994; **20**: 5S.

97 Woolf GM, Petrovic LM, Rojter SE *et al.* Acute liver failure due to lymphoma. A diagnostic concern when considering liver transplantation. *Dig. Dis. Sci.* 1994; **39**: 1351.

98 Wright TL. Etiology of fulminant hepatic failure: is another virus involved? *Gastroenterology* 1993; **104**: 640.

99 Zimmerman HJ, Maddrey WC. Acetaminophen (paracetamol) hepatotoxicity with regular intake of alcohol: analysis of instances of therapeutic misadventure. *Hepatology* 1995; **22**: 767.

Chapter 9
Ascites

Cirrhotic patients with ascites retain sodium avidly, urinary sodium excretion being less than 5 mmol daily. Serum sodium levels are somewhat reduced. This does not reflect sodium deficiency since, because of the greatly expanded extra-cellular sodium space, the actual body stores of sodium are increased.

Sodium retention is a cause rather than consequence of ascites formation. It precedes the accumulation of ascitic fluid. The localization of the fluid within the peritoneal cavity rather than in peripheral tissues is probably related to portal hypertension. Sodium retention is early as a result of hepatic venous outflow block and primary vasodilatation.

Sinusoidal portal hypertension correlates closely with both urinary sodium excretion and the degree of activation of the renin–angiotensin–aldosterone and sympathetic nervous systems. It results in increased hepatic lymph production. In cirrhotic patients, the rate of lymphatic return via the thoracic duct can reach 20 litres a day [71]. This hepatic lymph extravasates into the peritoneal cavity where it equilibrates with the intestinal capillaries. Ascitic fluid will be generated with essentially the same relative protein composition as that of the plasma but much diluted.

Mechanisms of ascites formation

Underfill theory

Traditionally, the kidney is believed to be responding to a contraction of the effective circulating plasma volume (that part of the total circulating volume that is effective in stimulating volume receptors) (fig. 9.1). High portal venous pressure, the dilatation of the *splanchnic* vascular bed, hypoalbuminaemia and peripheral vasodilatation associated with arteriovenous shunting all combine to sequester fluid away from the central arterial tree. The kidney therefore behaves as if it thinks its owner is underfilled and needs more salt and water [12]. Confirmation of this view has always been difficult as accurate measurements of effective circulating plasma volume in ascitic cirrhotic patients is difficult. Indirect confirmation comes from measuring the hormonal correlates of a reduced effective plasma volume. Such a reduction

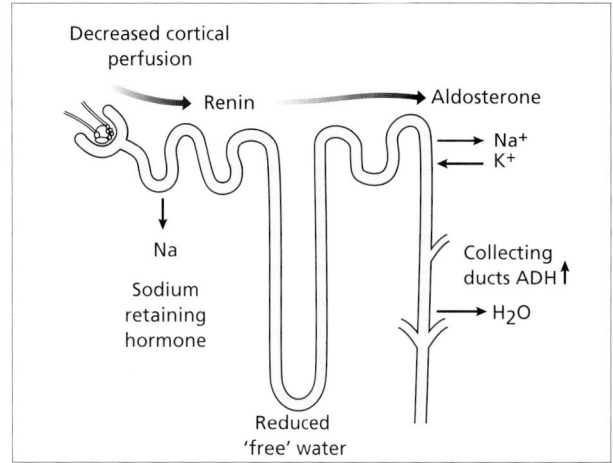

Fig. 9.1. Renal changes in ascites. Decreased renal cortical perfusion leads to renin release with aldosterone excess. Reduced extracellular fluid volume leads to sodium reabsorption. 'Free' water clearance is reduced. ADH plays a minor role.

would initiate a baroreceptor reflex and plasma noradrenaline, a marker of peripheral sympathetic activity, would rise. This has been shown in cirrhotic patients who were unable to excrete a water load normally [8, 9]. Increasing the effective plasma volume by body immersion [14] or by peritoneo-venous shunting may induce a diuresis.

Dilutional hyponatraemia, due to water retention, might be related to hypersecretion of arginine vasopressin which increases water absorption in the collecting renal tubules [3].

Reduction of the effective plasma volume has various consequences (fig. 9.2). The renin–angiotensin II system is stimulated with release of aldosterone. The sympathetic nervous system is enhanced with increased plasma noradrenaline levels. This may be responsible for renal vasoconstriction and some of the circulatory changes seen in cirrhosis.

Bradykinin and other kinins synthesized in the kidney modulate intrarenal blood flow and renal sodium handling and are low in cirrhosis.

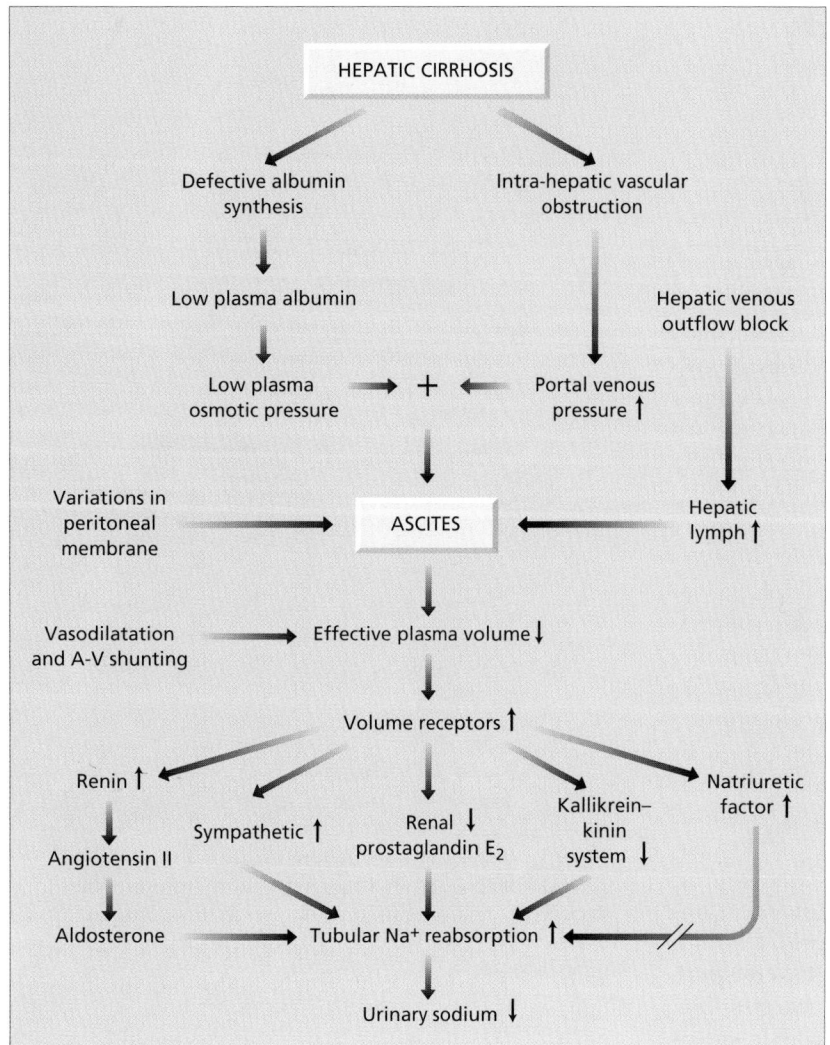

Fig. 9.2. The possible mechanisms of ascites formation in cirrhosis.

Overfill theory

Inappropriate renal sodium retention with expansion of the plasma volume is the primary event in ascites formation [30]. This is supported by the finding of sodium and water retention preceding ascites formation. The increased hepatic venous pressure is transmitted to the sinusoids which have a rich pre-sinusoidal innervation and are a suitable area for splanchnic baroreceptors. The main arguments in favour of this theory are that spontaneous diuresis occurs in the absence of a further increase in plasma volume, plasma volume expansion is frequently inefficient in provoking diuresis and haemodynamic alterations may not be detected in the very early sodium-retaining stage of the disease. This overfill theory may be correct in the early stages, when general and splanchnic vasodilatation results in increased vascular capacitance, arteriolar, capillary and venous. This is followed by arterial underfilling when renal sodium reabsorption cannot keep pace with the arterial vasodilatation.

Peripheral arterial vasodilatation hypothesis [57]

This hypothesis combines both the classical underfill and overfill views. Neither ascites formation and hypovolaemia-induced renal sodium and water retention (underfill), nor primary renal sodium and water retention, blood volume expansion and overflow ascites (overfill) are considered to be the initiating or primary mechanism of the renal sodium and water retention in cirrhosis. The cirrhotic patient is in a state of peripheral arterial vasodilatation and microscopic arteriovenous fistulae are frequent (fig. 9.3). There is decreased filling of the arterial vascular tree with an increase in cardiac output and hormonal stimulation, with rises in renin, aldosterone, noradrenaline and vasopressin. This leads to renal vasoconstriction and sodium and water retention. If severe and continued the hepato-renal syndrome results.

Vasodilatory factors. The hyperdynamic systemic and splanchnic circulation of chronic liver disease plays a key role in ascites formation. The vasodilators are often

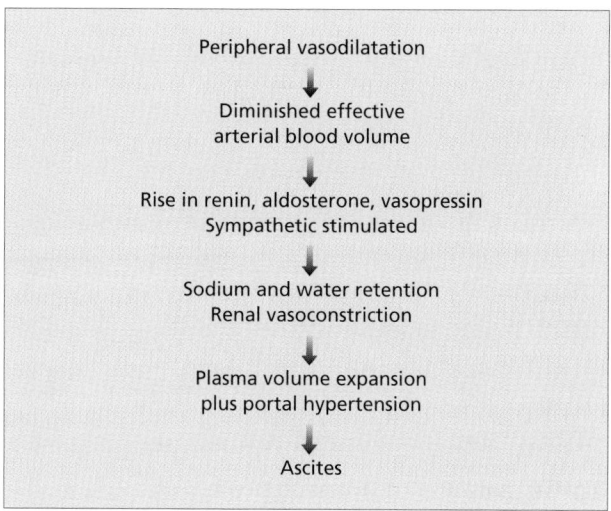

Peripheral vasodilatation

↓

Diminished effective
arterial blood volume

↓

Rise in renin, aldosterone, vasopressin
Sympathetic stimulated

↓

Sodium and water retention
Renal vasoconstriction

↓

Plasma volume expansion
plus portal hypertension

↓

Ascites

Fig. 9.3. The peripheral arterial vasodilatation hypothesis for ascites formation in cirrhosis [57].

of intestinal origin. They are produced by endothelial cells in response to endotoxin and cytokines which reach the circulation through a permeable gut or as a result of porto-systemic shunting (Chapter 6). They include nitric oxide [42] and substance P [16].

Renal changes

Atrial natriuretic factor (ANF) is a potent vaso-relaxant, natriuretic peptide released from the cardiac atria, probably in response to intravascular volume expansion [70]. In early compensated cirrhosis, ANF may maintain sodium homeostasis despite the presence of mild anti-natriuretic factors. In the later stages renal resistance to ANF develops, rendering it ineffective. ANF probably has no primary role in the sodium retention of cirrhosis.

Water excretion is defective because proximal tubular reabsorption of sodium is so great that none passes to the distal 'loop' site to allow 'free' water to be generated (fig. 9.1). It can be treated by giving an osmotic diuretic which flushes sodium distally and so allows free water to be cleared.

Serum potassium is normal or slightly depressed but the body's exchangeable potassium is decreased. This is due not only to excessive loss from secondary aldosteronism but to failure of the cells to maintain their potassium content (cellular depletion). Reduction in total muscle mass is contributory. Diarrhoea is a factor in alcoholics.

A normal renal circulation and glomerular filtration rate are necessary for sodium excretion. In patients with cirrhosis they may be depressed by intensive diuretic therapy, by complicating renal disease, by increased abdominal pressure of tense ascites on the renal veins, by

renal vaso-constriction or chronic liver failure with hypotension.

Non-steroidal anti-inflammatory drugs, such as indomethacin, which inhibit prostaglandin synthesis (cyclo-oxygenase activity) are contraindicated for they reduce glomerular filtration rate and renal water transport and lead to oliguria [36]. Conversely, infusion of arachidonic acid increases medullary blood flow by enhancing renal prostaglandin production (see fig. 9.2).

Circulation of ascites

Once formed, ascitic fluid can exchange with blood through an enormous capillary bed under the visceral peritoneum. This plays a vital, dynamic role, sometimes actively facilitating transfer of fluid into the ascites and sometimes retarding it. Ascitic fluid is continuously circulating, about half entering and leaving the peritoneal cavity every hour, there being a rapid transit in both directions. The constituents of the fluid are in dynamic equilibrium with those of the plasma.

Summary (figs 9.1, 9.2, 9.3)

The underfill hypothesis of ascites formation states that renal sodium and water retention is due to a reduced effective blood volume secondary to fluid drainage into an excessively filled splanchnic bed. The renal changes are mediated by stimulation of the renin–angiotensin–aldosterone system, an increase in sympathetic function, and a rise in prostaglandin E$_2$; the role of atrial natriuretic peptide is minor.

The overfill view suggests that renal retention of sodium is primary with expansion of the plasma volume and overflow into the extravascular space.

An active role of the peritoneal capillary membrane in controlling the passage of fluid is possible. The increase in intra-sinusoidal pressure found in cirrhosis and hepatic venous obstruction stimulates hepatic lymph formation and this adds to the ascites.

Clinical features

Onset

Ascites may appear suddenly or develop insidiously over the course of months with accompanying flatulent abdominal distension.

Ascites may develop suddenly when hepato-cellular function is reduced, for instance by haemorrhage, 'shock', infection or an alcoholic debauch. This might be related to the fall in serum albumin values and/or to intravascular fluid depletion. Occlusion of the portal vein may precipitate ascites in a patient with a low serum albumin level.

The insidious onset proclaims a worse prognosis, possibly because it is not associated with any rectifiable factor.

There is gradually increasing abdominal distension and the patient may present with dyspnoea.

Examination

The patient is sallow and dehydrated. Sweating is diminished. Muscle wasting is profound. The thin limbs with the protuberant belly lead to the description of the patient as a 'spider man'. The ascites may be classified into mild, moderate or tense.

The abdomen is distended not only with fluid but also by air in the dilated intestines. The fullness is particularly conspicuous in the flanks. The umbilicus is everted and the distance between the symphysis pubis and umbilicus seems diminished.

The increased intra-abdominal pressure favours the protrusion of hernias in the umbilical, femoral or inguinal regions or through old abdominal incisions. Scrotal oedema is frequent.

Distended abdominal wall veins may represent porto-systemic collateral channels which radiate from the umbilicus and persist after control of the ascites. Inferior vena caval collaterals result from a secondary, functional block of the inferior vena cava due to pressure of the peritoneal fluid. They commonly run from the groin to the costal margin or flanks and disappear when the ascites is controlled and intra-abdominal pressure is reduced. Abdominal striae may develop.

Dullness on percussion in the flanks is the earliest sign and can be detected when about two litres are present. The distribution of the dullness differs from that due to enlargement of the bladder, an ovarian tumour or a pregnant uterus when the flanks are resonant to percussion. With tense ascites it is difficult to palpate the abdominal viscera, but with moderate amounts of fluid the liver or spleen may be balloted.

A fluid thrill means much free fluid; it is a very late sign of fluid under tension.

The lung bases may be dull to percussion due to elevation of the diaphragm.

Secondary effects

A *pleural effusion* is found in about 6% of cirrhotics and in 67% of these it is right-sided. It is due to defects in the diaphragm allowing ascites to pass into the pleural cavity (fig. 9.4). This can be shown by introducing ^{131}I albumin or air into the ascites and examining the pleural space afterwards. A left-sided pleural effusion may indicate tuberculosis [35].

Right hydrothorax may be seen in the absence of ascites due to the negative intrathoracic pressure during

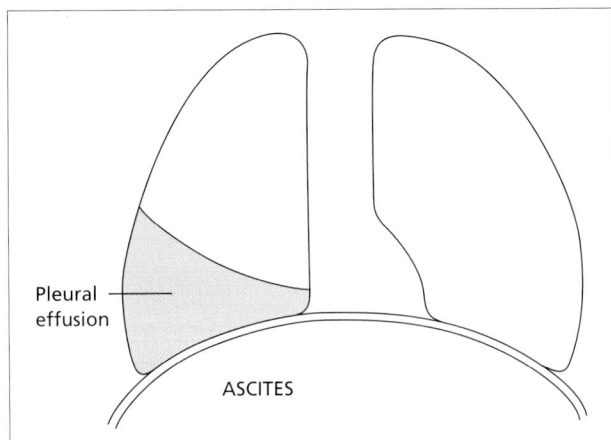

Fig. 9.4. A right-sided pleural effusion may accompany ascites and is related to defects in the diaphragm.

breathing, drawing the peritoneal fluid through the diaphragmatic defects into the pleural cavity [19].

The pleural fluid is in equilibrium with the ascites and control depends on medical control of the ascites. Thoracocentesis is followed by rapid filling up of the pleural space by ascitic fluid. Transjugular intra-hepatic portosystemic stent shunt (TIPS) has been successful [64].

Spontaneous bacterial empyema may be a complication [73].

Oedema usually follows the ascites and is related to hypoproteinaemia. A functional inferior vena caval block due to pressure of the abdominal fluid is an additional factor.

The *cardiac apex beat* is displaced up and out by the raised diaphragm.

The *neck veins* are distended. This is secondary to the increase in right atrial pressure and intrapleural pressure which follows tense ascites and a raised diaphragm. A persisting increase in jugular venous pressure after ascites is controlled implies a cardiac cause for the fluid retention.

Ascitic fluid

Diagnostic paracentesis (of about 50 ml) is always performed however obvious the cause of the ascites. Complications, including bowel perforation and haemorrhage, can develop, rarely, after paracentesis in patients with cirrhosis.

Protein concentration rarely exceeds 1–2 g/100 ml. Higher values suggest infection. Obstruction to the hepatic veins (Budd–Chiari syndrome) is usually, but not always, associated with a very high ascitic fluid protein. Pancreatic ascites is also found with a high ascitic protein value.

If the serum albumin minus ascites albumin *gradient* is

greater than 1.1 g/dl, the patient has portal hypertension.

Electrolyte concentrations are those of other extracellular fluids.

Ascitic fluid protein and white cell count, but not polymorph concentration, increase during a diuresis.

Fluid appears clear, green, straw-coloured or bile-stained. The volume is variable and up to 70 litres have been recorded. A blood-stained fluid indicates malignant disease or a recent paracentesis or an invasive investigation, such as liver biopsy or trans-hepatic cholangiography or TIPS.

Chylous ascites results from accumulation of fat, predominantly chylomicrons, in the ascitic fluid. It is a rare complication of advanced cirrhosis [11]. Intestinal lymph is probably the source.

The *protein content* and *white cell count* should be measured and a *film* examined for organisms. Aerobic and anaerobic *cultures* should be performed.

The percentage of positive cultures can be markedly increased if ascitic fluid is inoculated directly into blood culture bottles at the bedside.

Cytology. The normal endothelial cells in the peritoneum can resemble malignant cells, so leading to an over-diagnosis of cancer.

The *rate of accumulation of fluid* is variable and depends on the dietary intake of sodium and the ability of the kidney to excrete it. Rate of fluid reabsorption is limited to 700–900 ml daily.

The *pressure* exerted by the ascitic fluid rarely exceeds 10 mmHg above the right atrium. At high pressures, discomfort makes paracentesis obligatory. Vasovagal fainting may follow too rapid release of ascites.

A *low sodium state* may follow a large paracentesis, especially if the patient has been on a restricted sodium intake. Approximately 1000 mmol of sodium is lost in every 7 litres of ascites. This is rapidly replenished from the blood and the serum sodium level falls. Water may be retained in excess of sodium.

Urine

The urine volume is diminished, deeply pigmented and of high osmolarity.

The daily urinary output of sodium is greatly reduced, usually less than 5 mmol and in a severe case less than 1 mmol.

Radiological features

Plain X-ray of the abdomen shows a diffuse ground-glass appearance. Distended loops of bowel simulate intestinal obstruction. Ultrasound and CT scans show a space around the liver and these can be used to demonstrate quite small amounts of fluid (fig. 9.5).

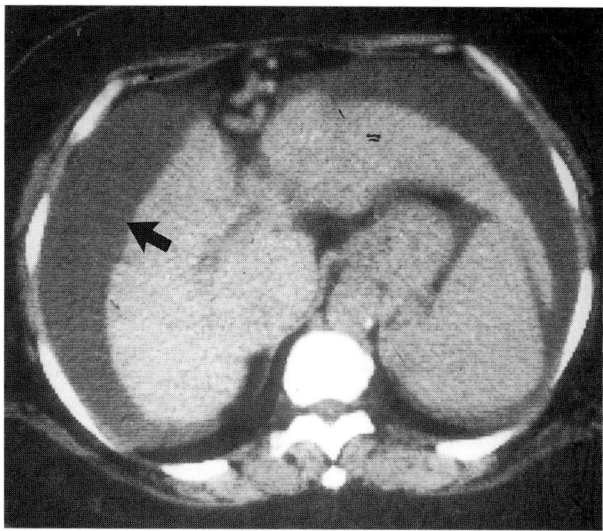

Fig. 9.5. CT scan showing an irregular cirrhotic small liver, splenomegaly and ascites (arrow).

Differential diagnosis

Malignant ascites. There may be symptoms and localizing signs due to the primary tumour. After paracentesis, the liver may be enlarged and nodular. The peritoneal fluid may be characteristic with a high protein content.

A low serum–ascites albumin gradient, less than 1.1 g/dl, suggests malignancy [1]. Lactic acid dehydrogenase levels are high.

Tuberculous ascites. This should be suspected particularly in the severely malnourished alcoholic. The patient is usually pyrexial. After paracentesis, lumps of matted omentum can be palpated. The ascitic fluid is of high protein content, usually with many lymphocytes and sometimes polymorphs. The deposit must always be stained for tubercle bacilli, and suitable cultures set up.

Constrictive pericarditis. Diagnostic points include the very high jugular venous pressure, the paradoxical pulse, the radiological demonstration of a calcified pericardium and the characteristic electrocardiogram and echocardiograph.

Hepatic venous obstruction (Budd–Chiari syndrome) must be considered, especially if the protein content of the ascitic fluid is high.

Ovarian tumour is suggested by resonance in the flanks. The maximum bulge is antero-posterior and the maximum girth is below the umbilicus.

Pancreatic ascites. This is rarely gross. It develops as a complication of acute pancreatitis. The amylase content of the ascitic fluid is very high.

Bowel perforation, with infected ascites, is shown by a low glucose and high protein concentration in the fluid.

Spontaneous bacterial peritonitis (table 9.1)

Infection of the ascitic fluid may be spontaneous or follow a previous paracentesis. The spontaneous type develops in about 8% of cirrhotic patients with ascites. It is particularly frequent if the cirrhosis is severely decompensated. In most cases the complication develops *after* the patient is admitted to hospital. These patients are more likely to have gastrointestinal bleeding and renal failure and to require invasive procedures or therapy.

The infection is blood-borne and in 90% monomicrobial (fig. 9.6). Gut permeability to bacteria is impaired in cirrhosis and the causative organisms are of gut origin. The mesenteric lymph nodes are positive for bacteria [53]. Host defences are abnormal with intra-hepatic shunting and impairment of bactericidal activity in the ascites. Reticulo-endothelial function is impaired. Neutrophils are abnormal in the alcoholic. Ascitic fluid favours bacterial growth and deficient ascitic opsonins lead to defective coating of bacteria which are indigestible by polymorphs. The opsonic activity of the ascitic fluid is proportional to protein concentration and spontaneous bacterial peritonitis is more likely if ascitic fluid protein is less than 1 g/dl [49].

Infection with more than one organism is likely to be associated with abdominal paracentesis, colonic perforation or dilatation, or any intra-abdominal source of infection.

Table 9.1. Spontaneous bacterial peritonitis

Suspect grade B and C cirrhosis with ascites
Clinical features may be absent and WBC normal
Ascitic protein usually <1g/dl
Usually monomicrobial and Gram-negative
Start antibiotics if ascites >250 mm polymorphs
50% die
69% recur in 1 year

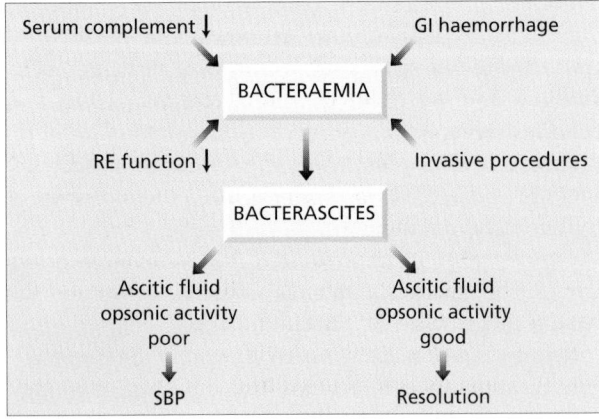

Fig. 9.6. The pathogenesis of spontaneous bacterial peritonitis (SBP) in patients with cirrhosis.

The ascitic polymorph count exceeds 250 cells per mm^3 and culture is positive. SBP should be suspected if a patient with known cirrhosis deteriorates, particularly with encephalopathy. It can develop in a fulminant form in a patient who previously had no ascites. Ascitic fluid protein less than 1 g/ml and a high serum bilirubin level independently predict the first spontaneous bacterial peritonitis [2]. Patients with variceal bleeding or with previous spontaneous bacterial peritonitis are at particular risk. Pyrexia, local abdominal pain and tenderness and systemic leucocytosis may be noted. These features, however, may be absent and the diagnosis is made on the index of suspicion with examination of the ascitic fluid.

Antibiotics should be started empirically in all those with more than 250 polymorphs per mm^3.

The bacterial count in the ascites is low. The infecting organisms are usually *Escherichia coli* or group D streptococci. Other causes include meningococci [7], *Campylobacter foetus* [65] and organisms of the *Pasteurella* group [18]. Anaerobic bacteria are rarely found. Opportunist organisms are identified in the immunosuppressed. Blood cultures are positive in 80%.

Monomicrobial, non-neutrocytic bacterascites may resolve without treatment but can progress to spontaneous bacterial peritonitis [50].

Prognosis

Deterioration is shown by marked increases in serum bilirubin and creatinine and by a very high white cell count in the blood.

50% of patients with spontaneous bacterial peritonitis will die during that hospital admission, and 69% will recur in 1 year, and again 50% will die [67].

The outlook depends on the association with recent gastrointestinal bleeding [10], the severity of the infection and the degree of renal and liver failure [33].

Treatment

Five days parenteral, third-generation cephalosporins such as cefotaxime, are usually effective [48, 52, 68]. An oral quinoline antibiotic, orofloxacin is less costly and effective in most patients.

Outpatient prophylaxis is with norfloxacin (400 mg daily) for 2–3 weeks, but resistant organisms are emerging and these might be important if a subsequent liver transplant becomes necessary. Trimethoprim-sulfamethoxazole is a less costly but effective alternative [60]. Although antibiotic prophylaxis has reduced the recurrence rate, the probability of survival is unaltered.

Diuretic therapy increases the total protein and ascitic opsonic activity [51]. Paracentesis does not have these effects, but it does not seem to increase the early and long-term risk of spontaneous bacterial peritonitis [61].

Recurrent spontaneous bacterial peritonitis is an indication, if other factors are suitable, for early hepatic transplantation.

Treatment of cirrhotic ascites

Therapy of ascites, whether by diuretics or paracentesis, is positive and the patient is grateful [51]. However, although the initial response may be excellent, the ultimate result may be a patient in renal failure or encephalopathy. Indications for treatment include the following.

Uncertain diagnosis. Control of ascites may allow such procedures as better abdominal examination, needle biopsy, scanning or venography to be performed.

Gross ascites, causing abdominal pain and/or dyspnoea.

Tense ascites so that an umbilical hernia has ulcerated and is near to rupture. This complication has a very high mortality. The patient may develop shock and pass into renal failure.

The control of ascites in patients with cirrhosis is more difficult than in other forms of fluid retention. Diuretic therapy is liable to be followed by electrolyte disturbances, encephalopathy and renal failure.

Restriction of physical activity reduces metabolites which have to be handled by the liver. Portal venous blood flow and renal perfusion increase in recumbency. The patient is weighed daily at the same time. Urine volume and body weight provide a satisfactory guide to progress. Urinary electrolyte determinations are helpful, but not essential. Serum electrolytes are measured twice weekly while the patient is in hospital. Treatment involves dietary sodium restriction, diuretics and abdominal paracentesis (table 9.2). The mild case is managed as an outpatient by diet and diuretics, but if admitted to hospital, paracentesis is usually a first procedure. In a recent survey of European hepatologists, 50% used paracentesis initially, to be followed by diuretics [1]. 50% regarded complete control of the ascites as

Table 9.2. General management of ascites

Bed rest. 22 mmol sodium diet. Restrict fluids to 1 litre daily. Check serum and urinary electrolytes. Weigh daily. Measure urinary volume. Sample ascites

If tense ascites consider paracentesis (see table 9.6)

Spironolactone 200 mg daily

After 4 days consider adding frusemide 80 mg daily. Check serum electrolytes

Stop diuretics if pre-coma ('flap'), hypokalaemia, azotaemia or alkalosis

Continue to monitor weight. Increase diuretics as necessary

desirable, whereas the other half were satisfied with symptomatic relief without removing all the ascites.

The cirrhotic patient who is accumulating ascites on an unrestricted sodium intake excretes less than 10 mmol (0.2 g) sodium daily in the urine. Extra-renal loss is about 0.5 g. Sodium taken in excess of 0.75 g will result in ascites, every gram retaining 200 ml fluid. If the ascites is to be absorbed the daily intake of sodium must be restricted to less than 22 mmol (0.5 g) daily. Fluid intake is restricted to 1 litre daily.

Diet: general remarks

1 Food to be cooked without added salt. No salt on table. Use salt substitute.

2 Use *salt-free* bread, crispbread, crackers or matzos and *salt-free* butter or margarine—as much as you like.

3 Seasonings such as lemon juice, orange peel, onion, vinegar, garlic, salt-free ketchup and mayonnaise, pepper, mustard, sage, parsley, thyme, marjoram, bay leaves, cloves or low-salt yeast extract, help to make salt-free foods more palatable.

4 *Omit* anything containing baking powder or baking soda. This includes pastry, biscuits, crackers, cake, self-raising flour and ordinary bread.

5 *Omit* pickles, olives, ham, bacon, corned beef, tongue, oyster, shellfish, canned fish and meat, chutney, salad cream, meat and fish paste, bottled sauces, sausages, kippers and all cheese and ice cream.

6 *Omit* dry cereals, except shredded wheat, puffed wheat or sugar puffs. *Omit* salted canned foods. Regular canned fruit may be used in place of fresh fruit.

7 Meat or poultry, rabbit, sweetbreads or fish — 4 oz (100 g) daily and one egg. Egg may be used as substitute for 2 oz (50 g) meat.

8 Do not use more than 10 fl. oz (0.50 pint, 0.25 litre) of milk daily. Heavy (double) cream is allowed.

9 Boiled rice (without salt) is permissible.

10 Eat fresh and home cooked fruit and vegetables of all kinds.

11 No candy, pastilles or milk chocolate.

Most protein-containing foods, such as meat, eggs and dairy produce, have a high sodium content and, to maintain a good protein intake, a low-sodium protein supplement should be taken. Salt-free bread and butter is used and all cooking is done without added salt. Many low-sodium foods are now available including soups, ketchups and crackers. It is possible to give a diet containing 1500–2000 calories, 70 g protein and only 22 mmol sodium (table 9.3). The patient should be virtually vegetarian.

Failure to adhere to a low-sodium diet is the usual reason for ascites to be termed 'resistant' or 'refractory'. In a severe case, even combinations of the newer diuretics in huge doses will not compensate for a high dietary sodium intake.

Table 9.3. Specimen salt-free diet

Calories 2000–2200
Protein 70 g (approx.)
Sodium 380–450 mg (18–20 mmol)

Breakfast
Shredded wheat with cream and sugar or stewed fruit
2 oz (60 g) salt-free bread or matzos or salt-free crispbread, unsalted
   butter, marmalade or jelly or honey
1 egg
Tea or coffee with milk from allowance

Lunch
2 oz meat or poultry, or 3 oz white fish
Potatoes
Green vegetables or salad
Fresh or stewed fruit

Tea
2 oz salt-free bread or matzos
Unsalted butter, jam, honey or tomato
Tea or coffee with milk from allowance

Dinner
Grapefruit or salt-free soup
Meat, fish or poultry as for lunch
Potatoes
Green vegetables or salad
Fresh or stewed fruit or jelly made with fruit juice and gelatine
Heavy cream
Coffee or tea with milk from allowance

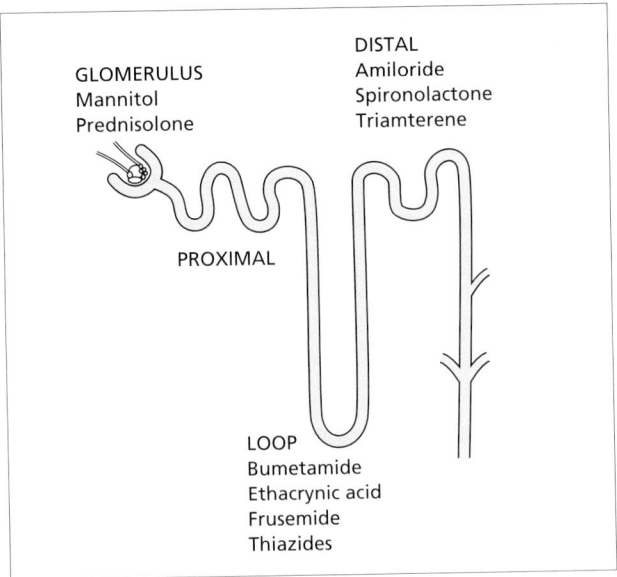

Fig. 9.7. The site of action of diuretics.

Table 9.4. Diuretics for ascites

Urine loss			
Loop diuretic			
Na++		K++	Frusemide
			Bumetamide
Distal diuretic			
Na+		K	Spironolactone
			Triamterene
			Amiloride

The patient may respond rapidly to this regime without the need for diuretics. Such *easy responders* are liable to be those:
• with ascites and oedema presenting for the first time—'virgin' ascites;
• with a 24-hour urine sodium excretion of more than 10 mmol;
• with a normal glomerular filtration rate (creatinine clearance);
• with underlying reversible liver disease such as fatty liver of the alcoholic;
• in whom the ascites has developed acutely in response to a treatable complication such as infection or bleeding;
• with ascites following excessive sodium intake, such as in sodium-containing antacids or purgatives, or spa waters with a high sodium content.

Diuretics

The dose and frequency of administration must be calculated for each individual patient.

Diuretics can be divided into two main groups (fig. 9.7; table 9.4). The first group comprises the thiazides, frusemide, bumetamide, muzolimine and ethacrynic acid. These are powerful natriuretic agents, but also powerful kaliuretics. Potassium chloride supplements are always necessary when these diuretics are given alone to cirrhotic patients.

The second group comprises spironolactone (an aldosterone antagonist), amiloride and triamterene. These are weakly natriuretic but conserve potassium. So potassium chloride supplements are usually unnecessary. In general it is advisable to start with one of these diuretics and then add a first group diuretic as required (table 9.5).

The ease of control and choice of diuretics can be related to the 24-hour urinary sodium content on admission to hospital (table 9.5).

The longer acting diuretics, such as the thiazides and ethacrynic acid, have disadvantages in patients with liver disease because the action may continue when electrolyte disturbances have already developed. The patient may thus continue to lose urinary potassium and become more alkalotic even after stopping the diuretic.

A start is usually made with spironolactone 200 mg daily, and this usually induces a diuresis. Long-term spironolactone causes painful gynaecomastia in cirrhotic males and should be replaced by 10–15 mg

Table 9.5. Treatment of ascites related to 24-hour urinary sodium excretion

24-hour urinary sodium (mmol)	Treatment
<5	Distal and loop diuretic
5–25	Distal diuretic
>25	Low-sodium diet only

amiloride daily. Then, if necessary, frusemide or bumetamide are added.

Frusemide may be ineffective in the presence of marked hyperaldosteronism when sodium that is not reabsorbed in the loop of Henle is taken up by the distal nephron.

Diuretic failures are in those with very poor hepato-cellular function who are usually dead within 6 months of starting therapy. In such refractory patients diuretics have eventually had to be withdrawn because of intractable uraemia, hypotension or encephalopathy.

The rate of ascitic fluid reabsorption is limited to 700–900 ml a day. If a diuresis of some 3 litres is induced, much of the fluid must have come from non-ascitic, extra-cellular fluids including oedema fluid and the intravenous compartment. This is safe as long as oedema persists. Indeed diuresis may be rapid (greater than 2 kg daily) until oedema disappears [46]. If the diuresis continues and exceeds the limits of ascites absorption in the absence of oedema, plasma volume will fall. Renal perfusion is reduced and the stage is set for the development of functional renal failure (*hepato-renal syndrome*).

In a few patients, on discharge from hospital, diuretics are no longer required. In the majority, however, the diuretic and dietetic regime has to be continued according to the individual needs.

Complications

Encephalopathy follows any profound diuresis. It is usually associated with hypokalaemia and hypochloraemic alkalosis.

A profound *serum electrolyte abnormality* with azotaemia indicates a very poor prognosis [59]. This probably reflects the severity of the underlying liver disease.

Hypokalaemia reflects diuretic effect and also secondary hyperaldosteronism. Levels of less than 3.1 mmol/litre necessitate stopping the diuretic and giving potassium chloride supplements.

Hyponatraemia reflects urinary excretion of sodium in excess of water in patients on a greatly restricted sodium diet. In the terminally ill, it may indicate the passage of sodium into the cells. When combined with other electrolyte abnormalities it indicates a particularly bad prog-

nosis [24]. It is treated by stopping the diuretic and restricting fluid intake to 500 ml/day. The clinician may be tempted to give sodium supplements, in fact body stores of sodium and water are excessive and giving more sodium will only lead to gaining weight and pulmonary oedema.

Azotaemia reflects altered renal circulation with contraction of the extra-cellular fluid volume. If it is part of a profound electrolyte disturbance the prognosis is poor as it predicts the development of the hepato-renal syndrome.

Follow-up advice

The patient should adhere to the strict low-sodium diet as far as possible. He should use bathroom scales and weigh himself daily, nude. A daily record should be kept and brought to the physician at each visit.

The dose of diuretics depends on the severity of the liver disease. A usual routine is 100–200 mg spironolactone or 10–20 mg amiloride daily with frusemide 40–80 mg every other day. Potassium chloride supplements, about 50 mmol potassium daily, are given. Serum electrolytes, blood urea nitrogen and liver function tests are monitored every 4 weeks. As liver function improves it may become possible to stop first the frusemide and then the spironolactone. Finally the low-sodium diet is relaxed, first to 'no added salt' and then to a normal diet.

Therapeutic abdominal paracentesis
(table 9.6)

This procedure was abandoned in the 1960s because of the fear of causing acute renal failure. Moreover, the loss of approximately 50 g of protein in a 5 litre paracentesis led to the patients becoming severely malnourished. New interest came with the observation that a 5 litre paracentesis was safe in fluid- and salt-restricted patients with ascites *and peripheral oedema* [26]. This work was extended to daily 4–5 litre paracenteses with 40 g

Table 9.6. Therapeutic paracentesis

Selection
Tense ascites
Preferably with oedema
Child's grade B
Prothrombin >40%
Serum bilirubin <10 mg/dl
Platelets >40 000/mm³
Serum creatinine <3 mg/dl
Urinary sodium >10 mmol/24 hours

Routine
Volume removed: 5–10 litres
i.v. salt-poor albumin: 6 g/litre removed

Table 9.7. Total paracentesis with intravenous albumin [66]

Volume: 10 litres
Time: 1 hour
i.v. Albumin (sodium-poor): 6 g/litre removed

Candidates (see table 9.6)

Advantages
Comfort
Shortened hospital stay

But
Relapse ⎤
Survival ⎦ unchanged
NOT in grade C patients

salt-poor albumin infused intravenously over the same period. Finally, a single large paracentesis, about 10 litres in 1 hour combined with intravenous albumin (6–8 g/litre ascites removed) was shown to be equally effective (table 9.7) [23, 66].

In a controlled trial, paracentesis resulted in a greater reduction in hospital stay compared with traditional diuretic treatment [22]. The probability of requiring readmission to hospital, survival and causes of death did not differ significantly between the paracentesis and diuretic groups. The procedure is contraindicated in grade C patients with serum bilirubin greater than 10 mg/dl (170 mmol/litre), prothrombin time less than 40%, platelets less than 40 000, creatinine greater than 3 mg/dl and urine sodium less than 10 mmol/day (table 9.6).

The complete, total, paracentesis results in hypovolaemia as reflected by a rise in plasma renin levels [20]. There is also some renal impairment proportional to the severity of the underlying liver disease. Its extent is a measure of survival.

Albumin replacement is effective in preventing the hypovolaemia. Less costly plasma expanders such as dextran 70 [15] or hemaccel are not so effective.

Conclusions

Paracentesis is a safe, cost-effective treatment for cirrhotic ascites [5]. It must not be done in end-stage cirrhotic patients or in those with renal failure. Intravenous salt-poor albumin replaces the protein lost in the ascitic fluid.

Sufficient ascitic fluid is removed to give the patient a flaccid, but not ascites-free, abdomen. The paracentesis must be followed by a good salt-free dietary and diuretic regime.

Refractory ascites [4]

This is defined as ascites that cannot be mobilized or the recurrence of which cannot be prevented by medical therapy. It is divided into diuretic-resistant ascites and diuretic-intractable ascites.

Diuretic-resistant ascites cannot be mobilized or the recurrence cannot be prevented (e.g. after therapeutic paracentesis) due to a lack of response (loss of weight, less than 200 g/day and urinary sodium excretion lower than 50 mmol/day) to a 50 mmol sodium diet with intensive diuretic therapy (spironolactone 400 mg, with frusemide 160 mg/day for 1 week).

Diuretic intractable ascites cannot be mobilized or the recurrence of which cannot be prevented due to the development of diuretic-induced complications that preclude the use of an effective diuretic dosage. Renal impairment, hepatic encephalopathy or electrolyte disturbances may be contraindications for commencing diuretic therapy.

Ascites ultrafiltration and re-infusion [44]

The automated ultrafiltration apparatus removes ascitic fluid via a peritoneal dialysis catheter and passes it over an ultrafilter which selects molecules of less than 50 000 mol.wt. The concentrate, which contains 2–4 times as much protein as the ascitic fluid, is returned to the patient intravenously. Up to 13 litres of ascites can be removed in 24 hours. The procedure demands special equipment but may reduce hospital stay.

Porto-systemic shunts

Porto-systemic shunts have been largely abandoned for the treatment of ascites because of the high encephalopathy rate.

TIPS will reduce diuretic needs, plasmin renin and plasma aldosterone activity [47, 62, 72]. Liver function may deteriorate and encephalopathy be induced [43].

Peritoneo-venous (Le Veen) shunt

The peritoneo-venous shunt system gives continuous treatment over many months [29]. It produces sustained expansion of the circulating blood volume by continuous passage of ascitic fluid from the peritoneal cavity to the general circulation (fig. 9.8). The expanded blood volume is confirmed by the fall in plasma levels of renin–angiotensin, noradrenaline, antidiuretic hormone and atrial natriuretic peptide. Renal function and nutrition improve.

The operation is performed under antibiotic cover with light general anaesthesia. The peritoneal cavity is drained by a long, perforated, plastic tube that reaches into the pelvis. This connects with a pressure-sensitive valve lying extra-peritoneally. This again connects with a silicone rubber tube which passes subcutaneously from

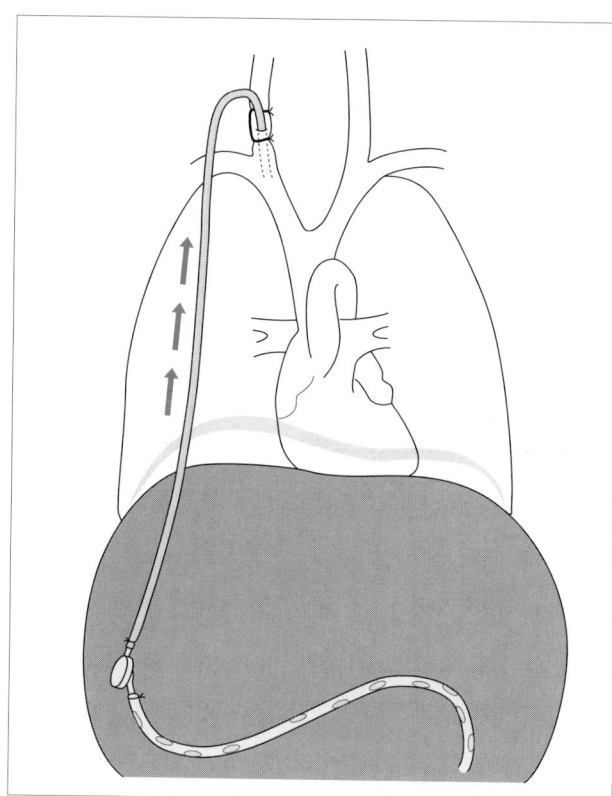

Fig. 9.8. The peritoneo-venous shunt.

the abdominal wound towards the neck and so into the internal jugular vein. The end of the tube is left in position in the superior vena cava. As the diaphragm descends during inspiration, the intra-peritoneal fluid pressure rises, whereas that in the intra-thoracic superior vena cava falls. Respiration provides the force which opens the valve and propels the fluid into the superior vena cava.

In a few good risk patients, the technique controls ascites for long periods. However, there are many complications. The peri-operative mortality is about 18% [39] and even as high as 52% [56]. Mild disseminated intravascular coagulation is constant but may be severe and fatal. It can be related to ascitic procoagulants and even collagen in the ascitic fluid [6]. Removal of ascites and replacement with saline before introducing the shunt may be a useful preventitive measure. Early complications include ascitic leaks, variceal bleeding and pulmonary oedema. Later infections, including right-sided endocarditis are common. There is a high readmission rate for shunt dysfunction. This is less than for repeated paracentesis. Time in hospital is the same as is the survival rate. The procedure is of no value in the hepato-renal syndrome [13].

In a multi-centre controlled study, treatment by the Le Veen shunt was not superior to paracentesis with or without diuretics. At 1 month, the shunt was more effec-

tive, but survival was reduced. At 1 year, reduction of ascites and survival were the same for both groups. The shunt may alleviate ascites more rapidly but survival is unaltered [63]. Grade C patients are not suitable for the procedure.

Prognosis

The prognosis is always grave after ascites develops in a patient with cirrhosis. It is better if the ascites has accumulated rapidly, especially if there is a well-defined precipitating factor such as gastrointestinal haemorrhage.

A patient with cirrhosis developing ascites has only a 40% chance of being alive 2 years later. Much depends on the major factor in the aetiology of the fluid retention. If liver cell failure, evidenced by jaundice and hepatic encephalopathy, is severe, the prognosis is poor. If the major factor is a particularly high portal pressure, the patient may respond well to treatment. The prognosis is also proportional to the ability to excrete a water load [58].

Ascites cannot be divorced from the underlying liver disease that caused it and, although it may be controlled, the patient is still liable to die from another complication such as haemorrhage, hepatic coma or primary liver cancer. It is questioned whether control of ascites *per se* increases lifespan. It certainly makes the patient more comfortable.

Functional renal failure (hepato-renal syndrome)

Hepato-renal syndrome occurs in patients with chronic liver disease (often alcoholic), severe hepatic failure and portal hypertension. It is characterized by impaired renal function and marked abnormalities in the arterial circulation and in the activity of endogenous vaso-active systems. In the kidney, there is marked renal vasoconstriction that results in a low glomerular infiltration rate [27]. In the extra-renal circulation, there is predominant arterial vasodilatation, which results in reduction of total systemic vascular resistance and arterial hypotension. A similar syndrome may occur in acute liver failure. The histology of the kidney is virtually normal and the failure is a functional one. Such kidneys have been successfully transplanted when they functioned normally [28]. Conversely, apparently moribund patients with this syndrome have returned to normal kidney function after liver transplantation.

The syndrome is marked by renal failure with normal tubular function (table 9.8). The patient is seldom admitted with the hepato-renal syndrome and its development is usually precipitated by events in hospital. These include reduction in the intravascular volume due to over-vigorous diuretic therapy, paracentesis or diar-

Table 9.8. Criteria for diagnosis of hepato-renal syndrome

Major
Chronic liver disease with ascites
Low glomerular filtration rate
   serum creatinine >1.5 mg/dl
   creatinine clearance (24 hour) < 4.0 ml/minute
Absence of shock, severe infection, fluid losses and
   nephrotoxic drugs
Proteinuria < 500 mg/day
No improvement following plasma volume expansion

Minor
Urine volume <1 litre/day
Urine sodium <10 mmol/litre
Urine osmolarity > plasma osmolarity
Serum sodium concentration <13 mmol/litre

Table 9.9. Iatrogenic hepato-renal syndrome

Drugs	Treatment
Diuretics	Volume expansion
Lactulose	Volume expansion
NSAID (prostaglandin inhibition)	Stop drug
Aminoglycosides	Diagnose urine β_2-microglobulins
Cyclosporin	Haemodialysis

rhoea. The classical features of uraemia are usually absent. The prognosis is extremely grave.

Hepato-renal syndrome may be classified into two different types. In type 1, the patients have a rapidly progressive (less than 2 weeks) reduction of renal function with doubling of the initial serum creatinine to greater than 2.5 mg/dl or a 50% reduction of the initial 24-hour creatinine clearance to less than 20 ml/minute.

In type 2 hepato-renal syndrome, the patients have the criteria for the diagnosis of hepato-renal syndrome but the renal failure does not progress rapidly.

In the mildest pre-azotaemic stage, renal dysfunction is shown by failure to excrete a water load, reduction in urinary sodium excretion and hyponatraemia. Hepatic dysfunction is usually severe and ascites is usual.

The more advanced stages are characterized by progressive azotaemia, usually with hepatic failure and ascites difficult to control. The patient complains of anorexia, weakness and fatigue. The blood urea concentration is raised. Hyponatraemia is invariable. Sodium is avidly reabsorbed by the renal tubules and urine osmolarity is increased. Fluid accumulates in spite of a normal urinary volume, dietary sodium restriction and diuretic therapy. In the later stages nausea, vomiting and thirst are added. The patient is drowsy. The picture may be indistinguishable from that of hepatic encephalopathy.

The serum urea and creatinine levels rise progressively. The serum sodium is usually less than 120 mmol/litre. Urinalysis is virtually normal. Urinary sodium excretion is very low. Acute tubular damage may coexist. Ascites is refractory. Terminally, coma deepens, blood pressure drops and urine volume falls even more. The terminal stages last from a few days to more than 6 weeks.

It may be difficult to distinguish hepatic from renal failure although the patients die with biochemical azotaemia rather than the full clinical picture of kidney failure. Death is due to liver failure; survival depends on the reversibility of the *liver* disease.

Iatrogenic renal failure in a cirrhotic patient must be diagnosed from genuine hepato-renal syndrome as the prognosis is different and effective treatment is possible (table 9.9). The causes include diuretic overdose and severe diarrhoea due, for instance, to lactulose. Nonsteroidal anti-inflammatory drugs reduce renal prostaglandin production, so reducing glomerular filtration rate and free water clearance [17]. Nephrotoxic drug effects, due to such drugs as cyclosporin, the aminoglycosides [31] or demeclocycline, are diagnosed by measuring urinary β_2-microglobulins. Glomerular mesangial IgA deposits, accompanied by complement deposition, complicate cirrhosis, usually in the alcoholic. They are diagnosed by finding proteinuria with microhaematuria and casts [41].

Duplex Doppler ultrasonography may be used to evaluate renal arterial resistance [54]. Values are already increased in the non-ascitic cirrhotic without azotaemia and identify patients with a high risk for the hepato-renal syndrome [45]. They are even higher in the ascitic phase and in the hepato-renal syndrome where they predict survival [34].

Mechanisms

The hepato-renal syndrome is marked by intense renal vasoconstriction even in the presence of systemic vasodilatation. The effective renal circulation is reduced. Cardiac output is normal or even increased, but is distributed to skin, splanchnic area, spleen and brain so that renal plasma flow is reduced. Glomerular filtration rate is reduced and plasma renin rises. Blood flow is diverted away from the renal cortex (fig. 9.9). This change in intrarenal distribution of blood flow can be shown even in well-compensated cirrhotic patients. It may explain their susceptibility to develop oliguric renal failure after haemorrhage not sufficiently large to reduce the blood pressure or after minor shifts of fluid within body compartments, such as with abdominal paracentesis or diuretic therapy. Reduced effective plasma volume may be a factor. Volume expansion may increase renal blood flow and institute a diuresis, but the response is not maintained and variceal haemorrhage may be precipitated.

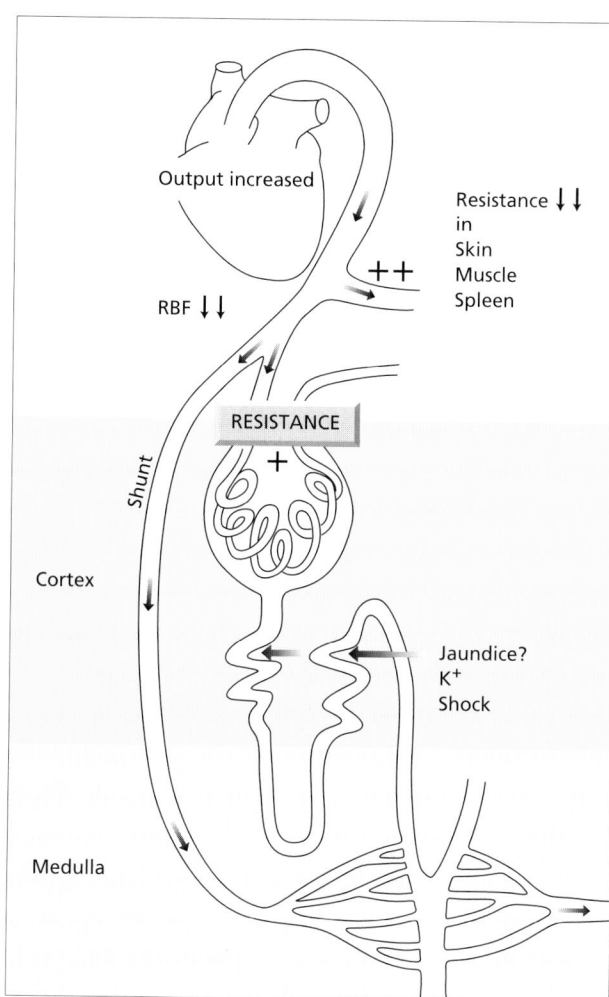

Fig. 9.9. Factors contributing to renal failure in cirrhosis ('hepato-renal syndrome').

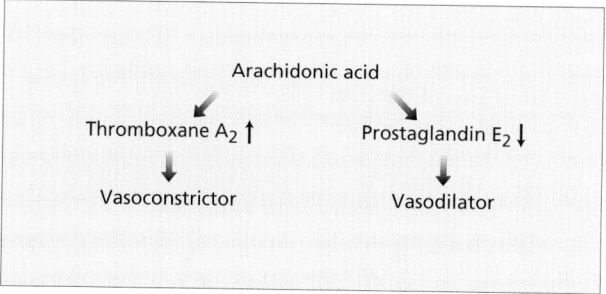

Fig. 9.10. Urinary changes in the hepato-renal syndrome.

renal syndrome [37]. They may be related to endotoxaemia [69]. They result in stimulation of platelet-activating factor, a potent phospholipid mediator in intercellular signalling [40]. Endothelin stimulates ANF release, aldosterone secretion and inhibits renin release.

There is particular sensitivity to the vaso-constrictor effect of endogenous adenosine [25, 32].

Nitric oxide, a potent vasodilator, may be related to the hyperdynamic circulation and hence to the hepato-renal syndrome (Chapter 6).

Treatment

The syndrome is prevented by avoiding diuretic over-dose, and by early recognition of any complication such as electrolyte imbalance, haemorrhage or infection. The conservative management is that of renal and hepatic failure whatever the cause. Hepatic failure holds the key to the problem and must be treated. Conservative measures include restriction of fluids, sodium, potassium and protein, and withdrawal of potentially nephro-toxic drugs such as the aminoglycosides. Blood cultures should be taken and any septicaemia treated appropriately. Mannitol is useless and may lead to intracellular acidosis. High doses of frusemide are unavailing. Renal dialysis does not improve survival and may precipitate gastrointestinal haemorrhage and shock.

Prostaglandins are not associated with significant improvement in renal function [21].

Vaso-constrictor drugs such as metaraminol, angiotensin II or ornipressin increase arterial resistance and lower cardiac output but have little effect on renal function [55]. Inhibitors of nitric oxide and other vasodilators are theoretically possible but are only being tested experimentally.

TIPS gives poor results in Child's grade C patients and should only be considered if hepatic transplant is an early option.

Hepatic transplantation can be safely managed and can be followed by return of renal function without increased rejection.

Terminal hyponatraemia [24] is in part dilutional (over-

Hepato-renal syndrome can be regarded as an imbalance between systemic vasodilators and renal vasoconstricting mechanisms (fig. 9.10) [74].

Thromboxane A_2, a metabolite of arachidonic acid, is a potent vasoconstrictor. Its metabolite thromboxane B_2 is markedly increased in the urine of patients with the hepato-renal syndrome. Prostaglandin E_2, another metabolite of arachidonic acid, is a vasodilator, and urinary excretion of this is decreased. An imbalance of the renal kallikrein–kinin system may also be involved in the maintenance of renal blood flow in cirrhotic patients with ascites. Impaired renal production of kallikrein and prostaglandins in the setting of activation of the renin–angiotensin and sympathetic nervous systems may lead to functional renal failure.

Increased production of vasoconstrictor cysteinyl leukotrienes may contribute [38].

Endothelin-1, formed in vascular endothelium and endothelin-2, formed in tissue, are long-acting vasoconstrictors. Plasma endothelins are increased in the hepato-

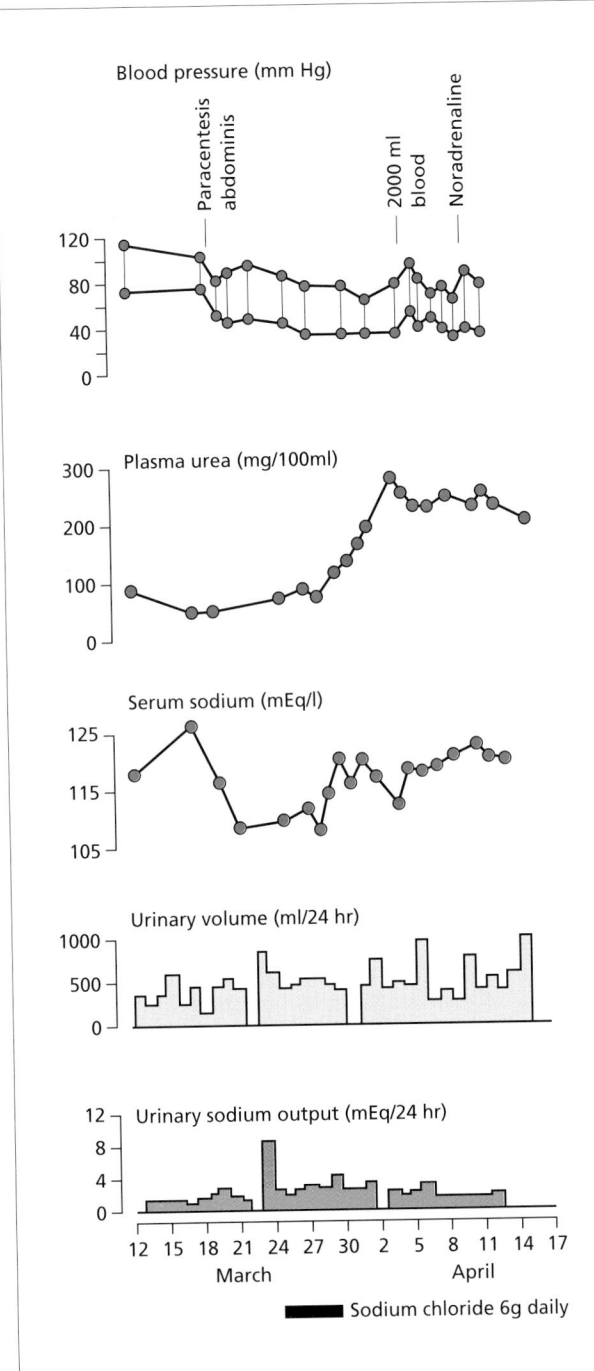

Fig. 9.11. Terminal sub-acute virus hepatitis. Note the low blood pressure which was only temporarily increased by blood transfusion and noradrenaline. Serum sodium values and urinary sodium excretion were profoundly depressed and were uninfluenced by oral sodium chloride. Blood urea rose progressively in the last 2 weeks [24].

hydration), in part due to over-administration of diuretics and in part due to redistribution of sodium, a raised proportion occurring in the intra-cellular compartments. It should not be treated with intravenous hypertonic sodium chloride as pulmonary oedema will develop and death will be accelerated (fig. 9.11).

The final combination of azotaemia, hyponatraemia and hypotension is terminal and quite unresponsive to all forms of therapy.

References

1 Albillos A, Cuervas-Mons V, Millan I *et al.* Ascitic fluid polymorphonuclear cell count and serum to ascites albumin gradient in the diagnosis of bacterial peritonitis. *Gastroenterology* 1990; **98**: 134.

2 Andreu M, Sola R, Sitges-Serra A *et al.* Risk factors for spontaneous bacterial peritonitis in cirrhotic patients with ascites. *Gastroenterology* 1993; **104**: 1133.

3 Arroyo V, Claria J, Saló J *et al.* Antidiuretic hormone and the pathogenesis of water retention in cirrhosis with ascites. *Semin. Liver Dis.* 1994; **14**: 44.

4 Arroyo V, Gines P, Gerbes AL *et al.* Definition and diagnostic criteria of refractory ascites and hepatorenal syndrome in cirrhosis. *Hepatology* 1996; **23**: 164.

5 Arroyo V, Ginès A, Saló J. A European survey on the treatment of ascites in cirrhosis. *J. Hepatol.* 1994; **21**: 667.

6 Baele G, Rasquin K, Barbier F. Coagulant, fibrinolytic, and aggregating activity in ascitic fluid. *Am. J. Gastroenterol.* 1986; **81**: 440.

7 Bar-Meir S, Chojkier M, Groszmann RJ *et al.* Spontaneous meningococcal peritonitis; a report of two cases. *Am. J. Dig. Dis.* 1978; **23**: 119.

8 Bichet D, Szatalowicz V, Chaimovitz C *et al.* Role of vasopressin in abnormal water excretion in cirrhotic patients. *Ann. Intern. Med.* 1982; **96**: 413.

9 Bichet DG, Van Putten VJ, Schrier RW. Potential role of increased sympathetic activity in impaired sodium and water excretion in cirrhosis. *N. Engl. J. Med.* 1982; **307**: 1552.

10 Blaise M, Pateron D, Trinchet J-C *et al.* Systemic antibiotic therapy prevents bacterial infection in cirrhotic patients with gastrointestinal haemorrhage. *Hepatology* 1994; **20**: 34.

11 Cheng WS, Gough IR, Ward M *et al.* Chylous ascites in cirrhosis: a case report and review of the literature. *J. Gastroenterol. Hepatol.* 1989; **4**: 95.

12 Epstein FH. Underfilling versus overflow in hepatic ascites. *N. Engl. J. Med.* 1982; **307**: 1577.

13 Epstein M. Peritoneovenous shunt in the management of ascites and the hepatorenal syndrome. *Gastroenterology* 1982; **82**: 790.

14 Epstein M (ed.) *The Kidney in Liver Disease*, 4th edn. Williams and Wilkins, Baltimore, 1996, p. 3.

15 Fassio E, Terg R, Landeira G *et al.* Paracentesis with dextran 70 versus paracentesis with albumin in cirrhosis and tense ascites. Results of a randomized study. *J. Hepatol.* 1992; **14**: 310.

16 Fernández-Rodriguez CM, Prieto J, Quiroga A *et al.* Plasma levels of substance P in liver cirrhosis: relationship to the activation of vasopressor systems and urinary sodium excretion. *Hepatology* 1995; **21**: 35.

17 Garella S, Matarese RA. Renal effects of prostaglandins and clinical adverse effects of nonsteroidal anti-inflammatory agents. *Medicine (Baltimore)* 1984; **63**: 165.

18 Gerding DN, Khan MY, Ewing JW *et al. Pasteurella multocida* peritonitis in hepatic cirrhosis with ascites. *Gastroenterology* 1976; **70**: 413.

19 Giacobbe A, Facciorusso D, Tonti P *et al*. Hydrothorax complicating cirrhosis in the absence of ascites. *J. Clin. Gastroenterol*. 1993; **16**: 271.

20 Ginès A, Planas R, Angeli P *et al*. Treatment of patients with cirrhosis and refractory ascites by Le Veen shunt with titanium tip: comparison with therapeutic paracentesis. *Hepatology* 1995; **22**: 124.

21 Ginès A, Salmerón JM, Ginès P *et al*. Oral misoprostol or intravenous prostaglandin E$_2$ do not improve renal function in patients with cirrhosis and ascites with hyponatremia or renal failure. *J. Hepatol*. 1993; **17**: 220.

22 Ginès P, Arroyo V, Quintero E *et al*. Comparison of paracentesis and diuretics in the treatment of cirrhotics with tense ascites. Results of a randomized study. *Gastroenterology* 1987; **93**: 234.

23 Ginès P, Arroyo V, Vargas V *et al*. Paracentesis with intravenous infusion of albumin as compared with peritoneovenous shunting in cirrhosis with refractory ascites. *N. Engl. J. Med*. 1991; **325**: 829.

24 Hecker R, Sherlock S. Electrolyte and circulatory changes in terminal liver failure. *Lancet* 1956; **ii**: 1121.

25 Jacobson ED, Pawlik WW. Adenosine regulation of mesenteric vasodilation. *Gastroenterology* 1994; **107**: 1168.

26 Kao HW, Rakov HE, Savage E *et al*. The effect of large volume paracentesis on plasma volume — a cause of hypovolemia? *Hepatology* 1985; **5**: 403.

27 Kew MC, Brunt PW, Varma RR *et al*. Renal and intrarenal blood-flow in cirrhosis of the liver. *Lancet* 1971; **ii**: 504.

28 Koppel MH, Coburn JW, Mims MM *et al*. Transplantation of cadaveric kidneys from patients with hepatorenal syndrome. *N. Engl. J. Med*. 1969; **280**: 1367.

29 Le Veen HH, Wapnick S, Grosberg S *et al*. Further experience with peritoneovenous shunt for ascites. *Ann. Surg*. 1976; **184**: 574.

30 Lieberman FL, Ito S, Reynolds TB. Effective plasma volume in cirrhosis with ascites: evidence that a decreased value does not account for renal sodium retention, a spontaneous reduction in glomerular filtration rate (GFR), and a fall in GFR during drug-induced diuresis. *J. Clin. Invest*. 1969; **48**: 975.

31 Lietman PS. Liver disease, aminoglycoside antibiotics and renal dysfunction. *Hepatology* 1988; **8**: 966.

32 Llach J, Ginès P, Arroyo V *et al*. Effect of dipyvaidamole on kidney function in cirrhosis. *Hepatology* 1993; **17**: 59.

33 Llovet JM, Planas R, Morillas R *et al*. Short-term prognosis of cirrhosis with spontaneous bacterial peritonitis: multivariate study. *Am. J. Gastroenterol*. 1993; **88**: 388.

34 Maroto A, Ginès A, Saló J *et al*. Diagnosis of function kidney failure of cirrhosis with Doppler sonography: prognostic value of resistive index. *Hepatology* 1994; **20**: 839.

35 Mirouze D, Juttner H-U, Reynolds TB. Left pleural effusion in patients with chronic liver disease and ascites: prospective study of 22 cases. *Dig. Dis. Sci*. 1981; **26**: 984.

36 Mirouze D, Zipser RD, Reynolds TB. Effect of inhibitors of prostaglandin synthesis on induced diuresis in cirrhosis. *Hepatology* 1983; **3**: 50.

37 Moore K, Wendon J, Frazer M *et al*. Plasma endothelin immunoreactivity in liver disease and the hepatorenal syndrome. *N. Engl. J. Med*. 1992; **327**: 1774.

38 Moore KP, Taylor GW, Maltby NH *et al*. Increased production of cysteinyl leukotrienes in hepatorenal syndrome. *J. Hepatol*. 1990; **11**: 263.

39 Moskovitz M. The peritoneovenous shunt: expectations

40 Mustafa SB, Gandhi CR, Harvey SAK *et al*. Endothelin stimulates platelet-activating factor synthesis by cultured rat Kupffer cells. *Hepatology* 1995; **21**: 545.

41 Newell GC. Cirrhotic glomerulonephritis: incidence, morphology, clinical features, and pathogenesis. *Am. J. Kidney Dis*. 1987; **9**: 183.

42 Niederberger M, Ginès P, Tsai P *et al*. Increased aortic cyclic guanosine monophosphate concentration in experimental cirrhosis in rats. Evidence for a role of nitric oxide in the pathogenesis of arterial vasodilation in cirrhosis. *Hepatology* 1995; **21**: 1625.

43 Ochs A, Rossle M, Haag K *et al*. The transjugular intrahepatic portosystemic stent–shunt procedure for refractory ascites. *N. Engl. J. Med*. 1995; **332**: 1192.

44 Parbhoo SP, Ajdukiewicz A, Sherlock S. Treatment of ascites by continuous ultrafiltration and reinfusion of protein concentrate. *Lancet* 1974; **1**: 949.

45 Platt JF, Ellis JH, Rubin JM *et al*. Renal duplex Doppler ultrasonography: a noninvasive predictor of kidney dysfunction and hepatorenal failure in liver disease. *Hepatology* 1994; **20**: 362.

46 Pockros PJ, Reynolds TB. Rapid diuresis in patients with ascites from chronic liver disease: the importance of peripheral oedema. *Gastroenterology* 1986; **90**: 1827.

47 Quiroga J, Sangro B, Nunez M *et al*. Transjugular intrahepatic portal–systemic shunt in the treatment of refractory ascites: effect on clinical, renal, humoral, and hemodynamic parameters. *Hepatology* 1995; **21**: 986.

48 Rimola A, Salmerón JM, Clemente G *et al*. Two different dosages of cefotaxime in the treatment of spontaneous bacterial peritonitis in cirrhosis: results of a prospective randomized, multicenter study. *Hepatology* 1995; **21**: 674.

49 Runyon BA. Patients with deficient ascitic fluid opsonic activity are predisposed to spontaneous bacterial peritonitis. *Hepatology* 1988; **18**: 632.

50 Runyon BA. Monomicrobial non-neutrocytic bacterascites: a variant of spontaneous bacterial peritonitis. *Hepatology* 1990; **12**: 710.

51 Runyon BA. Care of patients with ascites. *N. Engl. Med. J*. 1994; **330**: 337.

52 Runyon BA, McHutchinson JG, Antillon MR *et al*. Short-course versus long-course antibiotic treatment of spontaneous bacterial peritonitis. A randomized controlled study of 100 patients. *Gastroenterology* 1991; **100**: 1737.

53 Runyon BA, Squier S, Borzio M. Translocation of gut bacteria in rats with cirrhosis to mesenteric lymph nodes partially explains the pathogenesis of spontaneous bacterial peritonitis. *J. Hepatol*. 1994; **21**: 792.

54 Sacerdoti D, Bolognesi M, Merkel C *et al*. Renal vasoconstriction in cirrhosis evaluated by duplex Doppler ultrasonography. *Hepatology* 1993; **17**: 219.

55 Saló J, Inglada L, Quer JC *et al*. Ornipressin and ornipressin plus dopamine in cirrhotic patients with renal failure. *J. Hepatol*. 1993; **18**: S167.

56 Scholz DG, Nagorney DM, Lindor KD. Poor outcome from peritoneovenous shunts for refractory ascites. *Am. J. Gastroenterol*. 1989; **84**: 540.

57 Schrier RW, Arroyo V, Bernardi M *et al*. Peripheral arterial vasodilation hypothesis: a proposal for the initiation of renal sodium and water retention in cirrhosis. *Hepatology* 1988; **8**: 1151.

58 Schrier RW, Caramelo C. Hemodynamics and hormonal

and reality. *Am. J. Gastroenterol*. 1990; **85**: 917.

alterations in hepatic cirrhosis. In Epstein M, ed. *The Kidney in Liver Disease*, 3rd edn. Williams & Wilkins, New York, 1988.

59 Sherlock S, Senewiratne B, Scott A *et al.* Complications of diuretic therapy in hepatic cirrhosis. *Lancet* 1966; **i**: 1049.

60 Singh N, Gayowski T, Yu VL *et al.* Trimethoprim-sulfamethoxazole for the prevention of spontaneous bacterial peritonitis in cirrhosis: a randomized trial. *Ann. Intern. Med.* 1995; **122**: 595.

61 Solà R, Andreu M, Coll S *et al.* Spontaneous bacterial peritonitis in cirrhotic patients treated using paracentesis or diuretics: results of a randomized study. *Hepatology* 1995; **21**: 340.

62 Somberg KA, Lake JR, Tomlanovich SJ *et al.* Transjugular intrahepatic portosystemic shunts for refractory ascites: assessment of clinical and hormonal response and renal failure. *Hepatology* 1995; **21**: 709.

63 Stanley MM, Ochi S, Lee KK *et al.* Peritoneovenous shunting as compared with medical treatment in patients with alcoholic cirrhosis and massive ascites. *N. Engl. J. Med.* 1989; **321**: 1632.

64 Strauss RM, Martin LG, Kaufman SL *et al.* Transjugular intrahepatic portal systemic shunt for the management of symptomatic cirrhotic hydrothorax. *Am. J. Gastroenterol.* 1994; **89**: 1520.

65 Targan SR, Chow AW, Guze LB. Spontaneous peritonitis of cirrhosis due to *Campylobacter fetus. Gastroenterology* 1976; **71**: 311.

66 Titó L, Ginès P, Arroyo V *et al.* Total paracentesis associated with intravenous albumin management of patients with cirrhosis and ascites. *Gastroenterology* 1990; **98**: 146.

67 Titó L, Rimola A, Ginès P *et al.* Recurrence of spontaneous bacterial peritonitis in cirrhosis: frequency and predictive factors. *Hepatology* 1988; **8**: 27.

68 Toledo C, Salmerón J-M, Rimola A *et al.* Spontaneous bacterial peritonitis in cirrhosis: predictive factors of infection resolution and survival in patients treated with cefotaxime. *Hepatology* 1993; **17**: 251.

69 Uchihara M, Izumi N, Sato C *et al.* Clinical significance of elevated plasma endothelin concentration in patients with cirrhosis. *Hepatology* 1992; **16**: 95.

70 Warner L, Skorecki K, Blendis LM *et al.* Atrial natriuretic factor and liver disease. *Hepatology* 1993; **17**: 500.

71 Witte MH, Witte CL, Dumont AE. Progress in liver disease: physiological factors involved in the causation of cirrhotic ascites. *Gastroenterology* 1971; **61**: 742.

72 Wong F, Sniderman K, Liu P *et al.* Transjugular intra-hepatic portosystemic stent shunt: effects on hemodynamics and sodium homeostasis in cirrhosis and refractory ascites. *Ann. Intern. Med.* 1995; **122**: 816.

73 Xiol X, Castellote J, Baliellas C *et al.* Spontaneous bacterial empyema in cirrhotic patients: analysis of eleven cases. *Hepatology* 1990; **11**: 365.

74 Zipser RD, Radvan GH, Kronborg IJ *et al.* Urinary thromboxane B_2 and prostaglandin E_2 in the hepatorenal syndrome: evidence for increased vasoconstrictor and decreased vasodilator factors. *Gastroenterology* 1983; **84**: 697.

Chapter 10
The Portal Venous System and Portal Hypertension

The portal system includes all veins that carry blood from the abdominal part of the alimentary tract, the spleen, pancreas and gallbladder. The portal vein enters the liver at the porta hepatis in two main branches one to each lobe; it is without valves in its larger channels (fig. 10.1) [35].

The *portal vein* is formed by the union of the superior mesenteric vein and the splenic vein just posterior to the head of the pancreas at about the level of the second lumbar vertebra. It extends slightly to the right of the mid-line for a distance of 5.5–8 cm to the porta hepatis. The portal vein has a segmental intra-hepatic distribution, accompanying the hepatic artery.

The *superior mesenteric vein* is formed by tributaries

from the small intestine, colon and head of the pancreas, and irregularly from the stomach via the right gastro-epiploic vein.

The *splenic veins* (5–15 channels) originate at the splenic hilum and join near the tail of the pancreas with the short gastric vessels to form the main splenic vein. This proceeds in a transverse direction in the body and head of the pancreas, lying below and in front of the artery. It receives numerous tributaries from the head of the pancreas, and the left gastro-epiploic vein enters it near the spleen. The *inferior mesenteric vein*, bringing blood from the left part of the colon and rectum, usually enters its medial third. Occasionally, however, it enters the junction of superior mesenteric and splenic veins.

Portal blood flow in man is about 1000–1200 ml/minute.

Portal oxygen content. The fasting arterio-portal oxygen difference is only 1.9 volumes per cent (range 0.4–3.3 volumes per cent) and the portal vein contributes 40 ml/minute or 72% of the total oxygen supply to the liver.

During digestion, the arterio-portal venous oxygen difference increases due to increased intestinal utilization.

Stream-lines in the portal vein. There is no consistent pattern of hepatic distribution of portal inflow. Sometimes splenic blood goes to the left lobe and sometimes to the right lobe. Crossing-over of the bloodstream can occur in the human portal vein. Flow is probably stream-lined rather than turbulent.

Portal pressure is normally about 7 mmHg in man (fig. 10.2).

Collateral circulation

When the portal circulation is obstructed, whether it be within or outside the liver, a remarkable collateral circulation develops to carry portal blood into the systemic veins (figs 10.3, 10.28).

Intra-hepatic obstruction (cirrhosis)

Normally 100% of the portal venous blood flow can be recovered from the hepatic veins, whereas in cirrhosis

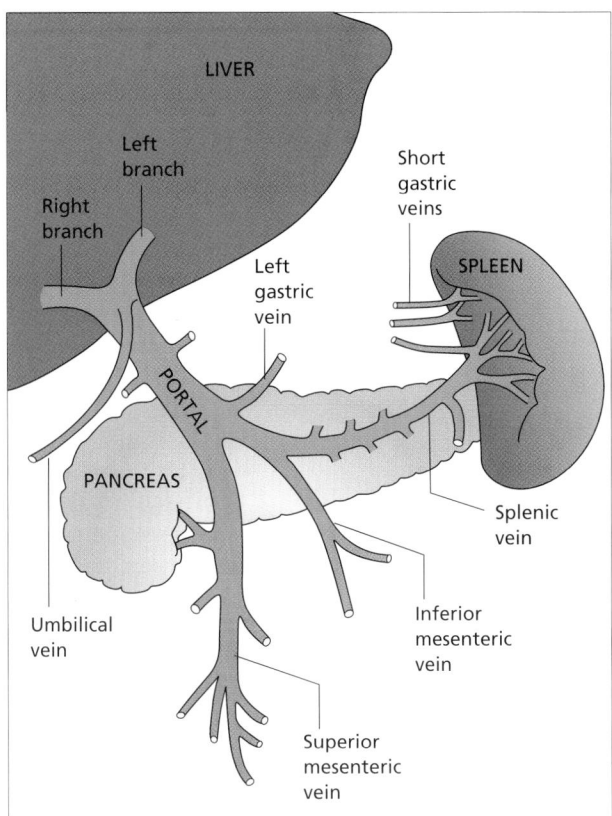

Fig. 10.1. The anatomy of the portal venous system. The portal vein is posterior to the pancreas.

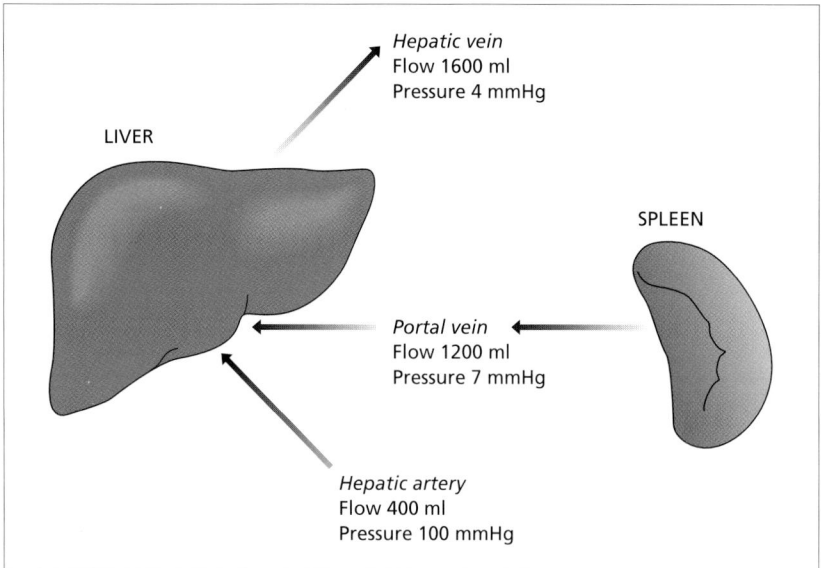

Fig. 10.2. The flow and pressure in the hepatic artery, portal vein and hepatic vein.

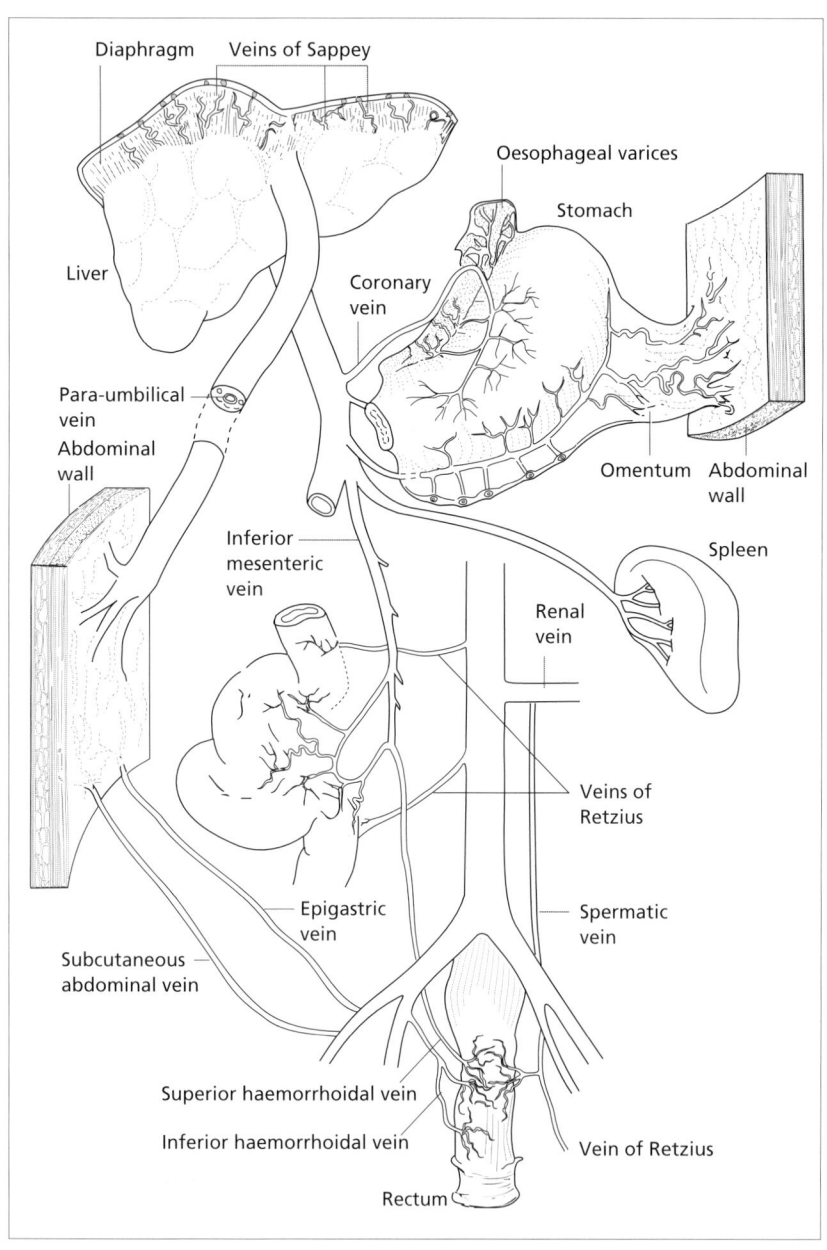

Fig. 10.3. The sites of the portal-systemic collateral circulation in cirrhosis of the liver [88].

only 13% is obtained [88]. The remainder enters collateral channels which form four main groups.

1 *Group I*: where protective epithelium adjoins absorptive epithelium:

(a) At the cardia of the stomach, where the left gastric vein, posterior gastric [65] and short gastric veins of the portal system anastomose with the intercostal, diaphragmo-oesophageal and azygos minor veins of the caval system. Deviation of blood into these channels leads to varicosities in the submucous layer of the lower end of the oesophagus and fundus of the stomach.

(b) At the anus, the superior haemorrhoidal vein of the portal system anastomoses with the middle and inferior haemorrhoidal veins of the caval system. Deviation of blood into these channels may lead to rectal varices.

2 *Group II*: in the falciform ligament through the paraumbilical veins relics of the umbilical circulation of the fetus (fig. 10.4).

3 *Group III*: where the abdominal organs are in contact with retro-peritoneal tissues or adherent to the abdominal wall. These collaterals run from the liver to diaphragm and in the spleno-renal ligament and omentum. They include lumbar veins and veins developing in scars of previous operations or in small or large bowel stomas.

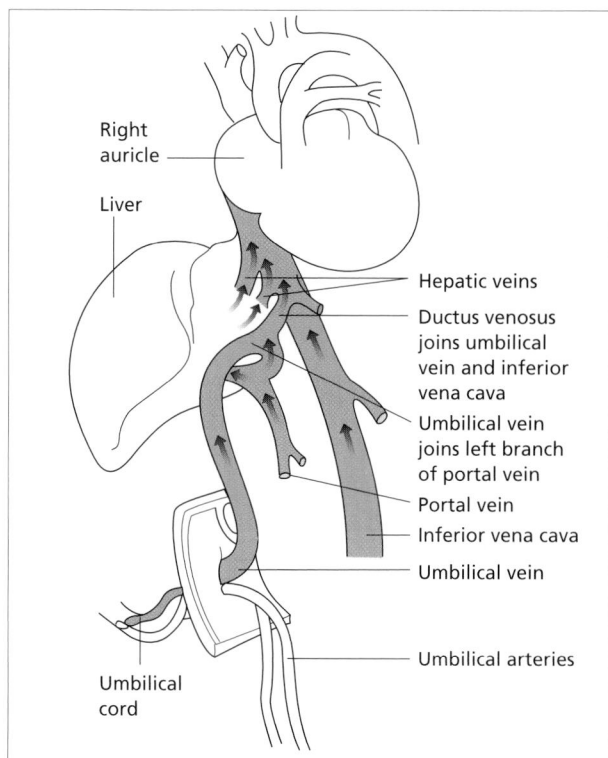

Fig. 10.4. The hepatic circulation at the time of birth.

4 *Group IV*: portal venous blood is carried to the left renal vein. This may be through blood entering directly from the splenic vein or via diaphragmatic, pancreatic, left adrenal or gastric veins.

Blood from gastro-oesophageal and other collaterals, ultimately reaches the superior vena cava via the azygos or hemiazygos systems. A small volume enters the inferior vena cava. An intra-hepatic shunt may run from the right branch of the portal vein to the inferior vena cava [112]. Collaterals to the pulmonary veins have also been described.

Extra-hepatic obstruction

With extra-hepatic portal venous obstruction, additional collaterals form, attempting to bypass the block and return blood *towards* the liver. These enter the portal vein in the porta hepatis beyond the block. They include the veins at the hilum, venae comitantes of the portal vein and hepatic arteries, veins in the suspensory ligaments of the liver and diaphragmatic and omental veins. Lumbar collaterals may be very large.

Effects

When the liver is cut off from portal blood by the development of the collateral circulation, it depends more on blood from the hepatic artery. It shrinks and shows impaired capacity to regenerate. This might be due to lack of hepatotrophic factors, including insulin and glucagon, which are of pancreatic origin.

Collaterals usually imply portal hypertension, although occasionally if the collateral circulation is very extensive portal pressure may fall. Conversely, portal hypertension of short duration can exist without a demonstrable collateral circulation.

A large portal-systemic shunt may lead to hepatic encephalopathy, septicaemias due to intestinal organisms, and other circulatory and metabolic effects.

Pathology of portal hypertension

Collateral venous circulation is disappointingly insignificant at autopsy. The oesophageal varices collapse.

The spleen is enlarged with a thickened capsule. The surface oozes dark blood (*fibro-congestive splenomegaly*). Malpighian bodies are inconspicuous. Histologically, sinusoids are dilated and lined by thickened epithelium (fig. 10.5). Histiocytes proliferate with occasional erythrophagocytosis. Peri-arterial haemorrhages may progress to siderotic, fibrotic nodules.

Splenic and portal vessels. The splenic artery and portal vein are enlarged and tortuous and may be aneurysmal. The portal and splenic vein may show endothelial haemorrhages, mural thrombi and intimal plaques and may

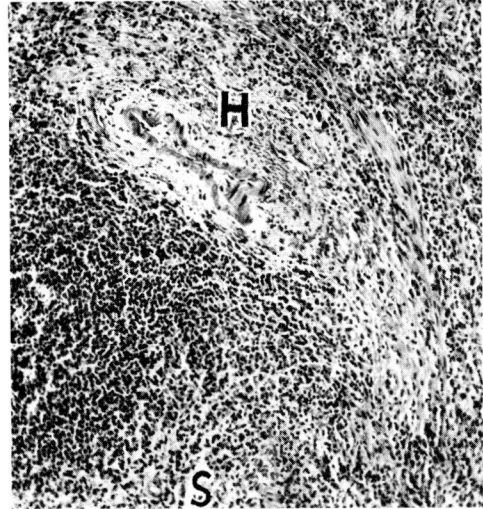

Fig. 10.5. The spleen in portal hypertension. The sinusoids (S) are congested and the sinusoidal wall is thickened. A haemorrhage (H) lies adjacent to an arteriole of a Malpighian corpuscle. (Stained H & E, ×70.)

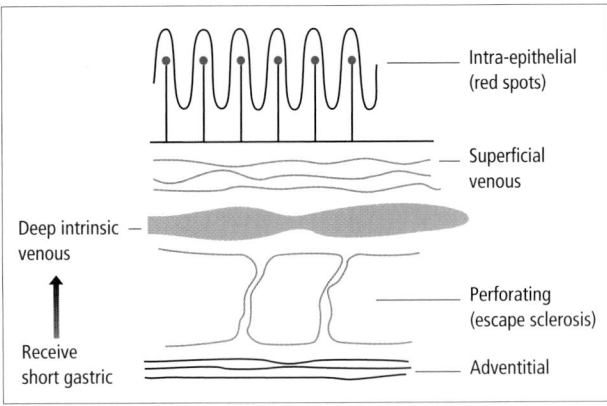

Fig. 10.6. Venous anatomy of the oesophagus.

calcify (see fig. 10.13). Such veins are usually unsuitable for portal surgery.

In 50% of cirrhotics small, deeply placed splenic arterial aneurysms are seen [89].

Hepatic changes depend on the cause of the portal hypertension.

The height of the portal venous pressure correlates poorly with the apparent degree of cirrhosis and in particular of fibrosis. There is a much better correlation with the degree of nodularity.

Varices

Oesophageal

If oesophago-gastric varices did not form and bleed portal hypertension would be of virtually no clinical significance [140]. The major blood supply to oesophageal varices is the left gastric vein. The posterior branch usually drains into the azygos system, whereas the anterior branch communicates with varices just below the oesophageal junction and forms a bundle of thin parallel veins that run in the junction area and continue in large tortuous veins in the lower oesophagus. There are four layers of veins in the oesophagus (fig. 10.6) [67]. *Intra-epithelial veins* may correlate with the red spots seen on endoscopy and which predict variceal rupture. The *superficial venous plexus* drains into larger, *deep intrinsic veins*. *Perforating veins* connect the deeper veins with the fourth layer which is the adventitial plexus. Typical large varices arise from the main trunks of the deep intrinsic veins and these communicate with gastric varices.

The connection between portal and systemic circula-

tion at the gastro-oesophageal junction is extremely complex [163]. Its adaptation to the cephalad and increased flow of portal hypertension is ill-understood. A palisade zone is seen between a gastric zone and the perforating zone (fig. 10.7). In the palisade zone flow is bidirectional and this area acts a water shed between portal and azygos systems. Turbulent flow in perforating veins between the varices and the peri-oesophageal veins at the lower end of the stomach may explain why rupture is frequent in this region [86]. Recurrence of varices after endoscopic sclerotherapy may be related to the communications between various venous channels or perhaps to enlargement of veins in the super-

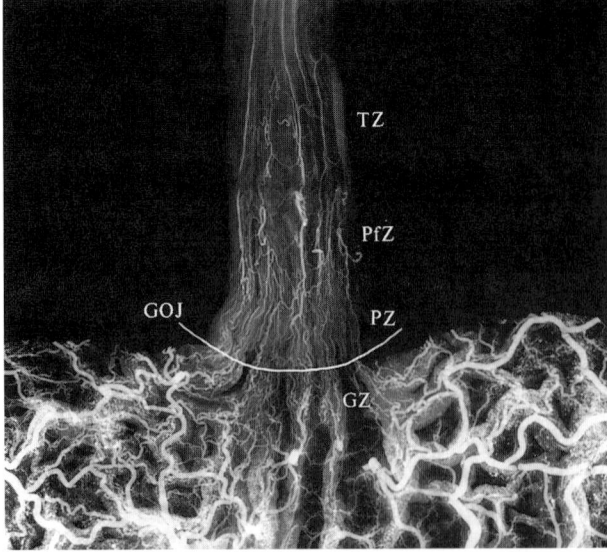

Fig. 10.7. Radiograph of a specimen injected with barium-gelatine, opened along the greater curvature. Four distinct zones of normal venous drainage are identified: gastric zone (GZ), palisade zone (PZ), perforating zone (PfZ) and truncal zone (TZ). A radio-opaque wire demarcates the transition between the columnar and stratified squamous epithelium. GOJ = gastro-oesophageal junction [163].

ficial venous plexus. Failure of sclerotherapy may also be due to failure to thrombose the perforating veins.

Gastric

These are largely supplied by the short gastric veins and drain into the deep intrinsic veins of the oesophagus. They are particularly prominent in patients with extra-hepatic portal obstruction.

Duodenal varices show as filling defects. Bile duct collaterals may be life-threatening at surgery [32].

Colo-rectal

These develop secondary to inferior mesenteric–internal iliac venous collaterals [55]. They may present with haemorrhage. They are visualized by colonoscopy. ^{99m}Tc-tagged red blood cell scans are useful for localizing bleeding. Colonic varices may become more frequent after successful oesophageal sclerotherapy.

Collaterals between the superior haemorrhoidal (portal) veins and the middle and inferior haemorrhoidal (systemic) veins lead to anorectal varices [174].

Portal hypertensive intestinal vasculopathy

Chronic portal hypertension may not only be associated with discrete varices but with a spectrum of intestinal mucosal changes due to abnormalities in the microcirculation [164].

Portal hypertensive gastropathy. Gastric vascularity is abnormal with increased submucosal arteriovenous communications between the muscularis mucosa and dilated pre-capillaries and veins—a vascular ectasia [115, 121]. Gastric mucosal perfusion is increased [110]. Gastric mucosa may be a particular risk of bleeding and of damage, for instance, by NSAIDs. These gastric changes may be increased after oesophageal sclerotherapy. They are relieved only by reducing the portal pressure [110].

Congestive jejunopathy and colonopathy. Similar changes are seen in duodenum and jejunum. Histology shows increase in size and number of vessels in jejunal villi [97]. The mucosa is oedematous, erythematous and friable [136].

Congestive colonopathy is shown by dilated mucosal capillaries with thickened basement membranes but with no evidence of mucosal inflammation [164].

Others

Portal systemic collaterals form in relation to bowel–abdominal wall adhesions secondary to previous surgery or pelvic inflammatory disease. Varices also form at mucocutaneous junctions, for instance, at the site of an ileostomy or colostomy.

Haemodynamics of portal hypertension

This has been considerably clarified by the development of animal models such as the rat with a ligated portal vein or bile duct or with carbon tetrachloride-induced cirrhosis. Portal hypertension is related both to vascular resistance and to portal blood flow (fig. 10.8). The fundamental haemodynamic abnormality is an increased resistance to portal flow. This may be mechanical due to the disturbed architecture and nodularity of cirrhosis or due to an obstructed portal vein. Other intra-hepatic factors such as collagenosis of the space of Disse [9], hepatocyte swelling [12] and the resistance offered by portal-systemic collaterals contribute. There is also a dynamic increase in resistance within the liver. Myofibroblasts can relax and sinusoidal endothelium and Ito cells contain contractile proteins.

As the portal venous pressure is lowered by the development of collaterals deviating portal blood into systemic veins, portal hypertension is maintained by increasing portal flow in the portal system which becomes hyperdynamic. It is uncertain whether the hyperdynamic circulation is the cause or the consequence of the portal hypertension or both. It is related to the severity of liver failure. Cardiac output increases and there is generalized vasodilatation (fig. 10.9). Arterial blood pressure is normal or low (Chapter 6).

Splanchnic vasodilatation is probably the most important factor in maintaining the hyperdynamic circulation.

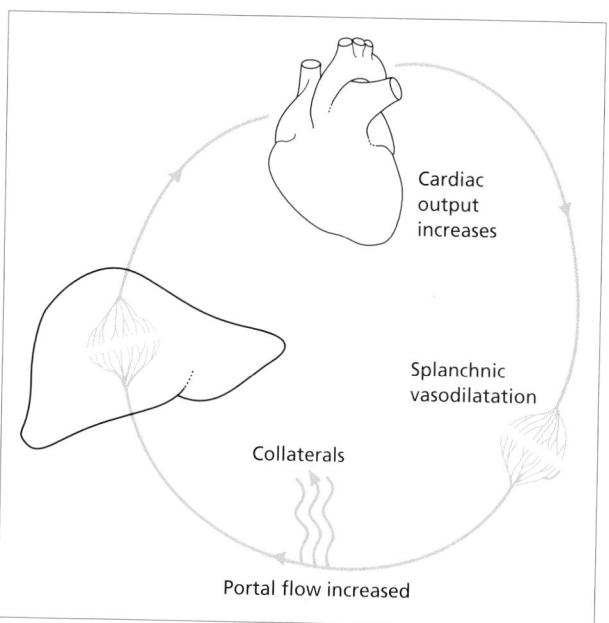

Fig. 10.8. Forward flow theory of portal hypertension.

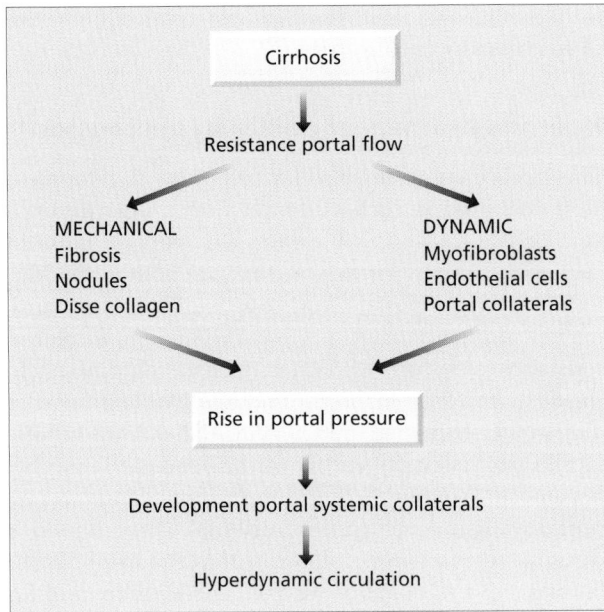

Fig. 10.9. The pathophysiology of portal hypertension in cirrhosis.

Azygous blood flow is increased. Gastric mucosal blood flow rises resulting in capillary vascular ectasia and congestive gastroscopy [121]. The increased portal flow raises the oesophageal variceal transmural pressure. The increased flow refers to *total* portal flow (hepatic and collaterals). The actual portal flow reaching the liver is, of course, reduced. The factors maintaining the hyperdynamic splanchnic circulation are multiple. There seems to be an interplay of vasodilators and vaso-constrictors. These might be formed by the hepatocyte, fail to be inactivated by it or be of gut origin and pass through intra-hepatic or extra-hepatic venous shunts.

Endotoxins and cytokines, largely formed in the gut, are important triggers [50]. Nitrous oxide (NO) and endothelin-1 are synthesized by vascular endothelium in response to endotoxin.

NO is a short-life, potent and important mediator of vascular relaxaton. The enzyme, NO synthase, is induced by endotoxins and cytokines, allowing the conversion of L-arginine to NO [13] (Chapter 6). Arginine analogues inhibit this conversion and cirrhotic rats are particularly sensitive to them and portal pressure increases [116].

Endothelin-1 is a vaso-constrictor and the high blood levels found in cirrhotics are believed to be useful for the maintenance of arterial pressure [2, 158]. It causes sinusoidal constriction in the isolated rat liver *in vivo* and increases portal pressure [106].

Prostacyclin is produced by portal vein endothelium and is a potent vasodilator [101]. It may play a major role in the circulatory changes of portal hypertension due to chronic liver disease.

Glucagon is secreted by pancreatic α-cells and inactivated by the liver. Hyperglucagonaemia in cirrhotic patients is probably related to portal venous shunting. Glucagon is vasodilatory after pharmacological doses but does not seem to be vaso-active at physiological doses. It is probably not a primary factor in the maintenance of the hyperkinetic circulation in established liver disease [109].

Clinical features of portal hypertension

History and general examination (table 10.1)

Cirrhosis is the commonest cause of portal hypertension. Any aetiological factor such as alcoholism or past hepatitis should be considered. Past abdominal inflammation, especially in the neonatal period, is particularly important in the aetiology of extra-hepatic portal block. Clotting diseases and some drugs such as sex hormones predispose to portal and hepatic venous thrombosis.

Haematemesis is the commonest presentation. The number and severity of previous haemorrhages should be noted, together with their immediate effects, whether there was associated confusion or coma and whether blood transfusion was required. Melaena, without haematemesis, may result from bleeding varices. The absence of dyspepsia and epigastric tenderness and a

Table 10.1. Investigation of a patient with suspected portal hypertension

History
Relevant to cirrhosis or chronic hepatitis (Chapter 19)
Gastrointestinal bleeding: number, dates, amounts, symptoms, treatment
Results of previous endoscopies
P/H: alcoholism, blood transfusion, hepatitis B, hepatitis C, intra-abdominal, neonatal or other sepsis, oral contraceptives, myeloproliferative disorder

Examination
Signs of hepato-cellular failure
Abdominal wall veins:
  site
  direction of blood flow
Splenomegaly
Liver size and consistency
Ascites
Oedema of legs
Rectal examination
Endoscopy of oesophagus, stomach and duodenum

Additional investigations
Aspiration liver biopsy
Hepatic vein catheterization
Selective splanchnic arteriography
Hepatic ultrasound, CT scan or MRI

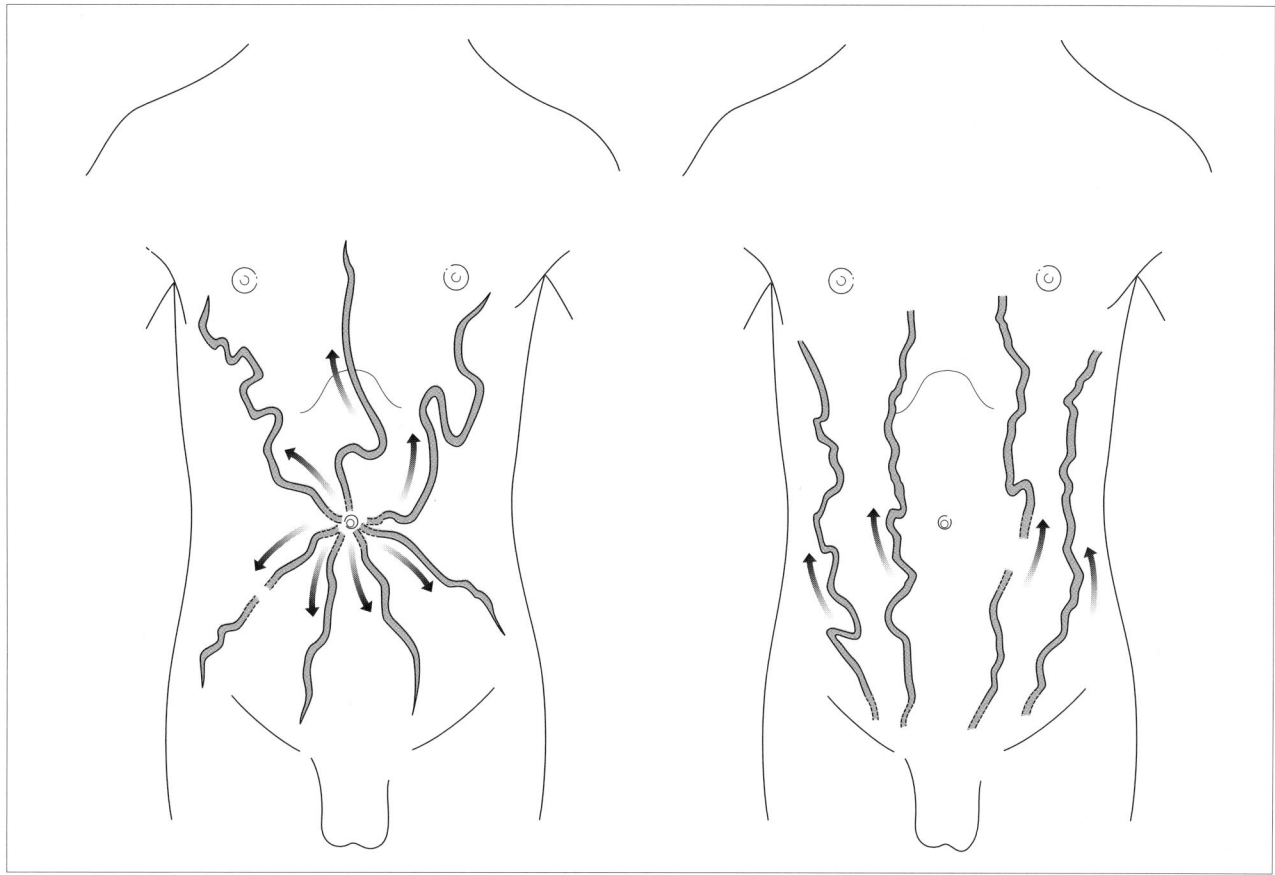

Fig. 10.10. Distribution and direction of blood flow in anterior abdominal wall veins in portal venous obstruction (left) and in inferior vena caval obstruction (right).

previously normal endoscopy help to exclude haemorrhage from peptic ulcer.

The stigmas of cirrhosis include jaundice, vascular spiders and palmar erythema. Anaemia, ascites and the prodromas of coma should be noted.

Abdominal wall veins

In intra-hepatic portal hypertension, some blood from the left branch of the portal vein may be deviated via para-umbilical veins to the umbilicus, whence it reaches veins of the caval system (fig. 10.10). In extra-hepatic portal obstruction, dilated veins may appear in the left flank.

Distribution and direction. Prominent collateral veins radiating from the umbilicus is termed *caput Medusae*. This is rare and usually only one or two veins, frequently epigastric, are seen (figs 10.10, 10.11). The blood flow is away from the umbilicus, whereas in inferior vena caval obstruction the collateral venous channels carry blood upwards to reach the superior vena caval system (fig. 10.10). Tense ascites may lead to functional obstruction of the inferior vena cava and cause difficulty in interpretation.

Abdominal veins can be visualized by *infra-red photography* (fig. 10.12).

Murmurs. A venous hum may be heard, usually in the region of the xiphoid process or umbilicus, occasionally radiating to the praecordium, sternum or over the liver. A thrill, detectable by light pressure, may be felt at the site of the maximum intensity. The sound may be accentuated during systole, in inspiration or in the erect or sitting positions. It is due to blood rushing through a large umbilical or para-umbilical channel in the falciform ligament from the left branch of the portal vein to the superior epigastric, internal mammary or inferior epigastric veins in the abdominal wall. A venous hum may also occasionally be heard over other large collaterals such as the inferior mesenteric vein. An arterial systolic murmur usually indicates primary liver cancer or alcoholic hepatitis.

The association of dilated abdominal wall veins and a loud abdominal venous murmur at the umbilicus with normal liver is termed the *Cruveilhier–Baumgarten*

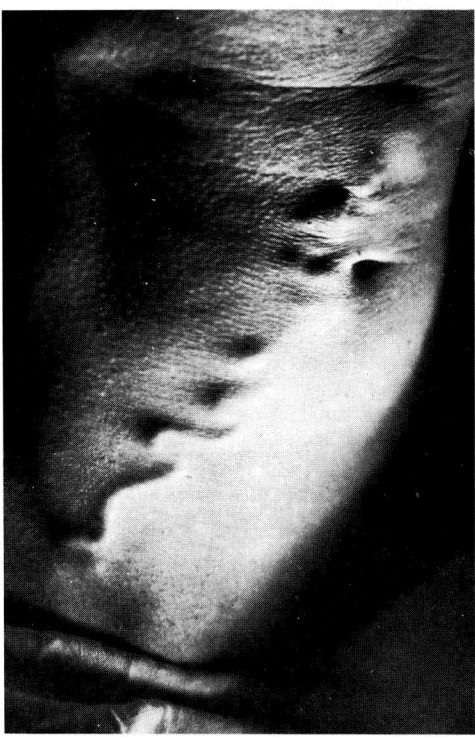

Fig. 10.11. Anterior abdominal wall vein in patient with cirrhosis of the liver.

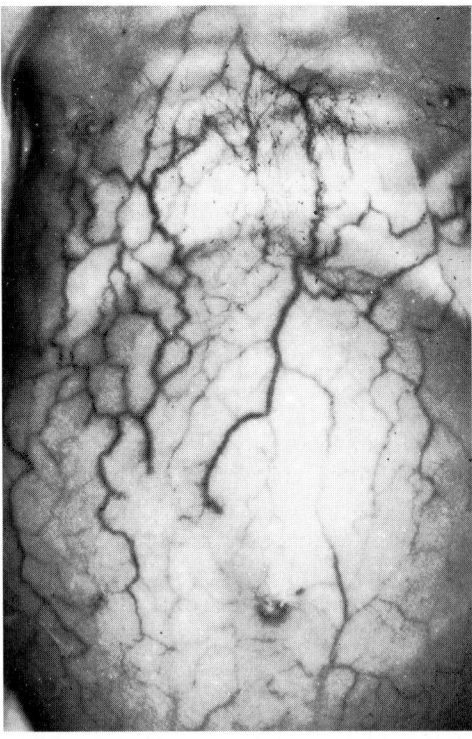

Fig. 10.12. Infra-red photograph of a patient with cirrhosis and ascites. The portal collateral circulation is demonstrated. Note the everted umbilicus.

syndrome [6, 29]. This may be due to congenital patency of the umbilical vein but more usually to a well-compensated cirrhosis [6, 10, 29].

The para-xiphoid umbilical hum and *caput Medusae* indicate the presence of portal obstruction beyond the origin of the umbilical veins from the left branch of the portal vein. They therefore indicate intra-hepatic portal venous hypertension (cirrhosis).

Spleen

The spleen enlarges progressively. The edge is firm. Size bears little relation to the portal pressure. It is larger in young people and in macronodular rather than micronodular cirrhosis.

An enlarged spleen is the single most important diagnostic sign of portal hypertension. If the spleen cannot be felt or is not enlarged on imaging, the diagnosis of portal hypertension is questionable.

The *peripheral blood* shows a pancytopenia associated with an enlarged spleen whatever the cause (*secondary 'hypersplenism'*). This is related more to the reticulo-endothelial hyperplasia than to the portal hypertension and is unaffected by lowering the pressure by porta-caval shunt.

Liver

A small liver may be as significant as a large one, and the size should be evaluated by careful percussion. Liver size correlates poorly with the height of the portal venous pressure.

Liver consistency, tenderness or nodularity should be recorded. A soft liver suggests extra-hepatic portal venous obstruction. A firm liver supports cirrhosis.

Ascites

This is rarely due to portal hypertension alone although a particularly high pressure may be a major factor. The portal hypertension raises the capillary filtration pressure, and determines fluid localization to the peritoneal cavity. Ascites in cirrhosis always indicates liver cell failure in addition to portal hypertension.

Rectum

Anorectal varices are visualized with the sigmoidoscope and may bleed. They are found in 44% of cirrhotic patients, increasing in those who have bled from oesophageal varices [62]. They must be distinguished from simple haemorrhoids which are prolapsed vascular cushions and which do not communicate with the portal system [174].

X-ray of the abdomen and chest

This is useful to delineate liver and spleen. Rarely, a calcified portal vein may be shown but CT is more sensitive [4] (fig. 10.13).

Branching, linear gas-shadows in the portal vein radicles, especially near the periphery of the liver and due to gas-forming organisms, may rarely be seen in adults with intestinal infarction or infants with enterocolitis. Portal gas may be associated with disseminated intravascular coagulation. CT and ultrasound may detect portal gas more often, for instance, in suppurative cholangitis when the prognosis is not so grave [33].

Tomography of the azygos vein may show enlargement (fig. 10.14) as the bulk of the collateral flow enters the azygos system.

A widened left paravertebral shadow may be due to lateral displacement of the pleural reflection between aorta and vertebral column by a dilated hemiazygos vein.

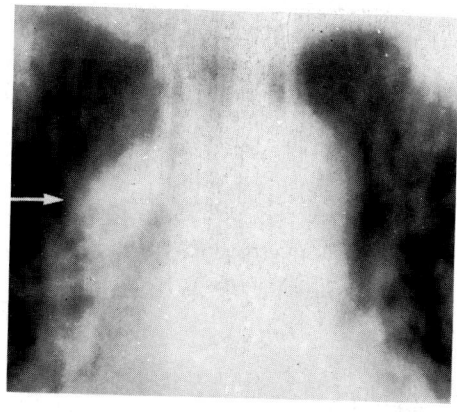

Fig. 10.14. Tomography of the mediastinum of a patient, with large porto-systemic collaterals shows enlargement of azygos vein (marked with arrow).

Massively dilated para-oesophageal collaterals may be seen on the plain chest radiograph as a retrocardiac posterior mediastinal mass.

Barium studies

These have largely been outmoded by upper endoscopy. For the oesophagus, small volumes of barium are required.

Normal oesophageal mucosa shows long, thin, evenly spaced lines. Varices show as filling defects in the regular contour of the oesophagus (fig. 10.15). They are most often in the lower third but may spread upwards so that the entire oesophagus is involved. Widening and finally gross dilatation are helpful signs.

Oesophageal varices are nearly always accompanied by gastric varices which pass through the cardia, line the fundus in a worm-like fashion and may be difficult to distinguish from mucosal folds. Occasionally gastric varices show as a lobulated mass in the gastric fundus simulating a carcinoma. Portal venography is useful in differentiation.

Endoscopy

This is the best method of visualizing oesophageal and gastric varices. The size of the varix must be graded (figs 10.16, 10.17) [100].

1 *Grade 1* (F1): the varices can be depressed by the endoscope.

2 *Grade 2* (F2): the varices cannot be depressed by the endoscope.

3 *Grade 3* (F3): the varices are confluent around the circumference of the oesophagus.

The larger the varix the more likely it is to bleed. Colour is extremely important. Varices usually appear white and opaque (fig. 10.18). Red colour correlates with blood flow through dilated sub-epithelial and commun-

(a)

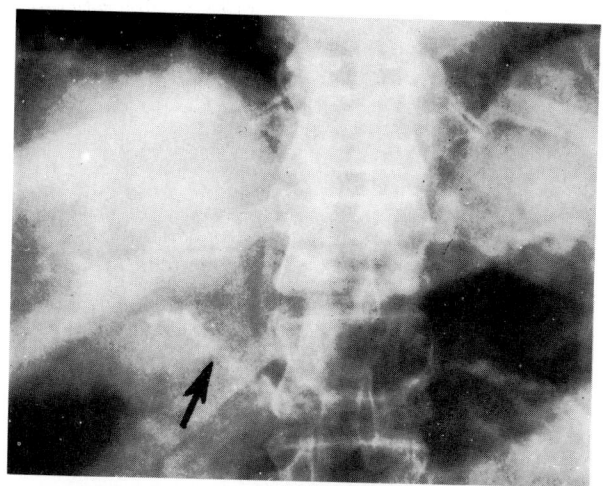

(b)

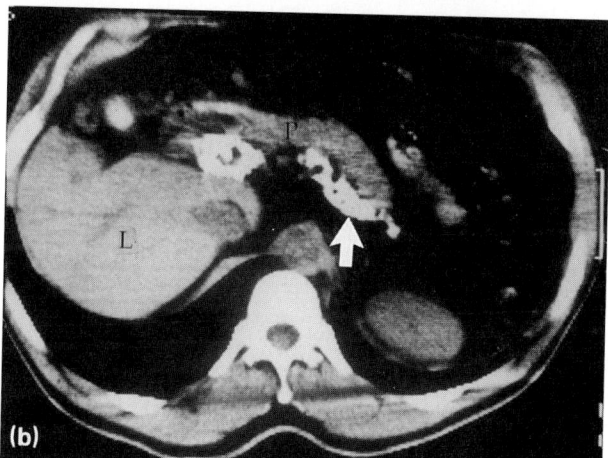

Fig. 10.13. (a) Plain X-ray of the abdomen. Calcification seen in the line of the splenic and portal vein (arrow). (b) CT scan confirms the calcified splenic vein (arrow).

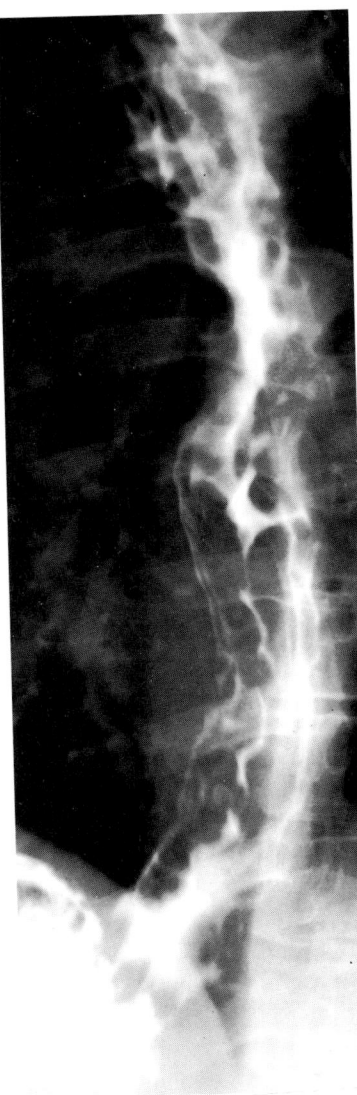

Fig. 10.15. Barium swallow X-ray shows a dilated oesophagus. The margin is irregular. There are multiple filling defects representing oesophageal varices.

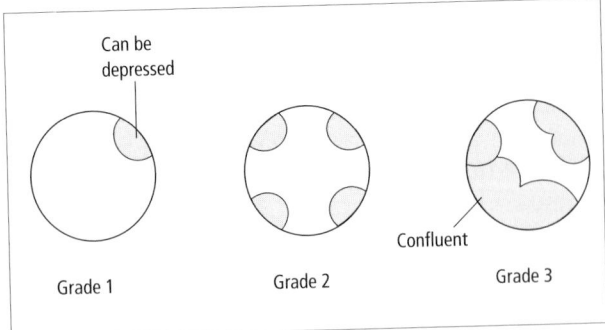

Fig. 10.16. Endoscopic classification of oesophageal varices (adapted from [100]).

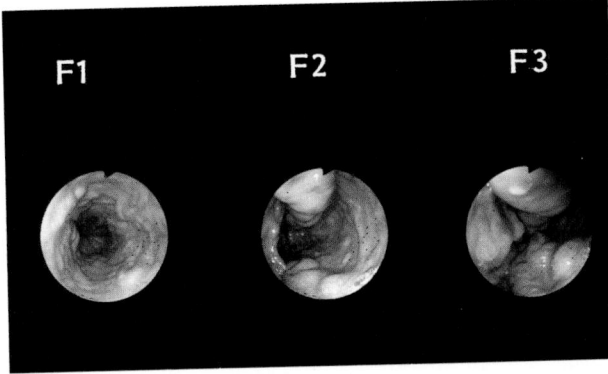

Fig. 10.17. The form of the oesophageal varices (from [100]).

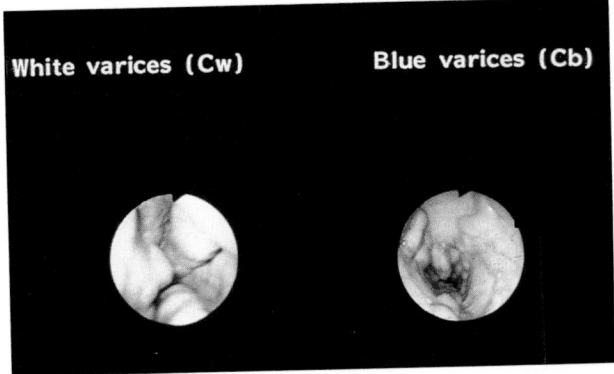

Fig. 10.18. Variceal colour through the endoscope (from [100]).

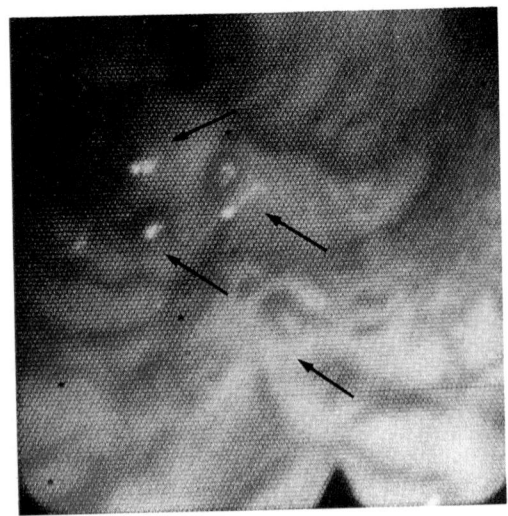

Fig. 10.19. Endoscopic view of cherry-red spots on oesophageal varices (arrows).

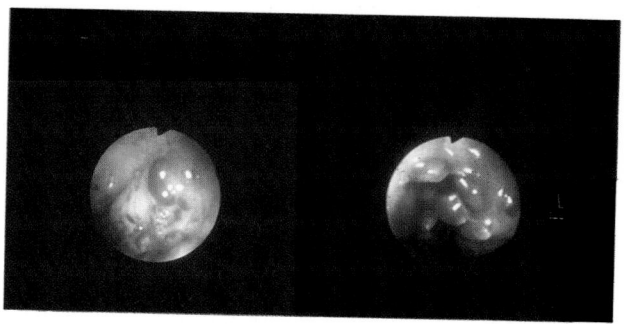

Fig. 10.20. Haemocystic spots on oesophageal varices (from [100]).

icating veins. Dilated sub-epithelial veins may appear as raised cherry-red spots (fig. 10.19) and red wheal markings (longitudinal dilated veins resembling whip marks). They lie on top of large sub-epithelial vessels. The haemocystic spot is approximately 4 mm in diameter (fig. 10.20). It represents blood coming from the deeper extrinsic veins of the oesophagus straight out towards the lumen through a communicating vein into the more superficial submucosal veins. Red colour is usually associated with larger varices. All these colour changes, and particularly the red colour sign, predict variceal bleeding. Intra-observer error may depend on the skill and experience of the endoscopist. On the whole, agreement is good for size and red signs [23].

Portal hypertensive gastropathy is seen largely in the fundus, but can extend throughout the stomach. It is shown as a mosaic-like pattern with small polygonal areas, surrounded by a whitish-yellow depressed border [149]. Red point lesions and cherry-red spots predict a

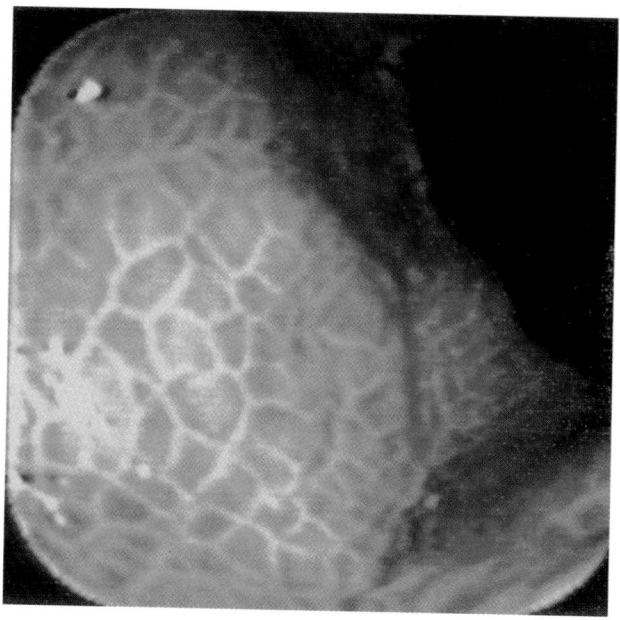

Fig. 10.21. Portal gastropathy. A mosaic of red and yellow is seen together with petechial haemorrhages.

high risk of bleeding. Black–brown spots are due to intra-mucosal haemorrhage (fig. 10.21). Sclerotherapy increases the gastropathy [31].

Variceal (azygos) blood flow can be assessed during diagnostic endoscopy by a Doppler ultrasound probe passed down the biopsy channel of the standard gastroscope.

Imaging the portal venous system

Non-invasive

The patency of the portal vein and the nature and extent of any collateral circulation must be established. Any space-ocupying lesion should be identified. The simplest initial investigation is ultrasound and/or CT. This can be followed by more definitive vascular imaging.

Ultrasound

Longitudinal scans at the sub-costal margins and transverse scans at the epigastrium are essential (fig. 10.22). The portal and superior mesenteric veins can always be seen. The normal splenic vein may be more difficult.

A large portal vein suggests portal hypertension, but this is not diagnostic. If collaterals are seen, this confirms portal hypertension. Portal vein thrombosis is accurately diagnosed and echogenic areas can sometimes be seen within the lumen.

Ultrasound has the advantage over CT in that any number of axes can be used.

Doppler ultrasound

Doppler ultrasound (US) may be used to demonstrate the anatomy of the portal veins and hepatic artery (table 10.2). Satisfactory results depend on meticulous attention to detail and on technical expertise. Small cirrhotic livers are difficult to see as are those of the obese. Colour-coded Doppler improves visualization (fig. 10.23). Portal venous obstruction is demonstrated by Doppler US as accurately as by angiography provided the Doppler is technically optimal.

Doppler US shows spontaneous hepato-fugal flow in portal, splenic and superior mesenteric veins in 8.3% of patients with cirrhosis [41]. Its presence correlates with severity of cirrhosis and with encephalopathy. Variceal bleeding is more likely if the flow is hepato-petal.

Abnormalities of the intra-hepatic portal veins can be shown. These are important if surgery is contemplated.

Colour Doppler is a good way of demonstrating portal-systemic shunts and the direction of flow in them. These include surgical shunts but also transjugular intrahepatic portal-systemic shunt (TIPS). Intra-hepatic portal-systemic shunts may be visualized [72].

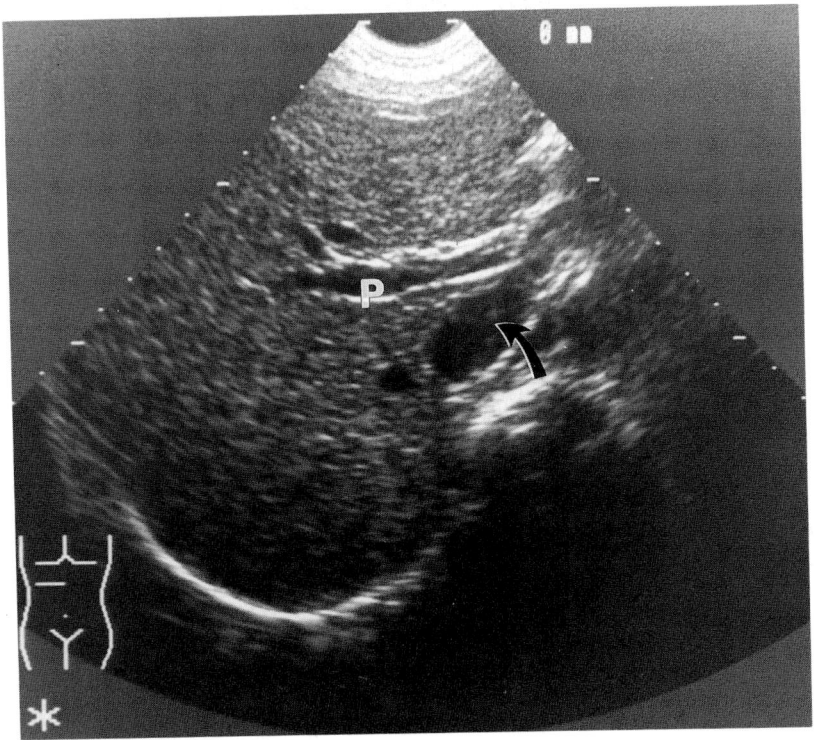

Fig. 10.22. Transverse ultrasound shows patent portal vein (P); arrow indicates inferior vena cava.

Table 10.2. Clinical uses of Doppler ultrasound

Portal vein
Patency
Hepato-fugal flow
Anatomical abnormalities
Portal-systemic shunt patency
Acute flow changes

Hepatic artery
Patency (post-transplant)
Anatomical abnormalities

Hepatic veins
Screening Budd–Chiari syndrome

Colour Doppler screening is useful for patients suspected of having the Budd–Chiari syndrome.

The hepatic artery is more difficult than the hepatic vein to locate because of its small size and direction. Nevertheless, duplex Doppler is the primary screening procedure to show a patent hepatic artery after liver transplantation.

Duplex Doppler has been used to measure portal blood flow. The average velocity of blood flowing in the portal vein is multiplied by the cross-sectional area of the vessel (fig. 10.24). There are observer errors in measurement particularly of velocity. The method is most useful in measuring rapid, large, acute changes in flow rather than monitoring chronic changes in portal haemodynamics.

Portal blood flow velocity correlates with the presence and size of oesophageal varices. In cirrhosis, the portal

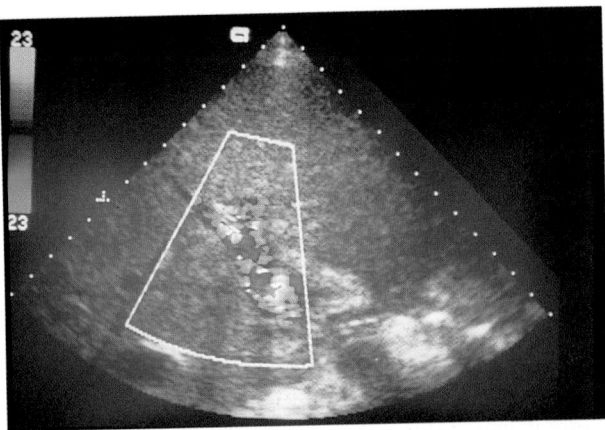

Fig. 10.23. Colour Doppler ultrasound of the porta hepatis shows hepatic artery in red and portal vein in blue.

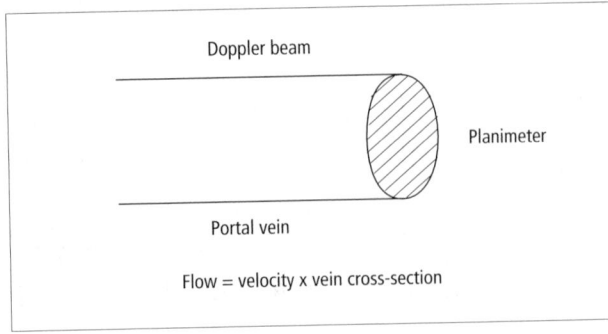

Fig. 10.24. The Doppler real-time ultrasound method of measuring portal venous flow.

vein velocity tends to fall and when less than 16 cm per second portal hypertension is likely. The portal vein calibre tends to increase and a *congestive index* may be calculated as the ratio between the cross-sectional area of the portal vein and the mean portal velocity. This is high in patients in varices and correlates with liver function [144].

CT scan

After contrast, portal vein patency can be established and retroperitoneal, perivisceral and para-oesophageal varices may be visualized (fig. 10.25). Oesophageal varices may be shown as intra-luminal protrusions enhancing after contrast. The umbilical vein can be seen (fig. 10.26). Gastric varices can be seen as rounded structures, indistinguishable from the gastric wall.

CT with arterial portography shows collateral pathways and arteriovenous shunts [154].

Magnetic resonance

This gives excellent depiction of blood vessels as regions of absent signal (fig. 10.27). It may be used to study vessels in a similar fashion to digital subtraction angiography. It has been used to show shunt patency and may be used to study portal blood flow. MR angiography is more reliable than Doppler [40].

Venography

In a patient with cirrhosis, if the portal vein is patent by scanning, confirmation by venography is not necessary

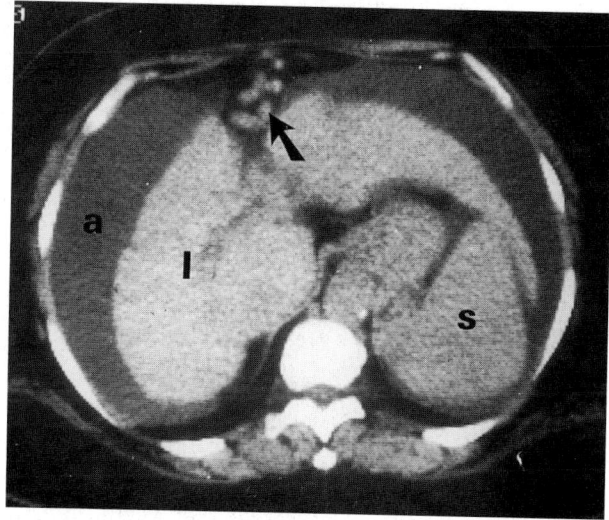

Fig. 10.26. CT scan (after enhancement) of a cirrhotic liver shows patency of the umbilical vein (arrow). l = liver; s = spleen; a = ascites.

unless portal surgery or hepatic transplantation is being considered. A probably thrombosed portal vein on scanning must be confirmed by venography.

Patency of the portal vein is important particularly in the diagnosis of splenomegaly in childhood and in excluding invasion by a hepato-cellular carcinoma in a patient with cirrhosis.

Anatomy of the portal venous system must be known before such operations as portal-systemic shunt, hepatic resection or hepatic transplantation. The patency of a surgical shunt may be confirmed.

The demonstration of a large portal collateral circulation is essential for the diagnosis of chronic hepatic encephalopathy (figs 10.25, 10.28). Its absence excludes it.

A filling defect in the portal vein or in the liver due to a space-occupying lesion may be demonstrated.

Venographic appearances

When the portal circulation is normal, the splenic and portal veins are filled but no other vessels are outlined (fig. 10.29). A filling defect may be seen at the junction of splenic and superior mesenteric veins due to mixing with non-opacified blood. The size and direction of the splenic and portal veins are very variable. The intra-hepatic branches of the portal vein show a gradual branching and reduction in calibre. Later the liver becomes opaque due to sinusoidal filling. The hepatic veins may rarely be seen in later films.

In cirrhosis, the venogram varies widely. It may be completely normal or may show filling of large numbers of collateral vessels with gross distortion of the intra-hepatic pattern ('tree in winter' appearance) (fig. 10.30).

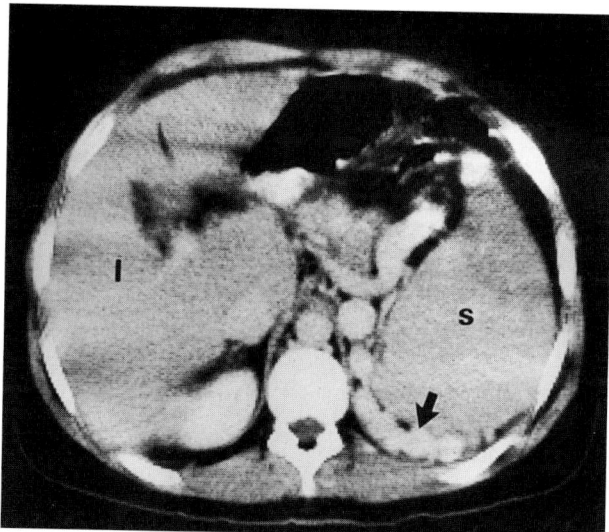

Fig. 10.25. Contrast-enhanced CT scan in a patient with cirrhosis and a large retroperitoneal retrosplenic collateral circulation (arrow). s = spleen; l = liver.

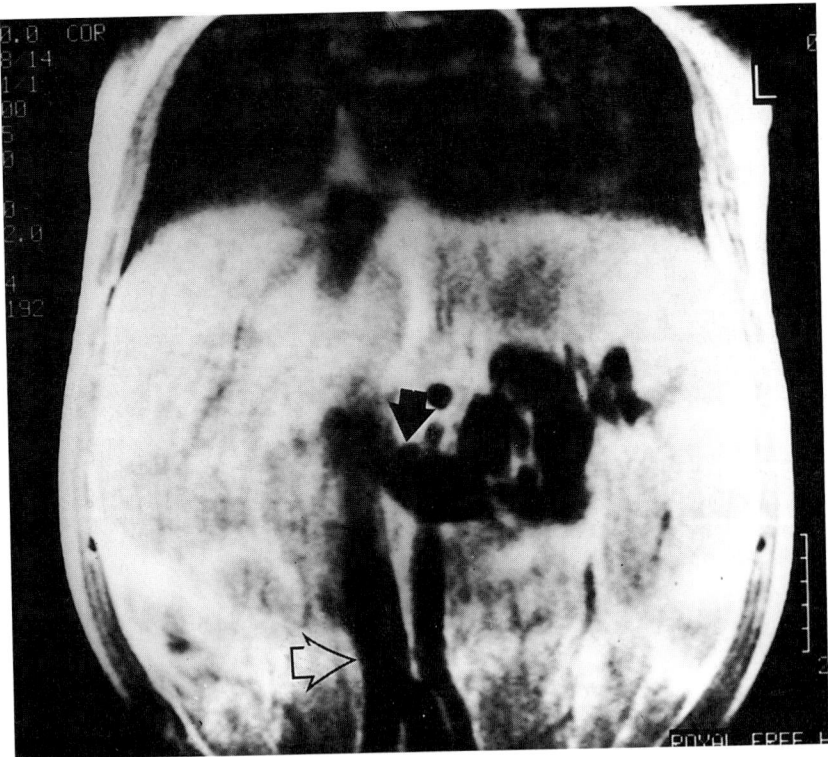

Fig. 10.27. MRI shows a spontaneous spleno-renal shunt to the inferior vena cava. Renal vein (black arrow), vena cava (open arrow).

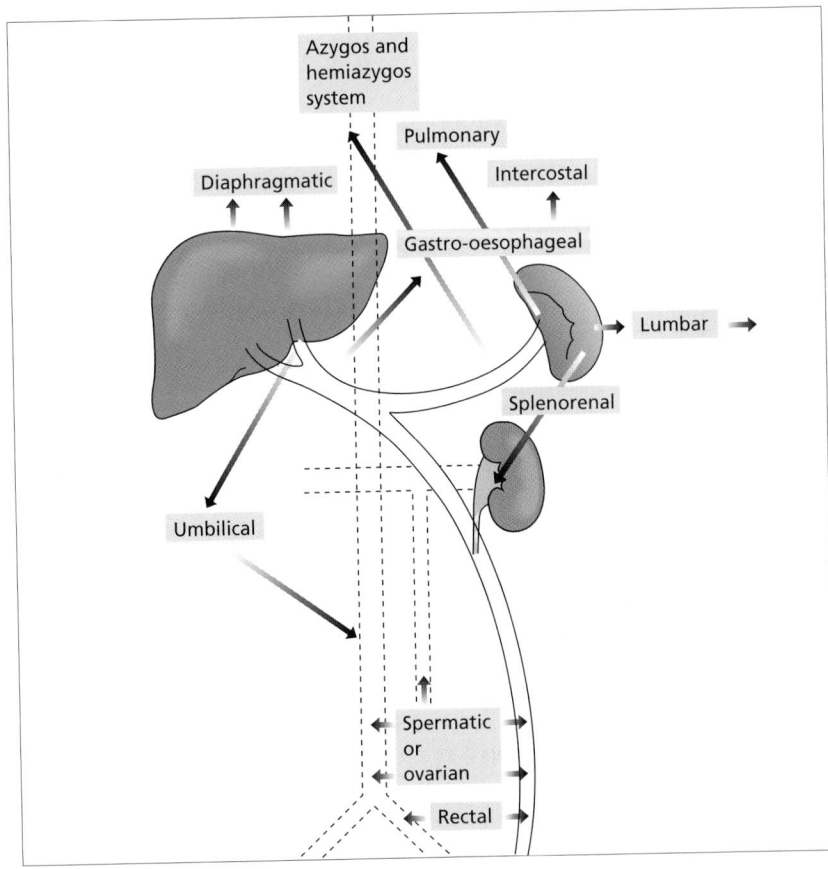

Fig. 10.28. The sites of the collateral circulation in the presence of intra-hepatic portal vein obstruction.

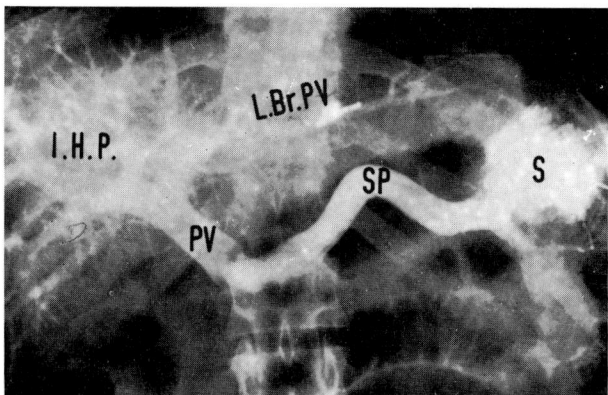

Fig. 10.29. Normal portal venogram obtained by percutaneous splenic puncture. All the dye injected into the spleen passes through the splenic and portal vein into the liver. S = pool of dye in spleen; SP = splenic vein; PV = portal vein; LBrPV = left branch of right portal vein; IHP = intra-hepatic pattern.

In extra-hepatic portal or splenic vein obstruction, large numbers of vessels run from the spleen and splenic vein to the diaphragm, thoracic cage and abdominal wall (fig. 10.31). Intra-hepatic branches are not usually seen although, if the portal vein block is localized, para-portal vessels may short-circuit the lesion and produce a delayed but definite filling of the vein beyond.

Visceral angiography

This technique is safe and is the one most commonly used for portal venography [34]. Safety has increased

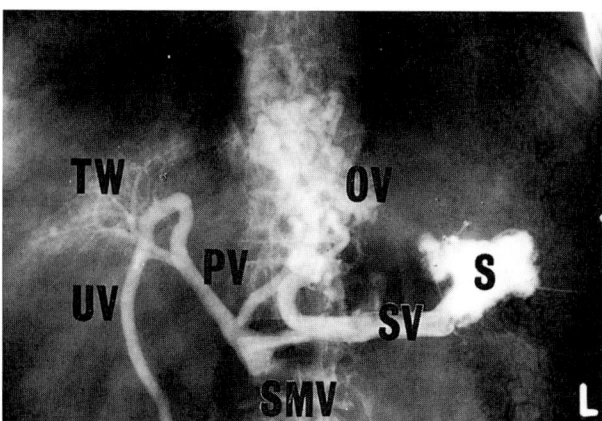

Fig. 10.30. Splenic venogram from a patient with cirrhosis of the liver. The gastro-oesophageal collateral circulation can be seen and the intra-hepatic portal vascular tree is distorted ('tree in winter' appearance). S = splenic pulp; SV = splenic vein; SMV = superior mesenteric vein; PV = portal vein; OV = oesophageal veins; UV = umbilical vein; TW = 'tree in winter' appearance.

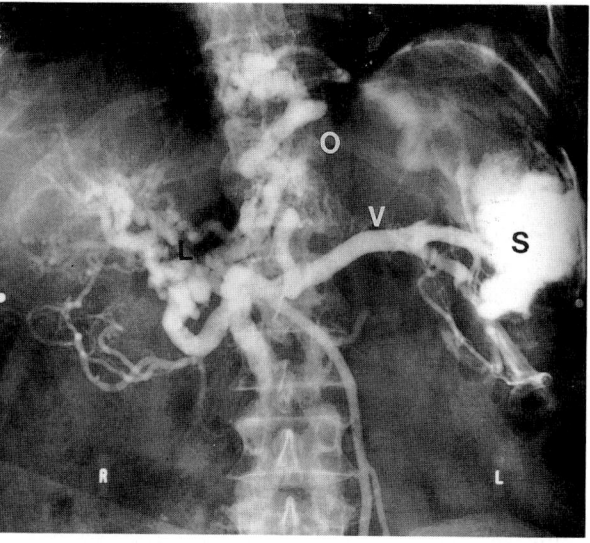

Fig. 10.31. Splenic venogram showing extra-hepatic portal venous obstruction. The portal vein is replaced by numerous small channels. S = spleen; V = splenic vein; L = leash of small collaterals; O = oesophageal collateral circulation.

with the use of smaller (French 5) arterial catheters. Contrast of low osmolarity is painless so that only local anaesthesia is needed. New contrast materials are less toxic to kidneys and other tissues and hypersensitivity reactions are rare.

The coeliac axis is catheterized via the femoral artery with a preformed opaque catheter and 50–60 ml contrast is injected. The contrast material that flows into the splenic artery returns through the splenic and portal veins and produces a splenic and portal venogram. Similarly, a bolus of contrast introduced into the superior mesenteric artery returns through the superior mesenteric and portal veins which can be seen in radiographs exposed at the appropriate intervals (figs 10.32, 10.33).

Visceral angiography demonstrates the hepatic arterial system so allowing space-filling lesions in the liver to be identified. A tumour circulation may diagnose hepato-cellular cancer or another tumour.

The markedly enlarged hepatic artery in a patient with cirrhosis carries a good prognosis compared with those showing a reduction in both hepatic arterial and portal venous flow. Knowledge of splenic and hepatic arterial anatomy is useful if surgery is contemplated. Haemangiomas, other space-occupying lesions and aneurysms may be identified. The portal vascular tree is not so well visualized as in splenic venography.

The portal vein may not opacify if flow in it is hepatofugal or if there is 'steal' by the spleen or by large collateral channels (fig. 10.34). A superior mesenteric angiogram will confirm that the portal vein is in fact patent.

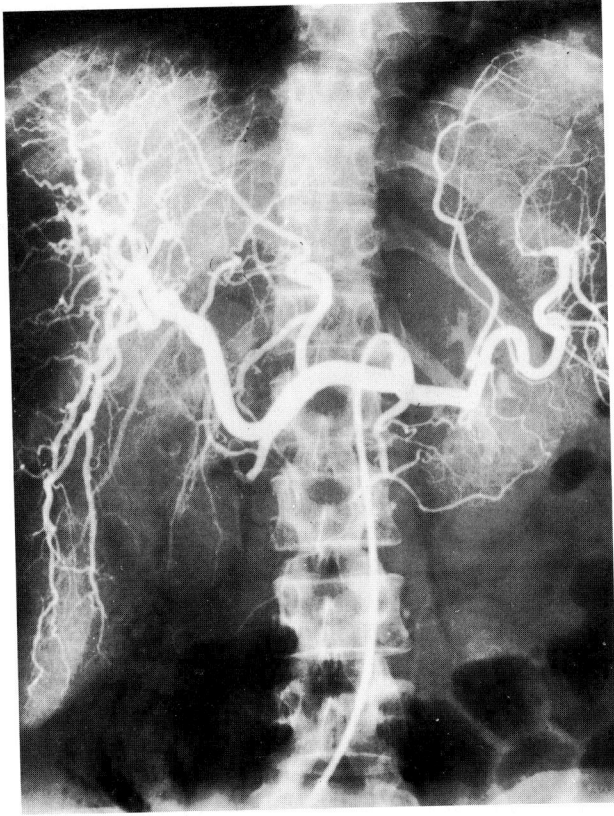

Fig. 10.32. Selective coeliac angiogram shows intra-hepatic arterial pattern. A Riedel's lobe is shown.

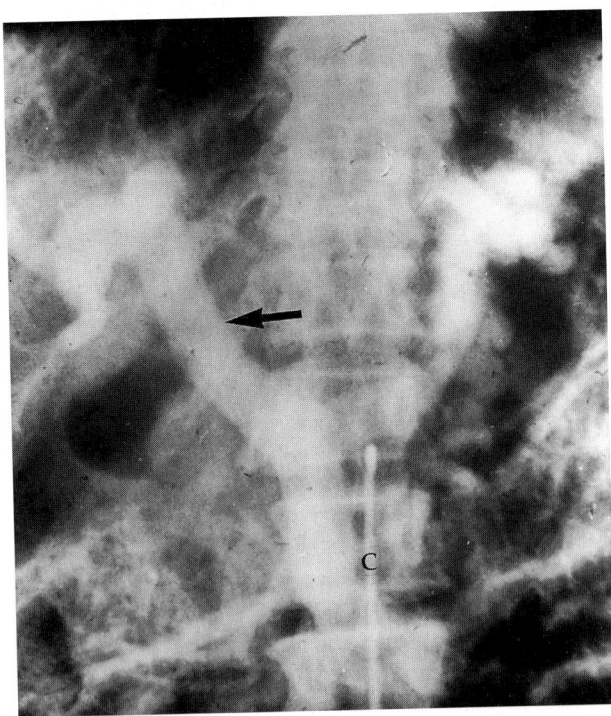

Fig. 10.33. Venous phase of selective coeliac angiogram shows patent portal (arrow) and splenic veins. C = catheter in coeliac axis.

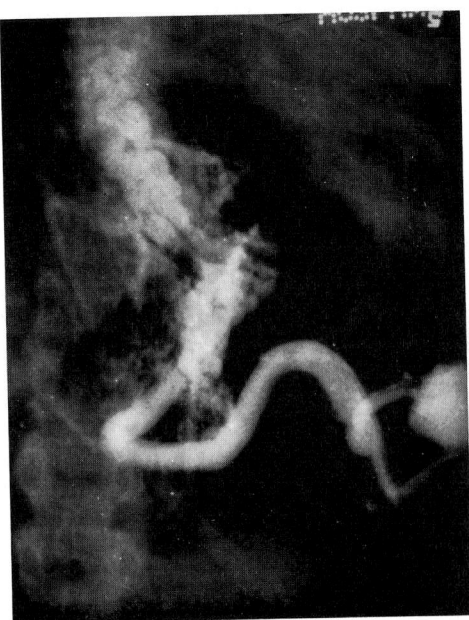

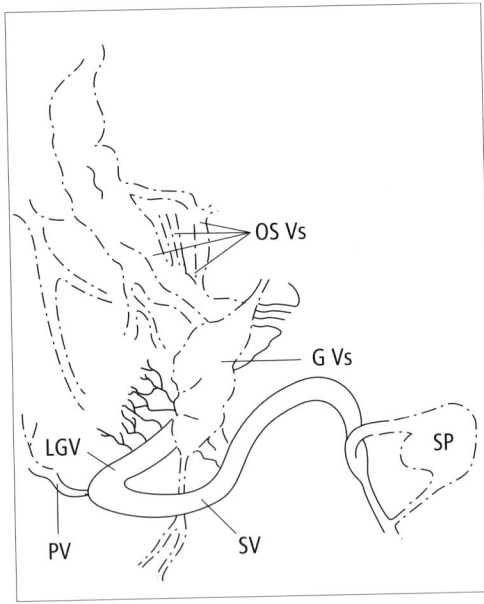

Fig. 10.34. Female patient with portal cirrhosis. Splenic venogram. The bulk of the contrast medium is diverted through the gastric and oesophageal veins and only a trickle enters the portal vein. The portal vein was patent. SP = splenic pulp; SV = splenic vein; PV = portal vein; LGV = left gastric vein; GVs, OSVs = gastric and oesophageal varices.

Digital subtraction angiography

The contrast is usually given by selective arterial injection with immediate subtraction of images although direct splenic injection has been used [17]. Less material is needed than for the conventional arterial technique and smaller catheters are used. The portal system is very well visualized free of other confusing images (fig. 10.35). Spatial resolution is poorer than with conven-

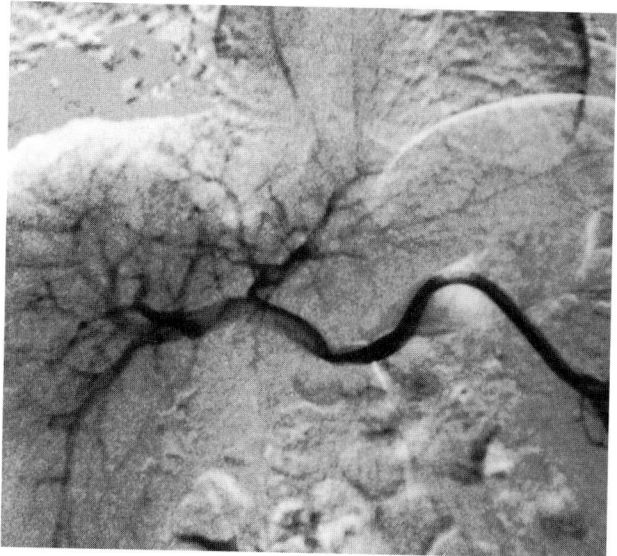

Fig. 10.35. Digital subtraction angiography shows a normal portal venous system.

tional film-based angiography. The technique is particularly valuable for the parenchymal phase of hepatic angiography and for the diagnosis of vascular lesions such as haemangiomas or arteriovenous malformations.

Splenic venography

Contrast material, injected into the pulp of the spleen, is absorbed into the portal bloodstream with sufficient rapidity to outline the splenic and portal veins.

The collateral circulation is particularly well visualized (see fig. 10.30) and it is the procedure of choice where extra-hepatic portal venous obstruction is suspected. Intrasplenic pressure may be measured [3].

Trans-hepatic portography [146]

This technique gives excellent visualization of the portal and splenic veins and the porto-systemic collateral circulation. It is, however, technically difficult and carries a greater risk than other procedures (fig. 10.36).

Portal venous pressure

Wedged hepatic venous pressure

A balloon catheter is introduced into a hepatic venous radicle via the femoral vein until it can go no further (fig. 10.37) [52]. It now prevents blood from flowing through the hepatic vein radical. The pressure measured represents that at the next point of free communication with the hepatic circulation and so measures the sinusoidal venous pressure. The catheter is properly wedged if the

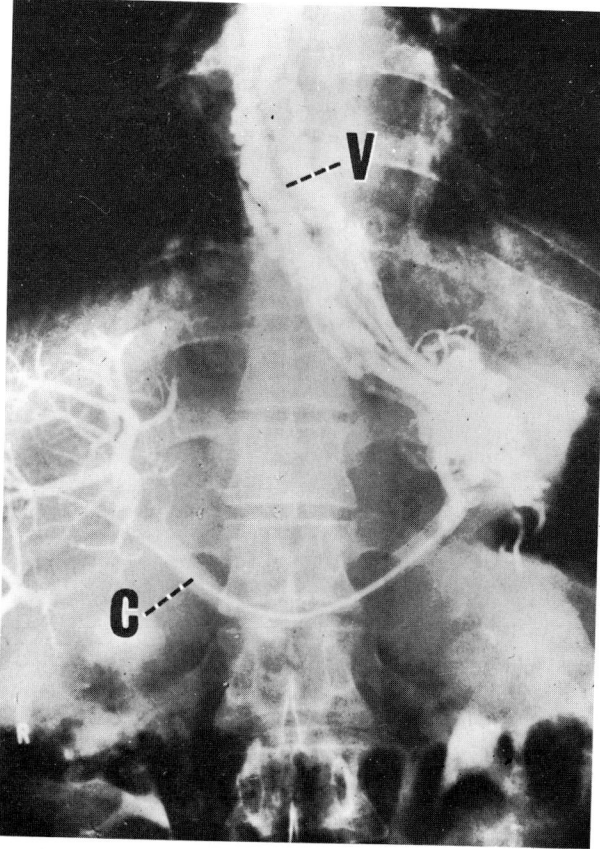

Fig. 10.36. Trans-hepatic portogram shows cannula passed through liver and portal vein into the left gastric vein. Contrast material has been injected and massive oesophageal varices filled. C = cannula; V = varices.

pressure tracing shows regular oscillations related to transmission of hepatic arterial pressure and, finally, a small amount of contrast material injected is seen to pass against the predominant flow into the sinusoidal bed. Measurements are then taken with the balloon deflated and reflect the free hepatic venous pressure.

The difference between 'wedged' and 'free' pressure is the portal (sinusoidal) venous pressure. The normal is 5–6 mmHg and values of about 20 mmHg are found in patients with cirrhosis. In alcoholic cirrhosis a gradient of 12 mmHg or greater is a requirement for the development of varices and hence haemorrhage.

The wedged hepatic venous pressure does not reflect portal venous pressure in pre-sinusoidal portal hypertension including that found in alcoholic liver disease. It may underestimate the true portal venous pressure.

The technique is relatively easy, safe, and can be performed in patients with a bleeding tendency or with ascites. It allows portal pressure to be measured in the splenectomized. Serial estimations are of value in following the effect of drugs on the portal system.

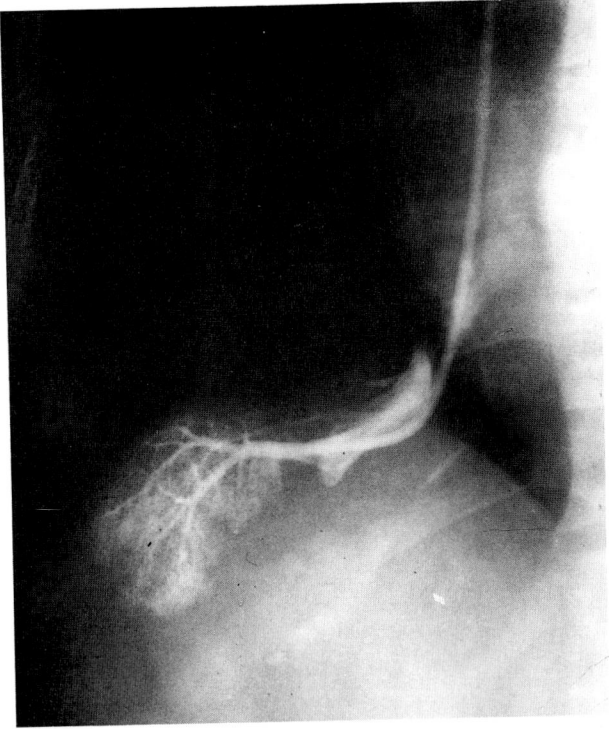

Fig. 10.37. A catheter has been inserted into a hepatic vein via the femoral vein. The wedged position is confirmed by introducing a small amount of contrast, which has entered the sinusoidal bed.

Trans-hepatic

This is safe if a 25-gauge needle is used under ultrasound guidance, the needle being replaced by a 5 French catheter which is placed in the main portal vein (figs 10.36, 10.38).

Operative

These measurements are unreliable, as they are affected by the anaesthetic, blood loss, position of the patient and duration of the operation.

Variceal pressure

Pressure in a varix may be estimated by a pneumatic pressure gauge fixed to the tip of an endoscope. The variceal pressure correlates with portal pressure and with variceal bleeding [123]. Unfortunately, the equipment is not readily available.

Direct puncture of varices at the time of sclerotherapy allows a pressure to be recorded. This is about 15.5 mmHg in cirrhotic patients, significantly lower than the main portal pressure of about 18.8 mmHg.

An endoscopic balloon has been developed to measure variceal pressure and this gives comparable results to direct puncture [44].

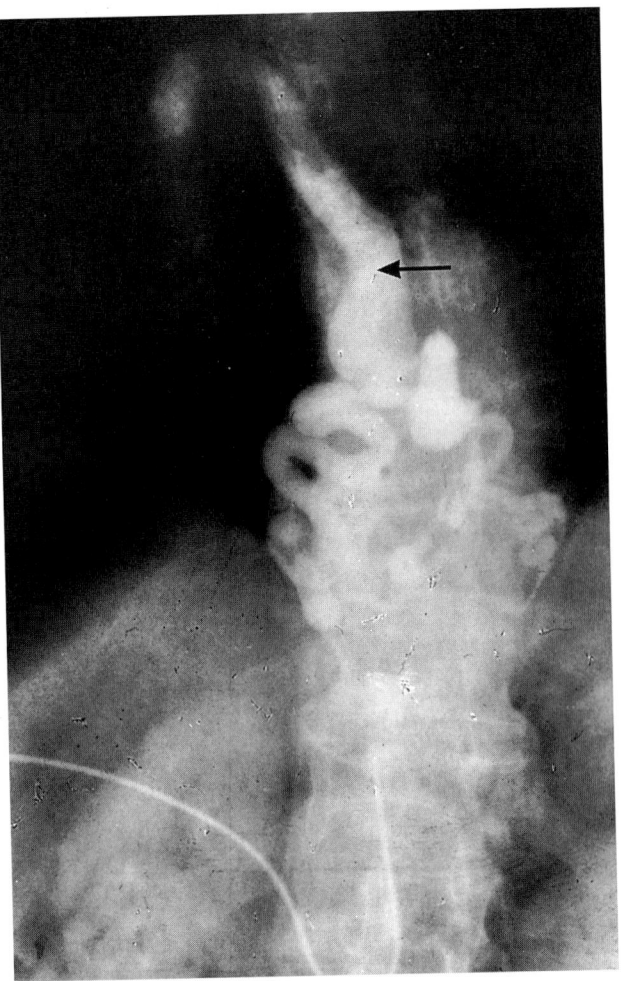

Fig. 10.38. Trans-hepatic catheterization of the azygos vein (arrow) via the portal vein and oesophageal collaterals.

Estimation of hepatic blood flow

Constant infusion method

Hepatic blood flow may be measured by a constant infusion of indocyanine green (ICG) and catheterization of the hepatic vein [16, 22]. Flow is calculated by the Fick principle.

This method depends on the dye being removed only by the liver at a steady rate shown by maintenance of constant arterial levels, and also on the absence of significant entero-hepatic circulation. It has been used to show a fall in hepatic blood flow in recumbency, fainting, heart failure, cirrhosis and exercise. Fever increases flow and it is unaltered in such high cardiac output states as thyrotoxicosis and pregnancy.

Plasma disappearance method

Hepatic blood flow can be measured after an intravenous injection of ICG followed by analysis of the disappearance curve in a peripheral artery and hepatic vein.

If the extraction of a substance is about 100%, for instance, using ^{131}I heat-denatured albumin colloidal complex, hepatic blood flow can be determined by peripheral clearance without hepatic vein catheterization.

In patients with cirrhosis, up to 20% of the blood perfusing the liver may not go through normal channels and hepatic extraction is reduced. In these circumstances, hepatic vein catheterization is necessary to estimate extraction and thus hepatic blood flow.

Electromagnetic flow meters

Flows in exposed vessels may be measured directly using the square-wave electromagnetic flow meter. This enables flow in portal vein and hepatic artery to be measured separately.

Azygos blood flow

Most of the blood flowing through gastro-oesophageal varices terminates in the azygos system. Azygos blood flow can be measured using a double thermo-dilution catheter directed under fluoroscopy into the azygos vein (fig. 10.38) [15]. Alcoholic cirrhotic patients who have bled from varices show a flow of about 596 ml/minute. Azygos flow is markedly reduced by propranolol.

EXPERIMENTAL PORTAL VENOUS OCCLUSION
AND HYPERTENSION

Survival following acute occlusion depends on the development of an adequate collateral circulation. In the rabbit, cat or dog this does not develop and death supervenes rapidly. In the monkey or man, the collateral circulation is adequate and survival is usual.

Acute occlusion of one branch of the portal vein is not fatal. The liver cells of the ischaemic lobe atrophy, but bile ducts, Kupffer cells and connective tissues survive. The unaffected lobe hypertrophies.

Experimentally, portal hypertension can be produced by occluding the portal vein, injecting silica into the portal vein, infecting mice with schistosomiasis, by any experimental type of cirrhosis, or by biliary obstruction. An extensive collateral circulation develops, the spleen enlarges but ascites does not form.

Classification of portal hypertension

Portal hypertension usually follows obstruction to the portal blood flow anywhere along its course. Intrasplenic pressure reflects pressure in the splenic vein. The trans-hepatic route can be used to measure pressure in

the main portal vein [146]. The wedged hepatic venous pressure represents sinusoidal pressure. Venography or visceral angiography show the site of obstruction and the nature of the collateral circulation. Liver biopsy helps in localization and diagnosis of the cause of obstruction. Using a selection of these techniques, portal hypertension has been classified into two groups: (i) *pre-sinusoidal* (extra-hepatic or intra-hepatic) and (ii) a big general group of *hepatic* causes (fig. 10.39, table 10.3). This distinction is a practical one. The pre-sinusoidal forms, which include obstruction to the sinusoids by Kupffer and other cellular proliferations are associated with relatively normal hepato-cellular function. Consequently, if patients with this type suffer a haemorrhage from varices, liver failure is rarely a consequence. In contrast, patients with the intra-hepatic type frequently develop liver failure after bleeding.

Extra-hepatic portal venous obstruction

This causes extra-hepatic pre-sinusoidal portal hypertension. The obstruction may be at any point in the course of the portal vein. The *venae comitantes* enlarge in an attempt to deliver portal blood to the liver, so assuming a leash-like cavernous appearance. The portal vein, represented by a fibrous strand, is recognized with difficulty in the multitude of small vessels. This cavernous change follows any block in the main vein (see fig. 10.31).

Aetiology

Infections

Umbilical infection with or without catheterization of the umbilical vein may be responsible in neonates (fig. 10.40) [156]. The infection spreads along the umbilical vein to the left portal vein and hence to the main portal vein. Acute appendicitis and peritonitis are causative in older children.

Portal vein occlusion is particularly common in India, accounting for 20–30% of all variceal bleeding. Neonatal dehydration and infections may be responsible.

Ulcerative colitis and Crohn's disease can be complicated by portal vein block.

Portal vein obstruction may be secondary to biliary infections due, for instance, to gallstones or primary sclerosing cholangitis.

Post-operative

The portal and splenic veins commonly block after splenectomy, especially when, pre-operatively, the patient had a normal platelet count. The thrombosis spreads from the splenic vein into the main portal vein. It

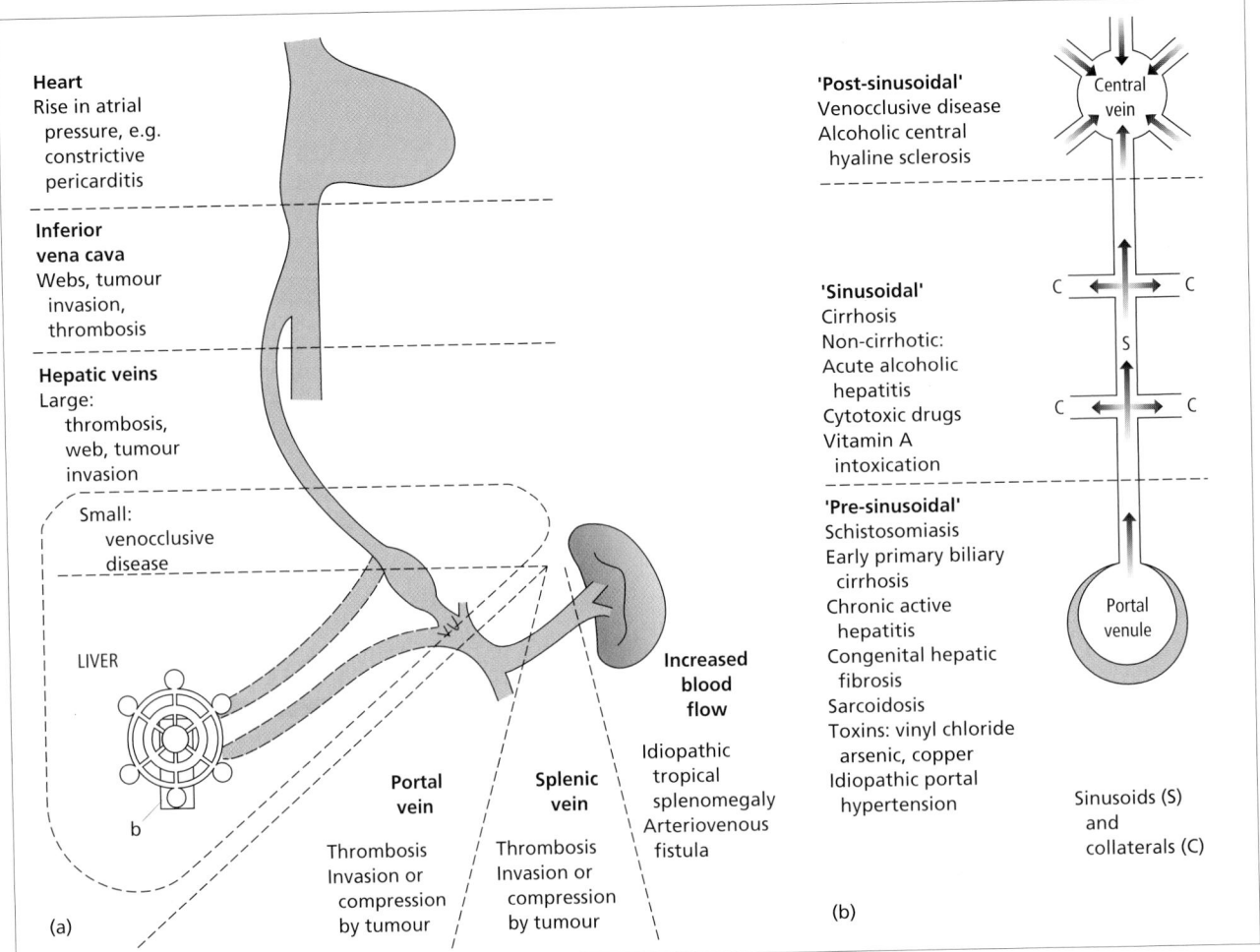

Fig. 10.39. Causes of portal hypertension. (a) Pre- and post-hepatic. (b) Intra-hepatic. (NB Overlap exists; wedge hepatic vein pressure may be high in patients with 'pre-sinusoidal' causes, especially as the disease progresses, indicating sinusoidal and/or collateral involvement. Some 'post-sinusoidal' conditions may also have a sinusoidal component.) [34].

Table 10.3. Classification of portal hypertension

Pre-sinusoidal	
Extra-hepatic	Blocked portal vein
	Increased splenic flow
Intra-hepatic	Portal zone infiltrates
	Toxic
	Hepato-portal sclerosis
Hepatic	
Intra-hepatic	Cirrhosis
Post-sinusoidal	Other nodules
	Blocked hepatic vein

is especially likely in patients with myeloid metaplasia [18]. A similar sequence follows occluded surgical porto-systemic shunts.

The portal vein may thrombose as a complication of major, difficult hepato-biliary surgery, for instance, repair of a stricture or removal of a choledochal cyst.

Trauma

Portal vein injury rarely follows automobile accidents or stabbing and is rare. Laceration of the portal vein is 50% fatal and ligation may be the only method to control the bleeding.

Hypercoagulable state

This is a frequent cause of portal vein thrombosis in adults. It is commonly due to a myeloproliferative disorder which may be in a latent from [159]. At autopsy, thrombotic lesions are frequently found in macroscopic and microscopic portal veins of patients dying with portal hypertension and myelometaplasia [170]. Ascites and oesophageal varices are associated.

Hereditary protein C deficiency can be complicated by portal vein thrombosis [159].

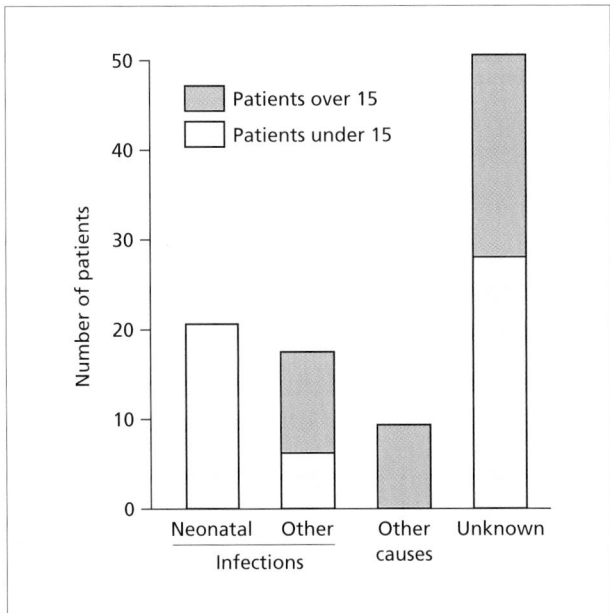

Fig. 10.40. Aetiology of portal vein occlusion in 97 patients over and under 15 years old [172].

Invasion and compression

The classic example is hepato-cellular carcinoma. Carcinoma of the pancreas, usually of the body, and of other adjacent organs may lead to portal vein block. Chronic pancreatitis is frequently associated with splenic vein obstruction, but involvement of the portal vein is rare (5.6%) [8].

Congenital

Congenital obstruction can be produced anywhere along the line of the right and left vitelline veins from which the portal vein develops. The portal vein may be absent with visceral venous return passing to systemic veins particularly the inferior vena cava [96]. Hilar venous collaterals are absent.

Congenital abnormalities of the portal vein are usually associated with congenital defects elsewhere [96, 104, 172].

Cirrhosis

The prevalence of portal vein thrombosis complicating cirrhosis is very low [105]. Invasion by a hepato-cellular carcinoma is the most frequent cause. Post-splenectomy thrombocytosis is another aetiological factor. Mural thrombi found at autopsy are probably terminal. It is easy to over-diagnose thrombosis by finding a non-filled portal vein on imaging. This usually represents 'steal' into massive collaterals or into a large spleen.

Miscellaneous

Portal vein thrombosis has very rarely been associated with pregnancy and with oral contraceptives, especially in older women and with long usage [24].

Portal vein block has been associated with general disease of veins and in particular with thrombophlebitis migrans.

In retro-peritoneal fibrosis, the portal venous system may be encased by dense fibrous tissue.

Unknown

In about half of patients the aetiology, even after the fullest investigation, remains obscure (fig. 10.40). Some of these patients have associated autoimmune disorders such as hypothyroidism, diabetes, pernicious anaemia, dermatomyositis or rheumatoid arthritis [172]. In some instances, the obstruction may have followed undiagnosed intra-abdominal infections such as appendicitis or diverticulitis.

Clinical features

The patient may present with features of the underlying disease, for instance, polycythaemia rubra vera or primary liver cancer.

Bleeding from oesophago-gastric varices is the most common presentation. In those of neonatal origin, the first haemorrhage is at about the age of 4 years (fig. 10.41). The frequency increases between 10 and 15 years and decreases after puberty. However, some patients with portal venous block never bleed and in others haemorrhage may be delayed for as long as 12 years. If blood replacement is adequate, recovery usually ensues in a matter of days. Apart from frank bleeds, intermittent minor blood loss is probably common. This is diagnosed only if the patient is having repeated checks for stool blood or if iron deficiency anaemia develops.

Especially in children, haemorrhage may be initiated by a minor, febrile, intercurrent infection. The mechanism is unclear. Aspirin or a similar drug may be the precipitating factor. Excessive exertion or swallowing a large bolus does not seem to initiate bleeding.

The spleen is always enlarged and symptomless splenomegaly may be a presentation, particularly in children. Peri-umbilical veins are not seen but there may be dilated abdominal wall veins in the left flank.

The liver is normal in size and consistency. Stigmas of hepato-cellular disease, such as jaundice or vascular spiders, are absent. With acute portal venous thrombosis, ascites is early and transient, subsiding as the collateral circulation develops. Ascites is usually related to an additional factor which has depressed hepato-cellular function, such as a haemorrhage or a surgical explora-

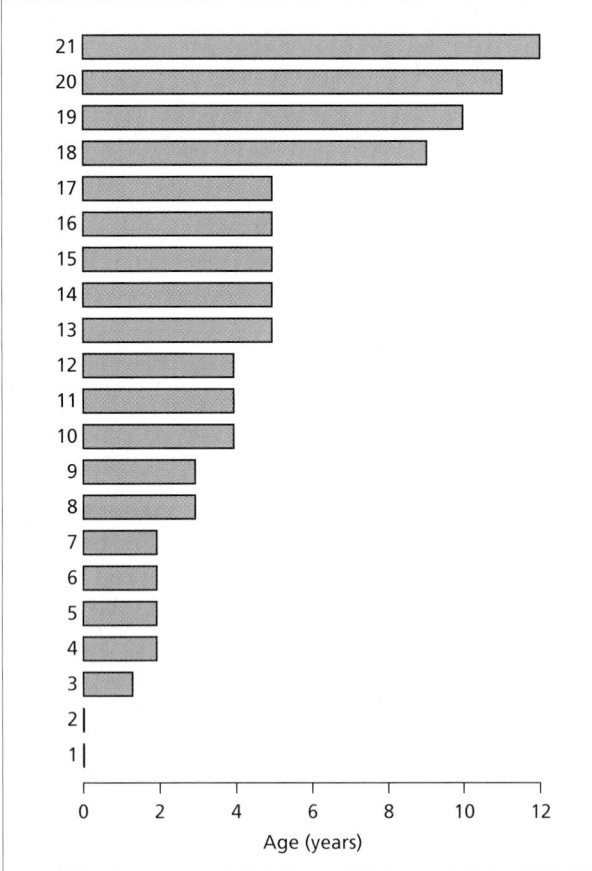

Fig. 10.41. Portal vein occlusion in neonates. Age at time of first haemorrhage in 21 patients in whom the portal vein block occurred in the neonatal period [172].

tion. It may be seen in the elderly where it is related to the deterioration of liver function with ageing [157].

Hepatic encephalopathy is not uncommon in adults, usually following an additional insult such as haemorrhage, infection or anaesthetic. Chronic encephalopathy may be seen in elderly patients with a particularly large portal-systemic collateral circulation.

Imaging

Ultrasound shows echogenic thrombus within the portal vein and colour Doppler shows no portal venous signal [113].

CT shows the thrombus as a non-enhancing filling defect within the lumen of the portal vein and dilatation of many small veins at the hilum (fig. 10.42).

MRI shows an area of abnormal signal within the lumen of the portal vein which appears iso-intense on T_1-weighted image with a more intense signal on T_2-weighted image.

Angiography in the portal venous phase shows a filling defect or non-opacification of the portal vein. However, the portal vein may not be visualized if blood is diverted away from it into extensive collaterals.

Haematology

Haemoglobin is normal unless there has been blood loss. Leucopenia and thrombocytopenia are related to the enlarged spleen. Circulating platelets and leucocytes, although in short supply, are adequate and function well.

Hypersplenism is not an indication for splenectomy. Blood coagulation is normal.

Serum biochemistry

All the usual tests of 'liver function' are normal. Elevation of serum globulin may be related to intestinal antigens, particularly *Escherichia coli* bypassing the liver through collaterals. Mild pancreatic hypofunction is presumably related to interruption of the venous drainage of the pancreas [173].

Prognosis

This depends on the underlying disease. The outlook is much better than for cirrhosis as liver function is normal. The prognosis is surprisingly good in the child and, with careful management of recurrent bleeding, survival to adult life is expected. The number of bleeds seems to reduce as time passes. Women may bleed in pregnancy but this is unusual; their babies are normal.

Treatment

Any underlying cause must be identified and treated. This may be more important than the portal hypertension. For instance, hepato-cellular carcinoma, invading the portal vein, precludes aggressive therapy for bleeding oesophageal varices. If the variceal bleeding is secondary to thrombosis of the portal vein related to polycythaemia rubra vera, reduction of the platelet count by venesection or cytotoxic drugs must precede any surgical therapy; anticoagulants may be needed.

Prophylactic treatment of varices is not indicated. They may never rupture and as time passes collaterals open up.

With acute portal vein thrombosis, anticoagulant therapy is usually too late as the clot will have undergone organization. If diagnosed early, anticoagulants may prevent spreading thrombosis.

Children should survive haemorrhage with proper management, including transfusion. Care must be taken to give compatible blood and to preserve peripheral veins. Aspirin ingestion should be avoided. Upper

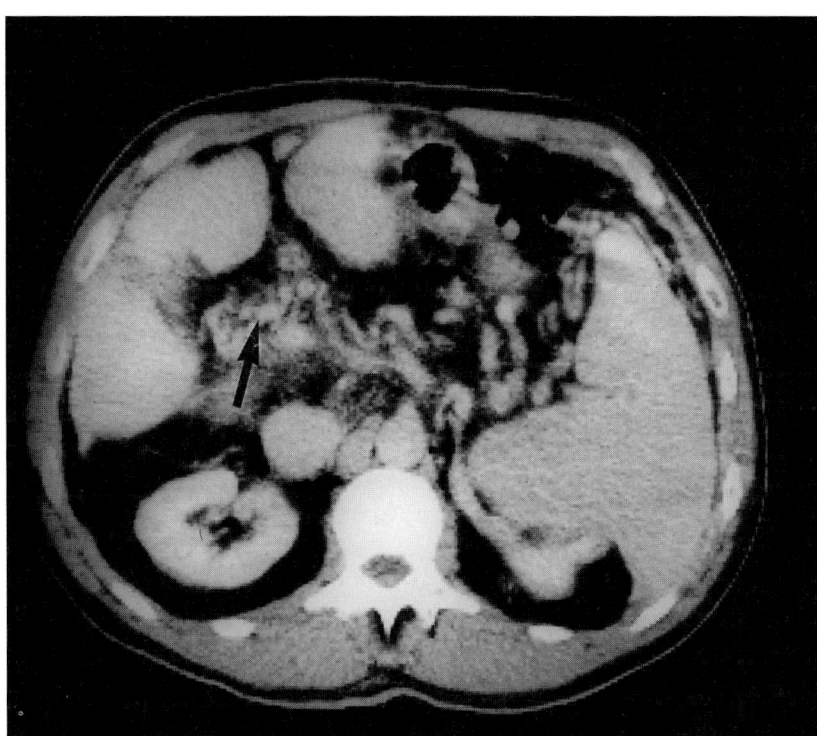

Fig. 10.42. Abdominal CT scan with contrast shows the main portal vein replaced by a leash of small veins (arrow).

respiratory infections should be treated seriously as they seem to precipitate haemorrhage.

Somatostatin infusions may be needed and occasionally the Sengstaken tube.

Endoscopic sclerotherapy is valuable as an emergency procedure.

Major or recurrent bleeds may be treated by later obliterative sclerotherapy. Unfortunately this does not treat the huge gastric fundal varices and the congestive gastropathy continues.

Definitive surgery to reduce portal pressure is usually impossible as there are no suitable veins for a shunt. Even apparently normal-looking veins seen on venography turn out to be in poor condition, presumably related to extension of the original thrombotic process. In children, veins are very small and difficult to anastomose. Myriads of collateral channels add to the technical difficulties.

Results for all forms of surgery are very unsatisfactory. Splenectomy is the least successful and has the highest complication rate. A shunt (porta-caval, meso-caval, or spleno-renal) is the most satisfactory treatment but usually proves impossible.

When the patient is exsanguinating, despite massive blood transfusion, an oesophageal transection may have to be performed using the stapling procedure. Here again gastric varices are not treated. Post-operative complications are common.

TIPS is usually impossible.

Splenic vein obstruction

Isolated splenic vein obstruction causes sinistral (left-sided) portal hypertension. It may be due to any of the factors causing portal vein obstruction. Pancreatic disease such as carcinoma (18%), pancreatitis (65%), pseudocyst and pancreatectomy are particularly important [8].

If the obstruction is distal to the entry of the left gastric vein, a collateral circulation bypasses the obstructed splenic vein through short gastric veins into the gastric fundus and lower oesophagus, so reaching the left gastric vein and portal vein. This leads to very prominent varices in the fundus of the stomach but few in the lower oesophagus.

Trans-hepatic venography, the selective venous phase of an angiogram (fig. 10.43), an enhanced CT scan or MRI are diagnostic. Splenectomy, by blocking arterial inflow, is usually curative but unnecessary if the patient has not bled from varices [83].

Hepatic arterio-portal venous fistulae

Portal hypertension results from increased portal venous flow. Increase in intra-hepatic resistance due to a rise in portal flow may also be important. The portal zones of the liver show thickening of small portal venous radicles with accompanying mild fibrosis and lymphocyte infiltration. The increased intra-hepatic resistance may persist after obliteration of the fistula.

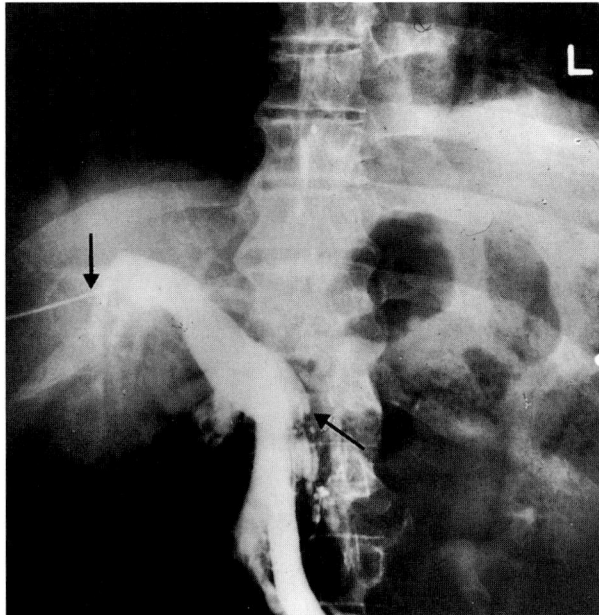

Fig. 10.43. A 64-year-old man with polycythemia rubra vera. Trans-hepatic portal venogram (arrow) shows thrombosed splenic vein marked by lower arrow with patent superior mesenteric and portal veins. This patient, after preliminary reduction of red cell and platelet count by radio-active phosphorus, was successfully treated by splenectomy.

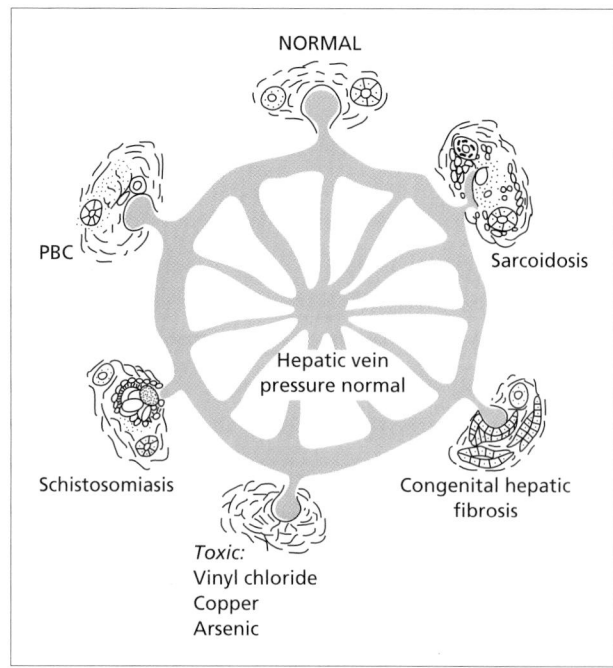

Fig. 10.44. The aetiology of pre-sinusoidal intra-hepatic portal hypertension (PBC = peripheral blood cells).

These fistulae are usually congenital, traumatic or related to adjacent malignant neoplasm [142]. Inferior mesenteric arteriovenous fistulae may be associated with acute ischaemic colitis.

With large fistulae, a loud arterial bruit is heard in the right upper abdomen. Pain may be pronounced. Others present with portal hypertension.

Ultrasound and enhanced CT show an enlarged hepatic artery and a dilated intra-hepatic portal vein. The diagnosis is confirmed by arteriography.

Selective non-invasive embolization of the fistula is the treatment of choice and has replaced surgery.

Portal-hepatic venous shunts

These are probably congenital and represent persistence of the omphalomesenteric venous system. They may be between the main portal and hepatic veins or between the right or left portal vein and hepatic veins [26]. They are diagnosed by ultrasound, enhanced CT scan, MRI and colour Doppler imaging and confirmed by arteriography.

Intra-hepatic pre-sinusoidal and sinusoidal portal hypertension (fig. 10.44)

Portal tract lesions

In *schistosomiasis*, the portal hypertension results from the ova causing a reaction in the minute portal-venous radicles.

In *congenital hepatic fibrosis* the portal hypertension is probably due to a deficiency of terminal branches of the portal vein in the fibrotic portal zones.

Portal hypertension has been reported with *myeloproliferative diseases* including myelosclerosis, myeloid leukaemia and Hodgkin's disease [37]. The mechanism is complex. In part it is related to infiltration of the portal zones with haemopoietic tissue, but thrombotic lesions in major and minor portal vein radicles and nodular regenerative hyperplasia contribute [170].

In *systemic mastocytosis*, portal hypertension is related to increased intra-hepatic resistance secondary to mast cell infiltration. Increased splenic flow, perhaps with splenic arteriovenous shunting and with histamine release, may contribute [53].

In *primary biliary cirrhosis*, portal hypertension may be a presenting feature long before the development of the nodular regeneration characteristic of cirrhosis (Chapter 14). The mechanism is uncertain, although portal zone lesions and narrowing of the sinusoids because of cellular infiltration have been incriminated. The portal hypertension of *sarcoidosis* may be similar. Massive fibrosis is usually associated.

Toxic causes

The injurious substance is taken up by endothelial cells, mostly lipocytes (*Ito cells*) in Disse's space; these are fibrogenic. Minute portal vein radicles are obstructed and intra-hepatic portal hypertension results.

Inorganic arsenic has caused portal hypertension in patients being treated for psoriasis.

Liver disease in vineyard sprayers in Portugal may be related to exposure to *copper*. Angiosarcoma may be a complication.

Exposure to the vapour of the polymer of *vinyl chloride* leads to sclerosis of portal venules with portal hypertension and angiosarcoma.

Reversible portal hypertension may follow *vitamin A intoxication* — vitamin A being stored in Ito cells [54]. Prolonged use of *cytotoxic drugs*, such as methotrexate, 6-mercaptopurine and azathioprine, can lead to perisinusoidal fibrosis and portal hypertension.

Hepato-portal sclerosis

This is marked by splenomegaly, hypersplenism and portal hypertension without occlusion of portal and splenic veins and with no obvious pathology in the liver [84]. It is a confused entity. It has also been termed noncirrhotic portal fibrosis, non-cirrhotic portal hypertension and idiopathic portal hypertension. *Banti's syndrome*, an obsolete term, probably fell into this group. Injury to intra-hepatic portal venous radicles and sinusoidal endothelial cells is the common denominator. In every case an increase in intra-hepatic resistance indicates an obstruction to hepatic blood flow. The injury may be infectious, toxic, or, in many instances, unknown (fig. 10.45). In childhood, intra-hepatic thrombosis of small portal veins could be the primary disorder.

In Japan it affects largely middle-aged women. Intra-hepatic portal veins show occlusive changes. The aetiology is unknown. A very similar condition in India, called *non-cirrhotic portal fibrosis*, largely affects young males [135]. It has been related to arsenic taken in drinking water and in unorthodox medicines. It is more likely to be due to the effects on the liver of multiple intestinal infections over many years.

Somewhat similar patients have been reported from the USA [93] and the UK [66].

Liver biopsy shows sclerosis and sometimes obliteration of the intra-hepatic venous bed but the changes, and especially the fibrosis, may be minimal. Large portal veins near the hilum may be thickened and narrow, but this is usually seen only at autopsy. Some of the changes seem to be secondary to partial thrombosis of small portal venous channels with recanalization. Perisinusoidal fibrosis is usually present but may be seen only by electron microscopy.

Portal venography shows small portal vein radicles to be narrowed and sparse. The peripheral branches may be irregular with acute-angle division. Some of the large intra-hepatic portal branches may be non-opacified with increase of very fine vasculature around large intra-hepatic portal branches. Hepatic venography confirms the vascular abnormalities and vein-to-vein anastomoses are frequent.

Tropical splenomegaly syndrome

This is marked by residence in a malarial area, splenomegaly, hepatic sinusoidal lymphocytosis and

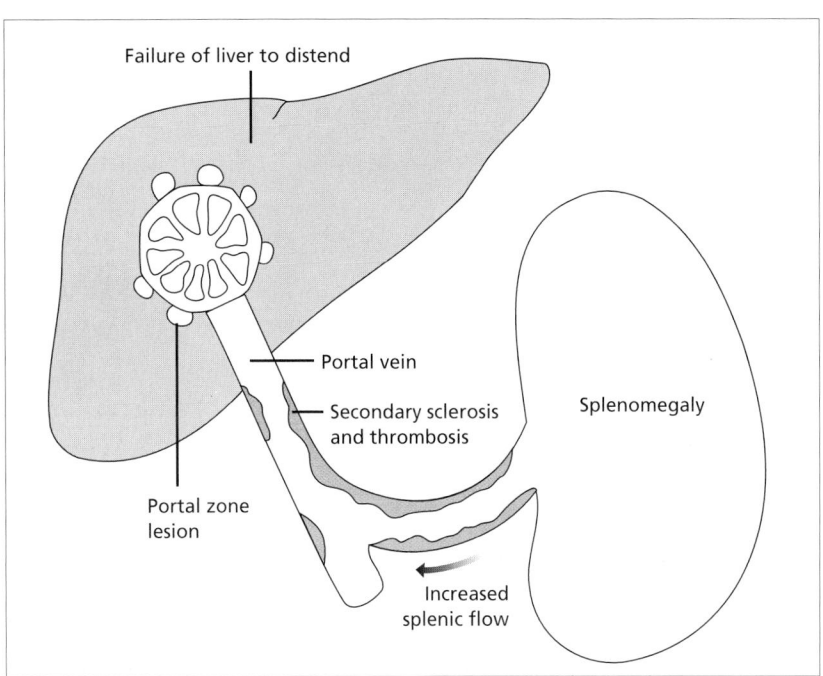

Fig. 10.45. Factors concerned in so-called idiopathic 'primary' portal hypertension.

Kupffer cell hyperplasia, raised serum IgM and malarial antibody titres and response to prolonged anti-malarial chemotherapy. Portal hypertension is not marked and variceal bleeding is rare [135].

Intra-hepatic portal hypertension

Cirrhosis

All forms of cirrhosis lead to portal hypertension and the primary event is obstruction to portal blood flow [88]. Portal venous blood is diverted into collateral channels and some bypasses the liver cells and is shunted directly into the hepatic venous radicles in the fibrous septa. These porto-hepatic anastomoses develop from pre-existing sinusoids enclosed in the septa (fig. 10.46) [118]. The hepatic vein is displaced further and further outwards until it lies in a fibrous septum linked with the portal venous radicle by the original sinusoid. The regenerating nodules become divorced from their portal blood supply and are nourished by the hepatic artery. Even larger portal hepatic venous anastomoses are found in the cirrhotic liver. About one-third of the total blood flow perfusing the cirrhotic liver may bypass sinusoids, and hence functioning liver tissue, through these channels [139].

The obstruction to portal flow is partially due to

Fig. 10.46. Cirrhosis of the liver. The formation of portal venous (PV), hepatic venous (HV) anastomoses or internal Eck fistulae at the site of pre-existing sinusoids (S). Note that the regeneration nodules are supplied by the hepatic artery (HA).

nodules which compress hepatic venous radicles (fig. 10.47) [64]. This would lead to a post-sinusoidal portal hypertension. However, in cirrhosis, the wedged hepatic venous (sinusoidal) and main portal pressures are virtually identical and the stasis must extend to the portal inflow vessels. Sinusoids probably provide the greatest resistance to flow. Changes in the space of Disse, particularly collagenization, result in sinusoidal narrowing and this may be particularly important in the alcoholic. Hepatocyte swelling in the alcoholic may also reduce sinusoidal flow [12]. Obstruction is therefore believed to be at all levels from portal zones through the sinusoids to the hepatic venous outflow (fig. 10.48).

The hepatic artery provides the liver with a small volume of blood at a high pressure. The portal vein delivers a large volume at a low pressure (see fig. 10.2). The two systems are equilibrated in sinusoids. In normals, the hepatic artery probably plays little part in maintaining portal venous pressure. In the cirrhotic, more direct arterio-portal shunting has been suspected. Hypertrophy of the hepatic artery and relative increase in flow help to maintain sinusoidal perfusion.

Non-cirrhotic nodules

Various non-cirrhotic nodular conditions of the liver lead to portal hypertension. They are difficult to diagnose, usually being confused with cirrhosis or with 'idiopathic' portal hypertension. A 'normal' needle liver biopsy does not exclude the diagnosis.

Nodular regenerative hyperplasia [30, 63]. Monoacinar nodules of cells resembling normal hepatocytes involve

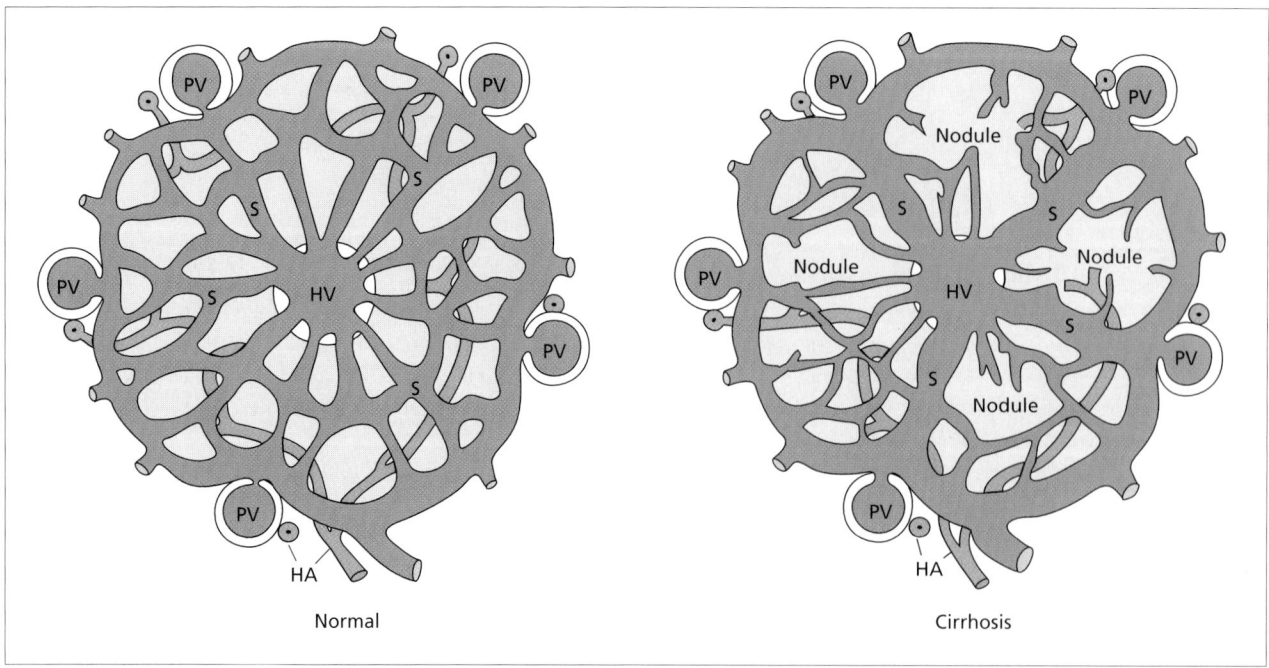

Normal   Cirrhosis

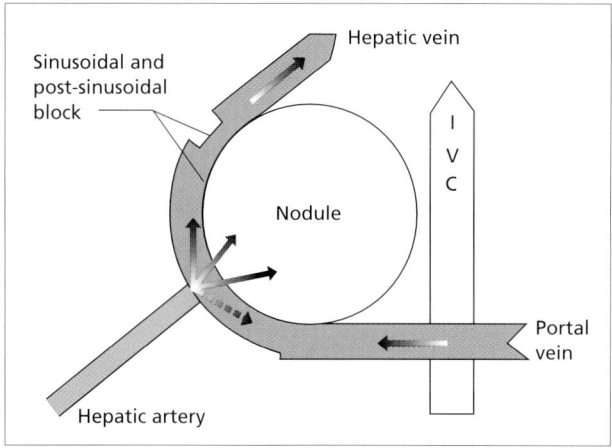

Fig. 10.47. The circulation in hepatic cirrhosis. A nodule obstructs the sinusoids and hepatic veins. The nodule is supplied mainly by the hepatic artery.

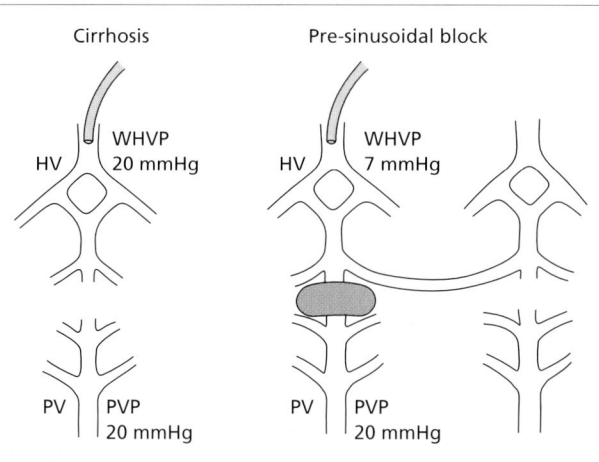

Fig. 10.48. In patients with cirrhosis the wedged hepatic venous pressure (WHVP) (20 mmHg) is equal to the pressure in the main portal vein (PVP) (20 mmHg) (measured via umbilical vein). Resistance to flow extends from the central hepatic vein, through the sinusoids to the portal vein. In pre-sinusoidal portal hypertension normal anastomoses exist between small vascular units and prevent the blocking catheter from producing a large area of stasis. WHVP (7 mmHg) is therefore less than the pressure in the main portal vein (20 mmHg) [122].

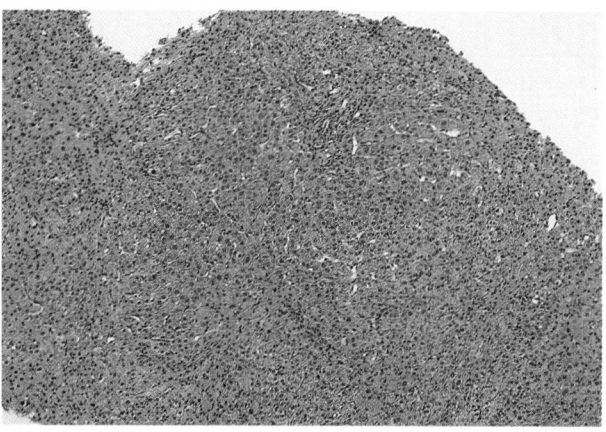

Fig. 10.49. Nodular regenerative hyperplasia. Surgical liver biopsy shows nodules of varying sizes resembling normal hepatocytes. (H & E, ×25).

the liver diffusely (fig. 10.49). They are not outlined by fibrous tissue. They are related to obliteration of small portal veins (less than 0.05 mm) at the level of the acinus. This causes atrophy of the involved acinus while adjacent acini, with intact blood supply, undergo compensatory hyperplasia causing micronodularity [171]. Portal hypertension is marked, and there is sometimes haemorrhage into a nodule.

Ultrasound shows hypoechoic or isoechoic masses with anechoic centres after bleeding. CT shows a hypodense pattern with no enhancement on contrast.

Liver biopsy is not diagnostic but shows two populations of hepatocytes differing in size.

The commonest association is with rheumatoid arthritis and Felty's syndrome. Nodules are also seen with myeloproliferative syndromes, hyperviscosity syndromes and as a reaction to drugs, particularly anabolic steroids and cytotoxics.

Porta-caval shunting for bleeding oesophageal varices is well tolerated.

Partial nodular transformation [141] is a very rare disease. The peri-hilar region is replaced by nodules. The periphery of the liver is normal or atrophic (fig. 10.50). Portal hypertension results from obstruction to hepatic blood flow by the nodules. Liver cell function remains good. Fibrosis is inconspicuous, diagnosis is difficult, confirmation often awaits autopsy. The cause is unknown.

Focal nodular hyperplasia (Chapter 18).

Veno-occlusive disease (Chapter 18).

Hepatic venous obstruction (Budd–Chiari syndrome) (Chapter 11).

Bleeding oesophageal varices

Predicting rupture

Sixty-five per cent of cirrhotic patients with varices will not bleed within 2 years of diagnosis but 50% will die of the first haemorrhage.

There is a strong correlation between variceal size, assessed endoscopically, and the probability of bleeding [23]. Intravariceal pressure is less important although a portal pressure above 12 mmHg appears necessary for varices to form and subsequently bleed [78].

'Red spots', danger signs seen at endoscopy, are valuable predictors of imminent haemorrhage [117].

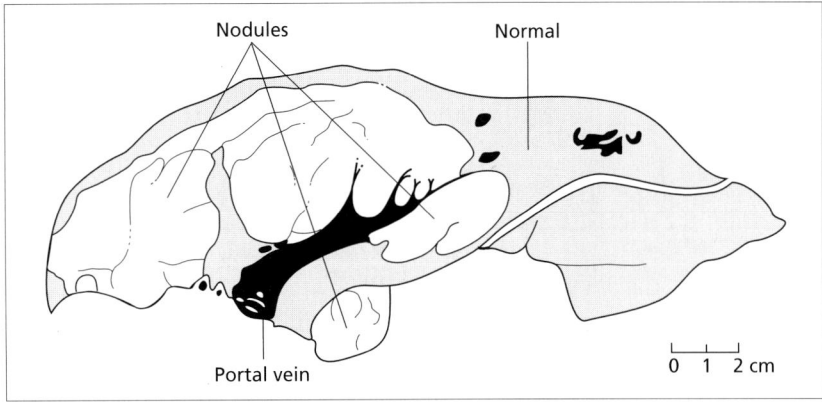

Fig. 10.50. Partial nodular transformation of the liver. Diagrammatic cross-section of the liver through the porta hepatis, in which nodules can be seen obstructing the portal vein. The rest of the liver appears normal.

Table 10.4. Child's classification of hepato-cellular function in cirrhosis

Group designation	A	B	C
Serum bilirubin (mg/dl)	Below 2.0	2.0–3.0	Over 3.0
Serum albumin (g/dl)	Over 3.5	3.0–3.5	Under 3.0
Ascites	None	Easily controlled	Poorly controlled
Neurological disorder	None	Minimal	Advanced coma
Nutrition	Excellent	Good	Poor 'wasting'

Child's grade is used to assess hepato-cellular function in cirrhosis (table 10.4). Every patient should be assigned a grade. It is the most important predictor of the likelihood of bleeding. It correlates with variceal size and with the presence of endoscopic red signs and with the response to treatment.

These three variables—size, presence of red signs and hepato-cellular function — are the best predictors of bleeding (fig. 10.51).

Patients with alcoholic cirrhosis may be at most risk [68].

Doppler sonography predicts likelihood of bleeding. This is based on velocity and diameter of the portal vein, spleen size and the presence of collaterals [137]. A high *congestive index* (the ratio between the area of the portal vein and the portal blood flow) predicts early bleeding [144].

Prevention of bleeding

Liver function must be improved, for instance, by abstaining from alcohol. Aspirin and NSAIDs should be avoided. No protection comes from avoiding certain foods such as spices or from taking long-term H_2-blockers.

Propranolol is a non-selective β-blocker which reduces portal pressure by splanchnic vaso-constriction and to a lesser extent by reducing cardiac output. Hepatic arterial

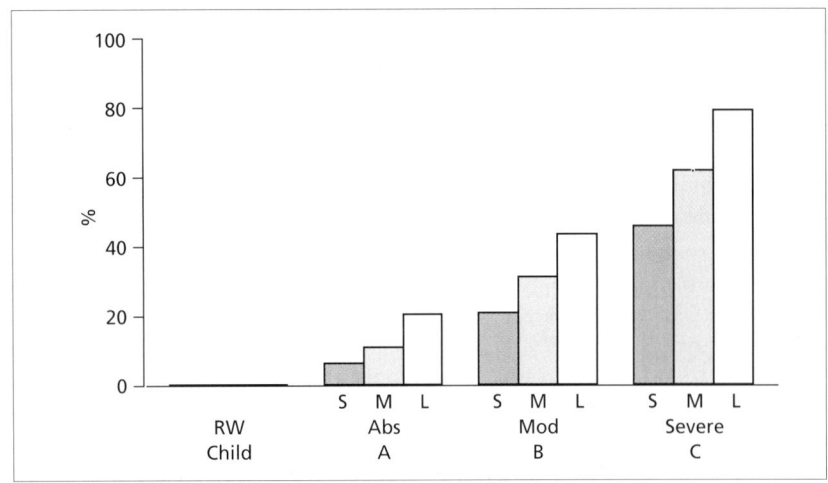

Fig. 10.51. Increasing variceal size (small, medium and large) combine with red wheals (RW) on varices (absent, moderate, severe) and Child's grade (A, B, C) to define probability of bleeding at 1 year (adapted from [100]).

blood flow falls [51, 91]. The drug is given in a dose which reduces the resting pulse rate by 25% 12 hours after taking it. There is marked individual variation in the lowering of the portal pressure [42]. Even with large doses, 20–50% of patients do not respond, especially those with advanced cirrhosis [42, 168]. The portal pressure must be maintained at 12 mmHg or lower [51]. If possible, wedged hepatic venous or endoscopic portal pressure should be monitored.

Propranolol should not be given to patients with restrictive airways disease. It may make resuscitation more difficult if the patient bleeds. Encephalopathy can also be induced. Propranolol is a high 'first pass effect' drug and might be expected to have unpredictable results in patients with advanced cirrhosis where hepatic clearance would be delayed. It causes some mental depression.

A meta-analysis of six trials showed a suggestively significant reduction in those bleeding but not in those dying [119] (fig. 10.52). Further meta-analysis of nine randomized trials showed the incidence of bleeding was significantly reduced by propranolol [108]. It is not easy to select those to treat as 70% of patients with varices will never bleed from them [14]. Propranolol is recommended for those with large varices and with red endoscopic danger signs [108]. Patients with hepatic venous pressure gradient greater than 12 mmHg should be treated whatever the size of the varices. *Nadolol* gives equivalent results. *Isosorbide-5-mononitrate* gives equivalent results to propranolol in survival and prevention of first bleed [1]. Liver function may be impaired in cirrhotic patients with ascites and isosorbide-5-

mononitrate should not be used in advanced cases [130, 167].

Meta-analysis of trials of *prophylactic sclerotherapy* showed generally unsatisfactory results. There was no clear evidence of prevention of first bleed or improvement in survival [108, 161]. Prophylactic sclerotherapy cannot be recommended.

Diagnosis of bleeding

The *clinical features* are those of gastrointestinal bleeding with the added picture of portal hypertension.

Bleeding may be a slow ooze with melaena, rather than a sudden haematemesis. The intestines may be full of blood before the haemorrhage is recognized and bleeding is liable to continue for days.

Bleeding varices in cirrhosis have injurious effects on the liver cells. These may be due to anaemia diminishing hepatic oxygen supply, or to increased metabolic demands resulting from the protein catabolism following haemorrhage. The fall in blood pressure diminishes hepatic arterial flow, on which the regenerating liver nodules depend, and necrosis may ensue. The increased nitrogen absorption from the intestines often leads to hepatic coma (Chapter 7). Deteriorating liver cell function may precipitate jaundice or ascites.

Non-variceal bleeding from duodenal ulcers, gastric erosions and the Mallory–Weiss syndrome is frequent.

Endoscopy is performed routinely to confirm the source of the bleeding (fig. 10.53). Routine ultrasound is used to determine patency of the portal and hepatic veins and to exclude a space-occupying lesion such as a hepato-cellular carcinoma.

Serum biochemical tests are not helpful in making the distinction between bleeding varix and bleeding ulcer.

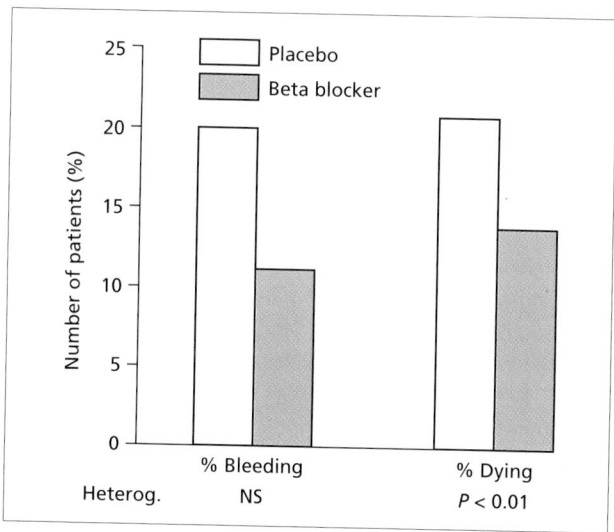

Fig. 10.52. Meta-analysis of six trials of prophylactic propranolol (β-blocker) therapy. Data on dying cannot be relied upon because of significant heterogeneity (Heterog.) in groups. There is, however, a significant reduction in those bleeding [119].

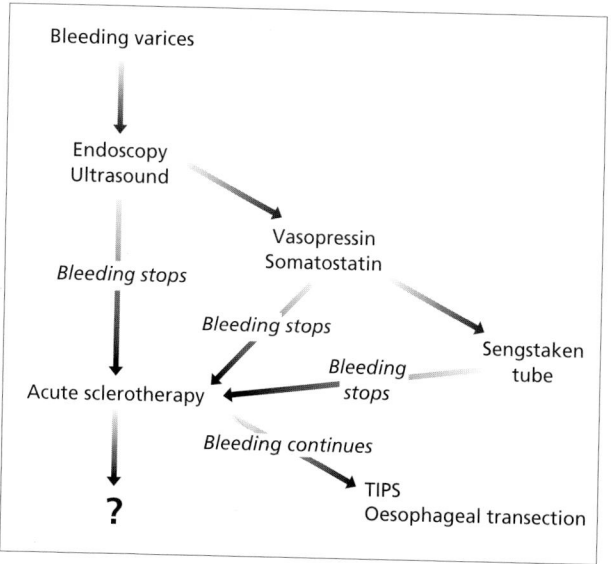

Fig. 10.53. The management of bleeding oesophageal varices.

Prognosis

In cirrhosis, the mortality of bleeding varices is about 40% with each episode. Recurrence during that hospital admission is 60% and long-term mortality is 60% after 2 years.

The prognosis is determined by the severity of the hepato-cellular disease. The ominous triad of jaundice, ascites and encephalopathy is associated with an 80% mortality. The 1-year survival in good-risk (Child grade A and B) patients is about 70% and in bad-risk (Child grade C) patients about 30% (table 10.5). The survival score can be based on encephalopathy, prothrombin time and the number of units transfused in the previous 72 hours [77]. Alcoholics have a worse prognosis as hepato-cellular disease is greater. Abstention from alcohol considerably improves the prognosis. Patients with continuing chronic hepatitis also do poorly. Patients with primary biliary cirrhosis tolerate the haemorrhage reasonably well.

A low portal blood velocity by Doppler predicts shorter survival [179].

The importance of hepato-cellular function is emphasized by the relatively good prognosis for bleeding in patients where hepato-cellular function is relatively well preserved, as in schistosomiasis, the non-cirrhotic portal hypertension of India and Japan, and portal vein thrombosis.

General measures

On admission to hospital, all cirrhotic patients with bleeding oesophageal varices should have their Child's grade recorded. Bleeding is likely to continue and observation must be close. If possible, the patient should be managed by an intensive care team, experienced in hepatology. A physician and a surgeon must be together in the picture from the start and subsequent management must be a joint undertaking.

Blood transfusion may need to be massive. The mean during the first 24 hours is 4 units and the mean total for a hospital admission about 10 units. Saline infusions must be avoided. Over-expansion of the blood volume may initiate re-bleeding. Animal studies suggest this is due to a rise in portal pressure over control levels

because of a post-bleeding increase in resistance in portal collaterals.

Clotting factors are liable to be deficient and if possible fresh blood or fresh packed red cells or fresh frozen plasma should be used. Platelet transfusions may be necessary. Vitamin K_1 intramuscularly should be routine.

Cimetidine or ranitidine is given. Although there is no controlled evidence of its benefit in patients with severe hepatic failure, stress-induced acute mucosal ulcers are frequent. Cirrhotic patients with gastrointestinal haemorrhage are at high risk of infection and should receive selective intestinal decontamination with an antibiotic such as norfloxacin [148].

Sedatives should be avoided and, if essential, oxazepam should be used. Chlordiazepoxide or heminevrin may be useful if the patient is an alcoholic and delirium tremens is a possible development. If the cause of the portal hypertension is pre-sinusoidal and hepato-cellular function is good, hepatic encephalopathy is unlikely and sedation may be liberal.

Routine measures in the cirrhotic patient to prevent hepatic encephalopathy include dietary protein abstention, lactulose, neomycin 4 g daily, gastric aspiration and phosphate enemas.

If ascites is very tense, intra-abdominal pressure may be reduced by a cautious paracentesis and the use of spironolactone.

The management of bleeding oesophageal varices requires the availability of many therapeutic options which can be combined in the individual patient (fig. 10.53). They include oesophageal sclerotherapy, which is the gold standard, vaso-active drugs, the Sengstaken tube, TIPS and emergency surgery. Controlled trials have failed to show conclusive benefit of one over the other although all can control oesophageal bleeding. There are remarkably few discrepancies between the results for variceal sclerotherapy and for vaso-active drugs.

Vaso-active drugs

These are used in acute variceal haemorrhage to lower portal venous pressure both before and as an adjunct to oesophageal sclerotherapy.

Vasopressin (Pitressin). This lowers portal venous pressure by constriction of the splanchnic arterioles, causing an increase in resistance to the inflow of blood to the gut. It controls variceal bleeding by lowering portal venous pressure.

Twenty units of vasopressin in a 100 ml 5% dextrose are given intravenously in 10 minutes. Portal pressure falls for 45–60 minutes (fig. 10.54). Alternatively, the vasopressin may be given by continuous intravenous infusion (0.4 iu/ml) for a maximum of 2 hours.

Vasopressin causes coronary vaso-constriction. An

Table 10.5. Pugh's (Child's) grading and hospital deaths at index bleed

Grade	No. patients	Hospital deaths
A	65	3 (5%)
B	68	12 (18%)
C	53	35 (68%)
Total	186	50 (27%)

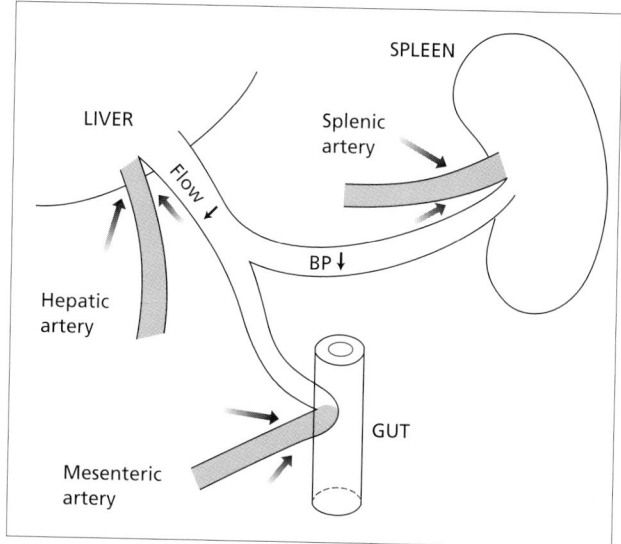

Fig. 10.54. The mode of action of vasopressin on the splanchnic circulation. Hepatic, splenic and mesenteric arteries are shown. Splanchnic blood flow (including hepatic blood flow) and portal venous pressure are reduced by arterial vaso-constriction (arrowed).

electrocardiogram should be taken before vasopressin is given. Abdominal colicky discomfort and evacuation of the bowels, together with facial pallor, are usual during the infusion.

Cessation of bleeding is related to the temporary drop in portal flow and blood pressure, allowing clotting at the bleeding point. The reduction in hepatic arterial flow in patients with cirrhosis is undesirable.

Efficacy drops with repeated use. Vasopressin may stop the bleeding but should be regarded as a preliminary to other forms of treatment. It may be less effective while the patient is bleeding due to the circulatory effects of bleeding [160].

Nitroglycerin is a powerful venous and mild arterial dilator. Combined with vasopressin it reduces transfusion needs and the use of oesophageal tamponade, but side-effects and hospital mortality are similar [47]. In treating bleeding varices, nitroglycerin intravenous (40 mg/min) or transdermally should be combined with vasopressin 0.4 iu/ml. If necessary, the doses are increased to maintain systolic pressure greater than 100 mmHg.

Glypressin (terlipressin) is more stable and has a longer action than vasopressin. It is given as a 2 mg bolus, and 1 mg every 4 hours for 24 hours. Oesophageal variceal pressure falls [25] with initial control of bleeding episodes [169].

Somatostatin. This reduces portal pressure by acting on smooth muscle and increasing splanchnic arterial resistance. It also inhibits a number of vasodilatory peptides including glucagon. There are few serious side-effects.

In a controlled study, re-bleeding was twice as frequent in those receiving placebo, and transfusion requirements and the use of tamponade were halved [20]. Patients with Child's grade C disease will not respond. In another trial, somatostatin controlled bleeding better than vasopressin [129], but another gave equivocal results [71]. Other trials suggested that somatostatin is safer and as effective as sclerotherapy [117].

An intravenous infusion has had adverse effects on the renal circulation and on the renal tubular handling of salt and water and it should be given cautiously in patients with ascites [48].

Octreotide is a synthetic analogue of somatostatin sharing four amino acids. It has a much longer half-life (1–2 hours). It has been shown as safe and as effective as sclerotherapy in controlling acute variceal bleeding [151] but does not decrease the incidence of early re-bleeding [120].

Sengstaken–Blakemore tube (figs 10.55, 10.56)

The use of oesophageal tamponade has decreased markedly with the advent of vaso-active drugs, oesophageal sclerotherapy and TIPS. Oesophageal tamponade is done with the Sengstaken–Blakemore tube. The four-lumen tube has an oesophageal and a gastric balloon, a tube in the stomach and a fourth lumen for continuous aspiration above the oesophageal balloon.

Two, but preferably three, assistants are required. The tube is easier to insert if it has been allowed to stiffen in the icebox of a refrigerator. The stomach is emptied. A new, tested and lubricated tube is passed through the mouth into the stomach. The gastric balloon is inflated with 250 ml of air and doubly clamped. The gastric tube is aspirated continuously. The whole tube is pulled back until resistance is encountered and the oesophageal tube is then inflated to a pressure of 40 mmHg, greater than that expected in the portal vein. The tube should be taped securely to the side of the face to provide skin traction. If necessary, a 500 ml bag of saline, taped to the tube and hung over the side of the bed, may be used for greater traction. Too little traction means that the gastric balloon falls back into the stomach. Too much causes discomfort with retching, and also potentiates gastro-oesophageal ulceration. The position of the tube is checked by X-ray (fig. 10.56). The head of the bed is raised.

The oesophageal tube has continuous low-pressure suction and occasional aspiration. Tube traction and oesophageal balloon pressure are checked hourly. After 12 hours, traction is released, and the oesophageal balloon deflated leaving the gastric balloon inflated. If bleeding recurs, the traction is reapplied and the oesophageal balloon re-inflated until emergency sclerotherapy, TIPS or surgery is performed.

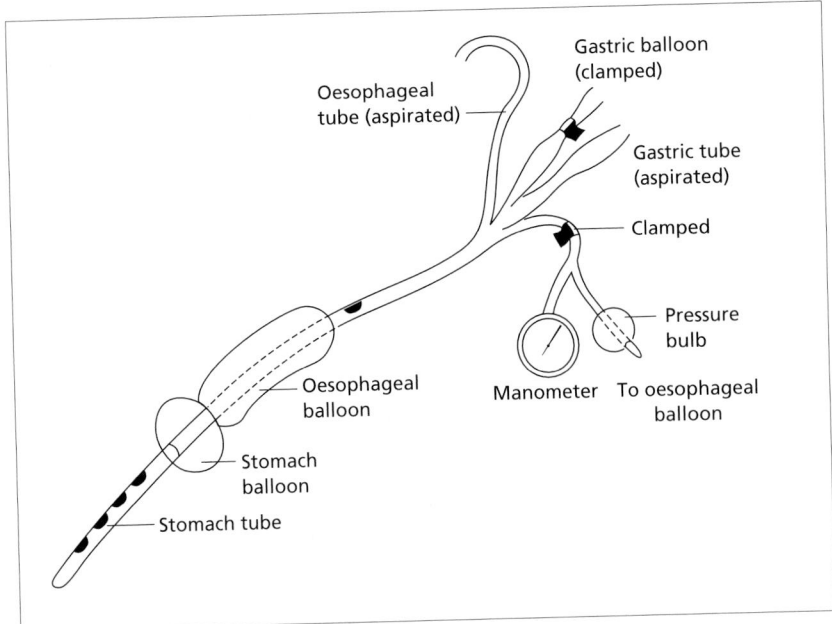

Fig. 10.55. Sengstaken–Blakemore oesophageal compression tube modified by Pitcher (1971). Note fourth oesophageal tube which aspirates the oesophagus above the oesophageal balloon.

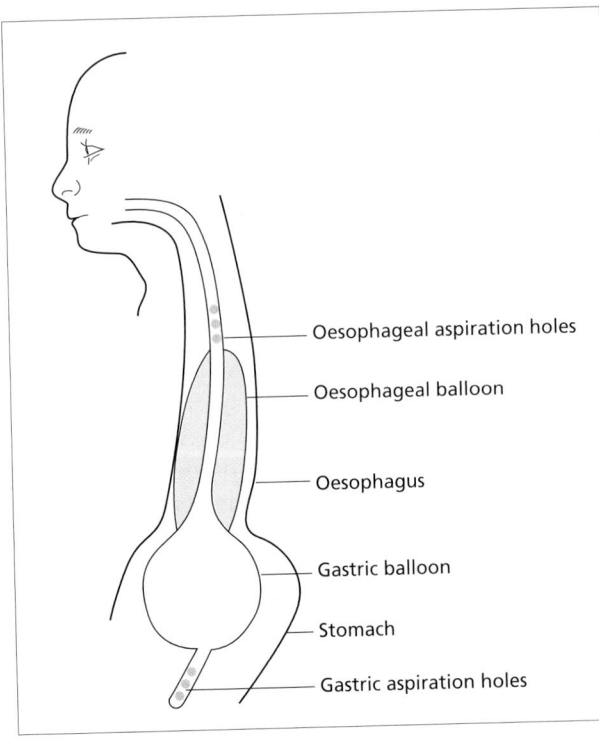

Fig. 10.56. The Sengstaken–Blakemore tube in position.

The compression tubes are successful. 10% of failures are due to fundal varices or non-variceal bleeding [111]. In 50%, re-bleeding follows tube withdrawal.

Complications include obstruction to upper airways. If the gastric balloon bursts or deflates, the oesophageal balloon may migrate into the oropharynx causing asphyxia. The oesophageal balloon must be deflated, and if necessary the tube transected with scissors.

Ulceration of the lower oesophagus complicates prolonged or repeated use. Aspiration of secretions into the lung is prevented by continuous suction above the oesophageal balloon but this still complicates 10% of insertions [111].

The Sengstaken tube is the most certain method for continued control of oesophageal bleeding over hours. Complications are frequent and are in part related to the experience of the operating team. It is unpleasant for the patient. It is useful when patients have to be transferred from one centre to another, when haemorrhage is torrential and when variceal sclerosis, TIPS or surgery are not immediately available. The oesophageal tube should not be kept inflated for more than 24 hours and preferably for not more than 10 hours.

Endoscopic sclerotherapy

This is the gold standard for emergency treatment of variceal bleeding [175]. In skilled hands it can be done while the patient is bleeding but preliminary somatostatin and tamponade may be necessary for clear vision. The varix is thrombosed by the injection of a sclerosing solution introduced via the endoscope (fig. 10.57). Routine sclerotherapy to obliterate the varices is much more controversial.

Technique (table 10.6)

The technique should be as sterile as possible with sterile needles, mouth washes and careful mouth hygiene. A conventional fibre endoscope is usual with local anaesthesia and sedation. The 23-gauge needle protrudes 3–4 mm beyond the catheter sheath (fig. 10.57). Large

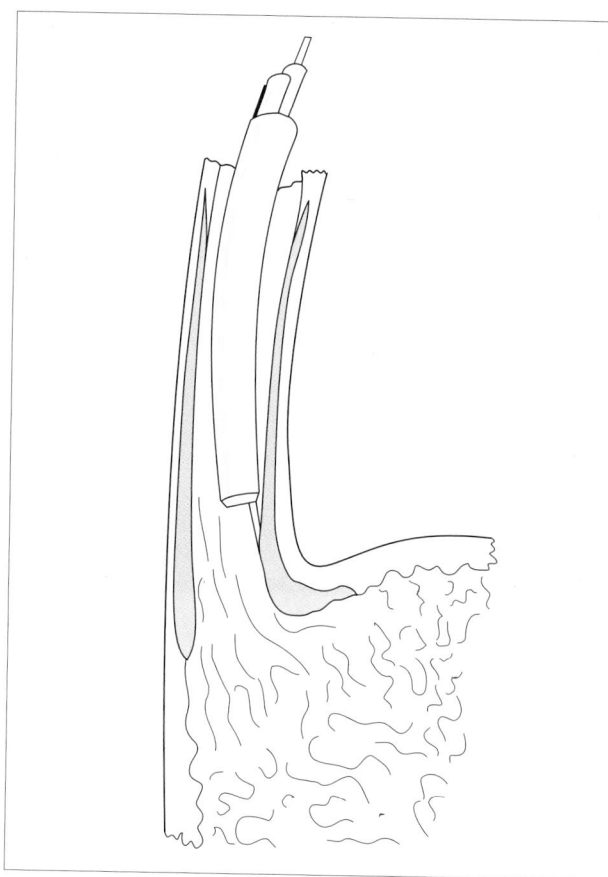

Fig. 10.57. Direct injection of oesophageal varices with an unmodified fibre-optic endoscope.

Table 10.6. Royal Free Hospital routine for oesophageal variceal sclerotherapy

Sedation (diazepam i.v.)
Local anaesthesia to throat
Endoscope (oblique viewing) (Olympus K10)
Intravariceal
1–4 ml 5% ethanolamine or 5% sodium morrhuate per varix
Maximum total sclerosant per session 15 ml
Omeprazole for chronic sclerosis ulcers

(3.7 mm channel) or double channel endoscopes allow a clear view and safer injection. They are of particular value in controlling acute bleeding.

The sclerosant may be 1% sodium tetradecyl sulphate or 5% ethanolamine oleate for intravariceal injection or polidocanol for paravariceal use. The injection is made just above the gastro-oesophageal junction and the volume should not exceed 4 ml in any one varix. Gastric varices within 3 cm of the gastro-oesophageal junction may be injected.

The sclerosant may be injected directly into the varix to obliterate the lumen or into the lamina propria to produce inflammation followed by fibrosis. The intravariceal technique seems more effective in controlling acute haemorrhage and has fewer variceal recurrences. However, if methylene-blue is added to the sclerosant it becomes apparent that most injections are both intra- and paravariceal.

Two sessions of emergency sclerotherapy may be required. If three are necessary, the salvage rate is poor and alternative therapy should be considered [21].

Gastric varices are difficult to treat if distant from the cardia.

Results

Control of bleeding is 71–88% successful with significant reduction in rebleeding [175]. Failure rate is 6%. In grade C patients, survival is probably unaltered [76]. Sclerotherapy is superior to tamponade [76] and to nitroglycerin and vasopressin although re-bleeding and survival may be no different [175]. Good results come from experienced groups. The occasional operator should not attempt to deal with bleeding oesophageal varices using the endoscope.

Patients who have large para-oesophageal venous collaterals, shown by CT, are less likely to respond to sclerotherapy.

Complications

These are greater with paravariceal than intravariceal injection. Other factors include the volume of sclerosant used and the Child's grade of cirrhosis. Complications are more likely with chronic, repeated sclerotherapy than with acute injection to stop bleeding.

Almost every patient will experience fever, dysphagia and chest pain. This is usually transient.

Bleeding is not usually from the puncture site but from remaining varices or deep ulcers that have opened in submucosal channels. Re-bleeding is seen in about 30% of patients before the varices have been obliterated. If the haemorrhage comes from varices, further sclerotherapy is indicated. If from an ulcer, omeprazole is the drug of choice [45].

Stricture formation is related to chemical oesophagitis, ulceration and acid reflux, impaired swallowing contributes [147]. Oesophageal dilatation is usually successful, but occasionally surgery becomes necessary [152].

Perforation (0.5% of procedures) is usually delayed 5–7 days and is probably an extension of the ulcerative process [114].

Pulmonary complications include chest pain, aspiration pneumonia and mediastinitis [7]. Pleural effusions are found in 50%. Sclerotherapy is followed, 1 day later, by a restrictive defect in respiratory function possibly due to sclerosant embolizing in the lungs [131]. Pyrexia is frequent and clinically significant bacteraemia complicates 13% of emergency endoscopic sessions [60].

Portal vein thrombosis complicates 36% of patients treated with sclerotherapy. This may be important if subsequent shunt or liver transplantation is required.

Varices increase at other sites including the stomach, ano-rectal area and percutaneously.

Other recorded complications include cardiac tamponade [153], pericarditis [69] and brain abscess.

Chronic oesophageal sclerotherapy

Chronic oesophageal variceal sclerotherapy is only moderately successful compared with acute sclerotherapy. Injections are performed at weekly intervals until all varices are thrombosed. Frequency of rebleeding is reduced (table 10.7) [176].

Thirty to 40% of varices return per year after sclerotherapy. Repeat sessions lead to a fibrotic oesophagus in which varices have been obliterated but gastric varices are marked and these may ooze continuously.

Endoscopic variceal ligation

This is based on a technique used for band ligation of haemorrhoids. The varices are ligated and strangulated by application of small elastic O rings (fig. 10.58) [46, 75, 150]. A standard end-viewing endoscope is inserted into the lower oesophagus and an overtube introduced. The endoscope is then removed and loaded with a banding device attached to its end. It is then reinserted to the distal oesophagus. A varix is identified and aspirated into the device followed by placement of an elastic band around it by pulling the trip wire. This process is repeated until all the varices are ligated. One to three bands are applied to each varix.

The technique is not difficult and has less morbidity than sclerotherapy with more sessions to eradication of varices [75, 150]. Transient dysphagia is the most usual complication and bacteraemia has been reported. The overtube can cause oesophageal perforation. Ulcers may develop at the site of previously applied bands. The bands can slip causing torrential haemorrhage.

Banding ligation is as effective as sclerotherapy for arresting acute variceal haemorrhage but is difficult to perform while the patient is bleeding. It prevents re-

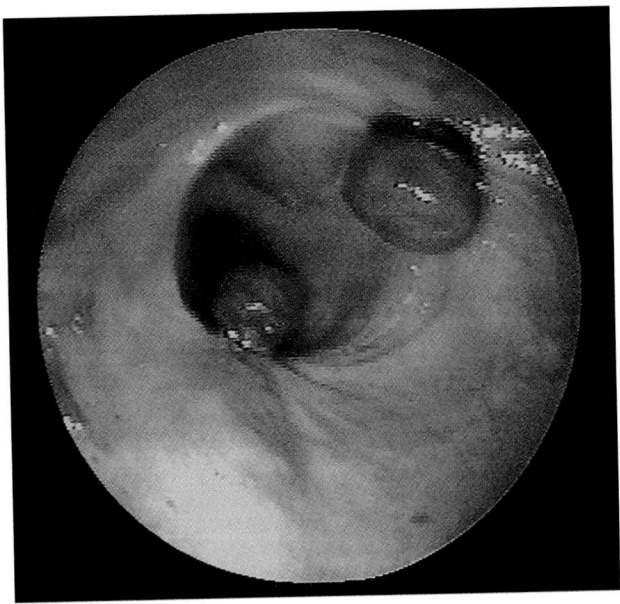

Fig. 10.58. Endoscopic variceal ligation. The varices have been strangulated by an elastic ring introduced via the endoscope.

bleeding but there is no difference in survival [46]. This technique will probably not replace the more generally available endoscopic sclerotherapy except in specialized centres. It should not be combined with sclerotherapy.

Emergency surgery

This has been remarkably reduced with the advent of sclerotherapy, vaso-active drugs, balloon tamponade and particularly TIPS. When these fail, or are not available, it must be considered. An emergency porta-caval shunt is effective in stopping bleeding [107]. Mortality is high in grade C patients, and the post-surgical encephalopathy rate is also high. If bleeding is torrential and recurs after two sclerotherapy sessions, TIPS is the best treatment. Alternatives are emergency mesocaval or narrow diameter (8 mm) porta-caval graft or oesophageal transection.

Emergency oesophageal transection using the staple gun

Under general anaesthesia, the staple gun is inserted into the lower oesophagus via an anterior gastrotomy (fig. 10.59). A ligature is tied just above the cardia, invaginating a section of oesophageal wall between the two parts of the gun. The stapler is closed and fired, and the oesophageal wall is transected and stapled. The gun with the segment of oesophagus is removed. The gastrotomy and anterior abdominal wall are closed. The stapling transection arrests haemorrhage in every patient. However, a third of the patients die during that hospital

Table 10.7. Sclerotherapy of varices

Prophylactic	Acute	Chronic
Benefit uncertain	Skill needed	Less deaths from bleeding
	Stops bleeding	Complications—many
	?Survival	Compliance
		Survival unaltered

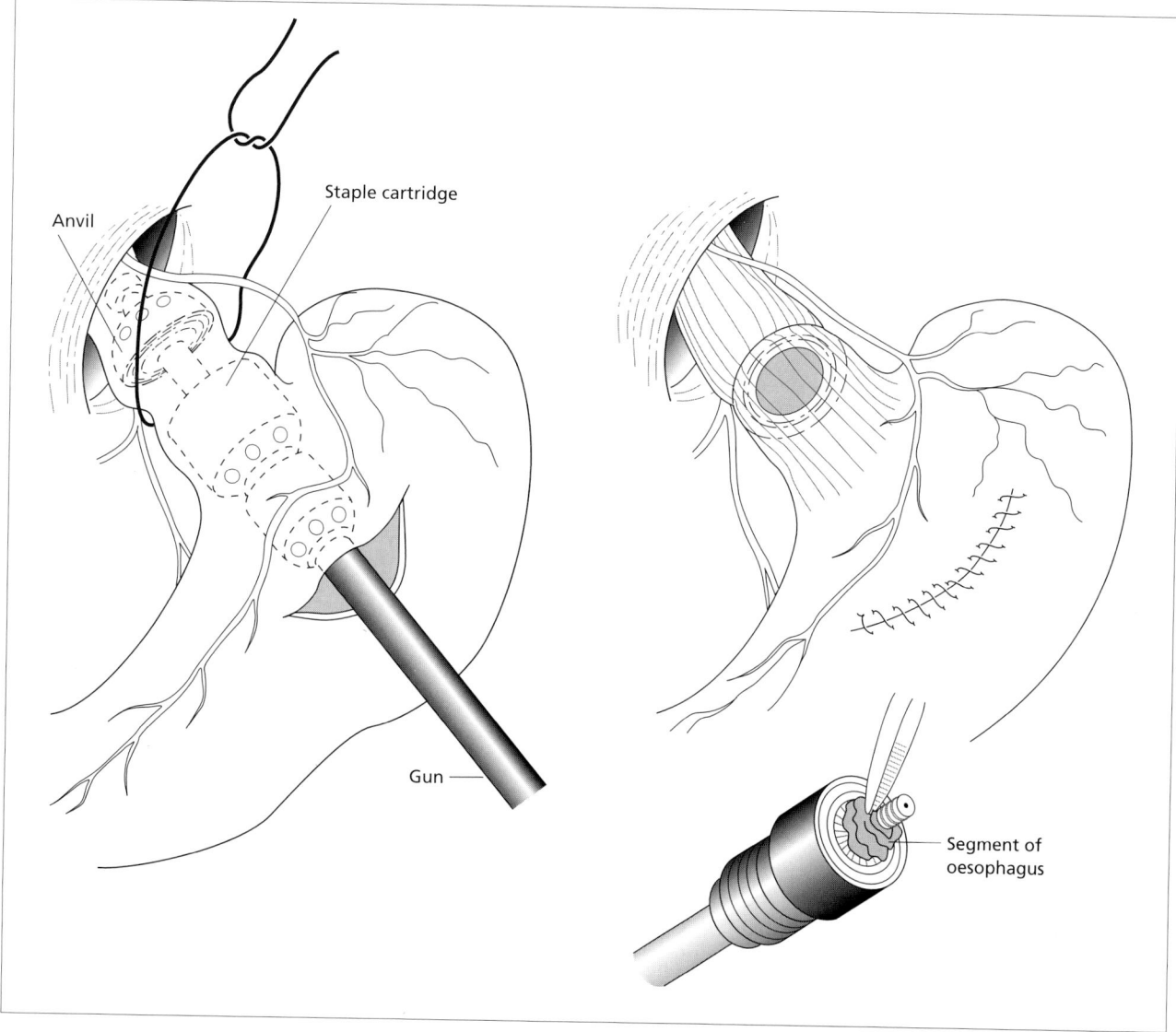

Fig. 10.59. Stapling transection of the lower oesophagus. The staple gun has been introduced into the lower oesophagus via a gastrotomy. A ligature has been tied just above the cardia invaginating a section of oesophageal wall between the two parts of the gun. When the gun is fired, a section of the oesophageal wall will be transected and stapled. (Courtesy K.E.F. Hobbs.)

admission, usually from hepatic failure. The staple gun procedure has a place in the emergency treatment of bleeding oesophageal varices [87]. Operative time is short, mortality low and complications few. It is not indicated as a prophylactic or elective procedure. Within 2 years, varices have often recurred, enlarged and frequently re-bled.

Prevention of re-bleeding

At 1 year, 25% of grade A, 50% of grade B and 75% of grade C patients with cirrhosis will have re-bled from varices. How can this be prevented? Propranolol is one possibility. In the first controlled trial, alcoholic cirrhotic patients with very large varices and in good condition showed marked reduction in re-bleeding [80]. Other trials gave variable results perhaps related to the type of cirrhosis and how many alcoholics were included [19]. Patients with decompensated cirrhosis do not respond to propranolol therapy. The longer the delay in starting treatment the better the results, for very bad risk patients will have already died [49]. In good risk patients, propranolol is as successful as sclerotherapy [177]. Propranolol decreases the risk of recurrent haemorrhage but probably has little effect on survival [108]. It is of value in portal gastropathy. Nadolol plus isosorbide mononitrate is better than sclerotherapy in reducing the risk of re-bleeding (165).

Chronic oesophageal variceal sclerotherapy is performed at weekly intervals until all varices are thrombosed. Three to five sessions will probably be needed and the procedure can be performed as an outpatient. After eradication, close endoscopic surveillance and repeated injections to ensure continued eradication are not indicated as survival is not increased. Sclerotherapy should be reserved for recurrent bleeding episodes [14]. Chronic oesophageal sclerotherapy reduces the rate of re-bleeding from varices and the transfusion requirement but has no long-term effect on survival [155, 162].

A shunt, either porta-caval or distal spleno-renal or TIPS is performed as a rescue when sclerotherapy has failed [59].

Portal-systemic shunt procedures (fig. 10.60)

The aim is to reduce portal venous pressure, maintain total hepatic and, particularly, portal blood flow and, above all, not have a high incidence of complicating hepatic encephalopathy. There is no currently available procedure that fulfils all these criteria satisfactorily. Hepatic reserve determines survival. Hepato-cellular function deteriorates after shunting.

Porta-caval

In 1877 Eck [38] first performed a porta-caval shunt in dogs and this remains the most effective way of reducing portal hypertension in man.

The portal vein is joined to the inferior vena cava either end-to-side, with ligation of the portal vein, or side-to-side, maintaining its continuity. The portal blood pressure falls, hepatic venous pressure falls and hepatic arterial flow increases.

The end-to-side shunt probably gives a greater fall in portal venous pressure than does the side-to-side procedure, of the order of 10 mmHg. Technically, it is easier to perform.

Porta-caval shunts are rarely performed nowadays because of the high incidence of post-shunt encephalopathy. Liver function deteriorates due to reduction of portal perfusion. A subsequent hepatic transplantation is made more difficult. It is still used, after the bleeding episode has been controlled, in patients with good liver reserves who do not have access to tertiary care or who may have bled from gastric varices. It is useful in some patients with early primary biliary cirrhosis, congenital hepatic fibrosis with good hepato-cellular function and those with portal vein obstruction of the hilum of the liver.

The probability of ascites, spontaneous bacterial peritonitis and hepato-renal syndrome is reduced.

Patients selected for any shunt should have had a haemorrhage from proven oesophageal varices. Portal

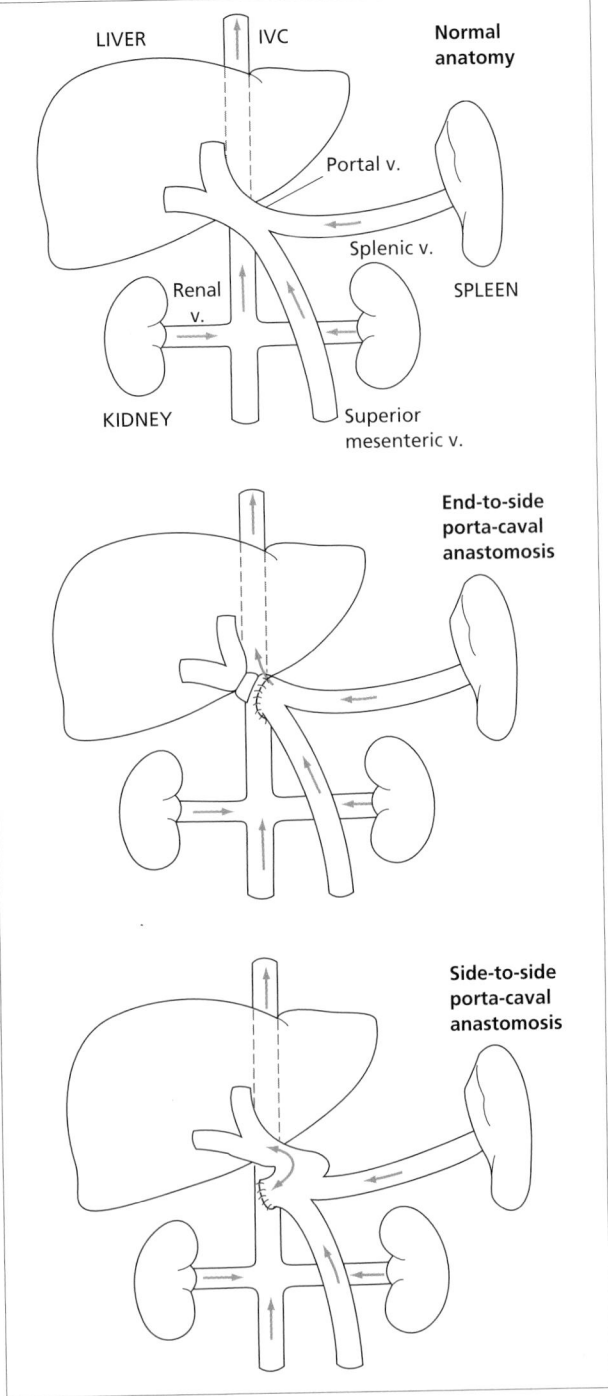

Fig. 10.60. The types of surgical portal-systemic shunt operation performed for the relief of portal hypertension.

hypertension must be established. The portal vein must be good and age preferably less than 50 years. After 40 years, survival is reduced and encephalopathy is twice as common.

The patient should not give a history of hepatic encephalopathy, and should be Child's grade A or B.

Meso-caval

This is made between the superior mesenteric vein and the inferior vena cava using a Dacron graft (fig. 10.61) [36]. It is technically easy. The portal vein remains patent but blood flow through it is uncertain. Shunt occlusion is usual with time and is followed by re-bleeding [36]. It does not interfere with subsequent hepatic transplantation.

Selective 'distal' spleno-renal (fig. 10.62)

Veins feeding the dangerous oesophago-gastric collaterals are divided while allowing drainage of portal blood

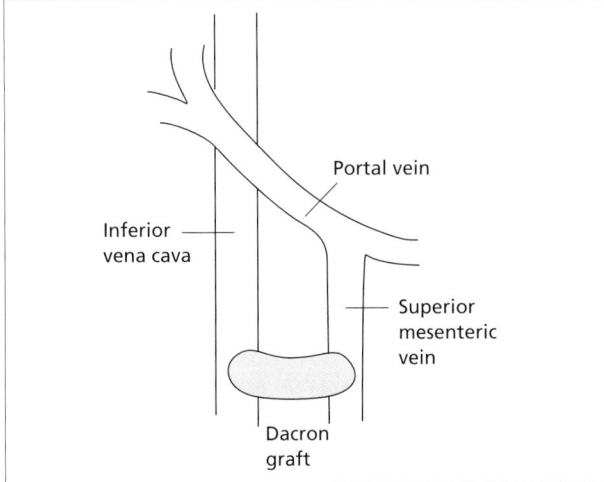

Fig. 10.61. The meso-caval shunt using a Dacron graft [9].

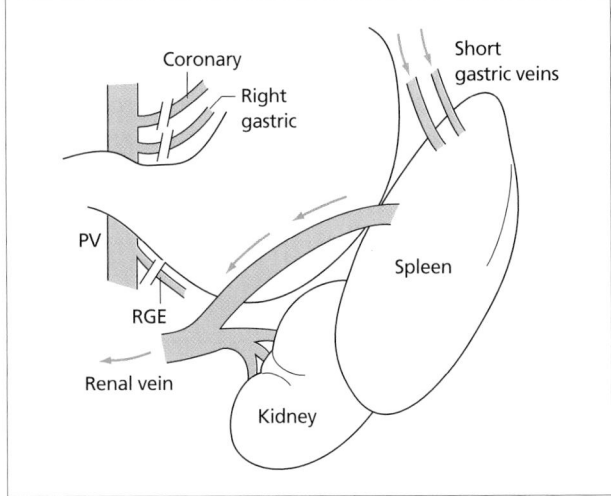

Fig. 10.62. The distal spleno-renal shunt. Veins feeding varices (coronary, right gastric, right gastro-epiploic—RGE) are ligated. A spleno-renal shunt is made, preserving the spleen; retrograde flow in the short gastric veins is possible. Portal blood flow to the liver is preserved. PV = portal vein.

through short gastric-splenic veins through a spleno-renal shunt to the inferior vena cava. It was hoped that portal perfusion would be maintained but this was not so.

Early results were good with 4.1% mortality, encephalopathy 12% and five-year survival 49%. However, a further randomized trial in largely alcoholic cirrhotic patients gave similar mortality and encephalopathy results as for non-selective spleno-renal shunts. Better results are recorded in non-alcoholic patients, and particularly where gastric varices are the main problem [94]. It is also useful in bleeding varices due to schistosomiasis or in patients with non-cirrhotic portal hypertension where the splenic vein is patent. The operation does not interfere with a subsequent hepatic transplant.

Distal spleno-renal shunt is a technically difficult operation and fewer and fewer surgeons are able or willing to perform it.

General results of portal-systemic shunts

Operative mortality in good-risk patients is about 5%. For poor-risk patients, the mortality is 50%.

Shunt closure is often due to operating on a diseased portal vein and is often fatal. Hepatic failure is the usual cause of death.

A patent end-to-side porta-caval anastomosis undoubtedly prevents bleeding from gastro-oesophageal varices.

After the shunt, abdominal wall collateral veins disappear and spleen size decreases. Endoscopy shows disappearance of varices within 6 months to 1 year of the operation.

Portal pressure and hepatic blood flow fall if the shunt is non-selective. This results in deterioration in hepatic function.

Post-operative jaundice is frequently related to haemolysis and reduction in hepatic function.

Oedema of the ankles is due to reduction in portal venous pressure while the serum albumin level remains low. Increased cardiac output with failure may contribute to the oedema.

Shunt patency is confirmed by ultrasound, CT scanning, MR, Doppler or angiography.

Hepatic encephalopathy may be transient. Chronic changes develop in 20–40% and personality deterioration in about one-third (Chapter 7). The incidence increases with the size of the shunt. Patients with progressive liver disease are at most risk. Encephalopathy is more common in older patients.

Myelopathy, with paraplegia and a Parkinsonian-cerebellar syndrome are other complications (Chapter 7).

Transjugular intra-hepatic portal-systemic shunt (TIPS)

Early attempts to establish intra-hepatic porto-systemic shunts in the dog [126] and man [27] were unsuccessful because the balloon tract between hepatic and portal vein did not remain patent. The use of a Palmaz expandable stent allowed maintenance of shunt patency and so the implantation of a metallic stent between an intra-hepatic branch of the portal vein and the hepatic vein radicle [28, 125, 128, 143, 178] (figs 10.63, 10.64).

The usual indication is control of bleeding from oesophageal or gastric varices. It is essential that full medical treatment including sclerotherapy and vaso-

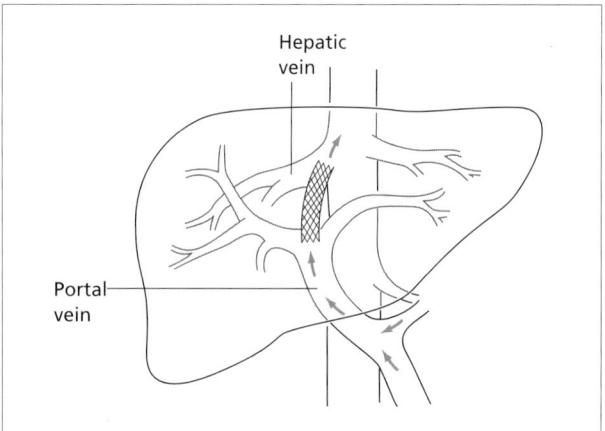

Fig. 10.63. TIPS. An expandable metal stent has been inserted between the portal vein and the hepatic vein producing an intra-hepatic porto-systemic shunt.

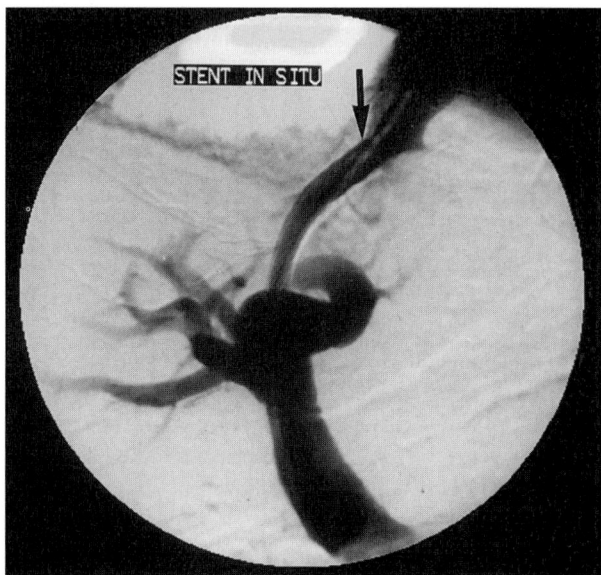

Fig. 10.64. TIPS. Portal venogram shows porto-hepatic venous shunt, the stent is *in situ* (arrow).

active drugs are given before TIPS is considered [58]. Results are poor if the patient is actively bleeding. The procedure is performed under sedation and with local anaesthesia. Under ultrasound control, the portal bifurcation is located. The middle hepatic vein is catheterized by the transjugular route, and a needle introduced through this catheter into a main portal vein branch. A guide wire is introduced through the needle and the catheter advanced into the portal vein. The needle is removed and portal venous pressure gradient measured. The needle track is balloon-dilated and angiography performed. A Palmaz metallic balloon expandable stent or a Wallstent (42–68) self-expanding metal stent is inserted and expanded to 8–12 mm [73]. Diameter is adjusted to achieve a portal pressure gradient of less than 12 mmHg. If portal hypertension persists, a second stent may be placed parallel to the first [57]. Ultrasound guidance is essential throughout. The time taken is 1–2 hours. A subsequent hepatic transplantation is not affected by a TIPS procedure.

TIPS is difficult. An experienced team which must include a skilled interventional radiologist can achieve a success rate of 95% [127]. However, in one series, technical difficulties, early re-bleeding and shunt stenosis or thrombosis led to a second TIPS in 30% in the same hospitalization [58]. In 8% of patients, bleeding was uncontrolled by two sessions.

The procedural mortality is less than 1% and at 30 days, it is between 3% [126] and 13% [74]. Complications include haemorrhage which may be intra-abdominal, biliary or through the liver capsule. The stent may dislocate and the Wallstent may have to be retrieved with a loop snare [132].

Infections are frequent and can be fatal. Prophylactic antibiotics should be given [11]. Renal failure is seen in those with impaired renal function and is due to the injection of large amounts of intravenous contrast. Intravascular haemolysis may be related to damage to erythrocytes by the steel mesh of the stent [134]. Hepatic infarction has followed misplacement of the stent into the right hepatic artery [81]. Hypersplenism is unaffected [133].

Stent stenosis and occlusion. The low pressure gradient between portal vein and hepatic vein favours occlusion. Shunt dysfunction is the most important cause of TIPS failure. Follow-up of shunt patency is essential. This may be done by routine portography, Doppler sonography [82] or Duplex sonography which gives semi-quantitative evaluation of shunt function [56]. Shunt occlusion usually results in variceal re-bleeding, although this is not always so.

Early shunt occlusion is seen in 12% and is usually thrombotic and related to technical problems in its introduction [58]. Later occlusion and stenosis are related to exuberant intimal changes at the hepatic venous end of the stent [28]. They are most frequent in Child grade C patients. Shunt stenosis and occlusion probably affect one-third of patients at 1 year and two-thirds at 2 years [82]. The prevalence probably depends on the enthusiasm with which the shunt patency is investigated. Shunt occlusion is treated by revision of the shunt under local anaesthesia. The shunt may be dilated by percutaneous catheterization or a further shunt may be inserted [74].

Control of bleeding. TIPS causes portal venous pressure to fall a mean of approximately 50%. It controls bleeding resulting from portal hypertension whether the source is oesophageal, gastric or intestinal. It is of particular value in refractory bleeding, not controlled by sclerotherapy, in a patient with poor liver function. TIPS seems more effective than sclerotherapy in preventing variceal re-bleeding [21]. TIPS seems to reduce the re-bleeding but have little effect on survival [92, 127]. The re-bleeding rate at about 6 months varies from 5% [134] to 19% [73] and at 1 year 18% [127].

TIPS encephalopathy. Surgical non-selective side-to-side portal-systemic shunt deprives the liver of portal blood and liver function falls post-TIPS [85]. TIPS is a side-to-side portal-systemic shunt and is not surprising that it is followed by encephalopathy in about the same percentage (25–30) as following surgically performed porta-caval shunts [138]. Nine of 30 patients having TIPS had 24 episodes of hepatic encephalopathy and in 12% it was *de novo* [134]. It is related to the age of the patient, Child's grade and shunt size [124]. It is worse in the first month. It may become less as stents develop spontaneous closure. It may be treated by the placement of a smaller stent within the intra-hepatic shunt. Resistant encephalopathy may be an indication for later transplant [85].

The hyperdynamic circulation of cirrhosis worsens. Cardiac output increases and there is an increase in systemic blood volume [5]. Splanchnic sequestration of blood is probable. A patient with underlying cardiac problems may be projected into heart failure.

Other indications. TIPS is an end-to-side portal-systemic shunt and effectively controls ascites in Child grade B patients. However, controlled trials show no benefit over conventional therapy and no difference in survival rates [79].

In the hepato-renal syndrome, TIPS has been useful in allowing prolongation of the waiting time so as to allow the performance of a hepatic transplant [13, 102].

Acute and chronic Budd–Chiari syndrome have been successfully treated by TIPS [103].

Conclusions. TIPS is an important method of treating acute oesophageal and gastric variceal bleeding where these are uncontrolled by sclerotherapy and vaso-active drugs. Its use in recurrent oesophageal bleeding should probably be confined to those with poor liver function who are candidates for liver transplantation.

Technical difficulties are many, particularly in inexperienced hands. Effective useful long-term control of portal hypertension is limited by problems of stent closure and hepatic encephalopathy. TIPS is easier and has less early complications than surgical portal-systemic shunts. We can however, expect the same long-term problems as for the surgical shunt.

Hepatic transplantation

Patients with cirrhosis and bleeding varices die because their hepatocytes fail, not from blood loss *per se*. The end-point has to be death or a liver transplant. Previous sclerotherapy or portal-systemic shunts does not affect post-transplant survival [61]. In fact, variceal sclerosis followed by transplantation gave better survival than for sclerotherapy alone [43] (fig. 10.65). However, there might have been selection bias favouring better risk patients for referral to transplant centres. Liver transplant must be considered for uncontrollable variceal bleeding and end-stage liver disease [39].

Previous surgical shunts make the transplant technically more difficult, particularly if there has been dissection at the hepatic hilum. Spleno-renal and meso-caval shunts and TIPS are not contraindications.

Most of the haemodynamic and humoral changes of cirrhosis are reversed by liver transplant [99]. Azygous blood flow is slow to normalize indicating slow closure of portal collateral vessels.

Pharmacological control of the portal circulation

Portal hypertension is a systemic disease, part of a hyperdynamic state with increased cardiac output and

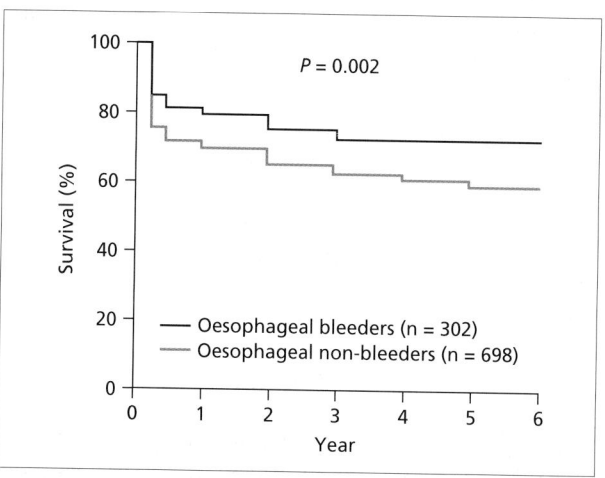

Fig. 10.65. Hepatic transplantation in cirrhotic patients who had and had not previously bled from oesophageal varices [43].

reduced peripheral resistance. There are profound changes in autonomic nervous system activity. The various hormonal factors probably involved make pharmacological control possible. Theoretically, portal blood pressure (and flow) could be reduced by lowering cardiac output, by reducing inflow through splanchnic vasoconstriction, by splanchnic venodilatation, by reducing intra-hepatic vascular resistance or, of course, by surgical porta-caval shunting (fig. 10.66). It is preferable to reduce pressure by lowering resistance rather than decreasing flow as hepatic blood flow and function will be maintained.

Reducing cardiac output

This could be achieved by blocking β_1-receptors in the myocardium. Propranolol acts partially in this way. Metoprolol and atenolol are cardioselective blockers but are less effective than propranolol in reducing portal pressure.

Reducing portal venous inflow

Vasopressin, glypressin, somatostatin and propranolol act as splanchnic vasoconstrictors and have already been discussed.

Portal and intra-hepatic vasodilators

The smooth muscle of the portal vein has α_1-receptors. Portal-systemic collaterals are probably already maximally dilated and have a poorly developed smooth muscle layer. They are less likely than main veins to respond to vasodilatatory stimuli. Serotonin is a potent vasoconstrictor in the portal bed, the effect mediated by S2-receptors. The collaterals may have increased sensitivity to its action. Ketanserin, a serotonin inhibitor, decreases portal pressure in patients with cirrhosis [166]. Complications, including encephalopathy, preclude its general use as a portal hypotensive drug.

In cirrhosis, there is a component of veno-motor tone which may be modified by drugs. The increased portal vascular resistance in the isolated perfused cirrhotic liver can be reduced by vasodilators including prostaglandin E_1 and isoprenaline [9]. The effect may be on contractile myofibroblasts. Nitroglycerin or 5-isosorbide dinitrate or mononitrate probably reduce portal venous pressure through systemic vasodilatation. They also cause a small reduction of intra-hepatic resistance in the isolated liver [90] and in cirrhotic patients [98].

Verapamil, a calcium channel antagonist, was shown to reduce hepatic venous pressure gradient and intra-hepatic resistance [70]. However, these beneficial results could not be confirmed in acute studies in cirrhotic patients. The sympathetic is hyperactive in patients with alcoholic cirrhosis. Intravenous clonidine, a centrally acting α-adrenergic-agonist, caused a fall in post-sinusoidal hepatic vascular outflow resistance in alcoholic cirrhotic patients [95]. The fall in systemic blood pressure has limited its use.

Conclusion: pharmacological control

Interactions between cardiac output, systemic resistance and flow, and portal resistance and flow are difficult to

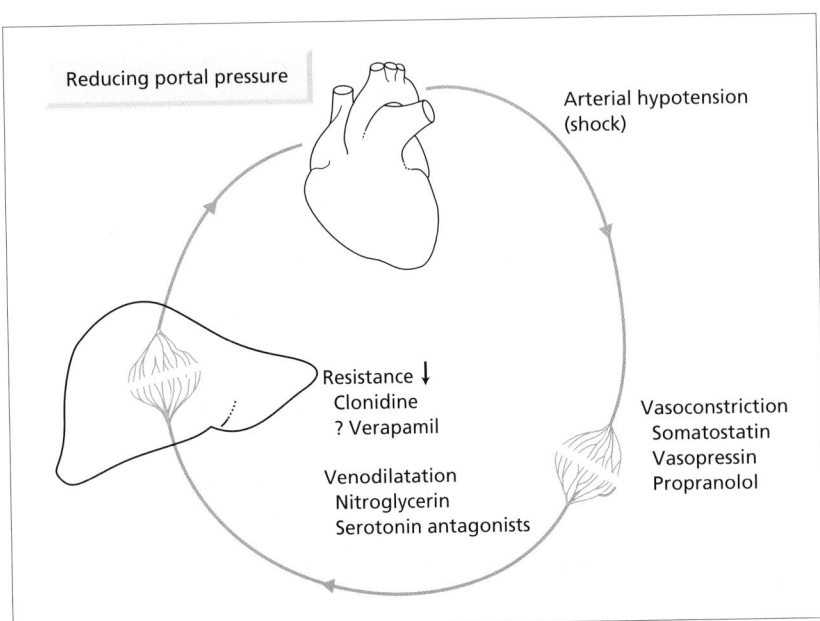

Fig. 10.66. The portal pressure can be reduced by arterial hypotension, splanchnic vaso-constriction, portal venodilatation or reduction in intra-hepatic resistance.

evaluate. A reciprocal relationship exists between the hepatic arterial and portal venous flow, one increasing when the other decreases.

The future will hold better agents for the pharmacological control of portal hypertension.

Conclusion

New treatments of gastro-oesophageal varices are usually variants of the old, such as anatomically different shunts or better methods of variceal obliteration. Their proponents are initially enthusiastic, but over the subsequent decade each method takes its place in the background with its forebears. Clinical trials must be interpreted cautiously, the type of patient being entered, the aetiology of the cirrhosis and of the portal hypertension, together with the degree of hepato-cellular failure (how many Child's grade C?) must be noted. The time of randomization is very important. The risk of further haemorrhage and death rapidly diminishes as the patient survives the first few days after a bleed (fig. 10.67).

Endoscopic or banding sclerotherapy, oesophageal tamponade, TIPS or oesophageal transection will usually stop acute variceal bleeding. Deaths from haemorrhage *per se* should no longer happen. All these procedures have complications and the varices may recur and will probably bleed again.

The problem of long-term control is difficult. All the surgical shunting procedures and TIPS have their complications, particularly encephalopathy. They also have their spectacular individual successes, usually in patients with well-compensated hepatic cirrhosis, where the main problem is the height of the portal pressure.

Controlled trials of long-term propranolol have given varied results. Many patients have a poor response especially those with grade C cirrhosis. Monitoring of portal pressure is essential. Endoscopic sclerotherapy to obliterate varices has many complications, but bleeding episodes are reduced. Both propranolol and sclerotherapy do not prolong survival. When these techniques fail, surgery must be considered, usually a meso-caval or distal spleno-renal shunt.

In the group with extra-hepatic portal obstruction, prognosis, even without surgery, is good provided adequate blood transfusion is given.

Medical measures such as bed rest and a good diet may be followed by a fall in portal pressure, especially in alcoholic subjects who lose fat from the liver. This makes assessment of surgical results even more difficult.

The ultimate treatment is hepatic transplantation [39]. This should be considered in a cirrhotic patient who has suffered at least two episodes of bleeding varices sufficient to require a blood transfusion.

References

1 Angelico M, Carli C, Piat C *et al*. Isosorbide-5-mononitrate versus propranolol in the prevention of first bleeding in cirrhosis. *Gastroenterology* 1993; **104**: 1460.

2 Asbert M, Ginès A, Ginès P *et al*. Circulating levels of endothelin in cirrhosis. *Gastroenterology* 1993; **104**: 1485.

3 Atkinson M, Sherlock S. Intrasplenic pressure as an index of the portal venous pressure. *Lancet* 1954; **i**: 1325.

4 Ayuso C, Luburich P, Vilana R *et al*. Calcifications in the portal venous system: comparison of plain films, sonography, and CT. *Am. J. Roentgenol.* 1992; **159**: 321.

5 Azoulay D, Castaing D, Dennison A *et al*. Transjugular intrahepatic portosystemic shunt worsens the hyperdynamic circulatory state of the cirrhotic patient: preliminary report of a prospective study. *Hepatology* 1994; **19**: 129.

6 Baumgarten P von. Über völlstandiges Offenbleiben der Vena umbilicalis: zugleichein Beitrag zur Frage des Morbus Bantii. *Arb. Path. Anat. Inst. Tübingen* 1907; **6**: 93.

7 Baydur A, Korula J. Cardiorespiratory effects of endoscopic esophageal variceal sclerotherapy. *Am. J. Med.* 1990; **89**: 477.

8 Bernades P, Baetz A, Lévy P *et al*. Splenic and portal venous obstruction in chronic pancreatitis. A prospective longitudinal study of a medical-surgical series of 266 patients. *Dig. Dis. Sci.* 1992; **37**: 340.

9 Bhathal PS, Grossman HJ. Reduction of the increased portal vascular resistance of the isolated perfused cirrhotic rat liver by vasodilators. *J. Hepatol.* 1985; **1**: 325.

10 Bisseru B, Patel JS. Cruveillier–Baumgarten disease. *Gut* 1989; **30**: 136.

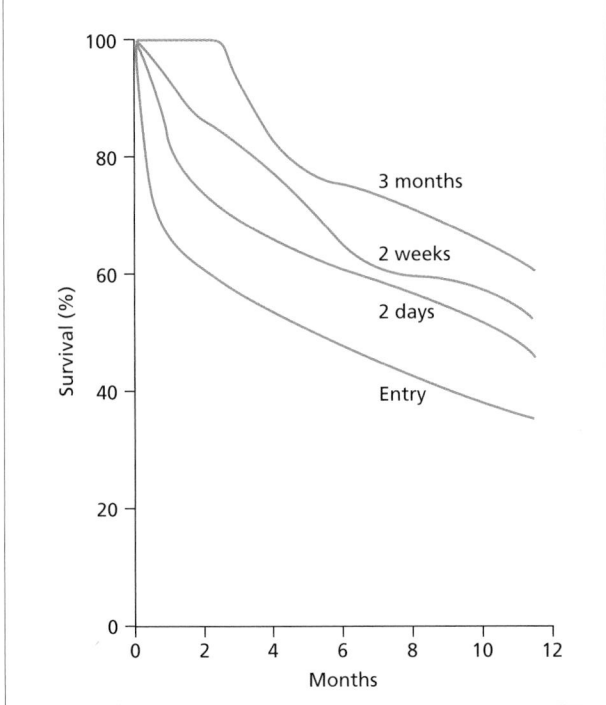

Fig. 10.67. In any trial, survival depends on the time elapsed between the bleed and entry into the trial [145].

11 Blaise M, Pateron D, Trinchet J-C *et al*. Systemic antibiotic therapy prevents bacterial infection in cirrhotic patients with gastrointestinal hemorrhage. *Hepatology* 1994; **20**: 34.

12 Blendis LM, Orrego H, Crossley IR *et al*. The role of hepatocyte enlargement in hepatic pressure in cirrhotic and non-cirrhotic liver disease. *Hepatology* 1982; **2**: 539.

13 Blum U, Rossle M, Haag K *et al*. Budd–Chiari syndrome: technical, hemodynamic, and clinical results of treatment with transjugular intra-hepatic portosystemic shunt. *Radiology* 1995; **197**: 805.

14 Bornman PC, Krige JEJ, Terblanche J. Management of oesophageal varices. *Lancet* 1994; **343**: 1079.

15 Bosch J, Groszmann RJ. Measurement of azygous venous blood flow by a continuous thermal dilution technique: an index of blood flow through gastroesophageal collaterals in cirrhosis. *Hepatology* 1984; **4**: 424.

16 Bradley SE, Ingelfinger FJ, Bradley GP *et al*. Estimation of hepatic blood flow in man. *J. Clin. Invest*. 1945; **24**: 890.

17 Braun SD, Newman GE, Dunnick NR. Digital splenoportography. *Am. J. Roentgenol*. 1985; **144**: 1003.

18 Broe PJ, Conley CL, Cameron JL. Thrombosis of the portal vein following splenectomy for myeloid metaplasia. *Surg. Gynecol. Obstet*. 1981; **152**: 488.

19 Burroughs AK, Jenkins WJ, Sherlock S *et al*. Controlled trial of propranolol for the prevention of recurrent variceal haemorrhage in patients with cirrhosis. *N. Engl. J. Med*. 1983; **309**: 1539.

20 Burroughs AK, McCormick PA, Hughes MD *et al*. Randomized, double-blind, placebo-controlled trial of somatostatin for variceal bleeding. Emergency control and prevention of early variceal rebleeding. *Gastroenterology* 1990; **99**: 1388.

21 Cabrera J, Maynar M, Granados R *et al*. Transjugular intra-hepatic portosystemic shunt versus sclerotherapy in the elective treatment of variceal hemorrhage. *Gastroenterology* 1996; **110**: 832.

22 Caesar J, Shaldon S, Chiandussi L *et al*. The use of indocyanine green in the measurement of hepatic blood flow and as a test of hepatic function. *Clin. Sci*. 1961; **21**: 43.

23 Calès P, Zabotto B, Meskens C *et al*. Gastroesophageal endoscopic features in cirrhosis. Observer variability, interassociations, and relationship to hepatic dysfunction. *Gastroenterology* 1990; **98**: 156.

24 Capron JP, LeMay JL, Muir JF *et al*. Portal vein thrombosis and fatal pulmonary thromboembolism associated with oral contraceptive treatment. *J. Clin. Gastroenterol*. 1981; **3**: 295.

25 Cestari R, Braga M, Missale G *et al*. Haemodynamic effect of triglycyl-lysine-vasopressin (glypressin) on intravascular oesophageal variceal pressure in patients with cirrhosis. A randomized placebo controlled trial. *J. Hepatol*. 1990; **10**: 205.

26 Chagnon SF, Vallee CA, Barge J *et al*. Aneurysmal portal hepatic venous fistula: report of two cases. *Radiology* 1986; **159**: 693.

27 Colapinto RF, Stronell RD, Birch SJ *et al*. Creation of an intrahepatic portosystemic shunt with a Gruntzig balloon catheter. *Can. Med. Assoc. J*. 1982; **126**: 267.

28 Conn HO. Transjugular intrahepatic portal-systemic shunts: the state of the art. *Hepatology* 1993; **17**: 148.

29 Cruveilhier J. Anatomie pathologique du corps humain. Vol. I. XVI livr. pl. vi-*Maladies du veines*. J.B. Ballière, Paris, 1829–35.

30 Dachman AH, Ros PR, Goodman ZD *et al*. Nodular regenerative hyperplasia of the liver: clinical and radiologic observations. *Am. J. Roentgenol*. 1987; **148**: 717.

31 D'Amico G, Montalbano L, Traina M *et al*. Natural history of congestive gastropathy in cirrhosis. *Gastroenterology* 1990; **99**: 1558.

32 Dan SJ, Train JS, Cohen BA *et al*. Common bile duct varices: cholangiographic demonstration of a hazardous portosystemic communication. *Am. J. Gastroenterol*. 1983; **78**: 42.

33 Dennis MA, Pretorius D, Manco-Johnson ML *et al*. CT detection of portal venous gas associated with suppurative cholangitis and cholecystitis. *Am. J. Roentgenol*. 1985; **145**: 1017.

34 Dick R, Dooley JS. Suspected portal hypertension. In Dooley JS, Dick R, Viamonte M *et al*. eds. *Imaging in Hepatobiliary Disease*. Blackwell Scientific Publications, Oxford, 1987; 147.

35 Douglass BE, Baggenstoss AH, Hollinshead WH. Variations in the portal systems of veins. *Proc. Mayo Clin*. 1950; **25**: 26.

36 Dowling JB. Ten years' experience with mesocaval grafts. *Surg. Gynecol. Obstet*. 1979; **149**: 518.

37 Dubois A, Dauzat M, Pignodel C *et al*. Portal hypertension in lymphoproliferative and myeloproliferative disorders: hemodynamic and histological correlations. *Hepatology* 1993; **17**: 246.

38 Eck NV. On the question of ligature of the portal vein (trans. title). *Voyenno Med. J. (St Petersburg)* 1877; **130**: Sect. 2.1.

39 Ewaga H, Keeffe EB, Dort J *et al*. Liver transplantation for uncontrollable variceal bleeding. *Am. J. Gastroenterol*. 1994; **89**: 1823.

40 Finn JP, Kane RA, Edelman RR *et al*. Imaging of portal venous system in patients with cirrhosis: MR angiography versus duplex Doppler sonography. *Am. J. Roentgenol*. 1993; **161**: 989.

41 Gaiani S, Bolondi L, Li Bassi S *et al*. Prevalence of spontaneous hepatofugal portal flow in liver cirrhosis. *Gastroenterology* 1991; **100**: 160.

42 Garcia-Tsao G, Grace ND, Groszmann RJ *et al*. Short-term effects of propranolol on portal venous pressure. *Hepatology* 1986; **6**: 101.

43 Garrett KO, Reilly JJ, Schade RR *et al*. Bleeding esophageal varices: treatment by sclerotherapy and liver transplantation. *Surgery* 1988; **104**: 819.

44 Gertsch P, Fischer G, Kleber G *et al*. Manometry of esophageal varices: comparison of an endoscopic balloon technique with needle puncture. *Gastroenterology* 1993; **105**: 1159.

45 Gimson A, Polson R, Westaby D *et al*. Omeprazole in the management of intractable esophageal ulceration following injection sclerotherapy. *Gastroenterology* 1990; **99**: 1829.

46 Gimson AES, Ramage JK, Panos MZ *et al*. Randomised trial of variceal banding ligation versus injection sclerotherapy for bleeding oesophageal varices. *Lancet* 1993; **342**: 391.

47 Gimson AES, Westaby D, Hegarty J *et al*. A randomized trial of vasopression and vasopressin plus nitroglycerin in the control of acute variceal hemorrhage. *Hepatology* 1986; **6**: 410.

48 Ginès A, Salmerón JM, Ginès P *et al*. Effects of somatostatin on renal function in cirrhosis. *Gastroenterology* 1992; **103**: 1868.

49 Graham DY, Smith JL. The course of patients after variceal hemorrhage. *Gastroenterology* 1981; **80**: 800.

50 Groszmann RJ. Hyperdynamic circulation of liver disease 40 years later: pathophysiology and clinical consequences. *Hepatology* 1994; **20**: 1359.

51 Groszmann RJ, Bosch J, Grace ND *et al.* Hemodynamic events in a prospective randomized trial of propranolol versus placebo in the prevention of a first variceal hemorrhage. *Gastroenterology* 1990; **99**: 1401.

52 Groszmann RJ, Glickman M, Blei AT *et al.* Wedged and free hepatic venous pressure measured with a balloon catheter. *Gastroenterology* 1979; **76**: 253.

53 Grundfest A, Cooperman AM, Ferguson R *et al.* Portal hypertension associated with systemic mastocytosis and splenomegaly. *Gastroenterology* 1980; **78**: 370.

54 Guarascio P, Portmann B, Visco G *et al.* Liver damage with reversible portal hypertension from vitamin A intoxication; demonstration of Ito cells. *J. Clin. Pathol.* 1983; **36**: 769.

55 Gudjonsson H, Zeiler D, Gamelli RL *et al.* Colonic varices. Report of an unusual case diagnosed by radionuclide scanning, with review of the literature. *Gatroenterology* 1986; **91**: 1543.

56 Haag K, Noeldge G, Sellinger M *et al.* Transjugular intrahepatic portosystemic stent-shunt (TIPS): monitoring of function by color duplex sonography. *Gastroenterology* 1992; **102**: A817.

57 Haskal ZJ, Ring EJ, LaBerge JM *et al.* Role of parallel transjugular intrahepatic portosystemic shunts in patients with persistent portal hypertension. *Radiology* 1992; **185**: 813.

58 Helton WS, Belshaw A, Althau S *et al.* Critical appraisal of the angiographic portacaval shunt (TIPS). *Am. J. Surg.* 1993; **165**: 566.

59 Henderson JM, Kunter MH, Millikan WJ *et al.* Endoscopic variceal sclerosis compared with distal splenorenal shunt to prevent recurrent variceal bleeding in cirrhosis. *Ann. Intern. Med.* 1990; **112**: 262.

60 Ho H, Zuckerman MJ, Wassem C. A prospective controlled study of the risk of bacteremia in emergency sclerotherapy of esophageal varices. *Gastroenterology* 1991; **101**: 1642.

61 Ho K-S, Lashner BA, Emond JC *et al.* Prior esophageal variceal bleeding does not adversely affect survival after orthotopic liver transplantation. *Hepatology* 1993; **18**: 66.

62 Hosking SW, Smart HL, Johnson AG *et al.* Anorectal varices, haemorrhoids and portal hypertension. *Lancet* 1989; **i**: 349.

63 International Working Party. Terminology of nodular hepatocellular lesions. *Hepatology* 1995; **22**: 983.

64 Kelty RH, Baggenstoss AH, Butt HR. The relation of the regenerated liver nodule to the vascular bed in cirrhosis. *Gastroenterology* 1950; **15**: 285.

65 Kimura K, Ohto M, Matsutani S *et al.* Relative frequencies of portosystemic pathways and renal shunt formation through the 'posterior' gastric vein: portographic study in 460 patients. *Hepatology* 1990; **12**: 725.

66 Kingham JGC, Levinson DA, Stansfeld AG *et al.* Noncirrhotic intrahepatic portal hypertension. A long-term follow-up study. *Q. J. Med.* 1981; **50**: 259.

67 Kitano S, Terblanche J, Kahn D *et al.* Venous anatomy of the lower oesophagus in portal hypertension: practical implications. *Br. J. Surg.* 1986; **73**: 525.

68 Kleber G, Sauerbruch T, Ansari H *et al.* Prediction of variceal hemorrhage in cirrhosis: a prospective follow-up study. *Gastroenterology* 1991; **100**: 1332.

69 Knauer CM, Fogel MR. Pericarditis: complication of esophageal sclerotherapy. A report of three cases. *Gastroenterology* 1987; **93**: 287.

70 Kong C-W, Lay C-S, Tsai Y-T. The hemodynamic effect of verapamil on portal hypertension in patients with postnecrotic cirrhosis. *Hepatology* 1986; **6**: 423.

71 Kravetz D, Bosch J, Teres J *et al.* Comparison of intravenous somatostatin and vasopressin infusions in treatment of acute variceal hemorrhage. *Hepatology* 1984; **4**: 442.

72 Kudo M, Tomita S, Tochio H *et al.* Intrahepatic portosystemic venous shunt: diagnosis by color Doppler imaging. *Am. J. Gastroenterol.* 1993; **88**: 723.

73 La Berge JM, Ring EJ, Gordon RL *et al.* Creation of transjugular intrahepatic portosystemic shunts with the Wallstent endoprosthesis: results in 100 patients. *Radiology* 1993; **187**: 413.

74 La Berge JM, Somberg KA, Lake JR *et al.* Two-year outcome following transjugular intra-hepatic portosystemic shunt for variceal bleeding: results in 90 patients. *Gastroenterology* 1995; **108**: 1143.

75 Laine L, Stein C, Sharma V. Randomized comparison of ligation versus ligation plus sclerotherapy in patients with bleeding esophageal varices. *Gastroenterology* 1996; **110**: 529.

76 Larson AW, Cohen H, Zweiban B *et al.* Acute esophageal variceal sclerotherapy. Results of a prospective randomized controlled trial. *JAMA* 1986; **255**: 497.

77 Le Moine O, Adler M, Bourgeois N *et al.* Factors related to early mortality in cirrhotic patients bleeding from varices and treated by urgent sclerotherapy. *Gut* 1992; **33**: 1381.

78 Lebrec D, de Fleury P, Rueff B. Portal hypertension, size of esophageal varices and risk of gastrointestinal bleeding in alcoholic cirrhosis. *Gastroenterology* 1980; **79**: 1139.

79 Lebrec D, Giuily N, Hadengue A *et al.* Transjugular intrahepatic portosystemic shunt (TIPS) vs paracentesis for refractory ascites. Results of a randomized trial. *Hepatology* 1994; **20**: 201A.

80 Lebrec D, Poynard T, Bernuau J *et al.* A randomized controlled study of propranolol for prevention of recurrent gastro-intestinal bleeding in patients with cirrhosis; a final report. *Hepatology* 1984; **4**: 355.

81 Lim HL, Abbitt PL, Kniffen JC *et al.* Hepatic infarction complicating a transjugular intrahepatic portosystemic shunt. *Am. J. Gastroenterol.* 1993; **88**: 2095.

82 Lind CD, Malisch TW, Chong WK *et al.* Incidence of shunt occlusion or stenosis following transjugular intrahepatic portosystemic shunt placement. *Gastroenterology* 1994; **106**: 1277.

83 Loftus JP, Nagorney DM, Ilstrup D *et al.* Sinistral portal hypertension. Splenectomy or expectant management. *Ann. Surg.* 1993; **217**: 35.

84 Ludwig J, Hashimoto E, Obata H *et al.* Idiopathic portal hypertension. *Hepatology* 1993; **17**: 1157.

85 Martin M, Zajko AB, Orons PD *et al.* Transjugular intrahepatic portosystemic shunt in the management of variceal bleeding: indications and clinical results. *Surgery* 1993; **114**: 719.

86 McCormack TT, Rose JD, Smith PM *et al.* Perforating veins and blood flow in oesophageal varices. *Lancet* 1983; **ii**: 1442.

87 McCormick PA, Kaye GL, Greenslade L *et al.* Esophageal staple transection as a salvage procedure after failure of acute injection sclerotherapy. *Hepatology* 1992; **15**: 403.

88 McIndoe AH. Vascular lesions of portal cirrhosis. *Arch. Path.* 1928; **5**: 23.

89 Manenti F, Williams R. Injection of the splenic vasculature in portal hypertension. *Gut* 1966; **7**: 175.

90 Marteau P, Ballet F, Chazouillères O *et al.* Effect of vasodilators on hepatic microcirculation in cirrhosis: a study in the isolated perfused rat liver. *Hepatology* 1989; **9**: 820.

91 Mastai R, Bosch J, Bruix J *et al.* β-Blockade with propranolol and hepatic artery blood flow in patients with cirrhosis. *Hepatology* 1989; **10**: 269.

92 Merli M, Riggio O, Capocaccia L *et al.* Transjugular intra-hepatic portosystemic shunt versus endoscopic sclerotherapy in preventing variceal rebleeding; preliminary results of a randomized controlled trial. *Hepatology* 1994; **20**: 107A.

93 Mikkelsen WP. Extrahepatic portal hypertension in children. *Am. J. Surg.* 1966; **111**: 333.

94 Millikan WJ, Warren WD, Henderson JM *et al.* The Emory prospective randomized trial: selective versus non selective shunt to control variceal bleeding. Ten year follow-up. *Ann. Surg.* 1985; **201**: 712.

95 Moreau R, Lee SS, Hadengue A *et al.* Hemodynamic effects of a clonidine-induced decrease in sympathetic tone in patients with cirrhosis. *Hepatology* 1987; **7**: 149.

96 Morse SS, Taylor KJW, Strauss EB *et al.* Congenital absence of the portal vein in oculoauriculo-vertebral dysplasia (Goldenhar syndrome). *Pediatr. Radiol.* 1986; **16**: 437.

97 Nagral AS, Joshi AS, Bhatia SJ *et al.* Congestive jejunopathy in portal hypertension. *Gut* 1993; **34**: 694.

98 Navasa M, Chesta J, Bosch J *et al.* Reduction of portal pressure by isosorbide-5-mononitrate in patients with cirrhosis. Effects on splanchnic and systemic hemodynamics and liver function. *Gastroenterology* 1989; **96**: 1110.

99 Navasa M, Feu F, García-Pagán JC *et al.* Hemodynamic and humoral changes after liver transplantation in patients with cirrhosis. *Hepatology* 1993; **17**: 355.

100 North Italian Endoscopic Club for study and treatment of esophageal varices. Prediction of the first variceal haemorrhage in patients with cirrhosis of the liver and esophageal varices. A prospective multicentre study. *N. Engl. J. Med.* 1988; **319**: 983.

101 Oberti F, Sogni P, Cailmail S *et al.* Role of prostacyclin in hemodynamic alterations in conscious rats with extrahepatic or intrahepatic portal hypertension. *Hepatology* 1993; **18**: 621.

102 Ochs A, Rössle M, Haag K *et al.* TIPS for hepatorenal syndrome. *Hepatology* 1994; **20**: 114A.

103 Ochs A, Sellinger M, Haag K *et al.* Transjugular intrahepatic portosystemic stent-shunt in the treatment of Budd–Chiari syndrome. *J. Hepatol.* 1993; **18**: 217.

104 Odièvre M, Pigé G, Alagille D. Congenital abnormalities associated with extrahepatic portal hypertension. *Arch. Dis. Child.* 1997; **52**: 383.

105 Okuda K, Ohnishi K, Kimura K *et al.* Incidence of portal vein thrombosis in liver cirrhosis. An angiographic study in 708 patients. *Gastroenterology* 1985; **89**: 279.

106 Okumura S, Takei Y, Kawano S *et al.* Vasoactive effect of endothelin-1 on rat liver *in vivo. Hepatology* 1994; **19**: 155.

107 Orloff MJ, Bell RH Jr, Orloff MS *et al.* Prospective randomized trial of emergency portacaval shunt and emergency medical therapy in unselected cirrhotic patients with bleeding varices. *Hepatology* 1994; **20**: 863.

108 Pagliaro L, D'Amico G, Sorensen TIA *et al.* Prevention of first bleeding in cirrhosis. A meta-analysis of randomized trials of nonsurgical treatment. *Ann. Intern. Med.* 1992; **117**: 59.

109 Pak J-M, Lee SS. Glucagon in portal hypertension. *J. Hepatol.* 1994; **20**: 825.

110 Panés J, Piqué JM, Bordas JM *et al.* Reduction of gastric hyperemia by glypressin and vasopressin administration in cirrhotic patients with portal hypertensive gastropathy. *Hepatology* 1994; **19**: 55.

111 Panés J, Terés J, Bosch J *et al.* Efficacy of balloon tamponade in treatment of bleeding gastric and esophageal varices. Results in 151 consecutive episodes. *Dig. Dis. Sci.* 1988; **33**: 454.

112 Park JH, Cha SH, Han JK *et al.* Intrahepatic portosystemic venous shunt. *Am. J. Roentgenol.* 1990; **155**: 527.

113 Parvey HR, Raval B, Sandler CM. Portal vein thrombosis: imaging findings. *Am. J. Roentgenol.* 1994; **162**: 77.

114 Pasricha PJ, Fleischer DE, Kalloo AN. Endoscopic perforations of the upper digestive tract: a review of their pathogenesis, prevention, and management. *Gastroenterology* 1994; **106**: 787.

115 Payen J-L, Calès P, Voigt J-J *et al.* Severe portal hypertensive gastropathy and antral vascular ectasia are distinct entities in patients with cirrhosis. *Gastroenterology* 1995; **108**: 138.

116 Pizcueta P, Piqué J-M, Fernandez M *et al.* Modulation of the hyperdynamic circulation of cirrhotic rats by nitric oxide inhibition. *Gastroenterology* 1992; **103** : 1909.

117 Planas R, Quer JC, Boix J *et al.* A prospective randomized trial comparing somatostatin and sclerotherapy in the treatment of acute variceal bleeding. *Hepatology* 1994; **20**: 370.

118 Popper H, Elias H, Petty DE. Vascular pattern of the cirrhotic liver. *Am. J. Clin. Path.* 1952; **22**: 717.

119 Poynard T, Cales P, Pasta L *et al.* Beta-adrenergic antagonist drugs in the prevention of gastrointestinal bleeding in patients with cirrhosis and esophageal varices. An analysis of data and prognostic factors in 589 patients from four randomized clinical trials. Franco Italian Multicenter Study Group. *N. Engl. J. Med.* 1991; **324**: 1532.

120 Primignani M, Andreoni B, Carpinelli L *et al.* Sclerotherapy plus octreotide versus sclerotherapy alone in the prevention of early rebleeding from esophageal varices: a randomized double-blind, placebo-controlled multicenter trial. *Hepatology* 1995; **21**: 1322.

121 Quintero E, Pique JM, Bombi JA *et al.* Gastric mucosal vascular ectasias causing bleeding in cirrhosis. *Gastroenterology* 1987; **93**: 1054.

122 Reynolds TB, Ito S, Iwatsuki S. Measurement of portal pressure and its clinical application. *Am. J. Med.* 1970; **49**: 649.

123 Rigau J, Bosch J, Bordas JM *et al.* Endoscopic measurement of variceal pressure in cirrhosis: correlation with portal pressure and variceal hemorrhage. *Gastroenterology* 1989; **96**: 873.

124 Riggio O, Merli M, Pedretti G *et al.* Hepatic encephalopathy after transjugular intra-hepatic portosystemic shunt. Incidence and risk factors. *Dig. Dis. Sci.* 1996; **41**: 578.

125 Ring EJ, Lake JR, Roberts JP *et al.* Using transjugular intrahepatic portosystemic shunts to control variceal bleeding before liver transplantation. *Ann. Intern. Med.* 1992; **116**: 304.

126 Rosch J, Hanafee WN, Snow H. Transjugular portal venography and radiologic portacaval shunt: an experimental study. *Radiology* 1969; **92**: 1112.

127 Rössle M, Deibert P, Haag K *et al.* TIPS versus sclerotherapy and β-blockade: preliminary results of a randomized study in patients with recurrent variceal hemorrhage. *Hepatology* 1994; **20**: 107A.

128 Rössle M, Haag K, Ochs A *et al.* The transjugular intrahepatic portosystemic stent-shunt procedure for variceal bleeding. *N. Engl. J. Med.* 1994; **330**: 165.

129 Saari A, Klvilaakso E, Inberg M *et al.* Comparison of somatostatin and vasopressin in bleeding esophageal varices. *Am. J. Gastroenterol.* 1990; **85**: 804.

130 Salmerón JM, del Arbol LR, Ginès A *et al.* Renal effects of acute isosorbide-5-mononitrate administration in cirrhosis. *Hepatology* 1993; **17**: 800.

131 Samuels T, Lovett MC, Campbell IT *et al.* Respiratory function after injection sclerotherapy of oesophageal varices. *Gut* 1994; **35**: 1459.

132 Sanchez RB, Roberts AC, Valji K *et al.* Wallstent misplaced during transjugular placement of an intrahepatic portosystemic shunt: retrieval with a loop snare. *Am. J. Roentgenol.* 1992; **159**: 129.

133 Sanyal AJ, Freedman AM, Purdum PP *et al.* The hematologic consequences of transjugular intra-hepatic portosystemic shunts. *Hepatology* 1996; **23**: 32.

134 Sanyal AJ, Freedman AM, Shiffman ML *et al.* Portosystemic encephalopathy after transjugular intrahepatic portosystemic shunt: results of a prospective controlled study. *Hepatology* 1994; **20**: 46.

135 Sarin SK. Progress report. Non-cirrhotic portal fibrosis. *Gut* 1989; **30**: 406.

136 Scandalis N, Archimandritis A, Kastanas K *et al.* Colonic findings in cirrhotics with portal hypertension. A prospective colonoscopic and histological study. *J. Clin. Gastroenterol.* 1994; **18**: 325.

137 Schmassmann A, Zuber M, Livers M *et al.* Recurrent bleeding after variceal hemorrhage: predictive value of portal venous duplex sonography. *Am. J. Roentgenol.* 1993; **160**: 41.

138 Sellinger M, Ochs A, Haag K *et al.* Incidence of hepatic encephalopathy and follow-up of liver function in patients with transjugular intrahepatic portosystemic stent-shunt. *Gastroenterology* 1992; **102**: A833.

139 Shaldon S, Chiandussi L, Guevara L *et al.* The measurement of hepatic blood flow and intrahepatic shunted blood flow by colloid heat denatured human serum albumin labelled with I¹³¹. *J. Clin. Invest.* 1961; **40**: 1346.

140 Sherlock S. Esophageal varices. *Am. J. Surg.* 1990; **160**: 9.

141 Sherlock S, Feldman CA, Moran B *et al.* Partial nodular transformation of the liver with portal hypertension. *Am. J. Med.* 1966; **40**: 195.

142 Shields SJ, Byse BH, Grace ND. Arterioportal fistula: a role for pre-TIPSS arteriography and hepatic venous pressure measurements. *Am. J. Gastroenterol.* 1992; **87**: 1828.

143 Shiffman ML, Jeffers L, Hoofnagle JH *et al.* The role of transjugular intra-hepatic protosystemic shunt for treatment of portal hypertension and its complications: a conference sponsored by the National Digestive Diseases Advisory Board. *Hepatology* 1995; **22**: 1519.

144 Siringo S, Bolondi L, Gaiani S *et al.* Timing of the first variceal hemorrhage in cirrhotic patients: prospective evaluation of Doppler flowmetry, endoscopy and clinical parameters. *Hepatology* 1994; **20**: 66.

145 Smith JL, Graham D. Variceal hemorrhage—a critical evaluation of survival analysis. *Gastroenterology* 1982; **82**: 968.

146 Smith-Laing G, Camilo ME, Dick R *et al.* Percutaneous transhepatic portography in the assessment of portal hypertension. *Gastroenterology* 1980; **78**: 197.

147 Snady H, Korsten MA. Esophageal acid — clearance and motility after endoscopic sclerotherapy of esophageal varices. *Am. J. Gastro.* 1986; **81**: 419.

148 Soriano G, Guarner C, Tomás A *et al.* Norfloxacin prevents bacterial infection in cirrhotics with gastrointestinal hemorrhage. *Gastroenterology* 1992; **103**: 1267.

149 Spina GP, Arcidiacono R, Bosch J *et al.* Gastric endoscopic features in portal hypertension: final report of a consensus conference, Milan, Italy, 19 September 1992. *J. Hepatol.* 1994; **21**: 461.

150 Stiegmann GV, Goff JS, Michaletz-Onody PA *et al.* Endoscopic sclerotherapy as compared with endoscopic ligation for bleeding esophageal varices. *N. Engl. J. Med.* 1992; **326**: 1527.

151 Sung JJY, Chung SCS, Lai C-W *et al.* Octreotide infusion or emergency sclerotherapy for variceal haemorrhage. *Lancet* 1993; **342**: 637.

152 Tabibian N, Alpert E, Refractory sclerotherapy-induced esophageal strictures. *Ann. Intern. Med.* 1987; **106**: 59.

153 Tabibian N, Schwartz JT, Lacey Smith J *et al.* Cardiac tamponade as a result of endoscopic sclerotherapy: report of a case. *Surgery* 1987; **102**: 546.

154 Taylor CR. Computed tomography in the evaluation of the portal venous system. *J. Clin. Gastroenterol.* 1992; **14**: 167.

155 Terés J, Bosch J, Bordas JM *et al.* Propranolol versus sclerotherapy in preventing variceal rebleeding: a randomized controlled trial. *Gastroenterology* 1993; **105**: 1508.

156 Thompson EN, Sherlock S. The aetiology of portal vein thrombosis with particular reference to the role of infection and exchange transfusion. *Q. J. Med.* 1964; n.s. **33**: 465.

157 Thompson EN, Williams R, Sherlock S. Liver function in extra-hepatic portal hypertension. *Lancet* 1964; **ii**: 1352.

158 Uchihara M, Izumi N, Sato C *et al.* Clinical significance of elevated plasma endothelin concentration in patients with cirrhosis. *Hepatology* 1992; **16**: 95.

159 Valla D, Casadevall N, Huisse MG *et al.* Etiology of portal thrombosis in adults. *Gastroenterology* 1988; **94**: 1063.

160 Valla D, Girod C, Lee SS *et al.* Lack of vasopressin action on splanchnic hemodynamics during bleeding; a study in conscious, portal hypertensive rats. *Hepatology* 1988; **8**: 10.

161 Van Ruiswyk J, Byrd JC. Efficacy of prophylactic sclerotherapy for prevention of a first variceal hemorrhage. *Gastroenterology* 1992; **102**: 587.

162 Veterans affairs cooperative variceal sclerotherapy group. Sclerotherapy for male alcoholic cirrhotic patients who have bled from esophageal varices: results of a randomized multicenter clinical trial. *Hepatology* 1994; **20**: 618.

163 Vianna A, Hayes PC, Moscoso G *et al.* Normal venous circulation of the gastroesophageal junction. A route to understanding varices. *Gastroenterology* 1987; **93**: 876.

164 Viggiano TR, Gostout CJ. Portal hypertensive intestinal vasculopathy: a review of the clinical, endoscopic, and histopathologic features. *Am. J. Gastroenterol.* 1992; **87**: 944.

165 Villanueva C, Balanzo J, Novella MT *et al.* Nadolzol plus isosorbide mononitrate compared with sclerotherapy for the prevention of variceal rebleeding. *N. Engl. J. Med.* 1996; **334**: 1624.

166 Vorobioff J, Garcia-Tsao G, Groszmann R *et al.* Long-term hemodynamic effects of ketanserin, a 5-hydrotryptamine

blocker, in portal hypertensive patients. *Hepatology* 1989; **9**: 88.

167 Vorobioff J, Picabea E, Gamen M *et al*. Propranolol compared with propranolol plus isosorbide dinitrate in portal-hypertensive patients: long-term hemodynamic and renal effects. *Hepatology* 1993; **18**: 477.

168 Vorobioff J, Picabea E, Villavicencio R *et al*. Acute and chronic hemodynamic effects of propranolol in unselected cirrhotic patients. *Hepatology* 1987; **7**: 648.

169 Walker S, Kreichgauer H-P, Bode JC. Terlipressin versus somatostatin in bleeding esophageal varices: a controlled, double-blind study. *Hepatology* 1992; **15**: 1023.

170 Wanless IR, Peterson P, Das A *et al*. Hepatic vascular disease and portal hypertension in polycythemia vera and agnogenic myeloid metaplasia: a clinicopathological study of 145 patients examined at autopsy. *Hepatology* 1990; **12**: 1166.

171 Wanless IR. Micronodular transformation (nodular regenerative hyperplasia). *Hepatology* 1990; **11**: 787.

172 Webb LJ, Sherlock S. The aetiology, presentation and natural history of extrahepatic portal venous obstruction *Q. J. Med.* 1979; **48**: 627.

173 Webb L, Smith-Laing G, Lake-Bakaar G *et al*. Pancreatic hypofunction in extrahepatic portal venous obstruction. *Gut* 1980; **21**: 227.

174 Weinshel E, Chen W, Falkenstein DB *et al*. Hemorrhoids or rectal varices: defining the cause of massive rectal hemorrhage in patients with portal hypertension. *Gastroenterology* 1986; **90**: 744.

175 Westaby D, Hayes PC, Gimson AES *et al*. Controlled clinical trial of injection sclerotherapy for active variceal bleeding. *Hepatology* 1989; **9**: 274.

176 Westaby D, MacDougall BRD, Williams R. Improved survival following injection sclerotherapy for esophageal varices: final analysis of a controlled trial. *Hepatology* 1985; **5**: 827.

177 Westaby D, Polson RJ, Gimson AES *et al*. A controlled trial of oral propranolol compared with injection sclerotherapy for the long-term management of variceal bleeding. *Hepatology* 1990; **11**: 353.

178 Zemel G, Katzen BT, Becker GJ *et al*. Percutaneous transjugular portosystemic shunts. *JAMA* 1991; **266**: 390.

179 Zoli M, Iervese T, Merkel C *et al*. Prognostic significance of portal hemodynamics in patients with compensated cirrhosis. *J. Hepatol.* 1993; **17**: 56.

Chapter 11
The Hepatic Artery and Hepatic Veins: the Liver in Circulatory Failure

The hepatic artery

The hepatic artery is a branch of the coeliac axis. It runs along the upper border of the pancreas to the first part of the duodenum where it turns upwards between the layers of the lesser omentum, lying in front of the portal vein and medial to the common bile duct. Reaching the porta hepatis it divides into right and left branches. Its branches include the right gastric artery and the gastro-duodenal artery. Aberrant branches are common. Surgical anatomy has been defined in donor livers [9]. The common hepatic artery usually rises from the coeliac axis to form gastro-duodenal and proper hepatic artery which divides into right and left branches. A replaced or accessory right hepatic artery may originate from the superior mesenteric artery. A replaced or accessory left hepatic artery may arise from the left gastric artery. Rarely the entire common hepatic artery arises as a branch of the superior mesenteric or directly from the aorta. Such anomalies are of great importance in liver transplantation.

Anastomoses occur between the right and left branches, with subcapsular vessels of the liver and with the inferior phrenic artery.

Intra-hepatic anatomy

The hepatic artery enters sinusoids adjacent to portal tracts [23]. Direct arterio-portal venous anastomoses are not seen in man [23].

The hepatic artery forms a capillary plexus around the bile ducts. Interference with this hepatic arterial supply leads to bile duct injury in such conditions as operative trauma, hepatic transplantation and intra-hepatic arterial cytotoxic therapy (fig. 11.1) [18]. Diseases of the hepatic artery, such as polyarteritis nodosa, may present as biliary strictures [2].

The connective tissue in the portal zones is supplied by the hepatic artery.

Hepatic arterial flow

In man, during surgery, the hepatic artery supplies 35% of the hepatic blood flow and 50% of the liver's oxygen

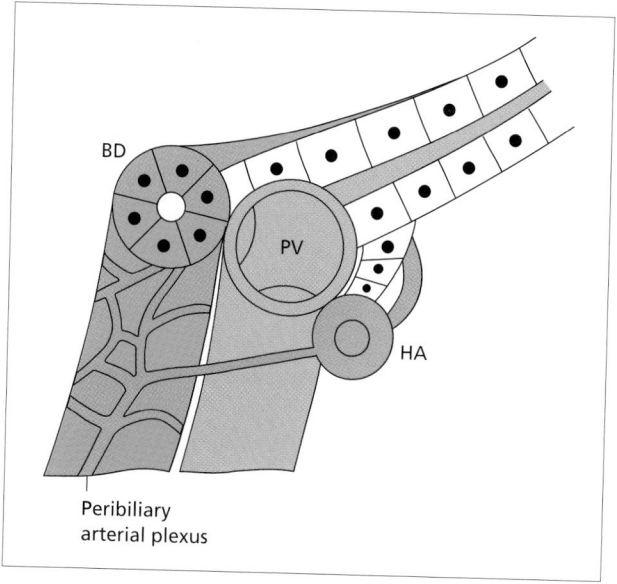

Fig. 11.1. The hepatic artery (HA) forms a peri-biliary plexus supplying the bile duct (BD). PV = portal vein.

supply [21]. The hepatic arterial flow serves to hold total hepatic blood flow constant. It is not regulated by the metabolic demands of the liver, but rather regulates blood levels of nutrients and hormones by maintaining blood flow, and thereby hepatic clearance, as steady as possible [13].

The proportion of hepatic arterial flow increases greatly in cirrhosis, related to the extent of portal–systemic venous shunting. It is the main blood supply to tumours. A drop in systemic blood pressure from haemorrhage, or any other cause, lowers the oxygen content of the portal vein and the liver becomes more and more dependent on the hepatic artery for oxygen. The hepatic artery and the portal vein adjust the volume of blood and of oxygen they supply to the liver according to demand [13].

Hepatic arteriography

The hepatic artery is cannulated via the aorta and coeliac axis. Hepatic arteriography is used for the diagnosis of space-occupying lesions including cysts, abscesses and benign and malignant tumours (Chapter 28), as well as vascular lesions such as aneurysms (fig. 11.2) or arterio-venous fistulae. Embolization via the catheter is used for treating tumours and hepatic trauma, and in the management of hepatic arterial aneurysm or arteriovenous fistulae (figs 11.3, 11.4).

Hepatic arterial catheterizaterion is used to introduce cytotoxic drugs into hepato-cellular neoplasms and for pump perfusion in patients with metastases, particularly from colo-rectal cancer (Chapter 26).

Spiral CT is of great value in diagnosing hepatic arterial thrombosis after liver transplant [14] and variations in intra-hepatic anatomy before liver resection [20].

Hepatic artery occlusion

The effects of hepatic artery occlusion depend on the site and on the extent of available collateral circulation. If the division is distal to the origins of the gastric and gastro-duodenal arteries the patient may die. Survivors develop a collateral circulation. Slow thrombosis is

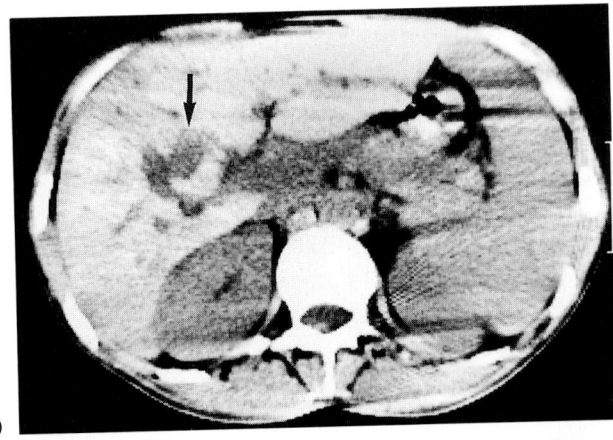

(a)

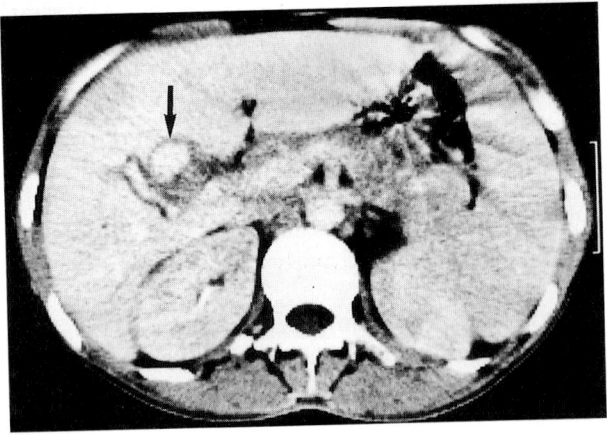

(b)

Fig. 11.2. Hepatic artery aneurysm in a patient with sub-acute bacterial endocarditis. CT scans of the upper abdomen: (a) before and (b) after contrast enhancement. The aneurysm shows as a filling defect (arrow) which highlights following contrast injection.

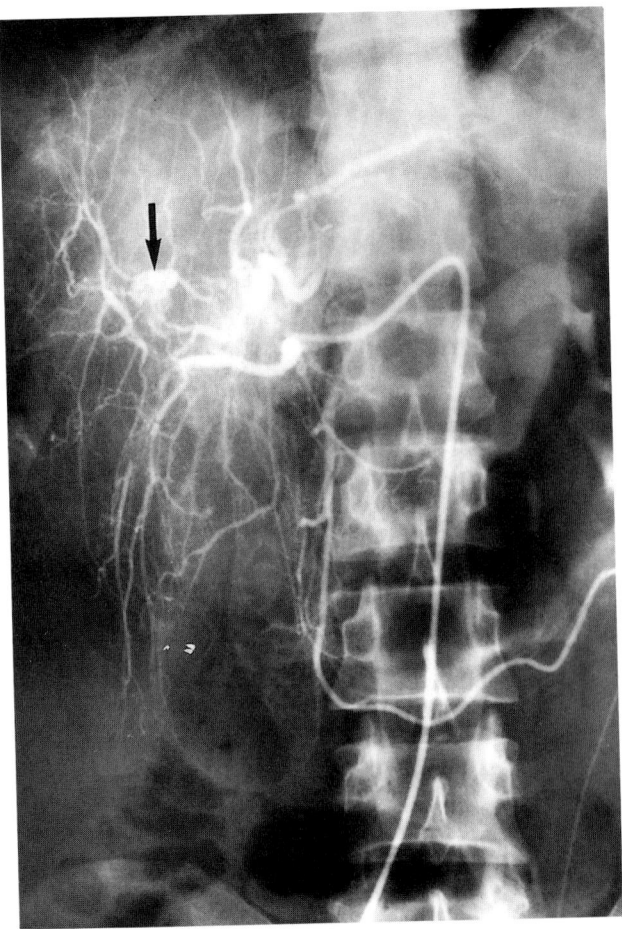

Fig. 11.3. Sub-acute bacterial endocarditis. Coeliac arteriogram showing a 3 cm false aneurysm (arrow) of one of the intra-hepatic branches of the right hepatic artery, 2.5 cm lateral to its major bifurcation.

better than sudden block. Simultaneous occlusion of the portal vein is nearly always fatal.

The size of the infarct depends on the extent of the collateral arterial circulation. It rarely exceeds 8 cm in diameter and has a pale centre with a surrounding congested haemorrhagic band. Liver cells in the infarcted area are jumbled together in irregular collections of eosinophilic, granular cytoplasm without glycogen or nuclei. Sub-capsular areas escape because they have an alternative arterial blood supply.

Hepatic infarction can develop without arterial occlusion in such conditions as shock, cardiac failure, diabetic ketosis, toxaemia of pregnancy [12] or systemic lupus erythematosus [10]. If sought by scanning, hepatic infarcts are frequent after percutaneous liver biopsy.

Aetiology

Occlusion of the hepatic artery is very rare. Hitherto it was regarded as a fatal condition. However, hepatic

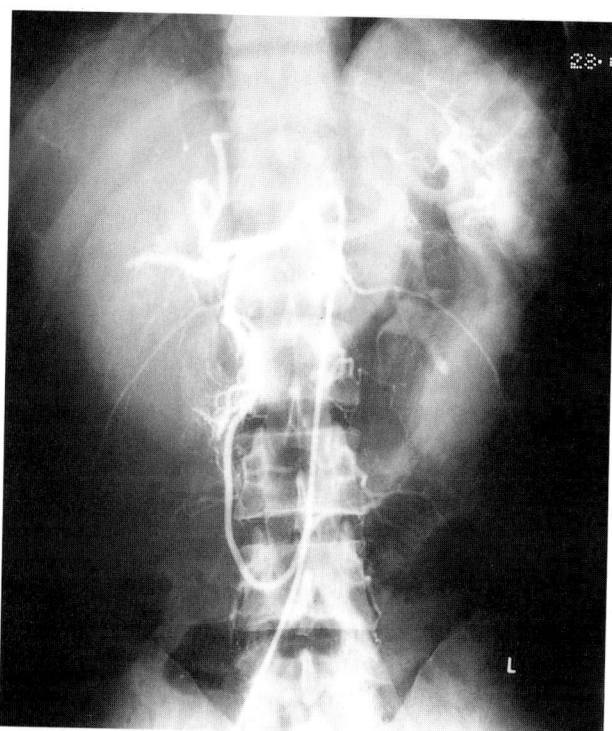

Fig. 11.4. Same patient as in fig. 11.3. Coeliac angiogram immediately post-embolization showing obliteration of the aneurysm and its feeding vessels [11].

angiography has allowed earlier diagnosis and the prognosis has improved. Some of the causes are polyarteritis nodosa, giant cell arteritis and embolism in patients with acute bacterial endocarditis. A branch of the artery may be tied during cholecystectomy but recovery is usual. Trauma to the right hepatic artery or cystic artery may complicate laparoscopic cholecystectomy [1]. Hepatic arterial dissection may follow abdominal trauma or hepatic arterial catheterization. Gangrenous cholecystitis can complicate hepatic artery embolization [19].

Clinical features

The condition is rarely diagnosed *ante mortem* and descriptions are meagre. The patient exhibits the features of the cause, such as bacterial endocarditis, or polyarteritis nodosa, or has undergone a difficult upper abdominal operation. Sudden pain in the right upper abdomen is followed by collapse and hypotension. Right upper quadrant tenderness develops and the liver edge is tender. Jaundice deepens rapidly. There is usually fever and leucocytosis and liver function tests show hepato-cellular damage. The prothrombin time rises precipitously and haemorrhages develop. With major occlusions the patient passes into coma and is dead within 10 days.

Hepatic arteriography is essential. The obstruction to the hepatic artery may be shown. Intra-hepatic arterial collaterals develop in the portal zones and subcapsular areas. Extra-hepatic collaterals form in the suspensory ligaments and with adjacent structures [3].

Scanning [15]. The infarcts are round or oval, rarely wedge-shaped and are centrally located. Early lesions are hypoechoic on ultrasound and CT shows a poorly demarcated low-density region which does not enhance with contrast. Later lesions are confluent with distinct margins. Magnetic resonance shows a lesion of low signal intensity on T_1-weighted images with high signal intensity on T_2-weighted images [12]. Bile lakes follow large infarcts and these may contain gas.

Treatment. The causative lesion must be treated. Antibotics may prevent secondary infection in the anoxic liver. The general management is that of acute hepato-cellular failure. Trauma to the artery is treated by percutaneous arterial embolization [22].

Hepatic arterial lesions following liver transplantation

The term *ischaemic cholangitis* is used to describe bile duct damage due to ischaemia [16]. It follows post-transplant-associated thrombosis or stenosis of the hepatic artery or occlusion of peri-biliary arteries [8]. It is difficult to diagnose as liver biopsy may show the picture of biliary obstruction without evidence of ischaemia.

After transplant, hepatic arterial thrombosis is diagnosed by visceral arteriography. Doppler sonography may not detect the abnormality or the result can be misinterpreted [6]. Spiral CT is highly accurate [14].

Aneurysms of the hepatic artery

These are rare but make up about one-fifth of all visceral aneurysms. The aneurysm may complicate bacterial endocarditis, polyarteritis nodosa or arteriosclerosis. Trauma is becoming increasingly important, including motor vehicle accidents and iatrogenic causes such as biliary tract surgery, liver biopsy and interventional radiological procedures. Pseudo-aneurysms may complicate chronic pancreatitis with pseudo-cyst formation [17]. Bile leaks are significantly associated with pseudo-aneurysms [5]. It may be congenital [4]. The aneurysm may be extra- or intra-hepatic and may vary in size from a pin point to a grapefruit. The aneurysm may be recognized by angiography, incidentally at operation or at autopsy.

Clinical presentation is varied. The classical triad of jaundice [24], abdominal pain and haemobilia is present in only about one-third of patients. Abdominal pain is a frequent feature and may last as long as 5 months before the aneurysm ruptures.

Sixty to 80% of patients present for the first time with rupture into the peritoneum, biliary tree or gastrointestinal tract with resultant haemoperitoneum, haemobilia or haematemesis.

The *diagnosis* is suggested by sonography and confirmed by hepatic arteriography and a CT scan after enhancement (see fig. 11.2) [11]. Pulsed Doppler ultrasound may show turbulent flow in the aneurysm [7].

Treatment. Intra-hepatic aneurysms are treated by angiographic embolization (see figs 11.3, 11.4). Aneurysms of the common hepatic artery are treated surgically by proximal and distal ligation.

Hepatic arteriovenous shunts

These are usually secondary to blunt trauma, liver biopsy or neoplasms, usually primary liver cancer. Multiple shunts may be part of hereditary haemorrhagic telangiectasia, when they can be so extensive that congestive heart failure follows.

Large shunts cause a bruit in the right upper quadrant. The diagnosis is confirmed by hepatic angiography. Embolization with gelfoam is the usual treatment.

References

1 Bacha EA, Stieber AC, Galloway JR *et al.* Non-biliary complication of laparoscopic cholecystectomy. *Lancet* 1994; **344**: 896.

2 Barquist ES, Goldstein N, Zinner MJ. Polyarteritis nodosa presenting as a biliary stricture. *Surgery* 1991; **109**: 16.

3 Charnsangavej C, Chuang VP, Wallace S *et al.* Angiographic classification of hepatic arterial collaterals. *Radiology* 1982; **144**: 485.

4 Cooper SG, Richman AH. Spontaneous rupture of a congenital hepatic artery aneurysm. *J. Clin. Gastroenterol.* 1988; **10**: 104.

5 Croce MA, Fabian TC, Spiers JP *et al.* Traumatic hepatic artery pseudoaneurysm with hemobilia. *Am. J. Surg.* 1994; **168**: 235.

6 Dravid VS, Shapiro MJ, Needleman L *et al.* Arterial abnormalities following orthotopic liver transplantation: arteriographic findings and correlation with Doppler sonographic findings. *Am. J. Roentgenol.* 1994; **163**: 585.

7 Falkoff GE, Taylor KJW, Morse S. Hepatic artery pseudoaneurysm: diagnosis with real-time and pulsed Doppler US. *Radiology* 1986; **158**: 55.

8 Fisher A, Miller CM. Ischemic-type biliary strictures in liver allografts: the Achilles heel revisited? *Hepatology* 1995; **21**: 589.

9 Hiatt JR, Gabbay J, Busuttil RW. Surgical anatomy of the hepatic arteries in 1000 cases. *Ann. Surg.* 1994; **220**: 50.

10 Khoury G, Tobi M, Oren M *et al.* Massive hepatic infarction in systemic lupus erythematosus. *Dig. Dis. Sci.* 1990; **35**: 1557.

11 Kibbler CC, Cohen DL, Cruickshank JK *et al.* Use of CT scanning in the diagnosis and management of hepatic artery aneurysm. *Gut* 1985; **26**: 752.

12 Kronthal AJ, Fishman EK, Kuhlman JE *et al.* Hepatic infarction in preeclampsia. *Radiology* 1990; **177**: 726.

13 Lautt WW, Greenaway CV. Conceptual review of the hepatic vascular bed. *Hepatology* 1987; **7**: 952.

14 Legmann P, Costes V, Tudoret L. Hepatic artery thrombosis after liver transplantation: diagnosis with spiral CT. *Am. J. Roentgenol.* 1995; **164**: 97.

15 Lev-Toaff AS, Friedman AC, Cohen LM *et al.* Hepatic infarcts: new observations by CT and sonography. *Am. J. Roentgenol.* 1987; **149**: 87.

16 Ludwig J, Batts KP, MacCarthy RL. Ischemic cholangitis in hepatic allografts. *Mayo Clin. Proc.* 1992; **67**: 519.

17 Pinsky MA, May ES, Taxler MS *et al.* Late manifestations of hepatic artery pseudo aneurysm: case presentation and review. *Am. J. Gastroenterol.* 1987; **82**: 467.

18 Sherlock S. The syndrome of disappearing intra-hepatic bile ducts. *Lancet* 1987; **ii**: 493.

19 Simons RK, Sinanan MN, Coldwell DM. Gangrenous cholecystitis as a complication of hepatic artery embolization: case report. *Surgery* 1992; **112**: 106.

20 Soyer P, Bluemke DA, Choit MA *et al.* Variations in the intrahepatic portions of the hepatic and portal veins: findings on helical CT scans during arterial portography. *Am. J. Roentgenol.* 1995; **164**: 102.

21 Tygstrup N, Winkler K, Mellengaard K *et al.* Determination of the hepatic arterial blood flow and oxygen supply in man by clamping the hepatic artery during surgery. *J. Clin. Invest.* 1962; **41**: 447.

22 Wagner WH, Lundell CJ, Donovan AJ. Percutaneous angiographic embolization for hepatic arterial haemorrhage. *Arch. Surg.* 1985; **120**: 1241.

23 Yamamoto K, Sherman I, Phillips MJ *et al.* Three-dimensional observations of the hepatic arterial terminations in rat, hamster and human liver by scanning electron microscopy of micro vascular casts. *Hepatology* 1985; **5**: 452.

24 Zachary K, Geier S, Pellecchia D *et al.* Jaundice secondary to hepatic artery aneurysm: radiological appearance and clinical features. *Am. J. Gastroenterol.* 1986; **81**: 295.

The hepatic veins

The hepatic veins begin as the zone 3 (central) veins. These join the sublobular veins and merge into larger hepatic veins, which enter the inferior vena cava while it is still partly embedded in the liver. The number, size and pattern of hepatic veins are very variable. Generally, there are three large veins, one draining the left lobe and the other two emerging from the right lobe (fig. 11.5). There are variable numbers of small accessory veins particularly from the caudate lobe [15].

In the normal liver there are no direct anastomoses between portal vein and hepatic vein which are linked only by the sinusoids. In the cirrhotic liver there are anastomoses between portal and hepatic veins so that the blood bypasses the regenerating liver cell nodules (see fig. 10.46). There is no evidence, either in the normal or cirrhotic liver, of anastomoses between the hepatic artery and the hepatic vein.

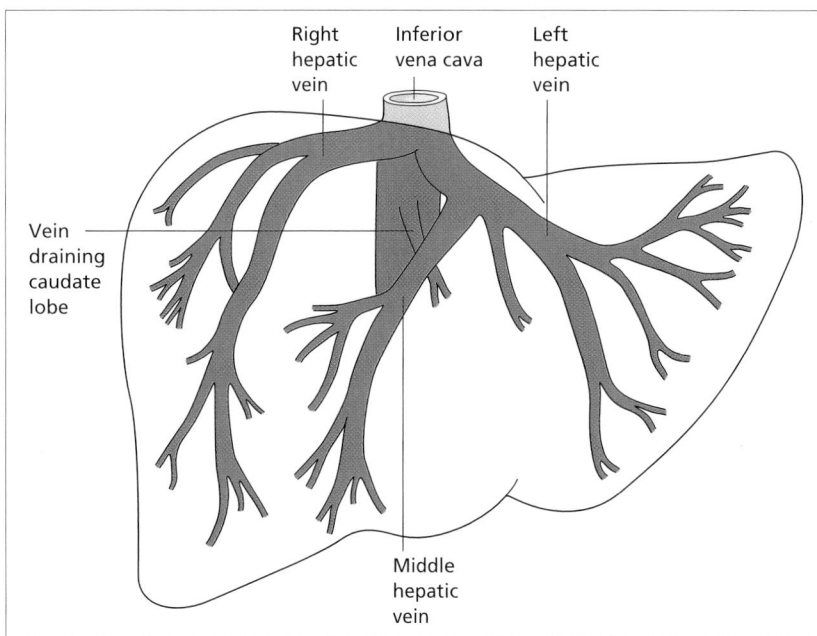

Fig. 11.5. The anatomy of the hepatic venous system. Note separate vein draining the caudate lobe.

Functions

The pressure in the free hepatic vein is approximately 6 mmHg.

The hepatic venous blood is only about 67% saturated with oxygen.

Dogs have muscular hepatic veins near their caval orifices which form a sluice mechanism. The hepatic veins in man have little muscle.

The hepatic venous blood is usually sterile since the liver is a bacterial filter.

Visualizing the hepatic vein

Hepatic venography is performed by slow injection of contrast material into a wedged hepatic vein radicle. This results in filling of the sinusoidal area draining into the catheter and also in retrograde filling of the portal venous system in that area. The portal radicle then carries the contrast medium to other parts of the liver and so other hepatic vein branches become opacified. Cirrhotic nodules and tumour deposits are surrounded by portal vein–hepatic vein anastomoses and may be outlined. In cirrhosis the sinusoidal pattern is coarsened, beady and tortuous, and gnarled hepatic radicles may be seen. The extent of filling of the main portal vein may indicate the extent to which the portal vein has become the outflow tract of the liver.

The hepatic veins may occasionally be seen after selective coeliac or hepatic arteriography, particularly when hepatic arterial blood flow is increased.

Scanning. The main hepatic veins may be visualized by ultrasound, by coloured Doppler imaging, by the enhanced CT scan and by MRI (see fig. 11.14). CT scan without contrast enhancement in a patient with a fatty liver shows excellent hepatic venous anatomy (fig. 11.6).

Experimental hepatic venous obstruction

Individual ligation of all the hepatic veins is impossible. The usual method is to constrict the inferior vena cava by a band placed above the entry of the hepatic veins, and so obstruct the venous return from the liver [4]. Centrizonal (zone 3) haemorrhage and necrosis with fibrosis follow.

The hepatic lymphatics dilate and lymph passes through the capsule of the liver forming ascites with a high protein content.

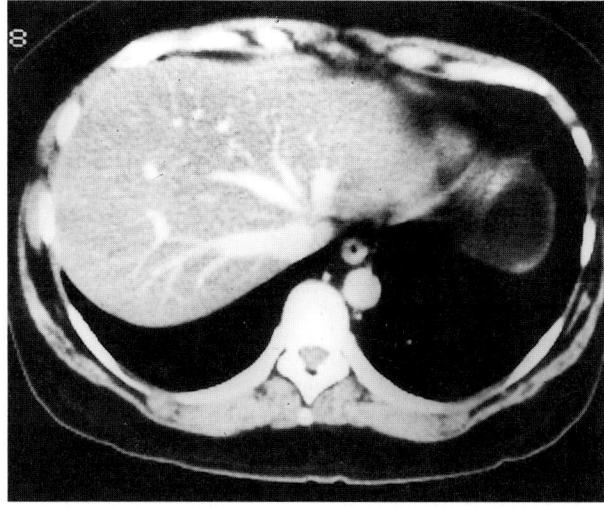

Fig. 11.6. CT scan, without contrast enhancement, in a patient with a fatty liver shows hepatic venous anatomy well.

Budd–Chiari (hepatic venous obstruction) syndrome (fig. 11.7) [9, 42, 44]

This condition is usually associated with the names of Budd and Chiari although Budd's description [5] omitted the features, and Chiari's paper [8] was not the first to report the clinical picture. The syndrome comprises hepatomegaly, abdominal pain, ascites and hepatic histology showing zone 3 sinusoidal distension and pooling. It may arise from obstruction to hepatic veins at any site from the efferent vein of the lobule to the entry of the inferior vena cava into the right atrium (fig. 11.7). A similar syndrome may be produced by constrictive pericarditis or right heart failure.

Myeloproliferative diseases, particularly polycythaemia rubra vera are associated in 60% of cases [45]. These may be overt and diagnosed only by the erythroid bone marrow colony test. The patient is often a young female.

The Budd–Chiari syndrome has been associated with systemic lupus erythematosus [14] and with circulating lupus anticoagulant [35], sometimes with disseminated intravascular coagulation. The antiphospholipid syndrome may be primary or secondary to systemic lupus [34]. Idiopathic granulomatous venulitis is another accompaniment which is treated successfully with corticosteroids [50].

Paroxysmal nocturnal haemoglobinuria may be asso-

ciated, the severity varying from the asymptomatic to a fatal Budd–Chiari syndrome [47].

The Budd–Chiari syndrome is associated with diseases having a deficiency of anticoagulant factors. These include antithrombin III deficiency whether primary or secondary to heavy proteinuria [10], protein S, and protein C deficiency [7]. It may complicate genetically determined resistance to the anticoagulant activated protein C (factor IV: Leiden) [12, 40].

Hepatic vein thrombosis complicating Behçet's disease is a sudden event usually related to extension of a caval thrombus to the osteum of the hepatic veins [1, 2].

There is double the risk in users of oral contraceptives. This is about the same as for other thrombotic complications [46]. Oral contraceptives may act synergistically in those predisposed to clotting.

Hepatic vein thrombosis has been reported in pregnancy [23].

Trauma (usually of blunt abdominal type) is often due to automobile accidents.

The hepatic veins may be mechanically compressed by severe, polycystic liver disease [43].

Obstruction to the inferior vena cava is secondary to thrombosis in malignant disease, for instance an adrenal or renal carcinoma or invasion by a hepato-cellular cancer [41] or angiosarcoma [37]. Rare tumours include leiomyosarcoma of the hepatic veins [27] and testicular lesions metastatic to the right atrium [16]. Wilm's tumour metastases may involve the inferior vena cava and hepatic veins [38].

Myxoma of the right atrium has caused hepatic venous obstruction. Invasion of hepatic veins by masses of aspergillosis has been reported.

Membranous obstruction of the supra-hepatic segment of the inferior vena cava by a web is particularly frequent in Japan and in South Africa and to a lesser extent in India [44]. It may affect children [20]. The web varies from a thin membrane to a thick fibrous band. The occluding and stenosing lesions are probably related to thrombosis and its sequelae [22]. A congenital malformation is unlikely, particularly in view of the presentation in adults.

The Budd–Chiari picture also follows central hepatic vein involvement in the alcoholic and in veno-occlusive disease (Chapter 18).

Liver transplantation may be followed by small hepatic vein stenosis with some of the features of veno-occlusive disease. It is usually associated with azathioprine and with cellular rejection [13].

In about one-quarter the cause remains unknown [9]. The Budd–Chiari syndrome is being diagnosed much more often and in milder forms, probably due to the routine use of imaging, especially ultrasound.

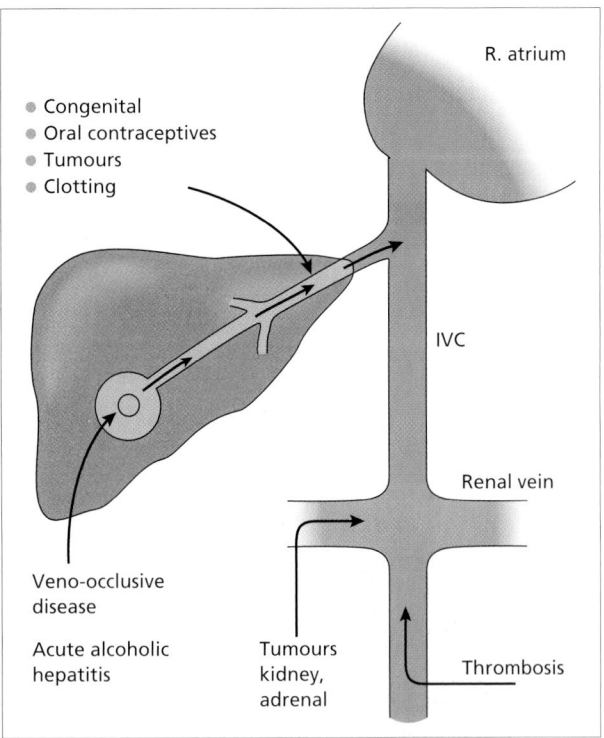

Fig. 11.7. Aetiological factors in the Budd–Chiari syndrome.

Pathological changes

The hepatic veins show occlusion at various points in their course from the ostia to the smaller radicles. Thrombus may have spread from an occluded inferior vena cava. Thrombus filling the veins may be purulent or may contain malignant cells, depending on the cause. In chronic cases, the vein wall is thickened and there may be some recanalization. In others it is replaced by a fibrous strand; a fibrous web may be seen.

Involvement of large hepatic veins is usually thrombotic. Isolated obstruction to the inferior vena cava or small hepatic veins is usually non-thrombotic [26].

The liver is enlarged, purplish and smooth. Venous congestion is gross and the cut surface shows a 'nutmeg' change. Hepatic veins proximal to the obstruction and, in the acute stage, subcapsular lymphatics, are dilated and prominent.

In the chronic case, the caudate lobe is enlarged (fig. 11.8) and compresses the inferior vena cava as it passes posterior to the liver (see fig. 11.12). Areas less affected by obstruction form nodules and nodular regenerative hyperplasia may be seen [11]. The spleen may enlarge and a portal-systemic collateral circulation develop. Mesenteric vessels may thrombose.

Histological sections show zone 3 venous dilatation and congestion with haemorrhage and necrosis (figs 11.9, 11.10). Blood cells in Disse's space could represent an extrasinusoidal circulation, attempting to circumvent the venous obstruction. Peri-portal areas are spared.

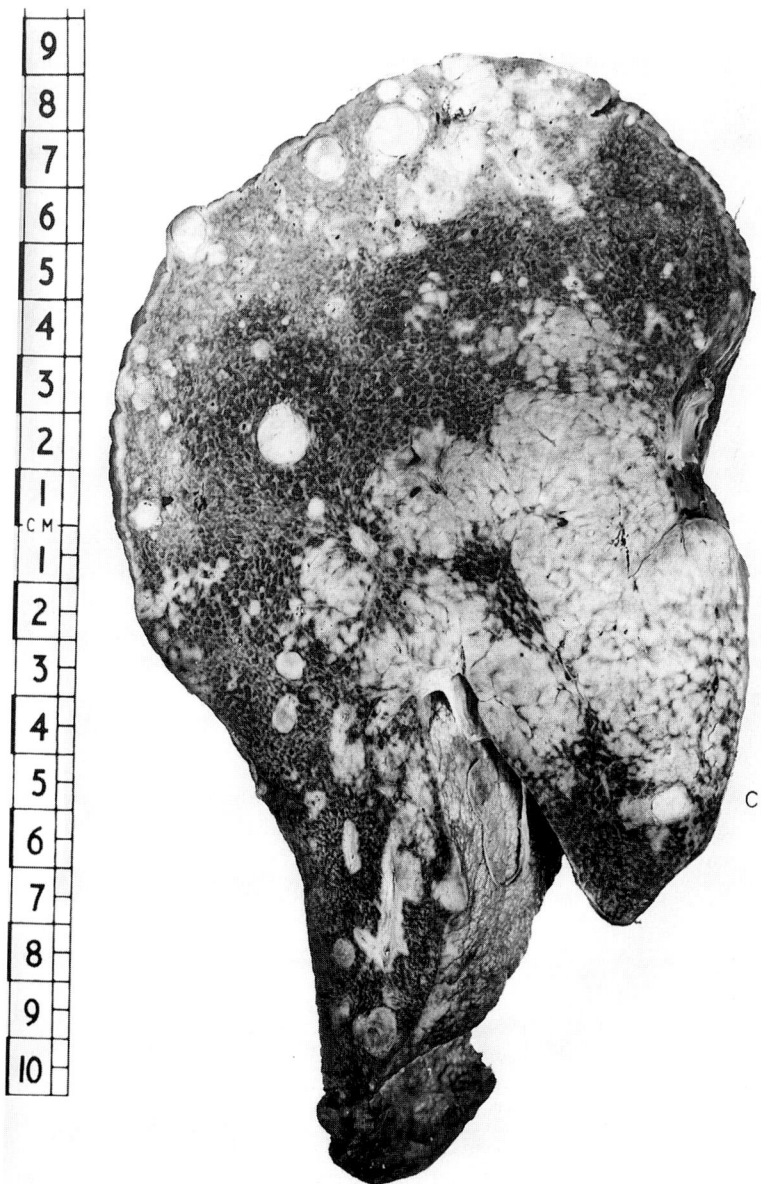

Fig. 11.8. Vertical section of the liver at autopsy in hepatic venous obstruction. The pale areas represent regeneration and the dark areas are congested. Note the marked hypertrophy of the caudate lobe (C).

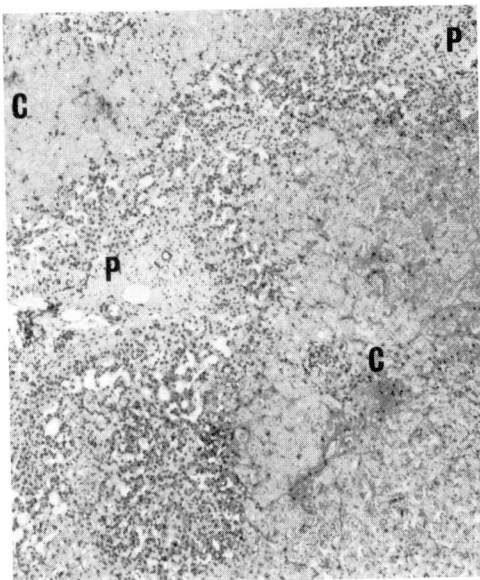

Fig. 11.9. Hepatic venous occlusion (Budd–Chiari syndrome). Hepatic histology shows marked zone 3 haemorrhage (C). The liver cells adjoining the portal zones (P) are spared. (Stained H & E, ×100.)

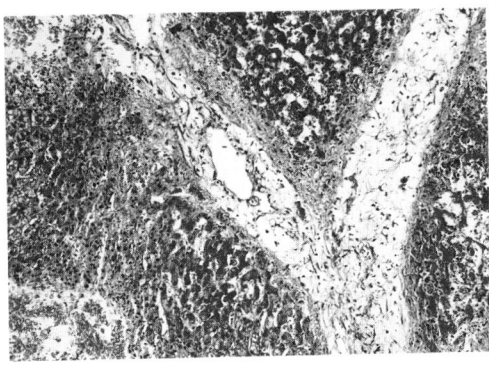

Fig. 11.10. Budd–Chiari syndrome. Longitudinal section of hepatic venules shows fibrosis in lumen, thickening of the wall and surrounding loss of hepatocyte. (Stained chromophobe aniline blue.)

Appearances are indistinguishable from those of any hepatic outflow obstruction, for instance cardiac failure or constrictive pericarditis.

In the later stages, zone 3 fibrosis develops and the picture becomes that of cardiac cirrhosis.

Clinical features

These depend on the speed of occlusion and the extent of the hepatic venous involvement. The picture varies all the way from a fulminant course, the patient presenting as encephalopathy and dying within 2–3 weeks, to presentation as chronic hepato-cellular disease, slowly developing and causing confusion with other forms of cirrhosis.

In the most *acute form* the picture is of an ill patient, often suffering from some other condition—for instance renal carcinoma, hepato-cellular cancer, thrombophlebitis migrans or polycythaemia. The presentation is with abdominal pain, vomiting, liver enlargement, ascites and mild icterus. Watery diarrhoea, following mesenteric venous obstruction, is a terminal, inconstant feature. If the hepatic venous occlusion is total, delirium and coma with hepato-cellular failure and death occurs within a few days.

In the more usual *chronic form* the patient presents with pain over an enlarged tender liver and ascites developing over 1–6 months. Jaundice is mild or absent, unless zone 3 necrosis is marked. Pressure over the liver may fail to fill the jugular vein (negative *hepato-jugular reflux*). As portal hypertension increases, the spleen becomes palpable. The enlarged caudate lobe, palpable in the epigastrium, may simulate a tumour.

Asymptomatic patients may have no ascites, hepatomegaly or abdominal pain [19]. Hepatic outflow is diagnosed fortuitously, either by imaging or by the investigation of abnormal liver function tests. It may be explained by remaining patency of one large hepatic vein or development of a large venous collateral.

If the inferior vena cava is blocked, oedema of the legs is gross and veins distend over the abdomen, flanks and back. Albuminuria is found.

The condition may develop over months as ascites and wasting.

Biochemical. Serum bilirubin rarely exceeds 2 mg/100 ml (34 μmol/l). The serum alkaline phosphatase level is raised and the albumin value reduced. Serum transaminase values increase and if very high concomitant blockage of the portal vein is suggested. The prothrombin time is markedly increased especially in the acute type. Hypoproteinaemia may be due to protein-losing enteropathy.

The protein content of the ascites should, theoretically, be high, but this is not always so.

Needle liver biopsy is essential. Speckled zone 3 areas can be distinguished from the pale portal areas. Histologically, the picture is of zone 3 congestion (figs 11.9, 11.10). Alcoholic hepatitis or phlebitis of the hepatic veins should be noted.

Hepatic venography may fail or show narrow occluded hepatic veins. Adjacent veins show a tortuous, lace-like spider-web pattern (fig. 11.11) [9]. This probably represents abnormal venous collaterals. The catheter cannot be advanced the usual distance along the hepatic vein and wedges 2–12 cm from the diaphragm.

Inferior vena cavography, both from above, via the right atrium, or below, via the femoral vein, or both, establishes the patency of the inferior vena cava. The hepatic

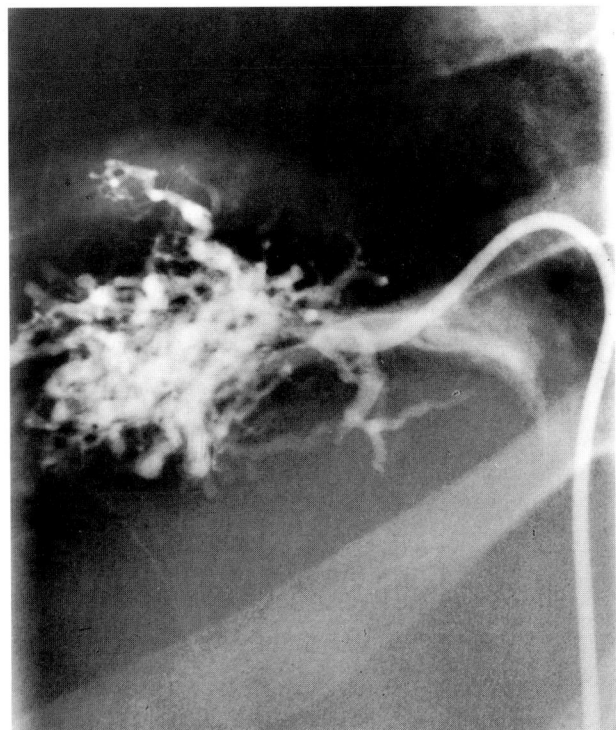

Fig. 11.11. Hepatic venogram in a patient with Budd–Chiari syndrome. Note lace-like spider-web pattern [9].

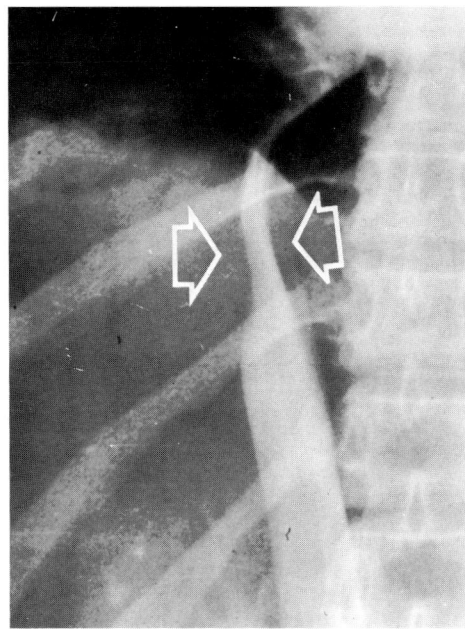

Fig. 11.12. Inferior venacavogram. Antero-posterior view showing side-to-side narrowing and distortion of the inferior vena cava (arrows). Extrinsic compression from the left is due to an enlarged caudate lobe [42].

segment may show side-to-side narrowing due to distortion from the enlarged caudate lobe (fig. 11.12). Pressure measurements should be taken in the inferior vena cava along its length to confirm its patency and to quantify the extent of any membranous or caudate lobe obstruction.

Selective coeliac arteriography. The hepatic artery appears small and the branches are of fine calibre. They appear stretched and displaced, producing the appearance of multiple space-occupying lesions simulating metastases [21]. The venous phase shows delayed emptying of the portal venous bed.

Ultrasound. This is the best method for emergency diagnosis. It shows hepatic vein abnormalities, caudate lobe hypertrophy, increased reflectivity and compression of the inferior vena cava. The appearances are hypoechogenic in the early stages of acute thrombosis and hyperechogenic with fibrosis in the later stages. Ascites is confirmed.

Pulsed Doppler sonography shows abnormalities in the direction of flow in hepatic vein and retro-hepatic inferior vena cava. The blood flow in the inferior vena cava and hepatic veins may be absent, reversed, turbulent or continuous. Colour Doppler imaging shows abnormalities in hepatic veins, portal vein and inferior vena cava and correlates well with venographic appearances [29].

Detection of intra-hepatic collateral vessels is important in the distinction from cirrhosis or where hepatic veins are inconspicuous on ultrasound [29].

CT scan (fig. 11.13) shows enlargement of the liver with diffuse hypodensity before and patchy enhancement after contrast. Heterogeneous hepatic parenchymal patterns are related to regional differences in portal flow [48]. Areas with complete hepatic vein obstruction remain hypodense after contrast probably due to portal flow inversion. Subcapsular areas may enhance.

In the unenhanced scan, the caudate lobe appears dense with surrounding underperfused parenchyma (fig. 11.13).

Thrombi in the inferior vena cava and/or hepatic vein may be seen as intraluminal filling defects that are not changed by contrast [30].

The CT appearances are easily confused with those of hepatic metastases.

MRI shows absence of normal hepatic venous drainage into the inferior vena cava, collateral hepatic veins and signal intensity alterations in the hepatic parenchyma [17] (fig. 11.14). The caudate lobe can be seen deforming the inferior vena cava.

Diagnosis

The condition should be suspected if a patient with a tendency to thrombosis, or with malignant disease in or near the liver, or on oral contraceptives, develops tender hepatomegaly with ascites. Diagnosis, prognosis and

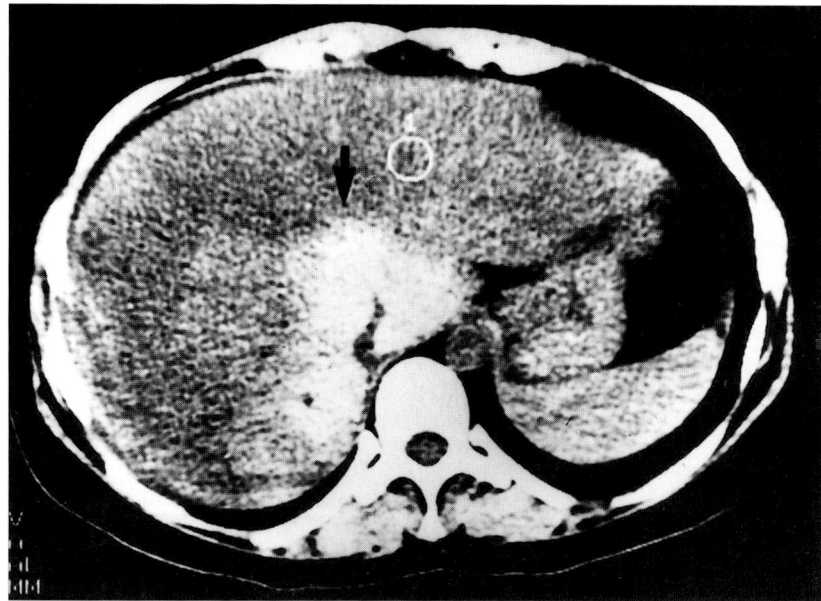

Fig. 11.13. CT scan (unenhanced) shows caudate lobe (arrow) with surrounding underperfused parenchyma.

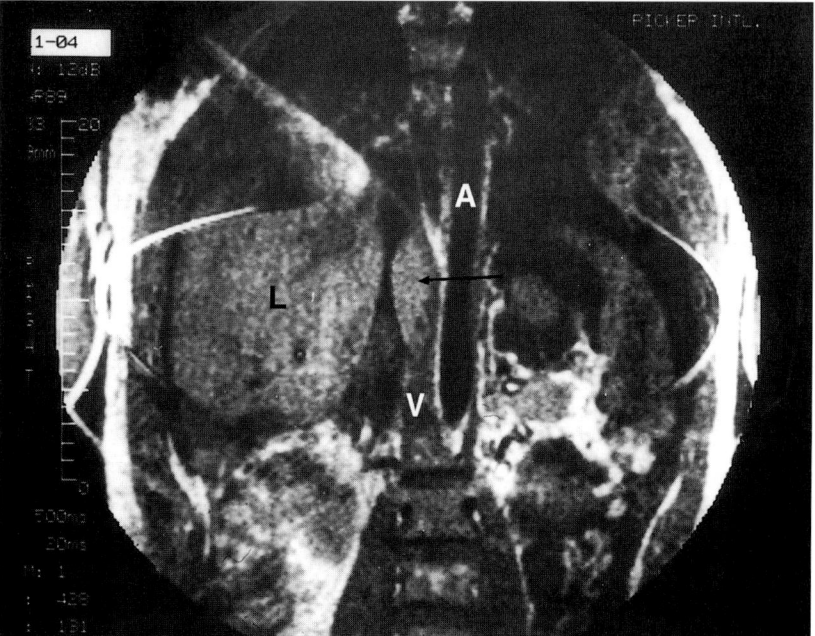

Fig. 11.14. Magnetic resonance scan in a patient with the Budd–Chiari syndrome shows a liver (L) which is dyshomogeneous, the aorta (A) and the inferior vena cava (V). The enlarged caudate lobe (arrow) is causing side-to-side narrowing of the inferior vena cava.

correct treatment are only possible if the block is localized by radiological and scanning techniques.

Heart failure and constrictive pericarditis must be excluded. Tense ascites *per se* can elevate the jugular venous pressure and displace the cardiac apex. Atrial myxoma may cause confusion.

Cirrhosis must be distinguished and liver biopsy is helpful. The ascitic fluid protein content is usually lower in cirrhosis.

Portal vein thrombosis rarely leads to ascites. Jaundice is absent and the liver is not very large.

Inferior vena caval thrombosis results in distended abdominal wall veins but without ascites. If the renal vein is occluded, albuminuria is gross. Hepatic venous and inferior vena caval thrombosis may, however, coexist.

Hepatic metastases are distinguished clinically and by the liver biopsy.

Prognosis

In the acute form, death in hepatic coma usually results. Thrombosis may spread to the portal and mesenteric veins with infarction of the bowel. In the more chronic and localized instances response to symptomatic therapy may allow prolongation of life for a few years [9].

Prognosis depends on the aetiology, on the extent of the occlusion and whether it can be corrected. Clotting diseases such as polycythaemia are usually found with multiple thrombosis of vessels of varying sizes. The inferior vena cava and portal vein may also be involved.

Haemorrhage from oesophageal varices is usually terminal.

Chronic cases may survive many months or even years and up to 22 years has been recorded.

Medical treatment is usually effective only for short periods.

Treatment

The value of fibrinolytic therapy in the early stages is uncertain. Later, anticoagulants may be used in those with underlying thrombosing disease.

In those with polycythaemia or thrombocytosis the haemoglobin and platelet count should be reduced by venesection and cytotoxic drugs.

Ascites is treated with a low sodium diet, diuretics and paracentesis. Severe cases demand ever-increasing doses of potent diuretics and eventually the patient is overtaken by inanition and renal failure. 17 of 19 patients treated with diet and diuretics were dead within 3.5 years [42]. Some milder cases, however, respond slowly and require less treatment with time. The peritoneo-jugular (Le Veen) shunt may be useful in some patients, although the shunt often clogs up.

The timing of surgery is difficult. On the one hand, some re-vascularization may continue. On the other, the long-term results of medical therapy are, in general, so poor that as time passes the patient's chances of surviving major surgery become less.

Surgical portal-systemic shunts

These are considered in patients with symptomatic Budd–Chiari syndrome who have a patent portal vein. The aim is to decompress the congested liver and reverse portal venous flow so allowing the portal vein to serve as an outflow channel.

Shunts are indicated only if there is no hepatic encephalopathy and hepatic synthetic function is preserved [39]. Results on the whole are unsatisfactory due to thrombosis of the shunt, especially in those with haematological disorders. In those whose shunt remains patent, 5-year actuarial survival rate is 87% falling to 38% if the shunt thromboses [33]. Thrombosis is more likely in long-standing cases.

Portal-systemic shunts are usually followed by slow deterioration of liver function making the patient a candidate for liver transplant [39].

The enlarged caudate lobe increases pressure in the infra-hepatic inferior vena cava so that it may exceed the portal venous pressure. If the pressure in the inferior vena cava exceeds 20 mmHg shunting is precluded [24]. The anatomic bulk of the caudate lobe makes a technical approach to the portal vein difficult. The shunt may stand a better chance of staying patent if the obstruction from the caudate lobe is first relieved by inserting, preoperatively and percutaneously, an expandable wire stent in the inferior vena cava [18].

If the portal vein is also occluded, shunts will not function. Transplantation becomes possible only if the mesenteric vein is patent.

Side-to-side porta-caval anastomosis. This has proved reliable and effective but may offer technical difficulties [32].

Meso-caval interposition shunt. This has given good results in some hands and does not affect a subsequent hepatic transplantation.

Meso-atrial shunt. This is used when the inferior vena cava is obstructed. The shunt is made between the super-

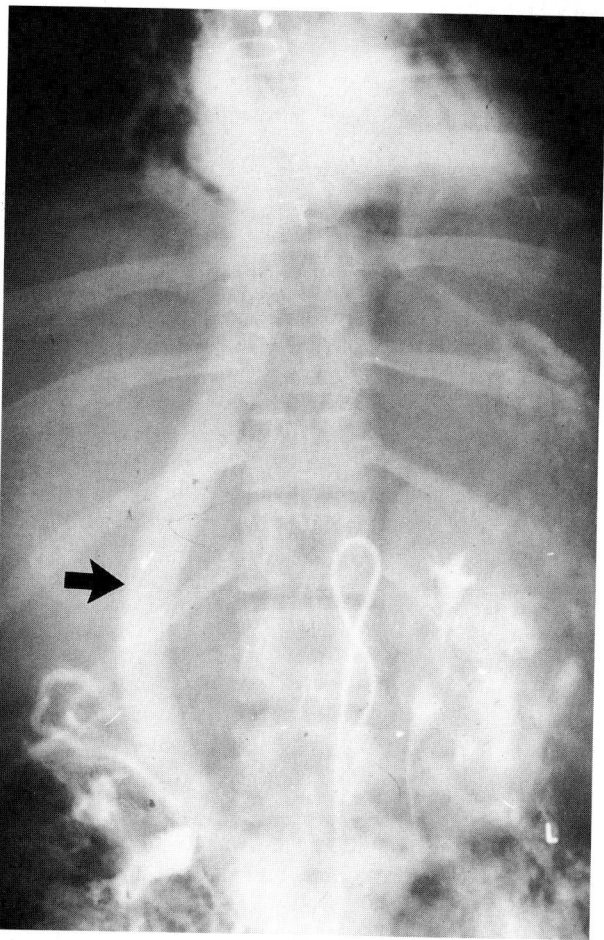

Fig. 11.15. Budd–Chiari syndrome. Surgical relief by meso-atrial stent (arrow).

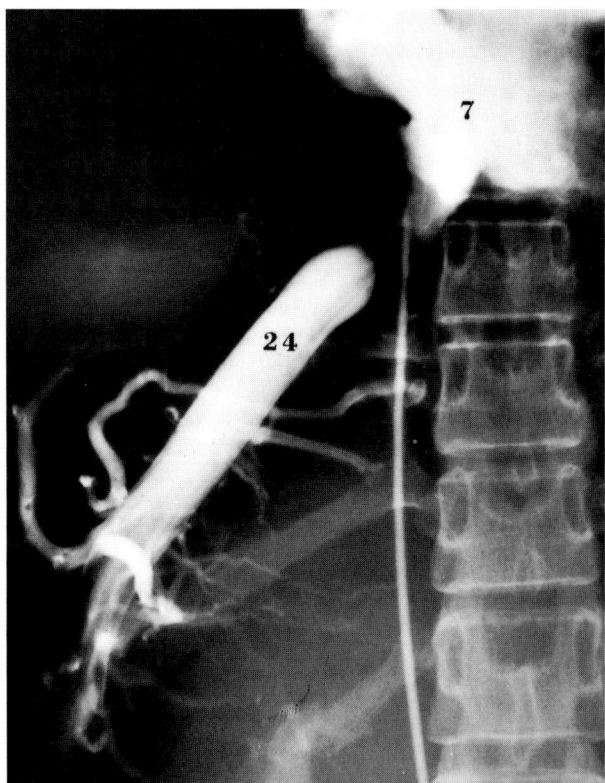

Fig. 11.16. Hepatic venogram in a patient with the Budd–Chiari syndrome due to obstruction of the right main hepatic vein. Right hepatic venous pressure 24 mmHg distal to the obstruction and 7 mmHg proximal to it. (Courtesy D.S. Zimmon.)

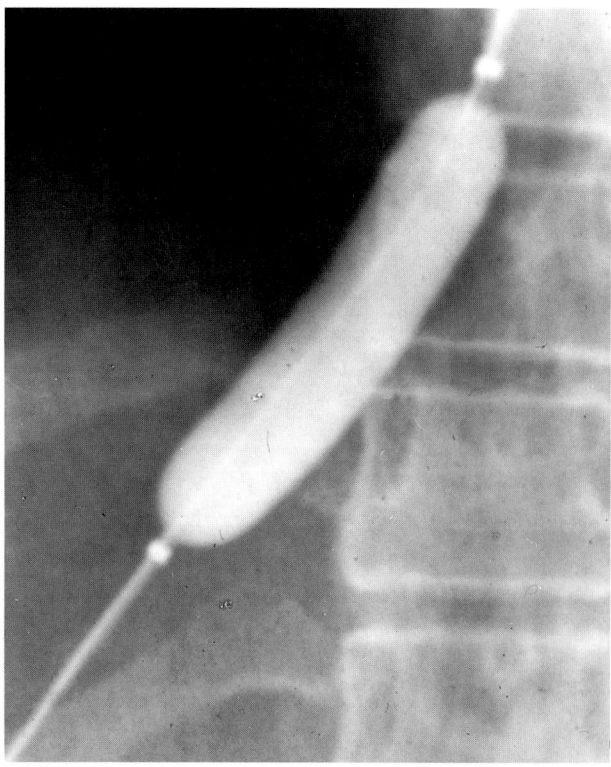

Fig. 11.17. Same patient as in fig. 11.16. A balloon inflated in the right hepatic vein is dilating the stricture.

ior mesenteric vein and the right atrium using a prosthetic graft (fig. 11.15) [24].

Trans-atrial membranotomy. Webs may be surgically corrected, either by resection or by fracturing with the finger.

Transjugular intra-hepatic portal-systemic shunt (TIPS) is technically feasible if the hepatic vein can be entered [31]. It may be useful in acute hepatic-vein thrombosis. In Budd–Chiari syndrome the shunt has an increased risk of later thrombosis.

Percutaneous transluminal angioplasty

This has been used to dilate webs (figs 11.16, 11.17, 11.18) and also for hepatic vein obstruction after liver transplant [51]. It is particularly useful if the supra-hepatic portion of the inferior vena cava is involved. Multiple dilatations are usually necessary [28]. Intravascular metallic stents may be introduced after the dilatation [49]. Stents are usually reserved for those in whom angioplasty has failed.

Balloon dilatation is particularly valuable if the inferior vena cava is obstructed [25].

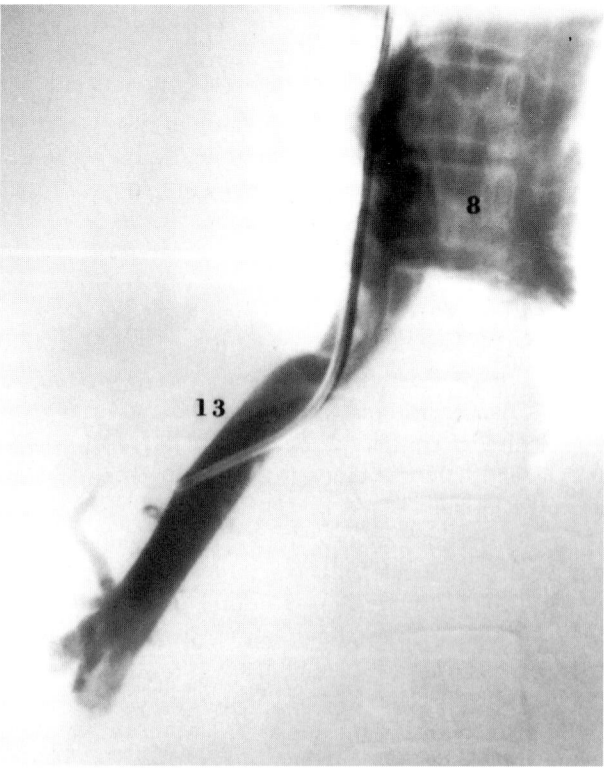

Fig. 11.18. Dilatation of the stricture in the right hepatic vein has resulted in a fall in distal right hepatic venous pressure to 13 mmHg while the pressure proximally is 8 mmHg.

Hepatic transplantation

This is usually indicated when medical treatment and angioplasty have failed. The patient has end-stage liver disease. The main difficulty is the underlying thrombotic condition which favours recurrence. Early post-operative anticoagulation is essential [3, 6]. Results are similar to those of portal-systemic surgical shunting for other conditions. 1-year actuarial survival is 86% and the 3-year survival 76% [39]. The preferred surgical approach must be integrated and based on the leading symptom. Venous decompression is indicated for predominant portal hypertension and transplant for predominant liver failure [36].

Veno-occlusive disease

See Chapter 18.

Spread of disease by the hepatic veins

The hepatic veins link the portal and systemic venous systems. Malignant disease of the liver is spread by the hepatic veins to the lungs and hence to other parts. Liver abscesses can burst into the hepatic vein and metastatic abscesses may result. Parasitic disease, including amoebiasis, hydatid disease and schistosomiasis, is spread by this route. The porto-hepatic venous anastomoses developing in cirrhosis may allow intestinal organisms to cause septicaemia.

References

1 Bayraktar Y, Balkanci F, Kansu E *et al.* Budd-Chiari syndrome: analysis of 30 cases. *Angiology* 1993; **44**: 541.

2 Bismuth E, Hadengue A, Hammel P *et al.* Hepatic vein thrombosis in Behçet's disease. *Hepatology* 1990; **11**: 969.

3 Bismuth H, Sherlock DJ. Portasystemic shunting versus liver transplantation for the Budd–Chiari syndrome. *Ann. Surg.* 1991; **214**: 581.

4 Bolton C, Barnard WG. The pathological occurrences in the liver in experimental venous stagnation. *J. Path Bact.* 1931; **34**: 701.

5 Budd G. *On Diseases of the Liver*, 3rd edn. Blanchard & Lea, Philadelphia, 1857.

6 Campbell DA Jr, Rolles K, Jamieson N *et al.* Hepatic transplantation with perioperative and longterm anticoagulation as treatment for Budd–Chiari syndrome. *Surg. Gynecol. Obstet.* 1988; **166**: 511.

7 Casella JF, Bontempo FA, Markel H *et al.* Successful treatment of homozygous protein C deficiency by hepatic transplantation. *Lancet* 1988; **i**: 435.

8 Chiari H. Ueber die selbständige Phlebitis obliterans der Hauptstämme der Venae hepaticae als Todesurache. *Beitr. Path. Anat.* 1899; **26**: 1.

9 Clain D, Freston J, Kreel L *et al.* Clinical diagnosis of the Budd–Chiari syndrome. *Am. J. Med.* 1967; **43**: 544.

10 Das M, Carroll SF. Antithrombin III deficiency: an etiology

of Budd–Chiari syndrome. *Surgery* 1985; **97**: 242.

11 De Sousa JMM, Portmann B, Williams R, Nodular regenerative hyperplasia of the liver and the Budd–Chiari syndrome. *J. Hepatol.* 1991; **12**: 28.

12 Denninger MH, Beldjord K, Durand F *et al.* Budd–Chiari syndrome and factor V Leiden mutation. *Lancet* 1995; **345**: 525 (letter).

13 Dhillon AP, Burroughs AK, Hudson M *et al.* Hepatic venular stenosis after orthotopic liver transplantation. *Hepatology* 1994; **19**: 106.

14 Disney TF, Sullivan SN, Haddad RG *et al.* Budd–Chiari syndrome with inferior vena cava obstruction associated with systemic lupus erythematosus. *J. Clin. Gastroenterol.* 1984; **6**: 253.

15 Dodds WJ, Erickson SJ, Taylor AJ *et al.* Caudate lobe of the liver: anatomy, embryology, and pathology. *Am. J. Roentgenol.* 1990; **154**: 87.

16 Feingold ML, Litwak RL, Geller SS *et al.* Budd–Chiari syndrome caused by a right atrial tumor. *Arch. Intern. Med.* 1971; **127**: 292.

17 Friedman AC, Ramchandani P, Black M *et al.* Magnetic resonance imaging diagnosis of Budd–Chiari syndrome. *Gastroenterology* 1986; **91**: 1289.

18 Gillams A, Dick R, Platts A *et al.* Dilatation of the inferior vena cava using an expandable metal stent in Budd–Chiari syndrome. *J. Hepatol.* 1991; **13**: 149.

19 Hadengue A, Poliquin M, Vilgrain V *et al.* The changing scene of hepatic vein thrombosis: recognition of asymptomatic cases. *Gastroenterology* 1994; **106**: 1042.

20 Hoffman H du P, Stockland B, von der Heyden U. Membranous obstruction of the inferior vena cava with Budd–Chiari syndrome in children: a report of nine cases. *J. Pediat. Gastroenterol. Nutr.* 1987; **6**: 878.

21 Hungerford GD, Hamlyn AN, Lunzer MR *et al.* Pseudometastases in the liver: a presentation of the Budd–Chiari syndrome. *Radiology* 1976; **120**: 627.

22 Kage M, Arakawa M, Kojiro M *et al.* Histopathology of membranous obstruction of the inferior vena cava in the Budd–Chiari syndrome. *Gastroenterology* 1992; **102**: 2081.

23 Khuroo MS, Datta DV. Budd–Chiari syndrome following pregnancy. Report of 16 cases with roentgenologic, hemodynamic and histologic studies of the hepatic outflow tract. *Am. J. Med.* 1980; **68**: 113.

24 Klein AS, Sitzmann JV, Coleman J *et al.* Current management of the Budd–Chiari syndrome. *Ann. Surg.* 1990; **212**: 144.

25 Kohli V, Pande GK, Dev W *et al.* Management of hepatic venous outflow obstruction. *Lancet* 1993; **342**: 718.

26 Ludwig J, Hashimoto E, McGill DB *et al.* Classification of hepatic venous outflow obstruction: ambiguous terminology of the Budd–Chiari syndrome. *Mayo Clin. Proc.* 1990; **65**: 51.

27 McMahon HE, Ball HG III. Leiomyosarcoma of hepatic vein and the Budd–Chiari syndrome. *Gastroenterology* 1971; **61**: 239.

28 Martin LG, Henderson JM, Millikan WJ Jr *et al.* Angioplasty for long-term treatment of patients with Budd–Chiari syndrome. *Am. J. Roentgenol.* 1990; **154**: 1007.

29 Millener P, Grant EG, Rose S *et al.* Color Doppler imaging findings in patients with Budd–Chiari syndrome: correlation with venographic findings. *Am. J. Roentgenol.* 1993; **161**: 307.

30 Mori H, Maeda H, Fukuda T *et al.* Acute thrombosis of

the inferior vena cava and hepatic veins in patients with Budd–Chiari syndrome: CT demonstration. *Am. J. Roentgenol.* 1989; **153**: 987.

31 Ochs A, Sellinger M, Haag K *et al.* Transjugular intrahepatic portosystemic stent-shunt in the treatment of Budd–Chiari syndrome. *J. Hepatol.* 1993; **18**: 217.

32 Orloff MJ, Girard B. Long-term results of treatment of Budd–Chiari syndrome by side to side portacaval shunt. *Surg. Gynecol. Obstet.* 1989; **168**: 33.

33 Panis Y, Belghiti J, Valla D *et al.* Portosystemic shunt in Budd–Chiari syndrome: long-term survival and factors affecting shunt patency in 25 patients in Western countries. *Surgery* 1994; **115**: 276.

34 Pelletier S, Landi B, Piette J-C *et al.* Antiphospholipid syndrome as the second cause of non-tumorous Budd–Chiari syndrome. *J. Hepatol.* 1994; **21**: 76.

35 Pomeroy C, Knodell RG, Swaim WR *et al.* Budd–Chiari syndrome in a patient with the lupus anticoagulant. *Gastroenterology* 1984; **86**: 158.

36 Ringe B, Lang H, Oldhafer K-J *et al.* Which is the best surgery for Budd–Chiari syndrome: venous decompression or liver transplantation? A single-center experience with 50 patients. *Hepatology* 1995; **21**: 1337.

37 Schluger LK, Cubukcu O, Klion F *et al.* Unexplained Budd–Chiari syndrome in a young man. *Hepatology* 1995; **21**: 584.

38 Schraut WH, Chilcote RR. Metastatic Wilm's tumor causing acute hepatic-vein occlusion (Budd–Chiari syndrome). *Gastroenterology* 1985; **88**: 576.

39 Shaked A, Goldstein RM, Klintmalm GB *et al.* Portosystemic shunt versus orthotopic liver transplantation for the Budd–Chiari syndrome. *Surg. Gynecol. Obstet.* 1992; **174**: 453.

40 Svensson PJ, Dahlback B. Resistance to activated protein C as a basis for venous thrombosis. *N. Engl. J. Med.* 1994; **330**: 517.

41 Takayasu K, Muramatsu Y, Moriyama N *et al.* Radiological study of idiopathic Budd–Chiari syndrome complicated by hepatocellular carcinoma. A report of four cases. *Am. J. Gastroenterol.* 1994; **88**: 249.

42 Tavill AS, Wood EJ, Kreel L *et al.* The Budd–Chiari syndrome: correlation between hepatic scintigraphy and the clinical, radiological and pathological findings in nineteen cases of hepatic venous outflow obstruction. *Gastroenterology* 1975; **68**: 509.

43 Uddin W, Ramage JK, Portmann B *et al.* Hepatic venous outflow obstruction in patients with polycystic liver disease: pathogenesis and treatment. *Gut* 1995; **36**: 142.

44 Valla D, Benhamou J-P. Obstruction of the hepatic veins or supra-hepatic inferior vena cava. *Dig. Dis.* 1996; **14**: 99.

45 Valla D, Casadevall N, Lacombe C *et al.* Primary myeloproliferative disorder and hepatic vein thrombosis: a prospective study of erythroid colony formation *in vitro* in 20 patients with Budd–Chiari syndrome. *Ann. Intern. Med.* 1985; **103**: 329.

46 Valla D, Le MG, Poynard T *et al.* Risk of hepatic vein thrombosis in relation to recent use of oral contraceptives: a case–control study. *Gastroenterology* 1986; **90**: 807.

47 Valla D, Dhumeaux D, Babany G *et al.* Hepatic vein thrombosis in paroxysmal nocturnal hemoglobinuria. *Gastroenterology* 1987; **93**: 569.

48 Van Beers B, Pringot J, Trigaux JP *et al.* Hepatic heterogeneity on CT in Budd–Chiari syndrome: correlation with regional disturbances in portal flow. *Gastrointest. Radiol.* 1988; **13**: 61.

49 Venbrux AC, Savader SJ, Mitchell SE *et al*: Interventional management of Budd–Chiari syndrome. *Semin. Intervent. Radiol.* 1994; **11**: 312.

50 Young ID, Clark RN, Manley PN *et al.* Response to steroids in Budd–Chiari syndrome caused by idiopathic granulomatous venulitis. *Gastroenterology* 1988; **94**: 503.

51 Zajko AB, Claus D, Clapuyt P *et al.* Obstruction to hepatic venous drainage after liver transplantation: treatment with balloon angioplasty. *Radiology* 1989; **170**: 763.

Circulatory failure

A rise in pressure in the right atrium is readily transmitted to the hepatic veins. Liver cells are particularly vulnerable to diminished oxygen supply, so that a failing heart, lowered blood pressure or reduced hepatic blood flow are reflected in impaired hepatic function. The left lobe of the liver may suffer more than the right.

Hepatic changes in acute heart failure and shock

Hepatic changes are common in acute heart failure and in shock due to trauma, burns, haemorrhage, sepsis, peritonitis or black water fever. Similar ischaemic changes follow cessation of hepatic blood flow during the course of hepatic transplantation or tumour resection [13].

Some patients show mild icterus. Jaundice has been recorded in severely traumatized patients. Serum transaminase levels increase markedly and the prothrombin time rises.

Light microscopy shows a congested zone 3 with local haemorrhage (fig. 11.19). Focal necrosis with eosinophilic hepatocytes, hydropic change and polymorph infiltration is usual. Mid-zonal necrosis may be due to tangential section cutting but in some instances is unexplained. The reticulin framework is preserved within the necrotic zone. With recovery, particularly after trauma, mitoses may be prominent. Diffuse hepatic calcification can follow shock [33]. This might be related to the disturbance of intra-cellular Ca^{2+} homeostasis as a result of ischaemic liver injury. It has been reported in a patient with cardiac ischaemia and chronic renal failure having a high calcium-phosphate product [25].

Mechanisms of the hepatic changes

The changes can be related to the duration of the shock. The fall in blood pressure leads to reduction in liver blood flow and hepatic arterial vasoconstriction. The oxygen content of the blood is reduced. The cells in zone 3 receive blood at a lower oxygen tension than the peripheral cells and therefore more readily become anoxic and necrotic. Intense selective splanchnic vaso-

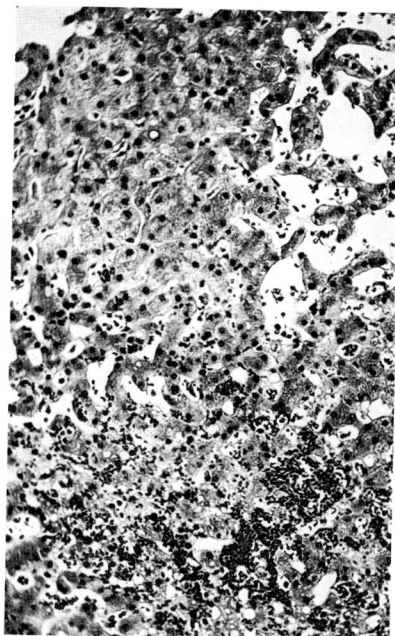

Fig. 11.19. Coronary thrombosis. Serum bilirubin 2.1 mg/100 ml. Liver cells have disappeared from zone 3 and are replaced by frank haemorrhage. (Stained H & E, ×120.)

constriction follows, perhaps in response to endogenous release of angiotensin II [4].

The hepatocyte injury is largely due to lack of oxygen. Insufficient substrates and accumulation of metabolites contribute. The mechanisms are multiple. The absence of available oxygen results in loss of mitochondrial oxidative phosphorylation. Impaired membrane function and reduced protein synthesis contribute [13]. There are alterations in hepato-cellular ion homeostasis [2]. Much of the tissue damage develops during reperfusion, when there is a large flux of oxygen-derived 'free' radicles [36]. These initiate lipid peroxidation with disruption of membrane integrity. Experimentally, superoxide, formed during reperfusion, may combine with nitric oxide (NO) to cause hepato-cellular injury [21]. Free radical peroxynitrate may be responsible. Lysosomal membranes may be peroxidized with the release of enzymes into the cytoplasm. Treatment is unsatisfactory. 'Free' radicle trapping agents such as vitamin E, glutathione and ascorbic acid are being evaluated.

Ischaemic hepatitis

This term is defined as marked and rapid elevation of serum transaminases in the setting of an acute fall in cardiac output [10]. *Acute hepatic infarction* or *hypoxic hepatitis* are alternative definitions. The picture simulates acute virus hepatitis.

The patient usually suffers from cardiac disease, often ischaemic or a cardiomyopathy. It is particularly fre-

quent in patients in coronary care units where it affects 22% of those with a low cardiac output, a decreased hepatic blood flow and passive venous congestion [14]. Zone 3 necrosis without inflammation, results. Clinical evidence of hepatic failure is absent. Congestive cardiac failure is inconspicuous. It may be associated with renal impairment and hyperglycaemia [11].

Severe arterial hypoxaemia due to obstructive sleep apnoea may be causative [24].

Serum bilirubin and alkaline phosphatase values increase slightly, but serum transaminases and lactic dehydrogenase values rise rapidly and strikingly [15]. Values return speedily towards recovery in less than 1 week. Mortality is high (58.6%) and depends on the underlying cause and not the liver injury [15]. If the liver has been previously damaged by chronic congestive heart failure, acute circulatory failure may lead to the picture of fulminant hepatic failure [27].

Post-operative jaundice

Jaundice developing *soon* after surgery may have multiple causes [17]. Increased serum bilirubin follows blood transfusion, particularly of stored blood. Extravasated blood in the tissues gives an additional bilirubin load.

Impaired hepato-cellular function follows operation, anaesthetics and shock. Severe jaundice develops in approximately 2% of patients with shock resulting from major trauma [28]. Hepatic perfusion is reduced particularly if the patient is in incipient circulatory failure and the cardiac output is already reduced. Renal blood flow also falls.

Halothane anaesthetics and other drugs used in the operative period must also be considered. Sepsis, *per se*, can produce deep jaundice which may be cholestatic.

Rarely a *cholestatic jaundice* may be noted on the first or second post-operative day. It reaches its height between the fourth and tenth day, and disappears by 14–18 days. Serum biochemical changes are variable. Sometimes, but not always, the alkaline phosphatase and transaminase levels are increased. Serum bilirubin can rise to levels of 23–39 mg/100 ml. The picture simulates extra-hepatic biliary obstruction. Patients have all had an episode of shock, and have been transfused. Zone 3 hepatic necrosis, however, is not conspicuous and hepatic histology shows only minor abnormalities. The mechanism of the cholestasis is uncertain. This picture must be recognized [17] and, if necessary, needle biopsy of the liver performed.

Severely ill patients in intensive care following severe trauma or post-operative intra-abdominal sepsis may develop jaundice, which reflects severe multiple organ failure and a poor prognosis [34]. The jaundice is usually of cholestatic type with raised conjugated serum bilirubin and alkaline phosphatase levels and only slightly increased transaminases.

Experimentally bile flow falls following haemorrhagic shock. Endotoxaemia and sepsis may activate inflammatory mediators leading to vascular damage, increased permeability and oedema and impaired oxygen transport [5].

Jaundice after cardiac surgery

Jaundice is frequent and develops in 20% of patients having cardio-pulmonary bypass surgery [6, 7]. It carries a bad prognosis. The jaundice is detected by the second post-operative day. Serum bilirubin is conjugated suggesting failure of canalicular biliary excretion and the level returns to normal in 2–4 weeks in those who survive. Serum alkaline phosphatase may be normal or only slightly increased and transaminases are raised, often to very high levels. Older patients are particularly at risk. Jaundice is significantly associated with multiple valve replacement, high blood transfusion requirements and a longer bypass time.

Many factors contribute. The liver may have already suffered from prolonged heart failure. Operative hypotension, shock and hypothermia contribute. Infections, drugs (including anticoagulants) and anaesthetics must be considered.

Liver blood flow drops by about 20% [12]. The serum bilirubin load is increased by blood transfusion. The pump may contribute by decreasing erythrocyte survival and by adding gaseous micro-emboli and platelet aggregates and debris to the circulation.

Virus B and C hepatitis are rare since blood donors have been screened. Cytomegalovirus hepatitis may develop after cardiac surgery.

Post-cardiac surgery tamponade may mimic acute hepatitis [29].

The liver in congestive heart failure

Pathological changes [20]

Hepatic autolysis is particularly rapid in the patient dying with heart failure [31]. Autopsy material is therefore unreliable for the assessment of the effects of cardiac failure on the liver in life.

Macroscopic changes. The liver is usually enlarged, and purplish with rounded edges. Nodularity is inconspicuous but nodular masses of hepatocytes (nodular regenerative hyperplasia) may be seen. The cut surface (fig. 11.20) shows prominent hepatic veins which may be thickened. The liver drips blood. Zone 3 is prominent with alternation of yellow (fatty change) and red (haemorrhage) areas.

Histological changes. The hepatic venule is always

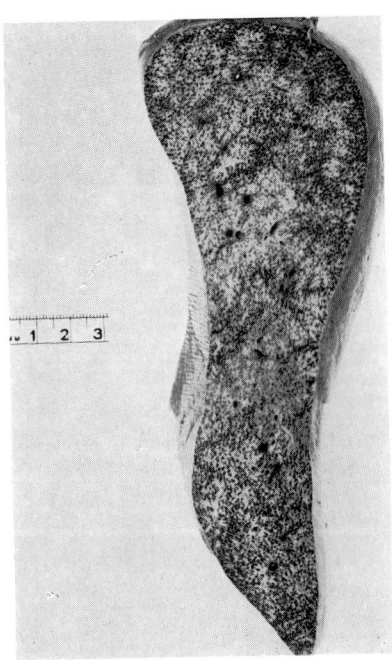

Fig. 11.20. Cut surface of the liver from a patient dying with congestive heart failure. Note dilated hepatic veins. Light areas corresponding to peripheral fatty zones alternate with dark areas corresponding to zone 3 congestion and haemorrhage.

dilated, and the sinusoids entering it are engorged for a variable distance towards the periphery (fig. 11.21). In severe cases, there is frank haemorrhage with focal necrosis of liver cells. The liver cells show a variety of degenerative changes but each portal tract is surrounded by relatively normal cells to a depth that varies inversely with the extent of the zone 3 atrophy. Biopsy sections show significant fatty change in only about a third. This contrasts with the usual post-mortem picture. Cellular infiltration is inconspicuous.

The zone 3 degenerating cells are often packed with brown lipochrome pigment. As they disintegrate, pigment lies free. Bile thrombi, particularly in zone 1, may be seen in deeply jaundiced patients. Zone 3 PAS-positive, diastase-resistant hyaline globules may be seen [18].

Zone 3 reticulin condenses. Collagen increases and the central vein shows phlebosclerosis (fig. 11.22). Eccentric thickening or occlusion of the walls of zone 3 veins and perivenular scars extends into the lobule [20]. If the heart failure continues or relapses, bridges develop between central veins so that the unaffected portal zone is surrounded by a ring of fibrous tissue (reversed lobulation) (fig. 11.23). Later the portal zones are involved and a complex cirrhosis results. A true cardiac cirrhosis is extremely rare.

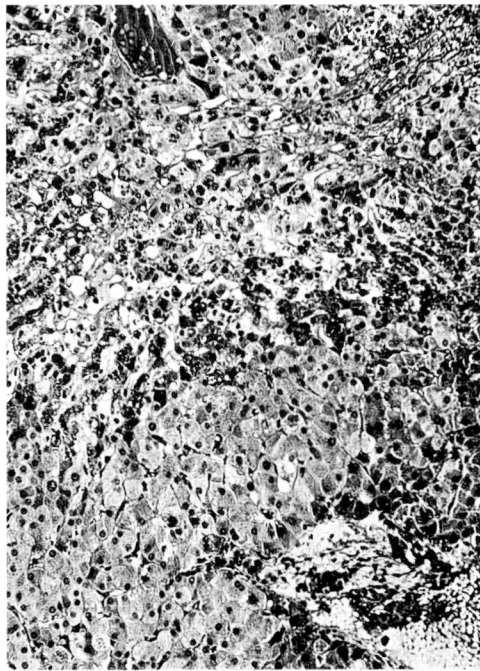

Fig. 11.21. Cor pulmonale. Serum bilirubin 3.4 mg/100 ml. Gross zone 3 congestion and liver cell necrosis. Pigment increase is seen in the degenerating liver cells. Liver cells in zone 1 are relatively normal. (Stained H & E, ×120.)

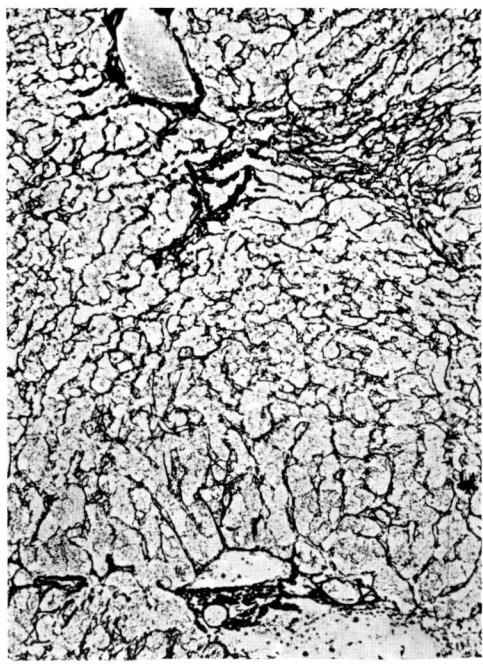

Fig. 11.22. Same section as in fig. 11.21. Reticulin stains show zone 3 condensation (×120).

Mechanism (fig. 11.24)

Hypoxia causes degeneration of the zone 3 liver cells, dilatation of sinusoids and slowing of bile secretion.

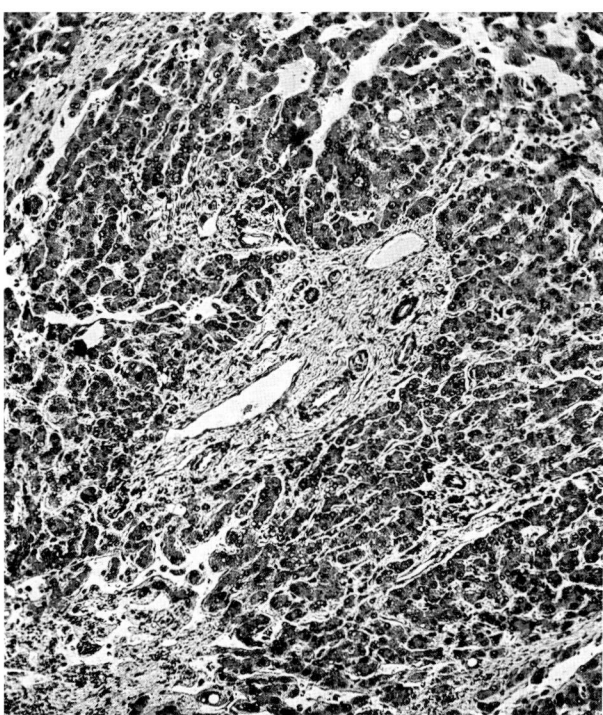

Fig. 11.23. Fibrous tissue bands pass from central vein to central vein. There is 'reversed lobulation' and a fully developed cardiac cirrhosis. Portal tracts show only slight fibrosis. (Stained H & E, ×90.)

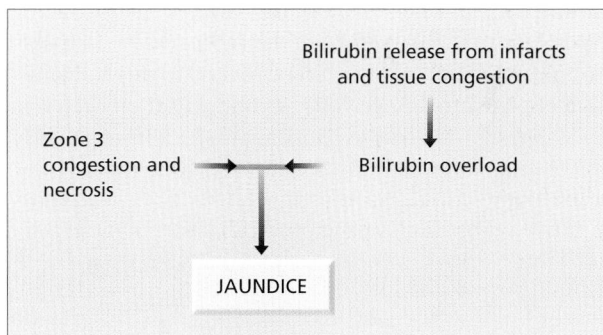

Fig. 11.24. Mechanisms of hepatic jaundice developing in patients with cardiac failure.

Endotoxins diffusing through the intestinal wall into the portal blood may augment this effect [32]. The liver attempts to compensate by increasing the oxygen extracted as the blood flows across the sinusoidal bed. Collagenosis of Disse's space may play a minor role in impairing oxygen diffusion.

Necrosis correlates with a reduced systemic blood pressure and hence with a low cardiac output [1]. The hepatic venous pressure increases in proportion to the rise in central venous pressure and this correlates with zone 3 congestion [1].

Thrombosis begins in sinusoids and may propagate to

hepatic veins with secondary local, portal vein thrombosis, ischaemia, parenchymal loss and fibrosis [35].

Clinical features

Mild jaundice is common but deeper icterus is rare and associated with chronic congestive failure due, for example, to coronary artery disease or mitral stenosis. In hospital inpatients, cardio-respiratory disease is the commonest cause of a raised serum bilirubin level. Jaundice increases with prolonged and repeated bouts of congestive failure. Oedematous areas escape, for bilirubin is protein-bound and does not enter oedema fluid with a low protein content.

Jaundice is partly hepatic, for the greater the extent of zone 3 necrosis the deeper the icterus (fig. 11.25) [31].

Bilirubin released from infarcts or simply from pulmonary congestion, provides an overload on the anoxic liver. Patients in cardiac failure who become jaundiced with minimal hepato-cellular damage usually have clear evidence of pulmonary infarction [31]. The serum shows unconjugated bilirubinaemia.

The patient may complain of right abdominal pain probably due to stretching of the capsule of the enlarged liver. The firm, smooth, tender lower edge may reach the umbilicus.

A rise in right atrial pressure is readily transmitted to the hepatic veins. This is particularly so in tricuspid incompetence when the hepatic vein pressure tracing resembles that obtained from the right atrium. Palpable systolic pulsation of liver can be related to this transmission of pressure. Pre-systolic hepatic pulsation occurs in tricuspid stenosis. The expansion may be felt bimanually with one hand over the liver anteriorly and the other over the right lower ribs posteriorly. This expansibility distinguishes it from the palpable epigastric pulsation due to the aorta or a hypertrophied right ventricle. Correct timing of the pulsation is important.

In heart failure, pressure applied over the liver increases the venous return and the jugular venous pressure rises due to the inability of the failing right heart to handle the increased blood flow. The hepato-jugular reflux is of value for identifying the jugular venous pulse and to establish that venous channels between the hepatic and jugular veins are patent. The reflux is absent if the hepatic veins are occluded or if the main mediastinal or jugular veins are blocked. It is useful for diagnosing tricuspid regurgitation [23].

Atrial pressure is reflected all the way to the portal system. Pulsed duplex Doppler sonography shows increased pulsatility in the portal vein depending on the severity of the heart failure [16]. However, patients with high atrial pressures do not always have pulsatile flow [9].

Ascites is associated with a particularly high venous pressure, a low cardiac output and severe zone 3 necrosis. This description applies to patients with mitral stenosis and tricuspid incompetence or constrictive pericarditis. In such patients the ascites may be out of proportion to the oedema and symptoms of congestive heart failure. The ascitic fluid protein content is raised to 2.5 g/dl or more, similar to that observed in the Budd–Chiari syndrome [30].

Confusion, lethargy and coma are related to cerebral anoxia. Occasionally the whole picture of impending hepatic coma may be seen. Splenomegaly is frequent. Other features of portal hypertension are usually absent except in very severe cardiac cirrhosis associated with constrictive pericarditis. However, at autopsy, 6.7% of 74 patients with congestive heart failure showed oesophageal varices, although in only one was there evidence of bleeding.

Bolus-enhanced CT shows retrograde hepatic venous opacification on the early scans and a diffusely mottled pattern of hepatic enhancement during the vascular phase of contrast administration [26].

Cardiac cirrhosis should be suspected in patients with prolonged, decompensated mitral valve disease with tricuspid incompetence or in patients with constrictive pericarditis. The prevalence has fallen since both these conditions are relieved surgically.

Biochemical changes

In general, the biochemical changes are small and proportional to the severity of the heart failure [19].

In congestive failure the serum bilirubin level usually exceeds 1 mg/dl and in about one-third it is more than

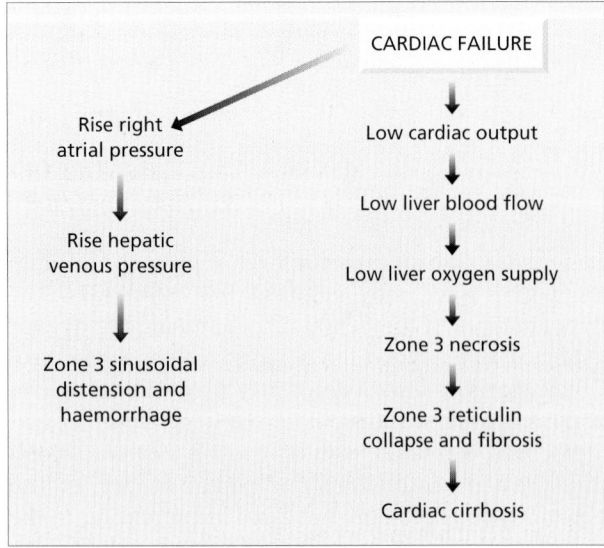

Fig. 11.25. Possible mechanisms of the hepatic histological changes in heart failure.

2mg/dl [31]. The jaundice may be deep, exceeding 5mg/dl and even up to 26.9mg. The serum bilirubin level corresponds to the degree of heart failure. Patients with advanced mitral valve disease and a normal serum bilirubin concentration have a normal hepatic bilirubin uptake but diminished capacity to eliminate conjugated bilirubin related to reduced liver blood flow [3]; this contributes to post-operative jaundice.

Serum alkaline phosphatase is usually normal or slightly increased. Serum albumin values may be mildly reduced. Protein loss from the intestine may contribute.

Serum transaminases are higher in acute than chronic failure and are proportional to the degree of shock and the extent of zone 3 necrosis. The association of very high values with jaundice may simulate acute viral hepatitis.

Prognosis

The prognosis is that of the underlying heart disease. Cardiac jaundice, particularly if deep, is always a bad omen.

Cardiac cirrhosis *per se* does not carry a bad prognosis and, if the heart failure responds to treatment, the cirrhosis can be expected to become compensated.

Hepatic dysfunction and cardiovascular abnormalities in paediatric patients

Infants and children with heart failure and cyanotic heart disease show liver dysfunction [22]. Hypoxaemia, systemic venous congestion and a low cardiac output are associated with increased prothrombin time, serum bilirubin and transaminase values. The most severe changes are found with a low cardiac output. Liver function correlates with cardiac status.

The liver in constrictive pericarditis

The clinical picture and hepatic changes are those of the Budd–Chiari syndrome.

Marked thickening of the liver capsule simulates sugar icing (*zuckergussleber*). Microscopically the picture is of cardiac cirrhosis.

Jaundice is absent. The liver is enlarged and hard and may pulsate [8]. Ascites is gross.

Diagnosis must be made from ascites due to cirrhosis or to hepatic venous obstruction. This is done by the paradoxical pulse, the venous pulse, the calcified pericardium, the echocardiogram, the electrocardiogram and by cardiac catheterization.

Treatment is that of the cardiac condition. If pericardectomy is possible, prognosis as regards the liver is good although recovery may be slow. Within 6 months of a successful operation, liver function tests improve and the liver shrinks. The cardiac cirrhosis cannot be expected to resolve completely, but fibrous bands become narrower and avascular.

References

1 Arcidi JM Jr, Moore GM, Hutchins GM. Hepatic morphology in cardiac dysfunction. A clinicopathologic study of 1000 subjects at autopsy. *Am. J. Pathol.* 1981; **104**: 159.

2 Berger ML, Reynolds RC, Hagler HK *et al.* Anoxic hepatocyte injury: role of reversible changes in elemental content and distribution. *Hepatology* 1989; **9**: 219.

3 Bohmer T, Kjekshus E, Nitter-Hauge S. Studies on the elevation of bilirubin preoperatively in patients with mitral valve disease. *Eur. Heart. J.* 1994; **15**: 10.

4 Bulkley GB, Oshima A, Bailey RW, Pathophysiology of hepatic ischemia in cardiogenic shock. *Am. J. Surg.* 1986; 151: 87.

5 Carrico JC, Meakins JL, Marshall JC *et al.* Multiple-organ-failure syndrome. *Arch. Surg.* 1986; **121**: 196.

6 Chu C-M, Chang C-H, Liaw Y-F *et al.* Jaundice after open heart surgery: a prospective study. *Thorax* 1984; **39**: 52.

7 Collins JD, Bassendine MF, Ferner R *et al.* Incidence and prognostic importance of jaundice after cardiopulmonary bypass surgery. *Lancet* 1983; **i**: 1119.

8 Coralli RJ, Crawley IS. Hepatic pulsations in constrictive pericarditis. *Am. J. Cardiol.* 1986; **58**: 370.

9 Duerinckx AJ, Grant EG, Perrella RR *et al.* The pulsatile portal vein in cases of congestive heart failure: correlation of duplex Doppler findings with right atrial pressures. *Radiology* 1990; **176**: 655.

10 Gibson PR, Dudley FJ. Ischemic hepatitis: clinical features, diagnosis and prognosis. *Aust. NZ J. Med.* 1984; **14**: 822.

11 Gitlin N, Serio KM. Ischemic hepatitis: widening horizons. *Am. J. Gastroenterol.* 1992; **87**: 831.

12 Hampton WW, Townsend MC, Schirmer WJ *et al.* Effective hepatic blood flow during cardiopulmonary bypass. *Arch. Surg.* 1989; **124**: 458.

13 Hasselgren P-O. Prevention and treatment of ischemia of the liver. *Surg. Gynecol. Obstet.* 1987; **164**: 187.

14 Henrion J, Descamps O, Luwaert R *et al.* Hypoxic hepatitis in patients with cardiac failure: incidence in a coronary care unit and measurement of hepatic blood flow. *J. Hepatol.* 1994; **21**: 696.

15 Hickman PE, Potter JM. Mortality associated with ischaemic hepatitis. *Aust. NZ J. Med.* 1990; **20**: 32.

16 Hosoki T, Arisawa J, Marukawa T *et al.* Portal blood flow in congestive heart failure: pulsed duplex sonographic findings. *Radiology* 1990; **174**: 733.

17 Kantrowitz PA, Jones WA, Greenberger NJ *et al.* Postoperative hyperbilirubinemia simulating obstructive jaundice. *N. Engl. J. Med.* 1967; **276**: 591.

18 Klatt EC, Koss MN, Young TS *et al.* Hepatic hyaline globules associated with passive congestion. *Arch. Pathol. Lab. Med.* 1988; **112**: 510.

19 Kubo SH, Walter BA, John DHA *et al.* Liver function abnormalities in chronic heart failure. Influence of systemic hemodynamics. *Arch. Intern. Med.* 1987; **147**: 1227.

20 Lefkowitch JH, Mendez L. Morphologic features of hepatic injury in cardiac disease and shock. *J. Hepatol.* 1986; **2**: 313.

21 Ma TT, Ischiropoulos H, Brass CA. Endotoxin-stimulated nitric oxide production increases injury and reduces rat liver chemiluminescence during reperfusion. *Gastroen-*

terology 1995; **108**: 463.

22 Mace S, Borkat G, Liebman J. Hepatic dysfunction and cardiovascular abnormalities. Occurrence in infants, children and young adults. *Am. J. Dis. Child*. 1985; **139**: 60.

23 Maisel AS, Atwood JE, Goldberger AL. Hepatojugular reflux: useful in the bedside diagnosis of tricuspid regurgitation. *Ann. Intern. Med*. 1984; **101**: 781.

24 Mathurin P, Durand F, Ganne N *et al*. Ischemic hepatitis due to obstructive sleep apnea. *Gastroenterology* 1995; **109**: 1682.

25 Milstein MJ, Moulton JS. Diffuse hepatic calcification after ischemic liver injury in a patient with chronic renal failure. *Am. J. Roentgenol*. 1993; **161**: 75.

26 Moulton JS, Miller BL, Dodd GD III *et al*. Passive hepatic congestion in heart failure: CT abnormalities. *Am. J. Roentgenol*. 1988; **151**: 939.

27 Nouel O, Henrion J, Bernuau J *et al*. Fulminant hepatic failure due to transient circulatory failure in patients with chronic heart disease. *Dig. Dis. Sci*. 1980; **25**: 49.

28 Nunes G, Blaisdell FW, Margaretten W. Mechanism of hepatic dysfunction following shock and trauma. *Arch. Surg*. 1970; **100**: 646.

29 Rex DK, Rogers DW, Mohammed Y *et al*. Post-cardiac surgery tamponade mimicking acute hepatitis. Report of two cases. *J. Clin. Gastroenterol*. 1992; **14**: 136.

30 Runyon BA. Cardiac ascites: a characterization. *J. Clin. Gastroenterol*. 1988; **10**: 410.

31 Sherlock S. The liver in heart failure; relation of anatomical, functional and circulatory changes. *Br. Heart J*. 1951; **13**: 273.

32 Shibayama Y. The role of hepatic venous congestion and endotoxaemia in the production of fulminant hepatic failure secondary to congestive heart failure. *J. Pathol*. 1987; **151**: 133.

33 Shibuya A, Unuma T, Sugimoto M *et al*. Diffuse hepatic calcification as a sequela to shock liver. *Gastroenterology* 1985; **89**: 196.

34 te Boekhorst Th, Urlus M, Doesburg W *et al*. Etiologic factors of jaundice in severely ill patients: a retrospective study in patients admitted to an intensive care unit with severe trauma or with septic intra-abdominal complications following surgery and without evidence of bile duct obstruction. *J. Hepatol*. 1988; **7**: 111.

35 Wanless IR, Liu JJ, Butany J. Role of thrombosis in the pathogenesis of congestive hepatic fibrosis (cardiac cirrhosis). *Hepatology* 1995; **21**: 1232.

36 Weisiger RA. Oxygen radicals and ischemic tissue injury. *Gastroenterology* 1986; **90**: 494.

Chapter 12
Jaundice

Bilirubin metabolism [2, 20, 50]

Bilirubin is the end product of haem, the majority (80–85%) coming from haemoglobin with only a small fraction derived from other haem-containing proteins such as cytochrome P450 (fig. 12.1). Approximately 300 mg bilirubin is formed daily. Production from haemoglobin takes place in reticulo-endothelial cells.

The enzyme that converts haem to bilirubin is microsomal haem oxygenase which has absolute requirements for oxygen and NADPH. Cleavage of the porphyrin ring occurs selectively at the alpha methane bridge (fig. 12.2). The alpha bridge carbon atom is converted to carbon monoxide and the original bridge function is replaced by two oxygen atoms which are derived from molecular oxygen. The resulting linear tetrapyrrole has the structure of the IX alpha biliverdin. This is converted further to IX alpha bilirubin by a cytosolic enzyme, biliverdin reductase. Such a linear tetrapyrrole should be water soluble, whereas bilirubin is lipid soluble. The lipid solubility is explained by the structure of IX alpha bilirubin which has six intramolecular stable hydrogen bonds [5]. This bonding can be broken by alcohol in the diazo (van den Bergh) reaction converting unconjugated (indirect) bilirubin to conjugated (direct) reacting bilirubin. *In vivo* the stable hydrogen bonds are altered by esterification of the propionic groups by glucuronic acid.

About 20% of circulating bilirubin is not formed from the haem of mature erythrocytes. A small proportion comes from immature cells in spleen and bone marrow. This component is increased in haemolytic states. The remainder is formed in the liver from haem proteins such as myoglobin, cytochromes and unknown sources. This component is increased in pernicious anaemia, congenital erythropoietic porphyria and the Crigler–Najjar syndrome.

Hepatic transport and conjugation of bilirubin
(fig. 12.3)

Unconjugated bilirubin is transported in the plasma tightly bound to albumin. A very small amount is dialysable, but this can be increased by substances such as fatty acids and organic anions which compete with bilirubin for albumin binding. This is important in the neonate where such drugs as sulphonamides and salicylates facilitate diffusion of bilirubin into the brain and so increase the risk of kernicterus.

The liver extracts such organic anions as fatty acids, bile acid and non-bile-acid cholephils, such as bilirubin, despite tight albumin binding. Studies suggest that bilirubin dissociating from albumin in the sinusoid diffuses across the unstirred water layer at the surface of the hepatocyte [55]. A previously proposed albumin receptor has not been substantiated. The mechanism for

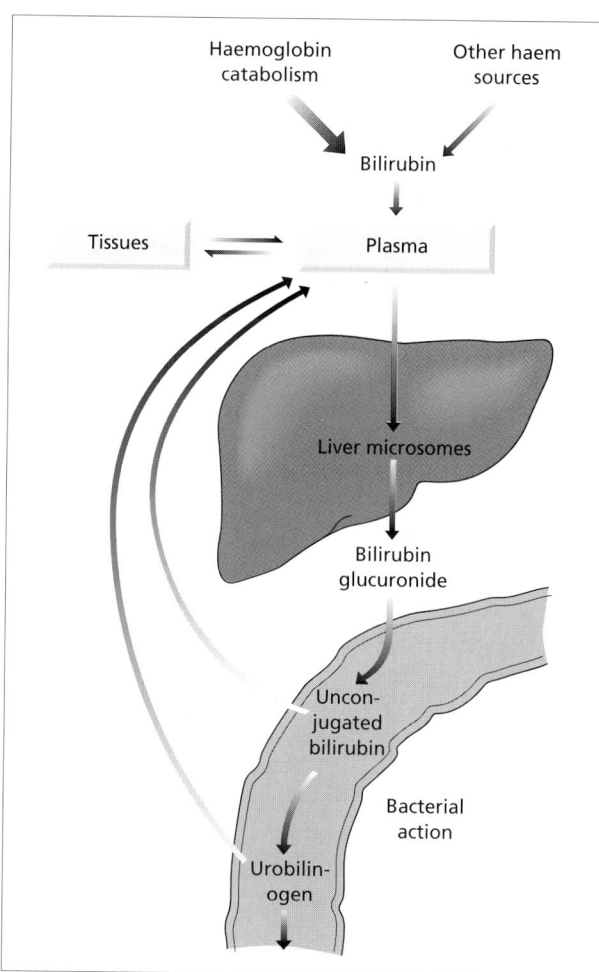

Fig. 12.1. The metabolism of bilirubin.

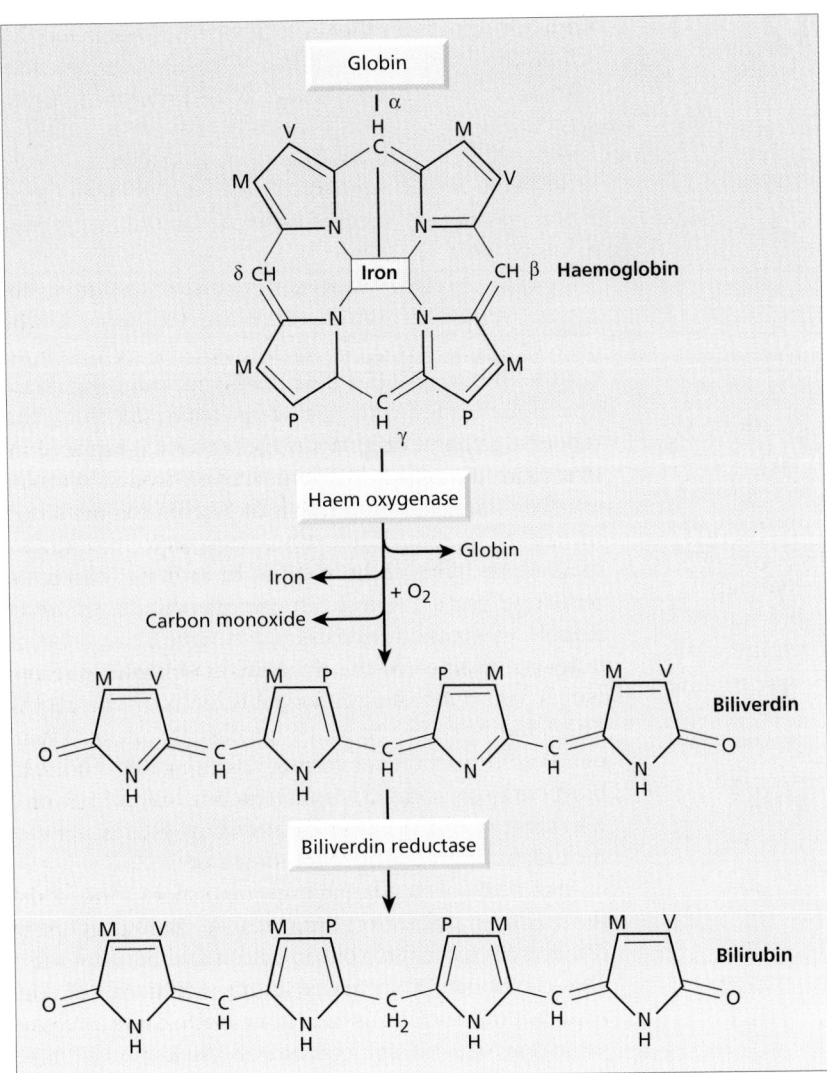

Fig. 12.2. The metabolism of haemoglobin to bilirubin (M = methyl; V = vinyl; P = propionate).

passage of bilirubin across the plasma membrane into the hepatocyte involves either transport proteins, such as the organic anion transporter [50], and/or bilirubin flip/flop across the membrane [55]. Uptake is highly effective because of the rapid hepatic metabolism by glucuronidization and excretion into bile, and also because of binding proteins in the cytosol such as ligandins (glutathione S-transferase).

Unconjugated bilirubin is non-polar (lipid soluble). It is converted to a polar (water soluble) compound by conjugation and this allows its excretion into the bile. This involves an enzyme in the microsomal fraction called bilirubin uridine-diphosphate glucuronosyl transferase (UGT) which converts unconjugated bilirubin to conjugated bilirubin mono- and diglucuronide. Bilirubin UGT is a one of several UGT enzyme isoforms that are responsible for the conjugation of many endogenous metabolites, hormones and neurotransmitters.

The gene expressing bilirubin UGT is on chromosome

2. The structure of the gene is complex (fig. 12.4) [2, 25]. Exons 2 to 5 at the 3′ end are constant components of all isoforms of UGTs. To complete the gene, one of several first exons can be employed. Exons 1A and 1D encode the variable region for bilirubin UGT1*1 and UGT1*2, respectively. UGT1*1 is responsible for virtually all bilirubin conjugation, with UGT1*2 playing little or any role [25]. Other first exons (exon 1F and 1G) encode the enzyme isoforms for phenol-UGTs. Thus selection of one of the exon 1 sequences gives different substrate specificity and enzyme characteristics.

Expression of UGT1*1 depends further on a promoter region in a 5′ position relative to each exon 1 [6]. This contains a TATAA box.

Detail of the gene structure is relevant to the pathogenesis of the unconjugated hyperbilirubinaemias (Gilbert's and Crigler–Najjar syndromes; see later section), where conjugating enzyme in the liver is reduced or absent.

Levels of UGTs are well maintained in hepato-cellular

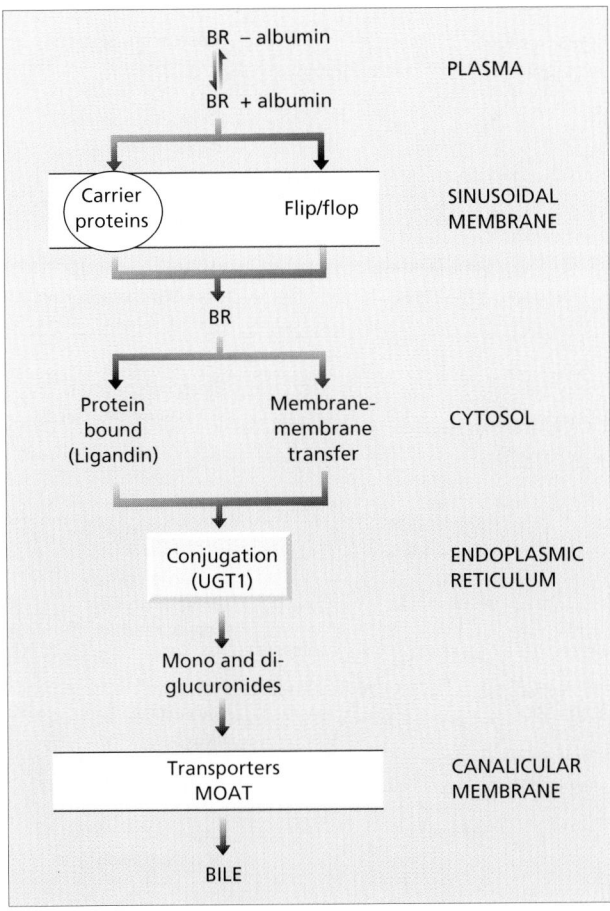

Fig. 12.3. Bilirubin (BR) uptake, metabolism and secretion by the hepatocyte (UGT1 = uridine-diphosphate glucuronosyl transferase –1; MOAT = multispecific organic anion transporter).

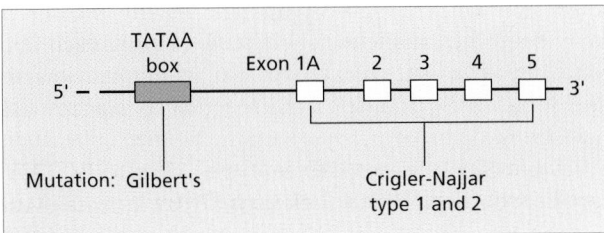

Fig. 12.4. Structure of gene for UGT1*1 with five exons and the promoter region (TATAA box). There are ten possible first exons (only one shown). Exon 1A (also called 1*1) is used for UGT1*1 (major active enzyme); exon 1D (=1*4) for UGT1*2.

jaundice and even increased in cholestasis [3]. They are reduced in the neonate.

The major bilirubin conjugate in human bile is the diglucuronide. A single microsomal glucuronyl system catalyses both the conversion of bilirubin to the monoglucuronide and also on to the diglucuronide [37].

With a high bilirubin load, as in haemolysis, monoglucuronide formation is favoured whereas if the bilirubin load is low or there is enzyme induction the diglucuronide increases.

Although conjugation as a glucuronide remains the most important mechanism, sulphate, xylose and glucose conjugation also occur to a small extent and may be increased in cholestasis [11].

In the late stages of cholestatic or hepato-cellular jaundice, despite high serum bilirubin levels, none can be detected in the urine. This is due apparently to a third type of bilirubin, a bilirubin mono-conjugate, covalently bound to albumin [54]. This would not be filtered by the glomerulus and hence would not reach the urine. This lessens the practical application of urinary bilirubin tests.

Biliary canalicular excretion of bilirubin is mediated by a family of ATP-dependent multispecific organic anion transporters (cMOAT) [27]. Bilirubin excretion of glucuronide is the rate-limiting factor in the transport of bilirubin from plasma to bile.

Bile acids are secreted into bile by another transporter. The separate mechanism for bilirubin and bile acid is exemplified by the Dubin–Johnson syndrome where there is a defect in the excretion of conjugated bilirubin while bile salt excretion is usually normal. A high proportion of the conjugated bilirubin in bile is incorporated into mixed micelles with cholesterol, phospholipids and bile salts. The role of the Golgi apparatus and of the microfilaments of the cytoskeleton in the intra-hepatic transport of conjugated bilirubin remains to be defined.

Bilirubin diglucuronide in bile is polar (water soluble) and hence is not absorbed from the small intestine. In the colon, bacterial beta-glucuronidases hydrolyse the conjugated bilirubin, which is then reduced to urobilinogens. In the presence of bacterial cholangitis some hydrolysis of the bilirubin glucuronide is possible in the biliary tree and unconjugated bilirubin is precipitated. This may be important in the production of bilirubin gallstones.

Urobilinogen is non-polar and is well absorbed from the small intestine, but only minimally from the colon. The little that is normally absorbed is re-excreted by the liver and kidneys (*entero-hepatic circulation*). With hepato-cellular dysfunction, re-excretion by the liver is impaired and more is excreted in the urine. This accounts for the urobilinogenuria of alcoholic liver disease, pyrexia, heart failure and the early stages of viral hepatitis.

Distribution of jaundice in the tissues

Circulating protein-bound bilirubin finds it difficult to enter protein-low tissue fluids. If the protein is increased, jaundice becomes more evident. Thus exudates tend to be more icteric than transudates.

The cerebrospinal fluid is more likely to be xanthochromic when meningitis is present, the classical example being Weil's disease with both jaundice and meningitis.

The basal ganglia may be stained yellow in the newborn (kernicterus). This is due to the high concentration of circulating, unconjugated bilirubin having an affinity for neural tissue.

Cerebrospinal fluid from jaundiced subjects contains a small amount of bilirubin, the level being one-tenth to one-hundredth of that found in the serum.

In deep jaundice, the ocular fluids are yellow, and this is considered to explain the extremely rare symptom of xanthopsia (seeing yellow).

Urine, sweat, semen and milk contain bile pigment in the deeply jaundiced patient. Bilirubin is a normal constituent of synovial fluid.

Paralysed parts and oedematous areas tend to remain uncoloured.

Bilirubin is readily bound to elastic tissue. Skin, ocular sclera and blood vessels have a high elastic tissue content, and easily become icteric. This also accounts for the disparity between the depth of skin jaundice and serum bilirubin levels during recovery from hepatitis and cholestasis.

Factors determining the depth of jaundice

Even with complete bile duct obstruction, the depth of jaundice is very variable. After an initial rapid increase, the serum bilirubin levels off after about 3 weeks although the obstruction persists. The level of jaundice depends on both bile pigment production and the capacity of the kidney for its excretion. Rates of bilirubin production may vary and products other than bilirubin, which do not give the diazo reaction, may be formed from haem catabolism. The intestinal mucosa may allow the passage of bilirubin, presumably unconjugated, from the blood.

In prolonged cholestasis the skin is greenish, possibly due to biliverdin, which does not give the diazo reaction for bilirubin. Other pigments may play a part.

Conjugated bilirubin, because of its water solubility and penetration of body fluids, produces more jaundice than unconjugated pigment. The extravascular space is greater than the vascular space. This accounts for the more intense colour of those with hepato-cellular and cholestatic rather than haemolytic jaundice.

Classification of jaundice

Jaundice might arise in four different ways (fig. 12.5). First, there may be an increased bilirubin load on the liver cell. Second, there may be a disturbance in uptake and transport of bilirubin within the hepatocyte. Third,

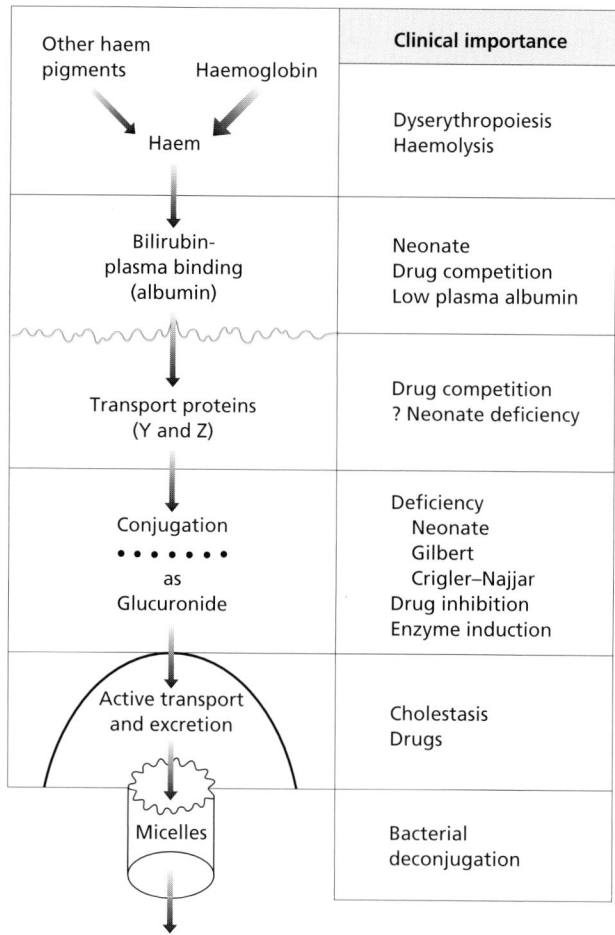

Fig. 12.5. The clinical importance of interference with the stages in the transport of bilirubin, from its production from haem through to its excretion in micellar form into the bile.

there may be defects in conjugation. Finally, the defect may be in the canalicular membrane altering excretion into the bile or there may be an obstruction to the larger bile channels before bilirubin reaches the intestines.

Classification is into three types (figs 12.6, 12.7): pre-hepatic, hepatic and cholestatic. There is much over-

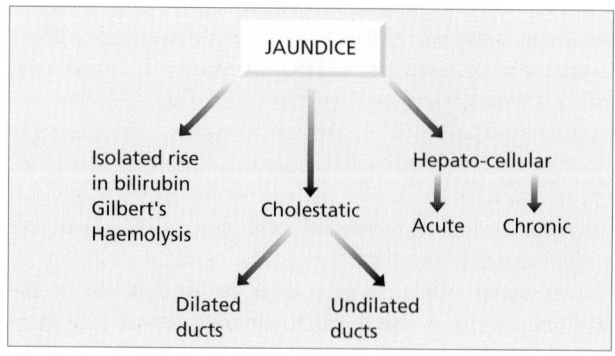

Fig. 12.6. Classification of jaundice.

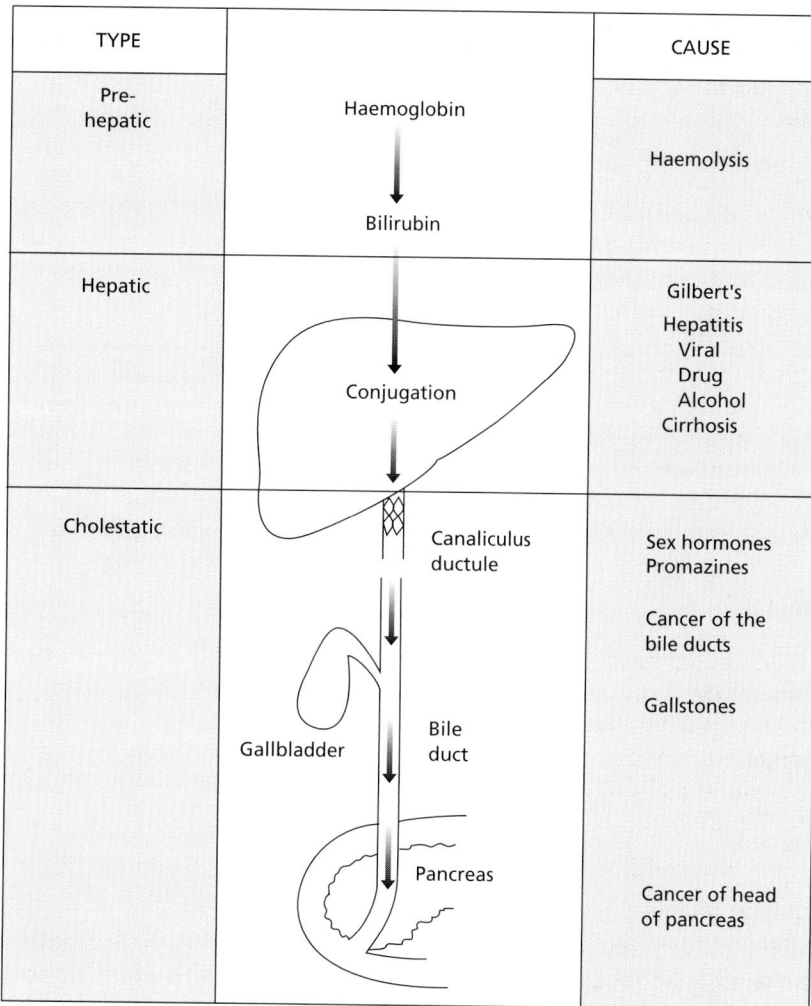

TYPE		CAUSE
Pre-hepatic	Haemoglobin ↓ Bilirubin	Haemolysis
Hepatic	Conjugation	Gilbert's Hepatitis Viral Drug Alcohol Cirrhosis
Cholestatic	Canaliculus ductule Gallbladder Bile duct Pancreas	Sex hormones Promazines Cancer of the bile ducts Gallstones Cancer of head of pancreas

Fig. 12.7. Classification and causes of jaundice.

lap, particularly between the hepatic and cholestatic varieties.

Pre-hepatic. Total serum bilirubin levels are increased with normal serum transaminases and alkaline phosphatase. The circulating serum bilirubin is largely unconjugated. Bilirubin cannot be detected in the urine. The cause may be haemolysis or a familial disturbance of bilirubin metabolism.

Hepatic (Chapters 16 and 18). The jaundice usually comes on rapidly and is of an orange tint. Fatigue and malaise are conspicuous. There are varying degrees of liver failure. These may be shown in a mild case as personality change and in the more severe as flapping tremor, confusion and coma. Fluid retention is shown in its mildest form by weight gain and in the more severe by oedema and ascites. Reduced hepatic synthesis of coagulation factors is shown by bruising in relation to venepunctures and also spontaneously. Serum biochemistry shows increases in transaminases. Serum albumin levels are reduced in the long-standing case.

Cholestatic (Chapter 13). This is due to failure of ad-

equate amounts of bile to reach the duodenum. The patient is relatively well, apart from the causative condition, and pruritus is prominent. The patient becomes increasingly pigmented. The serum shows increases in conjugated bilirubin, biliary alkaline phosphatase, gamma glutamyl transpeptidase (GT), total cholesterol

Table 12.1. First steps in the diagnosis of the jaundiced patient

Clinical history and examination
Urine, stools
Serum biochemical tests
  Bilirubin
  Transaminase ('AST', 'SGOT')
  Alkaline phosphatase, gamma GT
  Albumin
  Quantitative immunoglobulins
Haematology
  Haemoglobin, WBC, platelets
Blood film
Prothrombin time (before and after i.m. vitamin K)
X-ray chest

and conjugated bile acids. Steatorrhoea is responsible for weight loss and malabsorption of fat-soluble vitamins A, D, E and K, and calcium.

Diagnosis of jaundice (tables 12.1, 12.2)

A careful history and physical examination with routine biochemical and haematological tests are essential. The stool should be inspected and occult blood examination performed. The urine is tested for bilirubin and urobilinogen excess. The place of special tests such as ultrasound, liver biopsy and cholangiography—whether endoscopic or percutaneous — will depend on the category of jaundice.

Table 12.2. General features of the common types of acute jaundice

	Gallstones in common bile duct	Carcinoma peri-ampullary region	Acute viral hepatitis	Cholestatic drug jaundice
Antecedent history	Dyspepsia, previous attack	Nil	Contacts, injections, transfusion, or nil	Taking drug
Pain	Constant epigastric, biliary colic, or none	Constant epigastric, back, or none	Ache over liver or none	None
Pruritus	±	+	Transient	+
Rate of development of jaundice	Slow	Slow	Rapid	Rapid
Type of jaundice	Fluctuates or persistent	Usual but not always	Rapid onset, slow fall with recovery	Variable, usually mild
Weight loss	Slight to moderate	Progressive	Slight	Slight
Examination				
Diathesis	Frequently female obese	Over 40 years old	Young usually	Often older female, psychotic
Depth of jaundice	Moderate	Deep	Variable	Variable, rash sometimes
Ascites	0	Rarely with metastases	If severe and prolonged	0
Liver	Enlarged, slightly tender	Enlarged, not tender	Enlarged and tender	Slightly enlarged
Palpable gallbladder	0	+ (sometimes)	0	0
Tender gallbladder area	+	0	0	0
Palpable spleen	0	Occasionally	About 20%	0
Temperature	↑	Not usually	↑ onset only	↑ onset
Laboratory investigations				
Leucocyte count	↑ or normal	↑ or normal	↓	Normal
Differential leucocytes	Polymorphs ↑	—	Lymphocytes ↑	Eosinophilia at onset
Faeces				
Colour	Intermittently pale	Pale	Variable, light to dark	Pale
Occult blood	0	+	0	0
Urine: urobilin(ogen)	+	Absent	– Early + Late	– Early
Serum bilirubin (μmol/l)	Usually 50–170	Steady rise to 250–500	Varies with severity	Variable
Serum alkaline phosphatase (times normal)	> 3 ×	> 3 ×	< 3 ×	> 3 ×
Serum aspartate transaminase (times normal)	< 5 ×	< 5 ×	> 10 ×	> 5 ×
CT and ultrasound	Gallstones ± dilated duct	Dilated ducts ± mass	Splenomegaly	Normal

Clinical history

Occupation should be noted; particularly contact with rats carrying Weil's disease, or employment involving alcohol.

Place of origin (Mediterranean, African or Far East) may suggest carriage of hepatitis B or C.

Family history is important with respect to jaundice, hepatitis, anaemia, splenectomy or cholecystectomy. Positive histories are helpful in diagnosing haemolytic jaundice, congenital hyperbilirubinaemia, hepatitis and gallstones.

Contact with jaundiced persons particularly in nurseries, camps, hospitals and schools is noted. Close contact with patients on renal units or with drug abusers is recorded as is any *injection* in the preceding 6 months. 'Injections' include blood tests, drug abuse, tuberculin testing, dental treatment and tattooing as well as blood or plasma transfusions. The patient is asked about previous *drug treatment* with possible icterogenic agents. Consumption of *shellfish* and previous *travel* to areas where hepatitis is endemic should be noted.

Previous dyspepsia, fat intolerance and biliary colic suggest choledocholithiasis.

Jaundice after biliary tract surgery suggests residual calculus, traumatic stricture of the bile duct or hepatitis. Jaundice following the removal of a malignant growth may be due to hepatic metastases.

Alcoholics usually have associated features such as anorexia, morning nausea, diarrhoea and mild pyrexia. They may complain of pain over the enlarged liver.

Progressive failure of health and weight loss favour an underlying carcinoma.

The onset is extremely important. Preceding nausea, anorexia, aversion to smoking (in smokers), and jaundice, developing in a matter of hours and deepening rapidly, suggest viral hepatitis or drug jaundice. Cholestatic jaundice develops more slowly, often with persistent pruritus. Pyrexia with rigors suggests cholangitis associated with gallstones or biliary stricture.

Dark urine and pale stools precede hepato-cellular or cholestatic jaundice by a few days. In haemolytic jaundice the stools have a normal colour.

In hepato-cellular jaundice the patient feels ill; in cholestatic jaundice he may be inconvenienced only by the itching or jaundice, any other symptoms being due to the cause of the obstruction.

Persistent mild jaundice of varying intensity suggests haemolysis. The jaundice of cirrhosis is usually mild and variable and is associated with normal stools, although patients with superimposed acute 'alcoholic hepatitis' may be deeply jaundiced and pass pale stools.

Biliary colic may be continuous for hours rather than being intermittent. Back or epigastric pain may be associated with pancreatic carcinoma.

Examination (fig. 12.8)

Age and sex. A parous, middle-aged, obese female may have gallstones. The incidence of type A hepatitis decreases as age advances but no age is exempt from type B and C. The probability of malignant biliary obstruction increases with age. Drug jaundice is very rare in childhood.

General examination. Anaemia may indicate haemolysis, cancer or cirrhosis. Gross weight loss suggests cancer. The patient with haemolytic jaundice is a mild yellow colour, with hepato-cellular jaundice is orange and with prolonged biliary obstruction has a deep greenish hue. A hunched-up position suggests pancreatic carcinoma. In alcoholics, the stigmas of cirrhosis should be noted. Sites to be examined for a primary tumour include breasts, thyroid, stomach, colon, rectum and lung. Lymphadenopathy is noted.

Mental state. Slight intellectual deterioration with minimal personality change suggests hepato-cellular jaundice. Fetor and 'flapping' tremor indicate impending hepatic coma.

Skin changes. Bruising may indicate a clotting defect. Purpuric spots on forearms, axillae or shins may be related to the thrombocytopenia of cirrhosis. Other cutaneous manifestations of cirrhosis include vascular spiders, palmar erythema, white nails and loss of secondary sexual hair.

In chronic cholestasis, scratch marks, melanin pigmentation, finger clubbing, xanthomas on the eyelids (xanthelasmas), extensor surfaces and palmar creases, and hyperkeratosis may be found.

Pigmentation of the shins and ulcers may be seen in some forms of congenital haemolytic anaemia.

Malignant nodules should be sought in the skin. Multiple venous thromboses suggest carcinoma of the body of the pancreas. Ankle oedema may indicate cirrhosis, or obstruction of the inferior vena cava due to hepatic or pancreatic malignancy.

Abdominal examination. Dilated peri-umbilical veins indicate a portal collateral circulation and cirrhosis. Ascites may be due to cirrhosis or to malignant disease. A very large nodular liver suggests cancer. A small liver may indicate severe hepatitis or cirrhosis, and excludes extra-hepatic cholestasis in which the liver is enlarged and smooth. In the alcoholic, fatty change and cirrhosis may produce a uniform enlargement of the liver. The edge is tender in hepatitis, in congestive heart failure, with alcoholism, in bacterial cholangitis and occasionally in malignant disease. An arterial murmur over the liver indicates acute alcoholic hepatitis or primary liver cancer.

In choledocholithiasis the gallbladder may be tender and Murphy's sign positive. A palpable, and sometimes visibly enlarged, gallbladder suggests pancreatic cancer.

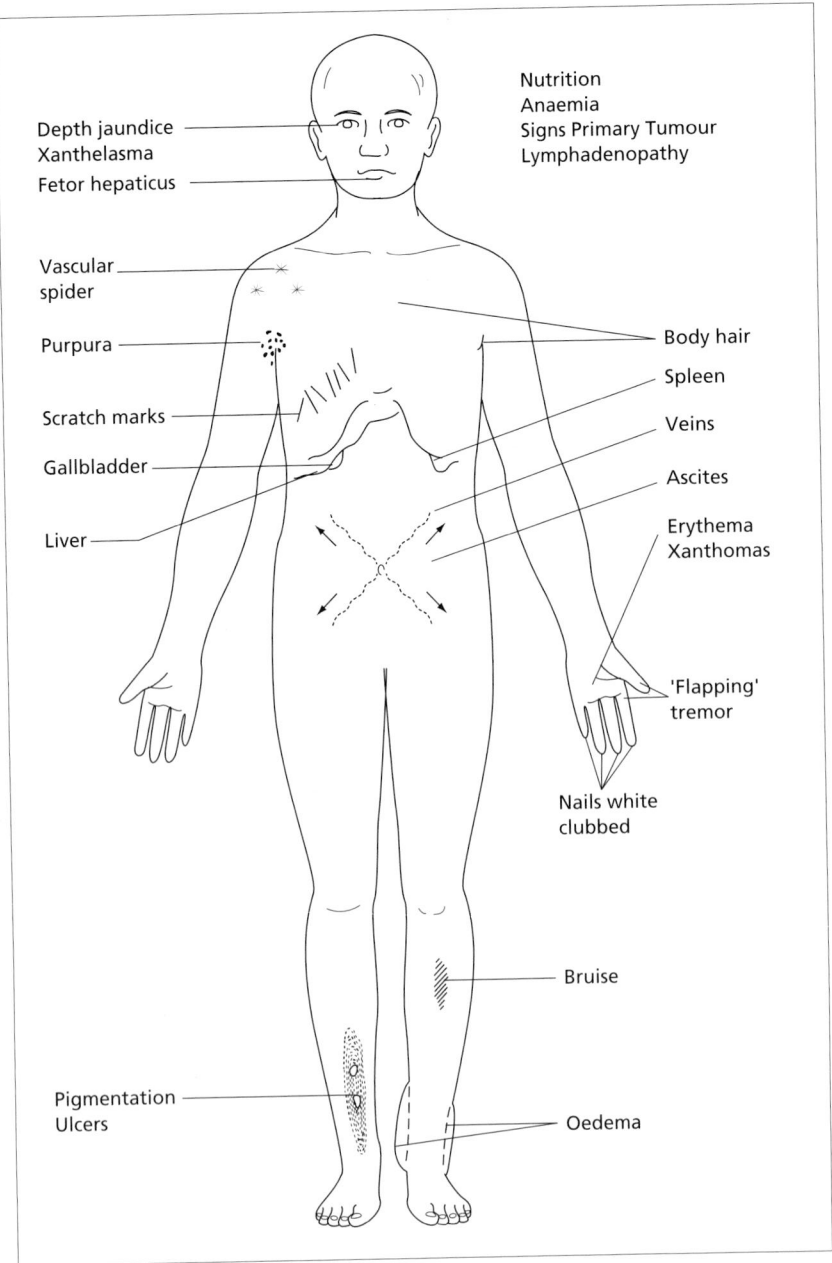

Fig. 12.8. Physical signs in jaundice.

The abdomen is carefully examined for any primary tumour. Rectal examination is essential.

Urine and faeces. Bilirubinuria is an early sign of viral hepatitis and drug jaundice. Persistent absence of urobilinogen suggests total obstruction of the common bile duct. Persistent excess of urobilinogen with negative bilirubin supports haemolytic jaundice.

Persistent acholic stools confirm biliary obstruction. Positive occult blood favours a diagnosis of ampullary, pancreatic or alimentary carcinoma or of portal hypertension.

Serum biochemical tests

Serum bilirubin confirms jaundice, indicates depth and is used to follow progress. Serum alkaline phosphatase values more than three times normal strongly suggest cholestasis if bone disease is absent and gamma GT is elevated; high values may also be found in patients with non-biliary cirrhosis.

Serum albumin and globulin levels are little changed in jaundice of short duration. In more chronic hepato-cellular jaundice the albumin is depressed and globulin increased. Electrophoretic analysis shows raised α_2- and β-globulins in cholestatic jaundice in contrast to γ-globulin elevation in hepato-cellular jaundice.

Serum transaminases increase in hepatitis compared with variable but lower levels in cholestatic jaundice. High values may sometimes be found transiently with acute bile duct obstruction due to a stone.

Haematology

A low total leucocyte count with a relative lymphocytosis suggests hepato-cellular jaundice. A polymorph leucocytosis may be found in alcoholic and severe viral hepatitis. Increased leucocyte counts are found with acute cholangitis or underlying malignant disease. If haemolysis is suspected, investigations should include a reticulocyte count, examination of the blood film, erythrocyte fragility, Coombs' test, and examination of the bone marrow.

If the prothrombin time is prolonged, vitamin K_1 10 mg intramuscularly for 3 days leads to return to normal in cholestasis, whereas patients with hepato-cellular jaundice show little change.

Diagnostic routine

Clinical evaluation allows the patient to be categorized into hepato-cellular, infiltrative, possible extra-hepatic biliary obstruction and likely extra-hepatic biliary obstruction [21]. Various algorithms are laid down (fig. 12.9). The sequence employed depends on the clinical evaluation, the facilities available and the risk of each investigation. Cost plays a part.

A small proportion of patients with extra-hepatic biliary obstruction are incorrectly diagnosed as having intra-hepatic cholestasis, whereas a larger proportion of patients with intra-hepatic disease are thought to have extra-hepatic obstruction.

Computer models are based on clinical history and examination with haematological and biochemical observations made during the first 6 hours in hospital [41]. These have a performance equalling that of the hepatologist and better than some non-specialist internists. One computer-based system had an overall diagnostic accuracy of 70%, which was the same as experienced hepatologists who, however, reached a correct diagnosis with fewer questions per consultation [10].

Radiology

A chest film is taken to show primary and secondary tumours and any irregularity and elevation of the right diaphragm due to an enlarged or nodular liver.

Visualization of the bile ducts

This is indicated if the patient is cholestatic (see Chapter 29). The first procedure in distinguishing hepato-cellular from surgical, main duct 'obstructive' jaundice is US or CT to show whether or not the intra-hepatic bile ducts are dilated (figs 12.6, 13.20). This is followed by endoscopic (ERCP) or percutaneous (PTC) cholangiography as indicated.

Viral markers

These are indicated for hepatitis A and B, cytomegala and Epstein–Barr infections (Chapter 16). The serum antibody to hepatitis C virus becomes positive only 2–4 months after infection.

Needle liver biopsy

Acute jaundice rarely merits liver biopsy which is reserved for the patient who presents diagnostic difficulty and where an intra-hepatic cause is suspected. The method carries extra risk in the jaundiced; the Menghini technique is safest. Deep jaundice is not a contraindication.

Trans-jugular or CT or US guided biopsy with plugging of the puncture site in the liver is useful if clotting defects preclude the routine percutaneous technique (Chapter 3).

Acute viral hepatitis is usually diagnosed easily. The greatest difficulty arises in the cholestatic group. However, in most instances an experienced histopathologist can distinguish appearances of intra-hepatic cholestasis, for instance due to drugs or to primary biliary cirrhosis, from the appearances of a block to main bile ducts. The cause of the cholestasis can be stated with much less certainty.

Laparoscopy

The appearance of a dark green liver with an enormous gallbladder favours extra-hepatic biliary obstruction. Tumour nodules may be seen and needle biopsy may

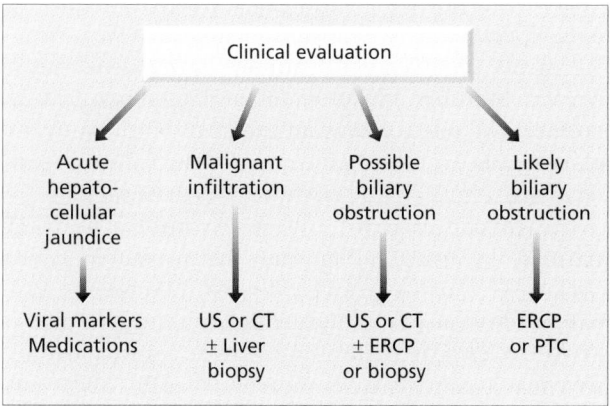

Fig. 12.9. An algorithm for diagnosing jaundice.

be made under direct vision. A pale yellow–green liver suggests hepatitis and cirrhosis is obvious. The method cannot be relied upon to distinguish extra-hepatic biliary obstruction, especially due to a carcinoma of the main hepatic ducts, from intra-hepatic cholestasis due to drugs.

A photographic record should be taken of the appearances. In the presence of jaundice peritoneoscopy is safer than needle biopsy but, if necessary, the two procedures may be combined.

Prednisolone test

In hepato-cellular jaundice, 30 mg prednisolone daily for 5 days leads to a 40% fall in serum bilirubin [49]. This may be useful in diagnosing cholestatic hepatitis A. Hepatitis B markers must be negative.

The corticosteroid 'white wash' cannot be accounted for by changes in the erythrocyte survival (reflecting changes in haemoglobin catabolism), faecal or urinary urobilinogen output, or urinary bilirubin. The bilirubin may take an alternative metabolic pathway.

Laparotomy

Jaundice is rarely a surgical emergency (see Chapter 13). If there is any diagnostic doubt, it is better to investigate further rather than to surgically explore the bile passages of a patient with hepatic jaundice and so run the very real risk of precipitating acute liver or renal failure. The patient rarely suffers from delay.

The familial non-haemolytic hyperbilirubinaemias (table 12.3)

Although the upper limit of serum bilirubin is usually taken to be 17 μmol/l (0.8 mg/dl), in some 5% of healthy blood donors higher values (20–50 μmol/l) may be found. When those suffering from haemolysis or from liver disease have been excluded there remain the patients with familial abnormalities of bilirubin metabolism [2]. The commonest is Gilbert's syndrome [22]. Other syndromes can also be identified. The prognosis is excellent. Accurate diagnosis, particularly from chronic liver disease, is important for it enables the patient to be reassured. It is based on family history, duration, absence of stigmas of hepato-cellular disease and of splenomegaly, exclusion of haemolysis, normal serum transaminases and, if necessary, by liver biopsy.

Primary hyperbilirubinaemia. This very rare condition is due to increased production of 'early-labelled' bilirubin in the bone marrow. The cause is probably the premature destruction of abnormal red cell precursors (ineffective erythrocyte synthesis). The clinical picture is of compensated haemolysis. Peripheral erythrocyte destruction is normal. The condition is probably familial [1].

Table 12.3. Isolated increases in serum bilirubin

Type	Diagnostic points
Unconjugated	
Haemolysis	Splenomegaly. Blood film. Reticulocytosis. Coombs' test
Gilbert's	Familial. Serum bilirubin increases with fasting and falls on phenobarbitone. Liver biopsy normal but conjugating enzyme reduced. Normal serum transaminases
Crigler–Najjar	
Type 1	No conjugating enzyme in liver. No response to phenobarbitone. Usually die young with kernicterus
Type 2	Absent or deficient conjugating enzyme in liver. Response to phenobarbitone
Conjugated	
Dubin–Johnson	Black-liver biopsy. No concentration of cholecystographic media. Secondary rise in BSP test
Rotor	Normal liver biopsy. Cholecystography normal. BSP test no uptake

Gilbert's syndrome

This is named after Augustin Gilbert (1858–1927) [22], a Parisian physician [53]. It is defined as benign, familial, mild, unconjugated hyperbilirubinaemia (serum bilirubin 17–85 μmol/l [1–5 mg/dl]) not due to haemolysis and with normal routine tests of liver function and hepatic histology. It affects some 2–5% of the population.

It may be diagnosed by chance at a routine medical examination or when the blood is being examined for another reason, for instance after viral hepatitis. It has an excellent prognosis. Jaundice is mild and intermittent. Deepening may follow an intercurrent infection or fasting and is associated with malaise, nausea and often discomfort over the liver. These symptoms are probably no greater than in normal abilirubinaemic controls [34]. There are no other abnormal physical signs; the spleen is not palpable.

Patients with Gilbert's syndrome have a deficiency in hepatic bilirubin glucuronidation [3], about 30% of normal. The bile contains an excess of bilirubin monoglucuronide over the diglucuronide. The Bolivian squirrel monkey is an animal model for this disorder [38].

The genetic basis for Gilbert's syndrome has been clarified by the finding that the promoter region (A(TA)$_6$TAA) of the gene encoding UGT1*1 (see fig. 12.4) has an additional TA dinucleotide, resulting in a change to (A(TA)$_7$TAA) [6, 31]. It is inherited as autosomal recessive; that is patients are homozygous for this abnormality. The lengthening of this promoter sequence is thought to interfere with the binding of the transcription factor

IID, resulting in reduced UGT1 enzyme production. However, although a reduced enzyme level is necessary for Gilbert's syndrome, it is not alone sufficient, and other factors such as hepatic transport abnormalities of bilirubin and occult haemolysis [40] may play a role in the development of hyperbilirubinaemia. Thus there is a mild impairment of bromsulphthalein (BSP) and tolbutamide clearance (a drug that does not need conjugation).

Peripheral blood cells show abnormalities resembling variegate porphyria, perhaps due to increased hepato-cellular bilirubin concentrations [29].

Familial increased serum intestinal alkaline phosphatase has been associated with Gilbert's syndrome [28].

Acetaminophen (paracetamol) is eliminated by glucuronidation which prevents its P450 catabolism to a hepatotoxic metabolite. A genetic deficiency of UDP-glucuronosyl transferase in Gilbert's syndrome may predispose to acetaminophen toxicity especially with overdose [13].

Specialist diagnostic tests include the increase in serum bilirubin on fasting (fig. 12.10) [35], the fall on taking phenobarbitone which induces the hepatic con-

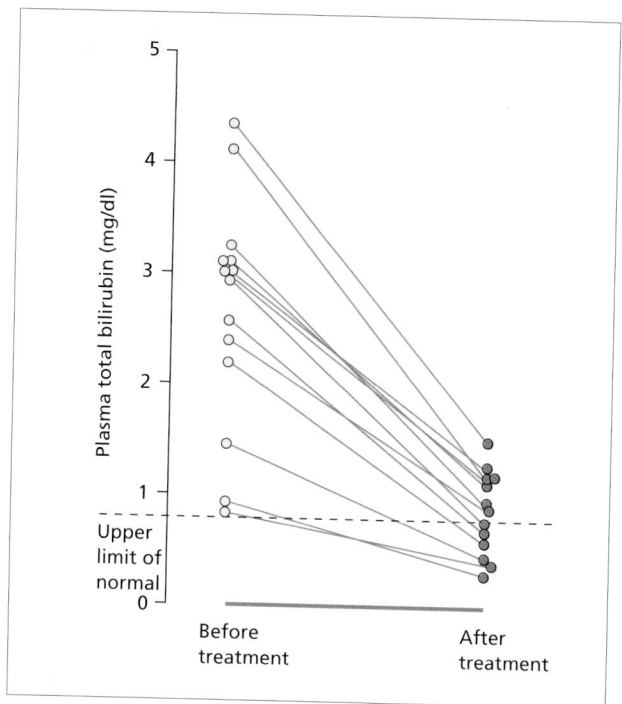

Fig. 12.11. Gilbert's syndrome. The effect of phenobarbitone (60 mg, three times a day) on the serum bilirubin level [4].

jugating enzyme (fig. 12.11) and the increase following intravenous nicotinic acid which raises the osmotic fragility of red blood cells [40].

Thin layer chromatography shows a significantly higher proportion of unconjugated bilirubin than in normals, chronic haemolysis or chronic hepatitis; this is diagnostic [45]. The fasting serum bile acids are normal or even low [52]. Low values for bilirubin conjugating enzyme are found in liver biopsies [3]. However, Gilbert's syndrome is usually diagnosed with ease without recourse to these specialist methods.

Gilbert's syndrome has a normal life expectancy and reassurance is the only necessary treatment. Hyperbilirubinaemia is life-long and not associated with increased morbidity [34].

Serum bilirubin may be reduced by phenobarbitone [4] but, as icterus is rarely obvious, few patients will gain cosmetic benefit from this treatment. 'Sufferers' should be warned that jaundice can follow an intercurrent infection, repeated vomiting or missed meals. The 'sufferer' is a normal risk for life insurance.

Crigler–Najjar type

This extreme form of familial non-haemolytic jaundice is associated with very high serum unconjugated bilirubin values [12]. Deficiency of conjugating enzyme can be demonstrated in the liver. Total pigment in bile is

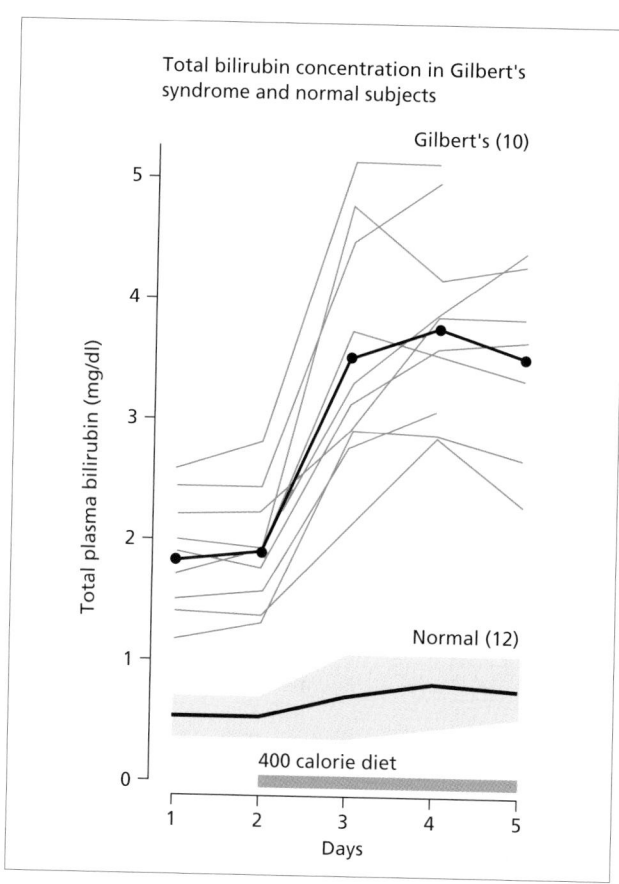

Fig. 12.10. Gilbert's syndrome. The serum unconjugated bilirubin level increases after a 400 calorie diet [35].

minimal. Bilirubin tolerance is impaired but the BSP test gives normal results.

Type 1

This is inherited as an autosomal recessive. No bilirubin conjugating enzyme can be detected in the liver. Conjugated bilirubin is absent from the bile. Bilirubin glucuronide is totally absent from serum [32]. Since the serum bilirubin levels eventually stabilize, the patient must have some alternative pathway of bilirubin metabolism.

The molecular defect is in one of the five exons (1A–5) of the bilirubin UGT1*1 gene (see fig. 12.4). Analysis of the Crigler–Najjar type 1 mutations by expression in COS cells or fibroblasts shows no bilirubin conjugating activity [25, 46].

Sufferers usually, but not always, die with kernicterus in the first year of life. There is no response to phenobarbitone. Phlebotomy and plasmapheresis have been used to reduce serum bilirubin but with only temporary success. Phototherapy can reduce the serum bilirubin by about 50% and may be carried out at home [19]. Encephalopathy (kernicterus) may develop any time in the first or second decade. Liver transplantation corrects the metabolic defect, cures hyperbilirubinaemia, and gives an excellent survival prospect [48]. It should be performed at a young age especially when reliable phototherapy cannot be guaranteed [51].

In *Gunn rats*, a mutant strain of the Wistar rat, bilirubin UGT is absent and there is unconjugated hyperbilirubinaemia. The genetic defect corresponds to that in Crigler–Najjar type 1, with a deletion in the gene common to all UGT enzymes resulting in premature stop codons which lead to the synthesis of truncated, inactive UGT isoforms [17]. Prenatal diagnosis has been done on placental DNA from rats [24] and this approach could be adapted for analysis of Crigler–Najjar type 1, although the range of mutations makes it far more complex than in this animal model. Experimentally, isolated microencapsulated hepatocytes introduced intraperitoneally have reduced serum bilirubin levels in the Gunn rat [14].

Type 2

This is also inherited as an autosomal recessive. Bilirubin conjugating enzyme is extremely reduced to less than 10% in the liver and, although present, is undetectable by the usual methods of analysis. The patients respond dramatically to phenobarbitone and survive into adult life [23].

DNA analysis of the bilirubin UGT1*1 gene (see fig. 12.4) has shown mutations in exons 1A–5 [7, 25]. However, expression analysis of these mutants has shown residual enzyme activity—explaining the lower serum bilirubin concentration than in Crigler–Najjar type 1, the presence of glucuronides in bile and the beneficial effect of phenobarbitone.

Some relatives of patients with Crigler–Najjar syndrome have an elevated serum bilirubin concentration, below that of true Crigler–Najjar but higher than Gilbert's syndrome [31]. Analysis of the UGT1*1 gene has suggested that these patients are compound heterozygotes, one allele having the Gilbert's TATAA box mutation, and the other having a Crigler–Najjar mutation [6].

Type 2 is not always benign and phototherapy and phenobarbitone should be given to keep the serum bilirubin level less than 450 µmol/l (26 mg/dl).

The distinction between type 1 and 2 Crigler–Najjar syndrome is not always easy. HPLC to estimate bilirubin fractions may be used to assess the effect of phenobarbitone treatment and should distinguish between the two types [36]. A distinction between the two types can also be drawn by measuring bile pigments in bile after phenobarbitone. In type 2, serum bilirubin falls with a decreased proportion of unconjugated bilirubin and an increase in biliary mono- and diconjugates. In type 1, serum bilirubin does not fall and unconjugated bilirubin predominates in bile [47]. In the future, *in vitro* expression of mutant DNA from patients with diagnostic problems could resolve the issue [46].

Dubin–Johnson type

This is a chronic, benign, intermittent jaundice with conjugated and some unconjugated hyperbilirubinaemia and with bilirubinuria [15, 16]. It is autosomal recessive, and is most frequent in the Middle East among Iranian Jews. There is reduced transport of many non-bile acid organic anions into bile due to a defective ATP-dependent canalicular transport system [33].

The liver, macroscopically, is greenish-black (black-liver jaundice) (figs 12.12, 12.13). In sections the liver cells show a brown pigment which is neither iron nor bile. There is no correlation between liver pigment and serum bilirubin levels. The chemical nature of the pigment is not certain. Previously thought due to melanin, recent data support the proposal that impaired secretion of anionic metabolites of tyrosine, phenylalanine and tryptophan is responsible [26].

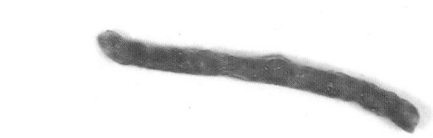

Fig. 12.12. Needle liver biopsy from patient with Dubin–Johnson syndrome is blackish-brown.

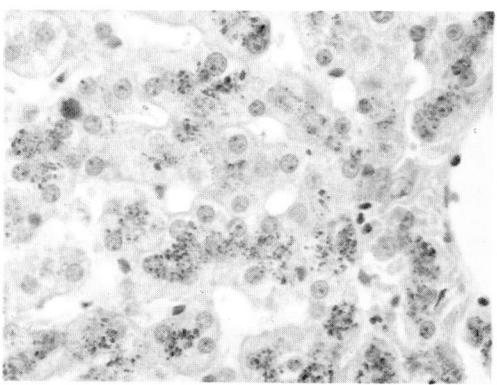

Fig. 12.13. Dubin–Johnson hyperbilirubinaemia. The liver cells and Kupffer cells are packed with a dark pigment which gives the staining reactions of lipofuscin. (H & E, ×275.)

Electron microscopy shows the pigment in dense bodies related to lysosomes (fig. 12.14).

An unrelated viral hepatitis leads to temporary mobilization of the hepatic pigment.

Pruritus is absent and the serum alkaline phosphatase and bile acid levels are normal.

Excretion of organic anions into bile is impaired. Hepatic uptake is usually normal. The contrast media used in intravenous cholangiography are not concentrated but ^{99m}Tc-HIDA excretion shows normal liver, biliary tree and gallbladder.

In patients a diagnostic pattern is seen in a prolonged BSP test. After an initial fall in serum level the BSP rises so that the value at 120 minutes exceeds that seen at 45 minutes (fig. 12.15) [30].

Urinary coproporphyrins are excreted in normal amounts but there is an increased proportion of coproporphyrin 1.

The condition may present as jaundice during pregnancy or after taking oral contraceptives, both of which reduce hepatic excretory function. Prognosis is excellent.

Rotor type

This is a similar form of chronic familial conjugated hyperbilirubinaemia. It resembles the Dubin–Johnson syndrome, the main difference being the absence of brown pigment in the liver cell [43]. The condition also differs from the Dubin–Johnson type in that the gallbladder opacifies on cholecystography and there is no secondary rise in the BSP test. The abnormality causing BSP retention appears to be related to a defect in hepatic uptake rather than excretion as originally demonstrated in the Dubin–Johnson syndrome. ^{99m}Tc-HIDA excretion gives no visualization of the liver, gallbladder or biliary tree.

Total urinary coproporphyrins are raised, as in cholestasis. The proportion of coproporphyrin 1 in urine is approximately 65% of the total [44]. Electron microscopy may show abnormalities of mitochondria and peroxisomes [18].

Family studies make an autosomal inheritance probable. The Rotor type has an excellent prognosis.

The group of familial non-haemolytic hyperbilirubinaemias

There is much overlap between the various syndromes of congenital hyperbilirubinaemia. Patients are found in the same family with conjugated hyperbilirubinaemia but with or without pigment in the liver cells. Pigmented livers have been found in patients with unconjugated hyperbilirubinaemia [9]. In one large family the pro-

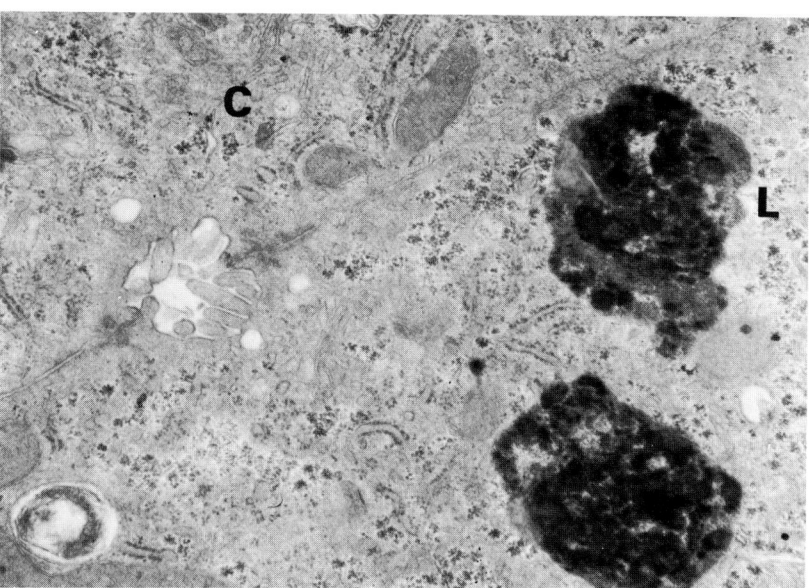

Fig. 12.14. Dubin–Johnson syndrome. Electron microscopy shows normal bile canaliculi with intact microvilli (C). Lysosomes (L) are enlarged, irregularly shaped and contain granular material and often membrane-bound lipid droplets.

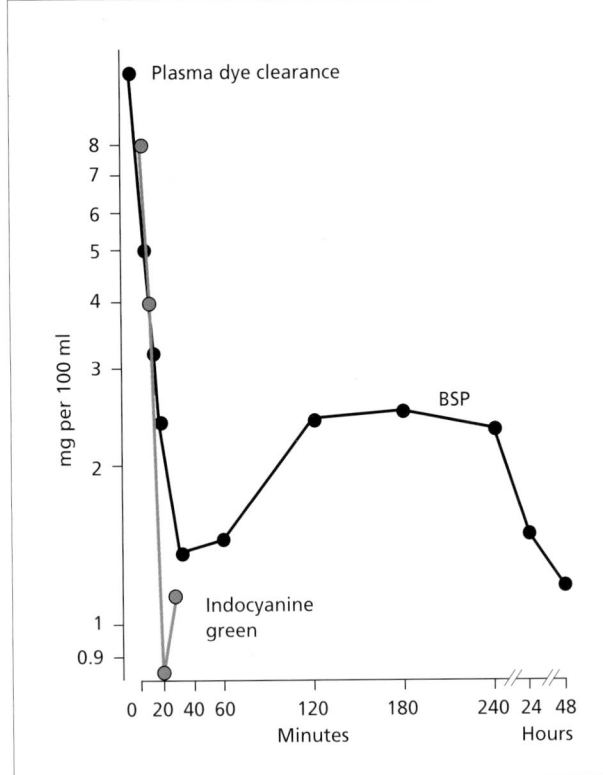

Fig. 12.15. Bromsulphthalein (BSP) tolerance test (5 mg/kg i.v.) in a patient with Dubin–Johnson syndrome. At 40 min, the BSP level has almost returned to normal. An increase is then seen at 120, 180 and 240 min. Dye can still be detected in the blood at 48 hours. The indocyanine green test is also shown and is normal at 20 min, but also has a tendency to increase at 30 min.

positi had the classic Dubin–Johnson picture, but the commonest abnormality in the family was unconjugated hyperbilirubinaemia [9]. In another family, conjugated and unconjugated hyperbilirubinaemia alternated in the same patient [42]. Such observations add to the confusion in separating the groups and in deciding the inheritance.

References

1 Arias IM. Chronic unconjugated hyperbilirubinaemia (CUH) with increased production of bile pigment not derived from the hemoglobin of mature, circulating erythrocytes. *J. Clin. Invest.* 1962; **41**: 1341.

2 Berk PD, Noyer C. Bilirubin metabolism and the hereditary hyperbilirubinaemias. *Semin. Liver Dis.* 1994; **14**: 323.

3 Black M, Billing BH. Hepatic bilirubin UDP-glucuronyl transferase activity in liver disease and Gilbert's syndrome. *N. Engl. J. Med.* 1969; **280**: 1266.

4 Black M, Sherlock S. Treatment of Gilbert's syndrome with phenobarbitone. *Lancet* 1970; **i**: 1359.

5 Bonnett R, Davies JE, Hursthouse MB. Structure of bilirubin. *Nature* 1976; **262**: 326.

6 Bosma PJ, Chowdhury JR, Bakker C *et al.* The genetic basis of the reduced expression of bilirubin UDP-glucuronosyltransferase 1 in Gilbert's syndrome. *N. Engl. J. Med.* 1995; **333**: 1171.

7 Bosma PJ, Goldhoorn B, Elferink RPJO *et al.* A mutation in bilirubin uridine 5′-diphosphate-glucuronosyltransferase isoform 1 causing Crigler–Najjar syndrome Type II. *Gastroenterology* 1993; **105**: 216.

8 Burchell B, Coughtrie MWH, Jansem PLM. Function and regulation of UDP glucuronosyltransferase genes in health and liver disease: report of the seventh international workshop on glucuronidation. September 1993, Pitlochry, Scotland. *Hepatology* 1994; **20**: 1622.

9 Butt HR, Anderson VE, Foulk WT *et al.* Studies of chronic idiopathic jaundice (Dubin–Johnson syndrome). II. Evaluation of a large family with the trait. *Gastroenterology* 1966; **51**: 619.

10 Camma C, Garofalo G, Almasio P *et al.* A performance evaluation of the expert system 'jaundice' in comparison with that of three hepatologists. *J. Hepatol.* 1991; **13**: 279.

11 Chowdhury JR, Chowdhury NR. Conjugation and excretion of bilirubin. *Semin. Liver Dis.* 1983; **3**: 11.

12 Crigler JF Jr, Najjar VA. Congenital familial non-hemolytic jaundice with kernicterus. *Pediatrics* 1952; **10**: 169.

13 De Morais SMF, Utrecht JP, Wells PG. Decreased glucuronidation and increased bioactivation of acetaminophen in Gilbert's syndrome. *Gastroenterology* 1992; **102**: 577.

14 Dixit V, Darvasi R, Arthur M *et al.* Restoration of liver function in Gunn rats without immunosuppression using transplanted microencapsulated hepatocytes. *Hepatology* 1990; **12**: 1342.

15 Dubin IN. Chronic idiopathic jaundice. A review of fifty cases. *Am. J. Med.* 1958; **24**: 268.

16 Dubin IN, Johnson FB. Chronic idiopathic jaundice with unidentified pigment in the liver cells: a new clinicopathological entity with a report of twelve cases. *Medicine (Baltimore)* 1954; **33**: 155.

17 Elawady M, Chowdhury RJ, Kesari K *et al.* Mechanism of the lack of induction of UDP-glucuronosyltransferase activity by 3-methylcholanthrene in Gunn rats. *J. Biol. Chem.* 1990; **265**: 10752.

18 Evans J, Lefkowitch J, Lim CK *et al.* Fecal porphyrin abnormalities in a patient with features of Rotor's syndrome. *Gastroenterology* 1981; **81**: 1125.

19 Farrell GC, Gollan JL, Stevens SM *et al.* Crigler–Najjar type 1 syndrome: absence of hepatic bilirubin UDP glucuronyl transferase activity and therapeutic responses to light. *Aust. NZ J. Med.* 1982; **12**: 280.

20 Fevery J, Vanstapel F, Blanckaert N. Bile pigment metabolism. *Clin. Gastroenterol.* 1989; **3**: 283.

21 Frank BB. Clinical evaluation of jaundice. A guideline of the patient care committee of the American Gastroenterological Association. *JAMA* 1989; **262**: 3031.

22 Gilbert A, Leerboullet P. La cholémie simple familiale. *Sem. Med. Paris* 1901; **21**: 241.

23 Gollan JL, Huang SN, Billing B *et al.* Prolonged survival in three brothers with severe type 2 Crigler–Najjar syndrome. Ultrastructural and metabolic studies. *Gastroenterology* 1975; **68**: 1543.

24 Huang T-J, Chowdhury JR, Lahiri P *et al.* Prenatal diagnosis of bilirubin-UDP-gluronosyltransferase deficiency in rats by genomic DNA analysis. *Hepatology* 1992; **16**: 756.

25 Jansen PLM. Genetic diseases of bilirubin metabolism: the inherited unconjugated hyperbilirubinaemias. *J. Hepatol.*

1996; **24** (in press).

26 Kitamura T, Alroy J, Gatmaitan Z *et al.* Defective biliary excretion of epinephrine metabolites in mutant (TR-) rats: relation to the pathogenesis of black liver in the Dubin–Johnson syndrome and Corriedale sheep with an analogous excretory defect. *Hepatology* 1992; **15**: 1154.

27 Kitamura T, Jansen PLM, Hardenbrook C *et al.* Defective ATP-dependent bile canalicular transport of organic anions in mutant (TR-) rats with conjugated hyperbilirubinemia. *Proc. Natl. Acad. Sci. USA* 1990; **87**: 3557.

28 Lieverse AG, van Essen GG, Beukeveld GJJ *et al.* Familial increased serum intestinal alkaline phosphatase: a new variant associated with Gilbert's syndrome. *J. Clin. Pathol.* 1990; **43**: 125.

29 McColl KEL, Thompson GG, El Omar E *et al.* Porphyrin metabolism and haem biosynthesis in Gilbert's syndrome. *Gut* 1987; **28**: 125.

30 Mandema E, De Fraiture WH, Nieweg HO *et al.* Familial chronic idiopathic jaundice (Dubin–Sprinz disease) with a note on bromsulphalein metabolism in this disease. *Am. J. Med.* 1960; **28**: 42.

31 Monaghan G, Ryan M, Seddon R *et al.* Genetic variation in bilirubin UDP-glucuronosyltransferase gene promoter and Gilbert's syndrome. *Lancet* 1996; **347**: 578.

32 Muraca M, Fevery J, Blanckaert N. Relationships between serum bilirubins and production and conjugation of bilirubin. Studies in Gilbert's syndrome, Crigler–Najjar disease, hemolytic disorders, and rat models. *Gastroenterology* 1987; **92**: 309.

33 Nishida T, Hardenbrook C, Gatmaitan Z *et al.* ATP-dependent organic anion transport system in normal and TR- rat liver canalicular membrane. *Am. J. Physiol.* 1992; **262**: G629.

34 Olsson R, Stigendal L. Clinical experience with isolated hyperbilirubinemia. *Scand. J. Gastroenterol.* 1989; **24**: 617.

35 Owens D, Sherlock S. The diagnosis of Gilbert's syndrome: role of the reduced caloric intake test. *Br. Med. J.* 1973; **iii**: 559.

36 Persico M, Romano M, Muraca M *et al.* Responsiveness to phenobarbital in an adult with Crigler–Najjar disease associated with neurological involvement and skin hyperextensibility. *Hepatology* 1991; **13**: 213.

37 Peters WHM, Jansen PLM. Microsomal UDP-glucuronyl-transferase-catalyzed bilirubin diglucuronide formation in human liver. *J. Hepatol.* 1986; **2**: 182.

38 Portman OW, Chowdhury JR, Chowdhury NR *et al.* A non-human primate model of Gilbert's syndrome. *Hepatology* 1984; **4**: 175.

39 Powell LW, Hemingway E, Billing BH *et al.* Idiopathic unconjugated hyperbilirubinaemia (Gilbert's syndrome). A study of 42 families. *N. Engl. J. Med.* 1967; **277**: 1108.

40 Röllinghoff W, Paumgartner G, Preisig R. Nicotinic acid test in the diagnosis of Gilbert's syndrome: correlation with bilirubin clearance. *Gut* 1981; **22**: 663.

41 Saint-Marc Girardin M-F, Le Minor M, Alperovitch A *et al.* Computer-aided selection of diagnostic tests in jaundiced patients. *Gut* 1985; **26**: 961.

42 Satler J. Another variant of constitutional familial hepatic dysfunction with permanent jaundice and with alternating serum bilirubin relations. *Acta Hepato-Splen.* 1966; **13**: 38.

43 Schiff L, Billing BH, Oikawa Y. Familial non-hemolytic jaundice with conjugated bilirubin in the serum. A case study. *N. Engl. J. Med.* 1959; **260**: 1314.

44 Shimizu Y, Naruto H, Ida S *et al.* Urinary coproporphyrin isomers in Rotor's syndrome: a study in eight families. *Hepatology* 1981; **1**: 173.

45 Seig A, Stiehl A, Raedsch R *et al.* Gilbert's syndrome: diagnosis by typical serum bilirubin pattern. *Clin. Chim. Acta* 1986; **154**: 41.

46 Seppen J, Bosma PJ, Goldhoorn, BG *et al.* Discrimination between Crigler–Najjar type I and II by expression of mutant bilirubin uridine diphosphate glucuronosyl transferase. *J. Clin. Invest.* 1994; **94**: 2385.

47 Sinaasappel M, Jansen PLM. The differential diagnosis of Crigler–Najjar disease, types 1 and 2 by bile pigment analysis. *Gastroenterology* 1991; **100**: 783.

48 Sokal EM, Silva ES, Hermans D *et al.* Orthotopic liver transplantation for Crigler–Najjar type I disease in six children. *Transplantation* 1995; **60**: 1095.

49 Summerskill WHJ, Clowdus BF II, Bollman JL *et al.* Clinical and experimental studies on the effect of corticotrophin and steroid drugs on bilirubinaemia. *Am. J. Med. Sci.* 1961; **241**: 555.

50 Tiribelli C, Ostrow JD. New concepts in bilirubin chemistry, transport and metabolism: report of the Second International Bilirubin Workshop, 9–11 April 1992, Trieste, Italy. *Hepatology* 1993; **17**: 715.

51 van der Veere CN, Sinaasappel M, McDonagh AF *et al.* Current therapy of Crigler–Najjar syndrome type I: report of a world registry. *Hepatology* 1996; **24**: 311.

52 Vierling JM, Berk PD, Hofmann AF *et al.* Normal fasting-state levels of serum cholyl-conjugated bile acids in Gilbert's syndrome: an aid to the diagnosis. *Hepatology* 1982; **2**: 340.

53 Watson KJR, Gollan JL. Gilbert's syndrome. *Clin. Gastroenterol.* 1989; **3**: 337.

54 Weiss JS, Gautam A, Lauff JJ *et al.* The clinical importance of a protein-bound fraction of serum bilirubin in patients with hyperbilirubinaemia. *N. Engl. J. Med.* 1983; **309**: 147.

55 Zucker SD, Goessling W, Gollan JL. Kinetics of bilirubin transfer between serum albumin and membrane vesicles. *J. Biol. Chem.* 1995; **270**: 1974.

Chapter 13
Cholestasis

Cholestasis is defined as failure of normal amounts of bile to reach the duodenum. This may be due to pathology anywhere between the hepatocyte and the ampulla of Vater. The term 'obstructive jaundice' is not used, as in many instances no mechanical block can be shown in the biliary tract.

Prolonged cholestasis produces biliary cirrhosis; the time taken for its development varies from months to years. The transition is not reflected in a sudden change in the clinical picture. The term 'biliary cirrhosis' is reserved for a pathological picture. It is diagnosed when there are features of cirrhosis such as nodule formation, encephalopathy or fluid retention.

Anatomy of the biliary system

Bile salts, conjugated bilirubin, cholesterol, phospholipids, proteins, electrolytes and water are secreted by the liver cell into the canaliculus (fig. 13.1). The bile secretory apparatus comprises the *canalicular membrane* with its carrier proteins, the *intra-cellular organelles* and the *cytoskeleton* of the hepatocyte (fig. 13.2). *Tight junctions* between hepatocytes seal the biliary space from the blood compartment.

The canalicular membrane contains carrier proteins which transport bile acids, bilirubin, cations and anions. The microvilli increase the surface area. The organelles include the Golgi apparatus and lysosomes. Vesicles carry proteins such as IgA from sinusoid to canaliculus, and newly synthesized cholesterol and phospholipid

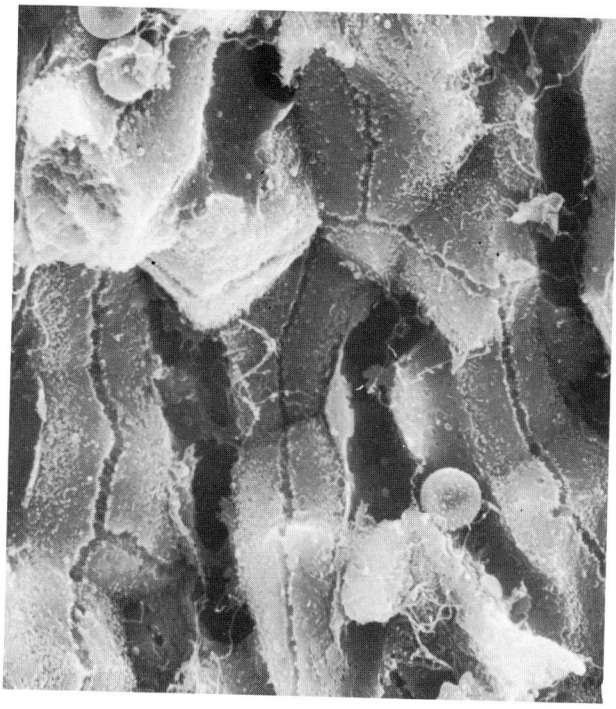

Fig. 13.1. Scanning electron micrograph of the canalicular biliary system.

and possibly bile acid membrane transporters [11] from the microsomes to the bile canalicular membrane.

The peri-canalicular cytoplasm contains elements of the *cytoskeleton* of the hepatocyte: *microtubules, microfilaments* and *intermediate filaments* [85]. Microtubules are

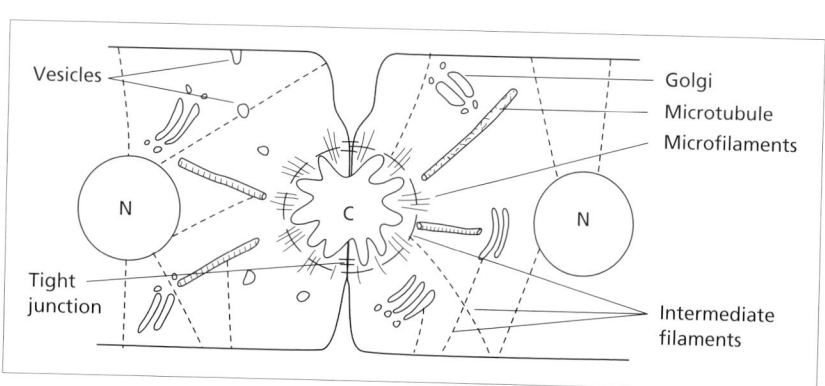

Fig. 13.2. The biliary secretory apparatus. Diagram of the ultrastructure of the bile canaliculus (C), cytoskeleton, and organelles (N = nucleus).

formed by the polymerization of tubulin and provide a network within the cell, particularly near the basolateral membrane and Golgi apparatus. They participate in receptor-mediated vesicular transcytosis, in the secretion of lipids, and under some conditions the secretion of bile acids. Their formation is inhibited by colchicine.

Microfilament formation involves the interaction between polymerized (F) and free (G) actin. Canalicular motility and contraction depend upon microfilaments which are clustered around the canalicular membrane. Phalloidin increases, and cytochalasin B reduces the polymerization of actin. Both inhibit canalicular motility and produce cholestasis.

Intermediate filaments are composed of cytokeratin. They form a network between plasma membrane, nucleus, intra-cellular organelles and other elements of the cytoskeleton. Disruption of intermediate filaments affects intra-cellular transport processes and obliterates the canalicular space.

The canalicular secretion is modified by water and electrolytes passing between hepatocytes across the tight junction (*paracellular flow*). This transfer is due to the osmotic gradient between the canalicular secretion and the intra-cellular fluid in continuity with the space of Disse. The integrity of the tight junction depends upon a 225 kDa protein (ZO-1) present on the inner surface of the plasma membrane [4]. Disruption of the tight junction leads to free passage of solute and larger molecules into the canaliculus with loss of the osmotic gradient and cholestasis. Canalicular bile may also regurgitate into the sinusoid.

The bile canaliculi empty into ductules sometimes called cholangioles or canals of Hering (fig. 13.3). These are found largely in the portal zones of the liver. The ductule passes into the interlobular bile duct which is the first bile channel to be accompanied by a branch of the hepatic artery and portal vein. These are also found in the portal triad. These channels unite with one another to form septal bile ducts and so on until the two main hepatic ducts emerge from the right and left lobes of the liver at the porta hepatis.

Secretion of bile (figs 13.4, 13.5)

Bile is formed by several different energy-dependent transport processes [61]. Secretion is relatively independent of perfusion pressure. The total bile flow in man is about 600 ml/day. The hepatocyte provides two components: bile salt dependent ($\simeq$ 225 ml/day) and bile salt independent ($\simeq$ 225 ml/day). Bile ductular cells contribute a further 150 ml/day.

The passage of bile salts into the biliary canaliculus is the most important factor promoting bile formation. This is the *bile salt dependent fraction*. Water follows the osmotically active bile salts and there is an excellent

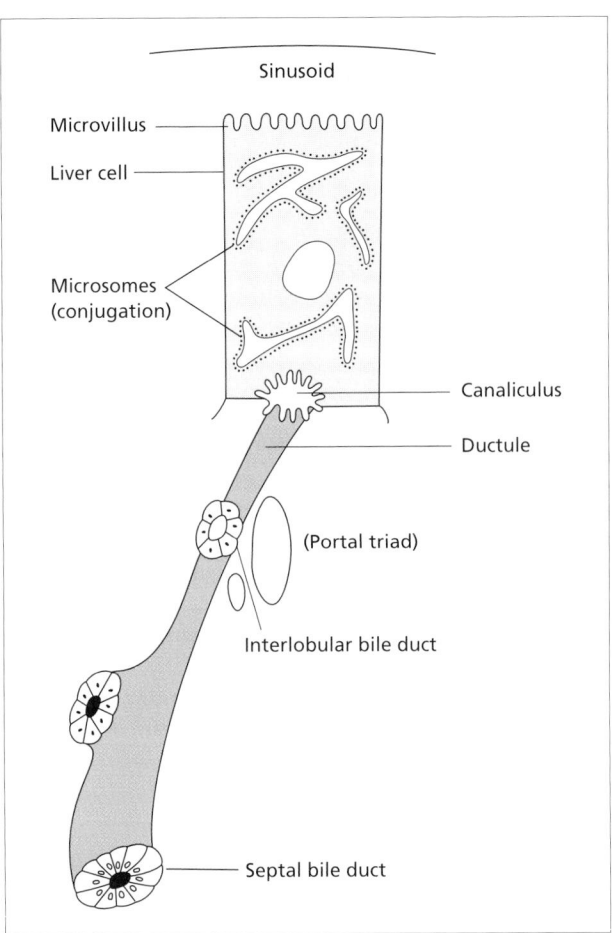

Fig. 13.3. The anatomy of the intra-hepatic biliary system.

correlation between bile flow and bile salt secretion. Changes in osmotic activity may be the regulatory mechanism for the flow of water into the bile.

Bile salt independent flow is shown by extrapolation of bile salt versus bile flow data to zero bile salt excretion when a positive intercept is shown. This indicates that flow would continue at zero bile salt excretion, presumably by a bile salt independent process. In this case osmotically active solutes such as glutathione and bicarbonate generate water flow.

Cellular mechanisms

The hepatocyte is a polarized secretory epithelial cell with a basolateral (sinusoidal and lateral) and apical (canalicular) membrane (fig. 13.5).

Bile formation requires the uptake of bile acids and other organic and inorganic ions across the basolateral (sinusoidal) membrane, transport through the hepatocyte and excretion across the canalicular membrane. This is followed by osmotic filtration of water from the hepatocyte and along the paracellular pathway. The iden-

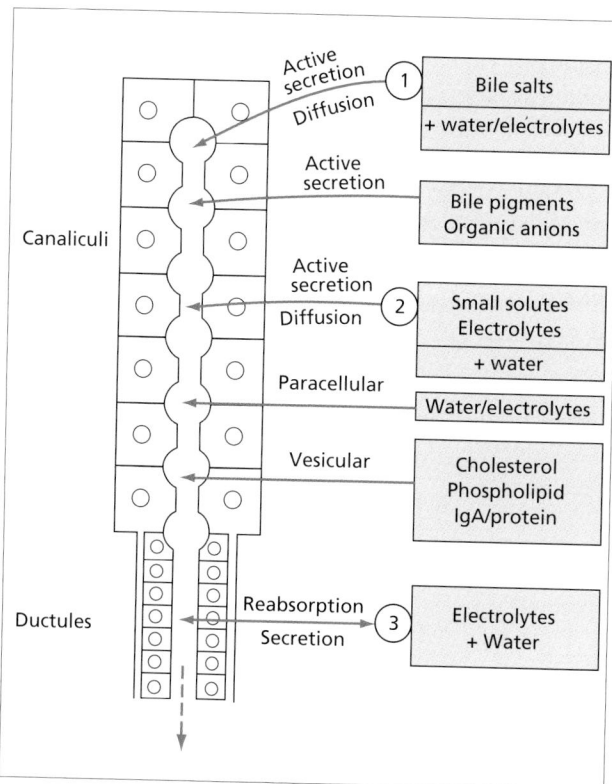

Fig. 13.4. Mechanisms of bile formation. (1) Bile salt dependent (≈225 ml/day). (2) Bile salt independent (≈225 ml/day). (3) Ductular flow (≈150 ml/day) stimulated by secretin.

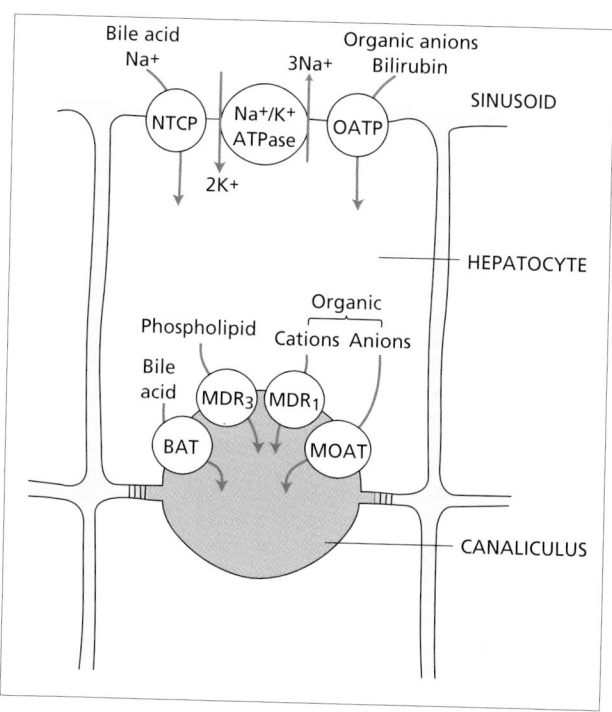

Fig. 13.5. Major transport systems in bile formation. Note the Na+–K+ ATPase or sodium pump (centre top), the sinusoidal Na+ taurocholate co-transporting protein (NCTP) and the sinusoidal multispecific organic anion transporter (OATP). The canalicular membrane transporters are: BAT, the ATP-dependent bile acid transporter; MOAT, the multispecific organic anion transporter; MDR1, the ATP-dependent transporter of organic cations; and MDR3, an ATP-dependent phospholipid transporter (flippase). Other transport systems include a sinusoidal Na+–H+ exchange, and canalicular bicarbonate transport.

tification and characterization of the sinusoidal and canalicular transporters is complicated. As can be imagined, investigation of the secretory apparatus for canalicular bile is difficult, but the development of hepatocyte couplet preparations in short-term culture has proved a powerful tool for many studies [35]. The recent cloning of transporters is allowing characterization of function in isolation [50].

The secretory process depends upon the presence of one set of carrier proteins in the basolateral membrane and another in the canalicular membrane (fig. 13.5). Driving the whole process is the Na+–K+ ATPase in the basolateral membrane which maintains a chemical gradient and potential difference between the hepatocyte and its surroundings. This transporter exchanges three intra-cellular sodium ions for two extra-cellular potassium ions, thus maintaining the sodium (high outside : low inside) and potassium (low outside : high inside) gradient. In addition, because of the imbalance of electrical exchange, the cell interior is negatively charged (−35 mV) compared with the exterior, favouring uptake of positively charged ions and excretion of those with a negative charge. The Na+–K+ ATPase is present on the basolateral membrane; it is not found on the canalicular

membrane [76]. This carrier, among others, is influenced by changes in membrane fluidity.

SINUSOIDAL UPTAKE

In the basolateral (sinusoidal) membrane of the hepatocyte there are multiple transport systems for organic anion uptake with partially overlapping substrate specificities (fig. 13.5) [58]. Characterization, previously dependent on the study of animal cells, has recently benefited from the cloning of human transporter proteins [50]. The organic anion transporting protein (OATP) is sodium independent and carries several molecules including bile acid, bromsulphthalein and probably bilirubin [49]. Other carriers are also thought to transport bilirubin into the hepatocyte [66]. Bile acids conjugated with taurine (or glycine) are predominantly taken up into the cell by the sodium/bile acid co-transporting protein (NCTP) [58].

Other ion transporters on the basolateral surface are the Na+–H+ exchanger involved in control of intra-cellular pH. A Na$^+$–HCO$_3^-$ co-transporter also serves this function. The basolateral membrane also contains uptake processes for sulphate, non-esterified fatty acids and organic cations [64].

Transport of bile acids across the cell involves cytosolic protein. The major protein is 3-α-hydroxysteroid dehydrogenase. Glutathione-S-transferase and fatty acid binding proteins are less important. The endoplasmic reticulum and Golgi apparatus are implicated in the transfer of bile acid. Vesicular transport only seems relevant at high, supraphysiological bile acid flux rates.

The transcytotic vesicular pathway transports fluid phase proteins and ligands such as IgA and LDL. Transfer from basolateral membrane to the region of the canaliculus takes about 10 minutes. This mechanism accounts for only a small percentage of total bile flow. It is microtubule dependent.

The canalicular membrane is a special part of the hepatocyte plasma membrane which contains transporters (mainly ATPase dependent) responsible for carrying molecules into bile against steep concentration gradients. It also contains enzymes such as alkaline phosphatase and gamma glutamyl transpeptidase. The canalicular multispecific organic anion transporter (cMOAT) carries glucuronide and glutathione-S-conjugates, for example bilirubin diglucuronide. The canalicular bile acid transporter (cBAT) carries bile acids and is in part driven by the negative intra-cellular electric potential. Bile acid independent flow probably depends upon glutathione transport as well as the canalicular secretion of bicarbonate, possibly by a Cl$^-$/HCO$_3^-$ exchanger.

Two members of the P-glycoprotein family are important in canalicular transport; both are ATP dependent [63]. Multiple drug resistance 1 (MDR1) is a transporter of organic cations, and derives its name from being responsible for transporting cytotoxic drugs out of cancer cells, rendering them resistant to these drugs. The endogenous substrate is not known. MDR3 is a phospholipid translocator that acts as a flippase for phosphatidylcholine, and is important in the secretion of phospholipid into bile. The function and importance of this protein has been clarified by the mouse knock-out model lacking the mdr2-P glycoprotein (equivalent to human MDR3) [79]. Without phospholipid in bile, bile acids damage the biliary epithelium and cause ductular inflammation and periductal fibrosis.

Water and inorganic ions (in particular sodium) enter canalicular bile by diffusion across the tight junctions because of the osmotic gradient. The tight junction is a negatively charged semi-permeable barrier.

Bile secretion is influenced by many hormones and second messengers including cyclic AMP and protein kinase C. An increase in cytosolic calcium inhibits bile secretion. Passage of bile down the canaliculus involves microfilaments which are responsible for canalicular motility and contraction (fig. 13.6) [81].

More distally bile ductular cells secrete a bicarbonate-rich solution—so-called *ductular bile flow*—which modifies canalicular bile. This is stimulated by secretin. The process involves generation of cyclic AMP, and several membrane transporters including the Cl$^-$/HCO$_3^-$ exchanger and the *cystic fibrosis transmembrane conductance regulator*, a cyclic AMP-regulated plasma membrane Cl$^-$ channel [16].

It is suggested that ursodeoxycholic acid is actively absorbed by the ductular cells and exchanged for bicarbonate and that the bile acid recirculates to the liver ('cholehepatic shunting') for further excretion. This may explain the choleretic effect of ursodeoxycholic acid associated with high biliary bicarbonate secretion which is preserved in experimental cirrhosis [25].

Bile is normally secreted at a pressure of about 15–25 cmH$_2$O. A rise to about 35 cm results in suppression of bile flow and so to jaundice. Bilirubin and bile acid secretion may stop, resulting in *white bile* which appears like a clear mucus-containing fluid.

The syndrome of cholestasis

Definition

Cholestasis is interference with bile flow or formation. This can occur anywhere between the basolateral (sinusoidal) membrane of the hepatocyte and the ampulla of Vater.

Functionally cholestasis is defined as a decrease in canalicular bile flow. There is a decreased hepatic secretion of water and/or organic anions (bilirubin, bile acid).

Morphologically cholestasis is defined as accumulation of bile in liver cells and biliary passages.

Clinically cholestasis is the retention in the blood of all substances normally excreted in the bile. Serum bile acids are increased. Clinical features are itching (not always present) and raised serum alkaline phosphatase (biliary isoenzyme) and gamma glutamyl transpeptidase.

Classification

Cholestasis may be classified as extra- or intra-hepatic, and acute or chronic.

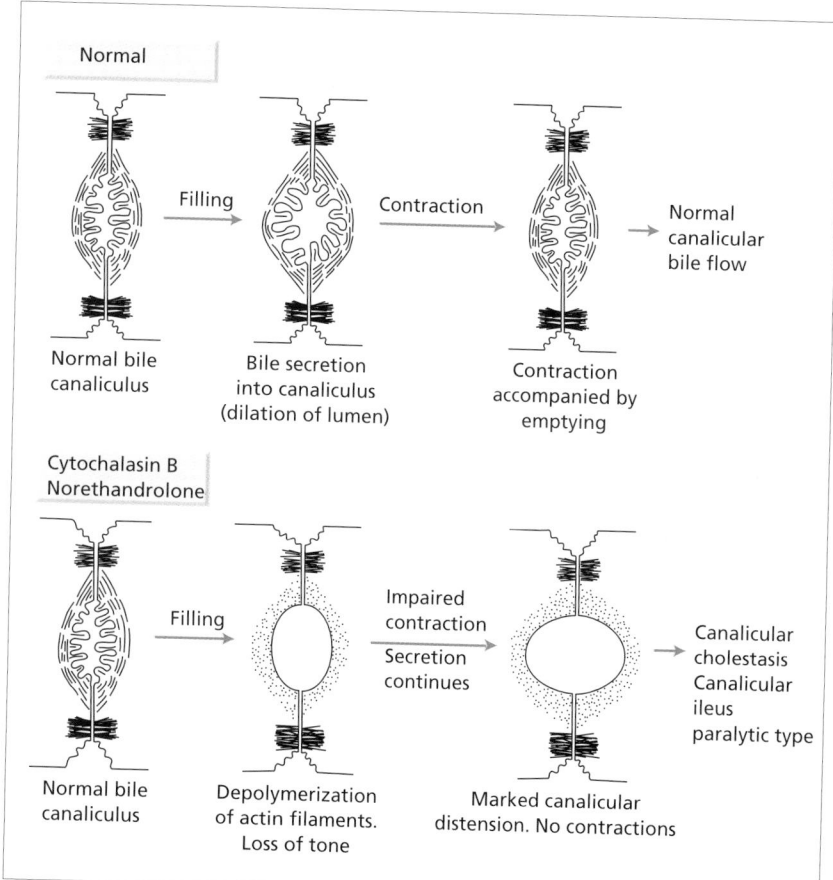

Fig. 13.6. A possible mechanism for intra-hepatic cholestasis. Normal canalicular bile secretion is accompanied by canalicular contraction and canalicular bile flow. Cytochalasin or norethandrolone depolymerizes actin filaments, resulting in loss of tone, canalicular distension and failure to contract, with consequent canalicular ileus and cholestasis. (Courtesy M.J. Phillips.)

Extra-hepatic cholestasis encompasses conditions where there is physical obstruction to the bile ducts. Usually this is outside the liver, but a hilar cholangiocarcinoma growing up main intra-hepatic ducts would be included. The most common cause is a stone in the common duct (Chapter 31); other causes are carcinoma of pancreas and ampulla (Chapter 33), benign bile duct stricture (Chapter 32) and cholangiocarcinoma (Chapter 34). Usually this group causes acute cholestasis.

Intra-hepatic cholestasis includes those conditions where there is no demonstrable obstruction (on cholangiography) to the major bile ducts. Causes are drug-induced cholestasis, cholestatic hepatitis (Chapter 18), hormones, primary biliary cirrhosis (Chapter 14) and septicaemia. Primary sclerosing cholangitis (Chapter 15) may produce both intra- and extra-hepatic cholestasis, depending on the size of duct involved and whether there is a 'dominant' stricture in the common duct. Rare causes of intra-hepatic cholestasis include Byler's disease, benign recurrent cholestasis, Hodgkin's disease and amyloid. Intra-hepatic cholestasis may be acute, for example drug related, or chronic as in primary biliary cirrhosis and primary sclerosing cholangitis.

The importance of the distinction between extra- and intra-hepatic cholestasis is that symptoms and biochem-istry may not separate them. There is a need for a diagnostic algorithm to differentiate between the two.

Patients with both acute and chronic cholestasis may itch, malabsorb fat and be vitamin K deficient. Chronic cholestatic patients may have in addition hyperlipidaemia and bone disease.

Pathogenesis

Physical obstruction to the bile duct by stone or stricture is straightforward. The pathogenesis of primary biliary cirrhosis and primary sclerosing cholangitis is described elsewhere (Chapters 14 and 15). Drugs, hormones and sepsis affect hepatocyte cytoskeleton and membrane (table 13.1).

Changes in *membrane fluidity* and *Na+–K+ ATPase activity* may give cholestasis [80]. Ethinyl oestradiol is known

Table 13.1. Possible cellular mechanisms of cholestasis

Membrane lipid/fluidity	Modified
Na+–K+ ATPase/other carriers	Inhibited
Cytoskeleton	Disrupted
Canalicular integrity (membrane, tight junction)	Lost

to decrease fluidity of the sinusoidal plasma membrane. In rats this can be prevented by the methyl donor, S-adenosyl methionine (SAME), which alters membrane fluidity [73]. *Escherichia coli* endotoxin, which decreases Na+–K+ ATPase activity, may act in a similar way.

Integrity of the canalicular membrane may be altered by disruption of either the *microfilaments* responsible for canalicular tone and contraction or *tight junctions*. Cholestasis due to phalloidin is related to depolymerization of the actin of microfilaments. Chlopromazine also affects the polymerization of actin. Cytochalasin B and androgens disrupt microfilaments, and canaliculi become less contractile [81] (fig. 13.6). Disruption of tight junctions leads to loss of the normal restrictive barrier between hepatocytes with subsequent passage of larger molecules directly into the canaliculus from the blood. There can also be regurgitation of solutes from bile to blood. Oestrogens and phalloidin disrupt tight junctions. Note that a single compound may affect several of the mechanisms contributing to bile formation.

Vesicular transport depends upon the integrity of microtubules and these can be disrupted by colchicine and chlorpromazine. If inadequate quantities of bile salts reach the canaliculus or leak from it the *bile salt dependent pump* fails. Interruption of the entero-hepatic circulation of bile salts may contribute. Cyclosporin A inhibits the ATP-dependent bile acid transporter in the canalicular membrane [9].

Ductular abnormalities such as inflammation and epithelial changes interfere with bile flow but are probably secondary rather than primary. The role of alterations in the cystic fibrosis transmembrane conductance regulator in ductular cells remains to be studied. Mutations in the gene are no more frequent in primary sclerosing cholangitis than controls [56].

Some *bile acids* that are retained due to cholestasis may cause cellular damage and exacerbate cholestasis. Administration of less toxic bile salts, such as tauro-ursodeoxycholate, is protective [74]. Oxygen-free radicals are produced by mitochondria when rat hepatocytes are exposed to hydrophobic bile acids, for example tauro-chenodeoxycholic acid [83]. Such damage may be reduced by the observed transposition of the canalicular bile salt transport protein to the basolateral membrane, resulting in a reversal of the bile salt secretory polarity of the hepatocyte [33]. This may prevent the accumulation of bile acids within the cytosol.

Pathology

Some changes are related to cholestasis itself and depend on its duration. Characteristic changes of specific diseases are not covered here but in the appropriate chapter.

Macroscopically the cholestatic liver is enlarged, green,

swollen and with a rounded edge. Nodularity develops late.

Light microscopy. Zone 3 shows marked bilirubin stasis in hepatocytes, Kupffer cells and canaliculi (fig. 13.7). Hepatocytes may show feathery degeneration, possibly due to retention of bile salts, with foamy cells and surrounding mononuclear accumulations. Cellular necrosis, regeneration and nodular hyperplasia are minimal.

Portal zones (zone 1) show ductular proliferation (fig. 13.8) due to the mitogenic effect of bile salts. Hepatocytes transform into bile duct cells and form basement membranes. Reabsorption of bile constituents by ductular cells can result in microlith formation.

Following bile duct obstruction the hepatic changes develop very rapidly. Cholestasis is seen within 36 hours. Bile duct proliferation is early; portal fibrosis develops later. After about 2 weeks, duration cannot be related to the extent of hepatic change. *Bile lakes* represent ruptured interlobular ducts.

With ascending cholangitis histology shows accu-

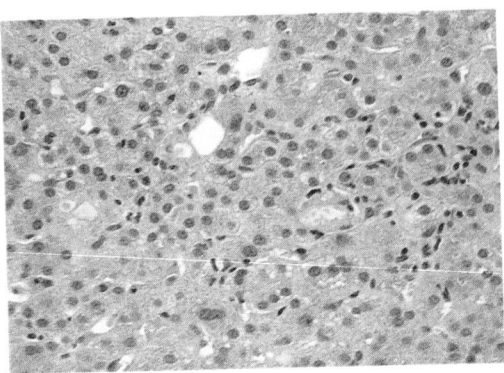

Fig. 13.7. Cholestasis: bile is seen in dilated canaliculi and hepatocytes.

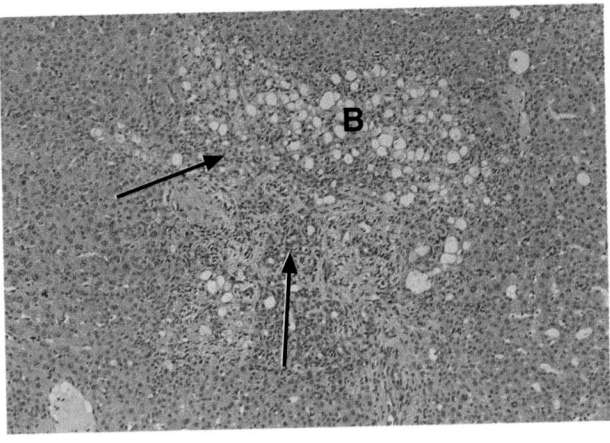

Fig. 13.8. Bile duct obstruction. There is portal tract expansion and ductular proliferation (arrows) with balloon ('feathery') degeneration of surrounding hepatocytes (B). (H & E, ×40.)

mulations of polymorphonuclear leucocytes related to bile ducts. The sinusoids also contain numerous polymorphs.

Fibrosis can be seen in zone 1. This is reversible if the cholestasis is relieved. The zone 1 fibrosis extends to meet bands from adjacent zones (fig. 13.9) so that eventually zone 3 is enclosed by a ring of connective tissue (fig. 13.10). In the early stages, the relationship of hepatic vein to portal vein is normal and this distinguishes the picture from biliary cirrhosis. Continuing periductular fibrosis may lead to disappearance of bile ducts and this is irreversible.

Zone 1 oedema and inflammation are related to biliolymphatic reflux and to leucotrienes. Mallory bodies can accompany the inflammation and fibrosis in zone 1. Copper-associated protein, demonstrated by orcein staining, is seen in periportal hepatocytes.

Class I HLA antigens are normally expressed on hepatocytes. Reports on the pattern of class II expression are conflicting. This HLA antigen seems to be absent on hepatocytes of normal children and present in some patients with autoimmune liver disease and primary sclerosing cholangitis [55].

Biliary cirrhosis follows prolonged cholestasis. Fibrous tissue bands in the portal zones coalesce and the lobules are correspondingly reduced in size. Fibrous bridges join

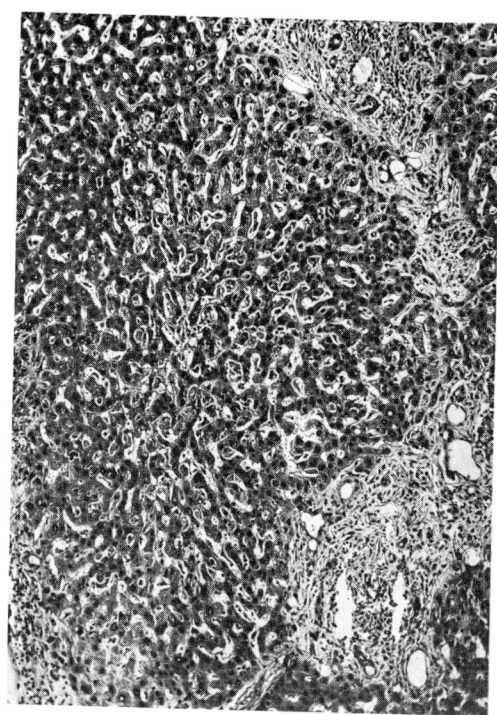

Fig. 13.9. Unrelieved common bile duct obstruction. Bile duct proliferation and fibrosis in the portal tracts which are becoming joined together. Bile pigment accumulations in the centrizonal areas. Hepatic lobular architecture normal. (H & E, ×67.)

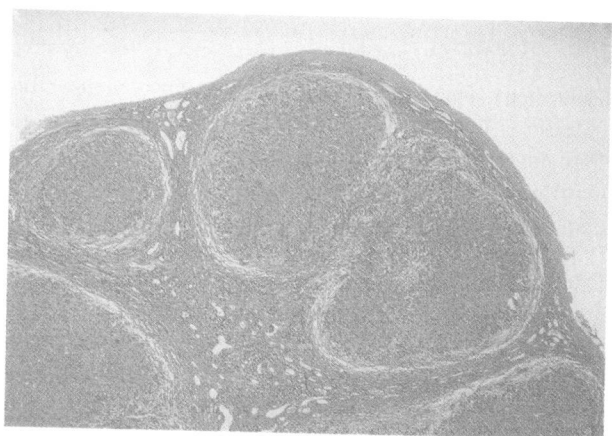

Fig. 13.10. Biliary cirrhosis. Low power showing marked perinodular oedema and partly coalescent nodules — features typical of this condition. (H & E, ×15.)

portal and centrizonal areas (fig. 13.10). Nodular regeneration of liver cells follows, but a true cirrhosis rarely follows biliary obstruction. In total biliary obstruction due to cancer of the head of the pancreas death ensues before nodular regeneration has had time to develop. Biliary cirrhosis is associated with partial biliary obstruction due for instance to biliary stricture or primary sclerosing cholangitis.

In biliary cirrhosis the liver is larger and greener than in non-biliary cirrhosis. Margins of nodules are clear cut rather than moth-eaten. If the cholestasis is relieved the portal zone fibrosis and bile retention disappear slowly.

Electron microscopy. The biliary canaliculi show changes irrespective of the cause. These include dilatation and oedema, blunting, distortion and sparsity of the microvilli. The Golgi apparatus shows vacuolization. Peri-canalicular bile-containing vesicles appear and these represent the 'feathery' hepatocytes seen on light microscopy. Lysosomes proliferate and contain copper bound as a metalloprotein.

The endoplasmic reticulum is hypertrophied; all these changes are non-specific for the aetiology of the cholestasis.

Changes in other organs. The spleen is enlarged and firm due to reticulo-endothelial hyperplasia and increase in mononuclear cells. Later, cirrhosis results in portal hypertension.

The intestinal contents are bulky and greasy; the more complete the cholestasis the paler the stools.

The kidneys are swollen and bile stained. Casts containing bilirubin are found in the distal convoluted tubules and collecting tubules. The casts may be heavily infiltrated with cells and the tubular epithelium is disrupted. The surrounding connective tissue may then show oedema and inflammatory infiltration. Scar formation is absent.

Clinical features

Prominent features of cholestasis, both acute and chronic, are itching and malabsorption. Bone disease (hepatic osteodystrophy) and cholesterol deposition (xanthomas, xanthelasmas) are seen with chronic cholestasis, which is also associated with skin pigmentation due to melanin. In contrast to the patient with hepato-cellular disease where there is malaise and physical deterioration, the cholestatic patient feels well. On examination, the *liver* is usually enlarged with a firm smooth non-tender edge. *Splenomegaly* is unusual except in biliary cirrhosis where portal hypertension has developed. Stools are pale.

Pruritus has been attributed to retained bile acids. However, even with the most sophisticated biochemical methods, pruritus did not correlate with the concentration of any naturally occurring bile acid in serum or in skin [32]. Moreover, in terminal liver failure, when pruritus is lost, serum bile acids may still be increased.

The association of pruritus with cholestasis suggests that it is due to some substance normally excreted in the bile. Disappearance of itching when liver cells fail indicates that the agent responsible may be manufactured by the liver. Cholestyramine binds many compounds and thus its success in treating the pruritus of cholestasis does not incriminate one particular agent.

Attention has turned towards agents that may produce itching by a central neurotransmitter mechanism [47]. There is evidence from animal studies and therapeutic trials that an endogenous opioid peptide may be responsible [8]. Cholestatic animals, in which endogenous opioids accumulate are in a state of analgesia which can be reversed by naloxone. Perception of itching in cholestatic patients is less during naloxone treatment [7]. However, ondansetron, a 5-HT3 serotonin receptor antagonist also improves itching in cholestatic patients [75]. Further studies are awaited to unravel the mechanism of this troublesome and occasionally devastating complication of cholestasis, and to find an effective reliable treatment without side-effects.

Steatorrhoea is proportional to the degree of jaundice. It is due to the lack of sufficient intestinal bile salts for the absorption of dietary fat and fat-soluble vitamins (A, D, K and E) (figs 13.11, 13.12). Micellar solution of lipid is inadequate. Stools are loose, pale, bulky and offensive. The colour gives a good indication of whether cholestasis is total, intermittent or decreasing.

Fat-soluble vitamins. In short-term cholestasis needing invasive techniques for investigation and treatment, vitamin K replacement may be necessary to correct the prolonged prothrombin time.

In prolonged cholestasis, plasma vitamin A levels fall. Hepatic storage is normal and the deficiency is due to poor absorption [62]. If cholestasis is sufficiently long,

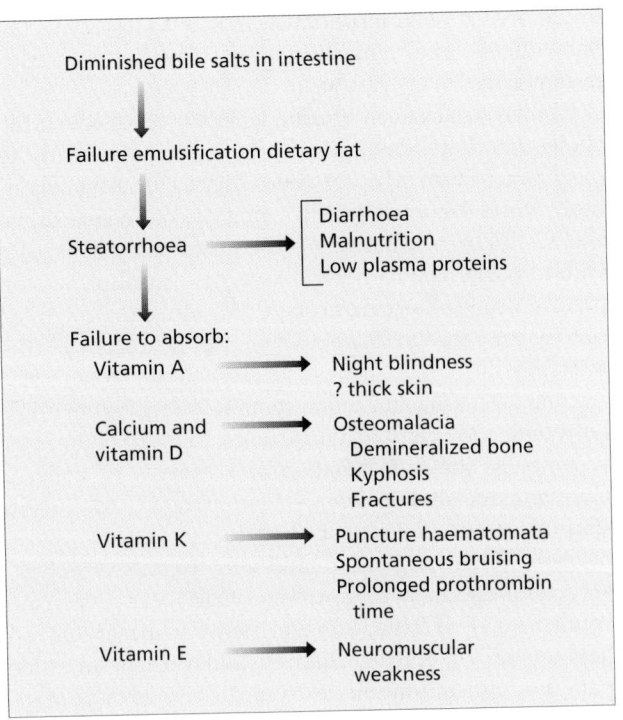

Fig. 13.11. The effects of lack of intestinal bile in chronic cholestatic jaundice.

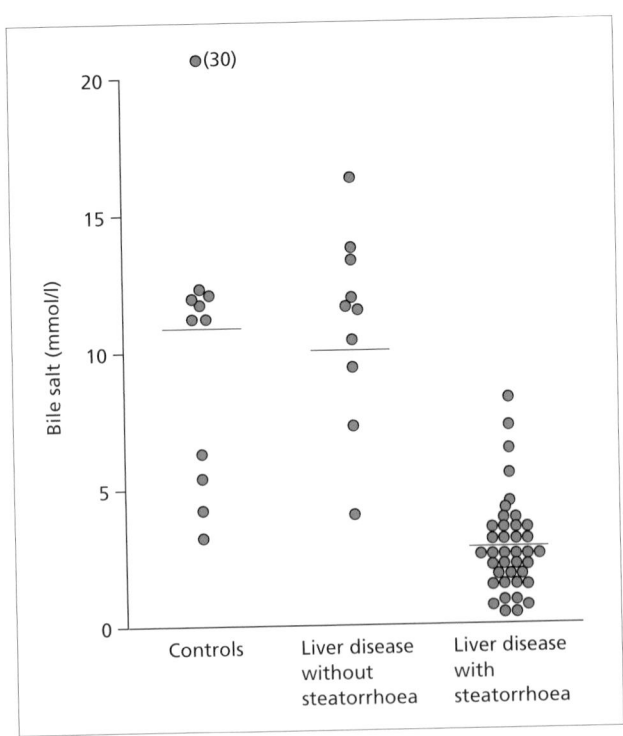

Fig. 13.12. Bile salt concentration of aspirated intestinal contents in patients with non-alcoholic liver disease with and without steatorrhoea [6].

hepatic reserves become exhausted and failure of dark adaption follows (night blindness) [86]. Vitamin D deficiency may also occur leading to osteomalacia.

Vitamin E deficiency has been reported in children with cholestasis [24, 82]. The picture is of cerebellar ataxia, posterior column dysfunction, peripheral neuropathy and retinal degeneration. If the serum bilirubin level exceeds 100 μmol/l (6 mg/dl) almost all adult patients with cholestasis will have subnormal vitamin E levels [46]. However, a specific neurological syndrome does not seem to develop in adults.

Xanthomas. These occur in chronic cholestasis but are seen less frequently than before because of treatment at an earlier stage with liver transplantation. The planous varieties (xanthelasma) are flat or slightly raised, yellow and soft and are usually noted around the eyes. They may also be seen in the palmar creases, below the breast and on the neck (figs 13.13, 13.14), chest or back. The tuberous lesions appear later and are found on extensor surfaces, especially the wrists, elbows, knees, ankles and buttocks (fig. 13.15), on pressure points and in scars. The xanthomas associated with cholestatic jaundice rarely affect tendon sheaths. They may involve bone or occasionally peripheral nerves [84]. Focal accumulations of xanthoma cells may be found in the liver.

Skin xanthomas develop in proportion to the height of the total serum lipids. The serum cholesterol value must be raised to over 450 mg/dl for longer than 3 months before skin xanthomas appear [51]. Skin xanthomas disappear if serum cholesterol levels fall after cholestasis is relieved or in the late stage of hepato-cellular failure.

HEPATIC OSTEODYSTROPHY [39]

Bone disease is a complication of chronic liver disease

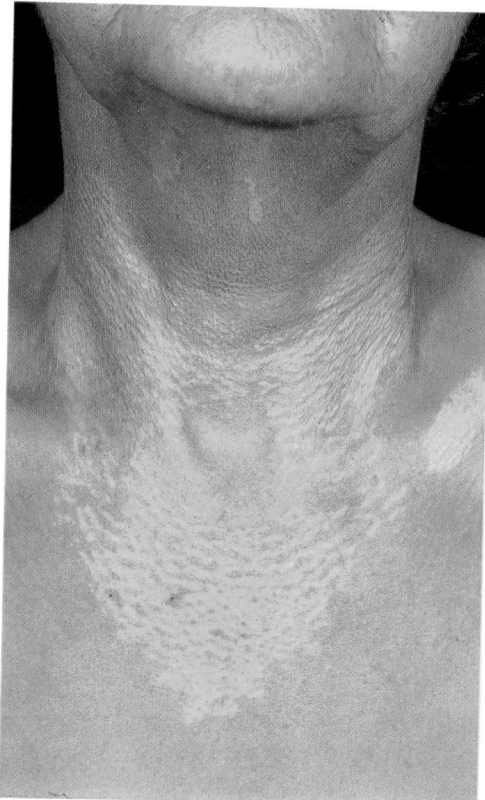

Fig. 13.14. Primary biliary cirrhosis. Xanthomatous skin lesions in the necklace area.

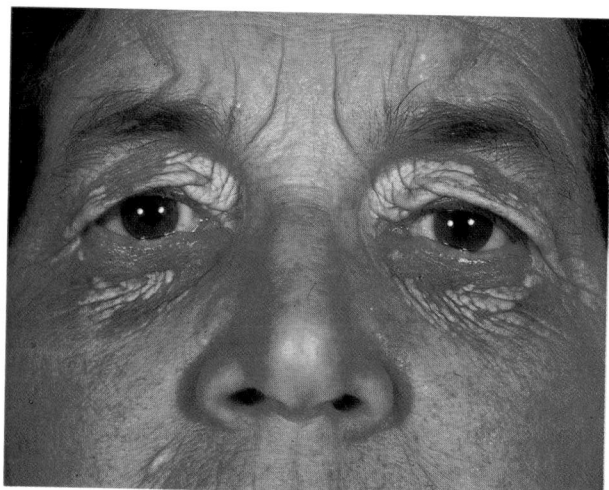

Fig. 13.13. Primary biliary cirrhosis. The patient shows xanthelasma and pigmentation.

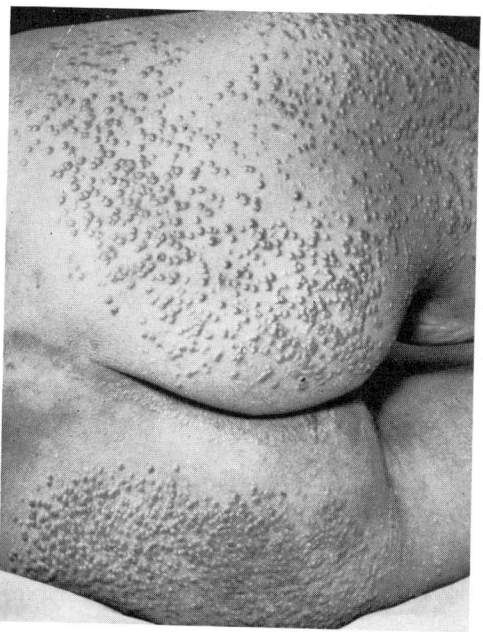

Fig. 13.15. Chronic obstructive jaundice. Xanthoma tuberosum affecting the buttocks.

and in particular chronic cholestasis where it has been studied in most detail. Bone pain and fractures occur. Possible mechanisms are *osteomalacia* and *osteoporosis*. Studies show that osteoporosis is responsible for the bone changes in the majority of patients with primary biliary cirrhosis and primary sclerosing cholangitis, although the potential for osteomalacia exists.

Bone disease manifests as loss of height, back pain (usually midthoracic or lumbar), collapsed vertebrae and fractures particularly of ribs with minimal trauma. Spinal X-rays may show vertebrae of low density, as well as compression (fig. 13.16).

Bone mineral density may be measured by dual photon absorptiometry. Using this method 31% of 123 women

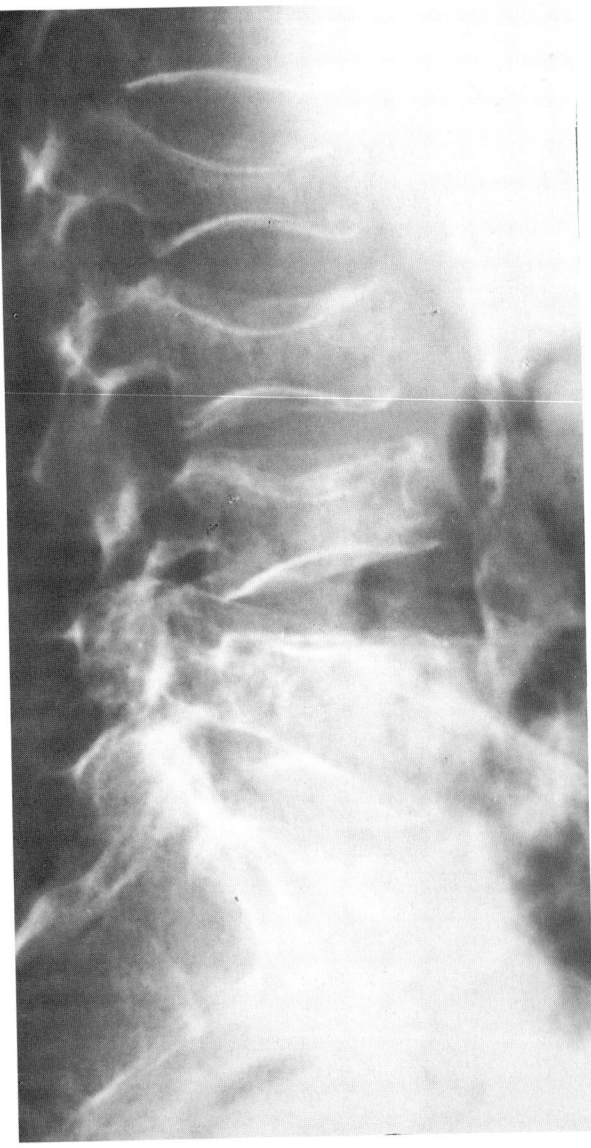

Fig. 13.16. Primary biliary cirrhosis jaundiced for 3 years. Lumbar spine shows very severe biconcave deformities and vertebral compression.

with primary biliary cirrhosis had severe bone disease. On follow-up 7% suffered fractures [14]. Reduced bone mineral density is also seen in patients with advanced primary sclerosing cholangitis and an elevated bilirubin (fig. 13.17) [41].

The pathogenetic mechanism of the bone disease is uncertain, but is likely to be multifactorial. Normal bone homeostasis depends on the correct balance between bone removal by osteoclasts and bone formation by osteoblasts. Remodelling begins with the retraction of cells from a quiescent area of bone. Osteoclasts attach and resorb bone, forming lacunae. These cells are then replaced by osteoblasts which fill the lacunae with new bone (osteoid), a matrix of collagen and other proteins. The osteoid is then 'mineralized', a process dependent on calcium, and therefore vitamin D. The two main forms of metabolic bone disease are osteoporosis and osteomalacia. In osteoporosis there is loss of bone (both matrix and its mineral). In osteomalacia there is defective mineralization of osteoid. To establish the process leading to bone disease in chronic cholestasis, bone biopsy with special analytical techniques was necessary.

Studies have shown that the majority of patients with hepatic osteodystrophy have *osteoporosis*. Both reduced bone formation and increased resorption have been found in chronic cholestatic liver disease. It has been suggested that reduced formation occurs in pre-cirrhotic patients, with increased resorption in those with advanced disease [39]. In post-menopausal women without liver disease both bone resorption and bone formation are increased, with resorption exceeding formation [57]. This will play a part in patients with primary biliary cirrhosis after the menopause.

The cause of osteoporosis in chronic cholestatic liver disease has not been established. Many factors involved in normal bone metabolism may play a role including vitamin D, calcitonin, parathyroid hormone, growth hormone and sex steroids. External influences in cholestatic patients include immobility, poor nutrition and reduced muscle mass. Vitamin D levels may be reduced due to malabsorption, inadequate diet and reduced exposure to the sun. Treatment with vitamin D, however, does not correct the bone disease [42]. Activation of vitamin D, by 25-hydroxylation in liver and 1-hydroxylation in the kidney, is normal.

Recent data show that plasma from patients with jaundice inhibits osteoblast proliferation; unconjugated bilirubin but not bile salts had an inhibitory effect [45]. This finding could explain reduced bone formation in chronic cholestasis, but awaits further study.

Treatment with ursodeoxycholic acid does not reduce the rate of bone loss in primary biliary cirrhosis [53]. Liver transplantation results in an improved bone density but this is delayed until 1–5 years after transplant [5, 40]. Before recovery spontaneous bone fractures

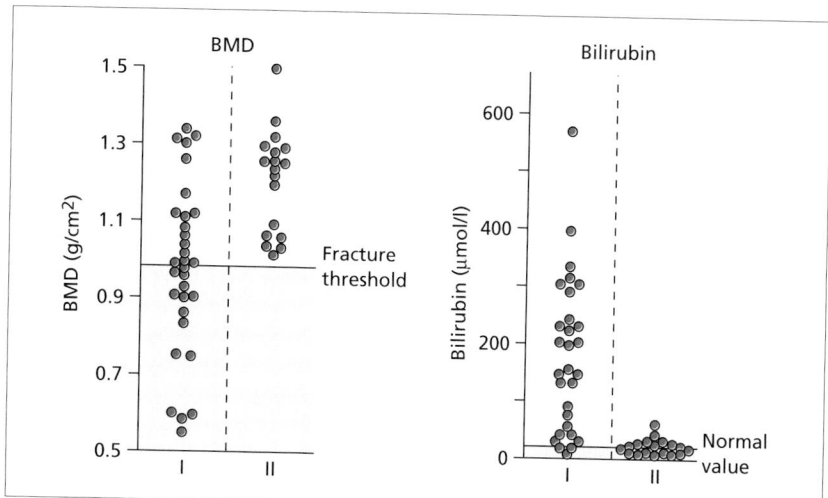

Fig. 13.17. Bone mineral density (BMD) and serum bilirubin concentration in patients with advanced sclerosing cholangitis (group I) and newly diagnosed primary sclerosing cholangitis (group II) [41].

are common [23] occurring in 35% of patients with primary biliary cirrhosis in the first year. Corticosteroids used for immunosuppression probably play a part in this increased fracture rate. Vitamin D levels may not return to normal for several months after transplantation and supplementation has been recommended [5].

It is important to measure vitamin D levels in patients with chronic cholestasis since although *osteomalacia* is unusual it may be present and is easily corrected. Isoenzyme analysis of serum alkaline phosphatase will show whether excess bone isoenzyme is present as well as the biliary/liver form. Bone changes cannot be predicted by serum calcium and phosphate values. X-rays may show changes of osteomalacia such as pseudofractures and Looser's zones. The hands show rarefaction. Bone biopsy shows wide, uncalcified osteoid seams surrounding the trabeculae. The cause of vitamin D deficiency is probably multiple. Cholestatic patients fail to go out in the sun or take an adequate diet. Absorption is poor due to steatorrhoea. Long-term cholestyramine use may exacerbate the deficiency.

Another manifestation of bone disease is painful *osteoarthropathy* in the wrists and ankles (fig. 13.18) [27]. This is a non-specific complication of chronic liver disease.

CHANGES IN COPPER METABOLISM

Approximately 80% of absorbed copper is normally excreted in the bile and lost in the faeces. In all forms of cholestasis, but particularly if it is chronic (as in primary biliary cirrhosis, biliary atresia or sclerosing cholangitis), copper accumulates in the liver to levels equal to or exceeding those found in Wilson's disease [78]. Pigmented corneal rings resembling the Kayser–Fleischer ring are seen rarely [30].

Hepatic copper may be measured in biopsies or

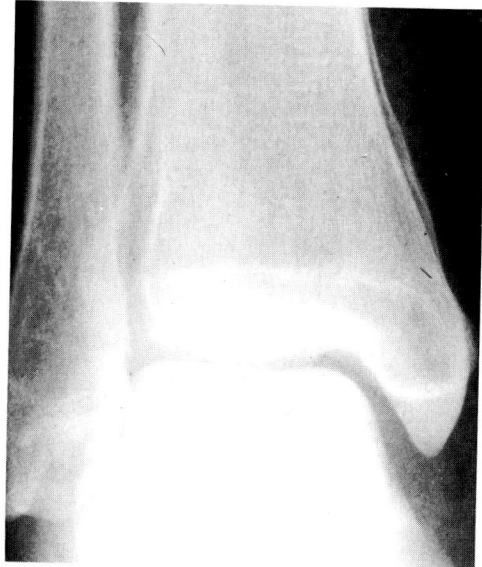

Fig. 13.18. Osteoarthropathy in chronic cholestasis. New subperiosteal bone is seen at the lower end of the tibia.

demonstrated histochemically by rhodanine staining. Copper-associated protein may be shown by orcein staining. These methods give circumstantial support to a diagnosis of cholestasis. In cholestasis the retained copper is probably not hepato-toxic [26]. Electron microscopy shows it in electron-dense lysosomes and the characteristic organelle changes associated with cytosolic copper, as in Wilson's disease, are not observed. In cholestasis, the copper is retained within the hepatocyte in a non-toxic form.

DEVELOPMENT OF HEPATO-CELLULAR FAILURE

This is slow, and it is remarkable how well the liver cells function in the presence of cholestasis. After 3–5 years of chronic jaundice, liver cell failure is indicated by rapidly deepening jaundice, ascites, oedema and a lowered serum albumin level. Pruritus lessens and the bleeding tendency is not controlled by parenteral vitamin K. Hepatic encephalopathy is terminal.

Microsomal drug oxidation. Patients with intra-hepatic cholestasis show a reduction in hepatic cytochrome P450 content in proportion to the severity of the cholestasis [48].

EXTRA-HEPATIC EFFECTS (fig. 13.19) [22]

Itching and jaundice are self evident, but there are numerous other less obvious effects of cholestasis. These have been studied mainly in the context of bile duct obstruction. They may result in serious complications when the patient is stressed by dehydration, blood loss or surgical or non-surgical procedures. Cardiovascular responses are abnormal and peripheral vasoconstriction in response to hypotension is impaired. The kidneys have an increased susceptibility to hypotension and hypoxic damage [31]. The processes involved in responding to sepsis and in wound healing are impaired. The prolonged prothrombin time is correctable with vitamin K but coagulation may still be abnormal through platelet dysfunction. The gastric mucosa is more susceptible to ulceration. The cause of these changes is multifactorial. Bile acids and bilirubin have been shown to alter cellular metabolism and function. Changes in serum lipids affect membrane structure and function. Endotoxaemia has many damaging effects. Thus although deeply jaundiced patients with cholestasis may appear well apart from itching, there are metabolic and functional changes that under the stress of surgical and non-surgical procedures may result in acute renal failure, haemorrhage, wound dehiscence and an increased risk of sepsis.

HAEMATOLOGY

Changes in cholestasis include the appearance of target cells on blood film related to an accumulation of cholesterol in the red cell membrane. This increases red cell surface area and leads to target cell formation.

In extra-hepatic cholestasis, anaemia implies infection, blood loss or malignant disease. A polymorphonuclear leucocytosis suggests cholangitis or underlying neoplastic disease.

BIOCHEMISTRY

All the constituents of the bile show an increased level in the serum. Conjugation of biliary substances is intact but excretion defective.

The *serum ('conjugated', 'ester') bilirubin level* is raised. In unrelieved cholestasis the level rises slowly for the first 3 weeks and then fluctuates, always tending to increase. When the cholestasis is relieved, serum bilirubin values fall slowly to normal. This is in part due to the formation of bili-albumin, in which bilirubin and albumin are covalently bound.

The *serum alkaline phosphatase level* is raised, usually to more than three times the upper limit of normal. *Serum γ-glutamyl transpeptidase levels* are raised. The rises are due to increased synthesis or release of enzymes from liver plasma membranes.

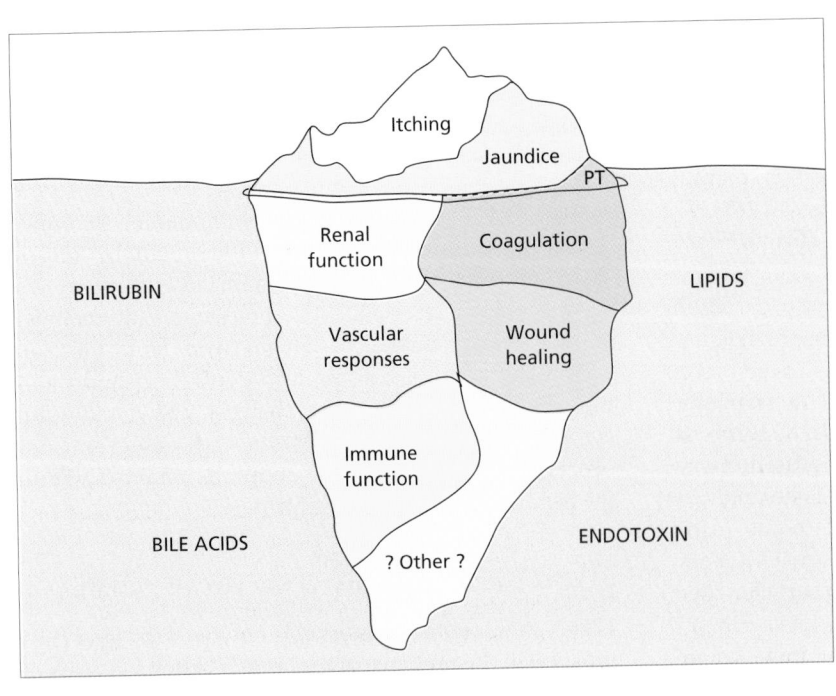

Fig. 13.19. Extra-hepatic effects of cholestasis. Itching and jaundice are obvious (the tip of the iceberg) but there are many other effects for which the clinician should make allowance. Pathogenic factors include bilirubin, bile acids, lipid changes and endotoxin.

The total *serum cholesterol* increases but not constantly. In chronic cholestasis the total serum lipids are greatly increased and this involves particularly phospholipid and total cholesterol. These changes probably reflect increased hepatic synthesis, regurgitation of biliary cholesterol and lecithin into the circulation, and reduced plasma lecithin cholesterol acyl transferase (LCAT) activity. Triglycerides are very slightly increased. In spite of the high lipid content, the serum is characteristically clear and not milky. This may be due to the surface action effect of phospholipid, which keeps the other lipids in solution. Serum cholesterol values fall terminally.

Serum lipoproteins are increased [51], due to a rise in the low density (α_2, β) fraction. The high-density lipoproteins are decreased.

The cholestatic liver secretes a variety of unusual lipoproteins and these can be related to low plasma LCAT levels [1]. The lipoproteins of cholestasis differ from those found in atherosclerosis. Atheroma is not a complication of prolonged cholestasis. The abnormal lipoproteins appear by electron microscopy as disc-shaped particles.

Lipoprotein-X (LP-X) is a spherical particle, 70 nm in diameter, associated with the low-density lipoprotein fraction [60]. It is increased in both intra-hepatic and extra-hepatic cholestasis but is of no practical diagnostic value.

Trihydroxy *bile salts* accumulate in the blood in cholestasis.

Serum albumin and globulin concentrations are normal in acute cholestasis. With the development of biliary cirrhosis the serum albumin tends to fall.

The *serum aspartate transaminase* is usually less than 100 i.u./l.

Urine. Conjugated bilirubin is present. Urinary urobilinogen is excreted in proportion to the amount of bile reaching the duodenum.

BACTERIOLOGY

In the febrile patient with bile duct obstruction or primary sclerosing cholangitis, blood cultures should be performed. Septicaemia, especially due to Gram-negative organisms, complicates patients with duct stones, and those with malignant obstruction or sclerosing cholangitis after invasive procedures. Patients with partial biliary obstruction and cholangitis have a high bacterial population in the bile, rivalling that in the colon. Whether this causes systemic sepsis depends on the biliary pressure and thus the degree of obstruction.

Diagnostic approach

The distinction between intra- and extra-hepatic cholestasis may be possible by an accurate history and physical examination. *Pain* can be related to duct stones, tumour or gallbladder disease. *Fever* and *rigors* may indicate cholangitis due to duct stone or traumatic stricture (*Charcot's intermittent biliary fever*). The patient may have taken *drug treatment* that coincides with the development of cholestasis. *Ulcerative colitis* raises the possibility of primary sclerosing cholangitis. On examination, hepatic nodularity may indicate metastatic *malignancy*. Other abdominal masses may indicate a primary lesion such as carcinoma of stomach or colon. Endoscopy, rectal examination and sigmoidoscopy may indicate carcinoma. An enlarged gallbladder suggests non-calculous biliary obstruction.

However, clinical and biochemical evaluation is not infallible. A small proportion of patients with extra-hepatic obstruction are incorrectly diagnosed as having intra-hepatic cholestasis, whereas a larger proportion of patients with intra-hepatic disease are thought to have extra-hepatic obstruction. A diagnostic algorithm is important (figs 13.20, 13.21). The first procedure should be real-time ultrasound, which allows the distinction between cholestasis with dilated bile ducts and cholestasis without duct dilatation. If ultrasound shows dilated ducts, direct cholangiography (Chapter 29) is necessary.

The endoscopic approach (ERCP) is the first choice, unless access to the duodenal papillary is impossible (e.g. hepatico-jejunostomy). If ERCP fails, the percutaneous route (PTC) should be taken. Drainage of an obstructed biliary system is possible by both approaches although there are fewer complications endoscopically. ERCP offers the added potential for endoscopic sphincterotomy for stones.

If ultrasound does not show dilated ducts the next

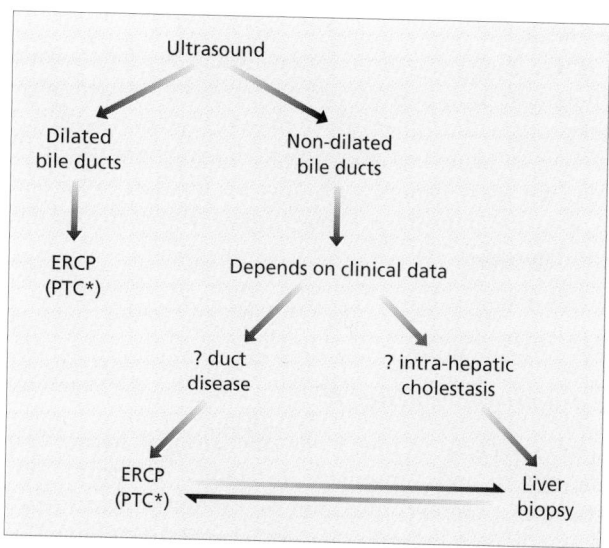

Fig. 13.20. Diagnosis of cholestasis. ERCP = endoscopic retrograde cholangiopancreatography; PTC = percutaneous transhepatic cholangiography; * = second choice.

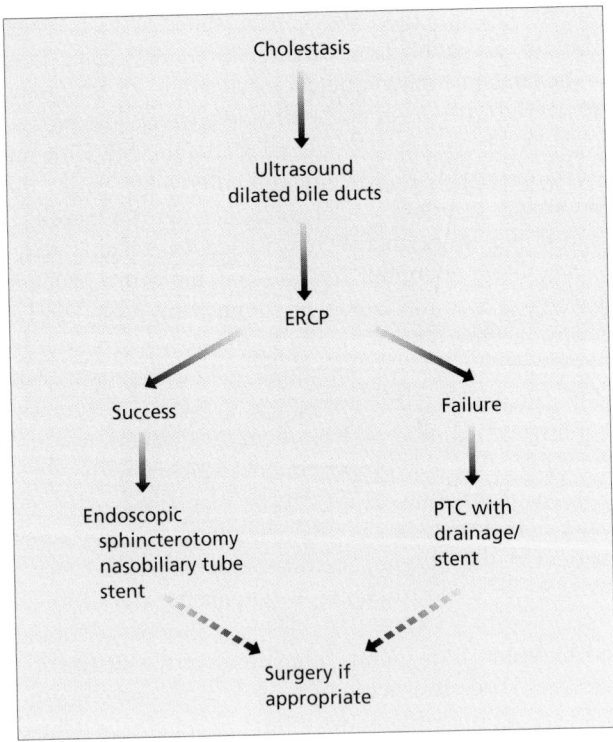

Fig. 13.21. Therapeutic options for bile duct obstruction.

step depends upon the clinical data. If duct disease such as stone or primary sclerosing cholangitis is suspected, ERCP is chosen. If the cholangiogram is normal then liver biopsy should be considered. If an intra-hepatic cholestasis due to a drug or primary biliary cirrhosis is likely, then liver biopsy is performed as the first approach. If this shows large bile duct disease ERCP is necessary.

Liver biopsy can be performed safely in patients with cholestatic jaundice, however deep, after correction of the prothrombin time with vitamin K. However, with the advent of scanning and direct cholangiography it is unusual for a patient with duct obstruction to have a biopsy, and indeed this should not be necessary to make the diagnosis.

DIAGNOSTIC POSSIBILITIES

Extra-hepatic cholestasis

Causes include common bile duct stone (Chapter 31), pancreatic and ampullary carcinoma (Chapter 33), cholangiocarcinoma (Chapter 34), benign bile duct stricture (Chapter 32) and bile duct infections (Chapter 27). Dominant benign strictures and cholangiocarcinoma can cause duct obstruction in primary sclerosing cholangitis (Chapter 15).

Large bile duct disease with undilated intra-hepatic ducts

Occasionally diseases that involve the main bile ducts do not result in intra-hepatic biliary dilatation and *simulate* intra-hepatic cholestasis. A common duct stone may be present without dilated intra-hepatic ducts if the stone is only causing intermittent obstruction. Ultrasound may mislead, but the history should indicate this possibility. There are also conditions that affect both intra- and extra-hepatic ducts and cross the diagnostic classification of intra- and extra-hepatic cholestasis. These include primary sclerosing cholangitis, sclerosing cholangitis complicating long-standing duct stones with sepsis, and rarely duct changes seen with sarcoidosis and histiocytosis-X (see Chapter 15).

Intra-hepatic cholestasis (fig. 13.22; table 13.2)

The cause of intra-hepatic cholestasis lies within the liver, somewhere distal to the hepato-cellular microsomes but above the major bile ducts. The general clinical and biochemical picture is the same as for extra-hepatic cholestasis. Febrile cholangitis is absent. The liver is not necessarily enlarged and is not tender. Bile ducts are not dilated within the liver.

Hepato-cellular

The cholestasis is complex. There is primary injury to intra-cellular membranes. Leakage of bile salts through defective canaliculi leads to a reduction of bile salt dependent bile flow. Inhibition of canalicular ATPase interferes with bile salt independent secretion. Impaired hydroxylation of cholesterol to bile acids in the endoplasmic reticulum reduces bile salt dependent flow.

Cholestatic viral hepatitis (Chapter 16). The history of exposure and the nature of the prodromal symptoms may be helpful. The liver biopsy appearances are those of acute viral hepatitis.

Acute alcoholic hepatitis (Chapter 20) can be cholestatic. The history of alcohol abuse, the large tender liver and, often, vascular spiders on the skin are helpful points. Liver biopsy appearances are diagnostic. Chronic pancreatitis may be associated.

In some patients with *cryptogenic macronodular cirrhosis* cholestasis may be prominent.

Canalicular membrane changes

Cholestatic reactions to oral contraceptives (Chapter 18) and in the last trimester of pregnancy (Chapter 25) fall into this group.

Drugs include the promazine group, long-acting sulphonamides, antibiotics and anti-thyroid drugs

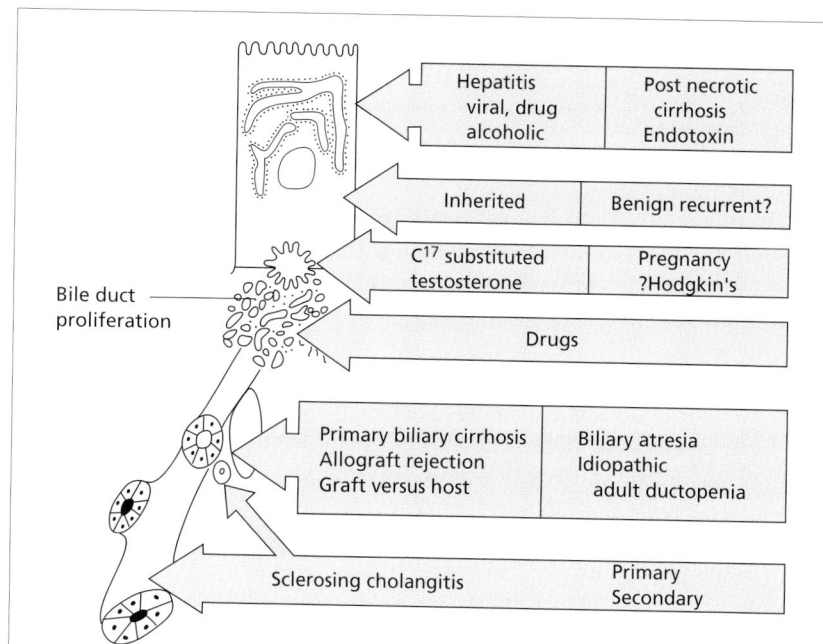

Fig. 13.22. Classification of intra-hepatic cholestasis according to possible major sites of involvement of the biliary tree.

Table 13.2. Intra-hepatic cholestasis

Type	Diagnostic points
Hepato-cellular	
Viral hepatitis	History; onset typical; viral A, B and C markers
Alcoholic hepatitis	History; large tender liver; spiders; liver biopsy
Drugs	History; onset 6 weeks of starting; liver biopsy
Sex hormones (canalicular)	Hormone therapy; remit on stopping; liver biopsy
Benign recurrent cholestasis	Repeated; cholangiography normal; normal liver between attacks
Bile acids	All rare; often familial
Biliary	
Intra-hepatic atresia	History; age; liver biopsy
Primary biliary cirrhosis	Female; onset pruritus; positive mitochondrial antibody; raised serum IgM; liver biopsy
Primary sclerosing cholangitis	Association ulcerative colitis; ERCP

(Chapter 18). The history is important and liver biopsy appearances are usually diagnostic.

Benign recurrent intra-hepatic cholestasis

This rare condition presents as multiple episodes of cholestatic jaundice [12, 88]. Main bile duct obstruction must be excluded by endoscopic or percutaneous cholangiography. Other causes known to produce cholestasis, such as drugs, should be ruled out. There should be symptom-free intervals of several months or years. The first patient described has now survived 22 episodes and three laparotomies [88]. Another patient had 27 attacks over 38 years.

The onset is with itching, occasionally with influenza-type illness and vomiting. Twenty-five to 50% of patients suffer abdominal pain [12]. There is often fatigue, anorexia and weight loss. Serum alkaline phosphatase levels increase but transaminases are virtually normal. Jaundice appears and persists for 3–4 months.

Hepatic histology shows cholestasis with bile plugs, portal zone expansion, mononuclear cells and some liver cell degeneration, mainly in zone 1. Hepatic histology and liver function are normal in remission [88].

Aetiology. In favour of a genetic origin is the early onset, usually starting before the age of 10, and the familial incidence. The disease is thought to be autosomal recessive carried on chromosome 18 [44]. It may be related to abnormal bile acid metabolism, or an intrinsic problem with bile secretion or one due to humoral factors.

Environmental factors are suggested by the allergic diathesis; some patients have rashes. The condition may recur at particular times of the year.

Treatment. The attacks are self-limiting and vary in duration. Corticosteroid treatment is probably of little benefit. S-adenosylmethionine is ineffective [28]. Results with ursodeoxycholic acid are conflicting.

Bile acid related

Toxic bile acids have detergent effects on canalicular membranes and are inadequate as micelle formers.

Lithocholic acid is a naturally occurring bile acid formed in the colon. The human liver probably metabolizes it when it is re-absorbed so preventing its injurious (cholestatic) action. However, it can reduce bile acid independent flow by inhibiting $Na^+–K^+$ ATPase and altering the canalicular membrane.

Monohydroxy bile acids, such as 3-β-hydroxy-5-cholenate, accumulate in canalicular membranes and are cholestatic. They have been found in the bile of infants with established cholestasis, but their role as cause or effect is uncertain.

Coprostanic acid [38]. Two children from two families with cholestasis from birth were found to have this C27 alligator bile acid in bile. They soon died of cirrhosis. An enzyme catalysing C24 hydroxylation may be defective.

Byler's disease. This fatal cholestasis has been reported in Amish kindreds named Byler [20]. Death is usual before the age of eight. Inheritance is autosomal recessive with the locus mapped to chromosome 18 [15] as in benign recurrent cholestasis. A defect in microfilament function or in the biliary canalicular membrane is postulated. Conjugated bile acids cannot be excreted and this may be related to the cholestasis. Hepatic transplantation has been tried with good results.

Zellweger's syndrome. This is very rare. There is defective formation of hepatic peroxisomes. Side-chain oxidation of bile acids does not occur normally, and C27 bile acids appear in serum and bile. There are other enzymatic defects, and infants die shortly after birth [59]. Oral bile acid therapy should be considered [77].

Miscellaneous

Cholestasis in *severe bacterial infections*, particularly in childhood or post-operatively, is presumably hepatocellular. It can also be related to the cholestatic effect of endotoxin on $Na^+–K^+$ ATPase.

Cholestasis develops with *prolonged parenteral nutrition* especially in neonates (Chapter 24) but also in adults [71]. It may be due to lithocholate formed by bacterial 7-α-dehydroxylation in the intestinal tract.

Hodgkin's disease may be complicated by deep cholestasis. This is not necessarily related to excess haemolysis, hepatic infiltration or invasion of major bile ducts. There may be loss of intra-hepatic bile ducts [43] (see Chapter 4).

Biliary precipitation of insoluble solutes. Unconjugated bilirubin may precipitate as intra-hepatic pigment stones or as inspissated bile in *cystic fibrosis* or *benoxyprofen toxicity* (Chapter 18).

Protoporphyrins in *erythrocytic protoporphyria* may lead to precipitation in the canalicular ducts.

The cholestasis of *intra-hepatic atresia* (infantile cholangiopathy) (Chapter 24) is probably related to viral injury to intra-hepatic bile ducts. Adults and adolescents with *paucity of intra-hepatic bile ducts* are being increasingly described [13, 29]. The condition may be familial or drug-induced [19], or a late onset form of the non-syndromic type seen in children [13].

The pathogenetic significance of high hepatic *zinc* levels in a small group of children with severe chronic cholestatic liver disease is uncertain [68].

Primary biliary cirrhosis (see Chapter 14).
Primary sclerosing cholangitis (see Chapter 15).

Treatment

BILIARY DECOMPRESSION: RESECTION

The choice between non-surgical and surgical treatment will depend upon the cause of obstruction and the clinical state of the patient. Common duct stones are treated by endoscopic sphincterotomy and removal (see Chapter 29). In malignant obstruction the resectability of the tumour should be assessed in the operable patient. If judged inoperable or irresectable, an endoscopic stent is inserted to drain the bile duct; the percutaneous route is taken if the endoscopic attempt fails. Surgical bypass is the alternative. Which approach is employed will depend upon the patient, the facilities, and the expertise available.

The preparation of the patient for any of these procedures is critical in order to avoid complications that include renal failure which may occur in 5–10% of patients [31], and sepsis. *Coagulation* is corrected with parenteral vitamin K. *Dehydration* and *hypotension*, which can lead to acute tubular necrosis, are prevented by intravenous hydration, usually with 0.9% NaCl, and close monitoring of fluid balance. *Mannitol* is given to protect renal function but patients must be well hydrated before its use. A recent trial has questioned its benefit [37]. Post-operative renal dysfunction may in part be caused by circulating endotoxin derived from increased intestinal absorption. To reduce absorption of endotoxin, oral deoxycholate or lactulose have been given and appear to protect against renal impairment after surgery [67]. There is no post-operative benefit if renal failure is already abnormal before surgery.

To reduce the risk of septic complications after both non-surgical and surgical intervention, antibiotic is given beforehand. The duration of treatment after the procedure will depend upon whether or not there is evidence of sepsis, and how successful biliary decompression has been.

The important factors associated with increased post-operative morbidity and mortality are an initial haematocrit of 30% or less, a serum bilirubin value exceeding 200 μmol/l (12 mg/dl) and a malignant lesion [21]. Deep jaundice can be relieved pre-operatively by percutaneous external drainage or endoscopy stenting but randomized controlled studies have not shown benefit [52].

MEDICAL

Pruritus (table 13.3) [72]

Biliary drainage. Pruritus is relieved in patients with biliary obstruction by external or internal biliary drainage. Itching disappears or is much improved after 24–48 hours.

Cholestyramine. This resin will stop itching in 4–5 days in patients with partial biliary obstruction. It is known to bind bile salts in the intestines so eliminating them in the faeces but until the pathogenesis of itching is better understood, its actual mechanism of action will remain speculative. One sachet (4 g) should be given before and one after breakfast so that the arrival of the drug in the duodenum coincides with gallbladder contraction. If necessary, a further dose may be taken before the midday and evening meals. The maintenance dose is usually about 12 g per day. The drug causes nausea and there is a reluctance to take it. It is particularly valuable for itching associated with primary biliary cirrhosis, primary sclerosing cholangitis, biliary atresia and biliary stricture. Serum bile acid levels fall. Serum cholesterol drops and skin xanthomas diminish or disappear.

Cholestyramine increases faecal fat even in normal subjects. The dose should be the smallest one that controls pruritus. Hypoprothrombinaemia has developed

Table 13.3. Drug treatment of pruritus

Routine	Cholestyramine
Variable effect	Anti-histamine; ursodeoxycholic acid; phenobarbitone
Careful use	Rifampicin
Experimental	Naloxone, nalmefene; ondansetron; S-adenosyl-L-methionine; propofol

due to failure to absorb vitamin K. This vitamin must be given by intra-muscular injection.

Cholestyramine may bind calcium, other fat-soluble vitamins and drugs having an entero-hepatic circulation, particularly digitoxin. Care must be taken that the cholestyramine and other drugs are given at separate times.

Ursodeoxycholic acid (13–15 mg/kg per day) can reduce itching in patients with primary biliary cirrhosis perhaps by a choleretic effect or by reducing toxic bile salts [70]. Although its use has been associated with biochemical resolution of drug-induced cholestasis [69], it is unproven as an antipruritic agent in this and other cholestatic syndromes.

Anti-histamines. These are of value only for their sedative action.

Phenobarbitone may relieve itching in patients resistant to other therapy.

Naloxone, an opiate antagonist given as an intravenous infusion, reduced itching in a randomized controlled trial [7], but is not appropriate for long-term use. An oral opiate antagonist, nalmefene, has produced promising results. It awaits further controlled trials [8] and is not currently commercially available.

Ondansetron, a 5-hydroxytryptamine type 3 receptor antagonist, reduced itching in a randomized trial [75]. Side-effects include constipation and changes in liver function tests, and further evaluation is needed.

Propofol, an hypnotic agent given intravenously, has improved itching in 80% of patients [10]. Only short-term benefit has been studied.

S-adenosyl-L-methionine, which among many effects improves membrane fluidity and acts as an antioxidant, has been used to treat cholestatic syndromes [65]. Results are inconsistent and currently this agent remains experimental.

Rifampicin (300–450 mg daily) relieves pruritus within 7 days [18, 34]. This may be by enzyme induction or by inhibition of bile acid uptake. Potential side-effects include increased risk of gallstone formation, reduction in 25-OH cholecalciferol levels, drug interactions and emergence of resistant organisms. Until the safety of long-term use of rifampicin is established, patients treated with this agent should be carefully selected and frequently monitored.

Steroids. Glucocorticoids will relieve itching, but at the expense of severe bone thinning particularly in post-menopausal women.

Methyltestosterone 25 mg sublingually daily relieves itching within 7 days [54] and is appropriate for men. Anabolic steroids such as stanazolol [87] (5 mg daily) are less virilizing and equally effective. These substances greatly increase jaundice and both can cause an intra-hepatic cholestasis in normal patients (Chapter 18). There are no ill effects on liver function, but these drugs should be given only for intractable pruritus and in the smallest effective dose.

Plasmapheresis. This has been used to treat intractable pruritus associated with hypercholesterolaemia and xanthomatous neuropathy. The procedure is temporarily effective but is costly and labour intensive.

Phototherapy. Ultraviolet radiation, 9–12 minutes daily, may relieve pruritus and decrease pigmentation.

Hepatic transplantation may be the only answer for some patients with chronic intractable pruritus.

Nutrition (table 13.4)

The problem is that of intestinal bile salt deficiency. Dietetic advice if available should be taken. Calorie intake should be maintained and protein must be adequate. In patients with clinically overt steatorrhoea, neutral fat will be poorly tolerated and badly absorbed with reduced calcium absorption. It should be restricted to 40 g daily. Additional fat is supplied by medium chain triglycerides (MCT) as an emulsion, for example in a milk shake. In the absence of luminal bile acids, MCT are digested and absorbed quite well into the portal vein as free fatty acids. They can be given as 'Liquigen' (Scientific Hospital Supplies Ltd, UK) or as MCT (coconut) oil for cooking or in salads. Calcium supplements should also be given.

In acute cholestasis, vitamin K deficiency may be shown by prolongation of the prothrombin time. Parenteral vitamin K (10 mg) should be given daily for 2–3 days; the prothrombin time characteristically corrects within a day or two.

In the chronic case, prothrombin time and serum vitamin A and D levels should be monitored, and vitamins A, D and K replaced as necessary. Replacement

Table 13.4. Management of chronic cholestasis

Dietary fat (if steatorrhoea)
reduce neutral fat (40 g daily)
add medium chain triglycerides (up to 40 g daily)

Fat-soluble vitamins*		
oral	K	10 mg/day
	A	25 000 U/day
	D	400–4 000 U/day
i.m.	K	10 mg/month
	A	100 000 U/3-monthly
	D	100 000 U/month

Calcium
extra low fat milk
oral calcium

* Initial dose and route depend on severity of deficiency and cholestasis, and compliance; Maintenance dose depends on response. See text for vitamin E.

may be done orally or parenterally depending on the severity of depletion, jaundice and steatorrhoea, and whether the deficiency is corrected. If testing of vitamin levels is not available, empirical replacement is appropriate particularly once the patient becomes jaundiced. Easy bruising suggests prothrombin and thus vitamin K deficiency.

Patients with night blindness may improve with oral rather than intramuscular vitamin A [86]. Vitamin E is not absorbed [3] and DL tocopherol, as the acetate 10 mg daily, is given by injection to children with chronic cholestasis. Others may take 200 mg daily by mouth.

Bone changes

The osteopenia of cholestatic liver disease is predominantly osteoporosis. Malabsorption of vitamin D with subsequent osteomalacia occurs but is less common. Monitoring of serum 25-hydroxy vitamin D levels is necessary; bone densitometry scans will show the degree of osteopenia.

When vitamin D deficiency is detected, treatment is with vitamin D, either 50 000 units orally three times a week [39], or 100 000 units intramuscularly monthly. If serum levels do not become normal on oral therapy, the dose should be increased, or the parenteral route used. Prophylaxis against vitamin D deficiency when vitamin D levels cannot be monitored is empirical but appropriate for the patient with jaundice or long-standing cholestasis without jaundice. Unless serum levels can be monitored, parenteral replacement of vitamin D is more appropriate than the oral route.

In patients with symptomatic osteomalacia, oral or parenteral 1,25-dihydroxy-D_3 appears to be the vitamin D metabolite of choice. It is biologically very active and has a short half-life. An alternative would be 1α vitamin D_3 but full metabolic activity only follows hepatic 25-hydroxylation.

Measures should be taken to prevent osteoporosis. These have been little studied in chronic cholestasis. A balanced diet is encouraged with calcium supplements. A daily oral intake of at least 1.5 g elemental calcium should be achieved using effervescent calcium (Sandoz) or calcium gluconate. Patients should be encouraged to take extra skimmed (fat-free) milk and expose themselves to safe levels of sunlight or ultraviolet light. They are also encouraged to be mobile and active, though if osteopenia is severe this may have to be moderated or an exercise programme planned under supervision.

Corticosteroids worsen the process of osteoporosis and should be avoided. In post-menopausal patients oestrogen-replacement therapy is worthwhile. Such treatment in a small group of patients with primary biliary cirrhosis showed no increase in cholestasis while there was a trend towards a reduction in bone loss [17].

Bisphosphonates and calcitonin have not been established as beneficial in cholestatic bone disease. Although a limited study of fluoride treatment showed improved bone density in patients with primary biliary cirrhosis [36] larger studies in post-menopausal osteoporosis show no reduction in fractures and question any overall benefit.

Severe bone pain may be controlled by intravenous calcium (15 mg calcium per kilogram of body weight as calcium gluconate in 500 ml 5% dextrose) given over 4 hours daily for about 7 days and repeated as necessary [2].

Hepatic bone disease worsens after liver transplantation and calcium and vitamin D supplementation should be continued.

No specific treatment is available for the painful periosteal reactions. Simple analgesics may be of use, and, if arthropathy is present, physiotherapy may be helpful.

References

1 Agorastos J, Fox C, Harry DS *et al.* Lecithin-cholesterol acyltransferase and the lipo-protein abnormalities of obstructive jaundice. *Clin. Sci. Molec. Med.* 1978; **54**: 369.

2 Ajdukiewicz AB, Agnew JE, Byers PD *et al.* The relief of bone pain in primary biliary cirrhosis with calcium infusions. *Gut* 1974; **15**: 788.

3 Alvarez F, Landrieu P, Laget P *et al.* Nervous and ocular disorders in children with cholestasis and vitamin A and E deficiencies. *Hepatology* 1983; **3**: 410.

4 Anderson JM, Glade JL, Stevenson BR *et al.* Hepatic immunohistochemical localization of the tight junction protein ZO-1 in rat models of cholestasis. *Am. J. Pathol.* 1989; **134**: 1055.

5 Argao EA, Balistreri WF, Hollis BW *et al.* Effect of orthotopic liver transplantation on bone mineral content and serum vitamin D metabolites in infants and children with chronic cholestasis. *Hepatology* 1994; **20**: 598.

6 Badley BWD, Murphy GM, Bouchier IAD *et al.* Diminished micellar phase lipid in patients with chronic nonalcoholic liver disease and steatorrhea. *Gastroenterology* 1970; **58**: 781.

7 Bergasa NV, Alling DW, Talbot TL *et al.* Effects of naloxone infusions in patients with pruritus of cholestasis: a double-blind randomized controlled trial. *Ann. Intern. Med.* 1995; **123**: 161.

8 Bergasa NV, Jones EA. The pruritus of cholestasis: potential pathogenic and therapeutic implications of opioids. *Gastroenterology* 1995; **108**: 1582.

9 Bohme M, Muller M, Leier I *et al.* Cholestasis caused by inhibition of the adenosine triphosphate-dependent bile salt transport in rat liver. *Gastroenterology* 1994; **107**: 255.

10 Borgeat A, Wilder-Smith OHG, Mentha G. Subhypnotic doses of propofol relieve pruritus associated with liver disease. *Gastroenterology* 1993; **104**: 244.

11 Boyer JL, Soroka CJ. Vesicle targeting to the apical domain regulates bile excretory function in isolated rat hepatocyte couplets. *Gastroenterology* 1995; **109**: 1600.

12 Brenard R, Geubel AP, Benhamou J-P. Benign recurrent intrahepatic cholestasis. *J. Clin. Gastroenterol.* 1989; **11**: 546.

13 Bruguera M, Llach J, Rodes J. Non-syndromic paucity of intrahepatic bile ducts in infancy and idiopathic ductopenia in adulthood: the same syndrome? *Hepatology* 1992; **15**: 830.

14 Camisasca M, Albisetti W, Grandinetti G *et al.* Bone disease in primary biliary cirrhosis: a large-scale prevalence study. *Eur. J. Gastroenterol. Hepatol.* 1991; **3**(Abstr): S26.

15 Carlton VEH, Knisely AS, Freimer NB. Mapping of a locus for progressive familial intrahepatic cholestasis (Byler disease) to 18q21–q22, the benign recurrent intrahepatic cholestasis region. *Hum. Mol. Genet.* 1995; **4**: 1049.

16 Cohn JA, Strong TV, Picciotto MR *et al.* Localization of the cystic fibrosis transmembrane conductance regulator in human bile duct epithelial cells. *Gastroenterology* 1993; **105**: 1857.

17 Crippin JS, Jorgensen RA, Dickson ER *et al.* Hepatic osteodystrophy in primary biliary cirrhosis: the effects of estrogen administration. *Gastroenterology* 1992; **102** (Abstract): A796.

18 Cynamon HA, Andres JM, Iafrate RP. Rifampin relieves pruritus in children with cholestatic liver disease. *Gastroenterology* 1990; **98**: 1013.

19 Degott C, Feldmann G, Larrey D *et al.* Drug-induced prolonged cholestasis in adults: a histological semiquantitative study demonstrating progressive ductopenia. *Hepatology* 1992; **15**: 244.

20 De Vos R, De Wolf-Peters C, Desmet V *et al.* Progressive intrahepatic cholestasis (Byler's disease): case report. *Gut* 1975; **16**: 943.

21 Dixon JM, Armstrong CP, Duffey SW *et al.* Factors affecting morbidity and mortality after surgery for obstructive jaundice: a review of 373 patients. *Gut* 1983; **24**: 845.

22 Dooley JS, Patel A. Extrahepatic biliary obstruction: systemic effects, diagnosis, management. In: *Oxford Textbook of Clinical Hepatology*, eds McIntyre N, Benhamou J-P, Bircher J, Rizzetto M, Rodes J. Oxford University Press, Oxford, 1991, p. 1139.

23 Eastell R, Dickson ER, Hodgson SF *et al.* Rates of vertebral loss before and after liver transplantation in women with primary biliary cirrhosis. *Hepatology* 1991; **14**: 296.

24 Elias E, Muller DPR, Scott J. Association of spino cerebellar disorders with cystic fibrosis or chronic childhood cholestasis and very low serum vitamin E. *Lancet* 1981; **ii**: 1319.

25 Elsing C, Sagesser H, Reichen J. Ursodeoxycholate-induced hypercholeresis in cirrhotic rats: further evidence for cholehepatic shunting. *Hepatology* 1994; **20**: 1048.

26 Epstein O, Arborgh B, Sagiv M *et al.* Is copper hepatotoxic in primary biliary cirrhosis? *J. Clin. Pathol.* 1981; **34**: 1071.

27 Epstein O, Dick R, Sherlock S. Prospective study of periostitis and finger clubbing in primary biliary cirrhosis and other forms of chronic liver disease. *Gut* 1981; **22**: 203.

28 Everson GT, Ahnen D, Harper PC *et al.* Benign recurrent intrahepatic cholestasis: treatment with S-adenosylmethionine. *Gastroenterology* 1989; **96**: 1354.

29 Faa G, Van Eyken P, Demelia L *et al.* Idiopathic adulthood ductopenia presenting with chronic recurrent cholestasis. *J. Hepatol.* 1991; **12**: 14.

30 Fleming CR, Dickson ER, Hollenhorst RW *et al.* Pigmented corneal rings in a patient with primary biliary cirrhosis. *Gastroenterology* 1975; **69**: 220.

31 Fogarty BJ, Parks RW, Rowlands BJ *et al.* Renal dysfunction in obstructive jaundice. *Br. J. Surg.* 1995; **82**: 877.

32 Freedman MR, Holzbach RT, Ferguson DR. Pruritus in cholestasis: no direct causative role for bile acid retention.

Am. J. Med. 1981; **70**: 1011.

33 Fricker G, Landmann L, Meier PJ. Extrahepatic obstructive cholestasis reverses the bile salt secretory polarity of rat hepatocytes. *J. Clin. Invest.* 1989; **84**: 876.

34 Ghent CN, Carruthers SG. Treatment of pruritis in primary biliary cirrhosis with rifampin. Results of a double-blind, crossover, randomized trial. *Gastroenterology* 1988; **94**: 488.

35 Graf J, Boyer JL. The use of isolated rat hepatocyte couplets in hepatobiliary physiology. *J. Hepatol.* 1990; **10**: 387.

36 Guanabens N, Pares A, del Rio L *et al.* Sodium fluoride prevents bone loss in primary biliary cirrhosis. *J. Hepatol.* 1992; **15**: 345.

37 Gubern JM, Sancho JJ, Simo J *et al.* A randomised trial on the effect of mannitol on postoperative renal function in patients with obstructive jaundice. *Surgery* 1988; **103**: 39.

38 Hanson RF, Isenberg JN, Williams GC *et al.* The metabolism of 3α, 7α, 12α-trihydroxy-5β-cholestan-26-oic acid in two siblings with cholestasis due to intrahepatic bile duct anomalies: an apparent inborn error of cholic acid synthesis. *J. Clin. Invest.* 1975; **56**: 577.

39 Hay JE. Bone disease in cholestatic liver disease. *Gastroenterology* 1995; **108**: 276.

40 Hay JE, Dickson ER, Wiesner RH *et al.* Long-term effect of orthotopic liver transplantation on the osteopenia of primary biliary cirrhosis. *Hepatology* 1990; **12**(Abstr): 838.

41 Hay JE, Lindor KD, Wiesner RH *et al.* The metabolic bone disease of primary sclerosing cholangitis. *Hepatology* 1991; **14**: 257.

42 Herlong HF, Becker RR, Maddrey WC. Bone disease in primary biliary cirrhosis: histologic features and response to 25-hydroxy-vitamin D. *Gastroenterology* 1982; **83**: 103.

43 Hubscher SG, Lumley MA, Elias E. Vanishing bile duct syndrome: a possible mechanism for intrahepatic cholestasis in Hodgkin's lymphoma. *Hepatology* 1993; **17**: 70.

44 Houwen RHJ, Baharloo S, Blankenship K *et al.* Genome screening by searching for shared segments: mapping a gene for benign recurrent intrahepatic cholestasis. *Nature Genet.* 1994; **8**: 380.

45 Janes CH, Dickson ER, Okazaki R *et al.* Role of hyperbilirubinaemia in the impairment of osteoblast proliferation associated with cholestatic jaundice. *J. Clin. Invest.* 1995; **95**: 2581.

46 Jeffrey GP, Muller DPR, Burroughs AK *et al.* Vitamin E deficiency and its clinical significance in adults with primary biliary cirrhosis and other forms of chronic liver disease. *J. Hepatol.* 1987; **4**: 307.

47 Jones EA, Bergasa NV. Why do cholestatic patients itch? *Gut* 1996; **38**: 644.

48 Kawata S, Imai Y, Inada M *et al.* Selective reduction of hepatic cytochrome P_{450} content in patients with intrahepatic cholestasis. A mechanism for impairment of microsomal drug oxidation. *Gastroenterology* 1987; **92**: 299.

49 Kullak-Ublick G-A, Hagenbuch B, Stieger B *et al.* Functional characterization of the basolateral rat liver organic anion transporting polypeptide. *Hepatology* 1994; **20**: 411.

50 Kullak-Ublick GA, Hagenbuch B, Stieger B *et al.* Molecular and functional characterization of an organic anion transporting polypeptide cloned from human liver. *Gastroenterology* 1995; **109**: 1274.

51 Kunkel HG, Ahrens EH Jr. The relationship between serum lipids and the electrophoretic pattern, with particular reference to patients with primary biliary cirrhosis. *J. Clin. Invest.* 1949; **28**: 1575.

52 Lai ECS, Mok FPT, Fan ST *et al.* Preoperative endoscopic

53 Lindor KD, Janes CH, Crippin JS *et al.* Bone disease in primary biliary cirrhosis: does ursodeoxycholic acid make a difference? *Hepatology* 1995; **21**: 389.

54 Lloyd-Thomas HGL, Sherlock S. Testosterone therapy for the pruritus of obstructive jaundice. *Br. Med. J.* 1952; **ii**: 1289.

55 Lobo-Yeo A, Senaldi G, Portmann B *et al.* Class I and Class II major histocompatibility complex antigen expression on hepatocytes: a study in children with liver disease. *Hepatology* 1990; **12**: 224.

56 McGill JM, Williams DM, Hunt CM. Survey of cystic fibrosis transmembrane conductance regulator genotypes in primary sclerosing cholangitis. *Dig. Dis. Sci.* 1996; **41**: 540.

57 Manolagas SC, Jilka RL. Bone marrow, cytokines, and bone remodelling: emerging insights into the pathophysiology of osteoporosis. *N. Engl. J. Med.* 1995; **332**: 305.

58 Meier PJ. Molecular mechanisms of hepatic bile salt transport from sinusoidal blood into bile. *Am. J. Physiol.* 1995; **269**: G801.

59 Moser AE, Singh I, Brown FR *et al.* The cerebrohepatorenal (Zellweger) syndrome. *N. Engl. J. Med.* 1984; **310**: 1141.

60 Narayanan S. Biochemistry and clinical relevance of lipoprotein X. *Ann. Clin. Lab. Sci.* 1984; **14**: 371.

61 Nathanson MH, Boyer JL. Mechanisms and regulation of bile secretion. *Hepatology* 1991; **14**: 551.

62 Ong DE, Amédée-Manesme O. Liver levels of vitamin A and cellular retinol-binding protein for patients with biliary atresia. *Hepatology* 1987; **7**: 253.

63 Oude Elferink RPJ, Groen AK. The role of mdr2 P-glycoprotein in biliary lipid secretion. Cross-talk between cancer research and biliary physiology. *J. Hepatol.* 1995; **23**: 617.

64 Oude Elferink RPJ, Meijer DKF, Kuipers F *et al.* Hepatobiliary secretion of organic compounds; molecular mechanisms of membrane transport. *Biochem. Biophys. Acta Rev. Biomembranes* 1995; **1241**: 215.

65 Osman E, Owen JS, Burroughs AK. Review article: S-adenosyl-L-methionine — a new therapeutic agent in liver disease? *Aliment. Pharmacol. Ther.* 1993; **7**: 21.

66 Ostrow JD, Mukerjee P, Tiribelli C. Structure and binding of unconjugated bilirubin: relevance for physiological and pathophysiological function. *J. Lipid Res.* 1994; **35**: 1715.

67 Pain JA, Cahill CJ, Gilbert JM *et al.* Prevention of postoperative renal dysfunction in patients with obstructive jaundice: a multicentre study of bile salts and lactulose. *Br. J. Surg.* 1991; **78**: 467.

68 Phillips MJ, Ackerley CA, Superina RA *et al.* Excess zinc associated with severe progressive cholestasis in Cree and Ojibwa-Cree children. *Lancet* 1996; **347**: 866.

69 Piotrowicz A, Polkey M, Wilkinson M. Ursodeoxycholic acid for the treatment of flucloxacillin-associated cholestasis. *J. Hepatol.* 1995; **22**: 119.

70 Poupon RE, Poupon R, Balkau B *et al.* Ursodiol for the long-term treatment of primary biliary cirrhosis. *N. Engl. J. Med.* 1994; **330**: 1342.

71 Quigley EMM, Marsh MN, Shaffer JL *et al.* Hepatobiliary complications of total parenteral nutrition. *Gastroenterology* 1993; **104**: 286.

72 Raiford DS. Pruritus of chronic cholestasis. *Q. J. Med.* 1995; **88**: 603.

73 Rosario J, Sutherland E, Simon FR. Protection by S-adenosyl-L-methionine against ethinyl estradiol induced

cholestasis is not due to alterations in sinusoidal membrane lipids. *Hepatology* 1986; **6**: 1201.

74 Scholmerich J, Baumgartner U, Miyai K *et al.* Tauroursodeoxycholate prevents taurolithocholate-induced cholestasis and toxicity in rat liver. *J. Hepatol.* 1990; **10**: 280.

75 Schwörer H, Hartmann H, Ramadori G. Relief of cholestatic pruritus by a novel class of drug: 5-hydroxytryptamine type 3 (5-HT3) receptor antagonists; effectiveness of ondansetron. *Pain* 1995; **61**: 33.

76 Sellinger M, Barrett C, Malle P *et al.* Cryptic Na+, K+–ATPase activity in rat liver canalicular plasma membranes: evidence for its basolateral origin. *Hepatology* 1990; **11**: 223.

77 Setchell KDR, Bragetti P, Zimmer-Nechemias L *et al.* Oral bile acid treatment and the patient with Zellweger syndrome. *Hepatology* 1992; **15**: 198.

78 Smallwood RA, Williams HA, Rosenoer VM *et al.* Liver-copper levels in liver disease: studies using neutron activation analysis. *Lancet* 1968; **ii**: 1310.

79 Smit JJM, Schinkel AH, Elferink RPJ *et al.* Homozygous disruption of the murine mdr2 P-glycoprotein gene leads to a complete absence of phospholipid from bile and to liver disease. *Cell* 1993; **75**: 451.

80 Smith DJ, Gordon ER. Membrane fluidity and cholestasis. *J. Hepatol.* 1987; **5**: 362.

81 Smith CR, Oshio C, Miyairi M *et al.* Coordination of the contractile activity of bile canaliculi. Evidence from spontaneous contractions *in vitro*. *Lab Invest.* 1985; **53**: 270.

82 Sokol RJ, Heubi JE, Iannaccone S *et al.* Mechanism causing vitamin E deficiency during chronic childhood cholestasis. *Gastroenterology* 1983; **83**: 1172.

83 Sokol RJ, Winklhofer-Roob BM, Devereaux MW *et al.* Generation of hydroperoxides in isolated rat hepatocytes and hepatic mitochondria exposed to hydrophobic bile acids. *Gastroenterology* 1995; **109**: 1249.

84 Thomas PK, Walker JG. Xanthomatous neuropathy in primary biliary cirrhosis. *Brain* 1965; **88**: 1079.

85 Tsukada N, Ackerley CA, Phillips MJ. The structure and organisation of the bile canalicular cytoskeleton with special reference to actin and actin-binding proteins. *Hepatology* 1995; **21**: 1106.

86 Walt RP, Kemp CM, Lyness L *et al.* Vitamin A treatment for night blindness in primary biliary cirrhosis. *Br. Med. J.* 1984; **288**: 1030.

87 Walt RP, Daneshmend TK, Fellows IW *et al.* Effect of stanazolol on itching in primary biliary cirrhosis. *Br. Med. J.* 1988; **296**: 607.

88 Williams R, Cartter MA, Sherlock S *et al.* Idiopathic recurrent cholestasis: a study of the functional and pathological lesions in four cases. *Q. J. Med.* 1964; **33**: 387.

Chapter 14
Primary Biliary Cirrhosis

Primary biliary cirrhosis (PBC) is a disease of unknown cause in which intra-hepatic bile ducts are progressively destroyed. It was first described in 1851 by Addison and Gull [1] and later by Hanot [40]. The association with high serum cholesterol levels and skin xanthomas led to the term 'xanthomatous biliary cirrhosis' [60]. Ahrens and co-workers [2] termed the condition 'primary biliary cirrhosis'. However, in the early stages nodular regeneration is inconspicuous and cirrhosis is not present. The term 'chronic non-suppurative destructive cholangitis' [89] is a better one although too cumbersome to replace the popular 'primary biliary cirrhosis'.

Aetiology

The disease is associated with a profound immunological disturbance which has been related to the bile duct destruction [29, 33]. Cytotoxic T-cells infiltrate the bile duct epithelium [118] as do class II restricted T4 lymphocytes. The final event is an attack by cytotoxic T-cells on biliary epithelium. Cytokines produced from the activated T-cells contribute to the liver cell damage [65]. Suppressor T-cells are reduced in number and function (fig. 14.1) [6]. Upregulated display of HLA class I antigens and *de novo* expression of HLA class II antigens are compatible with immune-mediated duct destruction [6].

The disease might represent a failure of immunoregulation, with loss of tolerance to tissues bearing a rich display of histocompatibility antigens. How and why the bile ducts are affected in this way, and the nature of the 'self' antigens presented, remains unknown. The triggers of the immunopathological cascade may be viral, bacterial or some other neoantigen, or simply defective immunoregulation alone.

In many respects, PBC is analogous to the graft-versus-host syndrome, as seen, for instance, after bone marrow transplant and where the immune system has become sensitized to foreign HLA proteins [26]. Structural changes in the bile ducts are similar. Other ducts with a high concentration of HLA class II antigens on their epithelium such as the lacrimal and pancreatic ducts are involved. The condition can be viewed as a dry gland syndrome.

Epithelioid granulomas suggest a delayed-type

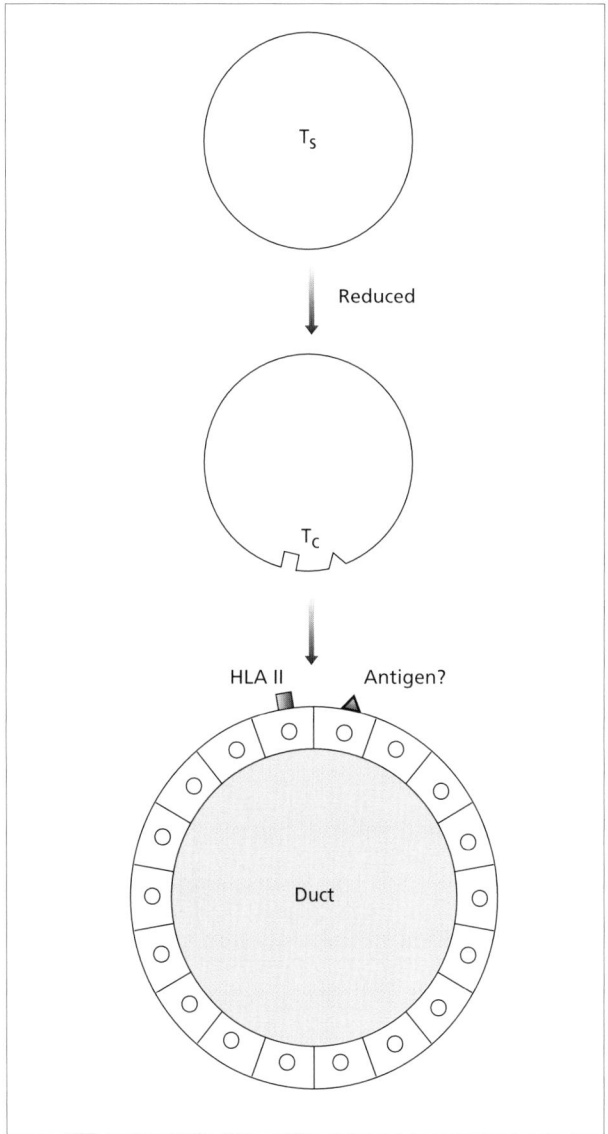

Fig. 14.1. Primary biliary cirrhosis: HLA class II antigens and another unknown antigen are displayed on the bile duct. T$_s$ lymphocytes are depressed and there is breach of tolerance to the biliary antigens.

hypersensitivity reaction. They are seen in the early, florid stage and may reflect an improved prognosis [55].

Copper is retained in the liver, but in a non-hepatotoxic form [23].

Mitochondrial antigens and antibodies

Circulating antibodies against mitochondria are found in virtually 100% of patients with PBC [70, 111]. They are non-organ and non-species specific. The antigens to which the antibodies are directed are localized on the inner mitochondrial membrane [102] (fig. 14.2). The antigenic component specific for PBC serum is M2. Four M2 antigen polypeptides have been identified, all components of the pyruvate dehydrogenase complex (PDC) of mitochondrial enzymes (fig. 14.2). E1 is a 50 kDa 2-oxoacid dehydrogenase complex, E2 is the 74 kDa complex of lipoamide acyl transferase, E3 is a 50 kDa 2-oxoglutarate complex. Protein X is a 52 kDa member of the PDC and cross-reacts with E2 [30, 31]. An ELISA test has been developed against E2 and components of the M2 complex. It is 88% sensitive and 96% specific for the diagnosis of PBC [7, 103]. PBC [56] is unlikely in the absence of serum anti-M2. The ELISA-specific sensitivity test is not generally available and the serum antimitochondrial test is usually performed by indirect immunofluorescence on rat kidney substrate. This is a difficult technique and can give false-negative results in inexperienced laboratories.

There are other mitochondrial antigens and antibodies. Anti-M9 is associated with early PBC and can be found in healthy relatives of sufferers and technicians handling PBC sera. 10–15% of normal persons are M9 positive. M4 and M8 are found only in those who are M2 positive, and may be associated with more progressive disease [113]. M3 is associated with drug reactions. M6 is related to iproniazid and M5 to collagen diseases.

An antinuclear antibody against a 200 kDa polypeptide gives a perinuclear fluorescence in 29% of patients with PBC with antibodies in 27%. Its relation to mitochondrial antibodies in PBC remains unclear.

Relation to aetiology

The relationship of mitochondrial antigens and antibodies to the pathogenesis of PBC has always been speculative. The responsible autoantigen might be related to mitochondria. The E2 component of the PDC complex has been expressed on bile duct epithelium of patients with early PBC [49, 108].

T-cell mediated mechanisms may be important. E2/X-specific T-cells have been demonstrated in the circulation and liver of PBC patients. They might be mediating biliary epithelial damage [48].

T-cell activation, if followed by B-cell recruitment and production of antibodies, may be responsible for the destruction of biliary epithelial cells [73].

There are some similarities between bacterial and

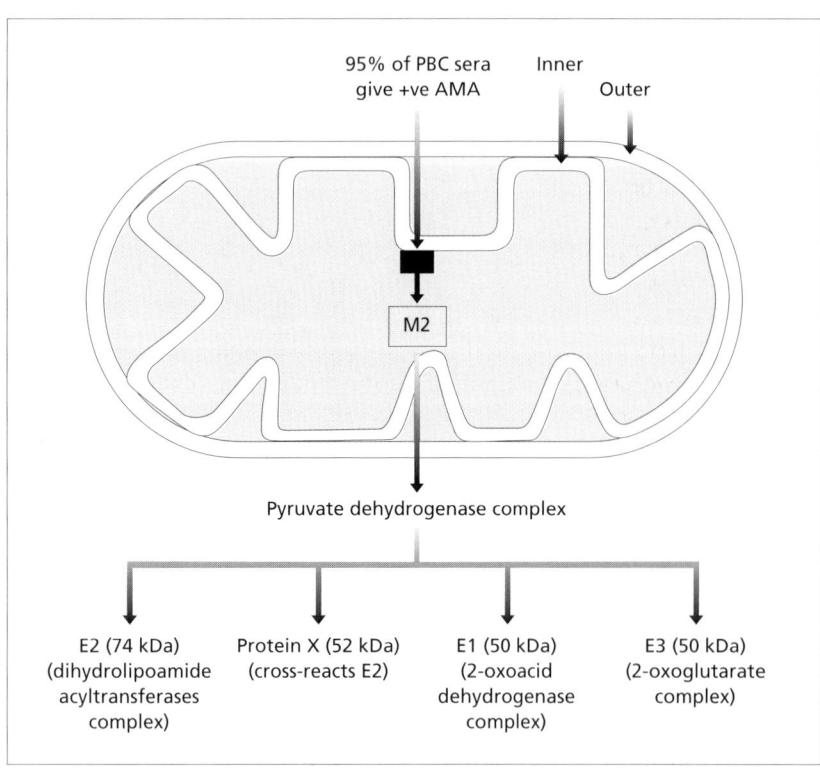

Fig. 14.2. Mitochondrial antibodies and antigens.

mammalian mitochondrial components. Cross-reactivity of the antigens between bile ducts and microorganisms is possible. The larger antigens such as E2 are highly conserved in evolution and are present in mammals, yeast and bacteria. AMA cross-reacts with subcellular constituents of Gram-negative and Gram-positive organisms [28].

PBC-specific AMA reactive proteins are present in several Enterobacteriaceae species, probably in the bacterial wall [101]. The AMA found in PBC may be primarily directed against enterobacterial antigens resulting from an intestinal infection [45]. Stool samples from patients with PBC show increased numbers of *Escherichia coli* R forms [45] and these contain PBC-AMA-specific proteins. Whether these R forms are aetiologically important and whether antigens released from the bacterial wall contribute to the disease remains uncertain. However, these observations might be linked with the increased incidence of Gram-negative urinary tract infections in patients with PBC [12, 15].

Epidemiology and genetics

The disease has been reported from all parts of the world. Asians, Caucasians, Jews, Black and Oriental people are affected. Prevalence varies widely between different countries and regions of the same country. Changing prevalence depends on increasing physician awareness, better diagnosis, especially the availability of the serum mitochondrial antibody test, and recognition of more asymptomatic patients. There is family clustering and PBC has been reported in sisters, twins, mothers and daughters [17, 105]. In New York, the familial frequency was 1.33% [3] and in London 5.5% [10]. Usually mothers and daughters are affected with presentation earlier in the second generation [10]. The prevalence of circulating mitochondrial antibodies is increased in relatives of patients [27, 32].

In one study from Sheffield, England, PBC was associated with a particular water supply [106]. Environmental factors in the water supply could not be identified. In Ontario, Canada, racial predisposition and geographic clustering were not seen [115]. More epidemiological studies are needed.

There are histocompatibility antigen associations. In a Caucasian population from the USA, HLA-DRw8 was associated with PBC [34].

C4A-QO, and HLA class 3 allele, is associated with many autoimmune diseases. Genetic typing revealed an increased incidence for C4A-QO alleles and a highly significant proportion of PBC patients carried DRw8 and C4A-QO alleles [63]. A mother and two sisters with PBC shared the same histocompatibility haplotype. Class 3 antigens are components of the complement system. This indicates a partial C4A deficiency in patients with

PBC. Other associations include HLA-DPB1*0301 in a German population [66] and DRB1*0803 in Japanese sufferers from PBC [77].

It is difficult to make a coherent story from these observations. They suggest a strong immunogenetic background for PBC that runs in families. Environmental factors, especially infections, cannot be ignored and these presumably act on a genetically predisposed host.

Clinical features

Presentation (table 14.1) [95, 98]

90% of patients with PBC are female. The cause for disease prevalence among women is unknown. The patient is usually 40–60 years of age, but can be as old as 80 or as young as 20 [69]. 10% are male in whom the disease runs a similar course. The disease starts insidiously, most frequently as pruritus without jaundice. Patients may be referred initially to dermatologists. Jaundice may never develop but in the majority appears within 6 months to 2 years of the onset of pruritus. In about a quarter, jaundice and pruritus start simultaneously. Jaundice preceding pruritus is extremely unusual and jaundice without pruritus at any time is very rare. The pruritus can start during pregnancy and be confused with cholestatic jaundice of the last trimester. Chronic right upper-quadrant pain is frequent (17%). This may persist or resolve [54]. Upper endoscopy may be necessary for diagnosis. Fatigue is frequent.

Examination shows a well-nourished, sometimes pigmented woman. Jaundice is slight or absent. The liver is usually enlarged and firm and the spleen palpable.

Table 14.1. Diagnosis of primary biliary cirrhosis at presentation [96]

Symptomatic
Middle-aged woman with pruritus followed by slowly progressive jaundice
Liver palpable
Serum bilirubin about twice normal serum alkaline phosphatase about 4 times normal: serum aspartate transaminase about twice normal; serum albumin normal
Serum mitochondrial antibody 1 : 40
Liver biopsy appearances compatible
ERCP (if diagnosis in doubt): normal intra-hepatic bile ducts

Asymptomatic
Routine laboratory screen
Increased serum alkaline phosphatase
Positive serum mitochondrial antibody
Investigation of other disease, especially collagen or thyroid
Hepatomegaly

The asymptomatic patient

Widespread use of automated biochemical screening has resulted in an increasing number of patients being diagnosed when asymptomatic usually by a raised serum alkaline phosphatase level. Liver biopsies performed after finding a positive mitochondrial antibody titre ≥1/40 are nearly always abnormal and usually show features consistent with primary biliary cirrhosis even if the patient is asymptomatic and the serum alkaline phosphatase is normal.

The diagnosis may be made in patients under investigation for a condition known to be associated with primary biliary cirrhosis, such as thyroid or collagen disease, or in the course of family surveys.

Abnormal physical signs may be absent. Mitochondrial antibody is always present. Serum alkaline phosphatase and bilirubin may be normal or only minimally increased. Serum cholesterol and transaminases can also be normal.

Course

Asymptomatic patients usually survive at least 10 years (fig. 14.3) [61]. In those with symptomatic disease and jaundice the survival is about 7 years [95].

Diarrhoea may be due to steatorrhoea. Weight loss is slow. Fatigue is the most disabling symptom but lifestyle is surprisingly normal. The course is afebrile and abdominal pain is unusual but may persist.

Skin xanthomas develop frequently and sometimes acutely, but many patients remain in the pre-xanthomatous state throughout their course; terminally xanthomas may disappear.

The skin may be thickened and tough over the fingers, ankles and legs. Pain in the fingers, especially on opening doors, and in the toes may be due to xanthomatous peripheral neuropathy [104]. There may be a butterfly area over the back which is inaccessible and escapes scratching [85].

The bone changes complicating chronic cholestasis are particularly profound in the deeply jaundiced (see figs 13.16, 13.17, 13.18). In the late stages the patient complains of backache and pain over the ribs, sometimes with pathological fractures.

Duodenal ulceration and haemorrhage are common.

Bleeding oesophageal varices may be a presenting feature even before nodules have developed [52]. At this stage the portal hypertension is probably pre-sinusoidal. Within 5.6 years, oesophageal varices have developed in 83 of 265 patients (31%), and in 40 (48%) have bled [35].

Hepato-cellular carcinoma is very rare perhaps because nodular cirrhosis develops so late [53].

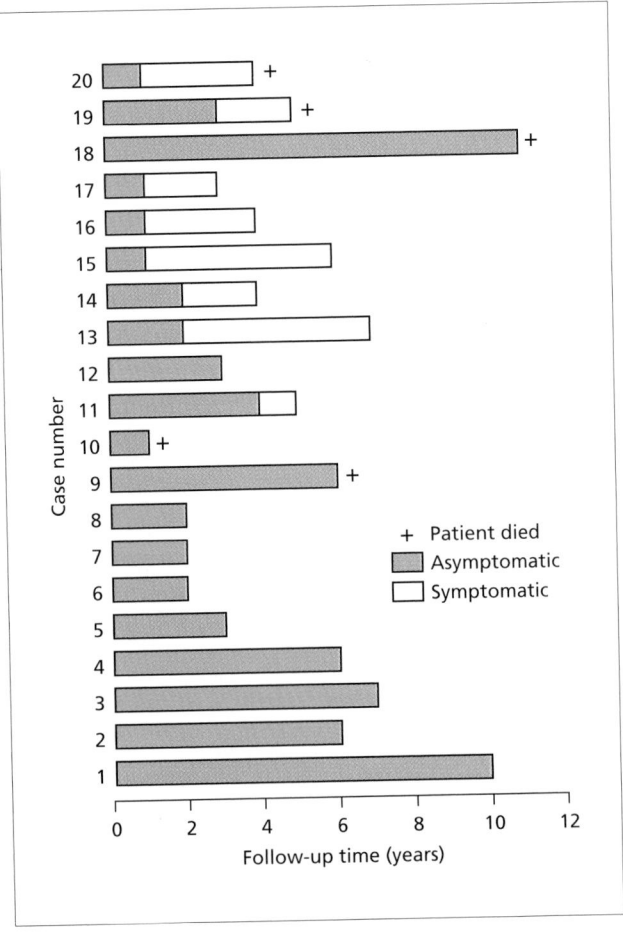

Fig. 14.3. The course of 20 patients with PBC diagnosed when asymptomatic. Note that one patient continued asymptomatic for 10 years [58].

Associated diseases

PBC is associated with almost any postulated autoimmune disease. The collagenoses, especially rheumatoid arthritis, dermatomyositis, mixed connective tissue disease and systemic lupus erythematosus [39], are particularly frequent.

PBC may be associated with scleroderma in 4% of patients and with the whole CREST syndrome [86]. The scleroderma is usually limited to sclerodactyly but occasionally involves face, arms and legs. Keratoconjunctivitis may be present [83]. These patients usually show 20–52 kDa Ro antibodies [21, 80]. A sicca complex of dry eyes and mouth, with or without the arthritis completing Sjögren's syndrome is found in about 75% of patients.

Other associated skin lesions include immune complex capillaritis and lichen planus [38]. Autoimmune thyroiditis affects about 20%. Graves' disease has also been reported [75].

PBC and jejunal villous atrophy, resembling coeliac

disease, have been reported [8]. Ulcerative colitis is another rare accompaniment [14].

PBC has been associated with autoimmune thrombocytopenia and insulin receptor autoantibodies [92].

Renal complications include IgM associated membranous glomerular nephritis [84].

Renal tubular acidosis is attributed to copper deposits in the distal renal tubule [79]. Hypouricaemia and hyperuricosuria are further expressions of renal tubular damage [46]. Bacteriuria develops in 35% of cases and may be asymptomatic [12, 15].

Association with selective immunoglobulin A deficiency has been reported [47]. This indicates that the pathogenesis does not require IgA-dependent immune mechanisms.

Breast cancer is increased 4.4 times over the rate prevailing in a comparable normal population [36, 116].

PBC has also been associated with transverse myelitis due to angiitis and necrotizing myelopathy [90]. Finger clubbing is common, and occasionally there is hypertrophic osteoarthropathy (see fig. 13.18) [24].

Pancreatic insufficiency is secondary to low bile flow [88] and perhaps to immunological damage to the pancreatic duct [26].

Gallstones, usually of pigment type, have been seen by ERCP in 39% of cases. They are occasionally symptomatic but rarely migrate to the common bile duct.

Abnormal pulmonary gas-transfer studies are associated with an abnormal chest X-ray showing nodules and interstitial fibrosis. Lung biopsies show interstitial lung disease. Pulmonary interstitial giant cell granulomas have also been described. These patients often have Sjögren's syndrome [107, 112] and positive Ro antibodies [21].

The CREST syndrome is accompanied by interstitial pneumonitis and pulmonary vascular abnormalities.

CT scanning shows 81% of patients to have enlarged nodes in the gastro-hepatic ligament and porta hepatis. Enlarged paracardiac and mesenteric nodes are also seen [78].

Biochemical tests

Initially, serum bilirubin values are rarely very high, usually less than 35 µmol/l (2 mg/100 ml) in symptomatic patients. Serum alkaline phosphatase and gamma-glutamyl transpeptidase are raised. The total serum cholesterol is increased but not constantly. The serum albumin level is usually normal at presentation and the total serum globulin only moderately increased. Serum IgM is usually raised. This is not reliable for diagnosis, although an increase may add some diagnostic weight.

Liver biopsy [89]

The only hepatic lesion diagnostic of PBC is the injured septal or interlobular bile duct. Such ducts are not often seen in needle biopsy specimens, but are usually well represented in surgical biopsies (fig. 14.4). However, such biopsies are decreasing because of less frequent surgery. The interpretation of a needle biopsy demands an experienced histopathologist.

The disease begins with damage to the epithelium of small bile ducts. Histometric examinations show that bile ducts less than 70–80 µm in diameter are destroyed, particularly in the early stages [72]. Epithelial cells are swollen, irregular and more eosinophilic. The bile duct lumen is irregular and the basement membrane is disrupted. The bile duct occasionally ruptures. Surrounding the damaged duct is a cellular reaction which includes lymphocytes, plasma cells, eosinophils and histiocytes. Granulomas commonly form, usually in zone 1 (fig. 14.4).

Bile ducts become destroyed. Their sites are marked by aggregates of lymphoid cells, and bile ductules begin to proliferate (fig. 14.5). Hepatic arterial branches can be identified in the portal zones but without accompanying bile ducts. Fibrosis extends from the portal zones and there is a variable degree of piecemeal necrosis. Substantial amounts of copper and copper-associated protein can be demonstrated histochemically. The fibrous septa gradually distort the architecture of the liver and regeneration nodules form (figs 14.6, 14.7). These are often irregular in distribution and cirrhosis may be seen in one part of a biopsy but not in another. In some areas lobular architecture may be preserved for some time. In the early stages, cholestasis is in zone 1 (portal).

Hepato-cellular hyaline deposits, similar to those of

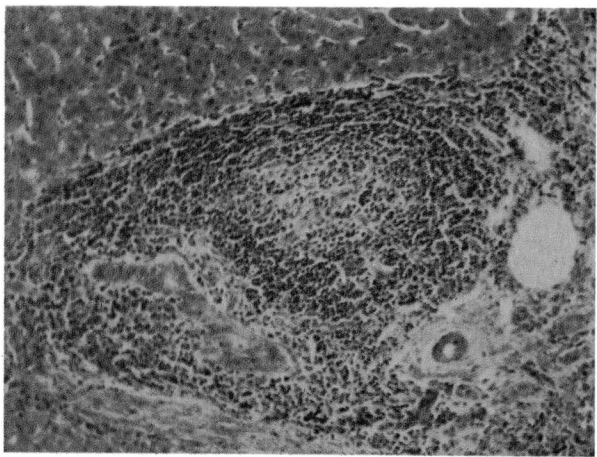

Fig. 14.4. The portal zone contains a well-formed granuloma. An adjacent bile duct shows damage.

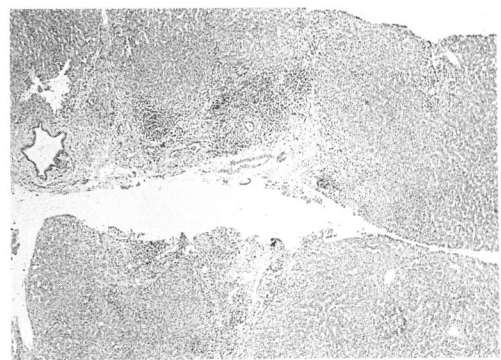

Fig. 14.5. Stage 2 lesion, marked by aggregates of lymphoid cells. Bile ducts begin to proliferate. (H & E, ×10.)

alcoholic disease, are found in hepatocytes in about 25% of cases.

The histological appearances have been divided into four stages: *stage I* florid bile duct lesions; *stage II* ductular proliferation; *stage III* scarring (septal fibrosis and bridging); and *stage IV* cirrhosis. Such staging is of limited value as the changes in the liver are focal and evolve at different speeds in different parts. Stages overlap. It is particularly difficult to separate stages II and III. The disease has a very variable course and advanced stage III lesions may be seen in the asymptomatic patient. Moreover, serial biopsies have shown that the same stage may persist for many years.

Diagnosis (table 14.2)

There are a number of PBC 'look-alikes', the chief difference being that they lack serum mitochondrial antibody.

Visualization of the bile ducts by endoscopic or percutaneous cholangiography may be necessary in atypical patients. These include males and those with a negative serum mitochondrial antibody test, with inconclusive liver biopsy findings or with marked abdominal pain. Surgical exploration of the bile ducts is not necessary.

Widespread tissue granulomas may suggest cholestatic sarcoidosis (table 14.3) [71] (Chapter 26). In sarcoidosis, however, the Kveim–Siltzbach skin test is positive (75%) and mitochondrial antibody is absent. Liver biopsy shows abundant well-formed granulomas and less bile duct damage than that seen in PBC.

T-lymphocytes (predominantly T4 positive cells) and activated alveolar macrophages are found by bronchoalveolar lavage in patients with PBC—similar findings to those of sarcoidosis [100]. There are overlaps and occasionally the distinction is impossible.

In later stages, the differentiation from autoimmune chronic active hepatitis may be difficult. The pattern of biochemical tests of liver function is usually different. Liver biopsy features favouring PBC include intact lobules, slight zone 1 necrosis and periseptal cholestasis.

Chronic hepatitis C virus infection is occasionally associated with prolonged cholestasis, but biochemical tests suggest hepatocellular disease and serological tests for hepatitis C virus are positive.

In immune cholangiopathy, the clinical features of biochemical tests and liver histology resembles that of PBC [9]. Serum mitochondrial antibody is always negative but antinuclear antibodies are present in high titre.

In primary sclerosing cholangitis, the mitochondrial antibody test is always negative or in low titre and cholangiography demonstrates the typical bile duct irregularities.

Idiopathic adult ductopenia is marked by absence of interlobular bile ducts. The aetiology is uncertain but some instances may represent small duct primary sclerosing cholangitis [11, 59].

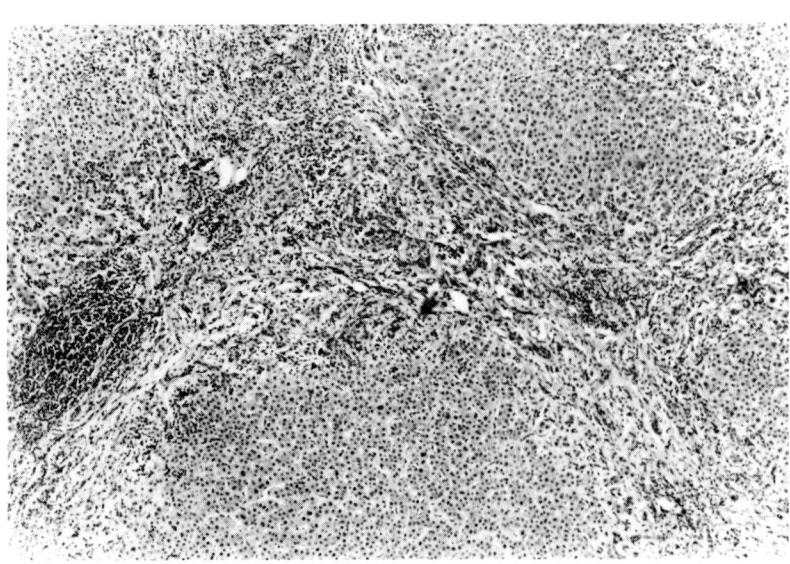

Fig. 14.6. There is scarring and septa contain lymphoid aggregates. Bile ducts are inconspicuous. Hyperplastic 'regeneration' nodules are beginning to develop. (H & E, × 48) [98].

Table 14.2. Differential diagnosis of primary biliary cirrhosis [96]

Disease	Features	MAb	Liver biopsy
Primary biliary cirrhosis	Female Pruritus High serum alkaline phosphatas	Positive	Bile duct damage Lymphoid aggregates Slight PMN Intact lobules Periseptal cholestasis
Primary sclerosing cholangitis	Males predominate Associated ulcerative cholitis Cholangiography is diagnostic	Negative or low titre	Ductular proliferation fibrosis Onion-skin duct fibrosis
Cholestatic sarcoidosis	Equal sexes Black patients Pruritus High serum alkaline phosphatase Chest X-ray changes	Negative	Many granulomas Modest bile duct changes
Autoimmune cholangiopathy	Females High serum alkaline phosphatase Serum ANA positive in high titre	Negative	Bile duct damage Lymphoid aggregates Slight PMN
Cholestatic drug reactions	History Usually within 6 weeks of starting drug Acute onset	Negative	Mononuclear portal reaction sometimes with eosinophils, granulomas and fatty change

ANA = antinuclear antibodies; MAb = mitochondrial antibodies; PMN = piecemeal necrosis.

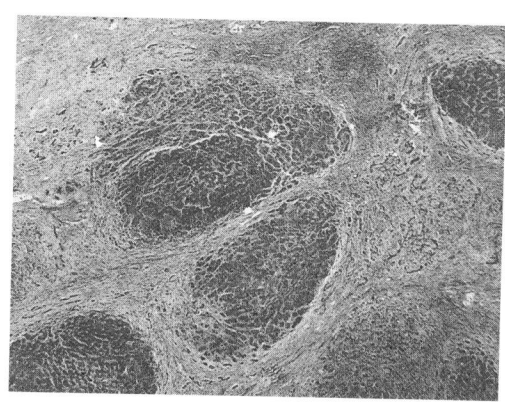

Fig. 14.7. Stage 4: biliary cirrhosis has developed.

Cholestatic drug reactions are excluded by the history and by the acute onset, with rapidly deepening jaundice developing 4–6 weeks after the drug is started.

Prognosis

The course of asymptomatic patients is variable and unpredictable and counselling the patient and her family is very difficult. Some will never become symptomatic and others will run a progressive downhill course (fig. 14.8). Nowadays, the patient with end-stage PBC faces not death, but possible liver transplantation.

The life expectancy of some asymptomatic patients may not differ from that of the general population.

Table 14.3. Cholestatic sarcoidosis compared with PBC

	Sarcoidosis	Primary biliary cirrhosis
Sex	Equal	80% female
Age	Young	Middle age
Pruritus	Yes	Yes
Jaundice	Yes	Yes
Respiratory complaints	Yes	No
Hepato-splenomegaly	Yes	Yes
Serum alkaline phosphatase	Raised	Raised
Hilar lymphadenopathy	Usual	Rare
Hepatic granulomas	Discrete Clustered	Poorly formed Surrounded by mixed cells
Serum angiotensin-converting enzyme	Raised	Raised
Mitochondrial antibody	No	Yes (98%)
Kveim–Siltzbach test	Positive	Negative
Broncho-alveolar lavage lymphocytosis activated macrophages	Present Present	Present Present

Reported results of the time taken to pass from the asymptomatic to the symptomatic stage are very variable and may depend on the patients studied and the mode of referral (table 14.4). Duration of disease depends on the time of first diagnosis. Patients seen at a referral centre such as the Mayo Clinic or Royal Free Hospital are usually more advanced and hence more

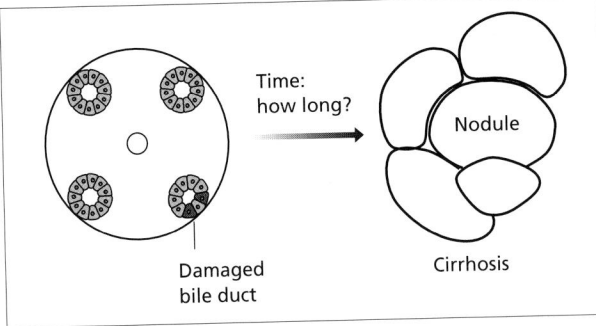

Fig. 14.8. Natural history of PBC: the time taken from acute bile duct damage to end-stage biliary cirrhosis is uncertain [97].

Table 14.4. Prognosis of asymptomatic primary biliary cirrhosis

Year	Centre	No.	Percent became symptomatic	Duration to symptoms (months)
1977	Royal Free (UK) [58]	20	50	27
1983	Yale [87]	37	42	54
1989	Uppsala [76]	56	37	89
1990	Mayo [5]	73	89	–
1990	Newcastle (UK) [68]	70	27	43
1990	Kings (UK) [68]	25	60	35
1990	Oslo [91]	13	38	60

likely to be symptomatic sooner than those in a regional referral centre such as Oslo or Newcastle. By and large, asymptomatic patients become symptomatic in 2–7 years when the course mirrors that of the patient who presents symptomatic [61].

In symptomatic patients prognosis is particularly important in determining the best time for hepatic transplantation. When serum bilirubin values are consistently greater than 100 µmol/l (6 mg/dl), the patient is unlikely to survive for more than 2 years (fig. 14.9) [25, 94]. Other features predicting decreased survival include symptoms, advanced age, hepatosplenomegaly, ascites and serum albumin less than 3 g/dl [18, 87]. Histologically, piecemeal necrosis, cholestasis, bridging fibrosis and cirrhosis correlate with the worst prognosis.

Within a median of 5.6 years, varices have developed in 31% of patients and 48% of these will have bled. Varices are more likely to develop in those with a high serum bilirubin and with an advanced histological stage of the disease. Once varices have developed, 83% survive 1 year and 59% 3 years. Survival after the initial bleed is 65% at 1 year and 46% at 3 years [35].

Autoimmune diseases such as thyroiditis, sicca syndrome or Raynaud's phenomenon correlate with decreased survival.

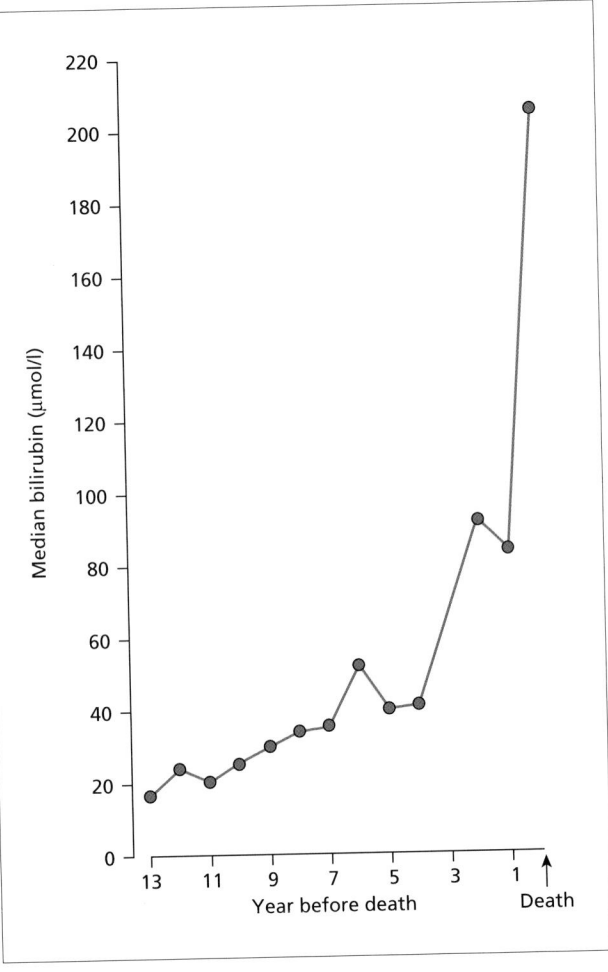

Fig. 14.9. The evolution of liver failure in PBC. This nomogram is derived from the medians of pooled serum bilirubin results in patients followed serially from diagnosis to death. Expected survival for any given bilirubin can be extrapolated from this nomogram [25].

Bilirubin (µmol/l)	Expected survival (years)
< 34	8–13
35–100	2–7
> 100	< 2
(17 µmol/l = 1 mg)	

Prognostic models are based on Cox's regression analysis. The Mayo Clinic model depends on age, serum bilirubin, albumin, and prothrombin time, and the presence or absence of oedema [20] (table 14.5). This predicts survival accurately and has the advantage of being independent of liver biopsy. A study from Glasgow included liver biopsy appearances [37]. Another European model uses age, serum bilirubin and albumin concentrations, presence of cirrhosis and the presence of cholestasis, and results agree with the Mayo Clinic model [18].

No model can yield a precise estimate of survival

Table 14.5. Mayo model for survival [20]

Age
Serum
   bilirubin
   albumin
Prothrombin time
Oedema

for the individual patient. These models do not take into account serial time-dependent factors. They cannot predict a life-threatening episode such as bleeding oesophageal varices.

The terminal stages last about 1 year and are marked by a rapid deepening of jaundice with disappearance of both xanthomas and pruritus. Serum albumin and total cholesterol levels fall. Oedema and ascites develop. The final events include episodes of hepatic encephalopathy with uncontrollable bleeding, usually from the oesophageal varices. An intercurrent infection, sometimes a Gram-negative septicaemia, may be terminal.

Treatment

General measures. Apply to all patients with cholestasis and include control of itching and management of steatorrhoea (Chapter 13).

Vitamin D and calcium loss, secondary to deficiency of bile, result in osteomalacia which is corrected by vitamin D and calcium supplements. Osteoporosis is much more frequent and important [41]. This is difficult to treat, but calcium supplements should be given and the patient encouraged to take adequate exercise and exposure to sunshine. Hormone replacement, perhaps by a patch method may be cautiously tried although the patient is at increased risk of breast cancer. Results with calcitonin proved disappointing [16].

Immunosuppressive drugs. These give only limited benefit and are not nearly so useful as in autoimmune chronic active hepatitis, where the response to corticosteroids is dramatic. Azathioprine [18], D-penicillamine and chlorambucil [44] have been abandoned. Corticosteroids reduce symptoms and improve serum biochemical changes but increased development of bone thinning contraindicates them [68].

In limited trials, *cyclosporin A* reduced symptoms and improved biochemical tests [114]. Liver biopsies showed less progression. However, nephrotoxicity and hypertension are serious complications and this therapy is unsafe for long-term use.

Methotrexate (15 mg by mouth once a week) reduces symptoms and serum alkaline phosphatase and bilirubin levels fall [51]. Liver biopsy shows reduction in inflammation. The Mayo prognostic score is unchanged.

Side-effects include a downward trend in white cell count and platelets, indicating reversible bone marrow toxicity. Interstitial pneumonitis develops in 12–15% of patients but responds to stopping the drug and the giving of corticosteroids [93]. There is probably little effect of methotrexate on survival. The effects in PBC are very variable. It should not be given to patients with PBC except in the context of continuing clinical trials.

Colchicine inhibits collagen synthesis and increases collagen degradation. Given to patients with PBC, hepatocellular function improves but there is no effect on survival. Colchicine is inexpensive and has virtually no side-effects but is of limited, if any, benefit in patients with PBC [50, 119].

Ursodeoxycholic acid is a non-hepatotoxic, hydrophilic bile acid that reverses the potential hepatotoxicity of endogenous bile acids. It is costly and is given in a total dose of 13–15 mg/kg body weight after the midday and evening meals. In a French, placebo-controlled, trial, ursodeoxycholic acid reduced the progression of disease and the probability of death or transplantation. Serum bilirubin levels fell. Results were less satisfactory if, on entry to the trial, the patient had a high serum bilirubin level and cirrhosis was present [82]. A Canadian trial did not give such impressive results. Serum bilirubin fell and biochemical tests improved but symptoms, liver histology and survival or time to transplant did not alter [42]. The Mayo Clinic placebo-controlled trial showed the only significant difference in the treated group was a reduction in the time taken to double the serum bilirubin level. There was no change in hepatic histology. Results were better in early than in advanced disease [19, 57]. The meta-analysis of results from all the trials has shown definite but modest reduction of time to death or transplant [43]. Ursodeoxycholic acid is certainly not a panacea for the treatment of PBC. Nevertheless, it should be given to all patients unless they have reached the end-stages and are approaching transplantation. The decision to treat the early, asymptomatic patient with ursodeoxycholic acid is a difficult one, and must be based on each individual patient, bearing in mind the cost.

Combination treatment, using smaller doses, may be more helpful, for instance a combination of colchicine with ursodeoxycholic acid [110] or ursodeoxycholic acid and methotrexate [13].

CONCLUSIONS

At present no satisfactory, specific medical treatment can be recommended for PBC. Ursodeoxycholic acid looks promising in early disease.

Reported trials have usually been too short, too small and poorly controlled. Statistically significant long-term benefits are difficult to establish in a disease with such a long and varied natural history [97]. Any trial must state the number of patients included in each grade. The group in the early, asymptomatic, excellent stage require no treatment. The ones with the poor outlook will be too end-stage to respond. The intermediate group should be included in trials. Evaluation of currently available measures should continue only in the context of large controlled clinical trials.

Haemorrhage from oesophageal varices may be early before a true nodular cirrhosis has developed. It is not surprising therefore that porta-caval shunting gives good results in these patients [99]. Hepatic encephalopathy is unusual. These encouraging results apply particularly to good-risk patients. Transjugular intra-hepatic portal-systemic stent shunt (TIPS) may be useful.

Gallstones should be left *in situ* unless causing severe symptoms or present in the common bile duct. Cholecystectomy is rarely indicated and is badly tolerated.

Hepatic transplantation

Transplantation should be considered when the patient's quality of life has been reduced to the level that he or she is virtually housebound. Uncontrollable itching, ascites, hepatic encephalopathy, bleeding oesophageal varices and recurrent infections are further indications. Results for the transplant are much better if referral is early and, in addition, the costs are considerably less. Patients should probably be referred to a transplant centre when the serum bilirubin approaches 9 mg/dl (150 mm/l).

The survival is considerably better than without transplant [64] (fig. 14.10). 1-year survival after liver transplant is about 85–90% and a 5-year survival rate of 60–70% is reported [109]. 25% will need a re-transplant, usually due to the development of the vanishing bile

duct syndrome [4, 81]. Rehabilitation after the operation is usually excellent (see Chapter 35).

Although antimitochondrial antibody titres fall in the first few months, the trend is then reversed. Disease probably recurs in the transplanted liver [4, 117]. In one series, 16% of patients studied for greater than 1 year after the transplant had hepatic histology suggesting recurrent disease. The patients were usually asymptomatic but some were already experiencing pruritus [4, 81].

For the first 1–3 months, bone density decreases and the results may be catastrophic. The worsening is probably related to bed-rest and corticosteroid therapy. After 9–12 months there is marked improvement in bone formation and density [22].

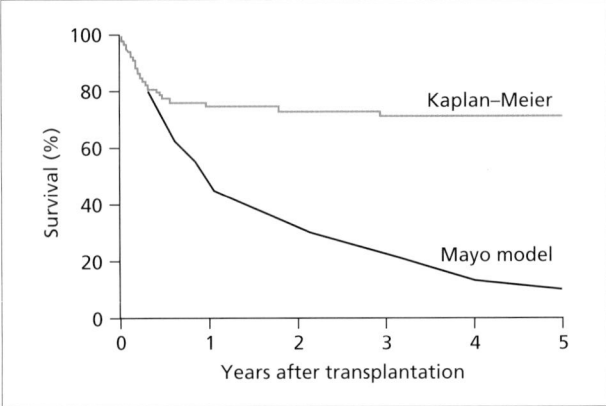

Fig. 14.10. Survival after transplantation in 161 patients with PBC and estimated survival without transplantation as predicted by the Mayo model (simulated control) [64].

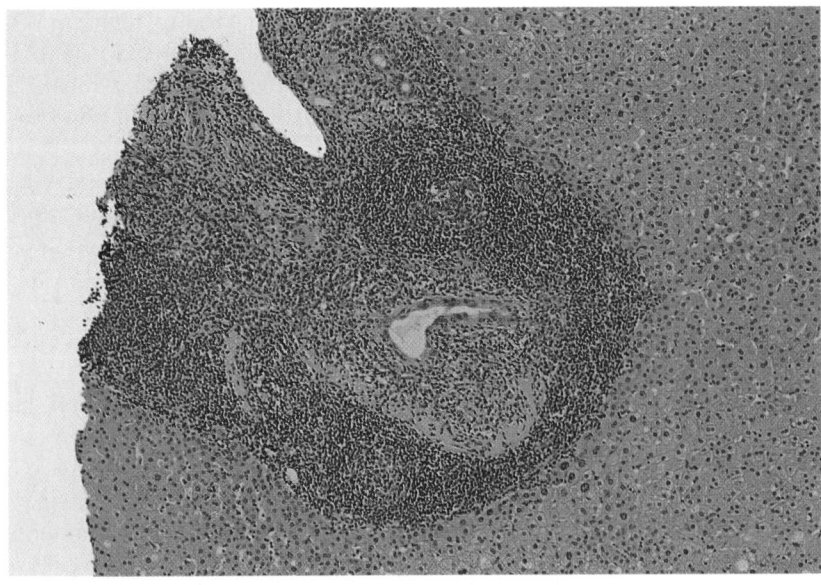

Fig. 14.11. Autoimmune cholangiopathy. Liver biopsy from a young man with mild pruritus, high serum alkaline phosphatase and gamma GT levels. Serum M2 was not detected. Serum ANA was present in high titre. Histology shows damaged zone 1 bile duct with marked inflammation. Appearances resemble PBC. (H & E, × 400.)

Immune cholangiopathy

About 5% of patients presenting as PBC have a negative serum mitochondrial antibody test. Serum antinuclear antibody and anti-actin antibody are usually present in high titre [9, 67]. The patients are usually asymptomatic. Liver histology is identical with that of PBC (fig. 14.11). Prednisolone results in some clinical and biochemical improvement. Liver histology shows less inflammation however bile duct lesions persist and serum gamma GT levels are very high. These patients provide an overlap between PBC and autoimmune chronic hepatitis.

References

1 Addison T, Gull W. On a certain affection of the skin — vitiligoidea — α plana, β tuberosa. *Guy's Hosp. Rep.* 1851; **7**: 265.

2 Ahrens EH Jr, Payne MA, Kunkel HG *et al.* Primary biliary cirrhosis. *Medicine (Baltimore)* 1950; **29**: 299.

3 Bach N, Schaffner F. Prevalence of primary biliary cirrhosis in family members of affected patients. *Gastroenterology* 1992; **102**: A776.

4 Balan V, Batts KP, Porayko MK *et al.* Histological evidence for recurrence of primary biliary cirrhosis after liver transplantation. *Hepatology* 1993; **18**: 1392.

5 Balasubramaniam K, Grambsch PM, Wiesner RH *et al.* Diminished survival in asymptomatic primary biliary cirrhosis. A prospective study. *Gastroenterology* 1990; **98**: 1567.

6 Ballardini G, Mirakian R, Bianchi FB *et al.* Aberrant expression of HLA-DR antigens on bile duct epithelium in primary biliary cirrhosis: relevance to pathogenesis. *Lancet* 1984; **ii**: 1009.

7 Bassendine MF, Yeaman SJ. Serological markers of primary biliary cirrhosis: diagnosis, prognosis and subsets. *Hepatology* 1992; **15**: 545.

8 Behr W, Barnert J. Adult celiac disease and primary biliary cirrhosis. *Am. J. Gastroenterol.* 1986; **81**: 796.

9 Ben-Ari Z, Dhillon AP, Sherlock S. Autoimmune cholangiopathy: part of the spectrum of autoimmune chronic active hepatitis. *Hepatology* 1993; **18**: 10.

10 Brind AM, Bray GP, Portmann BC *et al.* Prevalence and pattern of familial disease in primary biliary cirrhosis. *Gut* 1995; **36**: 615.

11 Bruguera M, Llach J, Rodés J. Nonsyndromic paucity of intrahepatic bile ducts in infancy and idiopathic ductopenia in adulthood: the same syndrome? *Hepatology* 1992; **15**: 830.

12 Burroughs AK, Rosenstein IJ, Epstein O *et al.* Bacteriuria and primary biliary cirrhosis. *Gut* 1984; **25**: 133.

13 Buscher H-P, Zietzschmnann Y, Gerok W. Positive responses to methotrexate and ursodeoxycholic acid in patients with primary biliary cirrhosis responding insufficiently to ursodeoxycholic acid alone. *J. Hepatol.* 1993; **18**: 9.

14 Bush A, Mitchison H, Walt R *et al.* Primary biliary cirrhosis and ulcerative colitis. *Gastroenterology* 1987; **92**: 2009.

15 Butler P, Valle F, Hamilton-Miller JMT *et al.* M2 mitochondrial antibodies and urinary rough mutant bacteria in patients with primary biliary cirrhosis and in patients with recurrent bacteriuria. *J. Hepatol.* 1993; **17**: 408.

16 Camisasca M, Crosignani A, Battezzati PM *et al.* Parenteral calcitonin for metabolic bone disease associated with primary biliary cirrhosis. *Hepatology* 1994; **20**: 633.

17 Chohan MR. Primary biliary cirrhosis in twin sisters. *Gut* 1973; **14**: 213.

18 Christensen E, Neuberger J, Crowe J *et al.* Beneficial effect of azathioprine and prediction of prognosis in primary biliary cirrhosis: final results of an international trial. *Gastroenterology* 1985; **89**: 1084.

19 Coombes B, Carithers RL Jr, Maddrey WC *et al.* A randomized, double-blind, placebo-controlled trial of ursodeoxycholid acid in primary biliary cirrhosis. *Hepatology* 1995; **22**: 759.

20 Dickson ER, Grambsch PM, Fleming TR *et al.* Prognosis in primary biliary cirrhosis: model for decision making. *Hepatology* 1989; **10**: 1.

21 Dörner T, Held C, Trebeljahr G *et al.* Serologic characteristics in primary biliary cirrhosis associated with sicca syndrome. *Scand. J. Gastroenterol.* 1994; **29**: 655.

22 Eastell R, Dickson ER, Hodgson SF *et al.* Rates of vertebral bone loss before and after liver transplantation in women with primary biliary cirrhosis. *Hepatology* 1991; **14**: 296.

23 Epstein O, Arborgh B, Sagiv M *et al.* Is copper hepatotoxic in primary biliary cirrhosis? *J. Clin. Pathol.* 1981; **34**: 1071.

24 Epstein O, Dick R, Sherlock S. Prospective study of periostitis and finger clubbing in primary biliary cirrhosis and other forms of chronic liver disease. *Gut* 1981; **22**: 203.

25 Epstein O, Fraga E, Sherlock S. Importance of clinical staging for prognosis in primary biliary cirrhosis. *Gut* 1985; **26**: A1126.

26 Epstein O, Thomas HC, Sherlock S. Primary biliary cirrhosis is a 'dry gland' syndrome with features of chronic graft-versus-host disease. *Lancet* 1980; **i**: 1166.

27 Feizi T, Naccarato R, Sherlock S *et al.* Mitochondrial and other tissue antibodies in relatives of patients with biliary cirrhosis. *Clin. Exp. Immunol.* 1972; **10**: 609.

28 Flannery GR, Burroughs AK, Butler P *et al.* Antimitochondrial antibodies in primary biliary cirrhosis recognize both specific peptides and shared epitopes of the M2 family of antigens. *Hepatology* 1989; **10**: 370.

29 Fox RA, Scheuer PJ, James DG *et al.* Impaired delayed hypersensitivity in primary biliary cirrhosis. *Lancet* 1969; **i**: 959.

30 Fregeau DR, Davis PA, Danner DJ *et al.* Antimitochondrial antibodies of primary biliary cirrhosis recognize dihydrolipoamide acyltransferase and inhibit enzyme function of the branched chain alpha-ketoacid dehydrogenase complex. *J. Immunol.* 1989; **142**: 3815.

31 Fussey SPM, Guest JR, James OFW *et al.* Identification and analysis of the major M2 autoantigens in primary biliary cirrhosis. *Proc. Natl. Acad. Sci. USA* 1988; **85**: 8654.

32 Galbraith RM, Smith M, Mackenzie RM *et al.* High prevalence of seroimmunologic abnormalities in relatives of patients with active chronic hepatitis or primary biliary cirrhosis. *N. Engl. J. Med.* 1974; **290**: 63.

33 Gershwin ME, Mackay IR. Primary biliary cirrhosis: paradigm or paradox for autoimmunity. *Gastroenterology* 1991; **100**: 822.

34 Gores GJ, Moore SB, Fisher LD *et al.* Primary biliary cirrhosis: associations with class II major histocompatibility complex antigens. *Hepatology* 1987; **7**: 889.

35 Gores GJ, Wiesner RH, Dickson ER *et al.* Prospective evaluation of esophageal varices in primary biliary cirrhosis:

development, natural history and influence on survival. *Gastroenterology* 1989; **96**: 1552.

36 Goudie BM, Burt AD, Boyle P *et al.* Breast cancer in women with primary biliary cirrhosis. *Br. Med. J.* 1985; **291**: 1597.

37 Goudie BM, Burt AD, Macfarlane GJ *et al.* Risk factors and prognosis in primary biliary cirrhosis. *Am. J. Gastroenterol.* 1989; **84**: 713.

38 Graham-Brown RAC, Sarkany I, Sherlock S. Lichen planus and primary biliary cirrhosis. *Br. J. Dermatol.* 1982; **106**: 699.

39 Hall S, Axelsen PH, Larson DE *et al.* Systemic lupus erythematosus developing in patients with primary biliary cirrhosis. *Ann. Intern. Med.* 1984; **100**: 388.

40 Hanot V. *Etude sur une Forme de Cirrhose Hypertrophique de Foie (Cirrhose Hypertrophique avec Ictère Chronique).* JB Baillière, Paris, 1876.

41 Hay JE. Bone disease in cholestatic liver disease. *Gastroenterology* 1995; **108**: 276.

42 Heathcote EJ, Cauch-Dudek K, Walker V *et al.* The Canadian multicenter double-blind randomized controlled trial of ursodeoxycholic acid in primary biliary cirrhosis. *Hepatology* 1994; **19**: 1149.

43 Heathcote EJ, Lindor KD, Poupon R *et al.* Combined analysis of French, American and Canadian randomized controlled trials of ursodeoxycholic acid therapy in primary biliary cirrhosis. *Gastroenterology* 1995; **108**: A1082.

44 Hoofnagle JH, Davis GL, Schafer DF *et al.* Randomized trial of chlorambucil for primary biliary cirrhosis. *Gastroenterology* 1986; **91**: 1327.

45 Hopf U, Möller B, Stemerowicz R *et al.* Relation between *Escherichia coli* R (rough) forms in gut, lipid A in liver, and primary biliary cirrhosis. *Lancet* 1989; **ii**: 1419.

46 Izumi N, Hasumura Y, Takeuchi J. Hypouricemia and hyperuricosuria as expressions of renal tubular damage in primary biliary cirrhosis. *Hepatology* 1983; **3**: 719.

47 James SP, Jones EA, Schafer DF *et al.* Selective immunoglobulin A deficiency associated with primary biliary cirrhosis in a family with liver disease. *Gastroenterology* 1986; **90**: 283.

48 Jones DEJ, Palmer JM, James OFW *et al.* T-cell responses to the components of pyruvate dehydrogenase complex in primary biliary cirrhosis. *Hepatology* 1995; **21**: 995.

49 Joplin RE, Johnson GD, Matthews JB *et al.* Distribution of pyruvate dehydrogenase dihydrolipoamide acetyltransferase (PDC-E2) and another mitochondrial marker in salivary gland and biliary epithelium from patients with primary biliary cirrhosis. *Hepatology* 1994; **19**: 1375.

50 Kaplan MM, Alling DW, Zimmerman HJ *et al.* A prospective trial of colchicine for primary biliary cirrhosis. *N. Engl. J. Med.* 1986; **315**: 1448.

51 Kaplan MM, Knox TA. Treatment of primary biliary cirrhosis with low-dose weekly methotrexate. *Gastroenterology* 1991; **101**: 1332.

52 Kew MC, Varma RR, Dos Santos HA *et al.* Portal hypertension in primary biliary cirrhosis. *Gut* 1971; **12**: 830.

53 Krasner N, Johnson PJ, Portmann B *et al.* Hepato-cellular carcinoma in primary biliary cirrhosis: report of four cases. *Gut* 1979; **20**: 255.

54 Laurin JM, DeSotel CK, Jorgensen RA *et al.* The natural history of abdominal pain associated with primary biliary cirrhosis. *Am. J. Gastroenterol.* 1994; **89**: 1840.

55 Lee RG, Epstein O, Jauregui H *et al.* Granulomas in primary biliary cirrhosis: a prognostic feature. *Gastroenterology* 1981; **81**: 983.

56 Leung PSC, Iwayama T, Prindiville T *et al.* Use of designer recombinant mitochondrial antigens in the diagnosis of primary biliary cirrhosis. *Hepatology* 1992; **15**: 367.

57 Lindor KD, Dickson ER, Jorgensen RA *et al.* The combination of ursodeoxycholic acid and methotrexate for patients with primary biliary cirrhosis: the results of a pilot study. *Hepatology* 1995; **22**: 1158.

58 Long RG, Scheuer PJ, Sherlock S. Presentation and course of asymptomatic primary biliary cirrhosis. *Gastroenterology* 1977; **72**: 1204.

59 Ludwig J, Rosen CB, Lindor KD *et al.* Chronic cholestasis in a young man. *Hepatology* 1994; **20**: 1351.

60 MacMahon HE, Thannhauser SJ. Xanthomatous biliary cirrhosis (a clinical syndrome). *Ann. Intern. Med.* 1949; **30**: 121.

61 Mahl TC, Shockcor W, Boyer JL. Primary biliary cirrhosis: survival of a large cohort of symptomatic and asymptomatic patients followed for 24 years. *J. Hepatol.* 1994; **20**: 707.

62 Makinen D, Fritzler M, Davis P *et al.* Anti-centromere antibodies in primary biliary cirrhosis. *Arthritis Rheum.* 1983; **26**: 9141.

63 Manns MP, Bremm A, Schneider PM *et al.* HLA DRw8 and complement C4 deficiency as risk factors in primary biliary cirrhosis. *Gastroenterology* 1991; **101**: 1367.

64 Markus BH, Dickson ER, Grambsch PM *et al.* Efficacy of liver transplantation in patients with primary biliary cirrhosis. *N. Engl. J. Med.* 1989; **320**: 1709.

65 Martinez OM, Villanueva JC, Gershwin ME *et al.* Cytokine patterns and cytotoxic mediators in primary biliary cirrhosis. *Hepatology* 1995; **21**: 113.

66 Mella JG, Roschmann E, Maier K-P *et al.* Association of primary biliary cirrhosis with the allele HLA-DPB1*0301 in a German population. *Hepatology* 1995; **21**: 398.

67 Michieletti P, Wanless IR, Katz A *et al.* Antimitochondrial antibody negative primary biliary cirrhosis: a distinct syndrome of autoimmune cholangitis. *Gut* 1994; **35**: 260.

68 Mitchison HC, Lucey MR, Kelly PJ *et al.* Symptom development and prognosis in primary biliary cirrhosis: a study in two centers. *Gastroenterology* 1990; **99**: 778.

69 Mistry P, Seymour CA. Primary biliary cirrhosis — from Thomas Addison to the 1990s. *Q. J. Med.* 1992; **82**: 185.

70 Munoz LE, Thomas HC, Scheuer PJ *et al.* Is mitochondrial antibody diagnostic of primary biliary cirrhosis? *Gut* 1981; **22**: 136.

71 Murphy JR, Sjögren MH, Kikendall JW *et al.* Small bile duct abnormalities in sarcoidosis. *J. Clin. Gastroenterol.* 1990; **12**: 555.

72 Nakanuma Y, Ohta G. Histometric and serial section observations of the intrahepatic bile ducts in primary biliary cirrhosis. *Gastroenterology* 1979; **76**: 1326.

73 Nakanuma Y, Tsuneyama K, Kono N *et al.* Biliary epithelial expression of pyruvate dehydrogenase complex in primary biliary cirrhosis: an immunohistochemical and immunoelectron microscopic study. *Hum. Pathol.* 1995; **26**: 92.

74 Neuberger JM, Gunson BK, Buckels JAC *et al.* Referral of patients with primary biliary cirrhosis for liver transplantation. *Gut* 1990; **31**: 1069.

75 Nieri S, Ricardo GG, Salvadori G *et al.* Primary biliary cirrhosis and Graves' disease. *J. Clin. Gastroenterol.* 1985; **7**: 434.

76 Nyberg A, Lööf L. Primary biliary cirrhosis: clinical fea-

tures and outcome with special reference to asymptomatic disease. *Scand. J. Gastroenterol.* 1989; **24**: 57.

77 Onishi S, Sakamaki T, Maeda T *et al.* DNA typing of HLA class II genes; DRB1*0803 increases the susceptibility of Japanese to primary biliary cirrhosis. *J. Hepatol.* 1994; **21**: 1053.

78 Outwater E, Kaplan MM, Bankoff MS. Lymphadenopathy in primary biliary cirrhosis: CT observations. *Radiology* 1989; **171**: 731.

79 Pares A, Rimola A, Bruguera M *et al.* Renal tubular acidosis in primary biliary cirrhosis. *Gastroenterology* 1981; **80**: 681.

80 Penner E. Demonstration of immune complexes containing the ribonucleoprotein antigen R_o in primary biliary cirrhosis. *Gastroenterology* 1986; **90**: 724.

81 Polson RJ, Portmann B, Neuberger J *et al.* Evidence for disease recurrence after liver transplantation for primary biliary cirrhosis. Clinical and histologic follow-up studies. *Gastroenterology* 1989; **97**: 715.

82 Poupon RE, Poupon R, Balkau B *et al.* Ursodiol for the long-term treatment of primary biliary cirrhosis. *N. Engl. J. Med.* 1994; **330**: 1342.

83 Powell FC, Schroeter AL, Dickson ER. Primary biliary cirrhosis and the CREST syndrome. A report of 22 cases. *Q. J. Med.* 1987; **62**: 75.

84 Rai GS, Hamlyn AN, Dahl MGC *et al.* Primary biliary cirrhosis, cutaneous capillaritis and IgM-associated membranous glomerulonephritis. *Br. Med. J.* 1977; **i**: 817.

85 Reynold TB. The 'butterfly' sign in patients with chronic jaundice and pruritus. *Ann. Intern. Med.* 1973; **78**: 545.

86 Reynolds TB, Denison EK, Frankl HD *et al.* Primary biliary cirrhosis with scleroderma, Raynaud's phenomenon and telangiectasia: new syndrome. *Am. J. Med.* 1971; **50**: 302.

87 Roll J, Boyer JL, Barry D *et al.* The prognostic importance of clinical and histologic features in asymptomatic and symptomatic primary biliary cirrhosis. *N. Engl. J. Med.* 1983; **308**: 1.

88 Ros E, Garcia-Puges A, Reixach M *et al.* Fat digestion and exocrine pancreatic function in primary biliary cirrhosis. *Gastroenterology* 1984; **87**: 180.

89 Rubin E, Schaffner F, Popper H. Primary biliary cirrhosis: chronic non-suppurative destructive cholangitis. *Am. J. Pathol.* 1965; **46**: 387.

90 Rutan G, Martinez AJ, Fieshko JT *et al.* Primary biliary cirrhosis, Sjögren's syndrome and transverse myelitis. *Gastroenterology* 1986; **90**: 206.

91 Rydning A, Schrumpf E, Abdelnoor M *et al.* Factors of prognostic importance in primary biliary cirrhosis. *Scand. J. Gastroenterol.* 1990; **12**: 119.

92 Selinger S, Tsai J, Pulini M *et al.* Autoimmune thrombocytopenia and primary biliary cirrhosis with hypoglycemia and insulin receptor auto-antibodies. *Ann. Intern. Med.* 1987; **107**: 686.

93 Sharma A, Provenzale D, McKusick A *et al.* Interstitial pneumonitis after low-dose methotrexate therapy in primary biliary cirrhosis. *Gastroenterology* 1994; **107**: 266.

94 Shapiro JM, Smith H, Schaffner F. Serum bilirubin: a prognostic factor in primary biliary cirrhosis. *Gut* 1979; **20**: 137.

95 Sherlock S. Primary biliary cirrhosis (chronic intrahepatic obstructive jaundice). *Gastroenterology* 1959; **31**: 574.

96 Sherlock S. Primary biliary cirrhosis: clarifying the issues. *Am. J. Med.* 1994; **96** (suppl 1A): 275.

97 Sherlock S. Therapeutic trials in primary biliary cirrhosis. *Q. J. Med.* 1994; **87**: 701.

98 Sherlock S, Scheuer PJ. The presentation and diagnosis of 100 patients with primary biliary cirrhosis. *N. Engl. J. Med.* 1973; **289**: 674.

99 Spisni R, Smith-Laing G, Epstein O *et al.* Results of portal decompression in patients with primary biliary cirrhosis. *Gut* 1981; **22**: 345.

100 Spiteri MA, Clarke SW. The nature of latent pulmonary involvement in primary biliary cirrhosis. *Sarcoidosis* 1989; **6**: 107.

101 Stemerowicz R, Hopf U, Möller B *et al.* Are antimitochondrial antibodies in primary biliary cirrhosis induced by R (rough) mutants of enterobacteriaceae? *Lancet* 1988; **ii**: 1166.

102 Surh CD, Roche TE, Danner DJ *et al.* Antimitochondrial autoantibodies in primary biliary cirrhosis recognize cross-reactive epitope(s) on protein X and dihydrolipoamide acetyltransferase of pyruvate dehydrogenase complex. *Hepatology* 1989; **10**: 127.

103 Teoh K-L, Rowley MJ, Zafirakis H *et al.* Enzyme inhibitory autoantibodies to pyruvate dehydrogenase complex in primary biliary cirrhosis: applications of a semiautomated assay. *Hepatology* 1994; **20**: 1220.

104 Thomas PK, Walker JG. Xanthomatous neuropathy in primary biliary cirrhosis. *Brain* 1965; **88**: 1079.

105 Tong MJ, Nies KM, Reynolds TB *et al.* Immunological studies in familial primary biliary cirrhosis. *Gastroenterology* 1976; **71**: 305.

106 Triger DR. Primary biliary cirrhosis: an epidemiological study. *Br. Med. J.* 1980; **281**: 772.

107 Tsianos EV, Hoofnagle JH, Fox PC *et al.* Sjögren's syndrome in patients with primary biliary cirrhosis. *Hepatology* 1990; **11**: 730.

108 Tsuneyama K, Van de Water J, Leung PSC *et al.* Abnormal expression of the E2 component of the pyruvate dehydrogenase complex on the luminal surface of biliary epithelium occurs before major histocompatibility complex class II and BB1/B7 expression. *Hepatology* 1995; **21**: 1031.

109 Tzakis AG, Carcassonne C, Todo S *et al.* Liver transplantation for primary biliary cirrhosis. *Semin. Liver Dis.* 1989; **9**: 144.

110 Vuoristo M, Farkkila M, Karvonen A-L *et al.* A placebo-controlled trial of primary biliary cirrhosis with colchicine and ursodeoxycholic acid. *Gastroenterology* 1995; **108**: 1470.

111 Walker JG, Doniach D, Roitt IM *et al.* Serological tests in diagnosis of primary biliary cirrhosis. *Lancet* 1965; **i**: 827.

112 Wallace JG Jr, Tong MJ, Ueli BH *et al.* Pulmonary involvement in primary biliary cirrhosis. *J. Clin. Gastroenterol.* 1987; **9**: 431.

113 Weber P, Brenner J, Stechemesser E *et al.* Characterization and clinical relevance of a new complement-fixing antibody—anti-M8—in patients with primary biliary cirrhosis. *Hepatology* 1986; **6**: 553.

114 Wiesner RH, Ludwig J, Lindor KD *et al.* A controlled trial of cyclosporine in the treatment of primary biliary cirrhosis. *N. Engl. J. Med.* 1990; **322**: 1419.

115 Witt-Sullivan H, Heathcote J, Cauch K *et al.* The demography of primary biliary cirrhosis in Ontario, Canada. *Hepatology* 1990; **12**: 98.

116 Wolke AM, Schaffner F, Kapelman B *et al.* Malignancy in primary biliary cirrhosis. High incidence of breast cancer in affected women. *Am. J. Med.* 1984; **76**: 1075.

117 Wong PYN, Portmann B, O'Grady JG *et al.* Recurrence of primary biliary cirrhosis after liver transplantation follow-

ing FK506-based immunosuppression. *J. Hepatol.* 1993; **17**: 284.

118 Yamada G, Hyodo I, Tobe K *et al.* Ultrastructural immuno-cytochemical analysis of lymphocytes infiltrating bile duct epithelia in primary biliary cirrhosis. *Hepatology*

1986; **6**: 385.

119 Zifroni A, Schaffner F. Long-term follow-up of patients with primary biliary cirrhosis on colchicine therapy. *Hepatology* 1991; **14**: 990.

Chapter 15
Sclerosing Cholangitis

This is a syndrome which has many causes (table 15.1). The end result is progressive fibrosis and ultimately disappearance of intra- or extra-hepatic ducts or both [64]. In the early stages the impact is on the biliary system and hepatocyte damage is minor; liver failure occurs late. Consequently the prognosis for sclerosing cholangitis is better than for diseases that affect primarily the hepatocyte. Ultimately, biliary cirrhosis and hepato-cellular failure evolve.

Primary sclerosing cholangitis (PSC)

The condition is of unknown cause. All parts of the biliary tree can be involved in a chronic, fibrosing, inflammatory process which results in obliteration of the biliary tree and ultimately in biliary cirrhosis [12, 38]. The extent of involvement of different parts of the biliary tree varies. The condition may be localized to intra- or extra-hepatic ducts. Eventually interlobular, septal and segmental bile ducts are replaced by fibrous cords. Involvement of very small ducts in the portal (zone 1) areas led to the term *pericholangitis* [73] or small duct PSC [6].

Diagnostic criteria are generalized beading and stenosis of the biliary tree on cholangiography. Bile duct cancer must be excluded, usually by prolonged follow-up. There is no specific diagnostic test.

Table 15.1. Types of sclerosing cholangitis

'Primary'
With or without ulcerative colitis
'Infective'
Bacterial
usually with biliary obstruction
'sump' syndrome
Opportunistic
usually with primary or secondary immunodeficiency
Vascular
Hepatic arterial obstruction
Hepatic artery cytotoxics

Aetiology

In about 70% the patient also suffers from ulcerative colitis (and very rarely from regional ileitis). Conversely the prevalence of sclerosing cholangitis among ulcerative colitis patients is approximately 5% amidst an overall 10–15% prevalence of hepatic abnormalities [55]. The cholangitis may even precede the colitis by as much as 3 years [67]. PSC and ulcerative colitis may be rarely familial [57]. There is an increased prevalence of the HLA haplotypes, A1, B8, DR3, DR4 and DRW52A classed as susceptibility markers [13, 21]. The course seems to be accelerated with DR4 [50].

There are signs of abnormal immunoregulation. Circulating antibodies to tissue components are present in low titre or absent. Perinuclear antineutrophil cytoplasmic antibodies (pANCA) are found in at least two-thirds [22]. They persist after liver transplant [26]. They are probably of no pathogenic significance and are epiphenomena [42]. Sera also contains autoantibodies against a cross-reactive peptide shared by colon and biliary epithelial cells [46]. PSC may be associated with other 'autoimmune' diseases including thyroiditis and type 1 diabetes.

Circulating immune complexes may be increased [7] and there is decreased immune complex clearance [51]. Complement metabolism is increased.

Cellular immune system is disturbed. Circulating T-cells are decreased but are increased in the portal tracts. The ratio of CD4 to CD8 lymphocytes in the circulation is increased as are the number and percentage of B-cells [66].

It is uncertain whether these immunological changes indicate a primary autoimmune disease or whether they are simply secondary to bile duct injury.

Similar cholangiographic and hepatic histological changes are found with known infections such as cryptosporidiosis and with immune deficiency diseases. This raises the possibility that primary sclerosing cholangitis might have an infectious basis. The association with ulcerative colitis could be through portal bacteraemia, but this cannot be confirmed. Bacterial products might be responsible. Toxic pro-inflammatory bacterial peptides introduced into the colon of rats with experimental colitis are increased in the bile and the liver shows pericholangitis [30]. Furthermore, genetically susceptible rats with blind loops and small bowel bacterial overgrowth develop hepatic injury with bile duct proliferation, fibrosis and zone 1 inflammation [40]. Finally, in rabbits, portal vein injection of killed nonpathogenic *Escherichia coli* leads to appearances in the liver somewhat resembling those of human pericholangitis [35].

In ulcerative colitis, the intestinal epithelium is leaky [5] so allowing endotoxin and toxic bacterial products to enter the portal vein and reach the liver (fig. 15.1).

This infective theory would not explain why ulcerative colitis is not constantly present and that the disease is unrelated to the severity of the colitis. It would not explain why the sclerosing cholangitis can precede the colitis, why antibiotics are ineffective and why proctocolectomy is not beneficial [10].

Conclusions

The aetiology of PSC is still unknown. It is difficult to fit together all these genetic, immunological and infective observations and the association with ulcerative colitis. An infective agent operating on a genetically and immunologically susceptible individual remains a possibility. A specific serological diagnostic test for the primary form of sclerosing cholangitis is urgently needed.

Clinical features (table 15.2) [12, 41]

Males are twice as commonly affected as females, usually between the ages of 25 and 45, but primary scle-

Table 15.2. Symptoms at presentation in 29 patients with PSC [12]. *n* = number of patients

Symptoms	n	%
Jaundice	21	72
Pruritus	20	69
Weight loss	23	79
Right upper quadrant pain	21	72
Acute cholangitis	13	45
Bleeding oesophageal varices	4	14
Malaise	1	3
Asymptomatic	2	7
Total	29	

rosing cholangitis can affect children as young as two (mean age 5) usually with associated chronic ulcerative colitis [23, 65, 76].

The majority present when asymptomatic, usually when a raised serum alkaline phosphatase level is found, particularly when screening patients with ulcerative colitis. However, PSC can be seen on a cholangiogram even if serum alkaline phosphatase is normal. The disease may even present as a raised serum transaminase value discovered at the time of blood donation [31]. Even if asymptomatic the patient may have underlying advanced liver disease, established cirrhosis and portal hypertension, usually pre-sinusoidal, without signs of cholangitis or cholestasis. The patient may have been treated for 'cryptogenic' cirrhosis for many years.

Presenting symptoms include weight loss, fatigue, right upper-quadrant abdominal pain and pruritus, and intermittent jaundice. Symptoms indicate advanced disease. Fever is unusual unless ascending cholangitis

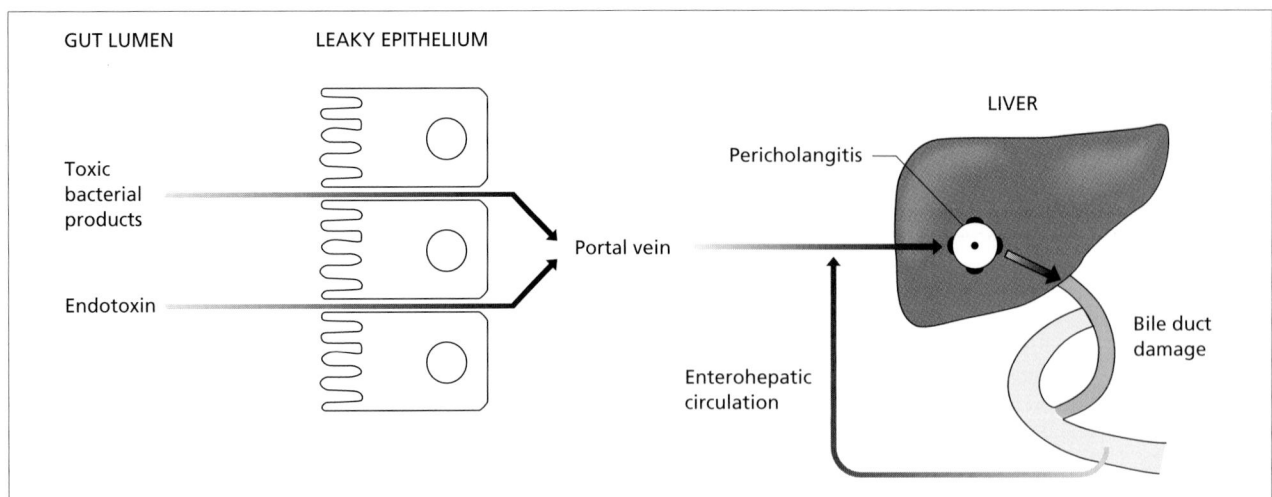

Fig. 15.1. In ulcerative colitis the colonic epithelium is leaky so allowing toxic bacterial products such as endotoxin to enter the lamina propria and ultimately reach the liver via the portal vein. These could cause pericholangitis, biliary excretion and larger bile duct injury. They probably have an enterohepatic circulation.

has complicated biliary surgery or endoscopy. However, occasionally the patient presents with fever, chills, right upper-quadrant pain, itching and jaundice resembling acute bacterial cholangitis [38]. Blood cultures are rarely positive and antibiotics are unhelpful.

Ulcerative colitis (rarely Crohn's disease) should be sought by sigmoidoscopy and rectal biopsy, even if there are no features of colonic disease. The colitis is usually chronic, diffuse and mild to moderate. The activity of the cholangitis is inversely related to that of the colitis. There are prolonged remissions. PSC may be diagnosed before or after the colitis. The course does not differ whether or not ulcerative colitis is associated.

Laboratory investigations

Serum tests show cholestasis with alkaline phosphatase three times above normal. Serum bilirubin values fluctuate markedly. They can exceed 10 mg/dl (170 mm/litre), but this is unusual. Serum copper, ceruloplasmin and liver copper content are increased, as in all patients with cholestasis. Serum gammaglobulin and IgM are increased in 40–50%.

Serum smooth muscle and antinuclear antibodies may be present in low titres but the mitochondrial antibody is absent.

Eosinophilia is a rare finding.

Liver pathology (table 15.3) [12, 39]

Perfusion studies of bile ducts in livers removed at the time of transplantation show intra-hepatic tubular and saccular cholangiectasia with transformation of bile ducts into fibrous cords and eventually complete loss of ducts [44].

The portal zones are infiltrated with small and large lymphocytes, polymorphs and occasional macrophages and eosinophils (fig. 15.2). The interlobular ductules show a periductular inflammation with occasional epithelial desquamation. Intralobular inflammatory cell

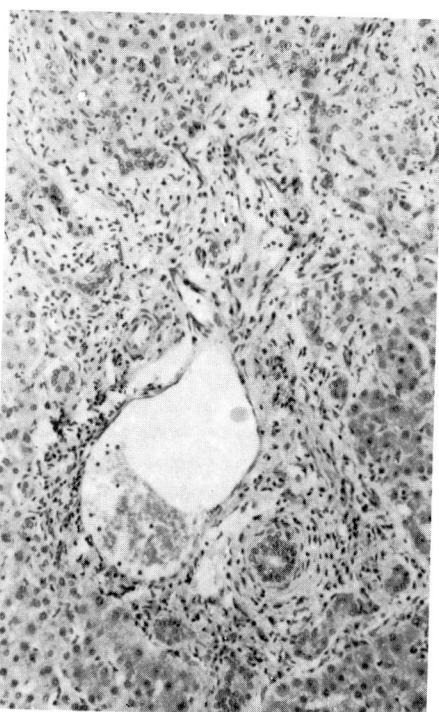

Fig. 15.2. Sclerosing cholangitis and pericholangitis. The portal zone is oedematous and expanded with proliferated bile ducts and an inflammatory cell infiltrate. (H & E, × 160.)

accumulations may be noted and the Kupffer cells are swollen and prominent. Cholestasis is inconspicuous unless jaundice is deep.

Eventually, fibrosis develops in the portal tracts until the small ducts are surrounded by a tuft of fibrous tissue ('onion-skin' appearance) (fig. 15.3). The remains of bile ducts may be shown only as a fibrous ring (fig. 15.4). The portal zones become stellate (fig. 15.5).

The appearances are not diagnostic, but the association of reduced numbers of bile ducts, ductular proliferation and substantial copper deposition with piecemeal necrosis is very suggestive of PSC and indicates the need for cholangiography [12].

Histology of the common bile duct shows non-diagnostic fibrosis and inflammation.

Cholangiography [12, 45]

ERCP is the most successful technique, although trans-hepatic cholangiography may be successful. The appearances are diagnostic with areas of irregular stricturing and dilatation (beading) of the intra- and extra-hepatic biliary tree (fig. 15.6).

The strictures are short (0.5–2 cm long) and angular with intervening segments of apparently normal or slightly dilated ducts. Diverticulum-like outpouchings may be seen along the common bile duct [45].

Cholangiograms may show involvement of the intra-

Table 15.3. Histological findings in 29 patients with PSC [12]

	−	+	++
Portal changes			
Inflammation	0	17	12
Bile duct diminution	12	10	7
Periductal fibrosis	18	9	2
Bile ductular proliferation	4	7	18
Lobular changes			
Piecemeal necrosis	10	8	11
Focal necrosis	11	18	0
Focal inflammation	12	17	0
Kupffer cell hyperplasia	5	11	13

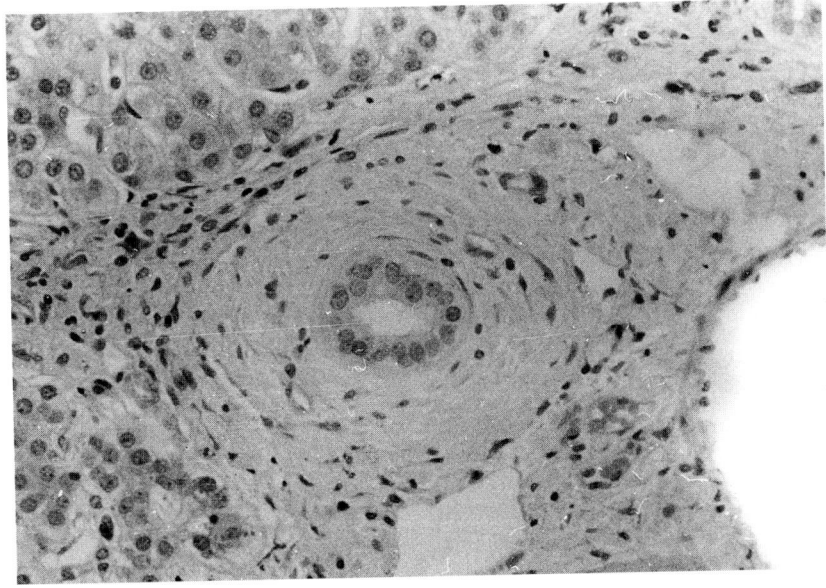

Fig. 15.3. Intra-hepatic bile duct shows abnormal epithelium and concentric periductal whorls of collagen ('onion-skin' appearance).

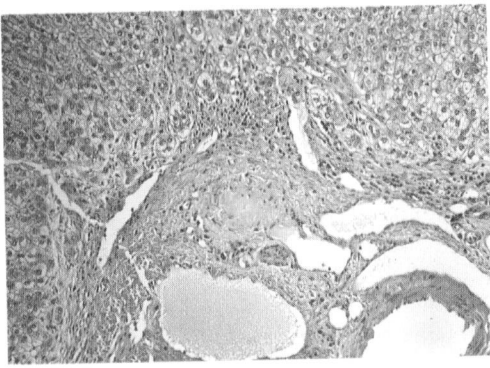

Fig. 15.4. A heavily fibrosed portal zone contains a ring representing an obliterated bile duct.

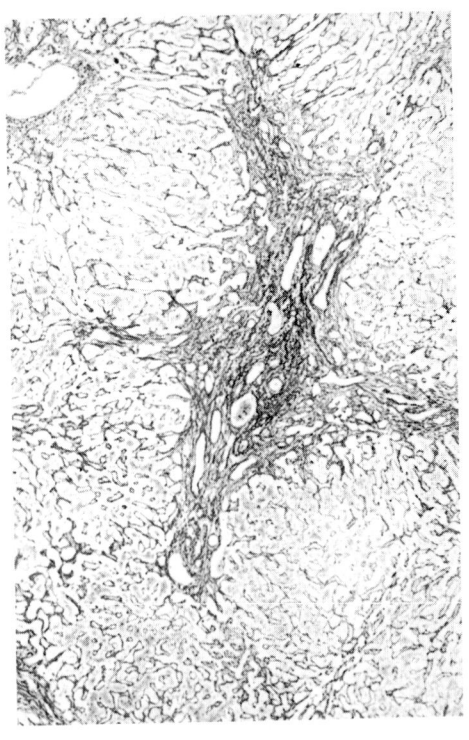

Fig. 15.5. Reticulin preparation of liver biopsy shows stellate expansion of portal zones.

hepatic ducts alone, the extra-hepatic ducts alone or even one hepatic duct.

Appearances are normal with small duct disease [6].

Imaging

Ultrasound shows thickening of the bile ducts. CT shows focal discontinuous minimal biliary dilatation, mimicked only by rare, diffuse cholangiocarcinoma [58].

Cholangiocarcinoma

Cholangiocarcinoma occurs in approximately 10% of patients with PSC. It may complicate large or small duct disease and usually in those with ulcerative colitis (fig. 15.7). Mean survival is 12 months.

Cholangiocarcinoma is extremely difficult to diagnose and should be suspected if the patient becomes progressively jaundiced. Suggestive cholangiographic features are localized biliary dilatation, progressive biliary stricture, and intra-duct polyps [45]. Superficial thrombophlebitis and dysplasia of the bile duct epithelium in areas free from tumour are also suggestive [48]. Cholangiography with bile and brush cytology and biopsy should be routine [36]. Serum tumour markers such as CA19/9 are useful [53]. Combinations of CA19/9 with carcinoembryonic antigen (CEA) give an accuracy of 86% [59].

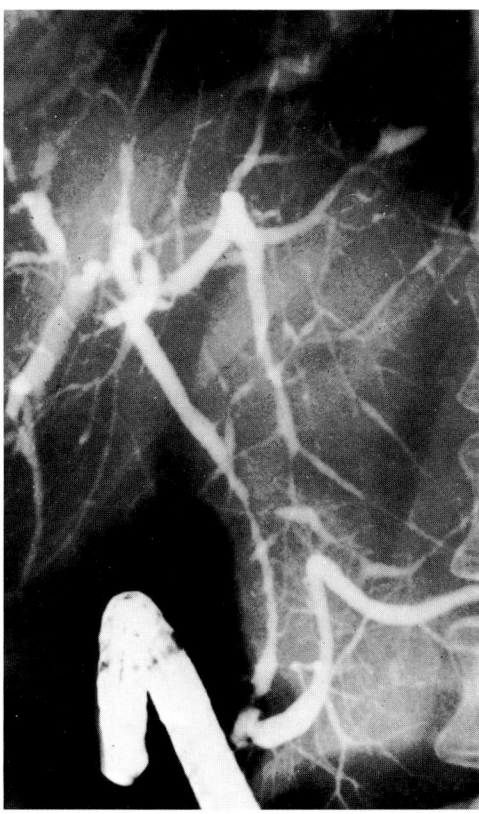

Fig. 15.6. ERCP in PSC shows an irregular common bile duct and beading irregularities in the intra-hepatic bile ducts.

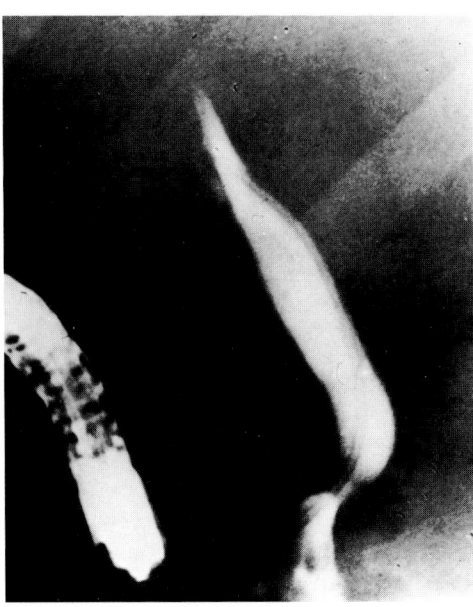

Fig. 15.7. ERCP in bile duct carcinoma shows the common bile duct terminating in a nipple-like deformity.

Diagnosis

Cholangiographic appearances and the negative mitochondrial antibody test distinguish PSC from PBC (table 15.4). PSC can present as chronic hepatitis especially in children [76] or as cryptogenic cirrhosis. The increased serum phosphatase level is the diagnostic clue and indicates confirmatory cholangiography.

The differentiation from secondary sclerosing cholangitis due to such conditions as post-operative biliary stricture or choledocholithiasis depends on the history of previous surgery or on the demonstration of gallstones.

Differentiation must be made from ischaemic bile duct damage due to intra-hepatic arterial floxuridine, from congenital biliary abnormalities, from infectious cholangiopathy in immunosuppressed AIDS patients or following liver transplantation, from bile duct neoplasms, and from histiocytosis X.

Prognosis

In one series the mean survival for patients with PSC from diagnosis was 11.9 years [74]. In another series, 75% were alive 9 years after diagnosis [28].

Six-year follow-up of asymptomatic patients showed 70% with disease progression and liver failure developing in one-third [56].

A subgroup may do well but the majority suffer deepening, cholestatic jaundice and progressive liver cell disease culminating in variceal bleeding, liver failure and cholangiocarcinoma [56].

Table 15.4. PSC and primary biliary cirrhosis (PBC)

	PSC	PBC
Sex	66% male	90% female
Presentation	Fatigue, jaundice, pruritus, cholangitis, weight loss, RUQ pain	Pruritus Jaundice
Serum mitochondrial antibody	−ve	+ve
Cholangiography (bile ducts)	Beaded, irregular	Pruned
Liver biopsy		
bile duct lesions	+	+
granulomas	−	+
copper	+	+
Associated diseases	Ulcerative colitis Retro-orbital and retroperitoneal fibrosis Immunodeficiency Cholangiocarcinoma	Arthritis Sicca syndrome Autoimmune diseases Thyroiditis

RUQ = right upper quadrant.

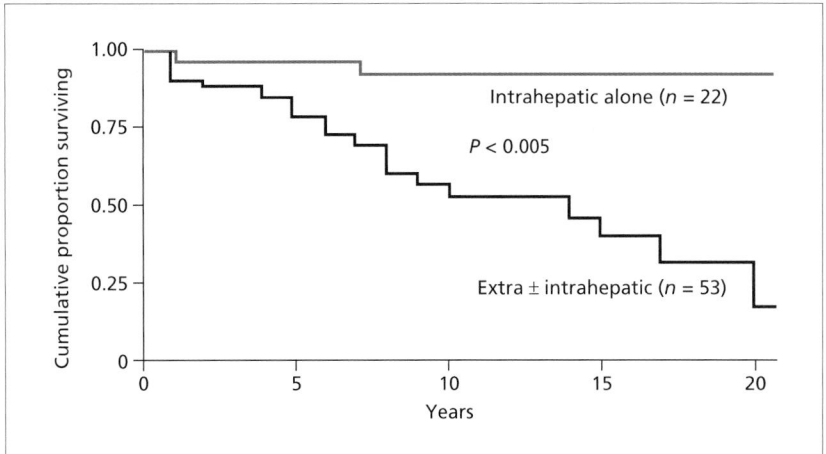

Fig. 15.8. Cumulative survival of patients with PSC according to distribution of cholangiographic changes.

Involvement of extra-hepatic ducts has a worse prognosis than intra-hepatic alone (fig. 15.8).

Peristomal varices may bleed after proctocolectomy [75].

Pericholangitis and sclerosing cholangitis are risk factors for dysplasia and colorectal cancer in patients with ulcerative colitis [16].

Survival models have been devised to evaluate therapy, to stratify patients in clinical trials and to define the time for liver transplantation. The Mayo Clinic model, based on 426 patients from five medical centres uses serum bilirubin concentration, histological stage, age and the presence of splenomegaly [17]. The possibility of surviving 5 years from diagnosis was 78%. Females had poorer survival than males [62]. Models are of less use in individual cases because of the great variability of the disease. Moreover, they do not identify the patient with cholangiocarcinoma [8].

Treatment

There is no specific treatment. In the jaundiced patient, the measures for chronic cholestasis and pruritus must be adopted (Chapter 13). Replacement of fat-soluble vitamins is particularly important. Systemic corticosteroids have not proved of value. Ursodeoxycholic acid improves serum biochemical tests and lessens disease activity on liver biopsy [4, 69]. Oral pulse methotrexate or colchicine is ineffective [35, 54]. Clinical treatment is difficult to assess because of the variable course and the long asymptomatic periods.

Cholangitis should be treated with broad-spectrum antibiotics.

Colectomy does not affect the course of PSC associated with ulcerative colitis [10].

Endoscopic treatment allows dilatation of dominant strictures and removal of small pigment stones or biliary debris [37]. Stents can be placed and naso-biliary tubes inserted. Liver function tests improve with variable results on cholangiographic appearances. Morbidity is low. There are no control trials of endoscopy in PSC.

Surgery such as resection of the extra-hepatic biliary tree with biliary reconstruction using trans-hepatic stents must be avoided because of the risk of complicating cholangitis [24].

The 3-year survival after *liver transplantation* in adults is 85% [49]. Strictures can develop in the transplanted bile ducts more commonly than with other transplant groups. Causes are multiple and include ischaemia, rejection and infection related to the biliary anastomosis. Recurrence in the transplanted liver is possible [27].

Cholangiocarcinoma was discovered at transplant in 11 of 216 patients and the survival was very bad [1] (fig. 15.9). Because of this transplant should be early [34].

Previous biliary surgery makes the transplant more

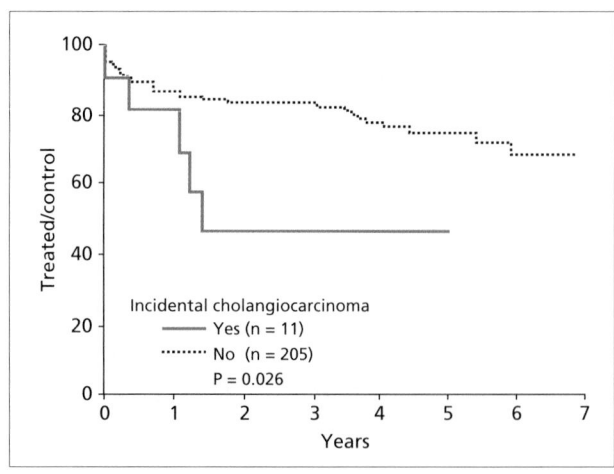

Fig. 15.9. Kaplan–Meier survival pilot after transplantation in patients with PSC with and without detection of cholangiocarcinoma in the excised liver. The difference was statistically significant with a 5-year survival rate of 0.47 ± 0.17 and 0.75 ± 0.04, respectively. (From [1].)

difficult, it takes longer and greater quantities of blood transfusion are required [47]. Because of the diseased recipient bile duct, a choledochojejunostomy is needed. Post-transplant biliary complications are therefore frequent.

Post-transplant the colitis usually improves. However, colon cancer can develop [29].

Infective sclerosing cholangitis

Patients having a well-recognized infective cause for their sclerosing cholangitis may show identical biochemical, hepatic histological and cholangiographic features to those of patients with PSC.

Bacterial cholangitis

Bacterial cholangitis is rare in the absence of mechanical, usually partial, biliary obstruction. The infection presumably ascends from the gut. The presence of a biliary stricture results in overgrowth of enteric organisms in the upper small intestine.

The damaged ducts show infiltration of their walls with polymorphs and destruction of the epithelium. Ultimately, the bile duct is replaced by a fibrous cord. The causes include choledocholithiasis, biliary strictures and stenosis of biliary-enteric anastomoses. The bile duct loss is irreversible and a point comes when, even if the cause of the biliary obstruction can be removed, for instance gallstones, the bile duct destruction with biliary cirrhosis persists.

If the common bile or hepatic duct is surgically anastomosed to a stagnant loop of duodenum, continued access of the biliary system to gut organisms can result in bacterial cholangitis without biliary obstruction (fig. 15.10) ('*sump syndrome*'). A similar sequence may follow sphincteroplasty.

The sclerosing cholangitis associated with infection by the Chinese liver fluke (*Clonorchis sinensis*) is related to secondary infection, usually with *Escherichia coli*, following biliary obstruction by the fluke.

Multiple pyogenic abscesses may lead to the picture of sclerosing cholangitis (figs 15.11, 15.12) [68].

Immunodeficiency-related opportunistic cholangitis

Opportunistic organisms can invade the bile ducts causing the picture of sclerosing cholangitis. There is usually a background of immunodeficiency which may be congenital or acquired.

In the neonate, cytomegalovirus and reovirus type III have a tropism for bile epithelium and obliterative cholangitis results.

Associated immunodeficiency syndromes include familial combined immunodeficiency [60], hyper-

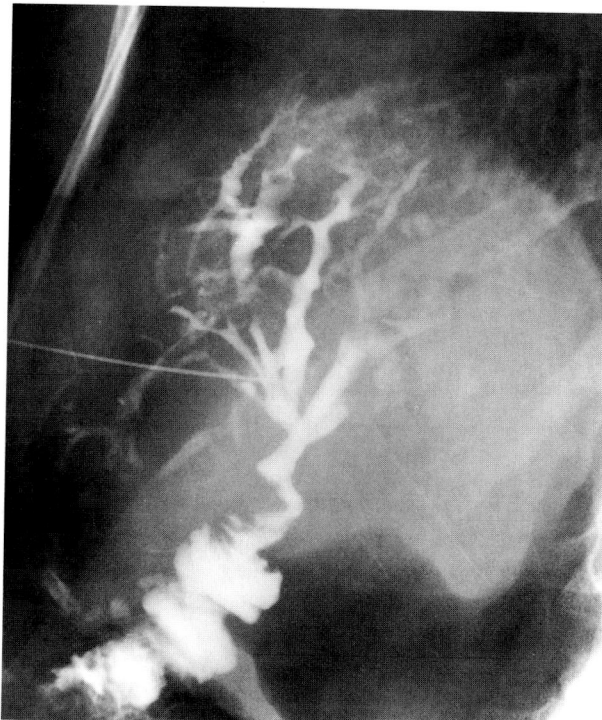

Fig. 15.10. Percutaneous cholangiography following choledochojejunostomy. There is no obstruction to flow of contrast into the jejunum but an intra-hepatic sclerosing cholangitis, marked by strictures and beading, has developed.

immunoglobulin M immunodeficiency [19], angioimmunoblastic lymphadenopathy [2], X-linked immunodeficiency [52] and immunodeficiency with transient T-cell abnormalities [15, 25]. The usual causative organism is cytomegalovirus or cryptosporidia alone or in combination. *Cryptococcus*, *Candida albicans* and *Klebsiella pneumoniae* may be associated [14].

Abnormalities of the biliary system are associated with AIDS [11]. In one series 20 of 26 patients with AIDS and biliary problems had markedly abnormal cholangiograms. In 14 of these, the pattern was of sclerosing cholangitis with or without papillary stenosis [11].

PSC and AIDS cholangiopathy differ in the inflammatory infiltration surrounding the diseased bile ducts. In primary sclerosing cholangitis, it is rich in T4-lymphocytes, the subpopulation specifically depleted in AIDS patients [61].

Graft-versus-host disease

Aberrant expression of HLA class II antigen on bile ducts is seen in the transplanted human liver undergoing rejection and in patients with graft-versus-host disease following allogenic bone marrow transplantation (fig. 15.13) [18]. Rejection is marked by progressive non-suppurative cholangitis culminating in disappearance of

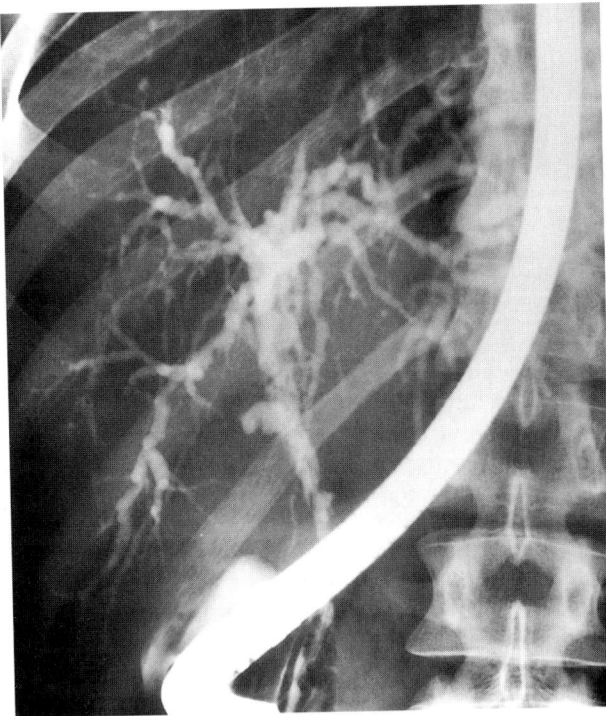

Fig. 15.11. ERCP shows distortion of the intra-hepatic biliary tree with irregularities in a patient with severe skin sepsis following burning. The picture resembles PSC.

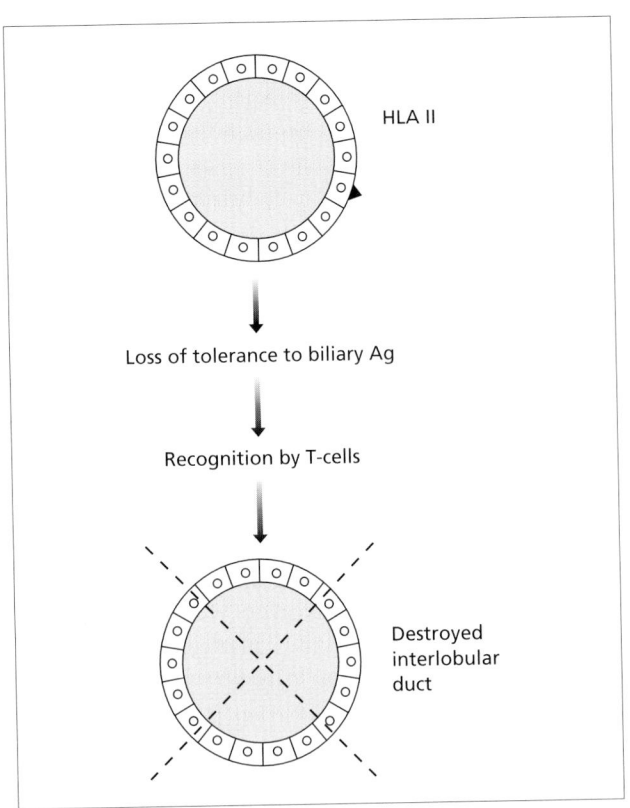

Fig. 15.13. Hepatic rejection (graft-versus-host disease). HLA class antigens are displayed on the bile duct. There is loss of tolerance to biliary antigens which are recognized by cytotoxic T-cells and the interlobular ducts are destroyed.

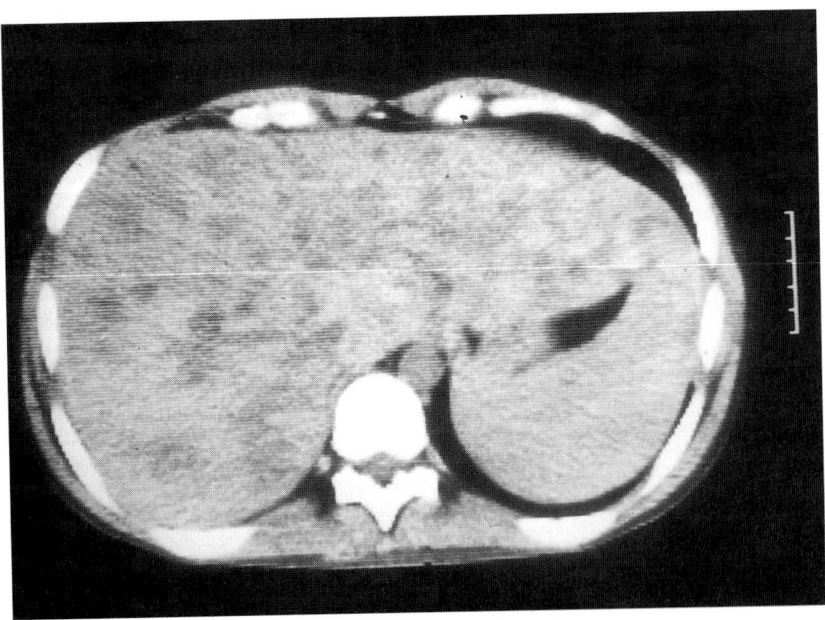

Fig. 15.12. CT from the same patient as in fig. 15.11 shows multiple space-occupying lesions due to metastatic bacterial abscesses.

interlobular bile ducts [72]. The bile duct epithelium is penetrated by mononuclear cells with focal necrosis and rupture of the epithelium. Similar lesions are found in graft-versus-host disease following allogenic bone marrow transplantation. In one such patient, marked cholestatic jaundice lasted 10 years, and serial liver biopsies confirmed progressive biliary-type fibrosis and cirrhosis [33]. She ultimately died in liver failure.

Sclerosing cholangitis following liver transplantation

Sclerosing cholangitis may be seen in failed grafts [63]. Liver biopsies may not be diagnostic and simply show evidence of large duct obstruction. The sclerosing cholangitis can be related to graft incompatibility, hepatic arterial thrombosis and chronic ductopenic arteriopathic rejection [20].

Vascular cholangitis

The bile ducts are richly supplied by the hepatic artery which forms a peri-biliary vascular plexus (Chapter 11). Interference leads to ischaemic necrosis of the bile ducts, both extra- and intra-hepatic, and to their ultimate disappearance [64]. Injury to major hepatic arterial branches, for instance during cholecystectomy, leads to ischaemia of the duct wall, damage to the ductal mucosa and entry of bile into the duct wall so causing fibrosis and stricture [70]. A similar sequence can complicate hepatic transplantation [77], especially if the segment of the recipient duct is too short and thus deprived of its arterial supply.

Biliary ischaemia secondary to intimal thickening of hepatic arterioles is a rare feature of chronic allograft rejection in man [72].

Diffuse small vessel arteritis, part of a systemic vasculitis, can be followed by bile duct loss.

Floxuridine (5-FUDR) can be infused by pump into the hepatic artery for the treatment of colo-rectal hepatic metastases. Biliary strictures can follow [43]. The picture resembles PSC [32]. The loss of bile ducts may be so severe that hepatic transplantation becomes necessary.

Drug-related cholangitis

Caustic cholangitis can be related to the injection of a scolicidal solution into a hydatid cyst. Only a part of the biliary tree is usually affected [3]. Within months the strictures result in jaundice, biliary cirrhosis and portal hypertension.

Histiocytosis X

A cholangiographic picture identical with that of PSC may complicate histiocytosis X [71]. The biliary lesions progress from a hyperplastic to a granulomatous, xanthomatous and, finally, a fibrotic stage. Clinically, the picture resembles PSC.

References

1 Abu-Elmagd KM, Malinchoc M, Dickson ER *et al.* Efficacy of hepatic transplantation in patients with primary sclerosing cholangitis. *Surg. Gyn. Obstet.* 1993; **177**: 335.

2 Bass NM, Chapman RW, O'Reilly A *et al.* Primary sclerosing cholangitis associated with angioimmunoblastic lymphadenopathy. *Gastroenterology* 1983; **85**: 420.

3 Belghiti J, Benhamou J-P, Heuly S *et al.* Caustic sclerosing cholangitis. A complication of the surgical treatment of hydatid disease of the liver. *Arch. Surg.* 1986; **121**: 1162.

4 Beurers, U, Spengler U, Kruis W *et al.* Ursodeoxycholic acid for treatment of primary sclerosing cholangitis: a placebo-controlled trial. *Hepatology* 1992; **16**: 707.

5 Bjarnason I, O'Morain C, Levi AJ *et al.* Absorption of 51 chromium-labeled ethylenediaminetetraacetate in inflammatory bowel disease. *Gastroenterology* 1983; **85**: 318.

6 Boberg KM, Schrumpf E, Fausa O *et al.* Hepatobiliary disease in ulcerative colitis. An analysis of 18 patients with hepatobiliary lesions classified as small-duct primary sclerosing cholangitis. *Scand. J. Gastroenterol.* 1994; **29**: 744.

7 Bodenheimer HC, LaRusso NF, Thayer WR *et al.* Elevated circulating immune complexes in primary sclerosing cholangitis. *Hepatology* 1983; **3**: 150.

8 Broomé U, Eriksson LS. Assessment for liver transplantation in patients with primary sclerosing cholangitis. *J. Hepatol.* 1994; **20**: 654.

9 Broome U, Lofberg R, Veress B *et al.* Primary sclerosing cholangitis and ulcerative colitis: evidence for increased neoplastic potential. *Hepatology* 1995; **22**: 1404.

10 Cangemi JR, Wiesner RH, Beaver SJ *et al.* Effect of proctocolectomy for chronic ulcerative colitis on the natural history of primary sclerosing cholangitis. *Gastroenterology* 1989; **96**: 790.

11 Cello JP. Acquired immunodeficiency syndrome cholangiopathy: spectrum of disease. *Am. J. Med.* 1989; **86**: 539.

12 Chapman RWG, Arborgh BAM, Rhodes JM *et al.* Primary sclerosing cholangitis — a review of its clinical features, cholangiography and hepatic histology. *Gut* 1980; **21**: 870.

13 Chapman RWG, Varghese Z, Gaul R *et al.* Association of primary sclerosing cholangitis with HLA-B8. *Gut* 1983; **24**: 38.

14 Cockerill FR, Hurley DV, Malagelada JR *et al.* Polymicrobial cholangitis and Kaposi's sarcoma in blood product transfusion-related acquired immune deficiency syndrome. *Am. J. Med.* 1986; **80**: 1237.

15 Davis JJ, Heyman MB, Ferrell L *et al.* Sclerosing cholangitis associated with chronic cryptosporidiosis in child with a congenital immunodeficiency disorder. *Am. J. Gastroenterol.* 1987; **82**: 1196.

16 D'Haens GR, Lashner BA, Hanauer SB. Pericholangitis and sclerosing cholangitis are risk factors for dysplasia and cancer in ulcerative colitis. *Am. J. Gastroenterol.* 1993; **88**: 1174.

17 Dickson ER, Murtaugh PA, Wiesner RH *et al.* Primary sclerosing cholangitis: refinement and validation of survival models. *Gastroenterology* 1992; **103**: 1893.

18 Dilly SA, Sloane JP. An immunohistological study of human hepatic graft-versus-host disease. *Clin. Exp. Immunol.* 1985; **62**: 545.

19 Di Palma JA, Strobel CT, Farrow JG. Primary sclerosing cholangitis associated with hyperimmunoglobulin M immuno-deficiency (dysgammaglobulinemia). *Gastroenterology* 1986; **91**: 464.

20 Donaldson PT, Alexander GJM, O'Grady J *et al.* Evidence for an immune response to HLA class 1 antigens in the vanishing-bile duct syndrome after liver transplantation. *Lancet* 1987; **i**: 945.

21 Donaldson PT, Farrant JM, Wilkinson ML *et al.* Dual associ-ation of HLA DR2 and DR3 with primary sclerosing cholangitis. *Hepatology* 1991; **13**: 129.

22 Duerr RH, Targan SR, Landers CJ *et al.* Neutrophil cytoplas-mic antibodies: a link between primary sclerosing cholangi-tis and ulcerative colitis. *Gastroenterology* 1991; **100**: 1385.

23 El-Shabrawi M, Wilkinson ML, Portmann B *et al.* Primary sclerosing cholangitis in childhood. *Gastroenterology* 1987; **92**: 1226.

24 Farges O, Malassagne B, Sebagh M *et al.* Primary sclerosing cholangitis: liver transplantation or biliary surgery. *Surgery* 1995; **117**: 146.

25 Gremse DA, Bucuvalas JC, Bongiovanni GL. Papillary stenosis and sclerosing cholangitis in an immunodeficient child. *Gastroenterology* 1989; **96**: 1600.

26 Haagsma EB, Mulder AHL, Gouw ASH *et al.* Neutrophil cytoplasmic autoantibodies after liver transplantation in patients with primary sclerosing cholangitis. *J. Hepatol.* 1993; **19**: 8.

27 Harrison RF, Davies MH, Neuberger JM *et al.* Fibrous and obliterative cholangitis in liver allografts: evidence of recur-rent primary sclerosing cholangitis. *Hepatology* 1994; **20**: 356.

28 Helzberg JH, Petersen JM, Boyer JL. Improved survival with primary sclerosing cholangitis. A review of clinicopatho-logic features and comparison of symptomatic and asymp-tomatic patients. *Gastroenterology* 1987; **92**: 1869.

29 Higashi H, Yanaga K, Marsh JW *et al.* Development of colon cancer after liver transplantation for primary sclerosing cholangitis associated with ulcerative colitis. *Hepatology* 1990; **11**: 477.

30 Hobson CH, Butt TJ, Ferry DM *et al.* Enterohepatic circula-tion of bacterial chemotactic peptide in rats with experi-mental colitis. *Gastroenterology* 1988; **94**: 1006.

31 Keeffe EB. Diagnosis of primary sclerosing cholangitis in a blood donor with elevated serum alanine aminotransferase. *Gastroenterology* 1989; **96**: 1358.

32 Kemeny MM, Battifora H, Blayney DW *et al.* Sclerosing cholangitis after continuous hepatic artery infusion of FUDR. *Ann. Surg.* 1985; **202**: 176.

33 Knapp AB, Crawford JM, Rappeport JM *et al.* Cirrhosis as a consequence of graft-versus-host disease. *Gastroenterology* 1987; **92**: 513.

34 Knechtle SJ, D'Alessandro AM, Harms BA. Relationships between sclerosing cholangitis, inflammatory bowel disease, and cancer in patients undergoing liver transplan-tation. *Surgery* 1995; **118**: 615.

35 Knox TA, Kaplan MM. A double-blind controlled oral-pulse methotrexate therapy in the treatment of primary sclerosing cholangitis. *Gastroenterology* 1994; **106**: 494.

36 Kurzawinski TR, Deery A, Dooley JS *et al.* A prospective study of biliary cytology in 100 patients with bile duct stric-tures. *Hepatology* 1993; **18**: 1399.

37 Lee JG, Schutz SM, England RE *et al.* Endoscopic therapy of sclerosing cholangitis. *Hepatology* 1995; **21**: 661.

38 Lee Y-M, Kaplan MM. Primary sclerosing cholangitis. *N. Engl. J. Med.* 1995; **332**: 924.

39 Lefkowitch JH. Primary sclerosing cholangitis. *Arch. Intern. Med.* 1982; **142**: 1157.

40 Lichtman SN, Sartor RB, Keku J *et al.* Hepatic inflammation in rats with experimental small intestinal bacterial over-growth. *Gastroenterology* 1990; **98**: 414.

41 Lindor KD, Wiesner RH, MacCarty RL *et al.* Advances in primary sclerosing cholangitis. *Am. J. Med.* 1990; **89**: 73.

42 Lo SK, Fleming KA, Chapman RW. A 2-year follow-up study of anti-neutrophil antibody in primary sclerosing cholangitis: relationship to clinical activity, liver biochem-istry and ursodeoxycholic acid treatment. *J. Hepatol.* 1994; **21**: 974.

43 Ludwig J, Kim CH, Wiesner RH *et al.* Floxuridine-induced sclerosing cholangitis: an ischemic cholangiopathy? *Hepa-tology* 1989; **9**: 215.

44 Ludwig J, MacCarty RL, LaRusso NF. Intrahepatic cholang-iectases and large duct obliteration in primary sclerosing cholangitis. *Hepatology* 1986; **6**: 560.

45 MacCarty RL, LaRusso NF, Wiesner RH *et al.* Primary sclerosing cholangitis: findings on cholangiography and pancreatography. *Radiology* 1983; **149**: 39.

46 Mandal A, Dasgupta A, Jeffers L *et al.* Autoantibodies in sclerosing cholangitis against a shared peptide in biliary and colon epithelium. *Gastroenterology* 1994; **106**: 185.

47 Martin FM, Rossi RL, Nugent FW *et al.* Surgical aspects of sclerosing cholangitis: results in 178 patients. *Ann. Surg.* 1990; **212**: 551.

48 Martins EBG, Fleming KA, Garrido MC *et al.* Superficial thrombophlebitis, dysplasia, and cholangiocarcinoma in primary sclerosing cholangitis. *Gastroenterology* 1994; **107**: 537.

49 Mc Entee G, Wiesner RH, Rosen C *et al.* A comparative study of patients undergoing liver transplantation for primary sclerosing cholangitis and primary biliary cirrhosis. *Trans-plant Proc.* 1991; **23**: 1563.

50 Mehal WZ, Dennis Lo Y-M, Wordsworth BP *et al.* HLA DR4 is a marker for rapid disease progression in primary scleros-ing cholangitis. *Gastroenterology* 1994; **106**: 160.

51 Minuk GY, Hershfield NB, Lee WY *et al.* Reticulo-endothelial system Fc receptor-mediated clearance of IgG-tagged erythrocytes from the circulation of patients with idiopathic ulcerative colitis and chronic liver disease. *Hepa-tology* 1986; **6**: 1.

52 Naveh Y, Mendelsohn H, Spira G *et al.* Primary sclerosing cholangitis associated with immunodeficiency. *Am. J. Dis. Child.* 1983; **137**: 114.

53 Nichols JC, Gores GJ, LaRusso NF *et al.* Diagnostic role of serum CA 19-9 for cholangiocarcinoma in patients with primary sclerosing cholangitis. *Mayo Clin. Proc.* 1993; **68**: 874.

54 Olsson R, Broomé U, Danielsson Å *et al.* Colchicine treat-ment of primary sclerosing cholangitis. *Gastroenterology* 1995; **108**: 1199.

55 Olsson R, Danielsson Å, Järnerot G *et al.* Prevalence of primary sclerosing cholangitis in patients with ulcerative colitis. *Gastroenterology* 1991; **100**: 1319.

56 Porayko MK, Wiesner RH, LaRusso NF *et al.* Patients with asymptomatic primary sclerosing cholangitis frequently have progressive disease. *Gastroenterology* 1990; **98**: 1594.

57 Quigley EMM, LaRusso NF, Ludwig J *et al.* Familial occur-rence of primary sclerosing cholangitis and ulcerative colitis. *Gastroenterology* 1983; **85**: 1160.

58 Rahn RH III, Koehler RE, Weyman PJ *et al.* CT appearance of sclerosing cholangitis. *Am. J. Roentgenol.* 1983; **141**: 549.

59 Ramage JK, Donaghy A, Farrant JM *et al.* Serum tumor markers for the diagnosis of cholangiocarcinoma in primary sclerosing cholangitis. *Gastroenterology* 1995; **108**: 865.

60 Record CO, Eddleston ALWF, Shilkin KB *et al.* Intrahepatic sclerosing cholangitis associated with a familial immunode-ficiency syndrome. *Lancet* 1973; **ii**: 18.

61 Roulot D, Valla D, Brun-Vezinet F *et al.* Cholangitis in the acquired immuno-deficiency syndrome: report of two cases and review of the literature. *Gut* 1987; **28**: 1653.

62 Schrumpf E, Abdelnoor M, Fausa O *et al.* Risk factors in primary sclerosing cholangitis. *J. Hepatol.* 1994; **21**: 1061.

63 Sebagh M, Farges O, Kalil A *et al.* Sclerosing cholangitis following human orthotopic liver transplantation. *Am. J. Surg. Pathol.* 1995; **19**: 81.

64 Sherlock S. The syndrome of disappearing intra-hepatic bile ducts. *Lancet* 1987; **ii**: 493.

65 Sisto A, Feldman P, Garel L *et al.* Primary sclerosing cholangitis in children: study of five cases and review of the literature. *Pediatrics* 1987; **80**: 918.

66 Snook JA, Chapman RW, Sachdev GK *et al.* Peripheral blood and portal tract lymphocyte populations in primary sclerosing cholangitis. *J. Hepatol.* 1989; **9**: 36.

67 Steckman M, Drossman DA, Lesesne HR. Hepatobiliary disease that precedes ulcerative colitis. *J. Clin. Gastroenterol.* 1984; **6**: 425.

68 Steinhart AH, Simons M, Stone R *et al.* Multiple hepatic abscesses: cholangiographic changes simulating sclerosing cholangitis and resolution after percutaneous drainage. *Am. J. Gastroenterol* 1990; **85**: 306.

69 Stiehl A, Waker S, Stiehl L *et al.* Effect of ursodeoxycholic acid on liver and bile duct disease in primary sclerosing cholangitis. A 3-year pilot study with a placebo-controlled study period. *J. Hepatol.* 1994; **20**: 57.

70 Terblanche J, Allison HF, Northover JMA. An ischemic basis for biliary strictures. *Surgery* 1983; **94**: 52.

71 Thompson HH, Pitt HA, Lewin KJ *et al.* Sclerosing cholangitis and histocytosis X. *Gut* 1984; **25**: 526.

72 Vierling JM, Fennell RH Jr. Histopathology of early and late human hepatic allograft rejection: evidence of progressive destruction of interlobular bile ducts. *Hepatology* 1985; **5**: 1076.

73 Wee A, Ludwig J. Pericholangitis in chronic ulcerative colitis: primary sclerosing cholangitis of the small bile ducts? *Ann. Intern. Med.* 1985; **102**: 581.

74 Wiesner RH, Grambsch PM, Dickson ER *et al.* Primary sclerosing cholangitis: natural history, prognostic factors and survival analysis. *Hepatology* 1989; **10**: 430.

75 Wiesner RH, LaRusso NF, Dozois RR *et al.* Peristomal varices after proctocolectomy in patients with primary sclerosing cholangitis. *Gastroenterology* 1986; **90**: 316.

76 Wilschanski M, Chait P, Wade JA *et al.* Primary sclerosing cholangitis in 32 children: clinical, laboratory, and radiographic features. *Hepatology* 1995; **22**: 1415.

77 Zajko AB, Campbell WL, Logsdon GA *et al.* Cholangiographic findings in hepatic artery occlusion after liver transplantation. *Am. J. Roentgenol.* 1987; **149**: 485.

Chapter 16
Virus Hepatitis

The first reference to epidemic jaundice has been ascribed to Hippocrates. The earliest record in Western Europe is in a letter written in 751 AD by Pope Zacharias to St Boniface, Archbishop of Mainz. Since then there have been numerous accounts of epidemics, particularly during wars. Hepatitis was a problem in the Franco-Prussian War, the American Civil War and World War I. In World War II huge epidemics occurred, particularly in the Middle East and Italy [14].

There are many varieties (table 16.1). Hepatitis A is a self-limited, faecally spread disease. Hepatitis B is a parenterally transmitted disease that often becomes chronic. Hepatitis D is parenterally spread and affects only those with a hepatitis B infection. Hepatitis C is a parenterally spread disease with a high chronicity rate. Hepatitis E is enterically spread, usually via water, and causes a self-limited hepatitis in underdeveloped countries. There is increasing evidence for another viral cause of hepatitis (non-A, B, C, D, E), [1, 2, 13]. Hepatitis G is one candidate and there will be others.

Pathology

All forms of viral hepatitis have a basic pathology. The essential lesion is an acute inflammation of the entire liver [4]. Hepatic cell necrosis is associated with leucocytic and histiocytic reaction and infiltration. Zone 3 shows the necrosis most markedly and the portal tracts the greatest cellularity (figs 16.1, 16.2, 16.3). The sinusoids show mononuclear cellular infiltration, polymorphs and eosinophils. Surviving liver cells retain their glycogen. Fatty change is rare. Zone 3 liver cells may show eosinophilic change (*acidophil bodies*), ballooning

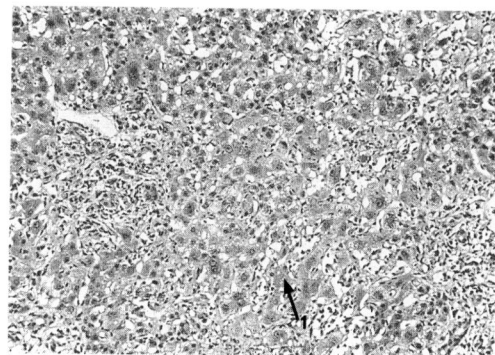

Fig. 16.1. Viral hepatitis: zone 3 (central) (arrow) shows marked loss of liver cells. Zone 1 (portal) shows expansion with cellular infiltration and bile duct proliferation. (H & E, ×40.)

Table 16.1. Viral hepatitis A, B, C, D and E contrasted

	HAV	HBV	HCV	HDV	HEV
Genome	RNA	DNA	RNA	RNA	RNA
Family	Picorna	Hepadna	Flavi : Pesti	Viroid	Calici
Incubation (days)	15–45	30–180	15–150	30–180	15–60
Transmission	Faecal	Blood	Blood	Blood	Faecal
	Oral	Saliva	Saliva		Oral
Acute attack	Depends on age	Mild or severe	Usually mild	Mild or severe	Usually mild
Rash	Yes	Yes	Yes	Yes	Yes
Serum diagnosis	IgM anti-HAV	IgM anti-HBc	Anti-HCV	IgM anti-HDV	IgM anti-HEV
		HBsAg	HCV RNA		
		HBV DNA			
Peak SGPT (ALT)	800–1000	1000–1500	300–800	1000–1500	800–1000
Up and down	No	No	Yes	No	No
Prevention	Vaccine	Vaccine	—	—	—
Treatment	Symptomatic	Symptomatic	Symptomatic	Symptomatic	Symptomatic
		?Antivirals	?Antivirals	?Antivirals	

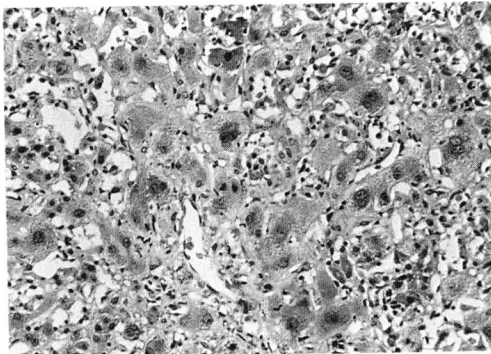

Fig. 16.2. Viral hepatitis: zone 3 shows swollen cells, mitoses and acidophilic bodies. (H & E, ×80.)

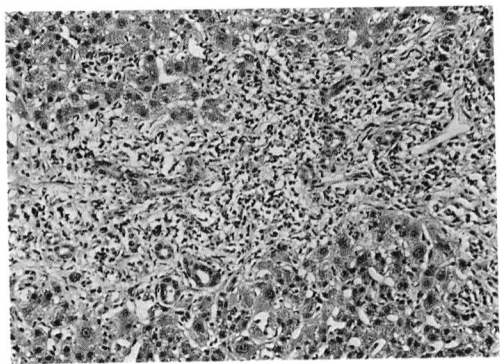

Fig. 16.3. Viral hepatitis: zone 1 (portal tract) shows an acute inflammatory reaction with ductular proliferation. (H & E, ×50.)

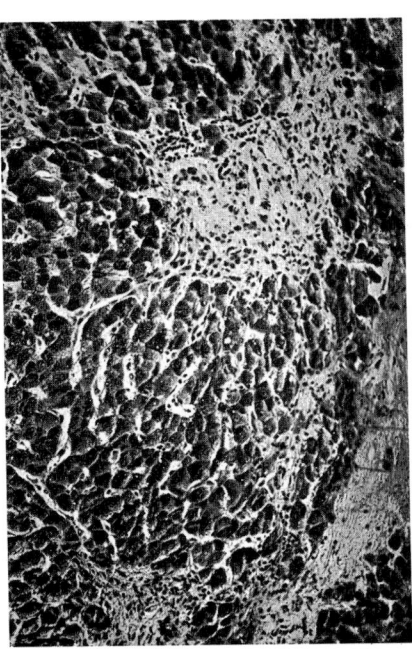

Fig. 16.4. Residual portal zone scarring seen 33 days after the onset of jaundice. (Best's carmine, ×100) [11].

pleomorphism and hyalinization, and giant multinucleated cells may be present. Mitoses are sometimes prominent. Zone 3 cholestasis may be found. Focal 'spotty' necrosis may be seen. Bile duct proliferation is usual and damage is an occasional feature [9]. Hepatitis is found even before the development of jaundice.

The reticulin framework is usually well preserved even in the midst of extreme disorganization. It provides a scaffolding when the liver cells regenerate. Inflammatory cells disappear gradually, and some new zone 1 portal connective tissue can often be found for many months (fig. 16.4). During recovery reticulo-endothelial activity increases throughout, apparently a 'scavenger' phenomenon. A slight increase in stainable fat is seen. The Kupffer cells contain lipofuscin pigment and iron.

Occasionally the necrosis may be *confluent* (submassive), affecting substantial groups of adjacent liver cells, usually in zone 3.

In massive fulminant necrosis the whole acinus is involved. Macroscopically the liver is reduced in size, being smallest in those who die the soonest. It is flaccid and shrunken and the left lobe may be disproportionately atrophied. Nodular regeneration is seen in those surviving for more than 2 weeks (fig. 16.5). The cut surface shows a 'nutmeg' appearance, red areas of haemorrhage alternating with yellow patches of necrosis. Necrosis in life is always less than that seen in autopsy material as autolysis proceeds particularly rapidly in the presence of acute hepatitis.

If the necrosis extends from zone 3 to zone 1 the reticulum collapses leaving connective tissue septa. This is termed *bridging* (fig. 16.6). This may be followed by the development of active fibrous septa, nodules and cirrhosis. More usually it is followed by scar formation (*post-necrotic scarring*) (fig. 16.7).

Acute viral hepatitis may be followed by chronic hepatitis (Chapter 17).

Changes in other organs

Regional lymph nodes are large. Splenomegaly is related to cellular proliferation and venous congestion. The bone marrow is moderately hypoplastic, but maturation is usually normal. In about 15% of fatal cases there is ulceration of the gastrointestinal tract — particularly caecal ulceration.

The brain shows an acute non-specific degeneration of ganglion cells. Occasionally acute pancreatitis and myocarditis have been noted. Haemorrhages are found in most organs.

Viral hepatitis is a multi-system infection involving many organs.

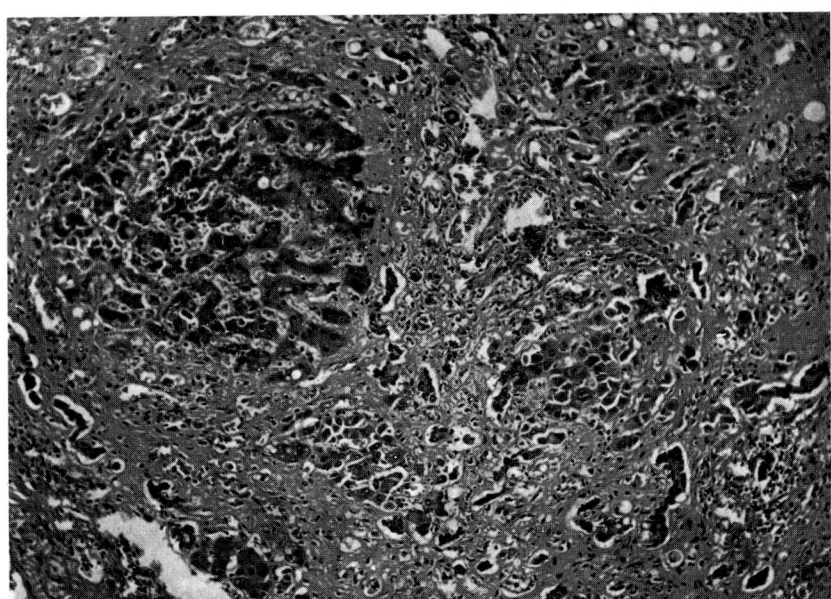

Fig. 16.5. Acute viral hepatitis. Sub-acute massive necrosis with nodular regeneration. (H & E, ×120.)

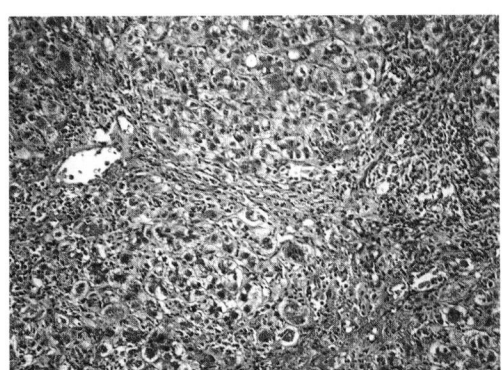

Fig. 16.6. Acute viral hepatitis. A passive septum (bridge) has formed between zones 1 and 2. (H & E, ×40.)

Clinical types

Acute hepatitis

Note is taken of ethnic origin, contacts, recent travel, injections, tattooing, dental treatment, transfusions, homosexuality or ingestion of shellfish. All drugs taken in the previous 2 months are listed.

In general, type A, B and C hepatitis run the same clinical course. Type B and C tend to be more severe and may be associated with a serum-sickness like syndrome.

The mildest attack is without symptoms and marked only by a rise in serum transaminase levels. Alternatively, the patient may be anicteric but suffer gastrointestinal and influenza-like symptoms. Such patients are likely to remain undiagnosed unless there is a clear history of exposure. Increasing grades of severity are then encountered, ranging from the icteric, from which recovery is usual, through to fulminant, fatal viral hepatitis.

The usual icteric attack in the adults is marked by a prodromal period, usually about 3 or 4 days, even up to several weeks, during which the patient feels generally unwell, suffers digestive symptoms, particularly anorexia and nausea, and may, in the later stages, have a mild pyrexia. Rigors are unusual. An ache develops in the right upper abdomen. This is increased by jolting movements. There is loss of desire to smoke or to drink

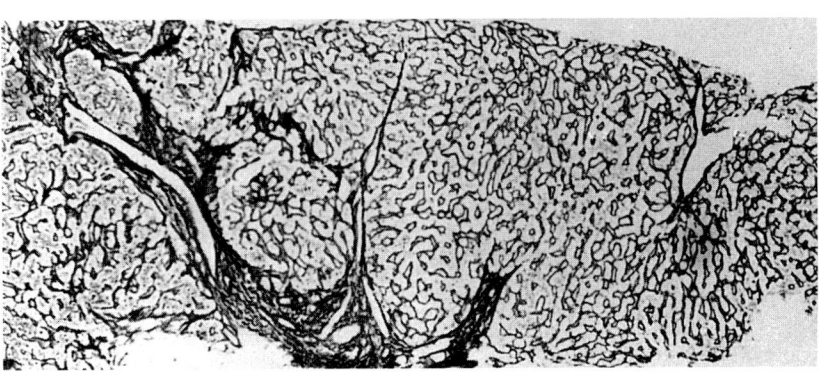

Fig. 16.7. Post-necrotic scarring. The liver biopsy specimen shows scarring, involving and extending from portal tracts. (Reticulin, ×34.)

alcohol. Malaise is profound and increases towards evening; the patient feels wretched.

Occasionally headache may be severe and, in children, its association with neck rigidity may suggest meningitis. Protein and lymphocytes in the CSF may be raised.

The prodromal period is followed by darkening of the urine and lightening of the faeces. This heralds the development of jaundice and symptoms decrease in severity. The temperature returns to normal and there may be bradycardia. Appetite returns and abdominal discomfort and vomiting cease. Pruritus may appear transiently for a few days.

The liver is palpable with a smooth, tender edge in 70% of patients. Heavy percussion over the right lower ribs posteriorly causes sickening discomfort. The spleen is palpable in about 20% of patients.

The adult loses about 4 kg in weight. A few vascular spiders may appear transiently.

After an icteric period of about 1–4 weeks the adult patient usually makes an uninterrupted recovery. In children, improvement is particularly rapid and jaundice mild or absent. The stools regain their colour. The appetite returns. After apparent recovery lassitude and fatigue persist for some weeks. Clinical and biochemical recovery is usual within 6 months of onset. However, chronic hepatitis may follow types B and C.

Neurological complications, including the Guillain–Barré syndrome, can complicate all forms of virus hepatitis [12].

Prolonged cholestasis

Occasionally, prolonged jaundice is of cholestatic type. Onset is acute; jaundice appears and deepens but, within 3 weeks, the patient starts to itch. After the first few weeks the patient feels well, gains weight and there are no physical signs apart from icterus and slight hepatomegaly. Jaundice persists for 8–29 weeks and recovery is then complete [10]. It is particularly associated with hepatitis A [6].

Liver biopsy shows conspicuous cholestasis which tends to mask the definite, usually mild, hepatitis.

This type must be differentiated from surgical obstructive jaundice [6]. The acute onset and only moderately enlarged liver are the most helpful points. Cholestatic drug jaundice is excluded by the history.

If doubt remains, ultrasound and liver biopsy are helpful.

The prognosis is usually excellent with complete clinical recovery and restitution of a normal liver [10].

Relapses

These occur in 1.8–15% of cases particularly with hepatitis A infection. In some the original attack is duplicated,

usually in a milder form. More often, the relapse is simply shown by an increase in serum transaminases and sometimes bilirubin. The relapse may be precipitated by premature activity. Multiple episodes may occur. Recovery is usually complete. In some patients relapses may indicate progression to chronic hepatitis.

Fulminant hepatitis (see Chapter 8)

This rare form of the disease usually overwhelms the patient within 10 days. It may develop so rapidly that jaundice is inconspicuous and the disease is confused with an acute psychosis or meningo-encephalitis. Alternatively, the patient, after a typical acute onset, becomes deeply jaundiced. Ominous signs are repeated vomiting, fetor hepaticus, confusion and drowsiness. The 'flapping' tremor may be only transient, but rigidity is usual. Coma supervenes rapidly and the picture becomes that of acute liver failure. Temperature rises, jaundice deepens and the liver shrinks. Widespread haemorrhages may develop.

Leucocytosis may be found in contrast to the usual leucopenia of virus hepatitis. The biochemical changes are those of acute liver failure (Chapter 8). The height of the serum bilirubin and transaminase are poor indicators of prognosis. Transaminase levels may actually fall as the patient's clinical condition worsens. Blood coagulation is grossly deranged and prothrombin is the best indicator of prognosis.

The time relationships and the course depend on whether the cause is A, B or non-A, non-B, non-C (table 16.2) [5].

Fulminant hepatitis is associated with viruses A, B and E. In the USA and Europe, HCV does not often seem to be related to fulminant hepatitis which may be due to another cause presumably viral [7].

The frequency of the fulminant course in the various types of viral hepatitis depends on the type of patient and the prevalence of hepatitis B carriage. In the UK and California the non-A, non-B, non-C type is more frequent, whereas in Denmark and Greece, hepatitis B predominates.

There are clinical differences in the fulminant course of the three main types [5]. Pyrexia is most frequent with

Table 16.2. Fulminant viral hepatitis in the UK: aetiology, duration from onset to fulminant, and survival [5]

	A	B	Non-A, non-B, non-C
Frequency (%)	31.5	24.7	43.8
Duration from onset (days)	10	7	21
Survival (%)	43.4	16.6	9.3

hepatitis A. The duration of illness before encephalopathy is longer with hepatitis non-A, non-B, non-C. The prothrombin time is greatest with hepatitis B. The bad prognosis in those with a longer duration from onset of illness to encephalopathy is probably related to the greater number of hepatitis non-A, non-B, non-C patients in that group (table 16.2).

Post-hepatitis syndrome

Adult patients feel below par for variable periods after acute hepatitis. Usually this is a matter of weeks but it may extend to months. This is termed the post-hepatitis syndrome [11]. Features are anxiety, fatigue, failure to regain weight, anorexia and alcohol intolerance, and right upper abdominal discomfort. The liver edge may be palpable and tender.

Serum transaminases may be raised up to three times normal. Continuing fluctuating transaminases may indicate the development of chronic hepatitis usually HCV or HBV.

Hepatic histology shows only mild, residual, portal zone cellularity and fibrosis with perhaps some fatty change in the liver cells. These features do not differ from those found in patients recovering normally who are now symptom-free. They rarely persist for longer than 1 year after the acute attack.

Treatment consists of reassurance after full investigation. If the acute attack has been type A, chronicity is excluded.

Investigations

Urine and faeces

Bilirubin appears in the urine before jaundice. Later it disappears although serum levels remain elevated.

Urobilinogenuria is found in the late pre-icteric phase. At the height of the jaundice, very little bilirubin reaches the intestine, so urobilinogen disappears. Its reappearance indicates commencing recovery.

The onset of jaundice is marked by lightening of the faeces. There is moderate steatorrhoea. Reappearance of stool colour denotes impending recovery.

Blood changes

Total serum bilirubin levels range widely. Deep jaundice generally implies a prolonged clinical course. An increase in conjugated pigment is early, even when the total bilirubin level is still normal.

Serum alkaline phosphatase level is usually less than three times the upper limit of normal. Serum albumin and globulin are quantitatively unchanged. The serum iron and ferritin levels are raised.

Serum immunoglobulins G and M are raised in about one-third of patients during the acute phase.

Serum transaminase estimations are useful in early diagnosis, in detecting the anicteric case, and for detection of inapparent cases in epidemics. The peak level is found 1 or 2 days before or after onset of jaundice. Later in the course the level falls, even if the clinical condition is worsening. The estimation cannot be used prognostically. Values may remain elevated for 6 months in those recovering completely.

Haematological changes

The pre-icteric stage is marked by leucopenia, lymphopenia and neutropenia. These revert towards normal as jaundice appears. Some 5–28% of patients show atypical lymphocytes (virucytes), resembling those seen in infectious mononucleosis. Acute Coombs' test positive haemolytic anaemia is a rare complication. Haemolysis may develop [8], especially in those with glucose-6-PD deficiency [3].

Aplastic anaemia is very rare. It appears weeks or months after the acute episode and is particularly severe and irreversible. It is not usually associated with A, B or C infection and may be due to a hitherto unidentified non-A, non-B, non-C type. It has been treated by bone marrow transplantation.

The *prothrombin time* is lengthened in the more severe cases and does not return completely to normal with vitamin K therapy.

The *sedimentation rate* of the red cells (ESR) is high in the pre-icteric phase, falls to normal with jaundice, and rises again when the jaundice subsides. It returns to normal with complete recovery.

Needle liver biopsy

This is rarely indicated in the acute stage. It may occasionally be needed in older patients to differentiate from extra-hepatic or other forms of intra-hepatic cholestasis and from drug jaundice. It may be used to diagnose the presence and type of chronic complications but should not be performed less than 6 months after the acute episode as the distinction between the picture of normal recovery and chronic hepatitis may be impossible.

Differential diagnosis

In the *pre-icteric stage*, hepatitis can be confused with other acute infectious diseases, with acute surgical abdomen, especially acute appendicitis, and with acute gastroenteritis. Bile in the urine, tender enlargement of the liver and a rise in serum transaminase values are the most helpful points. The distinction from infectious mononucleosis is given in table 16.16. Viral markers are essential.

In the *icteric stage*, the diagnosis must be made from surgical cholestasis. This is outlined in Chapter 12.

The diagnosis of acute viral hepatitis from drug reactions depends largely on the history.

Needle liver biopsy is valuable in the problem case. Attempts at a surgical diagnosis are disastrous.

The distinction from Weil's disease is discussed in Chapter 27.

In the *post-icteric stage*, the diagnosis of organic from non-organic complications necessitates routine investigations for the diagnosis of chronic hepatitis, and these may include needle biopsy.

Prognosis (table 16.2)

Type B infection is said to have the highest mortality. In a survey of 1675 cases in a group of Boston hospitals, one in eight sufferers from transfusion hepatitis (B and C) succumbed whereas only one in 200 died with the type A disease. Since many non-icteric cases are not included in the statistics the overall mortality rate is undoubtedly very much lower.

In the UK, non-A, non-B hepatitis, not due to hepatitis C but to another virus, has the poorest survival [5].

Those who are elderly or in poor general health have a poor prognosis. Fulminant hepatitis is rare in those less than 15 years old. Survival rate is the same for males as for females.

Treatment

Prevention

Compulsory notification leads to earlier detection and identification of methods of infection, for instance food or water contamination, sexual spread or carriage by blood donors. Vaccination is discussed later.

Treatment of the acute attack

Treatment has little effect in altering the course. At the outset this is unpredictable and it is wise to treat all attacks as potentially fatal and to insist upon bed rest with bathroom privileges. Traditionally this is enforced until the patient is free of jaundice. A less strict regime may be possible if the patients are young and previously healthy. They can be allowed up when they feel well, regardless of the degree of jaundice. They rest after each meal. If symptoms return, the patient is immediately returned to bed rest. Selected patients treated along these liberal lines do not show an increased incidence of later complications.

Convalescence is not allowed until the patient is symptom-free, the liver no longer tender, and the serum bilirubin less than 1.5 mg/100 ml. The period of convalescence should be twice the period spent in hospital or in bed at home.

The traditional low-fat, high-carbohydrate diet is popular because it has proved the most palatable to the anorexic patient. Apart from this, no benefit accrues from the rigid insistence upon a low-fat diet.

When the appetite returns, high protein intake may hasten recovery. Excess protein, however, is harmful to the severely ill patient in impending hepatic coma. The usual diet in hepatitis is composed of the food most appetizing to the patient. Supplementary vitamins, amino acids and lipotropic agents are not necessary.

Corticosteroids do not alter the degree of liver necrosis, accelerate the rate of healing or assist in immunity in virus hepatitis. Hepatitis tends towards spontaneous recovery and any benefit is not sufficient to justify their use except occasionally in cholestatic hepatitis A. The drug must be continued into convalescence because premature withdrawal leads to relapse. The steroid whitewash improves the morale of both patient and physician but probably has little effect on the healing process [10].

Patients showing signs of acute hepato-cellular failure with pre-coma require more active measures and the regime described in Chapter 8 must be instituted.

Follow-up

The patient should be seen 3–4 weeks after discharge, and if necessary at monthly intervals for the next 3 months. Special attention should be paid to recurrence of jaundice and to the size of the liver and spleen. Tests should include serum bilirubin, transaminase levels and hepatitis B and C markers if originally positive.

Exercise must be undertaken within the limits of fatigue. Alcohol must be denied for 6 months but preferably 1 year. The patient often has little inclination for it and excessive consumption leads to relapses. Diet can be unrestricted.

References

1 Alter MJ, Mast EE. The epidemiology of viral hepatitis in the United States. *Gastroenterol. Clin. North Am.* 1994; **23**: 437.

2 Buti J, Jardi R, Rodriguez-Frias F *et al.* Etiology of acute sporadic hepatitis in Spain: the role of hepatitis C and E viruses. *J. Hepatol.* 1994; **20**: 589.

3 Chan TK, Todd D. Haemolysis complicating viral hepatitis in patients with glucose-6-phosphate dehydrogenase deficiency. *Br. Med. J.* 1975; **i**: 131.

4 Dible JH, McMichael J, Sherlock SPV. Pathology of acute hepatitis. Aspiration biopsy studies of epidemic, arsenotherapy and serum jaundice. *Lancet* 1943; **ii**: 402.

5 Gimson AES, White YS, Eddleston ALWF *et al.* Clinical and prognostic differences in fulminant hepatitis type A, B, and non-A, non-B. *Gut* 1983; **24**: 1194.

6 Gordon SG, Reddy KR, Schiff L *et al.* Prolonged intrahepatic cholestasis secondary to acute hepatitis A. *Ann. Intern. Med.* 1984; **101**: 635.

7 Kuwada SK, Patel VM, Hollinger FB *et al.* Non-A, non-B fulminant hepatitis is also non-E, and non-C. *Am. J. Gastroenterol.* 1994; **89**: 57.

8 Lyons DJ, Gilvarry JM, Fielding JF. Severe haemolysis associated with hepatitis A and normal glucose-6-phosphate dehydrogenase status. *Gut* 1990; **31**: 838.

9 Poulsen H, Christoffersen P. Abnormal bile duct epithelium in liver biopsies with histological signs of viral hepatitis. *Acta Path. Microbiol. Scand.* 1969; **76**: 383.

10 Shaldon S, Sherlock S. Virus hepatitis with features of prolonged bile retention. *Br. Med. J.* 1957; **ii**: 734.

11 Sherlock S, Walshe VM. The post-hepatitis syndrome. *Lancet* 1946; **ii**: 482.

12 Tabor E. Guillain–Barré syndrome and other neurologic syndromes in hepatitis A, B, non-A, non-B. *J. Med. Virol.* 1987; **21**: 207.

13 Tassopoulos NC, Hatzakis A, Delladetsima I *et al.* Role of hepatitis C virus in acute non-A, non-B hepatitis in Greece: a 5-year prospective study. *Gastroenterology* 1992; **102**: 969.

14 Zuckerman AJ. The chronicle of viral hepatitis. *Bull. Hyg. Trop. Dis.* 1977; **54**: 113.

Hepatitis A Virus (HAV)

Hepatitis A accounts for 20–25% of clinical hepatitis in the developed world. It is due to a small, 27 nm cubically symmetrical RNA picorna virus (fig. 16.8) [5]. The capsid consists of 60 centromeres, each made of the same four

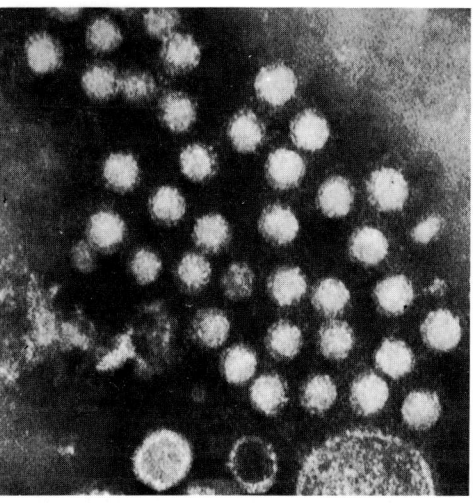

Fig. 16.8. Electron microscopy of hepatitis A antigen particles in faeces. These are shown as 22 nm spheres. (×250 000.)

viral proteins, VP1, VP2, VP3 and VP4. Only a single serotype has been identified. However, the genome has been cloned and characterized and minor differences have been found among isolates from different parts of the world [13].

The virus is absorbed from the gastrointestinal tract and reaches the liver where it is engulfed (fig. 16.9). Viral proteins are synthesized and packed into vesicles to be

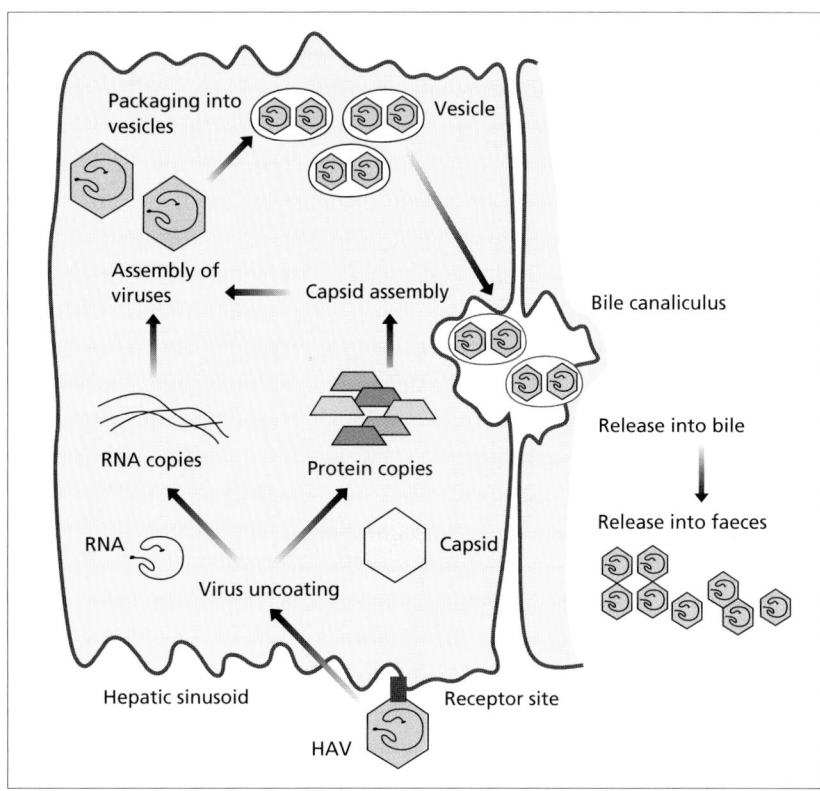

Fig. 16.9. The replication cycle of HAV.

released into the bile. The virus is not directly cytopathic and liver cell damage is not caused by viral replication but by T-cell mediated immune responses to infection.

The virus has been transmitted to marmosets and chimpanzees and cultivated *in vitro* (fig. 16.10). It grows in a variety of epithelial cell lines. DNA complementary to genomic hepatitis A virus RNA has been cloned in *Escherichia coli*.

A serum antibody (anti-HAV) appears as the stool becomes negative for virus, reaches a maximum in several months and is detectable for many years (fig. 16.11). IgG anti-HAV probably gives immunity from further infection with hepatitis A. The appearance of serum IgM anti-HAV is more helpful diagnostically and implies a recent infection. This antibody persists for only 2–6 months (fig. 16.11) and rarely, in low titre, up to 1 year.

Chronic carriers have not been identified.

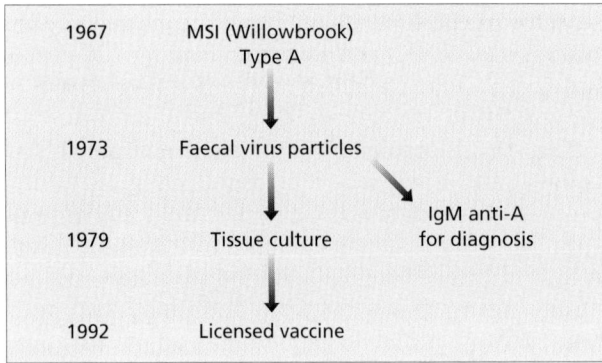

Fig. 16.10. Landmarks in hepatitis A.

Epidemiology

The disease occurs sporadically or in epidemic form and has an incubation time of 15–50 days. It is usually spread by the faecal–oral route. Parenteral transmission is extremely rare, but can follow transfusion of blood from a donor who is in the incubation stage of the disease [8].

Age 5–14 is the group most affected and adults are often infected by spread from children.

Spread is related to overcrowding, poor hygiene and poor sanitation. With an improved standard of living the prevalence is decreasing worldwide (fig. 16.12). In urban areas, 29% (Switzerland) to 96.9% (Yugoslavia) of adults show circulating IgG anti-HAV. In underdeveloped countries, 90% of children have the antibody by the age of 10. Young people not previously exposed, and visiting endemic areas, are increasingly becoming affected. Medical staff in developed countries are at risk. A large outbreak among nurses and mothers in a nursery spread from acute hepatitis A in a neonate with an ileostomy [1].

Outbreaks have been reported among haemophiliacs receiving solvent-detergent treated factor VIII concentrates and were presumably due to infection of plasma by blood donors who were incubating HAV [10].

Most sporadic cases follow person-to-person contact. Children in day-care centres and promiscuous homosexual men are at risk.

Explosive water-borne and food-borne epidemics are described. Use of human sewage for soil fertilization can result in frozen-fruit-related epidemics.

Ingestion of raw clams and oysters from polluted waters is known to have caused four epidemics. Steaming the clams may not kill the virus, for the temperature achieved inside the clams is not sufficiently high.

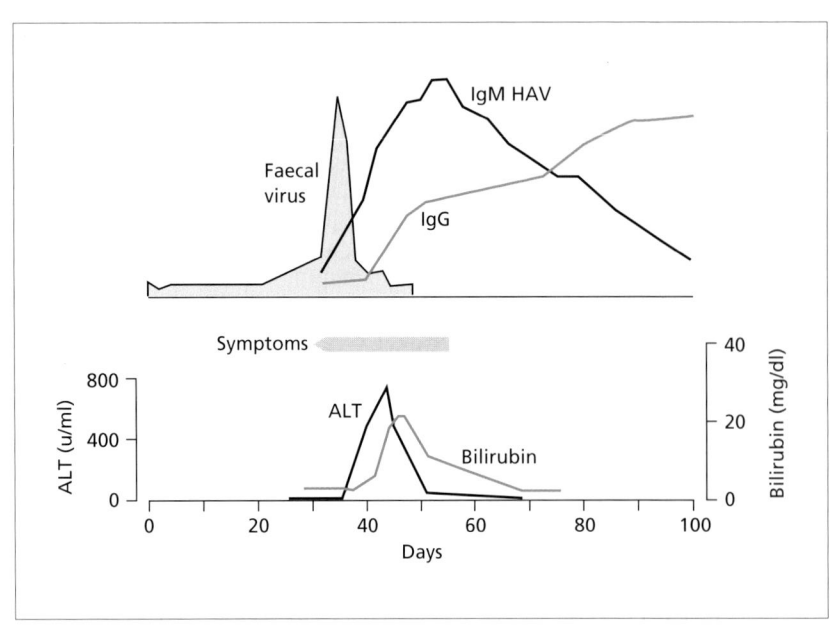

Fig. 16.11. The course of acute hepatitis A. ALT = alanine transferase (GPT).

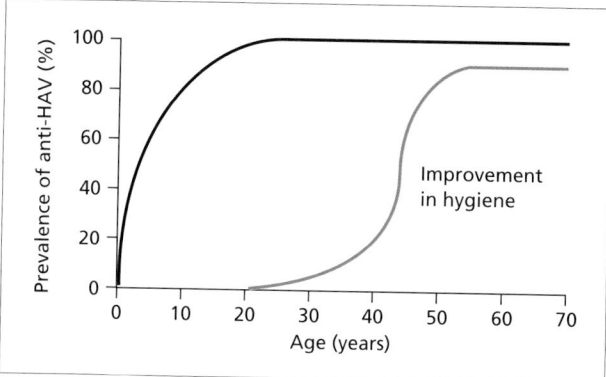

Fig. 16.12. Prevalence changes with improved hygiene. Older people lack immunity (IgG anti-HAV) to hepatitis A.

Contamination during preparation has resulted in transmission via other foods, including sandwiches, orange juice, potato salad and meat.

Clinical course

The hepatitis is usually mild, particularly in children where it is frequently subclinical or passed off as gastroenteritis. The disease is more serious and prolonged in adults.

Needle liver biopsy in patients with acute type A hepatitis shows a particularly florid portal zone lesion with expansion, marked cellular infiltration and erosion of the limiting plate. Cholestasis is marked. It is therefore surprising that hepatitis A infection never leads to ongoing chronic hepatitis or cirrhosis. Fibrin ring granulomas are described [11].

Cholestatic hepatitis A affects adults [6]. The jaundice lasts 42–110 days and itching is severe. Serum IgM anti-HAV is positive. The prognosis is excellent. A case can be made for cutting short the jaundice and relieving the itching by a short course of prednisolone 30 mg reducing to zero over about 3 weeks.

The *nephrotic syndrome* has been reported with immune complex, mesangial, proliferative glomerulonephritis [21].

Hepatitis A may trigger *chronic autoimmune hepatitis type 1* in genetically predisposed individuals [18]. This may be related to defects in T-cell suppressor-inducer cells.

Relapsing hepatitis A. Occasionally after 30–90 days the patient relapses. The serum transaminase levels have never returned to normal. The relapse resembles the original attack clinically and biochemically and virus A is found in the stools [16]. The relapse may last several months but recovery eventually ensues [5].

Rarely, the relapse can be associated with arthritis, vasculitis and cryoglobulinaemia [3].

Prognosis

This is excellent, and recovery is usually full. Mortality in large epidemics is less than 1 per 1000 and virus A accounts for less than 1% of cases of fulminant viral hepatitis. The average adult with icteric hepatitis can anticipate 6 weeks of illness and this will rarely exceed 3 months.

Chronicity does not develop. Follow-ups of large epidemics in World War I [2] showed no long-term sequelae. Viral carriage is usually but not always transient in faeces. The appearance of IgG anti-HAV marks long-term immunity to the disease.

Prevention

The virus is excreted in the faeces for as long as 2 weeks before the appearance of jaundice. The anicteric patient may excrete the virus for a similar period. The virus is therefore disseminated before the diagnosis is made. For this reason, isolation of patients and contacts cannot be expected to influence significantly the spread of hepatitis.

Virus A is relatively resistant to inactivation by heat, ether or acid, but it is inactivated by formalin 1 in 4000 at 37°C for 72 hours, chlorine 1 p.p.m. for 30 minutes and by microwaving.

Immune serum globulin (ISG) prophylaxis (table 16.7)

This can be used for short-term (about 6 months) prophylaxis. Efficacy depends on the antibody content and hence the source of the plasma. Its use has been largely replaced by vaccine.

ISG prevents HAV in 80–90% if given within 6 days of exposure. It is used for those with high risk exposure within 1 week, such as to a common source of infection or to close personal contact with sufferers.

ISG may be given with the first dose of vaccine but the resultant HAV antibody titres will be reduced [20].

Hepatitis A vaccines

Viral particles are obtained by culture and inactivated with formaldehyde. The vaccine has been licensed, is safe and immunogenic [7]. The only side-effect is mild soreness of the arm. A single 1 ml dose of vaccine is followed by a booster 6–12 months later. The single dose gives rapid protection within 15 days which lasts for 1 year. If followed by the booster, 95% seroconversion ensues with long-lasting protection [15]. Preliminary serum testing for HAV antibody is necessary only in those born after 1945, living in countries with low prevalence and who, presumably, have had a small chance of contracting the disease (fig. 16.12) [17].

A live, attenuated vaccine has been prepared from HAV in mammalian cell culture. It is inexpensive, effective and can be given orally. However, there is doubt concerning its safety and there is difficulty in obtaining fully attenuated strains.

In one dose, the formol inactivated vaccine was shown to be highly protective in children in a Jewish community in New York [19]. In a large study of children in Thailand, two doses protected against HAV for at least 1 year [9].

Application. Travellers to areas where hygiene is suspect are at risk. Unvaccinated, three to six visitors per 1000 per month will develop HAV.

The schoolchildren and staff in day-care units and their parents are at risk.

Nurses should be vaccinated, particularly those working in intensive care units.

Food handlers and sewage workers are candidates for vaccination [12].

The military should be vaccinated particularly if they are proceeding to areas where hygiene is poor [14].

Promiscuous homosexual males should be vaccinated.

References

1 Azimi PH, Roberto RR, Guralnik J *et al*. Transfusion acquired hepatitis A in a premature infant with secondary nosocomial spread in an intensive care nursery. *Am. J. Dis. Child.* 1986; **140**: 23.
2 Cullinan ER, King RC, Rivers JS. The prognosis of infective hepatitis. A preliminary account of a long-term follow-up. *Br. Med. J.* 1958; **i**: 1315.
3 Dan M, Yaniv R. Cholestatic hepatitis, cutaneous vasculitis and vascular deposits of immunoglobulin M and complement associated with hepatitis A virus infection. *Am. J. Med.* 1990; **89**: 103.
4 Feinstone SM, Kapikian AZ, Purcell RH. Hepatitis A: detection by immune electron microscopy of a virus-like antigen associated with acute illness. *Science* 1973; **182**: 1026.
5 Glikson M, Galun E, Oren R *et al*. Relapsing hepatitis A. Review of 14 cases and literature survey. *Medicine (Baltimore)* 1992; **71**: 14.
6 Gordon SG, Reddy KR, Schiff L *et al*. Prolonged intrahepatic cholestasis secondary to acute hepatitis A. *Ann. Intern. Med.* 1984; **101**: 635.
7 Hollinger FB. An overview of the clinical development of hepatitis A vaccine. *J. Infect. Dis.* 1995; **171**: S1.
8 Hollinger FB, Khan NC, Oefinger PE. Post-transfusion hepatitis type A. *JAMA* 1983; **250**: 2313.
9 Innis BL, Snitbhan R, Kunasol P *et al*. Protection against hepatitis A by an inactivated vaccine. *JAMA* 1994; **271**: 1328.
10 Mannuccio PM, Gdovin S, Gringeri A *et al*. Transmission of hepatitis A to patients with hemophilia by factor VIII concentrates treated with organic solvent and detergent to inactivate viruses. *Ann. Intern. Med.* 1994; **120**: 1.
11 Ponz E, Garcia-Pagán JC, Bruguera M *et al*. Hepatic fibrin-ring granulomas in a patient with hepatitis A. *Gastroenterology* 1991; **100**: 268.
12 Poole CJM, Shakespeare AT. Should sewage workers and carers for people with learning disabilities be vaccinated for hepatitis A? *Br. Med. J.* 1993; **306**: 1102.
13 Robertson BH, Khanna B, Nainan OV *et al*. Epidemiologic patterns of wild-type hepatitis A virus determined by genetic variation. *J. Infect. Dis.* 1991; **163**: 286.
14 Rubertone MV, DeFraites RF, Krauss MR *et al*. An outbreak of hepatitis A during a military field training exercise. *Mil. Med.* 1993; **158**: 37.
15 Sjögren MH, Hoke CH, Binn LN *et al*. Immunogenicity of an inactivated hepatitis A vaccine. *Ann. Intern. Med.* 1991; **114**: 470.
16 Sjögren MH, Tanno H, Fay O *et al*. Hepatitis A virus in stool during clinical relapse. *Ann. Intern. Med.* 1987; **106**: 221.
17 Steffen R, Kane MA, Shapiro CN *et al*. Epidemiology and prevention of hepatitis A in travellers. *JAMA* 1994; **272**: 885.
18 Vento S, Garofano T, Di Perri G *et al*. Identification of hepatitis A virus as a trigger for autoimmune chronic hepatitis type I in susceptible individuals. *Lancet* 1991; **337**: 1183.
19 Werzberger A, Mensch B, Kuter B *et al*. A controlled trial of a formalin-inactivated hepatitis A vaccine in healthy children. *N. Engl. J. Med.* 1992; **327**: 453.
20 Zaaijer HL, Leentvaar-Kuijpers A, Rotman H *et al*. Hepatitis A antibody titres after infection and immunization: implications for passive and active immunization. *J. Med. Virol.* 1993; **40**: 22.
21 Zikos D, Grewal KS, Craig K *et al*. Nephrotic syndrome and acute renal failure associated with hepatitis A viral infection. *Am. J. Gastroenterol.* 1995; **90**: 295.

Type B hepatitis (HBV)

In 1965, Blumberg and colleagues in Philadelphia found an antibody in two multiply-transfused haemophiliac patients which reacted with an antigen in a single serum in their panel which came from an Australian Aborigine [11]. Later the antigen was found in patients with viral hepatitis. Because of its discovery in an aboriginal serum the antigen was called Australia antigen. In 1977, Blumberg was awarded the Nobel prize for his discovery. Australia antigen is now known to be the surface of the hepatitis B virion and is termed hepatitis B surface antigen (HBsAg).

The virion of hepatitis B (Dane particle) consists of surface and core (fig. 16.13). The core is formed in hepatocyte nucleus and the surface particles are made in the cytoplasm. The core contains a DNA polymerase and the DNA has a molecular weight of $1.8-2.3 \times 10^6$. The DNA structure is double-stranded and circular. It is approximately 3200 nucleotides in length and has a single-stranded gap of 600–2100 nucleotides. The DNA polymerase reaction appears to repair the gap. The core contains a core antigen and another antigen, called 'e', is a protein sub-unit of the core.

The double-stranded DNA genome of HBV has been cloned and sequenced [59]. There are four major polypeptide reading frames (fig. 16.14). The S gene codes for an HBsAg polypeptide. The pre-S1 domain is

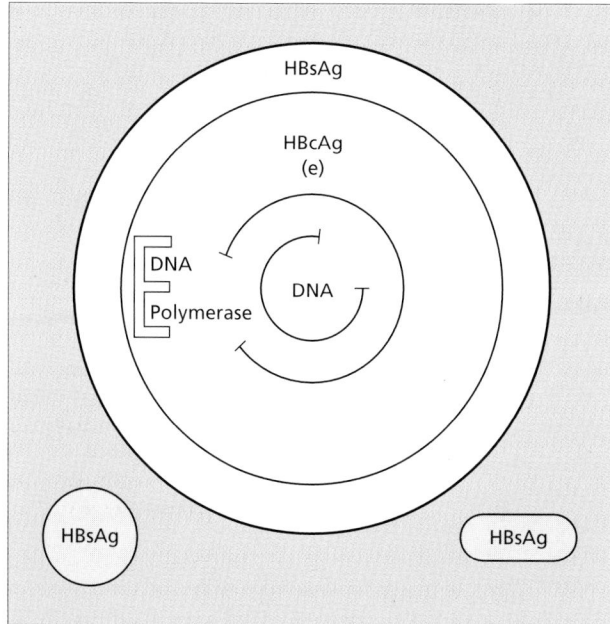

Fig. 16.13. Diagram of the virion of hepatitis B (HBV: Dane particle). The core contains DNA polymerase, double-stranded DNA, core antigen and e antigen. The surface consists of HBsAg. Spheres and tubules of HBsAg are free in serum.

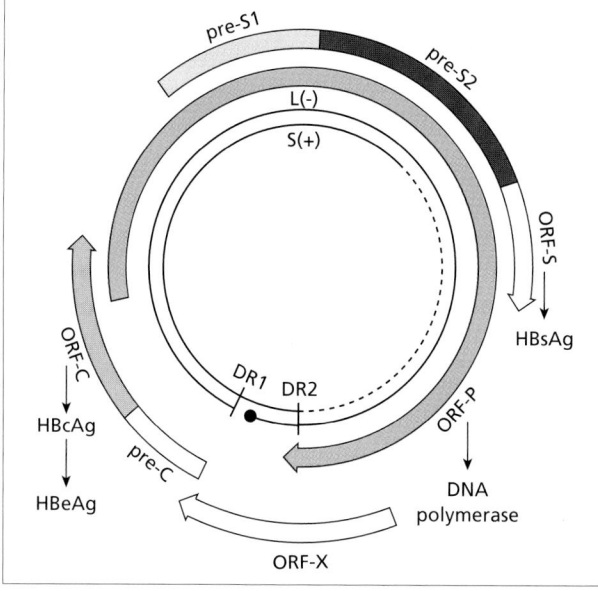

Fig. 16.14. Organization of the genome of the hepatitis B virus showing the four open reading frames (ORF), polymerase (P), surface antigen, core antigen and X, and the pre-S1 and pre-S2 regions.

involved in the recognition of hepatitis B virus by hepatocyte receptors. It evokes virus neutralizing antibody production (anti-pre-S1) and this can be detected in acute hepatitis B. A defect may participate in the development of chronic hepatitis B by allowing continuing

reinfection of hepatocytes by circulating virions [3]. Serum levels of pre-S1 antigen correlate with hepatitis B viral replication and may be useful in clinical assessment of chronic viral infection [68]. Pre-S2 is similar [46]. The C gene codes for a nucleocapsid protein bearing hepatitis B core antigen (HBcAg). The P gene codes for a putative DNA polymerase. The X gene codes for a protein with a transcriptional transactivating function, perhaps related to virus replication [33].

A similar disease affects woodchucks, ground squirrels and Peking ducks, and these animals have been extensively used for research [65, 69]. The whole group of agents have been termed *hepadna viruses*.

Sub-types of HBsAg

HBsAg particles have surfaces that are antigenically complex and this had led to the recognition of antigenic determinants. A common determinant is *a*. The other subdeterminants are designated *d*, *y*, *w* and *r*. The four major determinants are therefore *adw*, *adr*, *ayw* and *ayr*. They breed true and are very helpful epidemiologically.

Serological diagnosis (table 16.3)

HBsAg appears in the blood about 6 weeks after infection and has disappeared by 3 months (fig. 16.15). Persistence for more than 6 months implies a carrier state.

Table 16.3. Viral hepatitis: significance of serological markers

Marker	Significance
Hepatitis A	
IgM anti-HAV	Acute hepatitis A
IgG anti-HAV	Immune to hepatitis A
Hepatitis B	
HBsAg	Acute or chronic hepatitis B carriage
IgM anti-HBc	Acute hepatitis B (high titre)
	Chronic hepatitis B (low titre)
IgG anti-HBc	Past exposure to hepatitis B (with negative HBsAg)
	Chronic hepatitis B (with positive HBsAg)
Anti-HBs	Immune to hepatitis B
HBeAg	Acute hepatitis B. Persistence means continued infectious state
Anti-HBe	Convalescence or continued infectious state
HBV DNA	Continued infectious state
Delta	
IgM anti-delta	Acute or chronic infection with delta agent
IgG anti-delta	Chronic delta infection (high titre with positive IgM anti-delta)
	Past delta infection (low titre with negative IgM anti-delta)

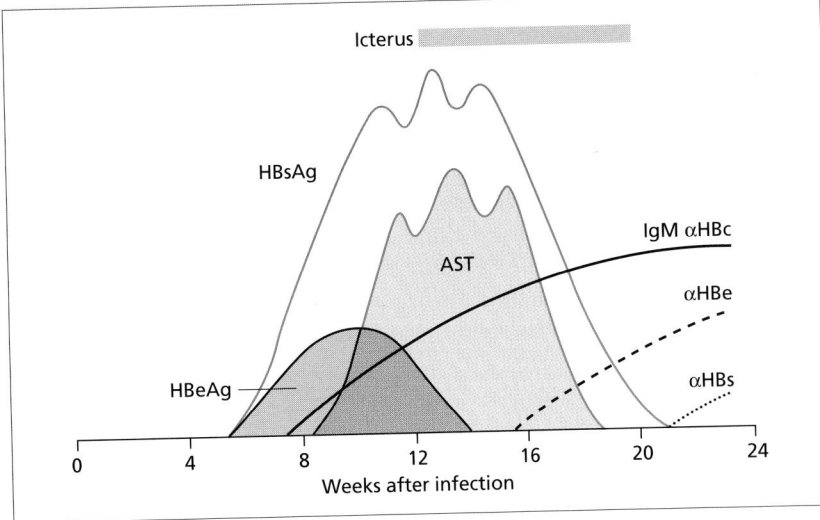

Fig. 16.15. The course of acute type B hepatitis. HBsAg = hepatitis B surface antigen; HBeAg = hepatitis Be antigen; AST = aspartate transaminase; IgM αHBc = IgM antibody against hepatitis B core antigen; αHBe = antibody against hepatitis e antigen; αHBs = antibody against hepatitis B surface antigen.

Anti-HBs appears late, some 3 months after the onset, and persists. Anti-HBs levels are rarely high and 10–15% of patients with acute type B hepatitis never develop the antibody. Anti-HBs accounts for recovery and immunity. In the past, HBsAg and HBsAb were believed to be mutually exclusive. However, as many as one-third of carriers of HBsAg also have HBsAb. The mechanism is uncertain, but it has been attributed to simultaneous infection with different sub-types.

HBeAg correlates with ongoing viral synthesis and with infectivity. It is transiently present during the acute attack. It is present for a shorter time than HBsAg. Persistence for more than 10 weeks strongly suggests the development of chronicity (Chapter 17).

Anti-HBe is a marker of relatively low infectivity. The appearance of anti-HBe is strong evidence that the patient will recover completely.

HBcAg cannot be detected in circulating blood, but its antibody (anti-HBc) can. High titres of IgM anti-HBc mark present acute virus hepatitis [17]. This antibody is detected after HBsAg has been cleared from the serum. This is true of 5–6% of cases with acute hepatitis B and is encountered particularly in fulminant hepatitis [73]. It is also useful in determining whether an acute attack of hepatitis is due to virus B or to superinfection with another virus. Persistence of *IgM anti-HBc* implies ongoing virus B-related chronic disease, usually chronic active hepatitis. Lower titres of *IgG anti-HBc* with anti-HBs mark hepatitis B infection in the remote past. Higher titres of IgG anti-HBc without anti-HBs indicate persistence of viral infection [40]. The significance of high titres of IgG anti-HBc without anti-HBs is uncertain. It may indicate the late phase of an acute attack. It may be due to inability to produce HBsAb. Some have immune complex-associated HBsAg and HBV DNA may be positive [40, 70]. Some still have ongoing HBV infection.

HBV DNA is the most sensitive index of viral replication. It is detected by polymerase chain reaction (PCR) [41]. Using PCR, HBV DNA can be found in serum and liver after the loss of HBsAg, particularly in those receiving antiviral treatment [55]. HBV DNA in serum detected by PCR is a good marker of the level of viraemia, can be correlated with serum transaminase levels and parallels the presence of HBsAg in serum [8]. Patients with an HBV precore mutant are HBeAg negative and HBV DNA positive.

Hepatitis B markers in hepatocytes

HBsAg may be stained orange with orcein (fig. 16.16) in the hepatocytes of carriers and chronic hepatitis patients, but not in those in the acute stage. Electron microscopy and immune histochemistry demonstrate the HBcAg to be in nuclei and the HBsAg in the membranes of liver cells. Core markers are not found in the liver in the acute stage.

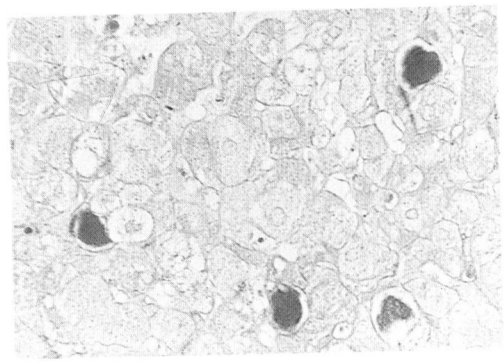

Fig. 16.16. Orcein staining shows liver cells containing HBsAg (brown).

Infectivity of body fluids

HBV-containing blood or any body fluid contaminated with blood is infectious. Mere positivity of a fluid for HBsAg is not synonymous with infectivity. However, saliva, urine and seminal fluid from HBeAg-positive males have shown the presence of HBV DNA.

Peripheral blood mononuclear cells can contain HBV DNA [9]. At autopsy, replicative viral intermediates have been found in lymph nodes, spleen, kidney pancreas, brain and some endocrine tissues [63, 85]. This extra-hepatic proliferation is particularly important in hepatitis-B-positive patients receiving hepatic transplant and accounts for re-infection of the graft.

Epidemiology (tables 16.4, 16.5)

The disease is transmitted parenterally or by intimate, often sexual, contact.

The carrier rate of HBsAg varies worldwide from 0.1 to 0.2% in Britain, the USA and Scandinavia to more than

Table 16.4. Approximate percentage carrier rate of HBsAg (by RIA) in 'healthy' blood donors

Scandinavia	0.1
UK	0.1
USA	0.1
Holland	0.2
Switzerland	0.2
Belgium	0.5
France	0.5
Spain	2.0
Southern Italy	3.0
Japan	3.0
Greece	5.0
South Africa	11.3
Taiwan	15.0
Singapore	15.0
Hong kong	15.0

Table 16.5. Groups in which acute and chronic type B hepatitis should be suspected

Immigrants from Mediterranean countries, Africa or the Far East
Drug abusers
Homosexuals
Neonates of HBsAg-positive mothers
Hospital staff
Patients with
   renal failure
   reticuloses
   cancer
   organ transplants
Staff and patients of hospitals for the mentally retarded
Post-transfusion

3% in Greece and southern Italy and even up to 10–15% in Africa and the Far East. If anti-HBs is measured, the rate of exposure to hepatitis B in any community is much higher. Carriage of HBsAg is even higher in some isolated communities: 45% in Alaskan Eskimos [54], and 85% in Australian Aborigines.

In high carriage rate areas, infection is acquired by passage from the mother to the neonate. The infection is usually not via the umbilical vein, but from the mother at the time of birth and during close contact afterwards. The chance of transmission increases as term approaches and is greater with acute than chronic carriers. The mother is HBsAg positive and also usually, but not always, HBeAg positive. Antigenaemia develops in the baby within 2 months of birth and tends to persist [12].

In high endemic areas such as Africa, Greece and the Far East, the transmission is in childhood and probably horizontal through kissing, shared utensils such as toothbrushes and razors, and injections [37, 38, 57]. Contact in preschool day-care centres is possible. Sexual contacts in the family are at risk [4].

Infection among homosexuals is related to duration of homosexual activity, number of sexual contacts and anal contact [71].

Blood-sucking arthropods such as mosquitoes or bed bugs may be important vectors, particularly in the tropics although insecticide spraying of dwellings had no effect on HBV infection [58].

The MHC class II allele DRB1*1302 is associated with protection against persistent HBV in children and adults in the Gambia [76].

Blood transfusion continues to cause hepatitis B in countries where donor blood is not screened. Transmission is more likely with blood from paid donors than from volunteer blood.

Opportunities for parenteral infection include the use of unsterile instruments for dental treatment, ear piercing and manicures, neurological examination, prophylactic inoculations, subcutaneous injections, acupuncture and tattooing.

Parenteral drug abusers develop hepatitis from using shared, unsterile equipment. The mortality may be very high in this group. Multiple attacks are seen and chronicity is frequent. Liver biopsy may show, in addition to acute or chronic hepatitis, foreign material, such as chalk, injected with the illicit drug.

Hospital staff in contact with patients, and especially patients' blood, usually have a higher carrier rate than the general community. This applies particularly to staff on renal dialysis or oncology units. Patients are immunosuppressed and, on contracting the disease, become chronic carriers. The patient's attendant is infected from contact with blood parenterally, such as from pricking or through skin abrasions. Surgeons and dentists are particularly at risk in operating on HBsAg-positive patients with a positive HBeAg. Holes in gloves and cuts on hands are common. Wire sutures may be a particular hazard in penetrating the skin.

Spread *from* a health-care worker is usually through a surgeon performing complex invasive procedures [82]. In the UK, proof of immunity (through vaccination or past infection) is required of all surgeons and other medical staff performing invasive procedures. Students have to show certificates of immunization and immunity on registration for a medical or dental course [27, 42].

Use of standard cleansing procedures means that HBV infection is not spread by endoscopes [81].

Institutionalized mentally retarded children (especially with Down's syndrome) and their attendants have a high carrier rate [45].

Worldwide, there are more than 350 million carriers of HBV, 60 million of whom will die from liver cancer and 45 million from cirrhosis.

The worldwide prevalence of HBV infection is falling. This is related not only to vaccination but to better hygiene and to the AIDS campaign which addresses the dangers of promiscuity and of shared syringes and needles [31] (fig. 16.17). The prevalence of all forms of hepatitis is tending to fall.

Clinical course

The course may be anicteric. The high carriage rate of serum markers in those who give no history of acute hepatitis B suggests that subclinical episodes must be extremely frequent. The non-icteric case is more liable to become chronic than the icteric one.

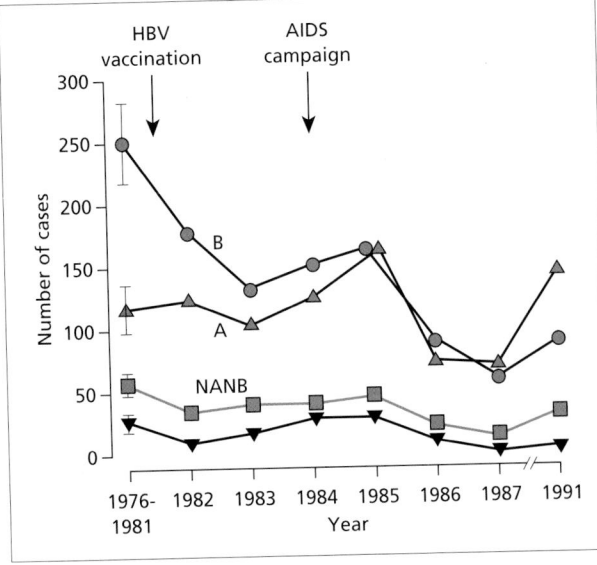

Fig. 16.17. Occurrence of acute hepatitis B in Zurich (1.1 million inhabitants) from 1976 to 1991. ● = Hepatitis B; ▲ = hepatitis A; ■ = non-A, non-B hepatitis; ▼ = unclassified. Modified from Grob *et al.* 1995.

The usual clinical attack diagnosed in the adult tends to be more severe than for virus A or C infections. The overall picture is, however, similar. The self-limited, benign icteric disease usually lasts less than 4 months. Jaundice rarely exceeds 4 weeks. Occasionally, a prolonged benign course is marked by increased serum transaminase values for more than 100 days. Relapses are rare. Cholestatic hepatitis with prolonged deep jaundice is unusual.

There may be features suggesting immune complex disease. This is shown in the prodromal period by a *serum sickness-like* syndrome. This develops about a week before jaundice. It can be associated with an icteric or an anicteric attack. The syndrome has also been described with chronic hepatitis B. Fever is usual. The skin lesion is urticarial, and rarely, in children, a papular acrodermatitis. The arthropathy is symmetrical, non-migratory and affects small joints. Serum rheumatoid factor is negative. It is usually transitory but can persist. These events can be related to circulating immune complexes.

A fulminant course of hepatitis B in the first 4 weeks is related to an enhanced immune response with more rapid clearing of virus. Antibodies to surface and 'e' antigen increase, and multiplication of virus ceases [13]. In fulminant hepatitis B, the surface antigen may be in low titre or undetectable. The diagnosis may be made only by finding serum IgM anti-HBc.

Another viral hepatitis, superimposed on the symptomless hepatitis B carrier, may precipitate a fulminant course. The new agent may be A or delta; hepatitis C has also been postulated.

Subacute hepatic necrosis is marked by increasing severe disease evolving over 1–3 months.

Chronic hepatitis can develop insidiously (see Chapter 17).

Extra-hepatic associations

These conditions are often associated with circulating immune complexes containing HBsAg. The accompanying liver disease is usually mild and at the most a chronic persistent hepatitis.

Acute and chronic type B hepatitis can develop in patients with *agammaglobulinaemia*.

Polyarteritis. This involves largely medium and small arteries and appears early in the course of the disease. Immune complexes containing HBsAg are found in the vascular lesions and their blood levels correlate with disease activity. Polyarteritis is a rare complication of hepatitis B [53]. Plasmaphoresis and adenine arabinoside have been used for treatment [78].

Glomerulonephritis. This has been associated with hepatitis B infection, largely in children [51]. Liver disease is minimal. The patients are usually HBeAg positive. Immune complexes of HBsAg and HBsAb, HBcAg and anti-HBc or HBeAg and anti-HBe are found in glomerular and papillary basement membranes [80]. In children, interferon treatment may lead to a remission [52]. The response to corticosteroids is poor [51]. Remission may precede HBe antigen seroconversion to anti-HBe. In children the glomerulonephritis usually resolves spontaneously in 6 months to 2 years. In adults the disease is slowly but relentlessly progressive in one-third and the response to interferon is disappointing [47].

Polymyalgia rheumatica has been connected with hepatitis B infection [7].

Essential mixed cryoglobulinaemia. A patient with peripheral neuropathy and cryoglobulinaemia showed a cryoprecipitate with a high concentration of HBsAg. However, anti-HBsAg and complement were not found [49]. The relationship of hepatitis B to this condition has not been proved [23].

The *Guillain–Barré syndrome* has been reported with HBsAg-containing immune complexes in serum and cerebrospinal fluid [67].

Myocarditis may have an immune complex basis [79].

Hepatitis B carriers

Approximately 10% of patients contracting hepatitis B as adults and 90% of those infected as neonates will not clear HBsAg from the serum within 6 months (fig. 16.18). Such patients become carriers and this is likely to persist. Reversion to a negative HBsAg is rare but may develop in old age. Males are six times more likely to become carriers than females.

The dilemma of a person, such as a hospital worker, carrying the antigen and coming from an area where it is prevalent is a very difficult one. Hospital staff who develop HBsAg-positive hepatitis and clear the antigen from the blood are immune to type B hepatitis. If they become carriers, the position is difficult.

'Healthy' carriers may show changes on liver biopsy ranging from non-specific minimal abnormalities

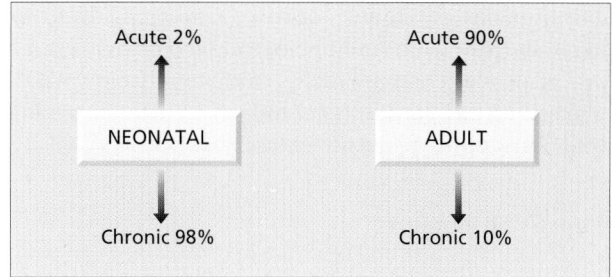

Fig. 16.18. The course of acute hepatitis B in the neonate and adult.

through to chronic hepatitis and cirrhosis. The extent of the changes is not reflected by serum biochemical tests and may only be revealed by liver biopsy. The carrier presenting by chance is likely to have minor hepatic changes compared to the patient presenting to a gastroenterology department where more serious liver disease is likely. In a survey of patients found to be HBsAg positive at blood donation, 95% had near normal liver biopsies and only 1.6% proceeded to chronic active hepatitis or cirrhosis [25]. 90% were serum HBeAg negative and anti-HBe positive.

In a carrier, a positive serum HBV DNA, IgM anti-HBc and HBeAg indicate infectivity and ongoing disease. Mechanisms of chronicity are discussed in Chapter 17.

Chronic organic sequelae

Exposure to HBV can have different results (fig. 16.19). Some are immune and have no clinical attack; they presumably have anti-HBs. In others, an acute attack develops varying from anicteric to fulminant. Previously normal people usually clear the antigen from the serum within about 4–6 weeks from the onset of symptoms. Chronic liver disease is associated with persistent antigenaemia. In general, the more florid and acute the original attack the less likely are chronic sequelae.

If the patient survives a fulminant attack of viral hepatitis, ultimate recovery is complete without the

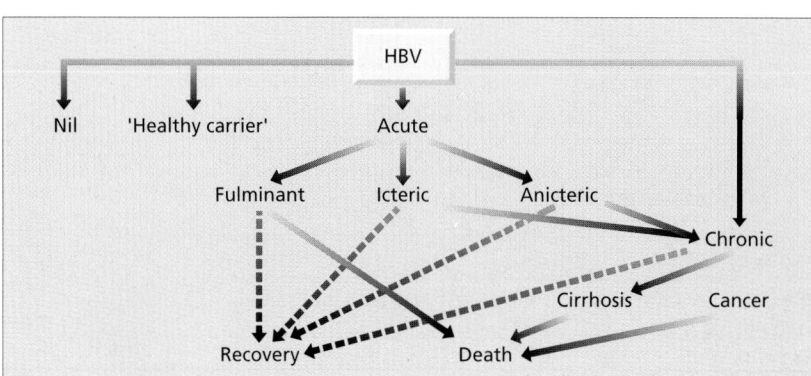

Fig. 16.19. The effect of exposure to hepatitis B virus (HBV).

development of chronic disease. Chronicity is more likely in those with immunological incompetence such as neonates, homosexuals, sufferers from AIDS, leukaemia and cancer, renal failure or those receiving immunosuppressive treatment (see Chapter 17) [26].

Hepatitis B mutants

Variants of the hepatitis B genome are described due to mutations in the various reading frames (fig. 16.20). Although more frequent with RNA viruses, HBV, a DNA virus, uses RNA and a reverse transcriptase for its replication and hence is associated with mutations. Nucleotide substitutions, deletions, duplications, insertions and rearrangements may have no consequences, may impair replication, may change host susceptibility or may lead to escape from host immune-attack. The effect of the various mutants is very variable, possibly related to the immune system of the patient or to the effect of interferons.

Patients are described with progressive liver disease, high serum HBV DNA levels and yet negative serum HBeAg. This variant is due to a mutation in the precore region resulting in disturbed secretion of HBeAg which is derived from continuous translation of the precore region [1, 14, 15]. There is a guanosine to adenine point mutation at nucleotide 83 resulting in a stop codon at 28 (fig. 16.20). Other point mutations contribute. The significance of this *precore mutation* is very variable. In Israel and Japan, it is associated with fulminant disease [44, 50, 64, 66]. However it has a low prevalence in fulminant hepatitis B in France [29] and in North America [48]. Activation of precore mutant hepatitis B may lead to fulminant liver failure following cytotoxic therapy [86]. The presence of the precore codon mutation is associated with a poor response to interferon in some studies but not in others. Core gene mutants occur predominantly at the time of HBeAg clearance when liver disease is most active [2].

The response to interferon in mutants may also be reduced by interference with T-cell function in advanced chronic HBV [62]. Appearance of precore mutants during therapy usually predicts failure to clear virus [28]. Precore mutants may be associated with severe recurrent disease after liver transplant [6]. Precore mutants can be detected in asymptomatic HBsAg-positive family members [2].

A mutation in the *surface region* has been associated with infants born to carrier mothers becoming HBsAg-positive despite apparently successful vaccination. This variant has been related to a substitution of arginine for glycine at amino acid 145, the 'a' determinant to which the vaccine promotes antibodies (fig. 16.21) [16].

Genetic mutations in the S gene outside the 'a' determinant may be responsible for failure to detect HBsAg in some Chinese patients with chronic HBV hepatitis [36].

Ever increasing numbers of escape mutants of HBV are being recognized. *X gene mutants* are described but their biological and clinical significance is not clearly defined [10].

A mutation in the *polymerase gene* has been described in a patient with HBV DNA in the liver but anti-HBc and anti-HBs positive [10].

The mutants may determine the clinical course and, by conferring an advantage to the virus, favour fulminant disease. Serum HBeAg becomes less useful as an indicator of infection. HBV vaccines may have to change so that some mutants are represented.

Prevention

Hepatitis B immunoglobulin (HBIG)

HBIG is a special hyperimmune serum globulin with a high antibody titre. It is effective for passive immunization against hepatitis B if given prophylactically or within hours of infection [72]. Hepatitis vaccine should always be given with HBIG, particularly if the subject is

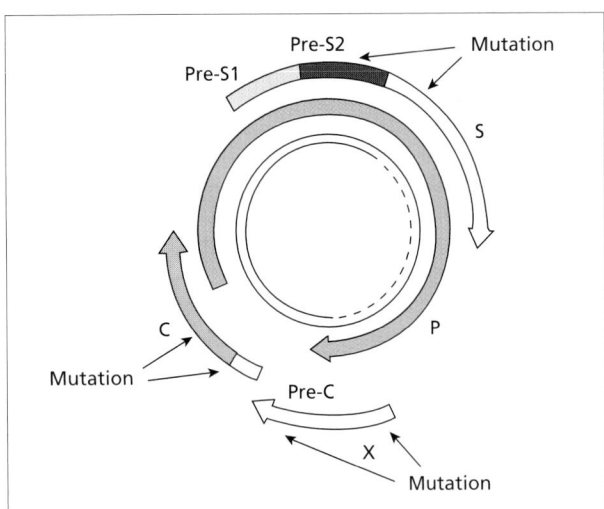

Fig. 16.20. The site of HBV mutations.

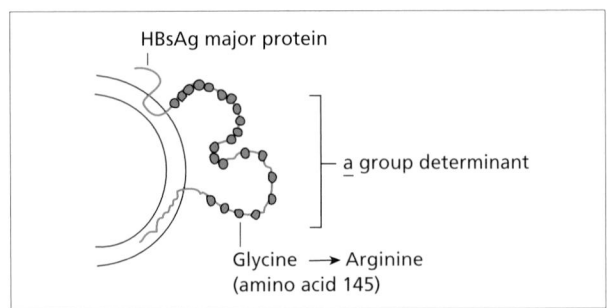

Fig. 16.21. HBV: vaccine-induced escape mutant.

Table 16.6. Immunoprophylaxis of viral hepatitis B

Type	Immunoglobulin	Indication	Regime
B (adults)	HBIG	Exposure to HBsAg-positive blood Sexual consorts	0.06 ml/kg as soon as possible combined first dose of vaccine*
B (neonates)	HBIG	HBsAg-positive mother	0.5 ml as soon as possible combined first dose of vaccine†

*Full course of vaccine given if subject is anti-HBc negative.
†Full course of vaccine given.

at risk of re-infection. It is indicated for sexual contacts of acute sufferers, babies born to HBsAg-positive mothers [84], and victims of parenteral exposure (needle stick) to HBsAg-positive blood (tables 16.6, 16.7, 16.8).

Repeated HBIG injections are being used to prevent reinfection of a donor liver inserted into an HBV DNA positive patient (see Chapter 35).

Hepatitis B vaccines

Vaccines are prepared from the uninfectious outer surface of the virus (HBsAg).

The *plasma-derived vaccine* comes from plasma of hepatitis B carriers. It is highly effective in preventing hepatitis B in high-risk groups. It is completely safe.

Table 16.7. Indications for hepatitis vaccination

Surgical and dental staff including medical students
Hospital and laboratory staff in contact with blood
Patients and staff in departments of oncology and haematology, kidney, mental subnormality and liver disease
Mental subnormality
Accidental exposure to HBsAg-positive blood
Close family and sexual contacts of HBsAg-positive carriers
Babies born to HBsAg-positive mothers
Children as part of EPI programme
Drug abusers
Homosexually active men
Travellers to high-risk areas

Table 16.8. Prophylaxis of persons accidentally exposed to possibly infectious blood
- **Check** donor blood for HBsAg; victim's blood for HBsAg and HBcAb
- **Give at once** 0.06 ml/kg HBIG plus first dose hepatitis B vaccine

	HBsAg	HBcAb	Further action to victim
Victim	+ve	+ve	None: immune
Donor	+ve		Continue vaccine course
	−ve		None or continue vaccine course if victim is at risk of further hepatitis B exposure

HBsAg has been expressed in yeast cells. The resultant *recombinant yeast vaccine* is free of human plasma. It is safe and as effective as the plasma-derived one [74].

Hepatitis B vaccines are effective in preventing hepatitis B in promiscuous homosexuals [75] (fig. 16.22), haemodialysis patients [22], Down's syndrome and other mentally retarded patients [34], health-care

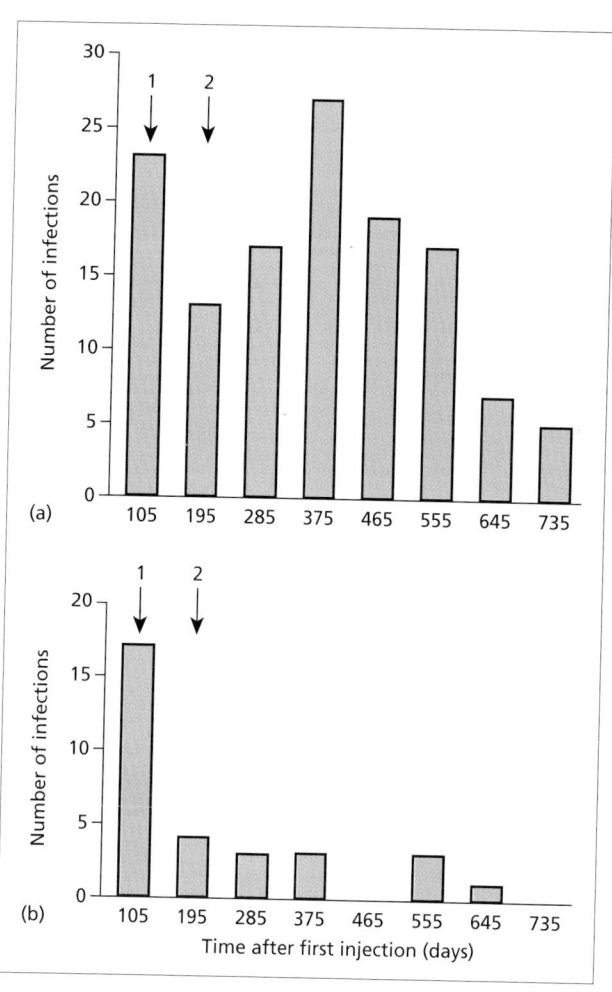

Fig. 16.22. Efficacy of hepatitis B vaccine. Results of a double-blind trial of the efficacy of hepatitis B vaccine in 1083 homosexual men. Distribution of infections in recipients of (a) placebo and (b) vaccine over 735 days. Arrows show time of first and second injections. Modified from [75].

workers [24], babies born to HBsAg-positive mothers [74, 84] and susceptibles in Alaska [54].

In the Gambia, vaccination of infants was 84% effective against HBV infection and 94% effective against chronic carriage (table 16.9) [30, 83]. A 12-year follow-up of infants vaccinated in Senegal, showed that 81% who received a booster at school age had anti-HBs. The protective efficacy of the vaccine was 88% [19].

In healthy individuals the recombinant vaccine is given in a dose of 10 μg (1 ml) intramuscularly at 0, 1 month and a booster at 6 months (fig. 16.23). This induces sufficient antibody response in at least 94% of individuals.

The vaccine is usually given intramuscularly into the arm. Intradermal administration is effective although antibody titres are not so high as with the intramuscular route [87].

Pre-testing. Vaccination is unnecessary if the person has a positive HBsAb or HBcAb.

The cost-effectiveness of pre-testing to save vaccine depends on the prevalence of serum B markers in a community.

The finding of an isolated serum anti-HBs does not necessarily mean immunity to hepatitis B. A positive serum anti-HBc is preferable as this detects infected as well as immune persons.

Duration of protection. This is uncertain, protection probably persists after the anti-HBs response has declined to undetectable levels. Immunological memory provides continued protection [77]. However, a booster should be considered at 5–7 years after the initial course if the subject is still being exposed to hepatitis B. Antibody levels at the time of the booster dose may give a good indication of a duration of adequate antibody titres [20].

Antibody response (table 16.10)

The long-term protection depends on the antibody response which is 85–100% in healthy young subjects. Anti-HBs should be measured 1–3 months after completion of the basic course of vaccine.

Non-responders have peak anti-HBs levels of ≤10 iu/litre and lack protection.

Low responders have peak anti-HBs levels of 10–100 iu/litre and generally lack detectable anti-HBs levels within about 5–7 years. They may respond to a further booster of double the dose of vaccine.

Good responders have peak anti-HBs ≥100 iu/litre and usually have long-term immunity.

Failure to develop adequate antibodies may be related to freezing the vaccine or giving it into the buttock rather than the deltoid region.

A poor antibody response is seen in the aged and in the immunocompromised including HIV-positive persons [18]. They should be given doses of 20 μg.

The subnormal response is significantly linked to a histocompatibility haplotype, HLA-B8, SCO1, DR3 [62].

Approximately 5–10% of normal persons have absent or poor antibody responses. Some may respond to a booster [21].

Indications (table 16.7) [60, 61]

The need for vaccination depends on the chance of being exposed to hepatitis B. Vaccination is mandatory for health-care staff in close contact with hepatitis B

Table 16.9. Hepatitis B vaccine in the Gambia (from [30])

	No.
Vaccinated	
Infancy	720
No	816
At 4 years	
Vaccine efficacy	84%
Prevention carriage	94%

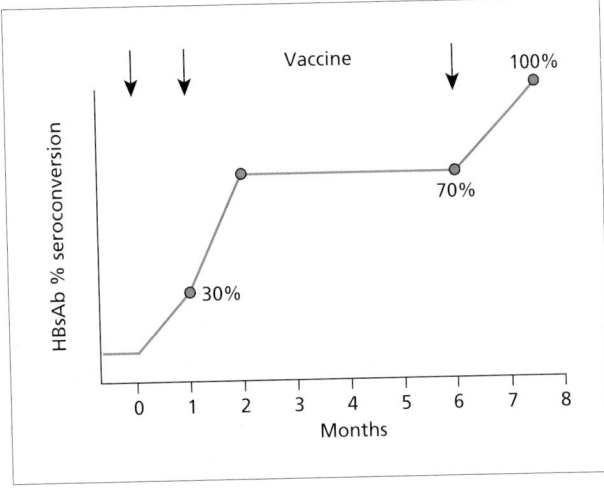

Fig. 16.23. The use of hepatitis B vaccine. Three injections result in about 93% seroconversion at 8 months in young healthy subjects.

Table 16.10. Failure of antibody response to hepatitis B vaccine

Age >50 years
Underlying disease
HIV positive
Genetics (HLA B8)
Buttock injection
Frozen vaccine
Unknown

patients, particularly those working on renal dialysis units, liver units, haemophilia and oncology units, genitourinary departments treating homosexuals or those working in homes for the mentally retarded [34]. Surgeons and dentists and their assistants, medical students and laboratory workers regularly exposed to blood are candidates. The vaccine should be given to medical personnel proceeding overseas to areas where the prevalence of hepatitis B is high.

Acute sufferers from hepatitis B are highly infectious and their sexual contacts should be vaccinated and given hyperimmune-globulin. Sexual and family contacts of hepatitis B carriers should be vaccinated after their antibody status has been determined.

Promiscuous homosexuals requesting vaccine should be screened for HBsAg and HBcAb and, if they are not immune, should be vaccinated. The same rules apply to drug abusers.

Babies born to HBsAg positive, and particularly HBe antigen positive mothers should be vaccinated and given immune globulin at birth [39].

Even in countries with a low carrier rate it is essential to screen *all* pregnant women for HBsAg and not only those with a high risk of being carriers. If possible, the pregnant woman should be tested at 14 weeks of gestation and supplemented at delivery by rapid screening of those who escaped routine prenatal care [32].

The problem of the health-care worker, accidentally exposed parenterally to blood which may be infectious, demands special consideration (table 16.8) [24].

The introduction of hepatitis B vaccination has had an effect on the epidemiology of hepatitis B in the USA [5]. The overall incidence has remained relatively constant, but there are changes in different groups [56]. The incidence in homosexuals has fallen, partly due to changing lifestyle (fig. 16.22). Intravenous drug abuse has increased and, with it, the spread to non-abuser social and sexual contacts. This may account in part for the increased percentage in those having a heterosexual exposure. Health care workers show a reduction, probably related to the acceptance of hepatitis B vaccination. Taken overall, these statistics are unsatisfactory. WHO decrees that universal vaccination of infants against HBV is mandatory [35]. This has already been done in 75 countries where the endemicity is high and it is hoped that, by 1997, this will also apply to countries with low endemicity. In children, transmission of HBV may be horizontal and a further dose of vaccine should be given at 10–12 years. Protection would thus be given before the individual has decided on his sexual lifestyle, become a drug abuser or joined the health-care professions. The 32% or so who acquire hepatitis without a recognized risk factor would also be protected.

In China, Italy, Korea, Taiwan, Malaysia, Singapore, Hong Kong, Saudi Arabia, Italy, Spain and the USA mass vaccination of neonates is performed irrespective of the hepatitis markers of the mother. Countries such as Australia, and the UK, where at present the chances of neonatal and childhood transmission of hepatitis B are small, should be included. The logistics, particularly cost, of universal vaccination in WHO's Extended Programme of Immunization (EPI) are difficult to face. The present low cost of vaccines supplied under government contracts to developing countries must also apply to developed countries where there is also need. A good example has been given by Italy which provides compulsory HBV vaccination to newborns and to adolescents at 12 years. Screening of pregnant women is compulsory and free vaccine is offered to risk groups.

Other vaccines

The most simple vaccine is derived from *heat-inactivated plasma containing HBsAg* and is based on the original observation of Krugman who boiled infectious hepatitis B-positive serum and showed it protected against hepatitis B [22]. This vaccine is relatively crude, highly immunogenic and inexpensive.

Polypeptide vaccines are composed of specific immunogenic antigenic determinants of HBsAg. So far they have not proved potent antibody stimulants and are uneconomical to produce.

The pre-S region. This is important for clearance of hepatitis B virus (fig. 16.14). Recombinant yeast vaccines are under investigation which will contain pre-S (pre-S1 and pre-S2) [43]. They may be effective in those failing to respond to conventional vaccination.

References

1 Akahane Y, Yamanaka T, Suzuki H *et al.* Chronic active hepatitis with hepatitis B virus DNA and antibody against e antigen in the serum. Disturbed synthesis and secretion of e antigen from hepatocytes due to a point mutation in the precore region. *Gastroenterology* 1990; **99**: 1113.

2 Akarca US, Greene S, Lok ASF. Detection of precore hepatitis virus mutants in asymptomatic HBsAg-positive family members. *Hepatology* 1994; **19**: 1366.

3 Alberti A, Cavalletto D, Chemello L *et al.* Fine specificity of human antibody response to the pre S1 domain of hepatitis B virus. *Hepatology* 1990; **12**: 199.

4 Alter MJ, Coleman PJ, Alexander WJ *et al.* Importance of heterosexual activity in the transmission of hepatitis B and non-A, non-B hepatitis. *JAMA* 1989; **262**: 1201.

5 Alter MJ, Hadler SC, Margolis HS *et al.* The changing epidemiology of hepatitis B in the United States. Need for alternative vaccination strategies. *JAMA* 1990; **263**: 1218.

6 Angus PW, Locarnini SA, McCaughan GW *et al.* Hepatitis B virus precore mutant infection is associated with severe recurrent disease after liver transplantation. *Hepatology* 1995; **21**: 14.

7 Bacon PA, Doherty SM, Zuckerman AJ. Hepatitis B antibody in polymyalgia rheumatica. *Lancet* 1975; **ii**: 476.

8 Baker BL, Di Bisceglie AM, Kaneko S *et al*. Determination of hepatitis B virus DNA in serum using the polymerase chain reaction: clinical significance and correlation with serological and biochemical markers. *Hepatology* 1991; **13**: 632.

9 Bartolomé J, Moraleda G, Molina J *et al*. Hepatitis B virus DNA in liver and peripheral blood mononuclear cells during reduction in virus replication. *Gastroenterology* 1990; **99**: 1745.

10 Bloom HE. Variants of hepatitis B, C and D viruses: molecular biology and clinical significance. *Digestion* 1995; **56**: 85.

11 Blumberg BS, Alter HJ, Visnich S. A 'new' antigen in leukemia sera. *JAMA* 1965; **191**: 541.

12 Bortolotti F, Cadrobbi P, Crivellaro C *et al*. Long-term outcome of chronic type B hepatitis in patients who acquire hepatitis B virus infection in childhood. *Gastroenterology* 1990; **99**: 805.

13 Brechot C, Bernuau J, Thiers V *et al*. Multiplication of hepatitis B virus in fulminant hepatitis. *Br. Med. J.* 1984; **288**: 270.

14 Brunetto MR, Stemler M, Schödel F *et al*. Identification of HBV variants which cannot produce precore derived HBeAg and may be responsible for severe hepatitis. *Ital. J. Gastroenterol.* 1989; **21**: 151.

15 Carman WF, Hadziyannis S, McGarvey MJ *et al*. Mutation preventing formation of hepatitis B e antigen in patients with chronic hepatitis B infection. *Lancet* 1989; **ii**: 588.

16 Carman WF, Zanetti AR, Karayiannis P *et al*. Vaccine-induced escape mutant of hepatitis B virus. *Lancet* 1990; **336**: 325.

17 Chau KH, Hargie MP, Decker RH *et al*. Serodiagnosis of recent hepatitis B infection by IgM class anti-HBC. *Hepatology* 1983; **3**: 142.

18 Collier AC, Corey L, Murphy VL *et al*. Antibody to human immunodeficiency virus (HIV) and suboptimal response to hepatitis B vaccination. *Ann. Intern. Med.* 1988; **109**: 101.

19 Coursaget P, Lebouilleux D, Soumare M *et al*. Twelve-year follow-up study of hepatitis B immunization of Senegalese infants. *J. Hepatol.* 1994; **21**: 250.

20 Coursaget P, Yvonnet B, Gilks WR *et al*. Scheduling of revaccination against hepatitis B virus. *Lancet* 1991; **337**: 1180.

21 Craven DE, Awdeh ZL, Kunches LM *et al*. Non-responsiveness to hepatitis B vaccine in health care workers. *Ann. Intern. Med.* 1986; **105**: 356.

22 Desmyter J, Colaert J, De Groote G *et al*. Efficacy of heat-inactivated hepatitis B vaccine in haemodialysis patients and staff: double-blind placebo-controlled trial. *Lancet* 1983; **ii**: 1323.

23 Dienstag JL, Wands JR, Isselbacher KJ. Hepatitis B and essential mixed cryoglobulinemia. *N. Engl. J. Med.* 1977; **297**: 946.

24 Dienstag JL, Werner BG, Polk BF *et al*. Hepatitis B vaccine in health care personnel: safety, immunogenicity, and indicators of efficacy. *Ann. Intern. Med.* 1984; **101**: 34.

25 Dragosics B, Ferenci P, Hitchman E *et al*. Long-term follow-up study of asymptomatic HBsAg-positive voluntary blood donors in Austria: a clinical and histologic evaluation of 242 cases. *Hepatology* 1987; **7**: 302.

26 Dudley FJ, Scheuer PJ, Sherlock S. Natural history of hepatitis-associated antigen-positive chronic liver disease. *Lancet* 1972; **ii**: 1388.

27 Editorial. Entry to medical school: by examination and vaccination? *Lancet* 1994; **343**: 927.

28 Fattovich G, McIntyre G, Thursz M *et al*. Hepatitis B virus precore/core variation and interferon therapy. *Hepatology* 1995; **22**: 1355.

29 Feray C, Gigou M, Samuel D *et al*. Low prevalence of precore mutations in hepatitis B virus DNA in fulminant hepatitis type B in France. *J. Hepatol.* 1993; **18**: 119.

30 Fortuin M, Chotard J, Jack AD *et al*. Efficacy of hepatitis B vaccine in the Gambian expanded programme on immunisation. *Lancet* 1993; **341**: 1129.

31 Grob P. Introduction to epidemiology and risk of hepatitis B. *Vaccine* 1995; **13**: S14.

32 Grosheide PM, Wladimiroff JW, Heijtink RA *et al*. Proposal for routine antenatal screening at 14 weeks for hepatitis B surface antigen. *Br. Med. J.* 1995; **311**: 1197.

33 Haruna Y, Hayashi N, Katayama K *et al*. Expression of X protein and hepatitis B virus replication in chronic hepatitis. *Hepatology* 1991; **13**: 417.

34 Heijtink RA, De Jong P, Schalm SW *et al*. Hepatitis B vaccination in Down's syndrome and other mentally retarded patients. *Hepatology* 1984; **4**: 611.

35 Hoofnagle JH. Toward universal vaccination against hepatitis B virus. *N. Engl. J. Med.* 1989; **321**: 1333.

36 Hou J, Karayiannis P, Waters J *et al*. A unique insertion in the S gene of surface antigen-negative hepatitis B virus Chinese carriers. *Hepatology* 1995; **21**: 273.

37 Hsu S-C, Change M-H, Ni Y-H *et al*. Horizontal transmission of hepatitis B virus in children. *J. Ped. Nutr.* 1993; **16**: 66.

38 Hurie MJ, Mast EE, Davis JP. Horizontal transmission of hepatitis B virus infection to United States born children of Hmong refugees. *Pediatrics* 1992; **89**: 269.

39 Ip HMH, Lelie PN, Wong VCW *et al*. Prevention of hepatitis B virus carrier state in infants according to maternal serum levels of HBV DNA. *Lancet* 1989; **i**: 406.

40 Joller-Jemelka HI, Wicki AN, Grob PJ. Detection of HBs antigen in 'anti-HBc alone' positive sera. *J. Hepatol.* 1994; **21**: 269.

41 Kaneko S, Miller RH, Di Bisceglie AM *et al*. Detection of hepatitis B virus DNA in serum by polymerase chain reaction. *Gastroenterology* 1990; **99**: 799.

42 Kingman S. Hepatitis B status must be known for medical school. *Br. Med. J.* 1994; **308**: 876.

43 Konriskern PJ, Hagopian A, Burke P *et al*. A candidate vaccine for hepatitis B containing the complete viral surface protein. *Hepatology* 1988; **8**: 82.

44 Kosaka Y, Takase K, Kojima M *et al*. Fulminant hepatitis-B-induction by hepatitis-B virus mutants defective in the precore region and incapable of encoding e-antigen. *Gastroenterology* 1991; **100**: 1087.

45 Krugman S, Overby LR, Mushahwar IK *et al*. Viral hepatitis type B: studies on natural history and prevention re-examined. *N. Engl. J. Med.* 1979; **300**: 101.

46 Kurai K, Iino S, Koike K *et al*. Serum titers of pre-S (2) antigen in patients with acute and chronic type B hepatitis: relation to serum aminotransferase activity and other hepatitis B virus markers. *Hepatology* 1989; **9**: 175.

47 Lai KN, Li PKT, Lui SF *et al*. Membranous nephropathy related to hepatitis B virus in adults. *N. Engl. J. Med.* 1991; **324**: 1457.

48 Laskus T, Persing DH, Nowicki MJ *et al*. Nucleotide sequence analysis of the precore region in patients with fulminant hepatitis B in the United States. *Gastroenterology* 1993; **105**: 1173.

49 Levo Y, Gorevic PD, Kassab HJ *et al*. Association between

hepatitis B virus and essential mixed cryoglobulinemia. *N. Engl. J. Med.* 1977; **296**: 1501.

50 Liang TJ, Hasegawa K, Rimon N *et al.* A hepatitis B virus mutant associated with an epidemic of fulminant hepatitis. *N. Engl. J. Med.* 1991; **324**: 1705.

51 Lin C-Y. Hepatitis B virus-associated membranous nephropathy: clinical features, immunological profiles and outcome. *Nephron* 1990; **55**: 37.

52 Lisker-Melman M, Webb D, Di Bisceglie AM *et al.* Glomerulonephritis caused by chronic hepatitis B virus infection: treatment with recombinant human alpha-interferon. *Ann. Intern. Med.* 1989; **111**: 479.

53 McMahon BJ, Heyward WL, Templin DW *et al.* Hepatitis B-associated polyarteritis nodosa in Alaskan Eskimos: clinical and epidemiologic features and long-term follow-up. *Hepatology* 1989; **9**: 97.

54 McMahon BJ, Rhoades ER, Heyward WL *et al.* A comprehensive programme to reduce the incidence of hepatitis B virus infection and its sequelae in Alaskan natives. *Lancet* 1987; **ii**: 1134.

55 Marcellin P, Martinot-Peignoux M, Loriot M-A *et al.* Persistence of hepatitis B virus DNA demonstrated by polymerase chain reaction in serum and liver after loss of HBsAg induced by antiviral therapy. *Ann. Intern. Med.* 1990; **112**: 227.

56 Matsuo A, Kusumoto Y, Ohtsuka E *et al.* Changes in HBsAg carrier rate in Goto Islands, Nagasaki prefecture, Japan. *Lancet* 1990; **335**: 955.

57 Mayans MV, Hall AJ, Inskip HM *et al.* Risk factors for transmission of hepatitis B virus to Gambian children. *Lancet* 1990; **336**: 1107.

58 Mayans MV, Hall AJ, Inskip HM *et al.* Do bedbugs transmit hepatitis B? *Lancet* 1994; **343**: 761.

59 Miller RH, Kaneko S, Chung CT *et al.* Compact organization of the hepatitis B virus genome. *Hepatology* 1989; **9**: 322.

60 MMWR. *Hepatitis Surveillance Report*, no. 52: Atlanta. Centers for Disease Control, Public Health Service 1989.

61 MMWR. Protection against viral hepatitis. *Recommendations of the Immunization Practices Advisory Committee (ACIP)* 1990; **39**: 1.

62 Naoumov NV, Thomas MG, Mason AL *et al.* Genomic variations in the hepatitis B core gene: a possible factor influencing response to interferon alfa treatment. *Gastroenterology* 1995; **108**: 505.

63 Omata M. Significance of extrahepatic replication of hepatitis B virus. *Hepatology* 1990; **12**: 364.

64 Omata M, Ehata T, Yokosuka O *et al.* Mutations in the precore region of hepatitis B virus DNA in patients with fulminant and severe hepatitis. *N. Engl. J. Med.* 1991; **324**: 1699.

65 Omata M, Uchiumi K, Ito Y *et al.* Duck hepatitis B virus and liver diseases. *Gastroenterology* 1983; **85**: 260.

66 Oren I, Hershow RC, Ben-Porath E *et al.* A common-source outbreak of fulminant hepatitis B in a hospital. *Ann. Intern. Med.* 1989; **110**: 691.

67 Penner E, Maida E, Mamoli B *et al.* Serum and cerebrospinal fluid immune complexes containing hepatitis B surface antigen in Guillain–Barré syndrome. *Gastroenterology* 1982; **82**: 576.

68 Petit M-A, Zoulim F, Capel F *et al.* Variable expression of pre S1 antigen in serum during chronic hepatitis B virus infection: an accurate marker for the level of hepatitis B virus replication. *Hepatology* 1990; **11**: 809.

69 Popper H, Shih JW-K, Gerin JL *et al.* Woodchuck hepatitis and hepatocellular carcinoma: correlation of histologic with virologic observations. *Hepatology* 1981; **1**: 91.

70 Sanchez-Quijano A, Jauregui JI, Leal M *et al.* Hepatitis B virus occult infection in subjects with persistent isolated anti-HBc reactivity. *J. Hepatol.* 1993; **17**: 288.

71 Schreeder MT, Thompson SE, Hadler SC *et al.* Hepatitis B in homosexual men: prevalence of infection and factors related to transmission. *J. Infect. Dis.* 1982; **146**: 7.

72 Seeff LB, Koff RS. Passive and active immunoprophylaxis of hepatitis B. *Gastroenterology* 1984; **86**: 958.

73 Shimizu M, Ohyama M, Takahashi Y *et al.* Immunoglobulin M antibody against hepatitis B core antigen for the diagnosis of fulminant type B hepatitis. *Gastroenterology* 1983; **84**: 604.

74 Stevens CE, Taylor PE, Tong MJ *et al.* Yeast-recombinant hepatitis B vaccine. Efficacy with hepatitis B immune globulin in prevention of perinatal hepatitis B virus transmission. *JAMA* 1987; **257**: 2612.

75 Szmuness W, Stevens CE, Harley EJ *et al.* Hepatitis B vaccine: demonstration of efficacy in a controlled trial in a high-risk population in the United States. *N. Engl. J. Med.* 1980; **303**: 833.

76 Thursz MR, Kwiatkowski D, Allsopp CEM *et al.* Association between an MHC class II allele and clearance of hepatitis B virus in the Gambia. *N. Engl. J. Med.* 1995; **332**: 1065.

77 Tilzey AJ. Hepatitis B vaccine boosting: the debate continues. *Lancet* 1995; **345**: 1000.

78 Trépo CG, Ouzan D. Successful therapy of polyarteritis due to hepatitis B virus by combination of plasma exchanges and adenine arabinoside therapy. *Hepatology* 1985; **5**: 1022 (abstract).

79 Ursell PC, Habib A, Sharma P *et al.* Hepatitis B virus and myocarditis. *Hum. Pathol.* 1984; **15**: 481.

80 Venkataseshan VS, Lieberman K, Kim DU *et al.* Hepatitis-B-associated glomerulonephritis: pathology, pathogenesis and clinical course. *Medicine (Baltimore)* 1990; **69**: 200.

81 Villa E, Pasquinelli C, Rigo G *et al.* Gastrointestinal endoscopy and HBV infection: no evidence for a causal relationship. *Gastrointest. Endosc.* 1984; **30**: 15.

82 Welch J, Webster M, Tilzey AJ *et al.* Hepatitis B infections after gynaecological surgery. *Lancet* 1989; **1**: 205.

83 Whittle HC, Maine N, Pilkington J *et al.* Long-term efficacy of continuing hepatitis B vaccination in two Gambian villages. *Lancet* 1995; **345**: 1089.

84 Wong VCW, Ip HMH, Reesink HW *et al.* Prevention of the HBsAg carrier state in newborn infants of mothers who are chronic carriers of HBsAg and HBeAg by administration of hepatitis-B vaccine and hepatitis-B immunoglobulin. *Lancet* 1984; **i**: 921.

85 Yoffe B, Burns DK, Bhatt HS *et al.* Extra hepatic hepatitis B virus DNA sequences in patients with acute hepatitis B infection. *Hepatology* 1990; **12**: 187.

86 Yoshiba M, Sekiyama K, Sugata F *et al.* Reactivation of precore mutant hepatitis B virus leading to fulminant hepatic failure following cytotoxic treatment. *Dig. Dis. Sci.* 1992; **37**: 1253.

87 Zoulek G, Lorbeer B, Jilg W *et al.* Evaluation of a reduced dose of hepatitis B vaccine administered intradermally. *J. Med. Virol.* 1984; **14**: 27.

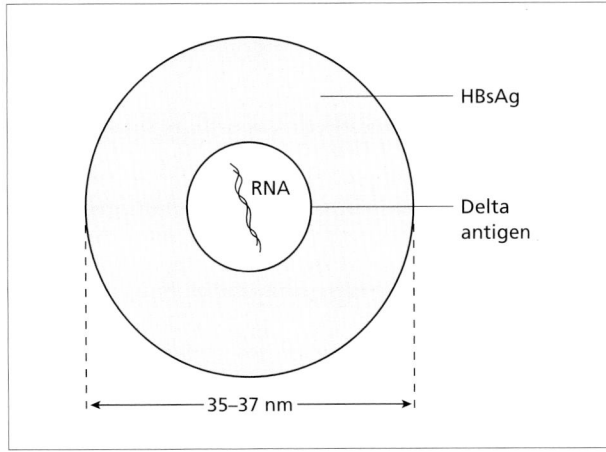

Fig. 16.24. Delta antigen is a small RNA particle coated by HBsAg.

Table 16.11. Characteristics of hepatitis delta virus infection

Satellite virus with hepatitis B
Worldwide
Particularly involves drug abusers
Suppresses replication of HBV
Poor response to interferon: relapses
Returns in transplanted liver

Delta virus (hepatitis D virus, HDV)

The delta agent is a very small (36 nm) RNA particle coated with HBsAg (fig. 16.24, table 16.11) [21]. It is not able to replicate on its own, but is capable of infection when activated by the presence of hepatitis B virus. It resembles satellite viruses of plants which cannot replicate without another specific virus. The interaction between the two viruses is very complex. Synthesis of delta virus may depress the appearance of hepatitis B viral markers in infected cells and even lead to elimination of active hepatitis B viral replication.

Delta virus is a single-stranded, circular, antisense RNA of 1.7 kilobases [19]. It is highly infectious and can induce hepatitis in an HBsAg-positive host. It has been transmitted to chimpanzees carrying hepatitis B [9].

Three genotypes of HDV have been cloned and sequenced. Genotype II is predominant in Taiwan and less frequently associated with fulminant hepatitis than genotype I which is more often associated with cirrhosis and hepatocellular cancer [28].

Hepatitis B and delta infection may be simultaneous (*co-infection*) or delta may infect a chronic HBsAg carrier (*superinfection*) (figs 16.25, 16.26).

Epidemiology

Delta virus infection is not a new disease. Analysis of

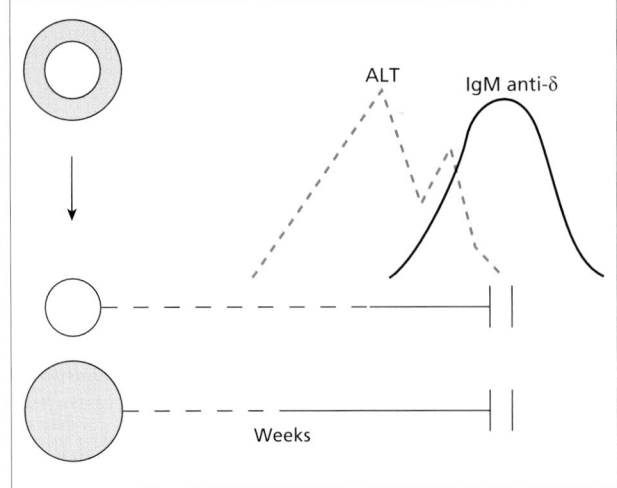

Fig. 16.25. Simultaneous infection with hepatitis B and delta results in acute hepatitis B with rise in ALT (alanine transaminase). Delta infection follows with a second peak of ALT and the appearance of IgM anti-delta in the blood. Clearing of HBsAg is associated with clearing of delta [21].

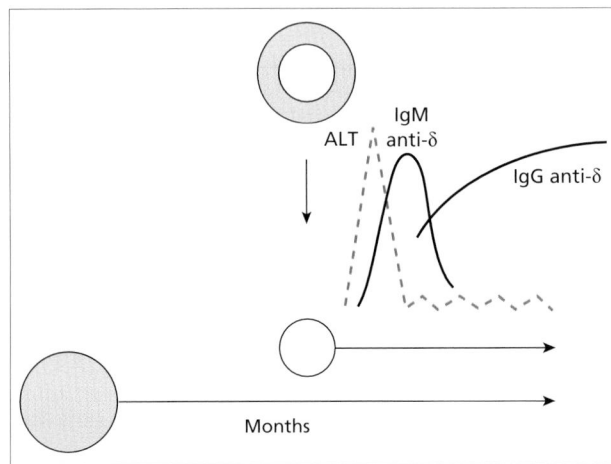

Fig. 16.26. Delta infection in an HBsAg carrier results in an attack of acute hepatitis with the appearance of IgM anti-delta followed by IgG anti-delta in the blood [21].

stored blood shows it among the American army in 1947, in Los Angeles since 1967 [8] and in liver specimens from Brazil in the 1930s.

Delta infection is strongly associated with intravenous drug abuse, but can affect all risk groups for hepatitis B infection. It is infrequent in homosexuals [26] but can affect health-care workers, transfusion recipients [16], haemophiliacs, immigrants and the developmentally disabled [14]. Delta can spread heterosexually [16]. Intra-family spread has been noted in Southern Italy [4]. Children can be affected. Delta infection may be reactivated by HIV infection.

HDV infection is worldwide, but particularly in

southern Europe, the Balkans, Middle East, South India, Taiwan and parts of Africa. An endemic area has been identified in Okinawa, Japan [23].

Epidemics of delta infection have been reported from the Amazon Basin, Brazil (Labrea fever) [3], Colombia (Santa Marta hepatitis) [5], Venezuela [13] and Equatorial Africa. In these areas children of the indigent population are affected and mortality is high.

In Italy, the incidence of early florid acute delta hepatitis is declining rapidly [25] and this will continue with mass vaccination against HBV.

Diagnosis (table 16.12)

Acute delta hepatitis is diagnosed by rising titres of serum IgG anti-delta.

Co-infection is diagnosed by finding serum IgM anti-delta in the presence of high-titre IgM anti-HBc. These markers appear at 1 week, and IgM anti-delta is gone by 5–6 weeks but may last up to 12 weeks [1]. When serum IgM anti-delta disappears, serum IgG anti-delta is found. There may be a window period between the disappearance of one and the detection of the other. Loss of IgM anti-HDV confirms resolution of delta infection, whereas persistence predicts chronicity [11].

HBsAg is positive, but often in low titre and may be undetectable. Serum IgM anti-HBc is also suppressed. Unless delta markers are sought, the patient may be misdiagnosed as acute C hepatitis.

Superinfection of a hepatitis B carrier with delta virus is marked by the early presence of serum IgM anti-delta, usually at the same time as early IgG anti-delta and both antibodies persist [6]. These patients are usually IgM anti-HBc negative, but may have low titres of this antibody. Sufferers of chronic delta infection with chronic hepatitis and active cirrhosis usually have a positive serum IgM anti-delta.

Serum and liver HDV RNA, by staining or PCR, are found in delta antibody-positive patients with acute and chronic HDV infection [7, 17, 27].

Table 16.12. The diagnosis of delta virus infection

	Acute co-infection		
	Early	Convalescence	Chronic
Serum			
IgG anti-HD	+	+ (low titre)	+ (high titre)
IgM anti-HD	+ (late)	–	+
HDAg	+	–	+
HDV RNA	+	–	+
Liver			
HDAg	+	–	–
HDV RNA	+	–	+

Clinical features (figs 16.25, 16.26)

With *co-infection*, the acute delta hepatitis is usually self-limited as the delta cannot outlive the transient HBs antigenaemia. The long-term outlook is therefore good. The clinical picture is usually indistinguishable from hepatitis due to hepatitis B alone. However, a biphasic rise in aspartate transaminase may be noted, the second rise being due to the acute effects of delta [10].

About a third of fulminant hepatitis B is related to coincidental delta infection. There are marked geographic differences in severity.

With *superinfection*, the acute attack may be severe and even fulminant, or may be marked only by a rise in serum transaminase levels. Delta infection should always be considered in any hepatitis B carrier, usually clinically stable, who has a relapse.

Delta infection reduces active hepatitis B viral synthesis and patients are usually HBeAg and HBV DNA negative. Two to 10% lose HBsAg. However, chronic delta hepatitis is usual and this results in acceleration towards cirrhosis.

Episodes of reactivation with delta viraemia can develop [12]. If hepatitis B viraemia persists, the outcome is worse for this favours the spread of delta virus from cell to cell and may increase its pathogenetic potential [24]. Hepato-cellular cancer seems less common in HBsAg carriers with delta. This may be due to inhibition of hepatitis B or rapid progression so that the patient dies before the cancer develops. However, when delta is found with late-stage chronic liver disease it does not seem to influence survival and hepatocellular cancer may be a complication in these patients.

Delta superinfection of healthy B carriers makes the liver disease more severe.

Hepatic histology

Histological severity is greater in delta-positive patients compared with the usual HBV carrier. Intralobular and periportal inflammation is marked. Focal, confluent and bridging necrosis may be seen. Acidophil bodies are noted in the hepatocytes.

The South American and Equatorial African epidemics are marked by microvesicular fat in hepatocytes, intense eosinophilic necrosis and large amounts of delta antigen within the liver [5] (fig. 16.27). These changes have also been noted in a New York drug abuser with delta infection [15]. Morula (plant-like) cells may be seen.

Using immunoperoxidase, delta antigen may be shown in the hepatocyte nuclei. This is reduced in acute delta hepatitis but increases with chronic liver disease and becomes low in the late stage of cirrhosis (fig. 16.28). It correlates with viraemia [27].

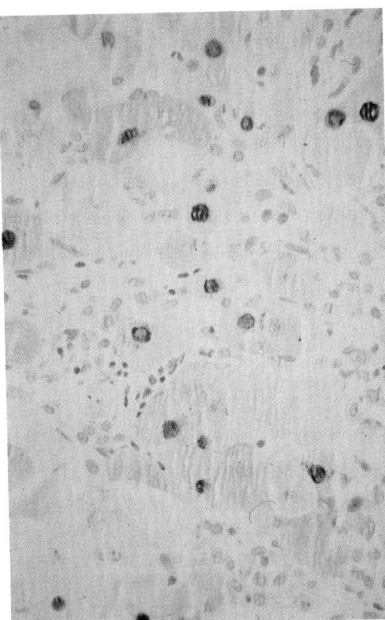

Fig. 16.27. Fulminant acute delta virus hepatitis (Labrea hepatitis) in a 3-year-old girl from Northern Brazil who died with fulminant hepatitis after 3 days' symptoms. An autopsy liver sample shows microvesicular fatty change in large hepatocytes with central nucleus (Morula-vegetable-type cells). (Immunoperoxidase, × 500.)

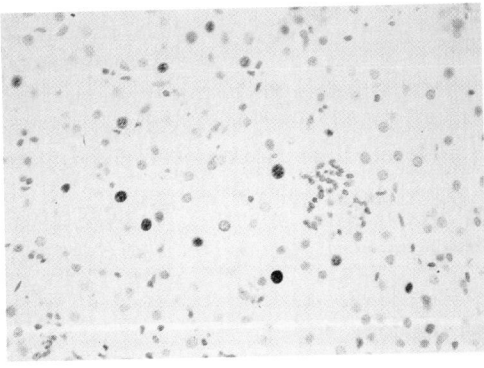

Fig. 16.28. Delta virus hepatitis: immunoperoxidase staining shows delta in hepatocyte nuclei (× 100).

Prevention

Vaccination against hepatitis B makes the recipient immune to hepatitis B virus infection and protects against delta virus infection. Patients likely to contract delta infection should be encouraged to have hepatitis B vaccine.

Hepatitis B carriers must be educated concerning the risks of acquiring delta by continued drug abuse.

Treatment

This is unsatisfactory. Interferon suppresses HDV replication but only transiently.

In a trial of 9 million units, three times a week for 12 months, transaminases normalized in 70% but side-effects were many [22]. 6 months later, 50% still had normal values. Larger doses over longer periods may be necessary [20]. The response is not influenced by concomitant active hepatitis B infection.

Patients treated with interferon who lose HBsAg also lose HDV RNA [2]. Patients receiving a liver transplant for HDV and HBV end-stage liver disease show reduced HBV recurrence [18], the hepatocytes contain large amounts of delta, but hepatitis only develops if there is persistent infection with HBV (see Chapter 35).

References

1 Aragona M, Macagno S, Caredda F *et al.* Serological response to the hepatitis delta virus in hepatitis D. *Lancet* 1987; **i**: 478.
2 Battegay M, Simpson LH, Hoofnagel JH *et al.* Elimination of hepatitis delta virus infection after loss of hepatitis B surface antigen in patients with chronic delta hepatitis. *J. Med. Virol.* 1994; **44**: 389.
3 Bensabath G, Hadler SC, Soares MCP *et al.* Hepatitis delta virus infection and labrea hepatitis. Prevalence and role in fulminant hepatitis in the Amazon Basin. *JAMA* 1987; **258**: 479.
4 Bonino F, Caporaso N, Dentico P *et al.* Familiar clustering and spreading of hepatitis delta virus infection. *J. Hepatol.* 1985; **1**: 221.
5 Buitrago B, Popper H, Hadler SC *et al.* Specific histologic features of Santa Marta hepatitis: a severe form of hepatitis delta-virus infection in Northern South America. *Hepatology* 1986; **6**: 1285.
6 Buti M, Amengual J, Esteban R *et al.* Serological profile of tissue autoantibodies during acute and chronic delta hepatitis. *J. Hepatol.* 1989; **9**: 345.
7 Buti M, Esteban R, Jardi R *et al.* Chronic delta hepatitis: detection of hepatitis delta virus antigen in serum by immunoblot and correlation with other markers of delta viral replication. *Hepatology* 1989; **10**: 907.
8 De Cock KM, Govindarajan S, Chin KP *et al.* Delta hepatitis in the Los Angeles area: a report of 126 cases. *Am. Intern. Med.* 1986; **105**: 108.
9 Fields HA, Govindarajan S, Margolis HS *et al.* Experimental transmission of the delta virus to a hepatitis B chronic carrier chimpanzee with the development of persistent delta carriage. *Am. J. Pathol.* 1986; **122**: 308.
10 Govindarajan S, De Cock KM, Redeker AG. Natural course of delta superinfection in chronic hepatitis B virus-infected patients: histopathologic study with multiple liver biopsies. *Hepatology* 1986; **6**: 640.
11 Govindarajan S, Gupta S, Valinluck B *et al.* Correlation of IgM anti-hepatitis D virus (HDV) to HDV RNA in sera of chronic HDV. *Hepatology* 1989; **10**: 34.
12 Govindarajan S, Smedile, A, De Cock KM *et al.* Study of reactivation of chronic hepatitis delta infection. *J. Hepatol.* 1989; **9**: 204.
13 Hadler SC, De Monzon M, Ponzetto A *et al.* Delta virus infection and severe hepatitis: an epidemic in the Yupca Indians of Venezuela. *Ann. Intern. Med.* 1984; **100**: 339.

14 Hershow RC, Chomel BB, Graham DR *et al.* Hepatitis D virus infection in Illinois state facilities for the developmentally disabled. *Ann. Intern. Med.* 1989; **110**: 779.

15 Lefkowitch JH, Goldstein H, Yatto R *et al.* Cytopathic liver injury in acute delta virus hepatitis. *Gastroenterology* 1987; **92**: 1262.

16 Lettau LA, McCarthy JG, Smith MH *et al.* Outbreak of severe hepatitis due to delta and hepatitis B viruses in parenteral drug abusers and their contacts. *N. Engl. J. Med.* 1987; **317**: 1256.

17 Madejón A, Castillo I, Bartolomé J *et al.* Detection of HDV-RNA by PCR in serum of patients with chronic HDV infection. *J. Hepatol.* 1990; **11**: 381.

18 Ottobrelli A, Marzano A, Smedile A *et al.* Patterns of hepatitis delta virus reinfection and disease in liver transplantation. *Gastroenterology* 1991; **101**: 1649.

19 Polish LB, Gallagher M, Fields HA *et al.* Delta hepatitis. Molecular biology and clinical and epidemiological features. *Clin. Microbiol. Rev.* 1993; **6**: 211.

20 Porres JC, Carreño V, Bartolomé J *et al.* Treatment of chronic delta infection with recombinant human interferon alpha 2c at high doses. *J. Hepatol.* 1989; **9**: 338.

21 Rizzetto M. The delta agent. *Hepatology* 1983; **3**: 729.

22 Rosina F, Pintus C, Meschievitz C *et al.* A randomized controlled trial of a 12-month course of recombinant human interferon-alpha in chronic delta (type D) hepatitis: a multicenter Italian study. *Hepatology* 1991; **13**: 1052.

23 Sakugawa H, Nakasone H, Shokita H *et al.* Seroepidemiological study of hepatitis delta virus infection in Okinawa, Japan. *J. Med. Virol.* 1995; **45**: 312.

24 Smedile A, Rosina F, Saracco G *et al.* Hepatitis B virus replication modulates pathogenesis of hepatitis D virus in chronic hepatitis D. *Hepatology* 1991; **13**: 413.

25 Stroffolini T, Ferrigno L, Cialdea L *et al.* Incidence and risk factors of acute delta hepatitis in Italy: results from a national surveillance system. *J. Hepatol.* 1994; **21**: 1123.

26 Weisfuse IB, Hadler SC, Fields HA *et al.* Delta hepatitis in homosexual men in the United States. *Hepatology* 1989; **9**: 872.

27 Wu J-C, Chen T-A, Huang Y-S *et al.* Natural history of hepatitis D viral superinfection: significance of viremia detected by polymerase chain reaction. *Gastroenterology* 1995; **108**: 796.

28 Wu J-C, Choo K-B, Chen C-M *et al.* Genotyping of hepatitis D virus by restriction-fragment length polymerase and relation to outcome of hepatitis D. *Lancet* 1995; **346**: 939.

Hepatitis C virus (HCV)

The availability of specific serological markers to diagnose hepatitis virus A and virus B infection did not resolve the diagnostic problem of acute and chronic hepatitis. A third, major category had always been suspected but, in the absence of a diagnostic test, had been designated non-A, non-B virus hepatitis. This third type has now been identified and called hepatitis C virus (HCV) (fig. 16.29). Worldwide, HCV infection is probably the most important liver disease. It is estimated that there are 300 million carriers of the virus, about 2.5 million in Europe. In the USA, it is conservatively estimated that approximately 170 000 cases of acute hepatitis C occur per year. Of these, between 70 and 80% will maintain infection and develop chronic hepatitis [3].

In the USA, it accounts for 8000–10 000 deaths per year from chronic liver disease and for 1000 people undergoing transplantation [63].

It was known that post-transfusion non-A, non-B hepatitis could be transmitted to chimpanzees, and from this animal and from the plasma of known infectious blood donors a plasma sample with high infectivity became available. The RNA from this plasma pellet was extracted and by reverse transcriptase a copy DNA prepared (fig. 16.29). A cDNA library was thus constructed by inserting pieces of the genome in a plasmid vector and cloning in *Escherichia coli*. Clones were prepared expressing different proteins, and these were screened against non-A, non-B convalescent serum assumed to contain antibody against the putative non-A, non-B agent. Finally, after testing millions of clones, and after 6

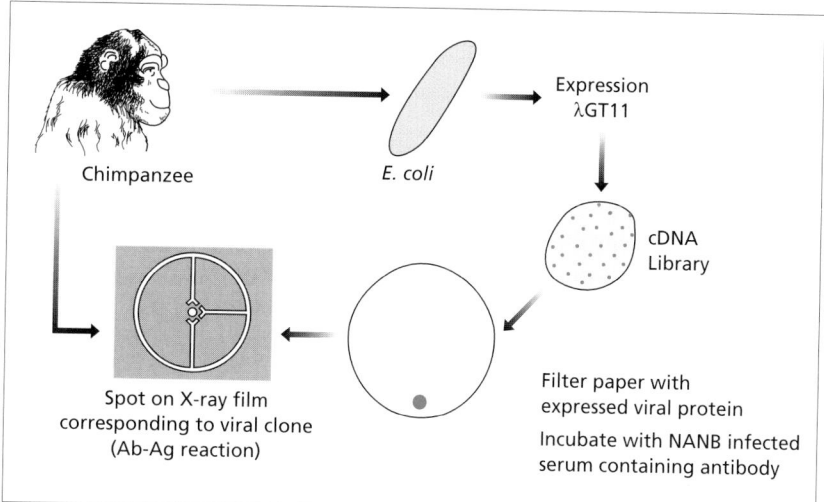

Fig. 16.29. The identification of a viral clone of the hepatitis C virus from chimpanzee liver infected with 'non-A, non-B' virus. This led to the development of antibody tests [68].

years hard work, a virus-specific clone was found which reacted with antibody in the convalescent serum [15]. This HCV cDNA was cloned in yeast and a serological assay developed which detected antibody to a part (c100 epitope) of the HCV virus [5, 68]. Results were validated by showing seroconversion in both the infected chimpanzee and in patients with the naturally occurring disease [5].

HCV is a single-stranded, enveloped RNA virus with one reading frame (fig. 16.30). It is 50–60 nm in size and contains 3011 amino acids and 9033 nucleotides. The agent is probably a distant relative of the flaviviruses of which yellow fever is one member [47].

Serological tests

Serological tests for HCV detect antibodies to viral antigens. The first-generation ELISA test used recombinant antigen c100 (fig. 16.30; table 16.13). Subsequent tests have used HCV recombinant and synthetic peptides and these have proved more sensitive and specific (table 16.14). The third-generation ELISA includes antigens from the putative core, NS3, NS4 and NS5 regions of the virus [18]. The original anti-c100 appeared only 4–6 months and even up to 1 year after the infection, whereas

the antibody to c33 appears early at 11 weeks and always within 20 weeks of the onset (fig. 16.31). False positives still occur and the mean period between infection and detection of antibody is 12 weeks [13]. ELISA blood donor screening is virtually 100% effective in preventing transmission of HCV to recipients [65]. Confirmatory third-generation RIBA assays have much reduced the number of false results [73], but these have not been eliminated [19].

A cDNA PCR has been used to show hepatitis C viral sequences (HCV RNA) in liver and serum. These are usually present in those who have a positive anti-HCV test and confirm infectivity [29]. They are also present in some patients negative for anti-HCV so that the antibody test may underestimate the prevalence of HCV infections. HCV RNA will determine whether positive anti-HCV implies ongoing infectivity or simply past infection. Measurements of HCV RNA should supersede such non-specific measures as the serum transaminases in the management of chronic HCV infection. PCR is a supersensitive technique too complicated, time-consuming, costly and subject to interlaboratory error [73] for routine general use.

A new quantitative method is branched DNA signal amplification [39]. This is costly, but generally available, easy to perform but less sensitive than PCR. Patients can be viraemic although the bDNA test is negative [11]. The specimen must be collected under optimal conditions, centrifuged within 2 hours of clot formation and separ-

Table 16.13. The % prevalence of anti-HCV among blood donors using ELISA and supplemental testing [3]

UK	0.075–0.01
Scandinavia	0.01–0.1
North America	0.3
Mediterranean	0.67
South America	2.0
Africa	1.4
Japan	2.2
Australia	0.06
Egypt	4
Other risk groups	
Haemophiliacs	70
Drug abusers	76
Homosexuals	43

Table 16.14. Serological tests for hepatitis C depend on antigen proteins from different domains of the viral genome

	Non-structural			Core
Antigen protein	c100	5-1-1	c33	c22
ELISA 1	+			
RIBA 2	+	+		
ELISA 2/RIBA 4	+	+	+*	+

* Appears early: 11–20 weeks.
Also HCV RNA by PCR.

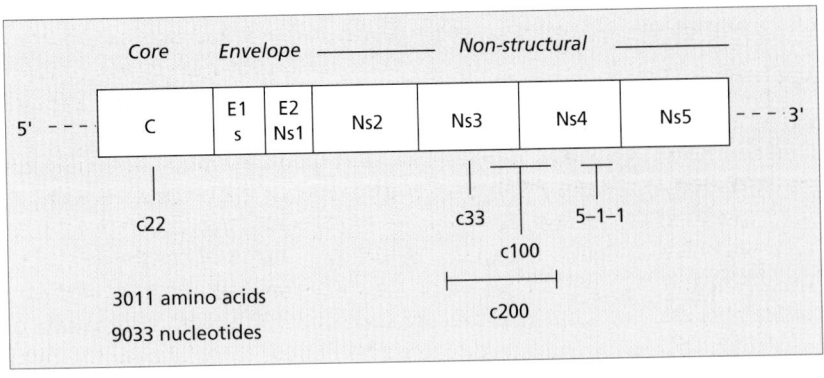

Fig. 16.30. Hepatitis C virus is a single-stranded, enveloped RNA virus, size 50–60 nm. It has core (C), envelope (E) and non-structural (Ns) domains. Schematic alignment of the polyproteins encoded by the HCV is shown. The relative locations of the individual viral proteins c22, c33 and c100 are shown. Putative domains in the HCV encoded polyproteins are indicated.

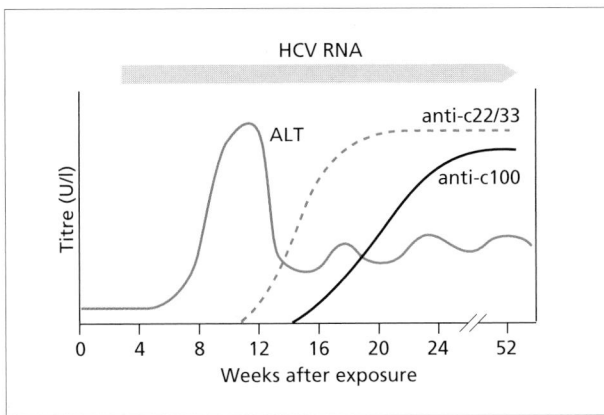

Fig. 16.31. The serological course of chronic hepatitis C infection. Note that HCV RNA appears early, before the rise in alanine transferase (ALT), and persists. Anti-c22/33 appears at 12 weeks and anti HCV-100 only appears about 20 weeks after exposure.

ated immediately. If possible, the specimen should be frozen within 2 hours of collection [20]. Using the bDNA HCV RNA test, most donors who are anti-HCV positive are positive by PCR which does not however, correlate with the serum transaminases [45]. Transaminases can be normal although circulating virus is present in high titre. The level of serum HCV RNA by bDNA signal amplification correlates with the histological severity [45]. The method is useful in assessing therapy [20].

Serum IgM anti-HCV correlates with active viral infection and biochemical evidence of active liver disease in acute and chronic HCV infection [12, 55].

The virus has not been cultured. Man and non-human primates seem the only susceptible species. The virus has been visualized by immune electron microscopy [34, 59].

Genotypes

There is considerable heterogeneity in HCV, particularly in the viral envelope region [60]. Core is relatively well preserved. The stable 5′ non-coding region has been amplified for genotyping. There are six phylogenic groups and at least 50 genotypes. There is considerable geographic variation in the prevalence of the various genotypes (table 16.15).

Genotype 1b is particularly serious. It is perhaps related to long duration of infection and is associated with a past blood transfusion or no obvious source of infection. It is found particularly in Australia, Europe and the USA. A sustained response to interferon is markedly reduced with genotype 1b [10, 45]. The response to interferon is much better with types 2a and 2b than with 1b [22]. Viral load and genotype are the best indications of a sustained response to interferon [6, 45].

Table 16.15. Geographic distribution of HCV genotypes

Area	Type
Europe	1, 2, 3
Australia	1, 2, 3
USA	1, 2, 3
Far East	1, 2
Middle East	4
North Africa	4
South Africa	5

Genotype 1b may favour recurrence after hepatic transplantation.

Type 4, largely found in the Middle East, is also associated with a poor response to interferon.

HCV quasi-species

RNA viruses are thought to consist of heterogeneous mixtures of closely related mutant genomes which result from the high error rates in RNA replication. This is referred to as a quasi-species nature. The degree of diversity is related to the progression of liver disease [32]. The quasi-species show different sensitivities to interferon [37, 49]. Lower heterogeneity increases the response to antiviral treatment for there are fewer variants to evade immune surveillance and so survive after antiviral treatment [37].

Epidemiology

Blood transfusion

Hepatitis C is carried by about 0.01–2% of blood donors worldwide (table 16.13) [3, 57]. The risk factors associated with acute hepatitis C in the USA are present or past injecting of drugs, transfusions in the past, health-care employment, sexual/household contact and a low socioeconomic status (fig. 16.32) [3]. Earlier studies using first-generation tests overestimated the prevalence of anti-HCV in blood donors. If supplemental testing is used, the prevalence in the UK and Scandinavia is only 0.01–0.1% and in the USA, only 0.3%. Egypt seems to have the highest prevalence in blood donors [1]. Anti-HCV was found in 12% of rural primary children, 22.1% of Army recruits and 16.4% in children with hepatosplenomegaly [1].

The introduction of second-generation screening for anti-HCV has greatly reduced the incidence of post-transfusion hepatitis. In Spain, it fell from 9.6 to 1.9% [31]. In Japan, the fall was 73% [33]. In the USA, the prevalence of post-transfusion hepatitis was reduced 73% in those screened for HCV with estimation of surrogate markers [24]. These (anti-HBc and alanine

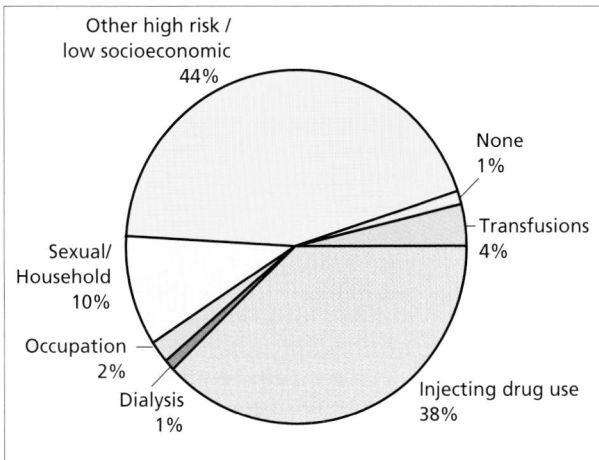

Fig. 16.32. Risk factors associated with acute hepatitis C in the USA (1990–1993). These include sexual or household contacts, health-care employment, multiple exposures to blood and injecting drug abuse. Other high-risk patients include low socio-economic status and multiple sexual partners. From the Sentinel Centers for Disease Control and Prevention [3].

transferase) are rarely performed now that anti-HCV screening is done. Their value has not been clearly established [9].

Other blood products

Those receiving repeated blood transfusions are at particular risk. Thalassaemics, because of repeated blood transfusions, have an anti-HCV prevalence of between 10 and 50% [42, 69].

Until about 1964, therapeutic coagulation factors contained HCV [41]. This has resulted in a prevalence of nearly 100% HCV in haemophiliac patients receiving unsterilized large-pool coagulation factors [67]. Introduction of vapour heated clotting factors has controlled this method of spread.

Patients with primary hypogammaglobulinaemia have developed hepatitis C after treatment with contaminated immunoglobulin [8, 71].

Contaminated anti-rhesus D immunoglobulin has caused large outbreaks of HCV in Ireland [54] and Germany [23]. Claims for compensation are being considered.

Parenteral exposure

The chances of HCV after a needle-stick exposure to a patient with a positive HCV RNA is 3–10% [48, 61].

Dentists are at risk of acquiring HCV, presumably from the blood and saliva of their patients. Thus, in New York City, anti-HCV was found in eight (1.75%) of 456 dentists compared with one (0.14%) of 723 control subjects. Oral surgeons are at particular risk [36]. An infected surgeon can transmit HCV to patients [26].

Dialysis patients develop HCV not only from blood transfusions but by negligent dialysis techniques [51]. The chances of infection increase with the years on dialysis.

Injecting drug users using shared needles and syringes account for 40% of acute HCV in the USA. The injection may have occurred many years ago, forgotten by the patient [17]. In an urban situation, 28% of injecting drug users will show anti-HCV positive after 2 years of injecting [64].

Sexual and intra-familial spread

This is debated but is generally believed to be very low [11]. Studies have tended to be based on few patients and to be uncontrolled. Results have depended on anti-HCV estimations rather than HCV RNA. In most population studies, anti-HCV does not appear until the age of 16 years. This would suggest that sexual transmission is important [62]. There are geographical differences in reported prevalence of sexual transmission. However, consorts of anti-HCV positive haemophiliac patients have tested positive and HCV has been linked with multiple sexual partners [4]. But in a Spanish study, only 6% of heterosexual contacts of injecting drug users were positive [25].

Serum samples of 94 husbands of women with HCV following contaminated immunoglobulin showed no HCV RNA [46]. Only three of their 231 children who were investigated showed serological evidence of HCV.

It is difficult to counsel couples where one member is HCV positive. Those with a steady sexual partner should not change their sexual practices. Those with multiple sexual partners should use safe sex. Prevalence in homosexuals is 3%, in prostitutes 6% and in heterosexuals attending a sexually transmitted disease clinic, 4%.

Intra-familial spread is rare but has been reported with the same strain of HCV [32].

Vertical transmission is infrequent. It is greater if the mother is serum HCV RNA positive [50]. Transmission may be increased by concomitant maternal HIV infection [74]. Infection is more likely if the mother suffers an acute attack in the last trimester. Breast milk does not seem to transmit HCV [43]. Babies born to anti-HCV positive mothers usually have circulating antibody for 6 months, presumably due to passive transfer, but HCV RNA is absent [56].

In those with no obvious risk factors

Where did the disease come from in the millions of carriers without risk factors? Family spread is possible but rare. Infection may be through sharing razors, toothbrushes or unsterile syringes and needles with infected people. Other possibilities include past abuse of intravenous drugs and folk remedies such as acupuncture and cutting skin using non-sterilized knives [35].

Hepatitis C is much less infectious than hepatitis B. The passage of large quantities of infective material is necessary for transmission.

Acute hepatitis C

The disease has an incubation period of 5–12 weeks. Only 25% of sufferers are jaundiced and the patient may be completely asymptomatic. The anti-HIV-positive patient may have a rapidly progressive course [44].

Fulminant hepatitis is variably associated with HCV. In the West, non-A, non-B fulminant hepatitis seems to be also non-C [38]. However, in Los Angeles, nine of 15 patients with fulminant acute hepatitis were HCV RNA positive [66]. In Japan and Taiwan, HCV is identified in about 50% of patients with fulminant hepatitis [16, 72].

Aplastic anaemia [7], agranulocytosis and peripheral neuropathy may be complications.

Serum transaminases are only moderately elevated — about 15 times the upper limit of normal. Serum hepatitis C RNA can be detected 1–2 weeks after infection [30]. Serum transaminases increase at 7–8 weeks. In those that recover completely, serum HCV RNA is lost but antibody persists for months.

At 1 year, the majority of sufferers from post-transfusion hepatitis will still have raised serum transaminase levels. Most of these patients will develop chronic hepatitis and 20% will proceed to cirrhosis. The disease is insidious and marked by fluctuant serum transaminases (see Chapter 17).

Hepatitis C infection is a frequent association of hepato-cellular cancer (see Chapter 17).

Associated conditions

HCV exerts a suppressor effect on HBV and HDV [53]. Nevertheless, patients having dual or triple viral infection with HCV plus HBV and HDV have more severe progressive liver disease, resistant to interferon [40].

HCV RNA levels are higher in HIV-infected haemophiliac patients [27], but this does not seem to predict survival [70]. Alcoholic liver disease may increase serum HCV RNA and so modulate interferon efficiency [52].

Prevention

Screening donor blood for anti-HCV has reduced post-transfusion hepatitis as has the reduction in the use of shared syringes and needles, an example from Egypt is the reduced used of tartar emetic to treat bilharzial infec-

tion using shared equipment. Vaccines will be difficult to prepare as the amounts of virus in the blood are very small. HCV vaccine development is in its infancy. The major problems are the heterogeneity of the virus and the lack of an identified neutralizing antibody. The highly conserved 5'-non-coding region is useful for PCR but not for vaccine development. There is a need to find a critical, conserved region that would code for an antigen capable of eliciting wide-based immunity. *In vitro* systems for propagating HCV are necessary to facilitate investigations into the cross-neutralization of different viral isolates. Envelope virus vaccines have been tested against chimpanzees but do not provide immunity to heterologous or homologous HCV infection [28]. Perhaps the patients with multiple episodes of HCV infection are in a similar position to the chimpanzees.

Another vaccine trial in chimpanzees was marred by the use of large doses of recombinant viral protein which would not be practical for widespread use [14]. Moreover, the challenge was performed with a low inoculum of virus and at the time of the expected peak level of antibody. The durability of the antibody response is uncertain.

Anti-HCV positive blood donors

Management is difficult as the natural history of any individual patient is difficult to predict. An algorithm is based on confirmation of anti-HCV by a second-generation test, serum HCV RNA and liver biopsy where necessary [21] (fig. 16.33). Most of anti-HCV positive

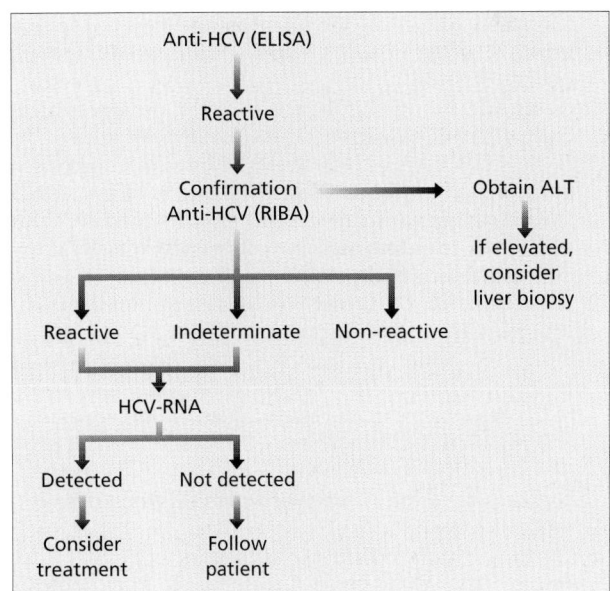

Fig. 16.33. Algorithm for further evaluation of anti-HCV enzyme-linked immunosorbent assay (ELISA) positive specimens [21].

donors harbour HCV RNA in serum and can transmit HCV regardless of whether serum transminases are elevated [2]. Most blood donors with anti-HCV have chronic HCV regardless of their serum ALT levels. Donors with normal ALT and no HCV RNA in the serum generally have normal histological findings or minimal changes and have probably recovered from HCV infection [58].

References

1 Abdel-Wahab MF, Zakaria S, Kamel M *et al*. High seroprevalence of hepatitis C infection among risk groups in Egypt. *Am. J. Trop. Med. Hyg.* 1994; **51**: 563.

2 Alberti A, Morsica G, Chemello L *et al*. Hepatitis C viraemia and liver disease in symptom-free individuals with anti-HCV. *Lancet* 1992; **340**: 697.

3 Alter MJ. Epidemiology of hepatitis C in the West. *Semin. Liver. Dis.* 1995; **15**: 5.

4 Alter MJ, Coleman PJ, Alexander WJ *et al*. Importance of heterosexual activity in the transmission of hepatitis B and non-A, non-B hepatitis. *JAMA* 1989; **262**: 1201.

5 Alter JH, Purcell RH, Shih JW *et al*. Detection of antibody to hepatitis C virus in prospectively followed transfusion recipients with acute non-A, non-B hepatitis. *N. Engl. J. Med.* 1989; **321**: 1494.

6 Aiyama T, Yoshioka K, Hirofuji H *et al*. Changes in serum hepatitis C virus RNA titer and response to interferon therapy in patients with chronic hepatitis C. *Dig. Dis. Sci.* 1994; **39**: 2244.

7 Bannister P, Miloszewski K, Barnard D *et al*. Fatal marrow aplasia associated with non-A, non-B hepatitis. *Br. Med. J.* 1983; **286**: 1314.

8 Bjøro K, Frøland SS, Yun Z *et al*. Hepatitis C infection in patients with primary hypogammaglobulinemia after treatment with contaminated immune globulin. *N. Engl. J. Med.* 1994; **331**: 1607.

9 Blajchman MA, Bull SB, Feinman SV. Post-transfusion hepatitis: impact of non-A, non-B hepatitis surrogate tests. *Lancet* 1995; **345**: 21.

10 Booth JCL, Brown JL, Thomas HC. The management of chronic hepatitis V virus infection. *Gut* 1995; **37**: 449.

11 Bresters D, Cuypers HTM, Reesink HW *et al*. Comparison of quantitative cDNA-PCR with the branched DNA hybridization assay for monitoring plasma hepatitis C virus RNA levels in haemophilia patients participating in a controlled interferon trial. *J. Med. Virol.* 1994; **43**: 262.

12 Brillanti S, Foli M, Gaiani S *et al*. Persistent hepatitis C viraemia without liver disease. *Lancet* 1993; **341**: 464.

13 Busch MP, Tobler LH, Francis B *et al*. Reinstatement of donors who test false-positive in second-generation hepatitis C virus enzyme immunoassay should await availability of licensed third-generation tests. *Transfusion* 1994; **34**: 278.

14 Choo Q-L, Kuo G, Ralston R *et al*. Vaccination of chimpanzees against infection by the hepatitis C virus. *Proc. Natl. Acad. Sci. USA* 1994; **91**: 1294.

15 Choo Q-L, Kuo G, Weiner AJ *et al*. Isolation of a cDNA clone derived from blood-borne non-A, non-B, viral hepatitis genome. *Science* 1989; **244**: 359.

16 Chu C-M, Sheen I-S, Liaw Y-F. The role of hepatitis C virus in fulminant viral hepatitis in an area with endemic hepatitis A and B. *Gastroenterology* 1994; **107**: 189.

17 Conry-Cantilena C, Van Raden M, Gibble J *et al*. Routes of infection, viremia, and liver disease in blood donors found to have hepatitis C virus infection. *N. Engl. J. Med.* 1996; **334**: 1691.

18 Couroucé A-M, Bouchardeau F, Girault A *et al*. Significance of NS3 and NS5 antigens in screening for HCV antibody. *Lancet* 1994; **343**: 853.

19 Craxi A, Valenza M, Fabiano C *et al*. Third-generation hepatitis C virus tests in asymptomatic anti-HCV-positive blood donors. *J. Hepatol.* 1994; **21**: 730.

20 Davis GL, Lau JYN, Urdea MS *et al*. Quantitative detection of hepatitis C virus RNA with a solid-phase signal amplification method: definition of optimal conditions for specimen collection and clinical application in interferon treated patients. *Hepatology* 1994; **19**: 1337.

21 De Medina M, Schiff ER. Hepatitis C: diagnostic assays. *Semin. Liver Dis.* 1995; **15**: 33.

22 Diodati G, Bonetti P, Tagger A *et al*. Relationship between serum HCV markers and response to interferon therapy in chronic hepatitis C. Evaluation of HCV genotypes during and after long-term follow-up. *Dig. Dis. Sci.* 1994; **39**: 2497.

23 Dittmann S, Roggendorf M, Dürkop J *et al*. Long-term persistence of hepatitis C virus antibodies in a single source outbreak. *J. Hepatol.* 1991; **13**: 323.

24 Donahue JG, Muñoz A, Ness PM *et al*. The declining risk of post-transfusion hepatitis C virus infection. *N. Engl. J. Med.* 1992; **327**: 369.

25 Esteban JI, Esteban R, Viladomiu L *et al*. Hepatitis C virus antibodies among risk groups in Spain. *Lancet* 1989; **2**: 294.

26 Esteban JI, Gomez J, Martell M *et al*. Transmission of hepatitis C virus by a cardiac surgeon. *N. Engl. J. Med.* 1996; **334**: 555.

27 Eyster ME, Fried MW, Di Besceglie AM *et al*. Increasing hepatitis C virus RNA levels in hemophiliacs: relationship to human immunodeficiency virus infection and liver disease. *Blood* 1994; **84**: 1020.

28 Farci P, Alter HJ, Govindarajan S *et al*. Lack of protective immunity against reinfection with hepatitis C virus. *Science* 1992; **258**: 135.

29 Farci P, Alter HJ, Wong D *et al*. A long-term study of hepatitis C virus replication in non-A, non-B hepatitis. *N. Engl. J. Med.* 1991; **325**: 98.

30 Garson JA, Tuke PW, Makris M *et al*. Demonstration of viraemia patterns in haemophiliacs treated with hepatitis-C-virus-contaminated factor VIII concentrates. *Lancet* 1990; **336**: 1022.

31 González A, Esteban JI, Madoz P *et al*. Efficacy of screening donors for antibodies to the hepatitis C virus to prevent transfusion-associated hepatitis: final report of a prospective trial. *Hepatology* 1995; **22**: 439.

32 Honda M, Kaneko S, Sakai A *et al*. Degree of diversity of hepatitis C virus quasispecies and progression of liver disease. *Hepatology* 1994; **20**: 1144.

33 Japanese Red Cross Non-A, non-B hepatitis research group. Effect of screening for hepatitis C virus antibody and hepatitis B virus core antibody on incidence of post-transfusion hepatitis. *Lancet* 1991; **338**: 1040.

34 Kaito M, Watanabe S, Tsukiyama-Kohara K *et al*. Hepatitis C virus particle detected by immunoelectron microscopic study. *J. Gen. Virol.* 1994; **75**: 1755.

35 Kiyosawa K, Tanaka E, Sodeyama T *et al*. Transmission of hepatitis C in an isolated area in Japan: community-acquired infection. *Gastroenterology* 1994; **106**: 1596.

36 Klein RS, Freeman K, Taylor PE *et al*. Occupational risk for hepatitis C virus infection among New York City dentists. *Lancet* 1991; **338**: 1539.

37 Koizumi K, Enomoto N, Kurosaki M *et al*. Diversity of quasispecies in various disease stages of chronic hepatitis C virus infection and its significance in interferon treatment. *Hepatology* 1995; **22**: 30.

38 Kuwada SK, Patel VM, Hollinger FB *et al*. Non-A, non-B fulminant hepatitis is also non-E and non-C. *Am. J. Gastroenterol*. 1994; **89**: 57.

39 Lau JYN, Davis GL, Kniffen J *et al*. Significance of serum hepatitis C virus RNA levels in chronic hepatitis C. *Lancet* 1993; **341**: 1501.

40 Liaw YF. Role of hepatitis C virus in dual and triple hepatitis virus infection. *Hepatology* 1995; **22**: 1101.

41 Makris M, Preston FE. Chronic hepatitis in haemophilia. *Blood Rev*. 1993; **7**: 243.

42 Makris M, Preston FE, Triger DR *et al*. Hepatitis C antibody and chronic liver disease in haemophilia. *Lancet* 1990; **335**: 1117.

43 Manzini P, Saracco G, Cerchier A *et al*. Human immunodeficiency virus infection as risk factor for mother-to-child hepatitic C virus transmission; persistence of anti-hepatitis C virus in children is associated with the mother's anti-hepatitis C virus immunoblotting patterns. *Hepatology* 1995; **21**: 328.

44 Martin P, Di Bisceglie AM, Kassianides C *et al*. Rapidly progressive non-A, non-B hepatitis in patients with human immunodeficiency virus infection. *Gastroenterology* 1989; **97**: 1559.

45 Martinot-Peignoux M, Marcellin P, Gournay J *et al*. Detection and quantitation of serum HCV-RNA by branched DNA amplification in anti-HCV positive blood donors. *J. Hepatol*. 1994; **20**: 676.

46 Meisel H, Reip A, Faltus B *et al*. Transmission of hepatitis C virus to children and husbands by women infected with contaminated anti-D immunoglobulin. *Lancet* 1995; **345**: 1209.

47 Miller RH, Purcell RH. Hepatitis C virus shares amino acid sequence similarity with pestiviruses and flaviviruses as well as members of two plant virus supergroups. *Proc. Natl. Acad. Sci. USA* 1990; **87**: 2057.

48 Mitsui T, Iwano K, Masuko K *et al*. Hepatitis C virus infection in medical personnel after needlestick accident. *Hepatology* 1992; **16**: 1109.

49 Mizokami M, Lau JYN, Suzuki K *et al*. Differential sensitivity of hepatitis C virus quasispecies to interferon-α therapy. *J. Hepatol*. 1994; **21**: 884.

50 Ohto H, Terazawa S, Sasaki N *et al*. Transmission of hepatitis C virus from mothers to infants. *N. Engl. J. Med*. 1994; **330**: 744.

51 Okuda K, Hayashi H, Kobayashi S *et al*. Mode of hepatitis C infection not associated with blood transfusion among chronic hemodialysis patients. *J. Hepatol*. 1995; **23**: 28.

52 Oshita M, Hayashi N, Kasahara A *et al*. Increased serum hepatitis C virus RNA levels among alcoholic patients with chronic hepatitis C. *Hepatology* 1994; **20**: 1115.

53 Pontisso P, Ruvoletto MG, Fattovich G *et al*. Clinical and virological profiles in patients with multiple hepatitis virus infections. *Gastroenterology* 1993; **105**: 1529.

54 Power JP, Lawlor E, Davidson F *et al*. Molecular epidemiology of an outbreak of infection with hepatitis C virus in recipients of anti-D immunoglobulin. *Lancet* 1995; **345**: 1211.

55 Quiroga JA, Binsbergen JV, Wang CY *et al*. Immunoglobulin M antibody to hepatitis C virus core antigen; correlations with viral replication, histological activity and liver disease outcome. *Hepatology* 1995; **22**: 1635.

56 Reinus J, Lelkin E, Alter H *et al*. Vertical transmission of hepatitis C virus. *Gastroenterology* 1991; A-789.

57 Sherlock S. Chronic hepatitis C. *Disease-a-month* 1994; **40**: 122.

58 Shakil AO, Conry-Cantilena C, Alter HJ *et al*. Volunteer blood donors with antibody to hepatitis C virus: clinical, biochemical and virologic and histologic features. *Ann. Intern. Med*. 1995; **123**: 330.

59 Shimizu YK, Feinstone SM, Kohara M *et al*. Hepatitis C virus: detection of intracellular virus particles by electron microscopy. *Hepatology* 1996; **23**: 305.

60 Simmonds P. Variability of hepatitis C virus. *Hepatology* 1995; **21**: 570.

61 Sodeyama T, Kiyosawa K, Urushihara A *et al*. Detection of hepatitis C virus markers and hepatitis C virus genomic-RNA after needlestick accidents. *Arch. Intern. Med*. 1993; **153**: 1565.

62 Tedder RS, Gilson RJC, Briggs M *et al*. Hepatitis C virus: evidence for sexual transmission. *Br. Med. J*. 1991; **302**: 1299.

63 Terrault N, Wright T. Interferon and hepatitis C. *N. Engl. J. Med*. 1995; **332**: 1509.

64 Thomas DL, Vlahov D, Solomon L *et al*. Correlates of hepatitis C virus infections among injection drug users. *Medicine (Baltimore)* 1995; **74**: 212.

65 Van der Poel CL, Cuypers HT, Reesink HW. Hepatitis C virus six years on. *Lancet* 1994; **344**: 1475.

66 Villamil FG, Hu K-Q, Yu C-H *et al*. Detection of hepatitis C virus with RNA polymerase chain reaction in fulminant hepatic failure. *Hepatology* 1995; **22**: 1379.

67 Watson HG, Ludlam CA, Rebus S *et al*. Use of several second-generation serological assays to determine the true prevalence of hepatitis C virus infection in haemophiliacs treated with non-virus inactivated factor VIII and IX concentrates. *Br. J. Haematol*. 1992; **80**: 514.

68 Weiner AJ, Kuo G, Bradley DW *et al*. Detection of hepatitis C viral sequences in non-A, non-B hepatitis. *Lancet* 1990; **335**: 1.

69 Wonke B, Hoffbrand AV, Brown D *et al*. Antibody to hepatitis C virus in multiply transfused patients with thalassemia major *J. Clin. Pathol*. 1990; **43**: 638.

70 Wright TL, Hollander H, Pu X *et al*. Hepatitis C in HIV-infected patients with and without AIDS: prevalence and relationship to patient survival. *Hepatology* 1994; **20**: 1152.

71 Yap PL, McOmish F, Webster ADB *et al*. Hepatitis C virus transmission by intravenous immunoglobulin. *J. Hepatol*. 1994; **21**: 455.

72 Yoshiba M, Dehara K, Inoue K *et al*. Contribution of hepatitis C virus to non-A, non-B fulminant hepatitis in Japan. *Hepatology* 1994; **19**: 829.

73 Zaaijer HL, Cuypers HTM, Reesink HW. Reliability of polymerase chain reaction for detection of hepatitis C virus. *Lancet* 1993; **341**: 722.

74 Zanetti AR, Tanzi E, Paccagnini S *et al*. Mother-to-infant transmission of hepatitis C virus. *Lancet* 1995; **345**: 289.

Hepatitis G virus (GBV)

For some time it has been believed that there was another non-A, non-B, non-C agent causing hepatitis in humans. The incubation periods for post-transfusion hepatitis is 14–145 days, too long for hepatitis B or C. In the USA, about 5% of chronic liver disease remains cryptogenic (non-A, non-B, non-C) and half the patients have been transfused [3]. Autoantibodies are absent.

In 1967, Friedrich Deinhardt showed that serum taken from a 34-year-old Chicago Surgeon with acute hepatitis induced hepatitis in tamarin monkeys [2]. The hepatitis could be passaged serially. The agent was designated HGBV, GB being the initials of the surgeon. The putative virus has now been investigated by a subtractive PCR method (representational difference analysis, RDA), and specific nucleotide sequences have been cloned from a GBV-infected tamarin monkey [7]. Three agents have been identified, HGBVA and HGBVB, which are probably tamarin viruses, and HGBVC which is a human virus.

Another recently identified agent, HGV was cloned from a patient with community-acquired chronic hepatitis whose plasma had transmitted hepatitis to tamarin monkeys [5]. Sequences of HGBVC and HGV are more than 95% homologous and the two are considered to be closely related isolates of the same virus.

The genomic structure of HGV/HGBVC has been sequenced and placed in the flaviviridae family. It has less than 25% sequence homology with HCV and other members of the flaviviridae family [4]. A PCR has been developed to monitor viraemia. A reliable antibody test is awaited.

The clinical significance of HGV remains uncertain [1]. The agent has been transmitted to chimpanzees with no resultant rises in transaminases or liver biopsy changes. 1–2% of blood donors in the United States are positive for HGV. It is more prevalent in the population than HCV [1]. Risk factors are similar to those for HCV. They include past-transfusion, non-A, non-E hepatitis, intravenous drug abuse, haemophiliacs receiving blood products and the multiply transfused.

The acute hepatitis is usually mild, with only modest or no rises in transaminase [1]. However, GBV has been associated with fulminant hepatitis of unknown aetiology in Japan [8].

HGV is detected in 3.1% of Japanese patients on haemodialysis, and those positive have more evidence of active disease [6]. It could persist in the blood for up to 16 years.

HGV is detected in 33% of patients after liver transplant and the effect may be more serious in the immunosuppressed. HGV is detected in 6% of patients with sporadic chronic hepatitis.

It remains to be determined whether HGV is an innocent bystander or a serious human pathogen. Serial observations on clinical features, hepatic histology and viral titres are not available. HGV will not be the last in the hepatitis alphabet and other hepatitis viruses remain to be identified [1].

References

1 Alter HJ. The cloning and clinical implications of HGV and HGBV-C. *N. Engl. Med. J.* 1996; **334**: 1536.
2 Deinhardt F, Holmes AW, Capps RB *et al.* Studies on the transmission of human viral hepatitis to marmoset monkeys. 1 Transmission of disease, serial passages and description of liver lesions. *J. Exp. Med.* 1967; **135**: 673.
3 Kodali VP, Gordon SC, Silverman AL *et al.* Cryptogenic liver disease in the United States: further evidence for non-A, non-B and non-C hepatitis. *Am. J. Gastroenterol.* 1994; **89**: 1836.
4 Leary TP, Muerhoff AS, Simon SJN *et al.* Sequence and genomic organization of GBV-C: a novel member of the flaviviridae associated with human non-A–E hepatitis. *J. Med. Virol.* 1996; **48**: 60.
5 Linnen J, Wages J Jr, Zhang-Keek ZY *et al.* Molecular cloning and disease association of hepatitis G virus: a transfusion-transmissible agent. *Science* 1996; **271**: 505.
6 Masuko K, Mitsui T, Iwano K *et al.* Infection with hepatitis GV virus C in patients on maintenance hemodialysis. *N. Engl. J. Med.* 1996; **334**: 1485.
7 Simons JN, Leary TP, Dawson GJ *et al.* Isolation of novel virus-like sequences associated with human hepatitis. *Nat. Med.* 1995; **1**: 564.
8 Yoshiba M, Okamoto H, Mishiro S. Detection of the GBV-C hepatitis virus genome in serum from patients with fulminant hepatitis of unknown aetiology. *Lancet* 1995; **346**: 1121.

Hepatitis E virus (HEV)

This accounts for sporadic and major epidemics of viral hepatitis in developing countries. Previously, many large epidemics of hepatitis believed due to HAV have now been identified as caused by HEV. The disease is enterically transmitted, usually by sewage-contaminated water. The virus has been successfully transmitted to monkeys but attempts at *in vitro* propagation have not met with success.

Hepatitis E is a 32–34 nm RNA virus, unenveloped and with three ORFs. It is probably a member of the calci virus group (such as the Norwalk virus) which are normally associated with severe diarrhoea.

It is difficult to obtain large quantities of virus from the stools as it is probably degraded in the gut. However, bile from acutely infected animals is a rich source. The first HEV nucleotide sequence was from an isolate from Burma [13]. Subsequently complete sequences have been reported from Mexico [16], Pakistan and China [7]. There is some sequence variation, particularly between the Mexican and Burmese strains. Sequence variability is evident particularly in one region of the non-structural ORF. Isolation of virus is difficult from stools and low faecal excretion of virus probably accounts for the low secondary spread [11]. Immunity probably wanes and longevity of protective antibody is uncertain.

Sequencing of the HEV genome has allowed the development of specific diagnostic tests. Recombinant proteins expressed from cloned HEV derived from Mexican and Burmese isolates are included in antibody tests. These detect both IgG and IgM antibodies [4]. More than one isolate is needed and the antibody tests are not completely satisfactory [10]. HEV RNA can be determined by PCR.

Positive antibody tests have been reported from almost all parts of the developing world [12]. They include Egyptian children [5], Kashmiris [6], Taiwanese [9] and migrant workers in Qatar [14]. HEV infection accounts for half the cases of non-A, non-B, non-C hepatitis in Hong Kong [10]. Sufferers diagnosed in Western countries have usually been recent visitors to developing areas [3, 15]. Infection is very unusual in residents in Western countries although antibody has been found in Italian injecting drug users [17] and 2% of American blood donors [10].

Clinical features

In general, hepatitis E resembles hepatitis A. It affects young adults and is rare in children [1]. It has a self-limited course. Human volunteer studies have given an incubation period of 22–46 days for blood and 34–46 days for faeces [2]. The onset is abrupt. 100% of patients are jaundiced and there are no extra-hepatic features. HEV accounts for acute liver failure in endemic regions [11]. It has also been associated with fulminant disease [8]. The course can be cholestatic. Chronicity does not develop. The mortality is very high (about 25%) in women in the last trimester of pregnancy when the picture is of an acute haemorrhagic syndrome with encephalopathy and renal failure [6].

Liver biopsy

This shows canalicular cholestasis, pseudoglandular formations, ballooning degeneration of hepatocytes and very prominent portal (zone 1) infiltrates which contain polymorphs (fig. 16.34).

Prevention

This is by clean water, better sanitation and better hygiene education. A vaccine may prove possible as there is a common genotype.

References

1 Arankalle VA, Tsarev SA, Chadha MS *et al*. Age-specific

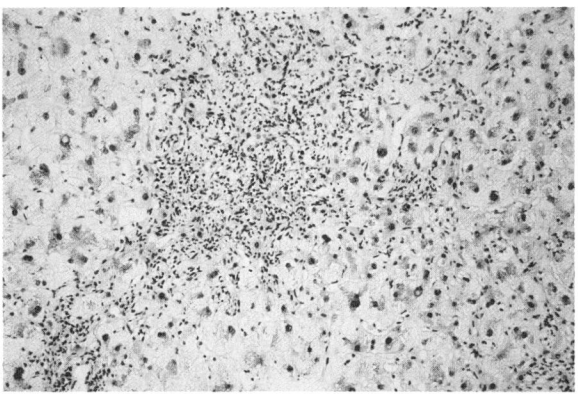

Fig. 16.34. Liver biopsy from a pregnant Arab girl suffering from acute hepatitis E shows cholestasis, pseudo-glandular formations, ballooning degeneration of hepatocytes and very prominent portal zone cellular infiltrates. She recovered. (H & E, ×100.)

prevalences of antibodies to hepatitis A and E viruses in Pune, India, 1982 and 1992. *J. Infect. Dis.* 1995; **171**: 447.
2 Chauhan A, Jameel S, Dilawari JB *et al*. Hepatitis E virus transmission to a volunteer. *Lancet* 1993; **341**: 149.
3 Coursaget P, Krawczynski K, Buisson Y *et al*. Hepatitis E and hepatitis C virus infections among French soldiers with non-A, non-B hepatitis. *J. Med. Virol.* 1993; **39**: 163.
4 DeGuzman LJ, Pitrak DL, Dawson GJ *et al*. Diagnosis of acute hepatitis E infection using enzyme immunoassay. *Dig. Dis. Sci.* 1994; **39**: 1691.
5 Goldsmith R, Yarbough PO, Reyes GR *et al*. Enzyme-linked immunosorbent assay for diagnosis of acute sporadic hepatitis E in Egyptian children. *Lancet* 1992; **339**: 328.
6 Khuroo MS, Rustgi VK, Dawson GJ *et al*. Spectrum of hepatitis E virus infection in India. *J. Med. Virol.* 1994; **43**: 281.
7 Krawczynski K. Hepatitis E. *Hepatology* 1993; **17**: 932.
8 Lau JYN, Sallie R, Fang JWS *et al*. Detection of hepatitis E virus genome and gene products in two patients with fulminant hepatitis E. *J. Hepatol.* 1995; **22**: 605.
9 Lee S-D, Wang Y-J, Lu R-H *et al*. Seroprevalence of antibody to hepatitis E virus among Chinese subjects in Taiwan. *Hepatology* 1994; **19**: 866.
10 Lok ASF, Soldevila-Pico C. Epidemiology and serologic diagnosis of hepatitis E. *J. Hepatol.* 1994; **20**: 567.
11 Nanda SK, Ansari IH, Acharya SK *et al*. Protracted viremia during acute sporadic hepatitis E virus infection. *Gastroenterology* 1995; **108**: 225.
12 Ray R, Aggarwal R, Salunke PN *et al*. Hepatitis E virus genome in stools of hepatitis patients during large epidemic in North India. *Lancet* 1991; **338**: 783.
13 Reyes GR, Purdy MA, Jungsuh PK *et al*. Isolation of a cDNA from the virus responsible for enterically transmitted non-A, non-B hepatitis. *Science* 1990; **247**: 1335.
14 Shidrawi RG, Skidmore SJ, Coleman JC *et al*. Hepatitis E—an important cause of important non-A, non-B hepatitis among migrant workers in Qatar. *J. Med. Virol.* 1994; **43**: 412.
15 Skidmore SJ, Yarbrough PO, Gabor KA *et al*. Imported hepatitis E in UK. *Lancet* 1991; **337**: 1541.
16 Velázquez O, Stetler HC, Avila C *et al*. Epidemic transmission of enterically transmitted non-A, non-B hepatitis in

Mexico, 1986–1987. *JAMA* 1990; **263**: 3281.
17 Zanetti AR, Dawson GJ and the Study Group of Hepatitis E. Hepatitis E in Italy: a seroepidemiological survey. *J. Med. Virol.* 1994; **42**: 318.

Yellow fever

This acute infection is due to a group B arbovirus transmitted to man by the bite of infected mosquitoes [3]. The virus cycle is a direct human one in urban yellow fever, or may involve wild monkeys in the jungle variety.

The two endemic regions are South America and Equatorial Africa.

Pathology

In humans, the liver histology shows predominantly midzonal acidophilic hepato-cellular necroses (Councilman bodies). Ceroid is abundant and inflammation scanty. Under electron microscopy viral particles are absent. The acidophilic bodies are composed of round cytoplasmic masses densely packed with organelles, fat vacuoles, ceroid pigment and residual bodies [2]. Appearance differs from acidophilic bodies found in other liver diseases. Inflammation is absent. Intranuclear inclusions (*Torres bodies*) are diagnostic. With recovery, regeneration is complete without chronicity.

Clinical features

Following an incubation period of 3–6 days, onset is sudden with fever, chills, headache, backache, prostration and vomiting, often of altered blood. The blood pressure falls, haemorrhages become widespread, jaundice and albuminuria are conspicuous and there is a relative bradycardia. Delirium proceeds to coma and death within nine days. With recovery the temperature becomes normal and convalescence progresses rapidly. There are no sequelae and life-long immunity follows. The majority of infections are probably milder, with no detectable jaundice and only a few constitutional symptoms.

Diagnosis. Laboratory confirmation is by demonstrating specific IgM antibodies to yellow fever virus. Yellow fever antigen may be detected in formalin-fixed, paraffin-embedded tissue cut from blocks as long as 8 years old [1].

Prothrombin deficiency parallels the severity of the liver lesion. The serum cholesterol and glucose levels fall in the fatal case. Serum transaminases are increased relative to severity.

Treatment

There is no specific treatment. Death results principally from renal damage. The hepatic lesion is self-limited and short and does not demand special treatment.

Prevention consists of vaccination at least 10 days before arrival in an endemic area and by control of mosquitoes.

References

1 Hall WC, Crowell TP, Watts DM *et al.* Demonstration of yellow fever and dengue antigens in formalin-fixed, paraffin-embedded human liver by immunohistochemical analysis. *Am. J. Trop. Med. Hyg.* 1991; **45**: 408.
2 Vieira WT, Gayotto LC, Dé Lima CP *et al.* Histopathology of the human liver in yellow fever with special emphasis on the diagnostic role of the Councilman body. *Histopathology* 1983; **7**: 195.
3 World Health Organization. Present status of yellow fever: memorandum from a PAHO meeting. *Bull. World Health Organ.* 1986; **64**: 511.

Infectious mononucleosis (Epstein–Barr virus)

This is due to human herpes IV (EBV) which excites a generalized reticulo-endothelial reaction [2].

Primary infection in children is usually asymptomatic. In adolescents and young people, it causes a hepatitis which may mimic HAV, HBV or HCV hepatitis. Presentation, particularly in adults, may be as fever with right, upper quadrant, abdominal discomfort. Pharyngitis and lymphadenopathy may be absent. It can cause fulminant hepatitis in elderly people [3]. It may be a trigger for autoimmune hepatitis in susceptible people [4]. In the immunosuppressed, whether congenital or recipients of solid organ or bone marrow transplants, or sufferers from AIDS, EB infection may be associated with lymphoproliferative disorders. This is especially so in children having liver transplants (see Chapter 35).

Hepatic histology (fig. 16.35)

The changes are seen within 5 days of the onset and reach their peak between the tenth and thirtieth days.

The sinusoids and portal tracts are infiltrated with large, mononuclear cells. Polymorphonuclear leucocytes and lymphocytes increase, and the Kupffer cells proliferate. The appearances may resemble leukaemia. The lesions resemble those of early A, B, or C viral hepatitis. The architecture of the liver is preserved.

Zone 3 focal necroses may be randomly distributed. The necroses are not bile stained and there is no surrounding cellular reaction.

In later biopsies, binucleate liver cells and mitoses are conspicuous. The features of regeneration are out of proportion to cell necrosis. After clinical recovery, abnormal cells disappear although this may take as long

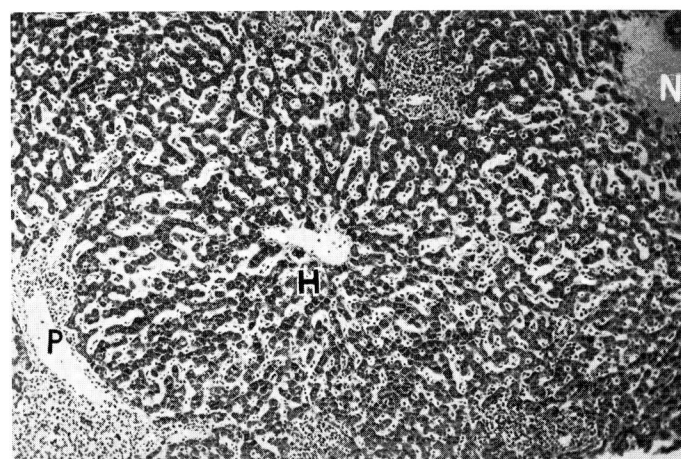

Fig. 16.35. Infectious mononucleosis. The sinusoids and portal tracts (P) are filled with mononuclear cells. H is a central hepatic vein. One small local necrosis (N) is seen in the upper right-hand corner. (Best's carmine, ×70.)

as 8 months. Chronic hepatitis and cirrhosis are not sequelae.

Clinical features

Occasionally jaundice can be deep [1]. Large glands in the portal hepatis do not compress the common bile duct.

Persistent infection is a cause of chronic ill health.

Immune responses determine the clinical and pathological expression. Using monoclonal antibodies, direct hepatic viral infection has been shown.

Diagnosis

The total serum albumin level may be slightly decreased and the serum globulin value slightly elevated.

Hyperbilirubinaemia is present in about one-half of patients. Serum transaminase values are raised to about 20 times the normal in 80% of patients. Values are usually less than those found in the early stages of an acute virus A, B or C hepatitis. In about one-third the serum alkaline phosphatase value is increased, often more so than that of bilirubin.

In the usual case of infectious mononucleosis, the monospot reaction is positive. The disease is diagnosed conclusively by an increase in serum IgM antibodies against Epstein–Barr capsid antigens.

In the immunosuppressed, particularly with post-transplant lymphoproliferative disease, EBV proteins may be shown by immunofluorescence on liver biopsy material. Specific RNA and DNA sequences may be demonstrated by Southern blot hybridization. PCR is used for DNA *in situ* hybridization in blood and tissues [2].

Distinction from viral hepatitis (table 16.16)

Although the diagnosis of viral hepatitis from infectious mononucleosis is usually easy, in an occasional patient with mild anicteric hepatitis or severe mononucleosis this may be impossible.

References

1 Fuhrman SA, Gill R, Horwitz CA *et al*. Marked hyperbilirubinemia in infectious mononucleosis. *Arch. Intern. Med.* 1987; **147**: 850.
2 Markin RS. Manifestations of Epstein–Barr virus-associated disorders in liver. *Liver* 1994; **14**: 1.
3 Papatheodoridis GV, Delladetsima JK, Kavallierou L *et al*. Fulminant hepatitis due to Epstein–Barr virus infection. *J. Hepatol.* 1995; **23**: 348.
4 Vento S, Guella L, Mirandola F *et al*. Epstein–Barr virus as a trigger for autoimmune hepatitis in susceptible individuals. *Lancet* 1995; **346**: 608.

Other viruses

All viruses may affect the liver in common with other organs. The histological changes are usually non-specific, consisting of fatty change, or focal necrosis and lymphocytic infiltration of the portal zones. Biochemical tests are usually unchanged or show mild rises in transaminases. Occasionally the patient may be frankly icteric when the picture of type A, B, or C hepatitis is closely simulated.

The upsurge of AIDS has increased the prevalence of hepatitis due to various, unusual viruses. These frequently prove fatal (Chapter 27). They are also important in those receiving large doses of immunosuppression, such as liver and bone marrow recipients, or patients with reticulosis. They are seen in neonates (Chapter 24) and may follow a blood transfusion.

Cytomegalovirus

In neonates it is usually inapparent. Confirmed disease in early infancy is rare. Sometimes, however, in asso-

Table 16.16. Comparison of infectious mononucleosis and viral hepatitis

	Infectious mononucleosis	Viral hepatitis
Epidemic history	Suggestive	Suggestive
Onset		
Fever	+	+
Anorexia	−	+
Sore throat	+	−
Rash	+	Rare
Pruritus	−	+
Physical signs		
Lymphadenopathy	++	±
Jaundice	Mild, transient	Well developed, persisting
Liver	Enlarged; not usually tender	Enlarged and tender
Spleen	Enlarged and tender	Enlarged but not tender
Pale stools	−	+
Dark urine	±	++
Peripheral blood		
Leucocytes	Usually increased. Characteristic cells	Decreased, with relative lymphocytosis
Monospot	Positive	Negative
IgM EB	Present	Absent
HBsAg	Negative	Positive, type B
IgM anti-hepatitis A	Negative	Positive, type A
Liver biopsy	Diffuse mononuclear infiltration. Focal necroses	Zone 3 'spotty' necrosis Mononuclear infiltration

ciation with the respiratory distress syndrome, cytomegalovirus may cause a devastating fatal pneumonitis [1]. In adults, the clinical picture can be very diverse.

Cytomegalovirus can cause a disease strongly resembling EBV-related mononucleosis [8]. Patients usually lack pharyngitis and posterior cervical lymphadenopathy. Serum transaminase and alkaline phosphatase levels are increased and atypical lymphocytes are found in the peripheral blood. The monospot test is usually negative.

The picture may simulate type A, type B or C hepatitis, having a similar onset but with failure of the pyrexia to subside with the onset of jaundice. Icterus lasts 2–3 weeks and even up to 3 months.

Occasionally, massive hepatic necrosis may be fatal.

Granulomatous hepatitis can develop in a previously normal adult with prolonged unexplained fever and without lymphadenopathy [3]. In these patients, liver biopsy shows non-caseating granulomas. The immunosuppressed show characteristic inclusions.

Cholangitis, papillary stenosis and sclerosing cholangitis can accompany cytomegalo infections in AIDS patients (see Chapter 15) [9, 15].

Cytomegalovirus infection is a rare cause of post-transfusion hepatitis.

Cytomegalovirus may cause disseminated disease, of which hepatitis is only a part, in the immunosuppressed, such as the leukaemic.

Cytomegalo hepatitis is a real problem in adult and paediatric recipients of kidney and, particularly, liver transplants [4, 10]. The infection is usually a primary one, rather than reactivation, and the donor is cytomegalovirus antibody positive (see Chapter 35).

Diagnosis is by isolation of virus from urine or saliva. Complement fixing antibodies rise and CMV IgM antibodies can be found. The virus cannot usually be shown in liver biopsy but direct hepatic involvement has been confirmed by demonstrating nuclear and cytoplasmic inclusions in hepatocytes by monoclonal antibodies, immunoperoxidase and immunofluorescent techniques [17].

Herpes simplex

Human herpes virus types I and II affect all humans at some time during their lives.

In *infants* herpes hepatitis may be part of generalized herpetic disease.

In *adults*, disseminated herpes simplex is very rare. It can affect those with underlying diseases, e.g. ulcerative colitis [18], with AIDS, receiving immunosuppressive treatment and having organ transplants. Fulminant hepatic failure can also affect the previously normal and immunocompetent [7]. It may complicate genital herpes [16] and be seen in pregnancy [11].

Herpetic mucocutaneous lesions are usually absent. The onset is with fever, prostration, marked elevation of transaminases and leucopenia [12]. Jaundice is absent. Fulminant liver failure with fatal coagulopathy can develop.

Liver biopsy shows patchy areas of coagulative necrosis with surrounding hepatocytes containing viral inclusions [7] (fig. 16.36). The virus can be shown by electron microscopy. It can be cultured from the liver and, using immunoperoxidase staining, may be shown in affected hepatocytes [12].

Acyclovir or gancyclovir is curative.

Other viruses

Coxsackie virus B may cause hepatitis in the adult. Coxsackie virus, group A, type IV, has been isolated from the plasma of a child with hepatitis, and complement fixing antibodies appeared in the serum during convalescence.

Adenovirus has caused fulminant hepatitis in a young immunosuppressed adult [2]. Intranuclear inclusions were confined to the liver.

Varicella and *varicella-zoster* may be complicated by hepatitis in both normal and immunologically compromised individuals [13]. In children the picture must be distinguished from Reye's syndrome [13].

Measles is affecting an older age group. 80% of adult sufferers have liver involvement — 5% becoming jaundiced [6]. It is most frequent in the seriously ill. Resolution is complete. A similar picture is seen with the atypical measles syndrome [5].

Rubella can be associated with serum transaminase

elevations and may be mistakenly diagnosed as hepatitis C [19].

Paramyxoma viruses. Severe sporadic hepatitis with, histologically, large syncytial giant hepatocytes may be related to the paramyxoma viruses [14]. Virological confirmation and classification is awaited.

References

1 Ballard RA, Drew L, Hufnagle KG *et al*. Acquired cytomegalovirus infection in preterm infants. *Am. J. Dis. Child*. 1979; **133**: 482.
2 Carmichael GP, Zarhadnik JM, Moyer GH *et al*. Adenovirus hepatitis in an immunosuppressed adult patient. *Am. J. Clin. Pathol*. 1979; **71**: 352.
3 Clarke J, Craig RM, Saffro R *et al*. Cytomegalovirus granulomatous hepatitis. *Am. J. Med*. 1979; **66**: 264.
4 Dummer JS. Cytomegalovirus infection after liver transplantation: clinical manifestations and strategies for prevention. *Rev. Infect. Dis*. 1990; **12**: S767.
5 Frey HM, Krugman S. Case report. Atypical measles syndrome: unusual hepatic, pulmonary, and immunologic aspects. *Am. J. Med. Sci*. 1981; **281**: 51.
6 Gavish D, Kleinman Y, Morag A *et al*. Hepatitis and jaundice associated with measles in young adults. *Arch. Intern. Med*. 1983; **13**: 674.
7 Goodman ZD, Ishak KG, Sesterhenn IA *et al*. Herpes simplex hepatitis in apparently immunocompetent adults. *Am. J. Clin. Pathol*. 1986; **85**: 694.
8 Horwitz CA, Henle W, Henle G *et al*. Clinical and laboratory evaluation of cytomegalovirus-induced mononucleosis in previously healthy individuals. *Medicine (Baltimore)* 1986; **65**: 124.
9 Jacobson MA, Cello JP, Sande MA. Cholestasis and disseminated cytomegalovirus disease in patients with the acquired immunodeficiency syndrome. *Am. J. Med*. 1988; **84**: 218.
10 King SM, Petric M, Superina R *et al*. Cytomegalovirus infections in pediatric liver transplantation. *Am. J. Dis. Child*. 1990; **144**: 1307.
11 Klein NA, Mabie WC, Shaver DC *et al*. Herpes simplex virus hepatitis in pregnancy. Two patients successfully treated with acyclovir. *Gastroenterology* 1991; **100**: 239.
12 Marrie TJ, McDonald ATJ, Conen PE *et al*. Herpes simplex hepatitis — use of immunoperoxidase to demonstrate the viral antigen in hepatocytes. *Gastroenterology* 1982; **82**: 71.
13 Myers MG. Hepatic cellular injury during varicella. *Arch. Dis. Child*. 1982; **57**: 317.
14 Phillips MJ, Blendis LM, Poucell S *et al*. Syncytial giant-cell hepatitis. Sporadic hepatitis with distinctive pathological features, a severe clinical course, and paramyxoviral features. *N. Engl. J. Med*. 1991; **324**: 455.
15 Roulot D, Walla D, Brun-Vezinet F *et al*. Cholangitis in the acquired immunodeficiency syndrome: report of two cases and review of the literature. *Gut* 1987; **28**: 1653.
16 Rubin MH, Ward DM, Painter J. Fulminant hepatic failure caused by genital herpes in a healthy person. *JAMA* 1985; **253**: 1299.
17 Sacks SL, Freeman HJ. Cytomegalovirus hepatitis: evidence for direct hepatic viral infection using monoclonal antibodies. *Gastroenterology* 1984; **86**: 346.

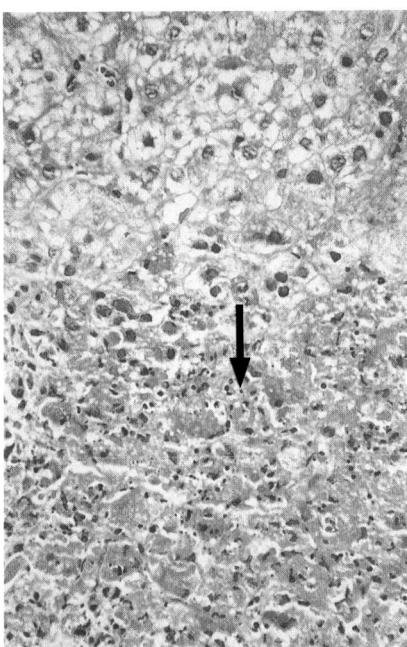

Fig. 16.36. Herpes virus II hepatitis. An area of coagulative necrosis can be seen (arrow). Adjacent liver cells were shown to have nuclear viral inclusions. (H & E, ×100.)

18 Shlien RD, Meyers S, Lee JA *et al.* Fulminant herpes simplex hepatitis in a patient with ulcerative colitis. *Gut* 1988; **29**: 257.

19 Zeldis JB, Miller JG, Dienstag JL. Hepatitis in an adult with rubella. *Am. J. Med.* 1985; **79**: 515.

Hepatitis due to exotic viruses

These very dangerous, newly identified and unusual viruses have the liver as the primary target [2]. They include Marburg, Lassa and Ebola viruses. They are becoming increasingly important as man encroaches into underdeveloped areas, as ecology changes and as a source of infection to medical or laboratory staff dealing with patients or their blood.

Lassa fever is due to an arena virus transmitted from rodents to man or from man to man. It is largely found in West Africa. The case fatality rate is 36–67%. Diagnosis is made by demonstrating virus in the blood during the first few days and by IgM antibodies from the fifth day. It has been successfully treated with ribavirin [3].

The liver shows eosinophilic necrosis of individual hepatocytes with little inflammation. Bridging necrosis is usual.

Marburg virus disease is due to an RNA virus transmitted by Vervet monkeys. In 1967, an outbreak of this disease occurred in persons in contact with monkeys in experimental institutes in Germany [4]. Further patients have been reported from South Africa and Kenya [5].

After an incubation period of 4–7 days the patients present with headache, pyrexia, vomiting, a characteristic rash, a haemorrhagic diathesis and central nervous system involvement. Serum transaminase levels are very high.

Liver pathology shows single-cell acidophilic necrosis and Kupffer cell hyperactivity. This is followed by eccentric and radial extension of the necrosis, cytoplasmic inclusions and portal zone cellularity. Steatosis is noted in the severely affected. Virus can persist in the body for 2–3 months after initial infection.

Ebola virus infection resembles Marburg in clinical course, hepatic histology and electron microscopy [1]. It has been reported from Zaïre and the Sudan and has been transmitted to biologists working with it.

Treatment

There is no specific treatment for these exotic virus infections. Symptomatic measures are used and very strict precautions are necessary to avoid spread to contacts.

References

1 Ellis DS, Simpson DIH, Francis DP *et al.* Ultra-structure of Ebola virus particles in human liver. *J. clin. Pathol.* 1978; **31**: 201.

2 Howard CR, Ellis DS, Simpson DIH. Exotic viruses and the liver. *Semin. Liv. Dis.* 1984; **4**: 361.

3 McCormick JB, King IJ, Webb PA *et al.* Lassa fever. Effective therapy with ribavirin. *N. Engl. J. Med.* 1986; **314**: 20.

4 Martini GA, Knauff HG, Schmidt HA *et al.* Uber eine bisher unbekannte von Affen eingeschleppte Infektions-krankheit: Marburg-Virus-Krankheit. *Dtsch. med. Wschr.* 1968; **57**: 559.

5 Smith DH, Johnson BK, Isaacson M. Marburg-virus disease in Kenya. *Lancet* 1982; **i**: 816.

Chapter 17
Chronic Hepatitis

The spectrum of chronic inflammatory diseases of the liver extends from acute hepatitis to chronic hepatitis and finally to cirrhosis. Whatever the aetiology, the same basic underlying liver histology is seen. However, before needle liver biopsy can be recommended, the physician must be aware of the mode of presentation and of the associated laboratory findings which suggest the diagnosis (table 17.1) [115].

Chronic hepatitis is defined as a chronic inflammatory reaction in the liver continuing without improvement for at least 6 months. However, where the diagnosis is obvious, as in autoimmune chronic hepatitis, it is not necessary to wait 6 months before commencing therapy.

Clinical presentation

The most important general symptom is fatigue. Viral causes (hepatitis B and C) may be identified at the time of a blood donation. Abnormal biochemical tests or viral markers may be found at the time of a routine check-up. Rarely the disease may be recognized when recovery fails following an attack of acute viral hepatitis.

Chronic hepatitis B is suggested by the ethnic origin of the patient, homosexuality, drug abuse or a likely contact with blood of persons carrying hepatitis B.

The history of receiving a blood transfusion or blood products, or of drug abuse, however distant, suggests hepatitis C. The patient may bring a chart recording up and down serum transaminase levels over many months or years.

An autoimmune aetiology may be suggested (page 308), but in some patients the cause is unknown.

Symptoms are difficult to grade [46]. They include nausea, upper abdominal pain, and muscle and joint aches. A patient questionnaire may be useful but difficult to interpret.

Clinical signs include jaundice, rarely vascular spiders, a large or small liver and splenomegaly.

The features of clinically diagnosable and symptomatic portal hypertension (ascites, bleeding oesophageal varices) are late.

Biochemical tests show a variably elevated serum bilirubin level. Serum transaminase values are usually increased and gamma-globulin concentration is also ele-

Table 17.1. The investigation of suspected chronic hepatitis

Presentation
Fatigue: generally unwell
Following blood donation—positive hepatitis B or C test
Following acute hepatitis—failure of recovery, whether clinical or biochemical or both
Abnormal liver function tests or positive hepatitis B or C markers at routine check-up
Abnormal physical findings—hepatomegaly, splenomegaly, jaundice
Blood transfusions in the past
Drug abuse in the past

Careful history and physical examination
Routine laboratory tests
Liver function tests
  Bilirubin
  Aspartate transaminase (SGOT)
  Alanine transferase (SGPT)
  Gamma-globulin
  Albumin
  Alkaline phosphatase
Haematology
  Haemoglobin
  White cell count
  Platelet count
  Prothrombin time
Hepatitis B surface antigen
Hepatitis C antibody

Special tests
Serum antibodies
  Nuclear
  Smooth muscle
  Mitochondrial
  Liver/kidney microsomal

Serum ceruloplasmin and copper
Slit lamp cornea
HBeAg
HBeAb
HBV DNA
Anti-HCV and HCV-RNA
Alpha-fetoprotein
Serum iron
Serum transferrin
Needle liver biopsy
Haematoxylin and eosin and connective tissue stains

Ultrasound
Liver

vated. Serum bilirubin, albumin and phosphatase are normal except in severe disease.

Serum transaminase levels do not always reflect the severity of the underlying liver disease as shown by liver biopsy, but can be used for an approximate grading [50].
• *Mild* less than 100 iu (three times the upper limit of normal).
• *Moderate* 100–400 iu (10 times the upper limit of normal).
• *Severe* more than 400 iu (over 10 times the upper limit of normal).

Hepatic histology

The liver shows varying degrees of hepatocellular necrosis and inflammation [46]. The portal zones are expanded by an inflammatory infiltrate primarily of lymphocytes and plasma cells (fig. 17.3). There is some fibrosis with increasing severity, the inflammation extends into the liver lobule causing erosion of the limiting plate and piecemeal necrosis (fig. 17.7). Individual hepatocytes show swelling (ballooning degeneration), shrinkage (acidophilic change) and the formation of acidophil bodies. Cholestasis is rare. There may be bile duct damage especially in hepatitis C viral-related cases. The histological picture may resemble acute viral hepatitis but the duration is longer and the picture is predominantly that of intralobular inflammation and necrosis. The necrosis may be focal (spotty) involving single cells or groups of cells.

The most severe form is marked by largely lobular areas of confluent necrosis with isolation of groups of liver cells in the form of rosettes (figs 17.4, 17.5, 17.6).

Confluent necrosis linking vascular structures is called bridging necrosis. This may be between portal zones or between portal tracts and terminal venules which is more serious (figs 17.6, 17.2).

Cirrhosis is defined as widespread fibrosis with nodule formation (Chapter 19). The normal zonal architecture of the liver cannot be recognized (fig. 17.1). This is a sequel of chronic hepatitis.

The role of liver biopsy

This is essential to confirm the diagnosis and indicate the possible aetiology. Activity may be graded and the stage of the disease evaluated. The presence of cirrhosis may be established. Treatment can be evaluated (table 17.2).

The liver lesion may vary in severity from place to place and this accounts for sampling errors which are particularly likely if the liver biopsy is small.

It can be difficult to distinguish peri-portal piecemeal necrosis from simple spill-over or inflammatory cells into the lobule, as in acute hepatitis.

In cholestatic diseases, peri-portal hepatocytes may swell and become necrotic. However, lymphocytes are usually sparse, neutrophils prominent and hepatocellular copper is often increased.

Difficulties in diagnosing cirrhosis on small samples are discussed in Chapter 19. An experienced histopathologist, armed with reticulin stains, is necessary.

Classification

The old classification into chronic persistent, chronic active and chronic lobular hepatitis has been replaced by a new nomenclature [36, 46]. This is based on aetiology, clinical grade, histological severity (necro-inflammatory activity) and the stage (extent of fibrosis) (tables 17.3, 17.4, 17.5, 17.6, 17.7).

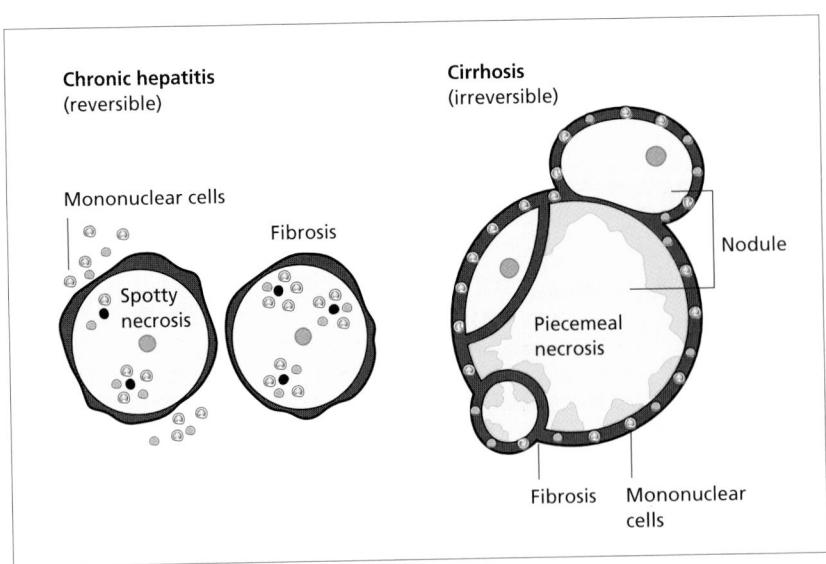

Fig. 17.1. In chronic hepatitis the zonal architecture of the liver is preserved. In cirrhosis, nodular regeneration leads to loss of the essential hepatic architecture. Chronic hepatitis is essentially reversible, cirrhosis is not.

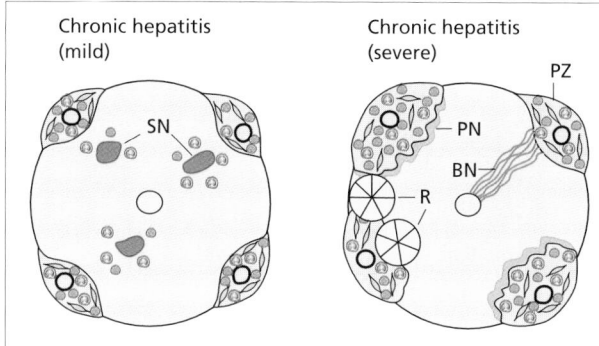

Fig. 17.2. Pattern of histological charges in chronic hepatitis. PZ = portal zone; SN = spotty necrosis; PN = piecemeal necrosis; BN = bridging necrosis; R = rosettes.

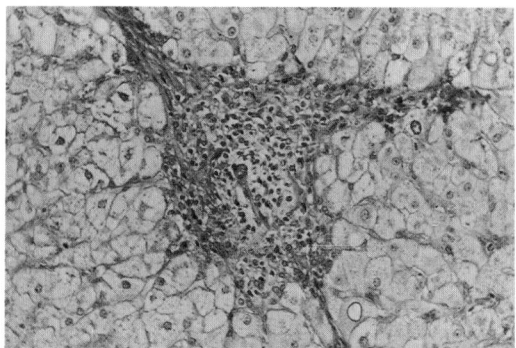

Fig. 17.3. Mild chronic hepatitis. Part of the liver biopsy shows an inflamed expanded portal zone but a well-defined limiting plate and no piecemeal necrosis. (H & E, ×100.)

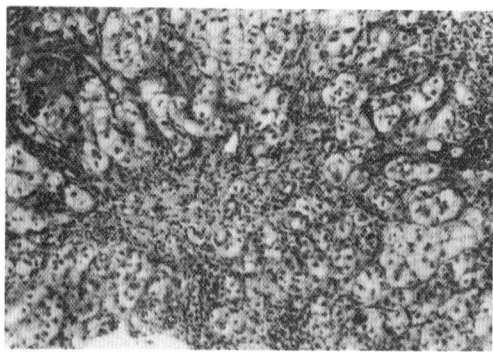

Fig. 17.4. Severe chronic hepatitis. The lobular architecture is completely disturbed. Isolated groups of liver cells, which often assume a rosette-like appearance, are separated by the septa of connective tissue. Remaining cells are large with clear cytoplasm. Lymphocytic and plasma cell infiltration is conspicuous. (H & E, ×40.)

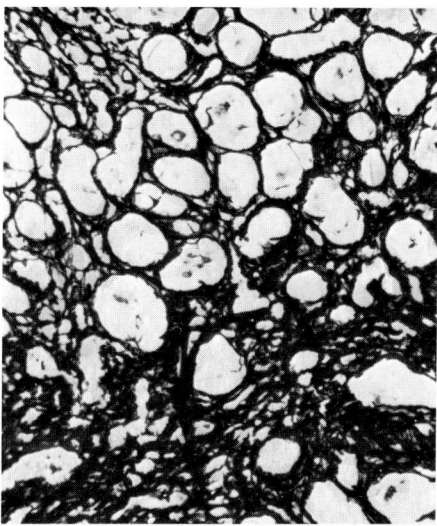

Fig. 17.5. Same case as fig. 17.4. Reticulin stains confirm the isolation of liver cells by bands of fibrous tissue (×120).

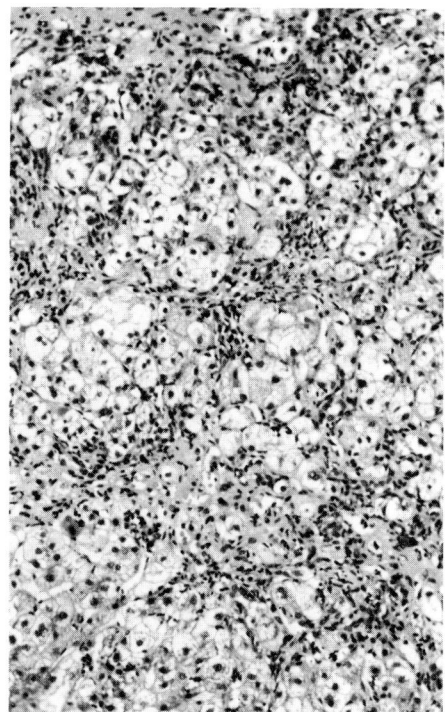

Fig. 17.6. Severe chronic hepatitis. Shown are isolation of cell groups, fibrosis and many plasma cells. (H & E, ×40.)

Table 17.2. Liver biopsy in chronic hepatitis

Confirms diagnosis
Suggests possible aetiology
Grades activity (inflammation)
Stages progress (fibrosis)
Confirms cirrhosis
Evaluates treatment

Table 17.3. Classification of chronic hepatitis [154]

Aetiology	Sex predominance	Age predominance	Associations	Diagnostic tests	Histological features
Hepatitis B and delta	M	All	Immigrants from Orient, Africa and Mediterranean, health-care workers, homosexuals, drug abusers, immunosuppressed	HBsAg HBeAg anti-HBe HBV DNA anti-HDV	Usually mild. Ground glass cells, orcein positive. Delta antigen in hepatocyte nuclei
Hepatitis C	Equal	All ages	Blood transfusion, blood products, drug abuse	Anti-HCV HCV-RNA	Fat, lobular component Lymphoid aggregates
Autoimmune	F	14–25 years and post-menopausal	Multi-system (diabetes, arthralgia, haemolytic anaemia, nephritis)	Antinuclear antibody +ve 70% Smooth muscle antibody +ve 70% Serum gamma-globulin high	Rosettes, plasma cell infiltrates, bridging Florid picture
Drug	F	Middle-aged and elderly	INAH, methyl dopa, furantoin, dantrolene anti-thyroid drugs, etc.	History, liver histology	Eosinophils, fat, granulomas
Wilson's	Equal	10–30 years	Family history, haemolysis, neurological signs	Kayser–Fleischer rings. Serum copper, ceruloplasmin, urinary copper, liver copper	Ballooned hepatocytes, glycogenic nuclei, fat

Table 17.4. Chronic hepatitis: prognosis and treatment [154]

Aetiology	Prognosis	Treated	Treatment
Hepatitis B	10–20% remission (HBeAg +ve → anti-HBe +ve), develop cirrhosis and primary liver cancer	?	?antivirals
Hepatitis C	Mild disease. May remit completely or develop cirrhosis and primary liver cancer	?	?antivirals
Autoimmune	60% dead in 5 years	15% dead in 5 years	Prednisolone
Drugs	Excellent		Withdraw drug

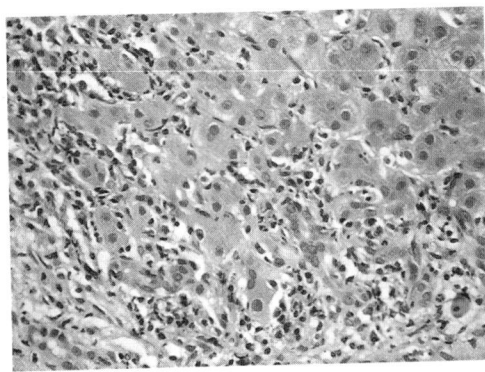

Fig. 17.7. Mild chronic hepatitis. Part of a liver biopsy specimen, showing necrosis of the limiting plate in the portal zone. (H & E, ×100.)

Table 17.5. Histological activity index (HAI) (excluding fibrosis) [100]

Component	Scores
Peri-portal necrosis with or without bridging necrosis	0–10
Intralobular degeneration and focal necrosis	0–4
Portal inflammation	0–4

Table 17.6. Chronic hepatitis: correlation of HAI score (excluding fibrosis) and diagnosis

HAI	Diagnosis
1–3	Minimal
4–8	Mild
9–12	Moderate
13–18	Severe

Table 17.7. Scoring system for staging of chronic hepatitis B on the basis of fibrosis and architectural alterations [46]

Score	Grade	Description
0	None	—
1	Mild	Portal expansion
2	Moderate	Portal–portal septa
3	Severe	Bridging with distortion
4	Cirrhosis	Cirrhosis

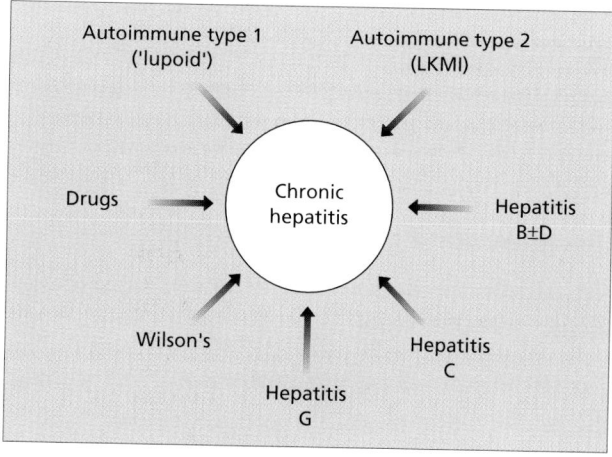

Fig. 17.8. The spectrum of chronic hepatitis.

Aetiology

A common clinical, biochemical and hepatic histological picture can be associated with more than one aetiological agent (figs 17.8, 17.9). Three main types have been identified (tables 17.2, 17.3, 17.5). One is associated with continuing hepatitis B infection, another is related to chronic hepatitis C infection and the third is termed 'lupoid' or 'autoimmune' because of the association with positive serum autoantibodies (table 17.8).

In the neonate, and occasionally in the immunosuppressed patient, other viral infections such as cytomegalovirus may lead to chronic hepatitis. Identical clinical, functional and morphological features may be found associated with some drug reactions (Chapter 18). α_1-Antitrypsin deficiency may lead to a chronic hepatitis but more often presents as cholestasis in the neonate (Chapter 23). A liver biopsy in the alcoholic occasionally shows the picture of chronic hepatitis (Chapter 20).

Clinical severity

Although generally regarded as unreliable, transaminases are commonly used to approximate clinical severity. Once cirrhosis has developed, the Child's grade is used related to bilirubin, albumin, prothrombin values and whether or not hepatic encephalopathy and ascites are present (see Chapter 10).

Histological severity

This is based on the severity of the necro-inflammatory process. The most widely used grading is the *histological activity index* (HAI) of Knodell [100] (table 17.5). Three separate scores for different components of the lesion have been included. The scores correlate reasonably well with brief descriptions of the lesion as given verbally by histopathologists (table 17.6).

Histological staging

This is related to the time course of the disease and is based on the extent of fibrosis and the development of cirrhosis (table 17.7).

Examples of classification

Suggestive profiles for two types of chronic hepatitis are shown in table 17.9. Activity score and staging are particularly important in predicting the development of cirrhosis [180].

Table 17.8. Chronic active hepatitis: comparison of types

	Autoimmune type 1	Hepatitis B	Hepatitis C
Sex predominance	Female	Male	Equal
Age preference	15–25	Older	All ages
	Menopause	Neonates	
Serum HBsAg	Absent	Present	Absent
Serum anti-HCV	Absent	Absent	Present
Autoimmune disease	Frequent	Rare	Occasional
Serum gamma-globulin increase	Marked	Moderate	Moderate
Smooth muscle antibody and ANF	High titre (70%)	Low or absent titre	Low or absent titre
Risk of primary liver cancer	Low	High	High
Response to corticosteroids	Good	Poor	Poor

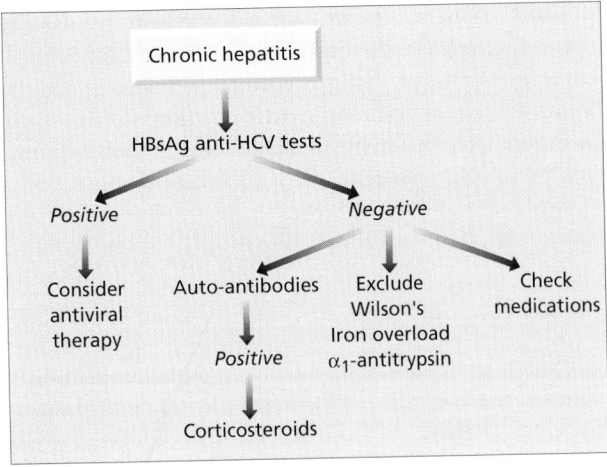

Fig. 17.9. The management of chronic hepatitis.

Table 17.9. Examples of the classification of chronic hepatitis

| | | Severity | | |
Aetiology	Clinical	Child's grade	Histology (score*)	Stage (score†)
Hepatitis C	Mild	A	Mild (5)	Mild (1)
Autoimmune	Moderate	B	Moderate (12)	Severe (3)

* See Table 17.6.
† See Table 17.7.

Immunological mechanisms of hepatotoxicity

Chronic hepatitis is the liver disease *par excellence* where immunological factors are invoked in the perpetuation of the liver cell injury.

Liver histology shows heavy infiltration by lymphocytes and plasma cells with peri-portal piecemeal necrosis. Hyperglobulinaemia and circulating tissue antibodies are often present. In chronic hepatitis, it is postulated that an immunological reaction is mounted against membrane constituents of the hepatocyte which serve as antigens. Cell-mediated immunity to liver cell antigens has been demonstrated in chronic hepatitis and this process is mediated by sensitized lymphocytes and mononuclear cells.

In autoimmune chronic hepatitis, various liver membrane proteins have been suggested as the postulated antigen. A membrane fixed IgG has been shown on hepatocytes and continuing necrosis of liver cells is seen in patients with this antibody which is not found in HBsAg-positive patients.

Chronic hepatitis is more a mode of progression than a disease entity.

Table 17.10. Chronic liver disease with circulating autoantibodies

| | Antibody | | | | | |
| | | | LKM | | | |
Type	DNA	SMA	I	II	III	AMA
I ('lupoid')	+++	+++	–	–	–	–
IIa	–	–	+++	–	–	–
IIb (HCV)	–	–	+	–	–	–
Tienilic acid	–	–	–	+	–	–
Hepatitis D	–	–	–	–	+	–
Autoimmune cholangiopathy	+++	+	–	–	–	–
Primary biliary cirrhosis	–	±	–	–	–	+++

ANA = antinuclear antibody; SMA = smooth muscle (actin) antibody; LKM = liver/kidney microsome antibody.

Autoimmune chronic hepatitis

An attempt at classification of autoimmune chronic hepatitis has been made on the basis of the pattern of circulating autoantibodies (table 17.10). Some types have no obvious aetiology, but others are associated with known entities such as tienilic acid (a diuretic) or viral hepatitis C or D. In general, those with no known aetiology are more florid clinically and have higher serum transaminase and gammaglobulin levels and liver histology is more active than those with a known aetiology and the response to corticosteroid therapy is better.

Type I (formerly called lupoid) is associated with high circulating titres of anti-DNA and anti-actin (smooth muscle). This type will be described in detail later as a prototype.

Type II autoimmune chronic hepatitis is associated with autoantibodies against liver/kidney microsomes type I. It is subdivided into type IIa and IIb.

Type IIa [81] LKM type I antibodies are found in high titre. It is associated with a severe chronic hepatitis. Other autoantibodies are usually absent. The disease largely affects girls, and there is a good response to corticosteroid treatment. Insulin-dependent diabetes, vitiligo and thyroiditis may be found. The disease can be fulminant in children. Treatment is with corticosteroids.

The major antigen is a cytochrome belonging to the P450-2D6 sub-family [69].

In type IIa autoimmune chronic hepatitis, antibodies to soluble liver antigen (SLA) may be found but do not define a distinct group of patients with autoimmune hepatitis [36].

Autoimmune chronic hepatitis type IIb. Antibodies to liver/kidney microsomes type I (LKM-I) are also found in some patients with chronic hepatitis C virus infection. This might be related to shared antigenic sites (molecular mimicry). However, more detailed analysis of the microsomal proteins showed that the anti-LKM-I autoantibody from patients with hepatitis C virus infection were directed against different antigenic sites on the P450-11D6 proteins than from those with autoimmune LKM positivity [179].

The differences between patients with type IIa (autoimmune) and type IIb (HCV-related) LKM-I positive chronic hepatitis are tabulated (see table 17.21). In particular, the treatment of the autoimmune group is with corticosteroids, while antivirals must be considered for the HCV-related disease.

Tienilic acid. A further LKM immunofluorescent pattern (LKM-II) is found in patients having a self-limited hepatitis following the administration of this diuretic, now withdrawn from clinical use.

Chronic hepatitis D

Some patients with chronic delta virus infection have a circulating autoantibody against liver/kidney microsomes type III (LKM-III) [32]. The microsomal target is uridine diphosphate glucuronyl transferase (GGT). These transferases play an important part in the elimination of toxic substances [142]. The relationship of this autoantibody to disease progression is uncertain.

Primary biliary cirrhosis and immune cholangiopathy

These cholestatic syndromes are marked by serum mitochondrial antibodies in the case of primary biliary cirrhosis (see Chapter 14) and to DNA and actin in the case of immune cholangiopathy (see Chapter 7) [7].

Chronic autoimmune hepatitis (type I)

In 1950, Waldenström [168] described a chronic hepatitis occurring predominantly in young people, especially women. The syndrome has since been given various titles [6, 104, 124, 174]; none are satisfactory and rather than dogmatize concerning aetiology, sex, age or pathology, all of which may vary, the term 'chronic autoimmune hepatitis' has been used. The frequency of the condition seems to be decreasing, but this may simply be due to more accurate diagnosis of other causes of chronic hepatitis, for instance drug-related or hepatitis B or C.

Aetiology

The aetiology is unknown. Immunological changes are conspicuous. Serum gamma-globulin levels are grossly elevated. The finding of a positive LE cell test in about 15% led to the term 'lupoid hepatitis'. Tissue antibodies are found in a high proportion of patients.

Chronic (lupoid) hepatitis is not the same as classical systemic lupus erythematosus [71] for the liver rarely shows any lesions in classical lupus. Moreover, the smooth muscle antibody and the mitochondrial antibody are not present in the blood of patients with systemic lupus erythematosus.

Immunological mechanisms and autoantibodies

Autoimmune chronic hepatitis is a disease of disordered immunoregulation marked by a defect in suppressor (regulatory) T-cells. This results in production of autoantibodies against hepatocyte surface antigens. It is uncertain whether the defect in the immune regulatory apparatus is primary or secondary to an acquired change in the antigenicity of the tissues.

The mononuclear infiltrate in the portal zones consists of B lymphocytes and helper T-cells with relatively fewer cytotoxic/suppressor cells [128]. This is consistent with the view that antibody-dependent cytotoxicity is the main effector mechanism (fig. 17.10).

Patients have persistently high titres of circulating measles antibodies. This is likely to be due to hyperfunction of the immune system and not to reactivation of persistent virus [94].

The nature of the target antigens on the hepatocyte membrane remains to be determined. One candidate, liver membrane protein (LMP) [173], seems largely related to piecemeal necrosis. Cell-mediated immunity to membrane proteins has been shown. Liver-membrane-specific activated T-cells in peripheral blood may be important in the autoimmune attack of chronic hepatitis.

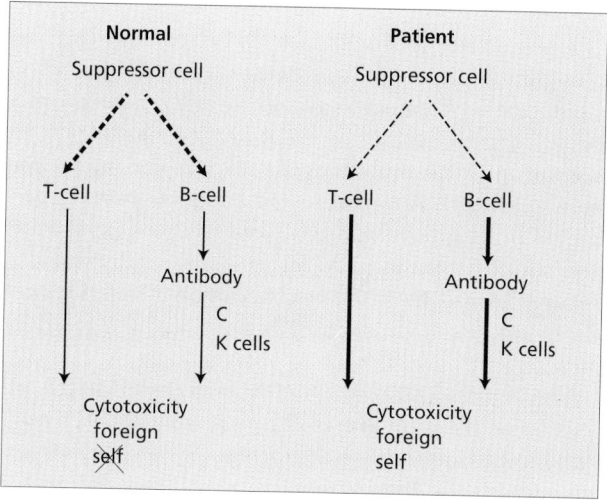

Fig. 17.10. The mechanism of immunological hepatocyte injury in autoimmune chronic hepatitis. In the patient, related to a defect in T-suppressor (regulatory) cells, cytotoxicity is directed not only against foreign antigens but also against self. C = cytotoxic T-cell; K = killer T-cell.

Patients show many serum autoantibodies. Their role in pathogenesis and course of the disease is not known but they are of great diagnostic value. There is no evidence that antibodies against cellular antigens can themselves mediate the autoimmune attack.

Antinuclear antibody is present in the serum of about 80% of patients. The homogeneous (diffuse) and speckled patterns of immunofluorescence are equal. The speckled form is more frequent in younger patients with higher serum transaminase values [39].

Double-stranded DNA is increased in all types of chronic hepatitis with highest titres in the autoimmune group where it disappears after corticosteroid therapy [57]. It is a non-specific manifestation of inflammatory activity [177].

Smooth muscle (actin) antibody is present in about 70% of patients and it is found in about 50% of patients with primary biliary cirrhosis. It is also present in low titre in patients with acute type A or B viral hepatitis or with infectious mononucleosis. Titres exceeding 1 : 40 are rare except in autoimmune chronic hepatitis type I. The antibody is of IgM type. The antigen is related to the S actin of smooth and skeletal muscle. It is also present in cell membranes and in the cytoskeleton of the liver cell. Smooth muscle antibody can therefore be regarded as a result of liver cell injury.

Human asialoglycoprotein receptor autoantibodies. The antigen is a component of liver specific protein (LSP). The presence is closely linked to inflammation and activity [164].

Mitochondrial antibody. This is usually absent or in only low titre.

Genetics [55, 119]

The female sex predominance (8 : 1) is similar to other autoimmune diseases. The disease can be familial [80].

Effector T lymphocytes recognize antigen only if presented on the surface of the damaged hepatocyte by autologous HLA molecules (fig. 17.11). The interaction between the HLA molecule, the antigenic peptide presented in its groove and the T-cell receptor are crucial. Certain alleles at the HLA loci predispose individuals to related disease. Only the predisposition is inherited not the disease itself which must be have been triggered by an antigen.

The major histocompatibility complex (MHC) are located on the short arm of chromosome 6. MHC class I and II genes are highly polymorphic [55, 119]. In autoimmune hepatitis type I, there is a dual association for white people with either HLA-A1-B8-DR3 or HLA-DR4. In Japanese patients the association is predominantly with HLA-DR4. Only limited data are available for autoimmune hepatitis type II. Analysis of the hypervariable region of HLA class II indicate that lysine at position 71 is crucial for autoimmune hepatitis type I in white

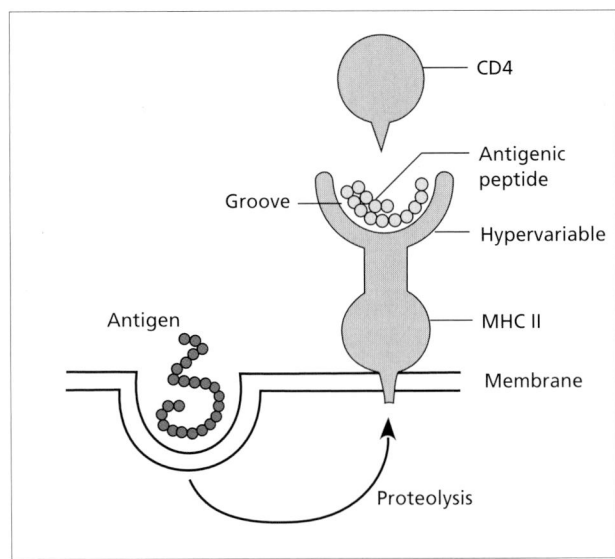

Fig. 17.11. Immunogenetics of autoimmune liver disease: the postulated antigen enters the liver cell by endocytosis. The HLA class II molecule fuses with the antigen-containing endosome and is cleared by proteolysis to peptides. The HLA class II peptide complex is transported to the plasma membrane expressed in a groove and presented to the CD4 lymphocyte. The hypervariability of HLA class II in the groove may predispose to autoimmune chronic hepatitis.

people, whereas the position 13 is important for Japanese.

The complement genes are also polymorphic and are known as HLA class III genes. The MHC class III allele C4A-QO is significantly increased in autoimmune hepatitis type I and II. In the future, HLA typing may be used to identify susceptibility to autoimmune chronic hepatitis. However, recognition of the nature of the antigenic peptide in the HLA groove which is presented to the lymphocyte is essential for further progress.

Hepatic pathology

The lesion is a severe chronic hepatitis. Activity is variable from place to place and some areas may be near normal.

Cellular infiltrates, largely lymphocytes and plasma cells, are seen in zone 1 and infiltrating between the liver cells. Aggressive septum formation isolates groups of liver cells as rosettes. Fatty change is inconspicuous. Areas of collapse may be seen. The connective tissue encroaches on the parenchyma. Cirrhosis develops rapidly and is usually of the macro-nodular type. The chronic hepatitis and the cirrhosis seem to develop almost simultaneously.

As time passes the activity subsides, the cellularity decreases, the piecemeal necrosis lessens and the fibrous tissue becomes denser. At necropsy in the long-standing case, the lesion is an inactive cirrhosis. In most cases, however, careful search will reveal areas of piecemeal necrosis and rosette formation remaining at the periphery of a nodule.

Although inflammation and necrosis may subside completely during remissions, and the disease remain inactive for a variable interval, regeneration appears inadequate as the perilobular architecture is not restored to normal and the pattern of injury remains detectable late in the disease.

Cirrhosis is present in only one-third early in the disease but is usually present 2 years after the onset [147]. Repeated episodes of necrosis with further stromal collapse and fibrosis lead to a more severe cirrhosis. Eventually the liver becomes small and grossly cirrhotic.

Clinical features

The condition is predominantly, but not exclusively, one of young people: half the patients present between the ages of 10 and 20 years. A further peak is seen about the menopause. Three-quarters are female.

The onset is usually insidious, the patient feels generally unwell and is noticed to be jaundiced. In about a quarter of cases the disease seems to present as a typical attack of acute viral hepatitis. It is only when the jaundice persists that the physician is alerted to the possibility of a more chronic liver disorder. It is unclear whether the disease can be initiated by acute viral hepatitis, or whether this is simply an intercurrent infection in a patient with long-standing chronic hepatitis.

In most instances, the hepatic lesion on presentation does not agree with the stated duration of symptoms. Chronic hepatitis must remain asymptomatic for some months or possibly years before jaundice becomes overt and the diagnosis is made. Patients may be recognized sooner if a routine examination reveals stigmas of liver disease or if biochemical tests of liver function are found to be abnormal.

Although the serum bilirubin level is usually increased, some are anicteric. Frank jaundice is often episodic. Rarely, deep cholestatic jaundice is seen.

Amenorrhoea is usual and regular menses is a good sign. However, if a period does occur it may be associated with increase of symptoms and deepening of jaundice. Epistaxis, bleeding gums and bruising with minimal trauma are other complaints.

Examination shows a tall girl, often above normal stature, well built and generally looking healthy (fig. 17.12). Spider naevi are virtually constant on face, necklace area or arms. They tend to be small and to come and go with changes in the activity of the disease. Livid cutaneous striae may sometimes be found on thighs, lateral aspect of the abdominal wall, and also, in severe cases, on upper arms, breasts and back (fig. 17.13). The face may be rounded even before administration of cortico-

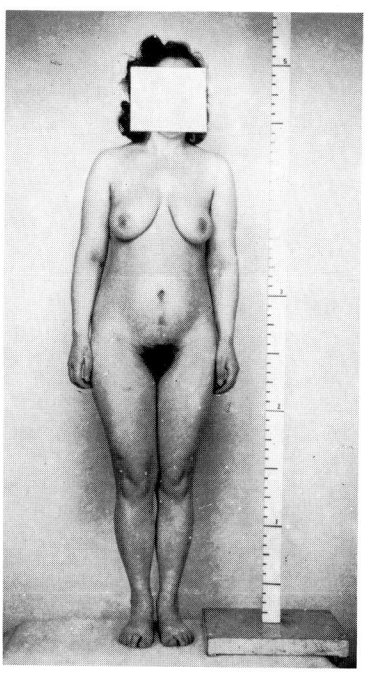

Fig. 17.12. Active juvenile cirrhosis. Well-developed girl with good nutrition.

steroids. Acne is prominent and hirsuties may be seen. The skin may show bruises.

Abdominal examination in the early stages shows a firm liver edge some 4 cm below the right costal margin. The left lobe may be disproportionately enlarged in the epigastrium; nodules are rarely palpable. In the later stages the liver shrinks and becomes impalpable. The spleen is almost universally enlarged. Ascites, oedema and hepatic encephalopathy are late features.

Recurrent episodes of active liver disease punctuate the course.

Associated conditions

Chronic autoimmune active hepatitis is not a condition confined to the liver (table 17.11).

In those who are particularly ill, there may be sustained pyrexia [147]. Such patients may also have an acute, recurrent, non-deforming, migrating polyarthritis of large joints. In most cases pain and stiffness are present without marked swelling. The changes usually resolve completely.

Associated skin conditions include allergic capillaritis, acne, erythema, LE type changes and purpura.

Splenomegaly may be present without portal hypertension, often with generalized lymphadenopathy, presumably part of the same process of lymphoid hyperplasia.

Renal biopsy often shows mild glomerulitis. Deposits of immunoglobulins and complement have been found in the glomeruli. Complexes containing small nuclear ribonucleoprotein and IgG are restricted to those with kidney disease [139]. Glomerular antibodies are present in about half the patients, but do not seem to relate to the extent of renal damage.

Pulmonary changes, including pleurisy and transitory pulmonary infiltrations and collapse, are found when the disease is active. The mottled chest radiograph may be related to dilated precapillary blood vessels. The high cardiac output of chronic liver disease would add to the pulmonary vascular plethora. Multiple pulmonary arteriovenous anastomoses are also found (Chapter 6). Fibrosing alveolitis is another possibility.

Primary pulmonary hypertension has been described in one patient with multi-system involvement [26].

Endocrine changes include the Cushingoid appearance, acne, hirsuties and cutaneous striae. Boys may develop gynaecomastia. Hashimoto's thyroiditis may be seen [147] and other thyroid abnormalities include myxoedema and thyrotoxicosis. Patients develop diabetes mellitus, before and after diagnosis of the chronic hepatitis [147].

Mild anaemia, leucopenia and thrombocytopenia are associated with the enlarged spleen ('hypersplenism'). A positive Coombs' test with haemolytic anaemia is another rare complication [147]. Rarely, a hypereosinophilic syndrome is associated [33].

Ulcerative colitis tends to present with the chronic active hepatitis or to follow it.

Hepato-cellular cancer is reported but it very rare [19, 88].

Biochemistry

This picture is of very active disease (table 17.12). Apart from the hyperbilirubinaemia of about 2–10 mg/dl (35–170 μmol/l), the serum gamma-globulin levels are very high — more than twice the upper limit of normal (fig. 17.14). Electrophoresis shows a polyclonal gammopathy, rarely monoclonal. Serum transaminases are very high, usually more than ten times increased. Serum albumin is maintained until the later stages of liver failure. During

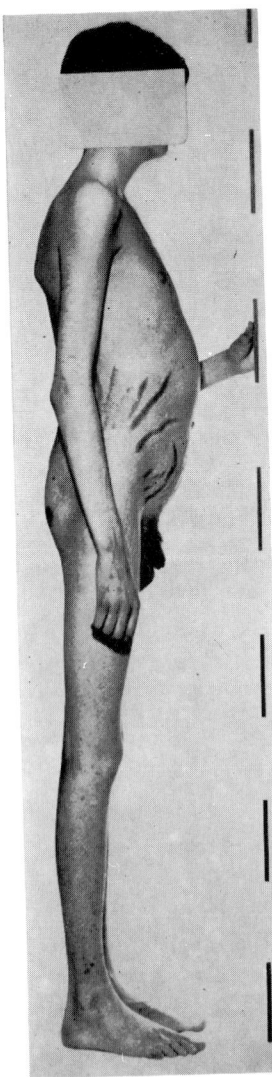

Fig. 17.13. Active chronic 'lupoid' hepatitis. Note tall boy with ascites and striae on the abdominal wall and upper arms.

Table 17.11. Associated lesions in 81 cases of autoimmune chronic hepatitis [147]

Purpura	2
Erythemas	4
Arthralgia	9
Lymphadenopathy	2
Pulmonary infiltrates	7
Pleurisy	2
Rheumatic heart disease	4
Ulcerative colitis	5
Diabetes	3
Hashimoto's thyroiditis	2
Renal tubular defects	3
Lupus kidney	3
Haemolytic anaemia	1

Table 17.12. Typical features of autoimmune chronic active hepatitis

Usually female
Age 15–25 years or menopause
Serum
transaminases ×10
gamma-globulin ×2
Liver biopsy: active, non-diagnostic
ANA > 1 : 40 diffuse
Anti-actin > 1 : 40
Dramatic response to corticosteroids

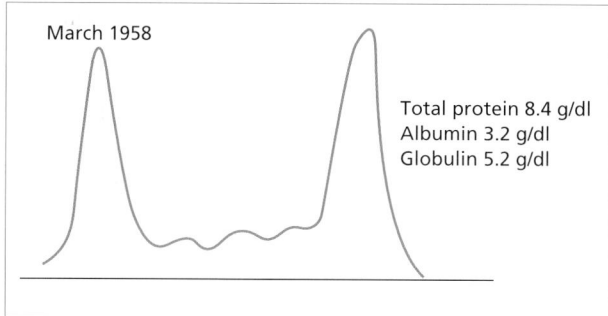

Fig. 17.14. Electrophoresis of the serum proteins. Note the very high gamma-globulin.

the course transaminases and gamma-globulin levels fall spontaneously.

Serum alpha-fetoprotein levels may be increased to greater than twice the upper limit of normal in about one-third of patients. Levels fall with corticosteroid therapy [37].

Haematology

Thrombocytopenia and leucopenia are frequent even before the late stage of portal hypertension and very large spleen. A mild normochromic normocytic anaemia is also usual. Prothrombin time is often prolonged even in the early stages when hepato-cellular function seems preserved.

Needle biopsy of the liver

This is very valuable, but may prove impossible to perform because of the coagulation defect. If biopsy is possible, classical severe chronic hepatitis is seen.

Differential diagnosis

Needle liver biopsy may be required to determine whether *cirrhosis* is also present.

The distinction from *hepatitis B-positive chronic hepatitis* is made by testing for hepatitis B markers.

Untreated patients with chronic hepatitis and antibody to the *hepatitis C virus* may have circulating tissue autoantibodies. Using first-generation testing some of these are false-positive results related to high serum globulin values, but even second-generation tests sometimes read positive. Patients with chronic hepatitis C viral infection may have circulating autoantibodies to LKM-II (see table 17.10).

The distinction from *Wilson's disease* is vital. A family history of liver disease is important. Presentation is often with haemolysis and ascites. Slit lamp examination of the cornea should be performed to look for Kayser–Fleischer rings. This should be done in all

patients under the age of 30 with chronic hepatitis. Confirmation of the diagnosis is made by finding a reduced serum copper and ceruloplasmin and increased urinary copper values. Live copper is increased.

Ingestion of *drugs*, such as nitrofurantoin, methyl dopa or isoniazid, must be excluded.

Chronic hepatitis may coexist with *ulcerative colitis*. Distinction must be made between the combination and *sclerosing cholangitis* where serum alkaline phosphatase values are usually increased and serum smooth muscle antibodies absent. ERCP is diagnostic.

Alcoholic liver disease. The history, stigmas of chronic alcoholism and large tender liver are helpful diagnostic points. Liver histology shows fat (a rare association of chronic hepatitis), alcoholic hyaline of Mallory, focal polymorph infiltration and maximally zone 3 liver damage.

Haemochromatosis should be excluded by serum iron determination.

Treatment

Controlled clinical trials have shown that corticosteroid treatment prolongs life in severe chronic type I hepatitis [30, 129, 158] (table 17.13).

Benefit is particularly seen in the first 2 years (figs 17.15, 17.16) [98]. Fatigue lessens, appetite improves, fever and arthralgias are controlled. The menses return. Serum bilirubin, transaminase and gamma-globulin levels usually fall. The changes are so dramatic as to be virtually diagnostic of autoimmune chronic hepatitis. Hepatic histology shows decreased inflammatory activ-

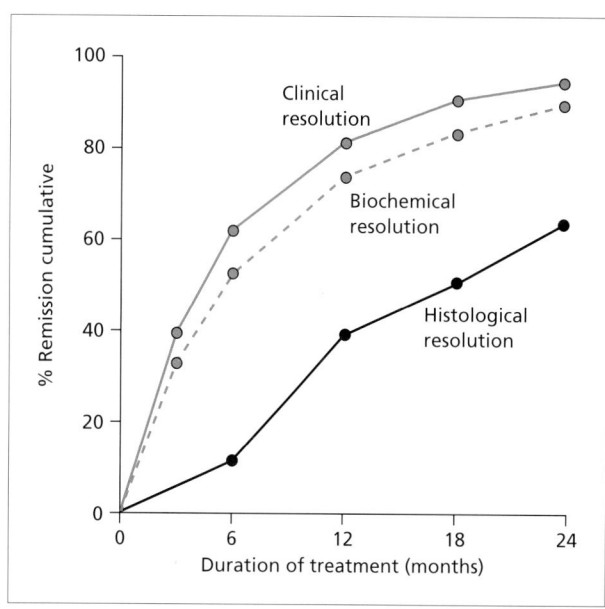

Fig. 17.15. The effect of prednisolone treatment in severe chronic autoimmune hepatitis.

Table 17.13. Significance between the difference in mortality in corticosteroid and control patients with chronic autoimmune hepatitis [30]

Group	Total no. patients	Deaths from liver failure	Deaths from other causes	Total deaths
Corticosteroid	22	3	0	3
Control	27	13	2	15
Significance (Xu21 with Yates' correction)		5.09 (*P* < 0.05)		7.45 (*P* < 0.01)

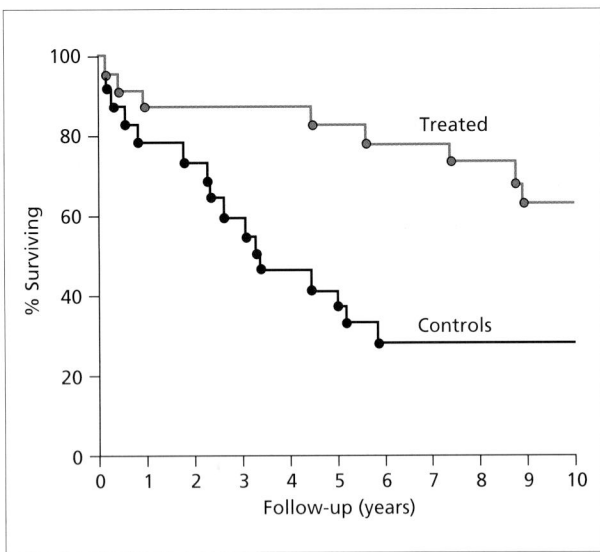

Fig. 17.16. Later results of the Royal Free Hospital trial of prednisolone in chronic autoimmune hepatitis. Note the improved survival in the treated group [98].

Table 17.14. Prednisolone in autoimmune chronic hepatitis

First week
10 mg prednisolone three times a day (30 mg/day)

Second and third weeks
Reduce prednisolone to maintenance dose (10–15 mg/day)

Every month
Clinical check—liver tests

At 6 months
Full check—clinical and biochemical
Liver biopsy

Full remission
Withdraw prednisolone slowly
Re-start if relapse

No remission
Continue maintenance dose for 6 more months, consider adding
    azathioprine (50–100 mg/day)
Maximum dose—20 mg prednisolone with 100 mg azathioprine

Table 17.15. Autoimmune chronic hepatitis: duration of prednisolone treatment

At least 2 years until:
    Serum
        ANA is negative
        Bilirubin
        Gamma-globulin   } normal
        Transaminase
    Liver biopsy inactive
    (usually more than 2 years)

ity but the progression from chronic hepatitis to cirrhosis is not prevented.

Liver biopsy must precede the commencement of therapy. If coagulation defects prohibit this procedure the biopsy must be done as soon as possible after a remission has been induced by corticosteroids.

The usual dose is 30 mg prednisolone for 1 week, reducing to a maintenance dose of 10–15 mg daily (table 17.14). The initial course lasts 6 months. If a remission has ensued, judged clinically, biochemically and if possible by a further liver biopsy, the drug should be tapered off slowly over about 2 months. In general, prednisolone therapy extends over 2–3 years and usually longer, often for life (table 17.15) [78]. Premature withdrawal leads to relapse. Although control is usually re-established within 1–2 months, there are occasional fatalities.

It is difficult to decide when to stop therapy. Long-term, low-dose (under 10 mg daily) prednisolone maintenance is probably preferable [35]. Prednisone may be used but in a slightly higher dose. Alternate day prednisolone is not recommended as the incidence of serious complications is higher and histological remission less frequent.

Complications of treatment include facial mooning,

acne, obesity, hirsuties and striae. These are particularly unwanted by female patients. More serious complications include growth retardation in those younger than 10 years, diabetes and serious infections.

Bone loss is found even with only 10 mg prednisolone daily and is related to duration of therapy.

Side-effects are rare if the dose of prednisolone is not more than 15 mg daily. If this is exceeded or serious complications have arisen, alternative measures must be considered.

If 20 mg prednisolone daily has not produced a remission, azathioprine 50–100 mg daily may be added. It is not given as a routine. Continual use of such a drug over many months or even years has obvious disadvantages.

Other indications for azathioprine include gross cushingoid features, associated diseases such as diabetes and other side-effects at doses required to induce remission.

Azothioprine in a higher dose (2 mg/kg body weight) has been given alone to those who have been in complete remission for at least 1 year on the combination [90]. Side-effects include arthralgias, myelosuppression and an increased risk of cancer.

Cyclosporine has been used in a patient resistant to corticosteroid therapy [86]. This toxic drug should not be given except as a last resort when conventional therapy has failed.

Hepatic transplantation is to be considered when corticosteroids have failed to induce a remission or in the late stages where the complications of cirrhosis have developed. The survival rate is comparable to that of patients who enter a remission after corticosteroids [149]. Successive liver biopsies have not shown recurrent autoimmune chronic hepatitis after the transplant.

Course and prognosis

This is extremely variable. The course is a fluctuant one marked by episodes of deterioration when jaundice and malaise are increased. The ultimate effect of this continuing chronic hepatitis is inevitably cirrhosis with very few exceptions.

The 10-year survival is 63% [98]. After an initial remission following 2 years of corticosteroid therapy, a third achieve a 5-year remission while two-thirds relapse and have to be re-treated. Further corticosteroids have more side-effects. The mean survival is 12.2 years. Mortality is greatest during the first 2 years when the disease is most active. Sustained remission is more likely if the patient is diagnosed early and if immunosuppression is adequate. Corticosteroid therapy prolongs life, but most patients eventually reach the end stage of cirrhosis.

Post-menopausal women respond to initial corticosteroid therapy but have more long-term complications [169].

Patients who are HLA-B8 positive tend to be younger and have more severe disease at presentation. They relapse more frequently [149].

Oesophageal varices are an uncommon initial finding. Nevertheless, bleeding from oesophageal varices and hepato-cellular failure are the usual causes of death.

Pregnancy in patients with chronic active hepatitis is discussed later (Chapter 25).

Syncytial giant-cell hepatitis

This chronic hepatitis was once considered to be related to paramyxoma infection [143]. However, this could not be confirmed. The condition is probably related to many forms of liver disease including autoimmune chronic hepatitis, primary sclerosing cholangitis and hepatitis C virus infection [47, 109].

Chronic hepatitis B virus infection

Chronic hepatitis is not usually preceded by a recognizable acute attack of hepatitis B (fig. 17.17). However, in

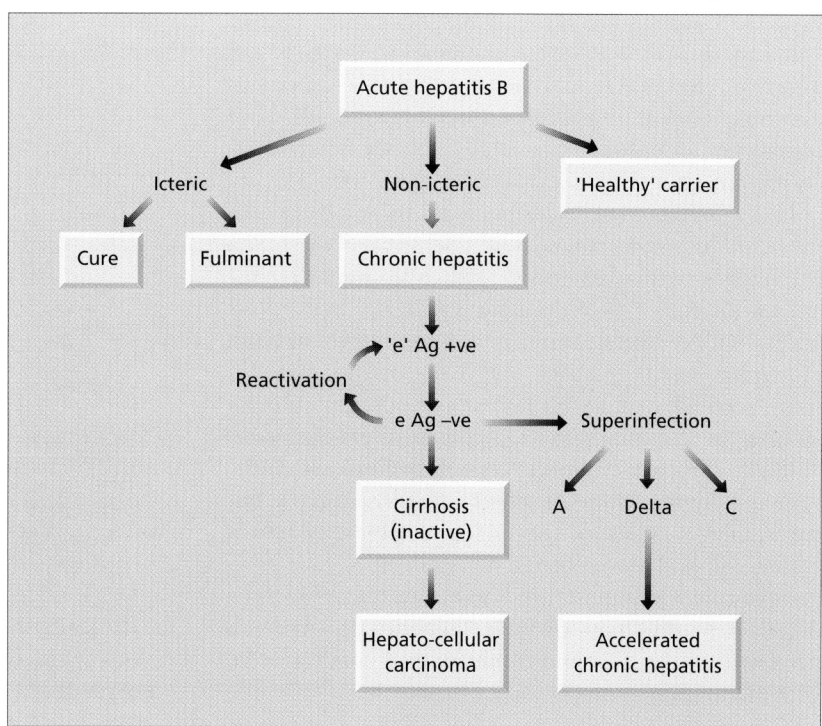

Fig. 17.17. The natural history of hepatitis B virus infection.

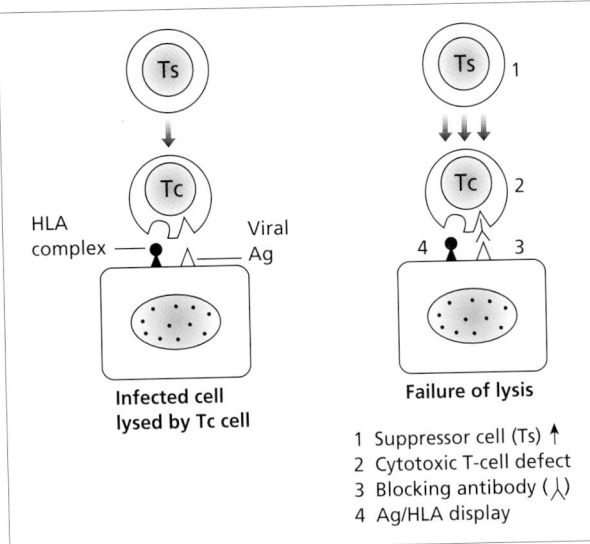

Fig. 17.18. T-lymphocyte lysis of infected hepatocytes and mechanisms of failure of lysis in chronic hepatitis. Ts = suppressor cell; Tc = cytotoxic cell.

some, the acute episode progresses directly to chronicity. In others, again, although the apparent onset is as an acute illness, chronic hepatitis already exists. About 10% of adult patients suffering from acute type B hepatitis fail to clear HBsAg from the blood in 12 weeks and become chronic carriers. Neonates acquiring hepatitis B have a 90% chance of becoming chronic carriers.

Mechanisms of chronicity

Progression depends on a combination of continuing viral replication in the liver and the status of the patient (particularly immunological status). The virus is not directly cytopathic and lysis of infected hepatocytes depends on the immune response of the host [56]. Viral persistence is probably related to a specific failure of T-cells to recognize HBV antigen [109] (fig. 17.18).

Those developing chronic hepatitis show a poor cell-mediated immune response to the virus [56]. If the response is particularly poor, little or no liver damage ensues and the virus continues to proliferate in the presence of normal liver function. Such a patient would be an apparently healthy carrier. The livers of such patients have been shown to contain enormous amounts of HBsAg in the absence of hepato-cellular necrosis. Patients with a slightly better cell-mediated immune response show continuing hepato-cellular necrosis, but the response is insufficient to clear the virus and a chronic hepatitis results [56].

Impairment of humoral and cell-based immunity thus determines the outcome in type B hepatitis. When this is defective, viral replication continues and a carrier state with or without chronic hepatitis results. This is particu-larly important in patients with leukaemia, renal failure or organ transplants, and in those receiving immuno-suppressive therapy, in homosexuals, sufferers from AIDS and neonates.

Failure of lysis of virally infected hepatocytes has various mechanisms (fig. 17.18). It could be due to increased suppressor (regulatory) T-cell function, to a defect in cytotoxic (K) lymphocytes, or to blocking anti-bodies on the cell membrane. In the neonatal disease, perpetuation may be related to maternal HBc antibody *in utero* blocking expression of viral core antigens on the hepatocyte membrane [24].

Some patients with adult acquired chronic hepatitis B show a reduced capacity to produce interferons with resultant defective expression of HLA class 1 antigens on the hepatocyte membrane.

However, IFN-α deficiency has not been proved. The nature of the viral antigen expressed on the hepatocyte membrane could be HBc, HBe or HBs.

Cytokines may be involved. IFN-α, interleukin-1 and tumour necrosis factor alpha (TNF-α) are produced locally in the liver in HBV-related active disease. However, this might be simply a non-specific reflection of inflammation.

Stages of HBV (tables 17.16, 17.17; figs 17.19, 17.20)

In the neonate, the baby is in a state of immune tolerance. There are large amounts of circulating HBV DNA and the baby is HBeAg positive, but the transaminases are normal and liver biopsy shows a mild chronic hepatitis.

In the child and young adult, the stage is immune clearance. Circulating HBV DNA falls but HBeAg remains positive. The zone III mononuclear cells are largely OKT3 (all T-cells) and T-8 (cytotoxic suppressor)

Table 17.16. The stages of infection with hepatitis B

	Replicating stage	Integrated stage
Infectivity	High	Low
Serum		
HBeAg	+ve	−ve
Anti-HBe	−ve	+ve
HBV DNA	+ve	−ve
Hepatocyte		
Viral DNA	Unintegrated	Integrated
Histology	Active CAH, C	Inactive CPH, C, HCC
Portal zone		
Suppressors	Increased	Normal
Inducers	Reduced	Reduced
Treatment	?Antivirals	?

CAH = chronic active hepatitis; C = cirrhosis; CPH = chronic persistent hepatitis; HCC = hepato-cellular carcinoma.

Table 17.17. Stages of hepatitis B viral infection

Age	Stage	HBV DNA	AST	Biopsy
Neonate	Immune tolerance	+++	Normal	CH (mild)
10–20 years	Immune clearance	++	+++	CH (severe)
Over 35 years	Quiescent	Low	Normal	Cirrhosis HCC

CH = chronic hepatitis; HCC = hepato-cellular carcinoma.

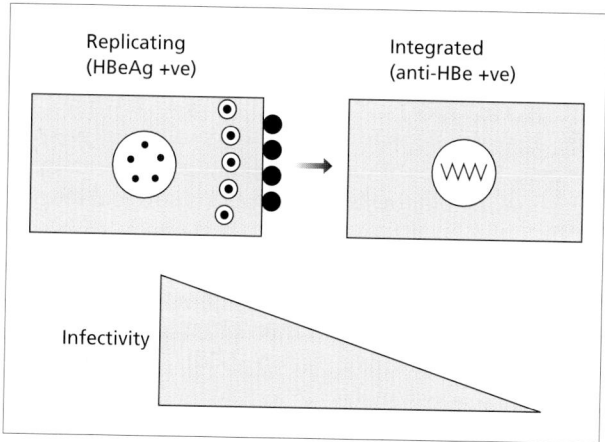

Fig. 17.19. Stages of hepatitis B viral infection. In the early replicative stages, the patient is HBeAg and HBV DNA positive. Core is seen on the hepatocyte membrane. With time, infectivity lessens and the patient becomes HBeAb positive and HBV DNA negative. The viral nuclear DNA has integrated with the host DNA.

cells [128]. Hepatitis B core antigen and possibly other viral antigens are displayed on the hepatocyte membrane. During this period the patient is highly infectious and there is rapid progression of hepatic inflammation.

Finally, in the older patient, the disease becomes quiescent, circulating HBV DNA is low, serum HBeAg is negative and serum HBeAb positive. The hepatocytes secrete HBsAg but core markers are not produced. Serum transaminases are normal or modestly increased and liver biopsy histology shows an inactive chronic hepatitis, cirrhosis or carcinoma. However in some young patients, viral replication is undoubtedly continuing as HBV DNA can be detected in the hepatocyte nuclei in integrated form [84]. The inflammatory infiltrate is similar to that found in autoimmune chronic hepatitis with more helper T-cells and more B-cells being present.

There are considerable differences in the time intervals between these various stages, both in the child and the adult. This differs worldwide. Asians are particularly likely to have a prolonged stage of viraemia with immunological tolerance, a positive circulating HBeAg and high HBV DNA levels. Europeans typically have a long asymptomatic period where HBeAg is negative, biochemical tests are normal and the risk of hepato-cellular cancer may be reduced.

Hepatitis B markers in the liver

HBsAg is usually found in largest amounts in the healthy carrier. In the replicative stage, HBcAg is invariably present in liver. It may be diffuse in asymptomatic carriers, the inactive and immunosuppressed, and focal

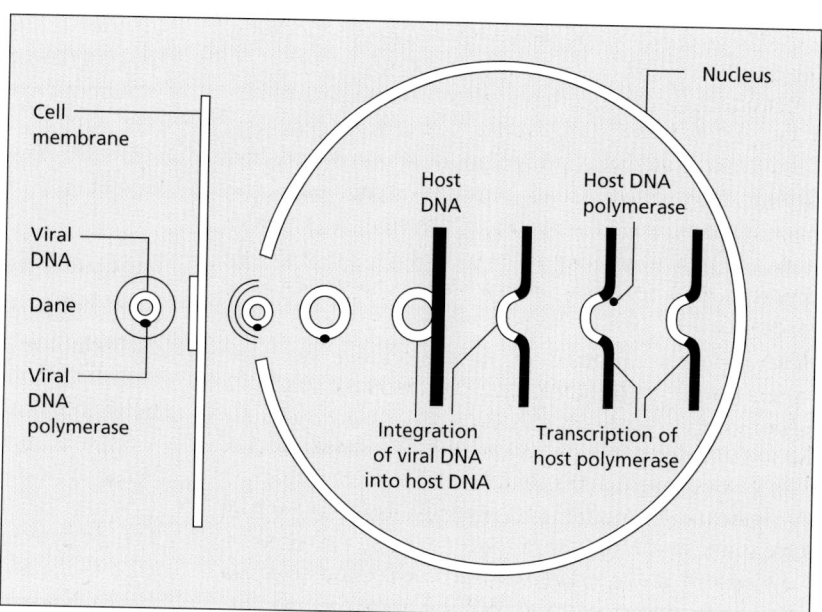

Fig. 17.20. The hepatitis B virion enters the hepatocyte and the core reaches the nucleus. At first the virus replicates using its own viral DNA. Then the viral DNA integrates with host DNA and the host DNA polymerase transcribes for the virus.

in those with much hepatic inflammation or with later disease.

The X protein of HBV may be shown in liver biopsies and correlates with viral replication [74].

HBV DNA can be demonstrated in formol-fixed, paraffin-embedded liver tissue by PCR [106, 157].

HBeAg may be demonstrated by immunoelectron microscopy in endoplasmic reticulum and cytosol [178].

Clinical features

Chronic hepatitis B is found predominantly in males.

Features suggesting an association with virus B include ethnic origin from a high carrier rate country, sexual contacts of sufferers, work in contact with human blood, patients having transplants or immunosuppressive treatment, drug abusers and homosexuals. Neonates born to an HBeAg carrier mother have an 80–90% chance of chronic infection. In healthy adults, the risk of chronicity after an acute attack is very low (about 5%) [87]. There may be none of these associations.

The condition may follow an unresolved acute hepatitis B. The acute attack is usually mild and of 'grumbling' type. The patient, having an explosive onset and deep jaundice, usually recovers completely. Similarly survivors of fulminant virus hepatitis seldom, if ever, develop progressive disease.

Following the attack, serum transaminase levels fluctuate with intermittent jaundice. The patient may be virtually symptom-free with only biochemical evidence of continued activity, and may simply complain of fatigue and being generally unwell, the diagnosis being made after a routine medical check.

The diagnosis may only be made at the time of a blood donation or routine blood screen when the HBsAg is found to be positive and serum transaminases modestly raised.

Chronic hepatitis is often a silent disease. Symptoms do not correlate with the severity of liver damage.

In about one-half, presentation is as established chronic liver disease with jaundice, ascites or portal hypertension. Encephalopathy is unusual at presentation. The patient usually gives no history of a previous acute attack of hepatitis. Some present as hepato-cellular carcinoma.

Clinical relapse and reactivation

An apparently stable patient with HBV-related chronic liver disease may have a clinical relapse. This is marked by increasing fatigue and usually rises in serum transaminase values.

Relapse may be related to seroconversion from an HBeAg-positive state to an HBeAg-negative one (fig.

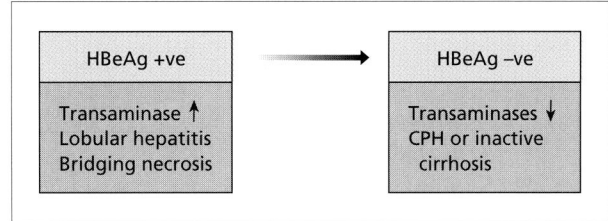

Fig. 17.21. Changes in a patient with chronic hepatitis B on conversion from HBeAg positive to HBeAg negative. CPH = chronic persistent hepatitis.

17.21). Liver biopsy shows an acute lobular type hepatitis which ultimately subsides and the serum transaminase values fall. Seroconversion may be spontaneous in 10–15% of patients per annum or it may follow antiviral therapy. HBV DNA can remain positive even when anti-HBe has developed [61]. In some HBeAg-positive patients, flare-ups of viral replication and transaminase elevation are found without eventual clearing of HBeAg [112].

Spontaneous reactivation from HBeAg negative to HBeAg and HBV DNA positive has also been described. The clinical picture ranges from absence of manifestations to fulminant liver failure [112]. Reactivation is particularly severe in those who are HIV positive.

Reactivation may be marked serologically simply by finding a positive IgM anti-HBc.

Reactivation can follow cancer chemotherapy, low dose methotrexate to treat rheumatoid arthritis [63], organ transplantation [45], or administration of corticosteroids to HBeAg-positive patients.

Severe exacerbations have been associated with mutations in the pre-core region of the virus [136] where HBV DNA is present but e antigen is absent.

The patient may be superinfected with delta virus (see Chapter 16) [66]. This leads to a marked acceleration in the progress of chronic hepatitis.

Superinfection with hepatitis A or C must also be considered.

Finally, any deterioration in a hepatitis B carrier should raise the possibility of hepato-cellular carcinoma.

Laboratory tests

Serum bilirubin, aspartate transaminase and gamma-globulin are only moderately increased (fig. 17.22). Serum albumin is usually normal. At time of presentation features of hepato-cellular disease are usually mild.

Smooth muscle antibody, if present, is in low titre. Serum mitochondrial antibody is negative.

Serum HBsAg is present. In the later stages, HBsAg may be detected with difficulty in the blood yet IgM anti-HBc is usually present. HBe antigen or antibody and HBV DNA are variably detected.

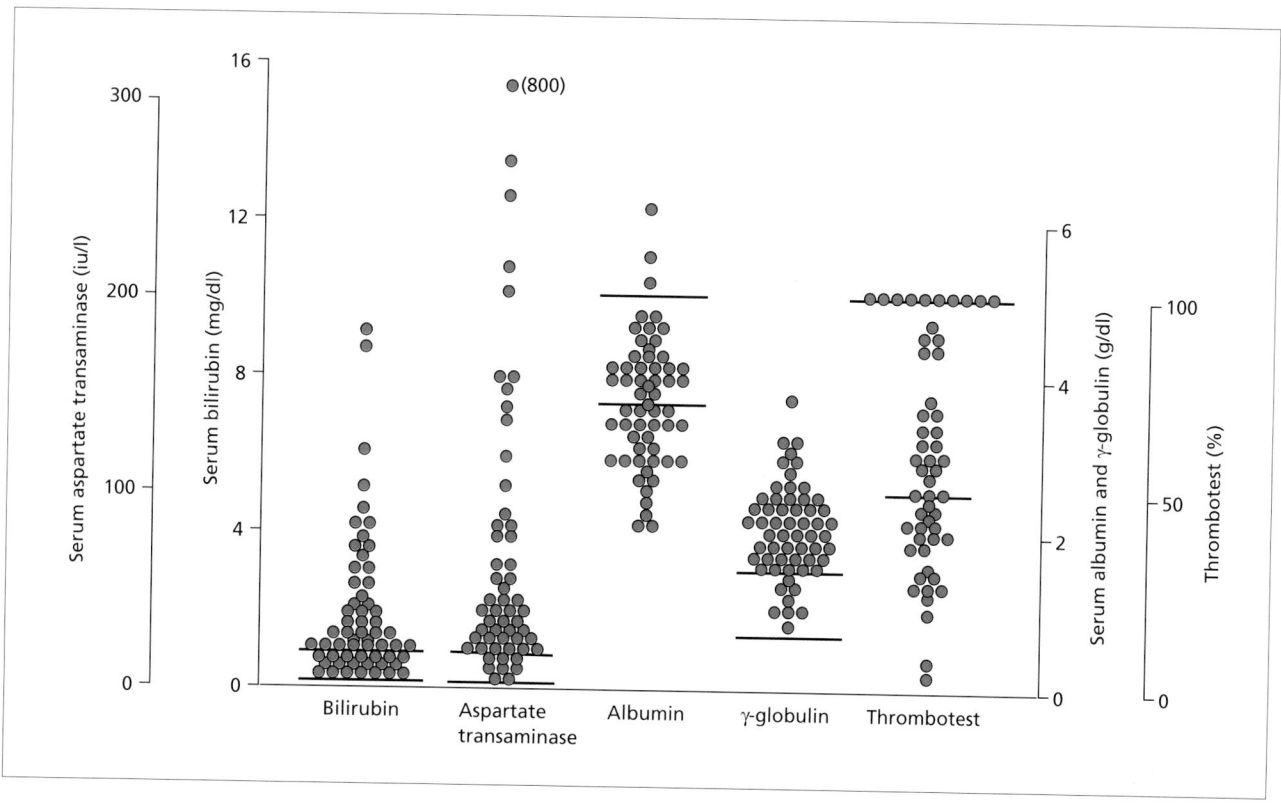

Fig. 17.22. Liver function tests of 59 hepatitis B antigen-positive patients when first seen at the Royal Free Hospital. Note that serum bilirubin, transaminase and gamma-globulin values are not particularly high and serum albumin is well maintained. Bars indicate upper and lower limit of normal range [56].

Hepatitis B virus DNA can be detected by the PCR technique even in the plasma of people negative for HBsAg [170].

Needle liver biopsy. Hepatic histology varies widely and includes chronic hepatitis, active cirrhosis and hepato-cellular carcinoma. There are no constant diagnostic features for distinguishing this from other forms of chronic active or persistent hepatitis unless HBsAg is demonstrated as 'ground glass' cells or by the orcein method or HBcAg by immunoperoxidase. Cirrhosis is less frequent at presentation than in the autoimmune type. The amount of replicating virus in the serum does not correlate with the degree of histological activity [126].

Treatment

The patient must be counselled concerning personal infectivity. This is particularly important if he or she is HBeAg positive. Close family and sexual contacts should be checked for HBsAb and HBcAb and, if negative, hepatitis B vaccination should be offered.

Bed rest is not helpful. Physical fitness is encouraged by graduated exercises. Diet is normal. Alcohol excess should be avoided as this enhances the effects of HBsAg carriage. However, one or two glasses of wine or beer a day are allowed if this is part of the patient's lifestyle.

The majority of patients with chronic hepatitis B lead normal lives. Strong reassurance will prevent introspection by the patient.

The patient's problem should be considered, whether largely of infectivity, of symptoms or of liver failure. Needle biopsy is usual before therapy is instituted. The presence of a severe, chronic hepatitis with cirrhosis will obviously make treatment more urgent. The patient in the infectious, replicating stage must be distinguished from the relatively non-infectious patient in the integrated stage (table 17.16).

HBeAg and HBV DNA positive patients

Treatment is aimed at controlling infectivity, eradicating the virus and preventing the development of cirrhosis and, possibly, hepato-cellular carcinoma (table 17.18). It is unusual with any treatment to actually rid the patient of the hepatitis B virus. However, successful antiviral therapy can reduce or stop inflammatory necrosis of hepatocytes.

Interferon-α

IFN-α, whether lymphoblastoid or recombinant, must

Table 17.18. Interferon for HBe Ag-positive patients: meta-analysis (15 studies) [175]

	Loss (%)	
	HBsAg	HBeAg
Interferon	7.8	33
Spontaneous	1.8	12

be considered. IFN enhances the display of HLA class I proteins and may increase interleukin-2 activity and so destroy diseased hepatocytes.

IFN-α is used only in patients with replicating HBV as shown by a positive HBeAg and HBV DNA, and if necessary, by HBcAg in hepatocytes [25, 49, 51].

The usual regime in the USA is 5 million units daily or 10 million units three times a week by subcutaneous injection for 16 weeks. This is a larger dose than is usually prescribed in Europe and has many side-effects so that there are many treatment drop-outs. Extending the duration of therapy or using higher doses does not seem to increase the response rate.

Early systemic side-effects usually temporary, occur 4–8 hours after the injection during the first week and are relieved by paracetamol (table 17.19). Later, psychiatric complications, especially in those with pre-existing nervous diseases, indicate cessation of interferon. A significant history of psychiatric disorder is a contraindication to giving interferon. Autoimmune changes develop 4–6 months after starting and include positive serum ANA, AMA and antithyroid antibodies. Pre-existing antibodies against thyroid microsomes are a contraindication to starting interferon. Bacterial infections develop especially in cirrhotics.

A positive response is shown by loss of HBeAg and

Table 17.19. Interferon side-effects

Early
Flu-like
Myalgia, usually temporary
Headaches
Nausea

Late
Fatigue
Muscle aches
Irritability
Anxiety and depression
Weight loss
Diarrhoea
Alopecia
Bone-marrow suppression
Bacterial infections
Autoimmune autoantibodies
Optic tract neuropathy
Lichen planus worsens

HBV DNA with a transient rise in transaminases at about 8 weeks as infected cells are lysed (figs 17.23, 17.24) [83]. Ultimately, liver biopsy appearances show less inflammation and hepato-cellular necrosis. Replicative forms of HBV disappear from the liver [116]. Serum HBeAb appears after about 6 months. HBsAg is cleared in only 5–10%, usually when the patient is treated very soon after acquiring the disease (fig. 17.24). Clearance may be delayed for many months.

Interferon treatment is undoubtedly effective [131]. A meta-analysis of 15 controlled studies of interferon for HBeAg-positive patients showed a fourfold increase in loss of HBsAg in those treated and a threefold loss of HBeAg [175] (tables 17.18, 17.21).

Patients with decompensated cirrhosis suffer side-effects, particularly infections which necessitate stopping IFN-α or reducing the dose. Those in Child's grade A may respond to a low dose (e.g. 1 million units three times a week) titratable IFN-α, but those in the more severe Child's B or C grades show poor responses and many side-effects [144].

IFN-α has resulted in long-term remission of liver disease in eight of 15 patients with chronic HBV and glomerulonephritis [29]. The renal disease usually improved.

These results apply to white adults, in good health and with compensated liver disease. Results are less satisfactory in Chinese patients where 25% of responders reactivate and only 17% of the patients who lost HBeAg became HBV DNA negative [115].

IFN can be effective in children [97]. A total of 7.5 million units/m² given three times a week for 6 months resulted in a 30% seroconversion rate of HBeAg to anti-HBe [5].

With such a small success rate, and in view of the cost [176] and discomfort, selection of patients is difficult. Candidates include health-care workers (surgeons, dentists, nurses, medical students, technicians) and the sexually promiscuous. The most likely to respond have a history of acute hepatitis, high serum ALT and low serum HBV levels [43] (table 17.20).

HBV mutations. Specific mutations in the core protein can interfere with T-cell function in advanced chronic HBV infection and may reduce the response to interferon. These mutations develop during the course of the disease and therapy to escape immune surveillance by the host [73]. Although some studies have shown that the presence of mutations is associated with a poor response to interferon, these results are not consistent and other workers have shown the opposite [9]. The appearance of precore mutants during therapy usually predicts failure to clear virus, but substitutions in the core do not influence the outcome [62]. Precore mutants may be associated with severe recurrent HBV disease after liver transplantation.

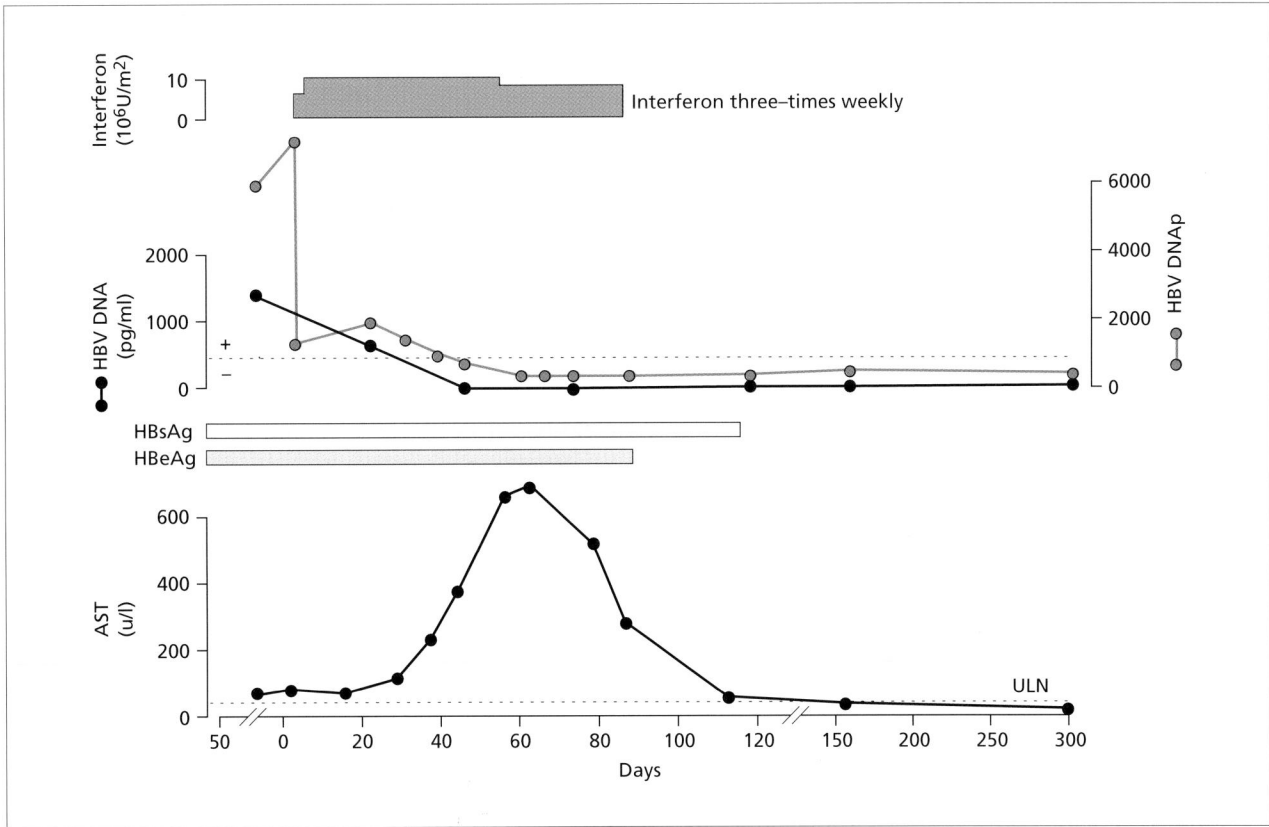

Fig. 17.23. Interferon (initially 10 million units/m²) was given three times a week for 12 weeks to this hepatitis B surface antigen (HBsAg) and hepatitis e antigen (HBeAg) positive patient with chronic hepatitis. HBV DNA and HBV DNAp fell to undetectable levels as did HBsAg and HBeAg. There was a rise in serum aspartate transaminase (AST, GOT) which then fell to below the upper limit of normal (ULN).

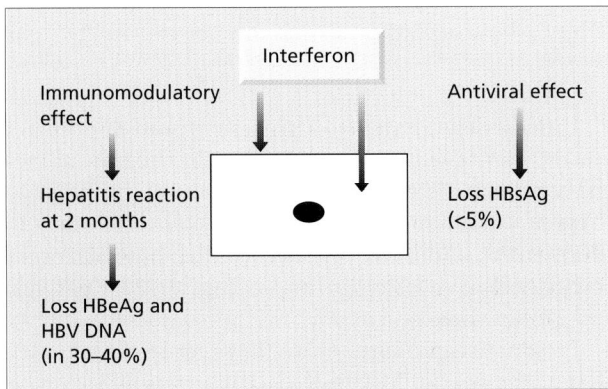

Fig. 17.24. Interferon, used to treat chronic hepatitis B, acts as an immunomodulatory agent resulting in loss of circulating HbeAg and HBV DNA in 30–40% of cases, and to a lesser extent as an antiviral agent resulting in loss of HBsAg in less than 5% of cases.

Table 17.20. Factors determining response of patients with chronic hepatitis B to antiviral therapy

Good
Female
Heterosexual
Compliant
Recent infection
High serum transaminases
'Active' liver biopsy
Low HBV DNA

Bad
Homosexual
HIV positive
Disease acquired early
Oriental

A 3–7 year follow-up of 23 patients responding to interferon therapy showed three relapsed while 20 remained HBeAg negative and asymptomatic; 13 became negative for HBsAg [101].

Nucleoside analogues

Nucleoside analogues are under trial for the treatment of chronic HBV infection. Adenine arabinoside-5-monophosphate (ARA-AMP) is a synthetic purine nucleoside that has antiviral activity against HBV. Early observations confirmed this effect but further trials were not undertaken because of neurotoxicity (myalgia, peripheral neuropathy) which was related to length of treatment. A more recent trial showed that ARA-AMP resulted in 37% of chronic HBV patients becoming negative for HBV DNA, but a complete and sustained response was found only in those with low HBV replication [122]. Myalgia led to withdrawal of treatment in 47%.

Nucleoside analogues have no intrinsic activity against HBV and they must be activated by enzymes present in cells [159]. These enzymes are highly dependent on host species (human or animal), cell type and stage in the cell cycle. This makes it difficult to extrapolate findings from experimental models such as using hepadna virus-infected animal cells, to effects in humans. The species may also play a major role in the different toxicities observed with these compounds.

New oral nucleoside analogues include fialuridine (FIAU), lamivudine and famcyclovir. The clinical toxicity profile is related to the ratio between their affinity for mitochondrial DNA and nuclear DNA. If the nuclear DNA affinity prevails, limited toxicity will become apparent within weeks. However, if the mitochondrial DNA affinity prevails, the development of clinically symptomatic toxicity may take months of exposure to become apparent. This can be explained by the large reserve capacity of mitochondrial function and the large number of DNA copies per cell organelle. The toxicity syndrome that can be expected in severe cases includes myopathy, neuropathy, pancreatitis, liver function disturbances and lactic acidosis.

FIAU initially gave promising results with marked reduction of HBV DNA. However, a prolonged study had to be stopped because of severe mitochondrial toxicity and deaths in volunteers [123].

Lamivudine inhibits the reverse transcriptase necessary to transcribe the HBV RNA pregenome into HBV DNA. Trials using a dose of 100–300 mg daily for 12 weeks have given promising results. HBV DNA becomes undetectable [53] and controlled trials are in progress. Careful watch must be kept for possible mitochondrial toxicity. Flare-ups may follow its withdrawal.

Lamivudine and famcyclovir have been used to prevent reinfection following transplantation in HBV DNA positive cirrhotic patients [67].

Corticosteroids

Corticosteroids enhance viral replication and, after withdrawal, an immunological rebound results in a fall of HBV DNA. Following the corticosteroids, a full course of interferon is given. This routine should not be used in ill patients as enhancement of the immune response may lead to hepato-cellular failure [107]. Moreover, a controlled trial comparing interferon alone with pred-nisolone followed by interferon showed no benefit for the combination therapy [140]. However, a sub-group with an initial serum transaminase less than 100 iu/litre may show improved results when prednisolone treatment is added.

HBeAg and HBV DNA negative patients

These patients tend to be older and have more advanced liver disease. Apart from general measures there is no well-defined treatment for this group. Conservative measures are all that should be offered. Ursodeoxycholic acid, a safe non-toxic hydrophilic bile acid, reduces the effect of more toxic bile acids retained in patients with hepato-cellular disease. In a dose of 500 mg daily, it lowers serum transaminases in patients with chronic hepatitis and is worth a trial [34]. Occasionally, HBeAb may be positive, but serum HBV DNA is present [10].

Screening for hepato-cellular carcinoma

Patients who are HBsAg positive with chronic hepatitis or cirrhosis, especially if male and more than 45 years old, should be screened regularly so that hepato-cellular carcinoma may be diagnosed early when surgical resection may prove possible (see Chapter 28). Serum α-fetoprotein should be measured and ultrasound examination performed at 6-monthly intervals.

Course and prognosis

Over 300 million carriers of hepatitis B are said to exist in the world. With these large numbers it is clear that the disease must, in most patients, be mild and only occasionally progressive.

The clinical course varies considerably (see fig. 17.19). Many patients remain in a stable, compensated state. This is particularly so in the asymptomatic and where hepatic histology shows only a mild, chronic hepatitis.

Clinical deterioration in a previously stable hepatitis B carrier can have varying explanations. The patient may be converting from a replicative to an integrated state. This is usually followed by a remission which may be permanent, serum enzyme levels falling into the normal range and liver histology improving; 10–20% per year may follow this course.

Prognosis is proportional to the severity of the underlying liver disease. Women have less severe liver disease. Age over 40 years and ascites are bad signs. There seem to be geographic and age-related differences in the natural history. HBV DNA positive Italian children have a 70% chance, before they are adults, of becoming HBeAb positive and HBV DNA negative with normalization of the transaminases; 29% will clear HBsAg [13]. In contrast, only 2% of healthy Chinese carriers or chronic hepatitis patients cleared HBsAg in a mean of 4.0 ± 2.3 years [114]. Patients over 40 years, HBeAg negative and with established cirrhosis are more likely to clear HBsAg.

In an Italian study of adults, 20% of patients presenting with chronic hepatitis developed active cirrhosis in 1–13 years [60]. Older age, presence of bridging hepatic necrosis on liver biopsy, persistence of serum HBV DNA and delta superinfection indicated a poor prognosis (see Chapter 16).

In general, the prognosis for the healthy HBV carrier is good. A 16-year follow-up of asymptomatic HBV carriers from Montreal, showed that they remained asymptomatic and the risk of death from HBV-related cirrhosis and/or hepato-cellular carcinoma was low. The annual negativation rate for HBsAg was 0.7% [167]. Similarly, HBsAg carriers with normal transaminase levels in Italy have an excellent prognosis.

A mortality follow-up of sufferers in the 1942 epidemic of HBV in the American Army, showed a slight excess for hepato-cellular cancer. However, the mortality from non-alcoholic chronic liver disease was less [50]. Very few immunocompetent adult males became carriers.

Recurrence of HBV in the graft is usual after liver transplantation in patients with HBV infection especially if HBV DNA, HBeAg positive (Chapter 35). Retransplant for recurrent HBV appears to be contraindicated due to the high mortality [31]. However, it can be considered in HBV-positive patients where the graft failure has other causes.

Chronic hepatitis C virus (HCV)

Worldwide, HCV accounts for more than 90% of post-transfusion chronic hepatitis and cirrhosis [55]. At the National Institutes of Health in the USA, acute post-transfusion hepatitis developed in 6.1% of patients transfused during heart surgery and became chronic in 60% [50]. Follow-up of 39 patients for 1–24 years showed cirrhosis developing in eight (20%). The average time to develop cirrhosis is believed to be about 20 years.

From Germany, follow-up on patients developing HCV infection due to contaminated immunoglobulin showed that of 56 sera, 52 (92.9%) were anti-HCV positive 6–12 months later and anti-HCV was present in 45 of 65 sera 9–10 years after the immunoglobulin [54]. However, 10 years after infection, most patients had not developed chronic disease and no longer had detectable antibodies.

Follow-up of patients with post-transfusion or community-acquired HCV showed an average of 67% with elevated ALT levels more than 6 months later [2].

Those with a raised transaminase and anti-HCV usually had positive virus in the blood (serum HCV RNA).

Chronic HCV accounts for 30% of liver transplants performed in the USA.

Worldwide, it seems that HCV is as important as HBV as a cause of chronic liver disease and hepato-cellular cancer. In certain countries, such as Japan, it may be more important.

The success of HCV in causing persistent infection is probably related to its extremely high mutation rate and its existence as multiple quasi-species, each slightly different in sequence from the other. Many patients have a clinical course characterized by peaks and depressions of clinical and biochemical activity suggesting that HCV may be capable of downregulation in order to reduce immune pressure [15, 82].

Mechanisms of liver injury

Direct viral cytopathic injury has been postulated. This is in contrast to HBV injury which is believed to be immune-mediated. There is increasing evidence that immune mechanisms may also be implicated in HCV chronicity [172].

Cytotoxic flaviviruses tend to cause direct hepato-cellular damage without much inflamation. In chronic HCV, hepatic histology shows minimal damage in spite of progression. The lymphocyte reaction response is weak and eosinophilic hepatic cytoplasm may be seen. In contrast to chronic HBV, treatment of chronic HCV with interferon results in a rapid fall in ALT levels and HCV RNA also falls [156].

There is a correlation of severity with viraemia. Very high levels and very severe liver damage are seen after hepatic transplantation in chronic HCV patients.

The immune response to HCV is weak as shown by repeated flares of serum ALT accompanied by increases in HCV RNA [105]. More severe liver disease is seen with a large viral inoculum (blood transfusion) than a small one (intravenous drug abuse).

Hepatitis C carriers are seen with persistent HCV viraemia but without clinical liver disease [16]. There is no correlation between hepatic HCV RNA and histological activity.

Immunosuppression reduces serum transaminase levels although viraemia increases [92].

Immune electron microscopy suggests that intralobular cytotoxic T-cells perpetuate the liver injury. Hepatitis C virus cytotoxic lymphocytes recognize epitopes in the core and protein envelope of HCV [103]. *In vitro* autologous hepatocytotoxicity assays have strongly suggested that HLA-1-restricted CD8+ T-cell-mediated toxicity is an important pathogenic mechanism in chronic HCV infection [113].

Positive serological tests for autoantibodies (antinuclear, smooth muscle and rheumatoid factor) are found [25]. However, these are unrelated to severity and have not been shown to have a causative role [118].

There is evidence for hepatic cytotoxicity in chronic HCV infection. The immune response to HCV has also been clearly documented but it is less clear how much of the response is protective and how much of it is causative in chronic infection.

Clinical features

Chronic HCV is an indolent disease extending over many years (figs 17.25, 17.26). The acute attack is usually unrecognized and has no clinical features which will predict chronicity. Nevertheless, 80% of patients will develop chronic hepatitis and 20% will go on to cirrhosis.

The patient may be completely asymptomatic, the diagnosis being made at the time of blood donation or a routine biochemical screen. Such patients may have prolonged periods of normal transaminases although

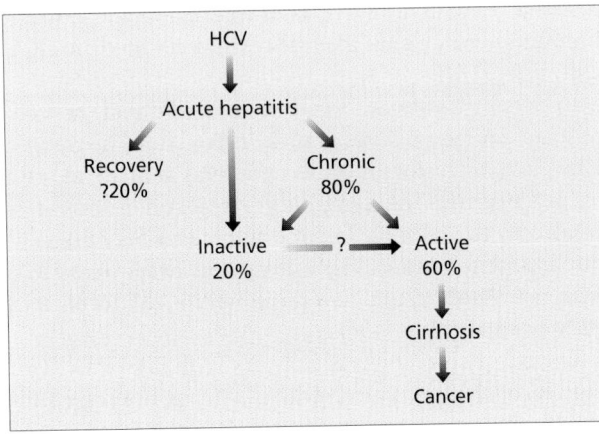

Fig. 17.25. The natural history of HCV infection.

chronic hepatitis is confirmed histologically [2]. Serum HCV RNA may be persistently positive.

Fatigue is a major symptom. The patient feels below par and this varies from time to time.

Direct questioning may reveal a risk factor such as a blood transfusion or intravenous drug abuse. There may be no significant relevant past history.

The course is a slow one, marked by fluctuating (yo-yo) transaminases over many years (fig. 17.27). Each elevation probably represents an episode of HCV viraemia perhaps due to quasi-species. Liver failure develops only after 10 or more years of disease. Before that, many patients, particularly post-transfusion, will have died from another condition [102]. Evidence of portal hypertension is rare, splenomegaly being present in only one-half of patients at presentation. Bleeding from oesophageal varices is unusual until late. Thrombocytopenia develops with the increase in spleen size.

Special investigations

At presentation, the serum transaminase levels rarely exceed six times the upper limit of normal and the mean is about three times (fig. 17.28). Transaminase levels do not predict liver pathology and significant changes can be found with repeatedly normal values [77]. However, results greater than ten times the upper limit of normal do suggest that chronic hepatitis with neuro-inflammation is present [72].

Serum albumin and bilirubin levels are usually normal at presentation and slowly deteriorate with time. Prothrombin is normal.

Serum HCV RNA is essential for measuring infectivity and monitoring the effects of treatment. Quantitative methods such as branch chain DNA (BDNA) assay are useful but insensitive. Confirmation will be necessary by

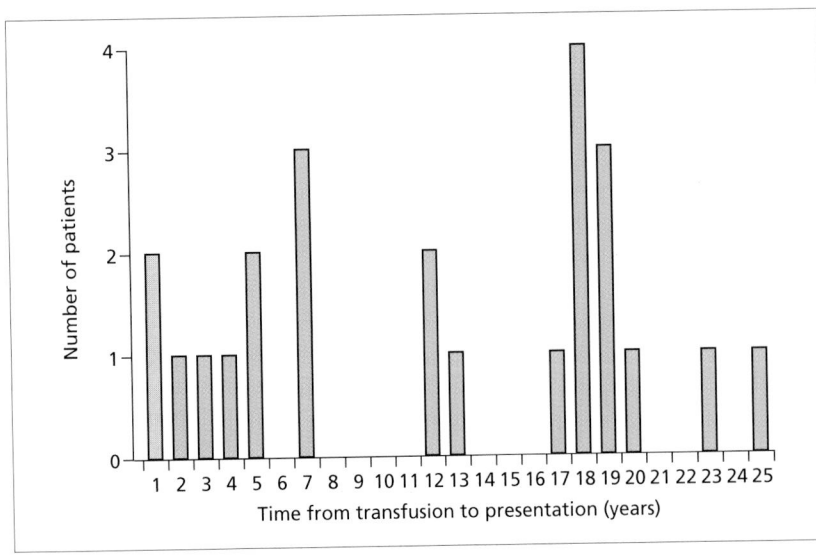

Fig. 17.26. In 25 patients with chronic liver disease after blood transfusion who were anti-HCV positive, the time from transfusion to presentation was very variable. The mean was 12 years, in 58% it was more than 10 years, and in one patient 25 years [137].

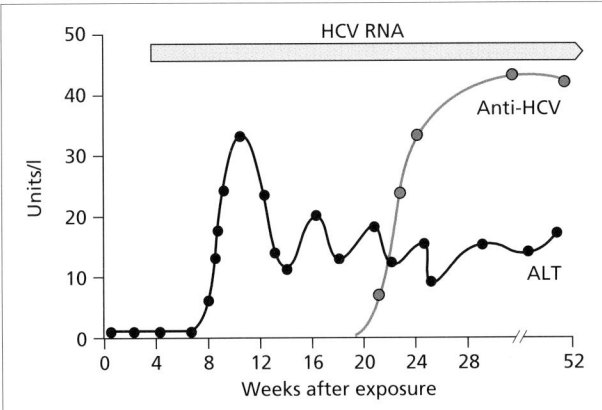

Fig. 17.27. The serological course of acute HCV infection. Serum HCV RNA appears very early. Anti-HCV positivity is delayed. ALT shows characteristic fluctuations as chronicity develops.

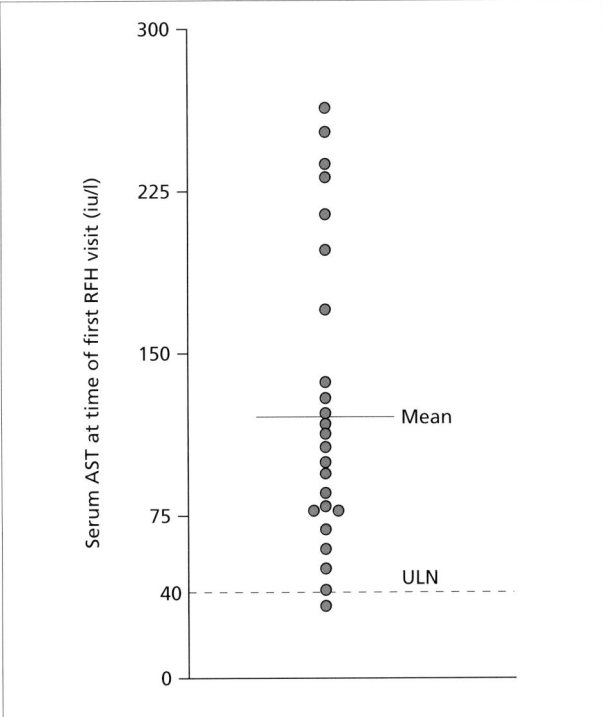

Fig. 17.28. Chronic anti-HCV-positive post-transfusion hepatitis. Serum aspartate transaminase (AST) values at time of referral to the Royal Free Hospital (RFH). Mean was 112 iu/litre and levels rarely exceeded six times the upper limit of normal (ULN) [137].

PCR [68]. If HCV RNA is positive, liver biopsy will be abnormal. A serum HCV RNA exceeding 10^5 molecular equivalents per millilitre correlates with active disease and with transaminase peaks.

The serum IgM anti-HCV core can be useful in monitoring therapy [146].

If possible, viral genotype should be checked (Chapter 16). Type 1b is related to increased severity, worse response to antivirals, recurrence after liver transplantation and the possible development of cancer. Type 4 is related to antiviral failure.

Serum autoantibodies should be sought for diagnosis from autoimmune chronic hepatitis and especially if interferon therapy is being considered.

Screening for hepato-cellular carcinoma by 6-monthly serum α-fetoprotein levels and ultrasound of the liver should be performed in cirrhotic patients, particularly if male and more than 40 years old (Chapter 28).

Hepatic histology (figs 17.29, 17.30)

This is not diagnostic but often makes a characteristic pattern [151]. The most striking feature is the presence of lymphoid aggregates or follicles in portal tracts, either alone or as part of a general inflammatory infiltration of the tracts [151]. The aggregates comprise a core of B-cells mixed with many T-helper/inducer lymphocytes. The outer ring is predominantly T-suppressor/cytotoxic

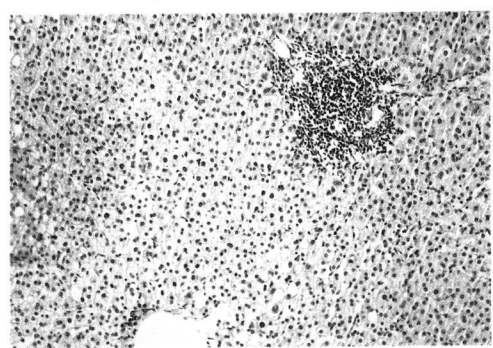

Fig. 17.29. Chronic hepatitis C. Liver biopsy shows a mild chronic active hepatitis with normal zonal architecture and expansion of the portal zone which contains a lymphoid aggregate. Sinusoids show cellular infiltration. (Stained H & E, ×70.)

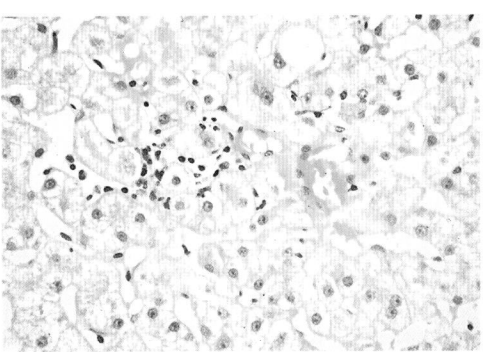

Fig. 17.30. Higher power view of liver biopsy shown in fig. 17.29 shows sinusoidal infiltration with lymphocytes, and acidophil bodies. (Stained H & E, ×100.)

lymphocytes [64]. The composition is similar to primary lymphoid follicles in lymph nodes. Their presence does not correlate with features of autoimmunity. The prevalence of bile duct damage varies amongst different series [4]. Interface hepatitis is mild but lobular cellular activity is usual. Fatty change is found in 75% of cases, the mechanism is unclear. The characteristic picture is of mild chronic hepatitis. Chronic hepatitis can exist with cirrhosis or the picture may simply be that of inactive cirrhosis. Appearances bear no relationship to duration or to the transaminase levels at presentation [137]. Liver biopsy is essential for diagnosis and for assessing activity and stage. Follow-up biopsies are essential in clinical trials but are probably unnecessary for individual patients being treated outside clinical trials.

HCV RNA may be detected in liver tissue by PCR assay [85].

Hepatatis C and serum autoantibodies

About 5% of patients with autoimmune hepatitis give false positive tests for anti-HCV and about 10% of patients with HCV have circulating autoantibodies. The two conditions however, are completely different [124] (table 17.21). Clinical features of HCV are not modified by the presence of autoantibodies.

An association has been found between HCV and a positive antibody test for LKM-I [8]. This might be related to shared antigenic sites between chronic HCV infection and LKM-I autoimmune chronic active hepatitis although detailed analysis has shown the sites to differ [179]. There are clinical differences between the two types. The HCV related patients are elderly, usually male and have a lower titre of LKM-I.

Anti-GOR is an autoantibody against a host protein found in patients with LKM-I positive HCV chronic hepatitis [125]. It is of no clinical significance.

Autoimmune hepatitis can be precipitated by interferon in patients with chronic HCV [65]. This cannot be predicted by pretreatment autoantibody levels. It is marked by sudden increases in serum ALT values and autoantibody titres. There is a good response to immunosuppressive therapy.

The finding of autoantibodies in a patient who is anti-HCV and HCV RNA positive can lead to difficulties in deciding treatment whether immunosuppressive to which genuine chronic autoimmune patients will respond, or antiviral in those infected with HCV.

Associated diseases

HCV-related chronic liver disease may be associated with various immunological disorders [138].

About one-third of patients with essential mixed cryoglobulinaemia have markers of HCV infection. The serum contains complexes including HCV virions and HCV AG/AB [1]. HCV antigen can also be found in liver and skin tissues [150]. It becomes clinically manifest as a systemic vasculitis with purpura, neuropathy, and Raynaud's phenomenon but in only a minority of cases [138]. Some patients respond to interferon therapy [127].

Membranous glomerulonephritis is associated with glomerular immune complexes containing HCV, anti-HCV, IgG, IgM and rheumatoid factors [89]. Interferon therapy may be of value [40].

A lymphocytic sialadenitis, resembling Sjögren's syndrome, has been described but without features of Sicca syndrome [138].

There is an association with thyroiditis even in patients not treated with interferon [163].

There is a strong association with porphyria cutanea tarda [58] and HCV may be the trigger in predisposed people [79].

Lichen planus is associated with chronic liver disease and HCV has been implicated [41, 70, 138].

Coexistence with alcoholic liver disease increases viraemia and accelerates liver damage [133].

The strong assciation of HCV with hepato-cellular carcinoma is discussed in Chapter 28.

Diagnosis

All possible *hepatotoxic drugs* must be sought.

Markers of present *hepatitis B* must be absent. However, some patients with chronic hepatitis due to B virus do get misdiagnosed as hepatitis C when titres of HBsAg and HBV DNA are too low to be detected.

Autoimmune chronic hepatitis is suggested by very high serum transaminase and gamma-globulin levels combined with high titres of autoantibodies.

Wilson's disease is excluded.

Prognosis

This is very variable. In some, the disease is benign with

Table 17.21. Comparison of autoimmune and hepatitis C chronic hepatitis

	Autoimmune	Hepatitis C
Age	Young and middle age	All ages
Sex	Predominantly female	Sexes equal
Transaminases		
AST—10 times	Usual	Rare
'yo-yo'	Very rare	Usual
HCV RNA	Absent	Present
Contact blood	Absent	Frequent
Corticosteroid response	Rapid fall of transaminases	None or modest

spontaneous improvement over 1–3 years. In others, chronic hepatitis tends to convert to more serious disease and on to cirrhosis. In an Italian study, 77% of 135 patients with post-transfusion hepatitis developed chronic hepatitis. By the end of 15 years 65 patients in whom a liver biopsy was performed had developed cirrhosis. Half of the cirrhotic patients progressed to life-threatening complications [165]. In a Japanese study, it took 20–25 years after transfusion hepatitis to develop cirrhosis and about 30 years to hepato-cellular carcinoma [99]. In a group of patients with chronic post-transfusion HCV infection referred to a tertiary care centre in the USA, the disease was progressive, leading to death from liver failure and hepato-cellular cancer [162].

In general, in spite of biochemical and hepatic histological disease, the patient is asymptomatic and the development of hepatic failure is late.

Hepato-cellular carcinoma has been associated with HCV in Spain [18], Italy [27], Japan [134] and the USA [75] (Chapter 28).

Factors indicative of a poor prognosis include very high serum transaminase levels, the presence of an active cirrhosis on liver biopsy, viral load (level of HCV RNA), genotype Ib and associated conditions such as alcoholic liver disease or HBV infection. A positive HCV RNA at the conclusion of interferon therapy predicts a relapse.

Treatment

There is no benefit from rest, diet or vitamin supplements. Older people with post-transfusion HCV infection usually die from some other cause before the HCV disease has progressed to liver failure. In such patients, reassurance may be all that is necessary. Others must be considered for antiviral treatment, usually with lymphoblastoid or recombinant IFN-α [160] (figs 17.31, 17.32). Sustained response is defined as a normal ALT and a negative HCV RNA a year after stopping IFN with histologically improved disease activity. Partial response is defined as improvement but not normalization of the

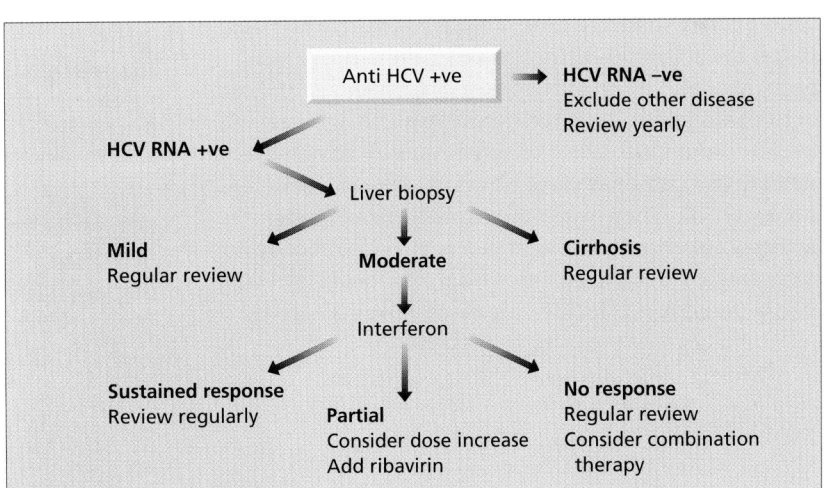

Fig. 17.31. Algorithm for management of the HCV-positive patient.

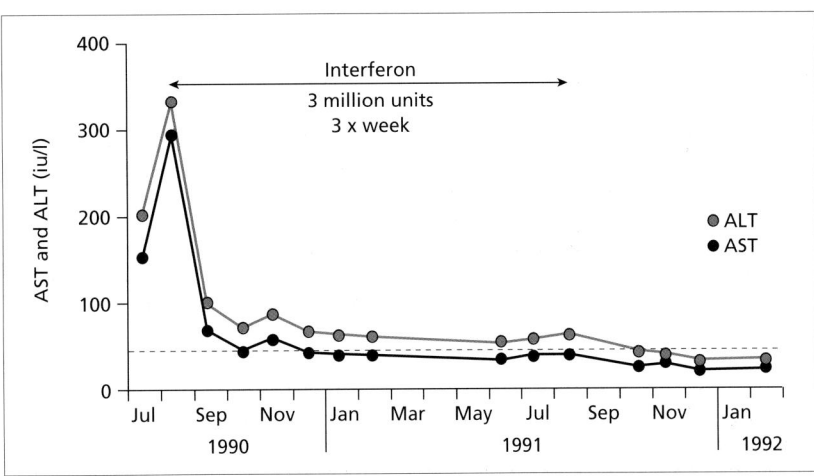

Fig. 17.32. This patient with HCV-related chronic hepatitis was treated with 3 million units recombinant IFN-α three times a week subcutaneously for 1 year. Serum transaminases (AST and ALT) fell to normal and this benefit was maintained when the interferon was stopped. Serum HCV RNA became negative.

serum ALT. Unfortunately, overall the results are unsatisfactory with 50% normalizing ALT during treatment but 50% relapsing, giving a 25% complete response (fig. 17.33) [43, 51, 121]. If serum HCV RNA levels are used for monitoring the response may be less good.

Results can be assessed by serial measurement of serum ALT. Unfortunately, this is not a sufficient indicator of therapeutic response [130]. Serial serum HCV RNA determinations have become essential [110]. Pretreatment liver biopsy is essential to confirm the diagnosis. Patients should not be treated if liver biopsy shows minimal disease and HCV RNA by PCR is negative. Those with cirrhosis are highly unlikely to respond.

Selection of patients for treatment is very difficult and many factors have to considered (table 17.22) [29, 153]. Favourable host factors include female sex, lack of obesity and a normal serum gamma GT [20], recent infection, and a non-cirrhotic liver biopsy [91]. Favourable viral factors include low level of viraemia [67], genotype II or III [166] and low viral diversity [95].

Disappointing results with genotype Ib have been related to mutations in the N55A gene [57].

The accepted routine treatment is IFN-α, 3 million units by injection three times a week for 6 months. There is still uncertainty whether results can be improved by changing the regime, for instance by increasing the dose or the duration. In a controlled trial, patients with non-A, non-B chronic hepatitis were given an initial course of 6 months of 3 million units of IFN three times a week [144] (table 17.23). They were then randomized into three groups: a further 6 months of therapy; a smaller dose for 12 months; or placebo. Follow-up was 19–42 months. Those receiving a further 12 months of therapy at 3

Table 17.22. Possible factors predicting a favourable response to antiviral therapy in chronic HCV infection

Host
Age less than 45 years
Female
Non-obese
Duration of infection less than 5 years
No coinfection with HBV
Not immunosuppressed
No alcoholism
ALT modestly increased
Normal gamma-glutamyl transpeptidase
Liver biopsy: low activity score
No cirrhosis
Liver iron low

Virus
Low serum HCV RNA
Genotype II or III
Viral diversity low

Table 17.23. Three IFN-α regimes for chronic non-A, non-B hepatitis (initially 3 million units three times a week for 6 months) [144]

Treatment group	Normal ALT (%)	Histology improved (%)	HCV RNA negative (%)
6 months more on initial dose	22.3	69	65
1 million units three times a week for 12 months	9.9	47	27
No further treatment	9.1	38	31

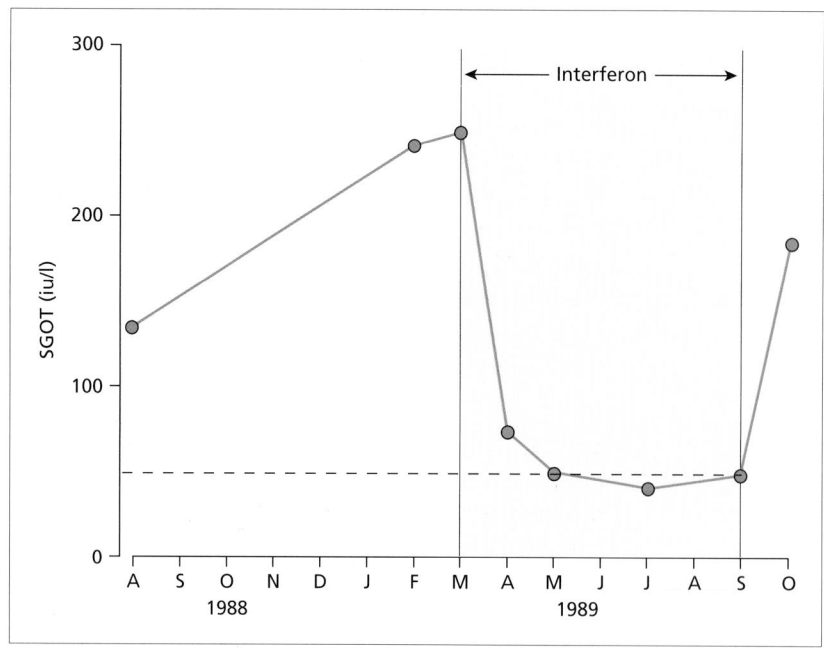

Fig. 17.33. Interferon 3 million units, three times a week for 6 months, to treat chronic hepatitis C resulted in a fall to normal of the serum transaminases within 2 months but with relapse on stopping interferon.

million units three times a week had a significant percentage of patients with a normal ALT, negative serum HCV RNA and improved hepatic histology. In another study, prolonging therapy from 28 to 52 weeks increased the sustained response from 33.3 to 53.5% [96]. However, 38% were resistant to prolonged IFN therapy. Prolonging therapy to 60 weeks has also increased the percentage of those with a sustained response [148]. Long-term treatment may be especially useful in those with a high pretreatment viral load [181].

The results of a randomized trial from Italy showed that a sustained response was significantly more likely if patients were treated with 6 million units three times a week for 6 months followed by dose modification according to ALT behaviour for a total of 12 months. Almost half of the patients had a sustained normalization of ALT and many of them cleared HCV RNA from the serum and hepatic histology improved [22]. The patients were relatively young with a recent diagnosis of HCV and a low rate of cirrhosis. The good results reported may not be generally applicable.

The most effective IFN dose and duration regime has not been decided. Meta-analysis of 20 randomized trials has shown that the best efficacy/risk ratio was in favour of 3 million units three times a week for at least 12 months giving a sustained response at 1 year [145]. Those not responding after 2 months of therapy should be withdrawn [11] (table 17.24). Little benefit follows increasing the dose.

In children, a sustained ALT normalization and HCV clearance may be induced in 43% of those given 5 million units/m^2 for 12 months [12].

By improving liver function, chronic HCV infection and cirrhosis may lead to a decreased incidence of hepato-cellular carcinoma [132].

Positivity for thyroid microsomal antibody before IFN therapy is a risk factor for subsequent thyroid dysfunction [171]. When anti-thyroid antibodies are not detectable, the risk of development of thyroid dysfunction is much lower [120].

HCV patients with anti-LKM may have an increased risk of an adverse hepatic reaction while being treated with IFN. However, the risk is minimal compared with the expected benefits. The patients, however, must be monitored closely for possible liver dysfunction [161].

Table 17.24. Levels of transaminase are measured after 2 months of treatment with interferon (3 million units three times a week) to determine the course of action

Value	Action
Normal	Continue 3×10^6
Partial fall	Increase to 6×10^6
No change	Stop

Management of those who relapse after IFN or who fail to respond is difficult. A few may benefit by an increase in IFN to 6 million units three times a week. In others, combination therapy with IFN plus ribavirin must be considered. In many, counselling and regular review are all that can be offered.

Interferon–ribavirin combinations

Ribavirin is a guanosine analogue with a broad spectrum of activity against RNA and DNA viruses including the flavivirus family. In patients with chronic HCV, it temporarily lowers ALT but has little effect on HCV RNA values, which may increase [52, 148].

Ribavirin has the advantage of oral administration, side-effects are minor and include mild abdominal discomfort and haemolysis (haemoglobin levels and serum bilirubin values must be monitored during therapy) and hyperuricaemia. The mild haemolysis may lead to increased hepatic iron stores [48].

Pilot studies suggested that when combined with IFN, the antiviral effect was enhanced, particularly in those who failed to achieve a sustained response with IFN alone [16, 23, 93, 152]. The ribavirin is given in a dose of 1000–1200 mg daily in two divided doses. The dose of IFN is 3 million units three times a week. Both are given for 24 weeks. Serum ALT falls, loss of serum HCV RNA is sustained in 40% and necro-inflammatory activity is reduced on liver biopsy. The combination has also been shown of value in non-cirrhotic IFN relapsers [22]. Comparison of IFN alone, ribavirin alone and the combination showed that ribavirin alone had only transient effects whereas the combination improved the rate of sustained complete response compared to IFN alone. In another study, 6 months IFN and ribavirin treatment resulted in 78% normal serum transaminase values, sustained for 5 months after therapy compared with 33% for IFN alone and 0% for ribavirin alone [108].

These trials have been small and multicentre trials are being set up to include IFN naive patients, IFN non-responders and IFN relapsers. These should clarify whether the combination, which will be costly, is effective antiviral therapy for chronic HCV and is better than that currently available.

Ursodeoxycholic acid

Ursodeoxycholic acid may improve liver function in patients with chronic hepatitis. It may have a particularly beneficial effect on the 'biliary' component with reduction in transaminases and serum gamma GT, ductular metaplasia, bile duct damage and cytokeratin changes [3].

The addition of ursodeoxycholic acid to IFN therapy significantly prolongs the period in which serum ALT remains in the normal range [14]. However, there are no effects on the clearance of HCV RNA or on liver histology.

Hepatic iron removal

Patients with chronic HCV who respond to IFN have a lower hepatic iron concentration than non-responders [135]. The higher iron content may result in a relative oxidative state and susceptibility to cellular injury [59]. Phlebotomy, to remove the iron, combined with IFN may improve the response in terms of serum ALT and HCV RNA and reduce the likelihood of relapse [21, 76].

New antiviral agents

The development of new antiviral agents and vaccines has been hampered by the failure of a reliable cell culture system for HCV. However, knowledge of the molecular biology of HCV has led to the identification of specific functions associated with particular regions of the virus [11]. These include a possible ribosomal entry site in the 5′ non-coding region, protease and helicase activity for the NS3 region, and an RNA-dependent RNA polymerase associated with the NS5 region. When the assays for these protein functions become available, compounds can be tested for specific inhibitory activity.

Drug-related chronic hepatitis

The whole picture of chronic active hepatitis can be related to drug reactions (Chapter 18) [111]. Such drugs include oxyphenisatin, methyl dopa, isoniazid, ketoconazole and nitrofurantoin. Older females are affected most frequently. Clinical features include jaundice and hepatomegaly. Serum transaminase and globulin levels are raised and LE cells may be found in the blood. Liver biopsy shows chronic active hepatitis and even cirrhosis. Bridging hepatic necrosis is not so serious in this group.

Clinical and biochemical improvement follows drug withdrawal. Exacerbations of hepatitis follow re-exposure to the drug. Drug reactions must be considered in the aetiology of any patient with the clinical syndrome of chronic hepatitis.

Hepatic transplantation

Clearly, transplantation should not be considered at the stage of chronic hepatitis but only when the stage of advanced cirrhosis is reached. Age, psychosocial status, economics, infections and previous upper abdominal surgery are among the pre-operative considerations (see Chapter 35). Transplant of the cirrhotic liver is difficult because of portal hypertension and poor blood clotting. Removal of a small cirrhotic liver may be difficult.

Hepatitis B usually recurs, largely due to extrahepatic replication [42]. Hepato-cellular carcinoma can develop after transplant for HBV disease [117]. Similarly, hepatitis C usually returns as does delta virus infection. Patients with autoimmune chronic active hepatitis rarely show recurrence.

References

1 Agnello V, Chung RT, Kaplan LM. A role for hepatitis C virus infection in type II cryoglobulinemia. *N. Engl. J. Med.* 1992; **327**: 1490.

2 Alter MJ, Margolis HS, Krawczynski K *et al.* The natural history of community-aquired hepatitis C in the United States. *N. Engl. J. Med.* 1992; **327**: 1899.

3 Attili AF, Rusticali A, Varriale M *et al.* The effect of ursodeoxycholic acid on serum enzymes and liver histology in patients with chronic active hepatitis. A 12-month double-blind, placebo-controlled trial. *J. Hepatol.* 1994; **20**: 315.

4 Bach N, Thung SN, Schaffner F. The histological features of chronic hepatitis C and autoimmune chronic active hepatitis: a comparative analysis. *Hepatology* 1992; **15**: 572.

5 Barbera C, Bortolotti F, Crivellaro C *et al.* Recombinant interferon-α (2a) hastens the rate of HBeAg clearance in children with chronic hepatitis B. Hepatology 1994; **20**: 287.

6 Bearn AG, Kunkel HG, Slater RJ. The problem of chronic liver disease in young women. *Am. J. Med.* 1956; **21**: 3.

7 Ben-Ari Z, Dhillon AP, Sherlock S. Autoimmune cholangiopathy: part of the spectrum of autoimmune chronic active hepatitis. *Hepatology* 1993; **18**: 10.

8 Bianchi FB. Autoimmune hepatitis: the lesson of the discovery of hepatitis C virus. *J. Hepatol.* 1993; **18**: 273.

9 Blum HE. Variants of hepatitis B, C and D viruses: molecular biology and clinical significance. *Digestion* 1995; **56**: 85.

10 Bonino F, Rosina F, Rizzetto M *et al.* Chronic hepatitis in HBsAg carriers with serum HBV-DNA and anti-HBe. *Gastroenterology* 1986; **90**: 1268.

11 Booth JCL, Brown JL, Thomas HC. The management of chronic hepatitis C virus infection. *Gut* 1995; **37**: 449.

12 Bortolloti F, Cadrobbi P, Crivellaro C *et al.* Long-term outcome of chronic type B hepatitis in patients who acquire hepatitis B virus infection in childhood. *Gastroenterology* 1990; **99**: 805.

13 Bortolotti F, Giacchino R, Vajro P *et al.* Recombinant interferon-alfa therapy in children with chronic hepatitis C. *Hepatology* 1995; **22**: 1623.

14 Boucher E, Jouanolle H, Andre P *et al.* Interferon and ursodeoxycholic acid combined therapy in the treatment of chronic virus C hepatitis: results from a controlled randomized trial in 80 patients. *Hepatology* 1995; **21**: 322.

15 Brechot C. Hepatitis C virus genetic variability: clinical implications. *Am. J. Gastroenterol.* 1994; **89**: S41.

16 Brillanti S, Foli M, Gaiani S *et al.* Persistent hepatitis C viraemia without liver disease. *Lancet* 1993; **341**: 464.

17 Brillanti S, Garson J, Foli M *et al.* A pilot study of combination therapy with ribavirin plus interferon alfa for interferon alfa-resistant chronic hepatitis C. *Gastroenterology* 1994; **107**: 812.

18 Bruix J, Barrera JM, Calvet X *et al.* Prevalence of antibodies to hepatitis C virus in Spanish patients with hepatocellular

carcinoma and hepatic cirrhosis. *Lancet* 1989; **2**: 1004.

19 Burroughs AK, Bassendine MF, Thomas HC *et al*. Primary liver cell cancer in autoimmune chronic liver disease. *Br. Med. J.* 1981; **282**: 273.

20 Camps J, Chrisostomo S, Garcia-Granero M *et al*. Prediction of the response of chronic hepatitis C to interferon alfa: a statistical analysis of pretreatment variables. *Gut* 1993; **34**: 1714.

21 Caraceni P, Fagiuoli S, Van Thiel DH. Iron reduction therapy: simply camouflage, or a real weapon? *Am. J. Gastroenterol.* 1994; **89**: 970.

22 Chemello L, Bonetti P, Cavalletto L *et al*. Randomized trial comparing three different regimens of alpha-2a-interferon in chronic hepatitis C. *Hepatology* 1995; **22**: 700.

23 Chemello L, Cavalletto L, Bernardinello E *et al*. Response to ribavirin, to interferon and to a combination of both in patients with chronic hepatitis C and its relation to HCV genotypes. *J. Hepatol.* 1994; **21**: S12.

24 Chu C-M, Shyu W-C, Kuo R-W *et al*. HLA class 1 antigen display on hepatocyte membrane in chronic hepatitis B virus infection: its role in the pathogenesis of chronic type B hepatitis. *Hepatology* 1987; **7**: 1311.

25 Clifford BD, Donahue D, Smith L *et al*. High prevalence of serological markers of autoimmunity in patients with chronic hepatitis C. *Hepatology* 1995; **21**: 613.

26 Cohen N, Mendelow H. Concurrent 'active juvenile cirrhosis' and 'primary pulmonary hypertension'. *Am. J. Med.* 1965; **39**: 127.

27 Colombo M, Kuo G, Choo L *et al*. Prevalence of antibodies to hepatitis C virus in Italian patients with hepatocellular carcinoma. *Lancet* 1989; **2**: 1006.

28 Conjeevaram HS, Everhart JE, Hoofnagle JH. Predictors of a sustained beneficial response to interferon alfa therapy in chronic hepatitis C. *Hepatology* 1995; **22**: 1326.

29 Conjeevaram HS, Hoofnagle JH, Austin HA *et al*. Long-term outcome of hepatitis B virus-related glomerulonephritis after therapy with interferon alpha. *Gastroenterology* 1995; **109**: 540.

30 Cook GC, Mulligan R, Sherlock S. Controlled prospective trial of corticosteroid therapy in active chronic hepatitis. *Q. J. Med.* 1971; **40**: 159.

31 Crippen J, Foster B, Carlen S *et al*. Retransplantation in hepatitis B—a multicenter experience. *Transplantation* 1994; **57**: 823.

32 Crivelli O, Lavarini C, Dhiaberce E *et al*. Microsomal autoantibodies in chronic infection with the HBsAg associated delta agent. *Clin. Exp. Immunol.* 1983; **54**: 32.

33 Croffy B, Kopelman R, Kaplan M. Hypereosinophilic syndrome. Association with chronic active hepatitis. *Dig. Dis. Sci.* 1988; **33**: 233.

34 Crosignani A, Battezzati PM, Setchell KDR *et al*. Effects of ursodeoxycholic acid in serum liver enzymes and bile acid metabolism in chronic active hepatitis: a dose-response study. *Hepatology* 1991; **13**: 339.

35 Czaja AJ. Low-dose corticosteroid therapy after multiple relapses of severe HBsAg-negative chronic active hepatitis. *Hepatology* 1990; **11**: 1044.

36 Czaja AJ. Chronic active hepatitis: the challenge for a new nomenclature. *Ann. Intern. Med.* 1993; **119**: 510.

37 Czaja AJ, Beaver SJ, Wood JR *et al*. Frequency and significance of serum alpha-fetoprotein elevation in severe hepatitis B surface antigen-negative chronic active hepatitis. *Gastroenterology* 1987; **93**: 687.

38 Czaja AJ, Carpenter HA, Manns MP. Antibodies to soluble liver antigen P450-IID5 and mitochondrial complexes in chronic hepatitis. *Gastroenterology* 1993; **105**: 1522.

39 Czaja AJ, Nishioka M, Morshed SA *et al*. Patterns of nuclear immunofluorescence and reactivities to recombinant nuclear antigens in autoimmune hepatitis. *Gastroenterology* 1994; **107**: 200.

40 D'Amico G, Fornasieri A. Cryoglobulinemic glomerulonephritis: a membranoproliferative glomerulonephritis induced by hepatitis C virus. *Am. J. Kidney Dis.* 1995; **25**: 361.

41 Daoud MS, Gibson LE, Daoud S *et al*. Chronic hepatitis C and skin diseases: a review. *Mayo Clin. Proc.* 1995; **70**: 559.

42 Davies SE, Portmann BC, O'Grady JG *et al*. Hepatic histological findings after transplantation for chronic B virus infection, including a unique pattern of fibrosing cholestatic hepatitis. *Hepatology* 1991; **13**: 150.

43 Davis GL, Balart LA, Schiff ER *et al*. Treatment of chronic hepatitis C with recombinant interferon alpha: a multicenter randomized, controlled trial. *N. Engl. J. Med.* 1989; **321**: 1501.

44 De Man RA, Heijtink RA, Niesters HGM *et al*. New developments in antiviral therapy for chronic hepatitis B infection. *Scand. J. Gastroenterol.* 1995; **30** (Suppl. 212): 100.

45 Degos F, Lugassy C, Degott C *et al*. Hepatitis B virus and hepatitis B-related viral infection in renal transplant recipients. A prospective study of 90 patients. *Gastroenterology* 1988; **94**: 151.

46 Desmet VJ, Gerber M, Hoofnagle JH *et al*. Classification of chronic hepatitis: diagnosis, grading and staging. *Hepatology* 1994; **19**: 1513.

47 Devaney K, Goodman ZD, Ishak KG. Post infantile giant-cell transformation in hepatitis. *Hepatology* 1992; **16**: 327.

48 Di Bisceglie AM, Bacon BR, Kleiner DE *et al*. Increase in hepatic iron stores following prolonged therapy with ribavirin in patients with chronic hepatitis C. *J. Hepatol.* 1994; **21**: 1109.

49 Di Bisceglie AM, Fong TL, Fried MW *et al*. A randomized, controlled trial of recombinant α-interferon therapy for chronic hepatitis B. *Am. J. Gastroenterol.* 1993; **88**: 1887.

50 Di Bisceglie AM, Goodman ZD, Ishak KG *et al*. Long-term clinical and histopathological follow-up of clinical post-transfusion hepatitis. *Hepatology* 1991; **14**: 969.

51 Di Bisceglie AM, Martin P, Kassianides C *et al*. Recombinant interferon alfa therapy for chronic hepatitis C. A randomized, double-blind, placebo-controlled trial. *N. Engl. J. Med.* 1989; **321**: 1506.

52 Di Bisceglie AM, Shindo M, Fong T-L *et al*. A pilot study of ribavirin therapy for chronic hepatitis C. *Hepatology* 1992; **16**: 649.

53 Dienstag JL, Perrillo RP, Schiff ER *et al*. A preliminary trial of lamivudine for chronic hepatitis B infection. *N. Engl. J. Med.* 1995; **333**: 1657.

54 Dittmann S, Roggendorf M, Durkop J *et al*. Long-term persistence of hepatitis C virus antibodies in a single source outbreak. *J. Hepatol.* 1991; **13**: 323.

55 Donaldson P, Doherty D, Underhill J *et al*. The molecular genetics of autoimmune liver disease. *Hepatology* 1994; **20**: 225.

56 Dudley FJ, Fox RA, Sherlock S. Cellular immunity and hepatitis associated (Australia) antigen liver disease. *Lancet* 1972; **i**: 743.

57 Enomoto N, Sakuma I, Asahina Y *et al.* Mutations in the non-structural protein 5A gene and response to interferon in patients with chronic hepatitis C virus 1b infection. *N. Engl. J. Med.* 1996; **334**: 77.

58 Fargion S, Piperno A, Cappellini MD *et al.* Hepatitis C virus and porphyria cutanea tarda: evidence of a strong association. *Hepatology* 1992; **16**: 1322.

59 Farinati F, Cardin R, De Maria N *et al.* Iron storage, lipid peroxidation and glutathione turnover in chronic anti-HCV positive hepatitis. *J. Hepatol.* 1995; **22**: 449.

60 Fattovich G, Brollo L, Giustina G *et al.* Natural history and prognostic factors for chronic hepatitis type B. *Gut* 1991; **32**: 294.

61 Fattovich G, Rugge M, Brollo L *et al.* Clinical, virologic and histologic outcome following sero-conversion from HBeAg to anti-HBe in chronic hepatitis type B. *Hepatology* 1986; **6**: 167.

62 Fattovich G, McIntyre G, Thursz M *et al.* Hepatitis B virus precore/core variation and interferon therapy. *Hepatology* 1995; **22**: 1355.

63 Flowers MA, Heathcote J, Wanless IR *et al.* Fulminant hepatitis as a consequence of reactivation of hepatitis B virus infection after discontinuation of low-dose methotrexate therapy. *Ann. Intern. Med.* 1990; **112**: 381.

64 Freni MA, Artuso D, Gerken G *et al.* Focal lymphocytic aggregates in chronic hepatitis C: occurrence, immuno-histochemical characterization, and relation to markers of autoimmunity. *Hepatology* 1995; **22**: 389.

65 Garcia-Buey L, Garcia-Monzon C, Rodriguez S *et al.* Latent autoimmune hepatitis triggered during interferon therapy in patients with chronic hepatitis C. *Gastroenterology* 1995; **108**: 1770.

66 Govindarajan S, De Cock KM, Redeker AG. Natural course of delta superinfection in chronic hepatitis B virus-infected patients: histopathologic study with multiple liver biopsies. *Hepatology* 1986; **6**: 640.

67 Grellier L, Brown D, McPhilips P *et al.* Lamivudine prophylaxis: a new strategy for prevention of reinfection in liver transplantation for hepatitis B DNA positive cirrhosis. *Hepatology* 1995; **22**: 224A.

68 Gretch DR, dela Rosa C, Carithers RL Jr *et al.* Assessment of hepatitis C viremia using molecular amplification technologies: correlations and clinical implications. *Ann. Intern. Med.* 1995; **123**: 321.

69 Gueguen M, Boniface O, Bernard O *et al.* Identification of the main epitope on human cytochrome P450-IID6 recognised by anti-liver kidney microsome antibody. *J. Autoimmun.* 1991; **4**: 607.

70 Gumber SC, Chopra S. Hepatitis C: a multifaceted disease. Review of extrahepatic manifestations. *Ann. Intern. Med.* 1995; **123**: 615.

71 Gurian LE, Rogoff TM, Ware AJ *et al.* The immunologic diagnosis of chronic active 'auto-immune' hepatitis: distinction from systemic lupus erythematosus. *Hepatology* 1985; **5**: 397.

72 Haber MM, West AB, Haber AD *et al.* Relationship of aminotransferases to liver histological status in chronic hepatitis C. *Am. J. Gastroenterol.* 1995; **90**: 1250.

73 Hamasaki K, Nakata K, Nagayama Y *et al.* Changes in the prevalence of HBeAg-negative mutant hepatitis B virus during the course of chronic hepatitis B. *Hepatology* 1994; **20**: 8.

74 Haruna Y, Hayashi N, Katayama K *et al.* Expression of X protein and hepatitis B virus replication in chronic hepatitis. *Hepatology* 1991; **13**: 417.

75 Hasan F, Jeffers LJ, De Medina M *et al.* Hepatitis C-associated hepatocellular carcinoma. *Hepatology* 1990; **12**: 589.

76 Hayashi H, Takikawa T, Nishimura N et al. Improvement of serum aminotransferase levels after phlebotomy in patients with chronic active hepatitis C and excess hepatic iron. *Am. J. Gastroenterol.* 1994; **89**: 986.

77 Healey CJ, Chapman RWG, Fleming KA. Liver histology in hepatitis C infection: a comparison between patients with persistently normal or abnormal transaminases. *Gut* 1995; **37**: 274.

78 Hegarty JE, Nouri Aria KT, Portmann B *et al.* Relapse following treatment withdrawal in patients with autoimmune chronic active hepatitis. *Hepatology* 1983; **3**: 685.

79 Herrero C, Vicente A, Bruguera M *et al.* Is hepatitis C virus infection a trigger of porphyria cutanea tarda? *Lancet* 1993; **341**: 788.

80 Hodges S, Loboyeo A, Donaldson P *et al.* Autoimmune chronic active hepatitis in a family. *Gut* 1991; **32**: 299.

81 Homberger JC, Abuaf JC, Bernard O *et al.* Chronic active hepatitis associated with anti-liver/kidney microsome antibody type I: a second type of 'autoimmune' hepatitis. *Hepatology* 1987; **7**: 1333.

82 Honda M, Kaneko S, Sakai A *et al.* Degree of diversity of hepatitis C virus quasispecies and progression of liver disease. *Hepatology* 1994; **20**: 1144.

83 Hoofnagle JH, Peters M, Mullen KD *et al.* Randomized, controlled trial of recombinant human alpha-interferon in patients with chronic hepatitis B. *Gastroenterology* 1988; **95**: 1318.

84 Hoofnagle JH, Shafritz DA, Popper H. Chronic type B hepatitis and the 'healthy' HBsAg carrier state. *Hepatology* 1987; **7**: 758.

85 Hosoda K, Omata M, Yukosuka O *et al.* Non-A, non-B chronic hepatitis is chronic hepatitis C: A sensitive assay for detection of hepatitis C virus RNA in the liver. *Hepatology* 1992; **15**: 777.

86 Hayams JS, Ballow M, Leichtner AM. Cyclosporine treatment of autoimmune chronic active hepatitis. *Gastroenterology* 1987; **93**: 890.

87 Hyams KC. Risks of chronicity following acute hepatitis B virus infection: a review. *Clin. Infect. Dis.* 1995; **20**: 992.

88 Jakobovits AW, Gibson PR, Dudley FJ. Primary liver cell carcinoma complicating auto-immune chronic acute hepatitis. *Dig. Dis. Sci.* 1981; **26**: 694.

89 Johnson RJ, Gretch DR, Yamabe H *et al.* Membranoproliferative glomerulonephritis associated with hepatitis C virus infection. *N. Engl. J. Med.* 1993; **328**: 465.

90 Johnson PJ, McFarlane IG, Williams R. Azathioprine for long-term maintenance of remission in autoimmune hepatitis. *N. Engl. J. Med.* 1995; **333**: 958.

91 Jouet P, Roudot-Thoraval F, Dhumeaux D *et al.* Comparative efficacy of interferon alfa in cirrhotic and non-cirrhotic patients with non-A, non-B, C hepatitis. *Gastroenterology* 1994; **106**: 686.

92 Kagawa T, Saito H, Tada S *et al.* Is hepatitis C virus cytopathic? *Lancet* 1993; **341**: 316.

93 Kakumu S, Yoshioka K, Wakita T *et al.* A pilot study of ribavirin and interferon beta for the treatment of chronic hepatitis C. *Gastroenterology* 1993; **105**: 507.

94 Kalland K-H, Endresen C, Haukenes G *et al*. Measles-specific nucleotide sequences and autoimmune chronic active hepatitis. *Lancet* 1989; **1**: 1390 (letter).

95 Kanazawa Y, Hayashi N, Mita E *et al*. Influence of viral quasispecies on effectiveness of interferon therapy in chronic hepatitis C patients. *Hepatology* 1994; **20**: 1121.

96 Kashara A, Hayashi N, Hiramatsu N *et al*. Ability of prolonged interferon treatment to suppress relapse after cessation of therapy in patients with chronic hepatitis C: a multicenter randomized controlled trial. *Hepatology* 1995; **21**: 291.

97 Kay MH, Wyllie R, Deimler C *et al*. Alpha interferon therapy in children with chronic active hepatitis B and delta virus infection. *J. Pediatr*. 1993; **123**: 1001.

98 Kirk AP, Jain S, Pocock S *et al*. Late results of Royal Free Hospital controlled trial of prednisolone therapy in hepatitis B surface antigen-negative chronic active hepatitis. *Gut* 1980; **21**: 78.

99 Kiyosawa K, Sodeyama T, Tanaka E *et al*. Interrelationship of blood transfusion, non-A, non-B hepatitis and hepatocellular carcinoma: analysis by detection of anti-body to hepatitis C virus. *Hepatology* 1990; **12**: 671.

100 Knodell RG, Ishak KG, Black WC *et al*. Formulation and application of a numerical scoring system for assessing histological activity in asymptomatic chronic active hepatitis. *Hepatology* 1981; **4**: 431.

101 Korenman J, Baker B, Waggoner J *et al*. Long-term remission of chronic hepatitis B after alpha-interferon therapy. *Ann. Intern. Med*. 1991; **114**: 629.

102 Koretz RL, Abbey H, Coleman E *et al*. Non-A, non-B posttransfusion hepatitis. Looking back in the second decade. *Ann. Intern. Med*. 1993; **119**: 110.

103 Koziel MJ, Dudley D, Afdhal N *et al*. Hepatitis C virus (HCV-specific, cytotoxic T lymphocytes recognise epitopes in the core and envelope proteins of HCV. *J. Virol*. 1993; **67**: 7522.

104 Krawitt EJ. Autoimmune hepatitis. *N. Engl. J. Med*. 1996; **334**: 897.

105 Lai MY, Yang PM, Kao JH *et al*. Combination therapy of α-interferon and ribavirin in patients with chronic hepatitis C: an interim report. *Hepatology* 1993; **18**: 93A.

106 Lampertico P, Malter JS, Colombo M *et al*. Detection of hepatitis B virus DNA in formalin-fixed, paraffin-embedded liver tissue by polymerase chain reaction. *Am. J. Pathol*. 1990; **137**: 253.

107 Laskus T, Slusarczyk J, Cianciara J *et al*. Exacerbation of chronic active hepatitis type B after short-term corticosteroid therapy resulting in fatal liver failure. *Am. J. Gastroenterol*. 1990; **85**: 1414.

108 Lau JYN, Konkoulis G, Mieli-Vergano G *et al*. Syncytial giant-cell hepatitis: a specific disease entity? *J. Hepatol*. 1992; **15**: 216.

109 Lau JYN, Mizokami N, Ohno T *et al*. Discrepancy between biochemical and virological responses to interferon-α in chronic hepatitis C. *Lancet* 1993; **342**: 1208.

110 Lau JYN, Wright TL. Molecular virology and pathogenesis of hepatitis B. *Lancet* 1992; **342**: 1335.

111 Lee WM. Drug-induced hepatotoxicity. *N. Engl. J. Med*. 1995; **333**: 1118.

112 Levy P, Marcellin P, Martinot-Peignoux M *et al*. Clinical course of spontaneous reactivation of hepatitis B virus infection in patients with chronic hepatitis B. *Hepatology* 1990; **12**: 570.

113 Liaw Y-F, Lee C-S, Tsai SL *et al*. T-cell-mediated autologous hepatocytotoxicity in patients with chronic hepatitis C virus infection. *Hepatology* 1995; **22**: 1368.

114 Liaw Y-F, Sheen I-S, Chen T-J *et al*. Incidence, determinants and significance of delayed clearance of serum HBsAg in chronic hepatitis B virus infection: a prospective study. *Hepatology* 1991; **13**: 627.

115 Lok AS, Chung HT, Liu VW *et al*. Long-term follow-up of chronic hepatitis B patients treated with interferon alfa. *Gastroenterology* 1993; **105**: 1883.

116 Lok ASF, Ma OCK, Lau JYN. Interferon alpha therapy in patients with chronic hepatitis B virus infection: effects on hepatitis B virus DNA in the liver. *Gastroenterology* 1991; **100**: 756.

117 Luketic VA, Shiffman ML, McCall JB *et al*. Primary hepatocellular carcinoma after orthotopic liver transplantation for chronic hepatitis B infection. *Ann. Intern. Med*. 1991; **114**: 212.

118 Lunel F. Hepatitis C virus and autoimmunity: fortuitous association or reality? *Gastroenterology* 1994; **107**: 1550.

119 Manns MP, Kruger M. Immunogenetics of chronic liver diseases. *Gastroenterology* 1994; **106**: 1676.

120 Marcellin P, Boyer N, Giostra E *et al*. Recombinant human alpha-interferon in patients with chronic non-A, non-B hepatitis: a multicenter, randomized controlled trial from France. *Hepatology* 1991; **13**: 393.

121 Marcellin P, Pouteau M, Benhamou J-P. Hepatitis C virus infection, alpha interferon therapy and thyroid dysfunction. *J. Hepatol*. 1995; **22**: 364.

122 Marcellin P, Pouteau M, Loriot MA *et al*. Adenine arabinoside 5′-monophosphate in patients with chronic hepatitis B: comparison of the efficacy in patients with high and low viral replication. *Gut* 1995; **36**: 422.

123 McKenzie R, Fried MW, Sallie R *et al*. Hepatic failure and lactic acidosis due to fialuridine (FIAU) an investigational nucleoside analogue for chronic hepatitis B. *N. Engl. J. Med*. 1995; **333**: 1099.

124 Meyer zum Buschenfelde K-H, Lohse AW. Autoimmune hepatitis. *N. Engl. J. Med*. 1995; **333**: 1004.

125 Michel G, Ritter A, Gerken G *et al*. Anti-GOR and hepatitis C virus in autoimmune liver diseases. *Lancet* 1992; **339**: 267.

126 Mills CT, Lee E, Perrillo R. Relationship between histology, aminotransferase levels, and viral replication in chronic hepatitis B. *Gastroenterology* 1990; **99**: 519.

127 Misiani R, Bellavita P, Fenili D *et al*. Interferon alfa-2a therapy in cryoglobulinemia associated with hepatitis C virus. *N. Engl. J. Med*. 1994; **330**: 751.

128 Montano L, Aranguibel F, Boffill M *et al*. An analysis of the composition of the inflammatory infiltrate in autoimmune and hepatitis B virus-induced chronic liver disease. *Hepatology* 1983; **3**: 292.

129 Murray-Lyon IM, Stern RB, Williams R. Controlled trial of prednisone and azathioprine in active chronic hepatitis. *Lancet* 1973; **i**: 735.

130 Naito M, Hayashi N, Hagiwara H *et al*. Serum hepatitis C virus RNA quantity and histological features of hepatitis C virus carriers with persistently normal ALT levels. *Hepatology* 1994; **19**: 871.

131 Niederau C, Heintges T, Lange S *et al*. Long-term follow-up of HBeAg-positive patients treated with interferon alfa for chronic hepatitis B. *N. Engl. J. Med*. 1996; **334**: 1422.

132 Nishiguchi S, Kuroki T, Nakatani S *et al*. Randomized trial of effects of interferon-α on incidence of hepatocellular car-

cinoma in chronic active hepatitis C with cirrhosis. *Lancet* 1995; **346**: 1051.

133 Nishiguchi S, Kuroki T, Yabusako T *et al.* Detection of hepatitis C virus antibodies and hepatitis C virus RNA in patients with alcoholic liver disease. *Hepatology* 1991; **14**: 985.

134 Nishioka K, Watanabe J, Furuta S *et al.* A high prevalence of antibody to the hepatitis C virus in patients with hepatocellular carcinoma in Japan. *Cancer* 1991; **67**: 429.

135 Olynyk JK, Reddy KR, Di Bisceglie AM *et al.* Hepatic iron concentration as a predictor of response to interferon alfa therapy in chronic hepatitis C. *Gastroenterology* 1995; **108**: 1104.

136 Omata M, Ehata T, Yokosuka O *et al.* Mutations in the precore region of hepatitis B virus DNA in patients with fulminant and severe hepatitis. *N. Engl. J. Med.* 1991; **324**: 1699.

137 Patel A, Sherlock S, Dusheiko G *et al.* Clinical course and histological correlations in post-tranfusion hepatitis C: The Royal Free Hospital experience. *Eur. J. Gastroenterol. Hepatol.* 1991; **3**: 491.

138 Pawlotsky J-M, Yahia MB, Andre C *et al.* Immunological disorders in C virus chronic active hepatitis: a prospective case–control study. *Hepatology* 1994; **19**: 841.

139 Penner E. Nature of immune complexes in auto-immune chronic active hepatitis. *Gastroenterology* 1987; **92**: 304.

140 Perillo RP, Schiff ER, Davis GL *et al.* A randomized controlled trial of interferon alfa-2b alone and after prednisone withdrawal for the treatment of chronic hepatitis B. *N. Engl. J. Med.* 1990; **323**: 295.

141 Perrillo R, Tamburro C, Regenstein F *et al.* Low-dose, titrable interferon-α in decompensated liver disease caused by chronic infection with hepatitis B virus. *Gastroenterology* 1995; **109**: 908.

142 Philipp T, Durazzo M, Trautwein C *et al.* Recognition of uridine diphosphate glucuronyl transferases by LKM-3 antibodies in chronic hepatitis D. *Lancet* 1994; **344**: 578.

143 Phillips MJ, Blendis LM, Paucell S *et al.* Syncytial giant-cell hepatitis. Sporadic hepatitis with distinctive pathologic features, a severe clinical course and paramyxoviral features. *N. Engl. J. Med.* 1991; **324**: 455.

144 Poynard T, Bedossa P, Chevallier M *et al.* A comparison of three interferon alfa-2b regimens for the long-term treatment of chronic non-A, non-B hepatitis. *N. Engl. J. Med.* 1995; **332**: 1457.

145 Poynard T, Leroy V, Cohard M *et al.* Meta-analysis of interferon randomized trials in the treatment of viral hepatitis C. Effects of dose and duration. *Hepatology* 1995; **22**: 113A.

146 Quiroga JA, Binsbergen J van, Wang CY *et al.* Immunoglobulin M antibody to hepatitis C virus core antigen: correlations with viral replication, histological activity, and liver disease outcome. *Hepatology* 1995; **22**: 1635.

147 Read AE, Harrison CV, Sherlock S. 'Juvenile cirrhosis'; part of a system disease. The effect of corticosteroid therapy. *Gut* 1963; **4**: 378.

148 Reichard O, Andersson J, Schvarcz R *et al.* Ribavirin treatment for chronic hepatitis C. *Lancet* 1991; **337**: 1058.

149 Sanchez-Urdazpal L, Czaja AJ, Van Hock B *et al.* Prognostic features and role of liver transplantation in severe corticosteroid-treated autoimmune chronic active hepatitis. *Hepatology* 1991; **15**: 215.

150 Sansonno D, Cornacchiulo V, Iacobelli AR *et al.* Localization of hepatitis C virus antigens in liver and skin tissues of chronic hepatitis C virus-infected patients with mixed cryoglobulinemia. *Hepatology* 1995; **21**: 305.

151 Scheuer PJ, Ashrafzadeh P, Sherlock S *et al.* The pathology of hepatitis C. *Hepatology* 1992; **15**: 567.

152 Schvarcz R, Yun ZB, Sonnerborg A *et al.* Combination treatment with interferon alfa-2b and ribavirin for chronic hepatitis C in patients who have failed to achieve sustained response to interferon alone: Swedish experience. *J. Hepatol.* 1996; **23** (Suppl. 2): 17–21.

153 Serfaty L, Giral P, Loria A *et al.* Factors predictive of the response to interferon in patients with chronic hepatitis C. *J. Hepatol.* 1994; **21**: 12.

154 Sherlock S. Chronic hepatitis and cirrhosis. *Hepatology* 1984; **4**: 25S.

155 Sherlock S. Chronic hepatitis C. *Dis. Month* 1994; **40**: 117.

156 Shindo M, Arai K, Sokawa Y *et al.* Hepatic hepatitis C virus RNA as a predictor of a long-term response to interferon-α therapy. *Ann. Intern. Med.* 1995; **122**: 586.

157 Shindo M, Okuno T, Arai K *et al.* Detection of hepatitis B virus DNA in paraffin-embedded liver tissues in chronic hepatitis B or non-A, non-B hepatitis using the polymerase chain reaction. *Hepatology* 1991; **13**: 167.

158 Soloway RD, Summerskill WH, Baggenstoss AH *et al.* Clinical, biochemical, and histological remission of severe chronic active liver disease: a controlled study of treatments and early prognosis. *Gastroenterology* 1972; **63**: 820.

159 Sommadossi J-P. Treatment of hepatitis B by nucleoside analogs: still a reality. *Curr. Opinion Infect. Dis.* 1994; **7**: 678.

160 Terrault N, Wright T. Interferon and hepatitis C virus infection. *N. Engl. J. Med.* 1995; **332**: 1509.

161 Todros L, Saracco G, Durazzo M *et al.* Efficacy and safety of interferon alfa therapy in chronic hepatitis C with autoantibodies to liver-kidney microsomes. *Hepatology* 1995; **22**: 1374.

162 Tong MJ, el-Farra NS, Reikes AR *et al.* Clinical outcomes after transfusion-associated hepatitis C. *N. Engl. J. Med.* 1995; **332**: 1463.

163 Tran A, Quaranta J-F, Benzaken S *et al.* High prevalence of thyroid autoantibodies in a prospective series of patients with chronic hepatitis C before interferon therapy. *Hepatology* 1993; **18**: 253.

164 Treichel U, Poralla T, Hess G *et al.* Autoantibodies to human asialoglycoprotein receptor in autoimmune-type chronic hepatitis. *Hepatology* 1990; **11**: 606.

165 Tremolada F, Casarin C, Alberti A *et al.* Long-term follow up of non-A, non-B (type C) post-transfusion hepatitis. *J. Hepatol.* 1992; **16**: 273.

166 Tsubota A, Chayama K, Ikeda K *et al.* Factors predictive of response to interferon-α therapy in hepatitis C virus infection. *Hepatology* 1994; **19**: 1088.

167 Villeneuve J-P, Desrochers M, Infante-Rivard C *et al.* A long-term, follow-up study of asymptomatic hepatitis B surface antigen-positive carriers in Montreal. *Gastroenterology* 1994; **106**: 1000.

168 Waldenström J. *Leber, Blutproteine und Nahrungsweiss Stoffwechs Krh*, Sonderband: XV, p 8. Tagung, Bad Kissingen, 1950.

169 Wang J-T, Wang T-H, Sheu J-C *et al.* Detection of hepatitis B virus DNA by polymerase chain reaction in plasma of volunteer blood donors negative for hepatitis B surface antigen. *J. Infect. Dis.* 1991; **163**: 397.

170 Wang KK, Czaja AJ. Prognosis of corticosteroid-treated

hepatitis B surface antigen-negative chronic active hepatitis in postmenopausal women: a retrospective analysis. *Gastroenterology* 1989; **97**: 1288.

171 Watanabe U, Hashimoto E, Hisamitsu T *et al.* The risk factor for development of thyroid disease during interferon-α therapy for chronic hepatitis C. *Am. J. Gastroenterol.* 1994; **89**: 399.

172 Wejstal R. Immune-mediated liver damage in chronic hepatitis C. *Scand. J. Gastroenterol.* 1995; **30**: 609.

173 Wiedmann KH, Bartholemew TC, Brown DJC *et al.* Liver membrane antibodies detected by immunoradiometric assay in acute and chronic virus-induced and autoimmune liver disease. *Hepatology* 1984; **4**: 199.

174 Willocx RG, Isselbacher KJ. Chronic liver disease in young people. Clinical features and course in thirty-three patients. *Am. J. Med.* 1961; **30**: 185.

175 Wong DKH, Chung AM, O'Rourke K *et al.* Effect of alpha-interferon in patients with hepatitis B antigen-positive chronic hepatitis B. A meta analysis. *Ann. Intern. Med.* 1993; **119**: 312.

176 Wong JB, Koff RS, Tinè F *et al.* Cost-effectiveness of interferon-α 2b treatment for hepatitis B e antigen-positive chronic hepatitis B. *Ann. Intern. Med.* 1995; **122**: 664.

177 Wood JR, Czaja AJ, Beaver SJ *et al.* Frequency and significance of antibody to double-stranded DNA in chronic active hepatitis. *Hepatology* 1986; **6**: 976.

178 Yamada G, Takaguchi K, Matsueda K *et al.* Immunoelectron microscopic observation of intra-hepatic HBeAg in patients with chronic hepatitis B. *Hepatology* 1990; **12**: 133.

179 Yamamoto AM, Cresteil D, Homberg JC *et al.* Characterization of anti-liver-kidney microsome antibody (anti-LKM I) from hepatitis C virus-positive and virus-negative sera. *Gastroenterology* 1993; **104**: 1762.

180 Yano M, Kumada H, Kage M *et al.* The long-term pathological evolution of chronic hepatitis C. *Hepatology* 1996; **23**: 1334.

181 Yuki N, Hayashi N, Kasahara A *et al.* Hepatitis B virus markers and antibodies to hepatitis C virus in Japanese patients with hepatocellular carcinoma. *Dig. Dis. Sci.* 1992; **37**: 65.

Chapter 18
Drugs and the Liver

The liver is particularly concerned with drug metabolism, and especially of drugs given orally (fig. 18.1). These must be lipid soluble to have passed the membrane of the intestinal cell. They must then be presented to the liver and converted to water-soluble (more polar) compounds for excretion via the urine or bile.

Drugs can cause toxic effects which can mimic almost every naturally occurring liver disease in man (table 18.1). About 2% of all cases of jaundice in hospitalized patients are drug induced. About one-quarter of cases of fulminant hepatic failure in the USA are thought to be medicament-related. In any patient with liver disease it is essential to know all drugs that have been taken over the last 3 months. The physician may have to be a detective to identify them all.

Early suspicion of a drug-related hepatic reaction, and, if possible, accurate diagnosis, are essential. Severity is greatly increased if the drug is continued after symptoms develop or after serum transaminases rise. This provides grounds for negligence claims.

The response of the liver to drugs depends on an interplay between absorption, environmental factors and genetics (fig. 18.2).

An individual drug may cause more than one type of reaction. There may be an overlap between hepatitic, cholestatic and hypersensitivity reactions. Halothane, for instance, can cause zone 3 necrosis and also an acute hepatitis-like picture. The promazines overlap between the hepatitic and cholestatic types. Methyl dopa can cause acute or chronic hepatitis, cirrhosis, hepatic granulomas or cholestasis.

Pharmacokinetics [93]

The hepatic clearance of drugs given by mouth depends on the efficiency of the drug metabolizing enzymes, the intrinsic clearance, the liver blood flow and the extent of plasma protein binding (fig. 18.3). Drugs vary in their pharmacological effects according to the relative importance of these different pharmacokinetic factors (table 18.2).

Drugs which are avidly taken up by the liver (high intrinsic clearance) are said to have a high *first-pass metabolism*. The rate-limiting factor in their hepatic uptake is liver blood flow and indeed their clearance can be used to measure liver blood flow. Indocyanine green is one such drug. These drugs are usually highly lipid soluble. If liver blood flow falls, for instance due to cir-

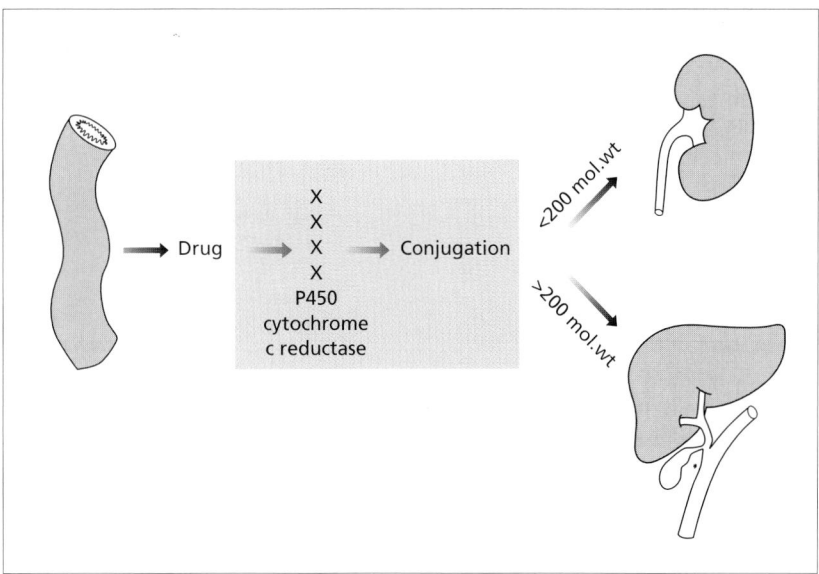

Fig. 18.1. Hepatic drug metabolism.

337

Table 18.1. Classification of hepatic drug reactions

Type	Features	Examples
Zone 3 necrosis	Dose dependent, multi-organ failure	Carbon tetrachloride Paracetamol Halothane
Mitochondrial cytopathies	Affects children Reye's-like syndrome Cirrhosis	Valproate
Steato-hepatitis	Long half-life Cirrhosis	Perhexiline Amiodarone
Acute hepatitis	Bridging necrosis Short term, acute Long term, chronic active hepatitis	Methyl dopa Isoniazid Halothane Ketoconazole
General hypersensitivity	Often with granulomas	Sulphonamides Quinidine Allopurinol
Fibrosis	Portal hypertension Cirrhosis	Methotrexate Vinyl chloride Vitamin A
Cholestasis		
canalicular	Dose dependent, reversible	Sex hormones
hepatocanalicular	Reversible 'obstructive' jaundice	Chlorpromazine Erythromycin Nitrofurantoin Azathioprine
ductular	Age related. Renal failure	Benoxyprofen
Vascular Veno-occlusive disease	Dose dependent	Irradiation Cytotoxics
Sinusoidal dilatation and peliosis		Azathioprine Sex hormones
Hepatic vein obstruction	Thrombotic effect	Sex hormones
Portal vein obstruction	Thrombotic effect	Sex hormones
Biliary Sclerosing cholangitis	Cholestasis	Hepatic arterial FUDR
Gallbladder sludge	Biliary colic	Ceftriaxone
Neoplastic Focal nodular hyperplasia	Benign. Presents space-occupying lesion	Sex hormones
Adenoma	May rupture. Usually regress	Sex hormones
Hepato-cellular carcinoma	Very rare Relatively benign	Danazol Sex and anabolic hormones

rhosis or heart failure, the systemic effect of the high first-pass rate drug will be enhanced. Administration of drugs such as propranolol or cimetidine which lower hepatic blood flow will have a similar effect.

Because of its high first-pass uptake, a drug such as glyceryl trinitrate has to be given sublingually to avoid entry into the portal vein. Similarly, lignocaine has to be given intravenously.

Drugs with a low intrinsic clearance, such as theophylline, depend on enzyme function. Changes in hepatic blood flow have little effect.

Plasma protein binding limits the presentation of the

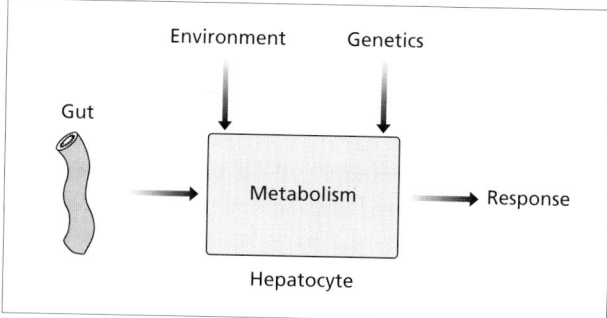

Fig. 18.2. The response of the liver to drugs depends on an interplay between absorption, environmental factors and genetics.

drug to hepatic enzymes. This will be affected by changes in the synthesis and degradation of plasma proteins.

$$CLH = QH \left[\frac{CLint.fb}{QH + CLint.fb} \right]$$

Fig. 18.3. Formula for calculating clearance (CLH) of a drug by the liver. QH = liver blood flow; CLint = intrinsic clearance; fb = plasma protein binding.

Hepatic drug metabolism

Phase 1. The main drug-metabolizing system resides in the microsomal fraction of the liver cell (smooth endoplasmic reticulum). The enzymes concerned are mixed function mono-oxygenases, cytochrome c-reductase and cytochrome P450. Reduced NADPH in the cytosol is a co-factor. The drug is rendered more polar by hydroxylation or oxidation. Alternative phase 1 drug-metabolizing

Table 18.2. Classification of drugs based on pharmacokinetic parameters obtained in normal subjects [93]

	Hepatic extraction	Protein binding	Effect of shunting on systemic availability	Examples
Enzyme limited, binding insensitive	Low	High	0	Antipyrine Amobarbital Caffeine Theophylline Aminopyrine
Enzyme limited, binding sensitive	Low	High	0	Chlordiazepoxide Diazepam Diphenylhydantoin Indomethacin Phenylbutazone Rifampicin Tolbutamide Warfarin
Flow and enzyme sensitive	Medium	Medium	+	Acetaminophen Chlorpromazine Isoniazid Merperidine Metoprolol Nortriptyline Quinidine
Flow limited	High	Medium	+++	Galactose Indocyanine green Labetalol Lidocaine Morphine Pentazocine Propoxyphene Propranolol Verapamil

reactions include the conversion of alcohol to acetaldehyde by alcohol dehydrogenases found mainly in the cytosolic fraction.

Enzyme inducers include barbiturates, alcohol, anaesthetics, hypoglycaemic and anticonvulsant agents, griseofulvin, rifampicin, glutethimide, phenylbutazone and meprobamate. Enlargement of the liver following the introduction of drug therapy can be related to enzyme induction.

Phase 2. These biotransformations involve conjugation of the drug or drug metabolite with a small endogenous molecule. The enzymes concerned are usually not confined to the liver, but are present there in high concentration.

Active transport. This system is located at the biliary pole of the hepatocyte. The mechanism is energy dependent and can be saturated.

Biliary and urinary excretion. Factors determining whether the metabolized drug will be excreted ultimately in bile or urine are multiple and many are unclear. Highly polar substances are excreted unaltered in the bile and also those which become more polar after conjugation. Those with a molecular weight exceeding 200 tend to be excreted in the bile. As the molecular weight falls, the urinary route becomes more important (fig. 18.1).

The P450 system

Drug metabolism and the production of toxic metabolites is performed by the P450 system of haemoproteins situated in the endoplasmic reticulum of the hepatocyte. At least 50 P450s have been identified and there are undoubtedly more. Each P450 protein is encoded by a unique gene [217]. The human P450s concerned with drug metabolism are members of the three families, P450-I, P450-II and P450-III (fig. 18.4). Each P450 has a unique 'substrate' binding site, capable of binding some, but not all, drugs. Each P450 can metabolize many drugs. Genetic differences in the catalytic activity of the P450s may determine idiosyncratic, untoward reactions to drugs. This is exemplified by the poor metabolism of debrisoquine (an anti-arrhythmic drug) due to abnormal expression of P450-II-D6 [54]. This enzyme system also metabolizes most β-blockers and neuroleptics. Poor metabolism of debrisoquine can be identified by PCR amplification of parts of the mutant genes for cytochrome P450-II-D6. This raises the possibility that in the future patients who will react abnormally to a drug can be identified [67].

P450-II-E1 is involved in the production of electrophilic metabolites of acetaminophen.

P450-III-A is concerned with the metabolism of cyclosporin and other drugs, especially erythromycin, steroids and ketoconazole. P450-II-C polymorphism affects the metabolism of mephenytoin, diazepam and many other drugs.

Enzyme induction and drug interactions

Enzyme induction, by increasing the P450 enzymes, leads to enhanced production of toxic metabolites (table 18.3). Expression of P450s and induction by phenobarbitone are maintained in transplanted hepatocytes without reference to acinar position or zonal sinusoidal microenvironment [117].

Two active drugs competing for an enzyme binding site may lead to the drug with the lower affinity being

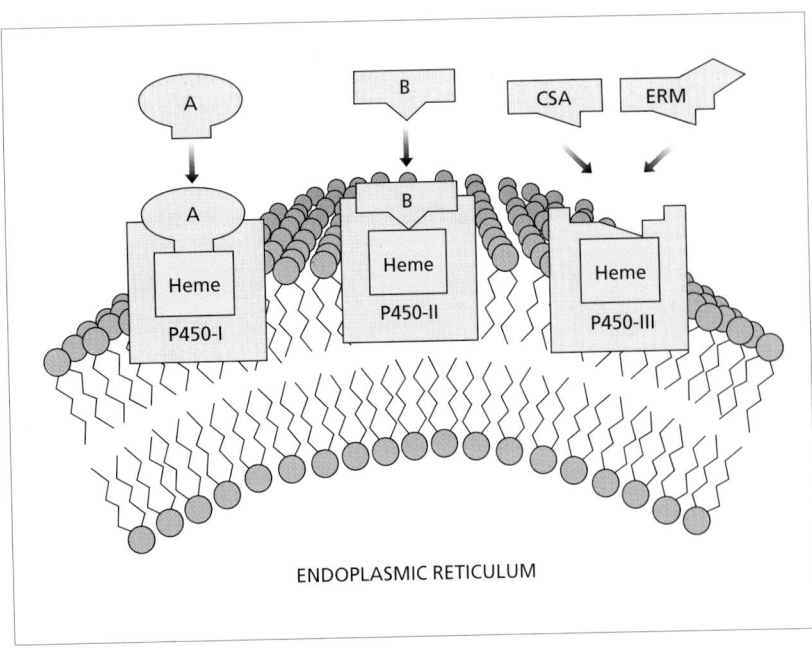

Fig. 18.4. P450s involved in drug metabolism are members of three gene families: P450-I, P450-II and P450-III. Individual P450s have distinct catalytic properties. Cyclosporin (CSA) and erythromycin (ERM) bind to and are metabolized by P450s within the P450-III family [217].

Table 18.3. Characteristics of some human liver P450s [217]

P450	Drug substrates	Probable inducers
I-A1	Carcinogens	Omeprazole
I-A2	Caffeine Theophylline	Cigarette smoke Acetaminophen
II-C*	Mephenytoin Tienylic acid Diazepam Tolbutamide Phenylbutazone	None identified
II-D*	Debrisoquine Most beta-blockers Many neuroleptics Encainide Codeine	None identified
II-E1	Acetaminophen Ethanol	Ethanol Isoniazid
III*	Cyclosporin A Erythromycin Ketoconazole Nifedipine Oestrogens Midazolam/triazolam Lidocaine	Anti-seizure medications Rifampicin Glucocorticoids

*Multiple subfamily members exist which may have differing catalytic properties and regulation.

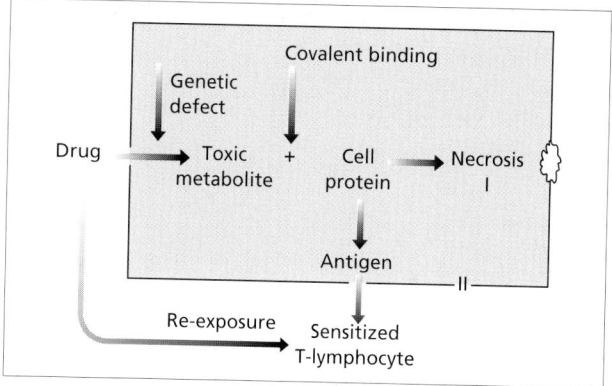

Fig. 18.5. The mechanisms of hepatotoxicity, direct metabolic-related and immunological hypersensitivity.

inducing immunological liver injury (fig. 18.5). The P450s can be involved. Several P450 isoenzymes are present and inducible on the membranes of hepatocytes and immunization against them might lead to immunological destruction of the liver cell [110].

Patients with halothane hepatitis have serum antibodies that recognize halothane-altered liver microsomal proteins [121].

An idiosyncratic reaction to the diuretic, tienilic acid, is associated with autoantibodies that react with both liver and kidney microsomes (anti-LKM-II). The antigen recognized is within the P450-II-C family which is also involved in the metabolism of tienilic acid [8].

metabolized more slowly and thus having a more prolonged action.

Ethanol induces P450-II-E1 and so enhances the toxicity of acetaminophen (see fig. 18.8). Similarly, patients treated with isoniazid which also induces P450-II-E1 have increased acetaminophen toxicity [129].

P450-III-A which metabolizes cyclosporin is induced by rifampicin and steroids. This explains the reduced blood cyclosporin levels when these drugs are given. Cyclosporin, F506, erythromycin and ketoconazole compete for binding and metabolism by P450-III-A and cyclosporin levels rise after they are given.

Omeprazole induces P450-I-A [35]. This is important in the biotransformation of procarcinogens, carcinogens and many drugs. An increased tendency to malignancy after omeprazole is possible.

In the future, it should be possible to determine P450 profiles and detect those likely to develop an adverse drug reaction. Selective inhibitors or inducers may be used to alter the P450 profile [217].

Immunological hepatotoxicity

The metabolite may act as a hapten with cell protein so

Risk factors for hepatic drug injury [99]

Liver disease

The impaired metabolism is proportional to the extent of hepato-cellular failure and is greatest in cirrhosis. A correlation exists between the half-life of a drug and the prothrombin time, serum albumin level, hepatic encephalopathy and ascites [43].

The causes of the impaired drug metabolism are multiple. Reduced hepatic blood flow leads to impaired metabolism particularly of high first-pass drugs [23]. Impaired oxidative metabolism is seen particularly with barbiturates and with chlordiazepoxide. Glucuronidation is preserved so that morphine, which is a high-clearance drug normally inactivated in this way, is eliminated normally. However, glucuronidation of some drugs may be impaired in patients with liver disease [73].

Reduced plasma protein binding follows failure of hepatic albumin synthesis. Benzodiazepines, for instance, are eliminated almost solely by hepatic biotransformation, highly protein bound, and this restricts their elimination. In hepato-cellular disease there is a decrease in drug clearance from plasma, and an increase in its volume of distribution which is accounted for by decreased protein binding.

Increased cerebral sensitivity, particularly to sedatives, may be related to an increase in cerebral receptors in liver disease.

Age and sex

Hepatic drug reactions are rare in children, apart from accidental overdose. They may even be resistant, since children with paracetamol overdose have much less liver damage than an adult with an equivalent paracetamol serum concentration [108]. Valproate hepatotoxicity, however, does affect children, as rarely does halothane [83] and salazopyrine [19].

Old age is associated with decreased disposition of drugs undergoing phase 1 but not phase 2 biotransformation [171]. This is not related to a fall in cytochrome P450 activities but rather to diminished hepatic volume and liver blood flow [224].

Hepatic drug reactions are more frequent in females.

In the fetus, P450 enzymes are very low, if present at all. After birth, they increase and their intralobular distribution changes [152].

Drugs causing interference with bilirubin metabolism

Drugs can affect bilirubin metabolism at any stage. The reactions are predictable, reversible and not serious in the adult. In the neonate, however, a rise in unconjugated bilirubin in the brain potentiates bilirubin encephalopathy (*kernicterus*). This is enhanced by drugs such as salicylates or sulphonamides which compete with bilirubin for its attachment to albumin. In adults, with such conditions as Gilbert's syndrome, chronic active hepatitis or primary biliary cirrhosis, bilirubinaemia is enhanced by drugs which interfere with bilirubin metabolism.

Haemolytic reactions increase the bilirubin load on the liver cell. This is rare as a single defect and is usually combined with a hypersensitivity reaction which decreases in hepato-cellular function. Sulphonamides, phenacetin or quinine can cause such reactions. Such drugs may also precipitate haemolysis in those with glucose 6PD deficiency.

The offending drug may be transmitted in the mother's milk. The toxic effects of synthetic vitamin K preparations in neonates may be partially due to increased haemolysis.

Certain drugs interfere with the uptake and transport of bilirubin in the hepatocyte. They include cholecystographic media and rifampicin. Transport proteins may be decreased in neonates making them susceptible to drugs that compete with bilirubin for transport. These drugs would potentiate kernicterus.

Cholestasis follows interference by drugs, such as sex hormones, with bilirubin canalicular excretion.

Diagnosis of drug-induced liver disease (table 18.4)

Common causes of drug-related hepatic reactions are antibiotics, non-steroidal anti-inflammatory drugs, cardiovascular drugs and central nervous modifiers — in fact the whole range of modern pharmacotherapeutics. Every drug should be suspected and the manufacturer and the Safety of Medicines Organization should be contacted.

History must include dose, route of administration, duration, previous administration and any concomitant drugs.

The onset (*challenge*) is usually within 5–90 days of starting. A positive *de-challenge* is a 50% fall in serum transaminases within 8 days of stopping the drug. Deliberate *re-challenge* is usually ethically impossible. However, *inadvertent re-challenge* gives valuable evidence that the drug was indeed hepatotoxic.

Other causes of a hepatic reaction such as hepatitis A, B or C, autoimmune liver disease or biliary obstruction must be excluded.

In difficult cases, liver biopsy can be valuable. A drug-related reaction is suggested by fatty change, granulomas, bile duct lesions, zonal hepatic necrosis and general hepato-cellular unrest.

Hepato-cellular zone 3 necrosis

Hepato-cellular injury is rarely due to the drug itself and a toxic metabolite is usually responsible (fig. 18.5). The drug-metabolizing enzymes activate chemically stable drugs to produce electrophilic metabolites. These potent alkylating, arylating or acylating agents bind covalently to liver molecules which are essential to the life of the hepatocyte, and necrosis ensues (fig. 18.6). This follows

Table 18.4. Investigation of drug-related liver disease

	Notes
Suspect any drug	Contact manufacturer and safety medicines organization
Drug history	All medicines, dose, duration, previous administration
De-challenge	Rapid fall transaminases
Re-challenge	Inadvertent. Deliberate usually impossible
Exclude other liver diseases	Hepatitis A, B and C; autoimmune; biliary obstruction
Liver biopsy	If necessary, fat, granulomas, zonal hepatitis, bile duct lesions

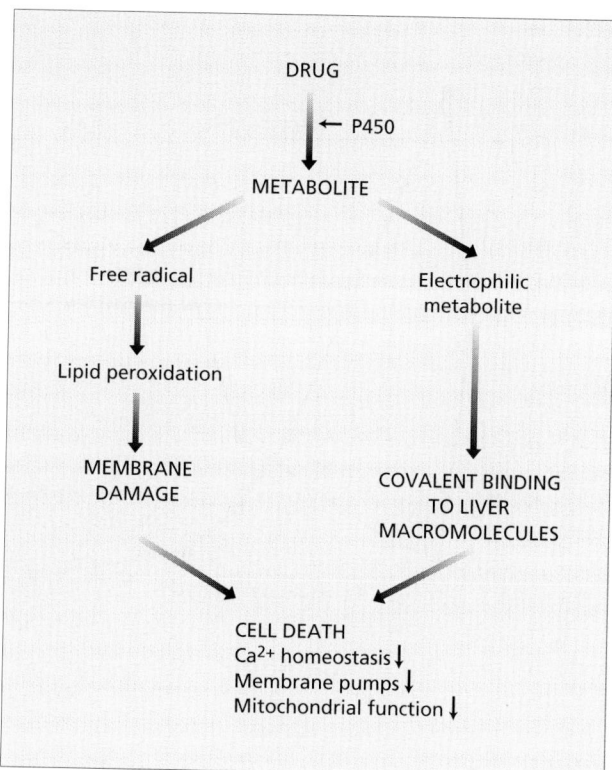

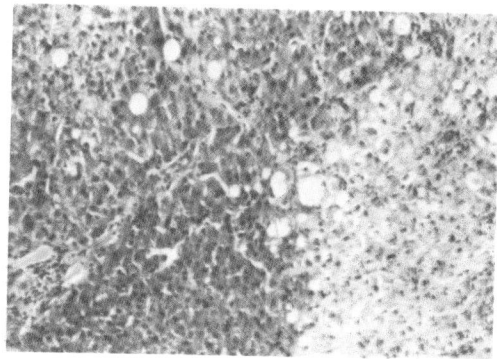

Fig. 18.7. Accidental carbon tetrachloride poisoning. To the right of the section liver cells are necrotic and show hydropic degeneration and fatty change. Surviving liver cells to the left of the section show occasional fatty change. The portal zones are unaffected.

Fig. 18.6. The mechanism of metabolite-related direct hepatocellular necrosis.

exhaustion of intra-cellular substances such as glutathione which are capable of preferentially conjugating with the toxic metabolite. In addition, metabolites with an unpaired electron are produced by oxidative reactions of cytochrome P450. These *free radicals* can also bind covalently to proteins and to unsaturated fatty acids of cell membranes. This results in *lipid peroxidation* and membrane damage. The end result is hepatocyte death related to failure to pump calcium from the cytosol and to depressed mitochondrial function (fig. 18.6). Necrosis is greatest in zone 3, where drug metabolizing enzymes are found in highest concentration and where the oxygen tension is lowest in sinusoidal blood [28]. Fatty change is also seen but the inflammatory reaction is slight.

The hepatic necrosis is dose dependent. Animal models exist. Other organs also suffer and renal damage is often the most important. In mild cases, jaundice may be mild, slight and transient. Serum biochemical tests show marked rises in transaminases. Prothrombin time increases rapidly. Light microscopy shows clear-cut zone 3 necrosis, with scattered fatty change and little inflammatory reaction (fig. 18.7). Peri-portal fibrosis may sometimes be marked. Paracetamol (acetaminophen) is a good example of this type.

Some drugs cause zone 3 hepatic necrosis, but in only a small proportion of those exposed. The mechanism

cannot be straightforward dose-dependent toxicity, and metabolic idiosyncrasy is postulated. Halothane occasionally causes confluent zonal or massive necrosis as well as an hepatitic reaction [10]. The products of reductive metabolism are reactive as are the oxidative ones. The metabolites produced by either mechanism could bind to cellular macro-molecules and cause lipid peroxidation and inactivation of drug-metabolizing and other enzymes.

Effects of enzyme induction and inhibition

Due to enzyme induction, rats pre-treated with phenobarbital show increased zone 3 necrosis following carbon tetrachloride.

Alcohol ingestion considerably enhances paracetamol toxicity so that as little as 4–8 g can cause serious liver damage (fig. 18.8) [177, 230]. This is apparently due to the induction by alcohol of P450-3a (P450-II-E1) which is important in generating toxic metabolites. It is also concerned in oxygenation of nitrosamines at the α-carbon (fig. 18.9). Theoretically, this could increase the risk of cancer in alcoholics. Cimetidine inhibits P450 mixed-function oxidase activities and modifies the hepatotoxic effects of paracetamol. Omeprazole acts similarly [59]. Ranitidine in high doses reduces metabolic activation of paracetamol but at low doses it potentiates hepatotoxicity [102].

The administration of drugs which induce microsomal enzymes, for instance phenytoin, results in increases in serum γ-glutamyl transpeptidase [82].

Carbon tetrachloride

This may be taken accidentally or suicidally. It may be inhaled, for instance in dry-cleaning or in filling fire extinguishers, or mixed in drinks.

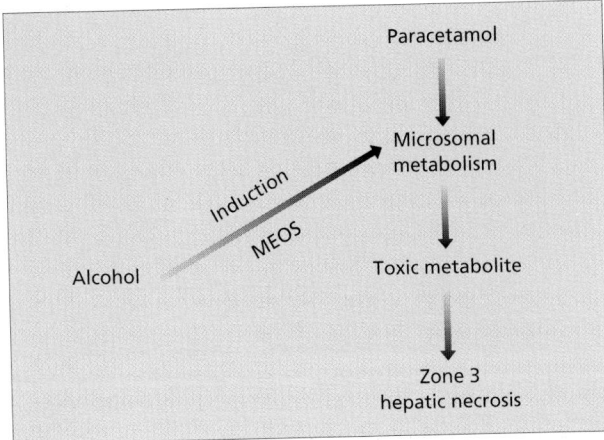

Fig. 18.8. Alcohol, as an enzyme-inducing agent, increases the production of toxic metabolites of paracetamol, so potentiating hepatic necrosis. MEOS = microsomal enzyme oxidizing system.

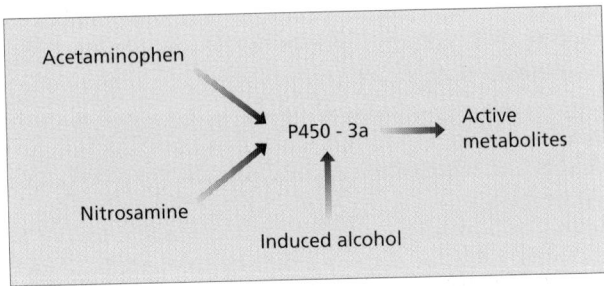

Fig. 18.9. Alcohol, by inducing P450-3a (P450-II-E1) drug-metabolizing enzymes, enhances the toxicity of paracetamol (acetaminophen) and the carcinogen nitrosamine.

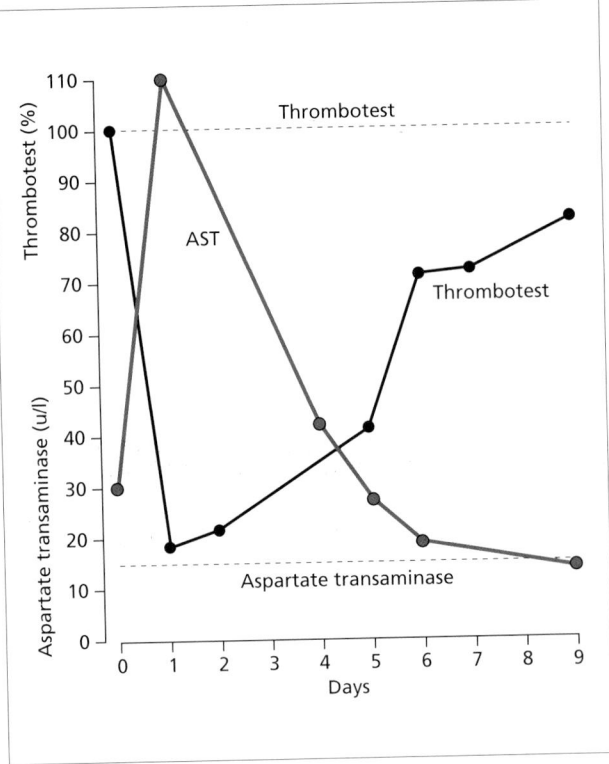

Fig. 18.10. Suicidal inhalation of carbon tetrachloride in a young male. Note the rapid fall in thrombotest with rise in transaminase (AST) values. At 6 days they have virtually returned to normal.

The liver injury is induced by a toxic metabolite. This depends on a cytochrome P450-dependent mono-oxygenase which is located in the smooth endoplasmic reticulum of peri-venular hepatocytes [3]. The effect is enhanced by enzyme-inducers such as alcohol and barbiturates and reduced by protein malnutrition which depresses drug-metabolizing enzymes.

Clinical features

Vomiting, abdominal pain and diarrhoea are followed within 48 hours by jaundice. The liver may be enlarged and tender. Spontaneous haemorrhages reflect the profound hypoprothrombinaemia. Serum transaminase values are very high (fig. 18.10); the serum albumin level falls.

In severe cases acute renal failure overshadows hepatic destruction. Acute haemorrhagic gastritis is prominent. Since carbon tetrachloride is an anaesthetic the patient becomes increasingly drowsy.

Pathology

Zone 3 cells show hydropic degeneration marked by clear cytoplasm and pyknotic nuclei (fig. 18.7). Fatty change varies from a few droplets to diffuse involvement of liver cells. Polymorphonuclear infiltration of the portal zones is slight, fibrosis is uncommon. With recovery the liver pattern returns to normal.

Prognosis

Death in the acute stage is due to kidney failure. If the patient survives the acute episode there are no late hepatic sequelae. In rats repeated administration leads to cirrhosis. This sequence is not seen in man. Liver cells may even be more resistant with prolonged exposure. Carbon tetrachloride is not an aetiological factor in hepatic cirrhosis in man.

Treatment

Screening tests in workers should include routine examination for liver enlargement and tenderness, urine testing for urobilinogen, and serum transaminase and γ-glutamyl transpeptidase estimations.

Acute poisoning is treated by a high-calorie, high-carbohydrate diet and along the usual lines for acute hepato-renal failure including dialysis. Prompt treatment with acetyl cysteine may minimize hepato-renal damage [167].

Related compounds

Teenagers sniffing cleaning fluid, which contains trichlorethylene, or glue containing toluene [136], suffer jaundice with liver necrosis and renal failure.

Industrial exposure to the solvent, 1,1,1-trichlorethane, can cause a somewhat similar picture to carbon tetrachloride [72].

Benzene derivatives include trinitrotoluene (TNT), dinitrophenol and toluene. The maximum effect is on the bone marrow with aplasia. The liver may be involved acutely, but chronic sequelae are rare.

Industrial exposure to organic solvents can lead to abnormal transminase values. Short exposure (less than 3 months) to the solvent dimethylformamide results in digestive symptoms, marked rise in transaminases, focal hepato-cellular necrosis and microvesicular steatosis [155]. With longer exposure (greater than 1 year) symptoms are minimal and transaminase elevations modest. Liver biopsies show microvesicular steatosis and prominent smooth endoplasmic reticulum. Electron microscopy shows PAS-positive inclusions and abnormal mitochondria.

Occupational exposure to 2-nitropropane may be fatal [64].

Industrial liver injury may be under-diagnosed. The prognosis of those exposed chronically remains uncertain.

Amanita mushrooms

Acute liver failure follows ingestion of various *Amanita* mushrooms, including *A. phalloides* and *A. verna*. Three stages of illness can be recognized. The first, starting 8–12 hours after ingestion, consists of nausea, cramping abdominal pain and rice-water diarrhoea and lasts for 3–4 days. The second phase is characterized by apparent improvement. The third stage includes hepato-renal and central nervous system degeneration with massive cell destruction. The liver shows zone 3 necrosis without much inflammation. Fatty change is seen in fatal cases [220]. The condition is life-threatening although recovery can occur.

The mushroom toxin, phalloidin, inhibits actin polymerization and causes cholestasis. Amanitine inhibits protein synthesis by RNA inhibition.

Supportive measures are all that can be offered. Haemodialysis may be helpful. Hepatic transplantation has been successfully employed [25].

Paracetamol (acetaminophen)

In an adult, a minimum of 7.5–10 g produces hepatic necrosis but the dose is difficult to assess because of early vomiting and unreliable histories.

Alcohol, as an enzyme-inducer, enhances hepatotoxicity and as little as 4–8 g paracetamol a day may produce liver damage in an alcoholic and even less if there is underlying liver disease [230].

The electrophilic metabolite of paracetamol preferentially conjugates with hepatic glutathione. When the glutathione is exhausted, the paracetamol metabolite arylates essential nucleophilic macromolecules, so producing hepatic necrosis (fig. 18.11).

Clinical features

Within a few hours of ingestion, the patient becomes nauseated and vomits. Consciousness is preserved. After about 48 hours recovery seems in progress; then about on the third or fourth day the patient deteriorates and becomes jaundiced when the liver is tender. Serum transaminase and prothrombin levels are enormous. In the more seriously affected, deterioration is then rapid with the signs of acute hepatic necrosis. Acute tubular necrosis develops in 25–30% of those untreated. Myocardial damage and hypoglycaemia are prominent.

Hepatic histology. Shows zone 3 necrosis, some fatty change and very little inflammation. Reticulin collapse may be confluent and massive, but cirrhosis is not a sequel.

Chronic injury. Long-term (about 1 year) exposure to paracetamol (3–4 g daily) can lead to chronic liver injury. Underlying liver disease and alcoholism may potentiate the effect.

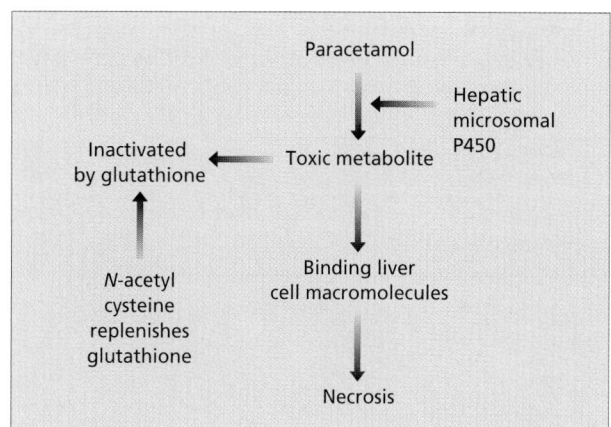

Fig. 18.11. The mechanism of paracetamol (acetaminophen) liver injury and of *N*-acetyl cysteine treatment.

Prognosis

The overall mortality for 201 patients admitted to a general hospital was 3.5%. Prognosis is related to late presentation, coma, prothrombin elevation, metabolic acidosis and renal dysfunction [130].

Severity can be assessed using a nomogram relating blood level versus time after ingestion. Death occurs between 4 and 18 days after ingestion.

Cardiopulmonary and renal insufficiency in elderly patients increases the risk of damage after modest doses of paracetamol [17].

Treatment

The stomach is washed out. The patient is admitted to hospital. Features of hepatic necrosis are delayed and early improvement should not give a false sense of security.

Forced diuresis and renal dialysis do not increase the excretion of paracetamol or its metabolites already bound to tissues. The treatment of acute liver failure is outlined in Chapter 8.

Treatment is aimed at replenishing the glutathione reserves of the liver cell. Unfortunately the penetration of glutathione itself into liver cells is poor. Precursors of glutathione and glutathione-like substances have therefore been employed. Therapy is assessed by plasma levels. The patient's value is plotted against a line joining $200\,\mu g/ml$ at 4 hours, and $60\,\mu g/ml$ at 12 hours on a semi-log graph of concentration versus time. If the patient's concentration is below this line, liver damage will be clinically insignificant and treatment can be stopped.

Intravenous acetylcysteine (Mucomist, Parvolex) [147] is rapidly hydrolysed to cysteine. The dose is $150\,mg/kg$ in $200\,ml$ 5% glucose over 15 minutes, followed by $50\,mg/kg$ in $500\,ml$ 5% dextrose over 4 hours and $100\,mg/kg$ in 1 litre 5% dextrose over the next 16 hours (total dose $300\,mg/kg$ in 20 hours). It should be given to *all* patients with hepatic damage due to paracetamol even if delayed more than 15 hours from ingestion [62]. It may be useful in other forms of fulminant liver failure [63].

When given within 16 hours of ingestion, *N*-acetylcysteine is so effective that liver injury is now rare after paracetamol self-poisoning [20, 118].

In fulminant cases, hepatic transplantation may be necessary. Survival is good and psychological rehabilitation has not proved difficult [130].

Salicylates

Patients on salicylate therapy for acute rheumatic fever, juvenile and adult rheumatoid arthritis, and systemic lupus erythematosus, may develop acute hepatic injury and even chronic active hepatitis. This may develop even with serum salicylate levels below $25\,mg/100\,ml$.

Cocaine

Fifty-nine per cent of patients with acute cocaine intoxication and rhabdomyolysis will have biochemical evidence of liver damage [183].

Liver histology shows zone 1, 2 or 3 necrosis with zone 1 microvesicular fat [78, 213].

The hepatotoxic metabolite is norcocaine nitroxide produced by *N*-methylation and catalysed by P450. The highly reactive metabolites cause liver injury by peroxidation, free radical formation and covalent binding to hepatic proteins. Enzyme induction by phenobarbitone or other inducers enhances the effect.

Hyperthermia [65]

Heat stroke is accompanied by hepato-cellular damage, in 10% severe and contributing to death. Pathologically it is marked by microvesicular fat, congestion, cholestasis (sometimes ductal), haemosiderosis and sinusoidal infiltration with primitive cells. Dilatation of portal venules is prominent in fatal cases. Biochemically there may be jaundice, increased transaminase levels and a fall in prothrombin and albumin levels. The damage is due to hypoxia and to direct thermal injury. Some of the changes may be related to endotoxaemia. Obesity is a risk factor.

Exertional heat stroke is marked by collapse, convulsions, hypotension and hyperpyrexia. Rhadomyolysis and neuronal cerebellar damage are complications. Treatment is by core cooling and rehydration. Liver transplant may have to be considered.

MDMA (*ecstasy*) can lead to a malignant hyperthermia syndrome with hepato-cellular necrosis [70] which can mimic viral hepatitis. Transplant may be indicated [40].

Hypothermia

Although the changes in experimental animals are impressive, in man they are inconspicuous. The effect of low temperatures on the liver is unlikely to be of serious consequence.

Burns

Within 36–48 hours of burning, the liver shows changes very similar to those seen in carbon tetrachloride poisoning. These are reflected in minor changes in liver function tests.

Hepato-cellular zone 1 necrosis

This type of injury resembles that of zone 3 but is maximal in zone 1 (peri-portal) areas.

Ferrous sulphate

Accidental ingestion of large quantities of ferrous sulphate is followed by zone 1 coagulative degeneration with nuclear pyknosis and karyorrhexis with little or no inflammation.

Phosphorus

The red form is relatively non-toxic but the yellow is extremely lethal — as little as 60mg being fatal. It is usually taken accidentally or suicidally as rat poison or in fire crackers.

Poisoning causes acute gastric irritation. Phosphorus may be found by gastric lavage. The patient's breath has a characteristic garlic odour and the faeces are frequently phosphorescent. Jaundice appears on the third or fourth day. The course may be fulminating with coma and death within 24 hours or, more usually, within the first 4 days.

The liver biopsy shows zone 1 necrosis with macro- and medium-sized fat droplets. Inflammation is minimal.

About one-half of patients recover, and ultimate recovery will probably be complete. There is no specific treatment.

Mitochondrial cytopathies

Some drugs seem to have a predominant effect on mitochondrial function causing inhibition of respiratory chain enzymes. Clinically they are marked by vomiting and apathy. Lactic acidosis, hypoglycaemia and metabolic acidosis are seen. Mitochondrial β-oxidation of fatty acids is associated with microvesicular fatty liver. Electron microscopy shows mitochondrial damage. The diseases are multi-system.

Sodium valproate

Asymptomatic rises in serum transaminases, which subside on withdrawing the drug or reducing the dose, are reported in about 11% of patients receiving valproate. However, a more severe, even fatal, hepatic reaction may develop [146]. The patients are usually young, between 2.5 months and 34 years with 69% being 10 years old or less. Males are particularly affected. Presentation is usually within 1–2 months of starting the drug and is not seen after 6–12 months therapy. Vomiting and disturbed consciousness are seen with hypoglycaemia and clotting defects. Other features of the microvesicular fat syndrome are also found.

Liver biopsy shows microvesicular fat mainly in zone 1. Variable hepato-cellular necrosis is seen in zone 3. Electron microscopy shows obvious mitochondrial changes.

Valproate or one of its metabolites, particularly 2-propyl-pentanoic acid, interfere with mitochondrial function, particularly β-oxidation of fatty acids [230]. Polypharmacy, presumably by enzyme induction, may be a risk factor for fatal hepatotoxicity in young children. Blood ammonia levels rise, indicating inhibition of mitochondrial urea-cycle enzymes. Even in healthy subjects valproate induces inhibition of urea synthesis with hyperammonaemia [71]. Patients having severe reactions to valproate might have an inborn deficiency of urea-cycle enzymes, but this has never been proved, although one patient with inherited carbamoyl transferase deficiency died when receiving valproate [71].

Tetracyclines

Tetracycline inhibits production of the transport proteins which excrete phospholipids from the hepatocyte, so resulting in fatty liver.

Deaths due to hepato-renal failure have followed large doses of intravenous tetracycline to pregnant women with pyelonephritis [173]. Tetracyclines also have been associated with acute fatty liver of pregnancy. Tetracyclines should be avoided during pregnancy although large intravenous doses are probably necessary for significant hepatotoxicity.

Antiviral nucleoside analogues

Clinical trials of *FIAU*, a fluorinated pyridine nucleoside analogue originally approved for the treatment of AIDS, had disastrous consequences when used to treat chronic hepatitis B infection [115]. After 8–12 weeks, volunteers developed hepatic failure, lactic acidosis, hypoglycaemia, coagulopathy, neuropathy and renal failure. Three patients died of multi-organ failure, four proceeded to liver transplantation of whom two died and two survived. Liver biopsies showed microvesicular steatosis and abnormal mitochondria. The mechanism is probably the incorporation of FIAU into the mitochondrial genome in place of thymidine [140].

Fulminant hepatitis with severe lactate acidosis has been reported in HIV infected patients on *didanosine (ddI)* [12]. Some of the side-effects of *AZT* and *23-dideoxycitidine (ddC)* are probably due to inhibition of mitochondrial DNA synthesis. *Lamivudine*, a nucleoside analogue currently under trial for hepatitis B virus infections has not resulted in serious toxicity but does not inhibit mito-chondrial DNA replication in intact cells [203].

Steato-hepatitis

The reaction termed *non-alcoholic steato-hepatitis* (*NASH*) histologically resembles acute alcoholic hepatitis with sometimes, in addition, electron microscopical evidence of lysosomal phospholipidosis. Mallory's hyaline is found in zone 3 in distinction to true alcoholic hepatitis.

Perhexiline maleate

Perhexiline maleate, an anti-anginal drug now with-drawn, has been associated with hepatic histology resembling acute alcoholic hepatitis. Patients with this reaction lack a gene concerned with the oxidation of debrisoquine. The defect leads to a deficiency of a monoxygenase reaction in liver microsomes [66].

Amiodarone

This anti-cardiac-arrhythmia drug has caused toxic damage to lung, cornea, thyroid, peripheral nerves and liver. Abnormal biochemical tests of liver function are found in 15–50% of patients receiving it [159].

Hepatic toxicity usually develops more than 1 year after starting therapy but can occur within 1 month. The spectrum is wide, from isolated asymptomatic transam-inase elevations to a fulminant fatal disorder. Hepa-totoxicity is usually marked by an increase in serum transaminases and rarely by jaundice. Symptoms may be absent and toxicity detected only by routine monitor-ing; hepatomegaly is not constant [158]. Severe cholest-asis may be a feature [126]. Fatal cirrhosis can develop. Children can be affected [225].

Amiodarone has a very large volume of distribution and a very long half-life, so that blood levels may remain raised for many months after withdrawal of therapy (fig. 18.12). Amiodarone and its major metabolite, *N*-desethylamiodarone, are present in the liver for several months after stopping the drug [185]. The incidence and severity of side-effects correlates with the serum concen-tration and the daily dose must be kept between 200 and 600 mg daily.

Amiodarone is iodinated and this results in an increased density on a CT scan [53]. This does not corre-late with hepatic injury.

Hepatic histology shows an acute alcoholic hepatitis-like picture with fibrosis and, sometimes, pronounced bile-ductular proliferation. Fatal cirrhosis can develop. Electron microscopy shows phospholipid-laden lysoso-mal lamellar bodies containing myelin figures (fig. 18.13) [103]. These are constantly found in amiodarone-treated patients and signify drug exposure, not drug toxicity

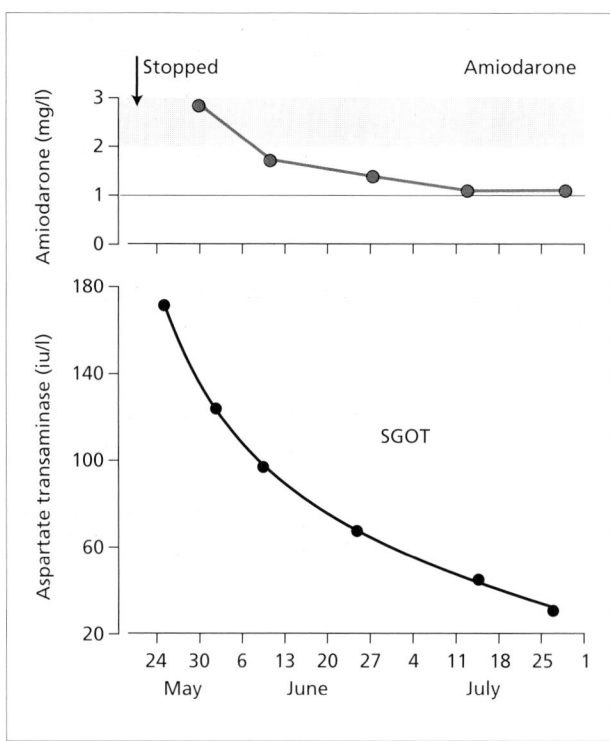

Fig. 18.12. AST (SGOT) and blood amiodarone levels in a 63-year-old physician. Note persistence of blood amiodarone levels 2 months after stopping therapy.

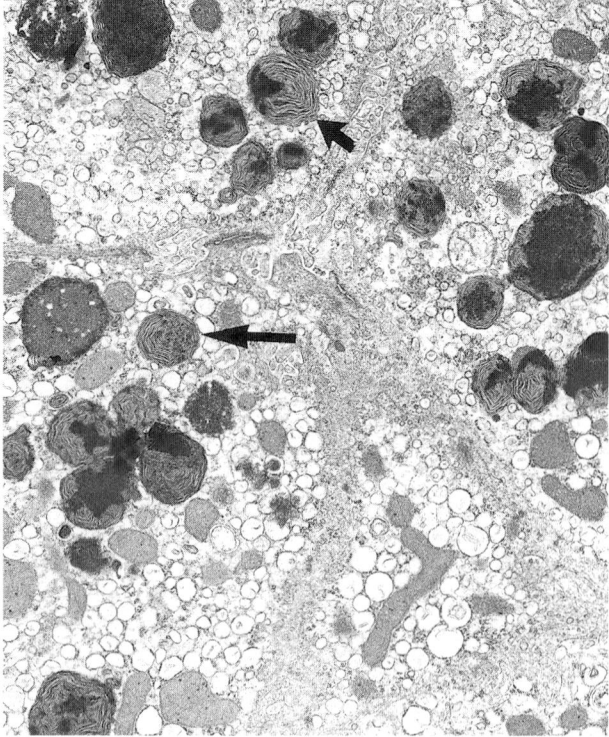

Fig. 18.13. Amiodarone hepatotoxicity: electron microscopy of the liver shows lysosomal lamellar bodies containing myelin figures (arrows).

[60]. Cultured rat hepatocytes exposed to amiodarone and desethylamiodarone develop similar inclusion bodies [187]. Swollen granular zone 3 macrophages, presumably iodine-laden lysosomal bodies, may be an early marker of amiodarone hepatotoxicity. Either the drug itself or its main metabolite probably inhibit lysosomal phospholipases responsible for catabolizing phospholipids.

A similar phospholipidosis can be found with *parenteral nutrition* and complicating *trimethoprimcotrimoxazole* therapy (*Septrin, Bactrim*) [128].

Synthetic oestrogens

A picture of 'alcoholic hepatitis' has been associated with massive doses of synthetic oestrogen used to treat prostatic cancer [178].

Calcium channel blockers

Nifedipine and dilatiazem have been associated with steato-hepatitis but more evidence is required [5].

Amodiaquine

This antimalarial drug may lead to a hepatic reaction of variable severity 4–15 weeks after starting [11]. It is dose and duration dependent. It is no longer used for malaria prophylaxis. Amodiaquine inhibits protein synthesis in cultured mammalian cells.

Cyanamide

This aldehyde dehydrogenase inhibitor is used for alcohol-aversion therapy. Liver biopsy from asymptomatic recipients shows ground glass hepatocytes in zone 3 resembling those of hepatitis B surface antigen carriers but negative to orcein and positive to PAS staining. The cells disappear when the drug is stopped.

Fibrosis

Fibrosis forms part of most drug reactions, but in some it may be the predominant feature. The fibrous tissue is deposited in the Disse space, where it obstructs sinusoidal blood flow, causing non-cirrhotic portal hypertension and hepato-cellular dysfunction. The lesion is related to toxic drug metabolites and is usually in zone 3, an exception being methotrexate where the damage is in zone 1.

Methotrexate

Hepatotoxicity results from a toxic metabolite of microsomal origin which induces fibrosis and ultimately cirrhosis (fig. 18.14). Primary liver cancer can develop. Hepatotoxicity is likely to follow long-term therapy, usually for psoriasis, rheumatoid arthritis or leukaemia. Risk seems to be lower in rheumatoid patients than in those with psoriasis [222]. Symptomatic liver disease is rare. Serial liver biopsies usually show benign appearances but three of 45 patients with rheumatoid arthritis developed serious liver disease [144]. Fibrosis may be graded from mild which is probably insignificant to significant and even to cirrhosis when the drug should be stopped [88, 161] (fig. 18.14).

Fibrosis is dose and duration dependent. When given in three 5 mg doses at 12-hour intervals each week (i.e. 15 mg a week), it seems safe [92]. Baseline liver biopsies are only indicated in those at particular risk, having significant alcohol intake or a history of liver disease [87]. Serum transaminases are a poor reflection of underlying liver disease but should be monitored monthly; increases indicate liver biopsy. In all cases a routine liver biopsy should be performed at 2 years or when the cumulative dose of methotrexate exceeds 1.5 g [104].

Ultrasound may be useful in detecting fibrosis and indicating stopping therapy. Hepatic transplantation has been performed for severe methotrexate hepatotoxicity [52].

Other cytotoxic drugs

These have a wide range of hepatotoxicity [143]. The liver, however, is surprisingly resistant to injury by cytotoxic drugs, perhaps due to its low proliferative rate and extensive detoxifying capabilities.

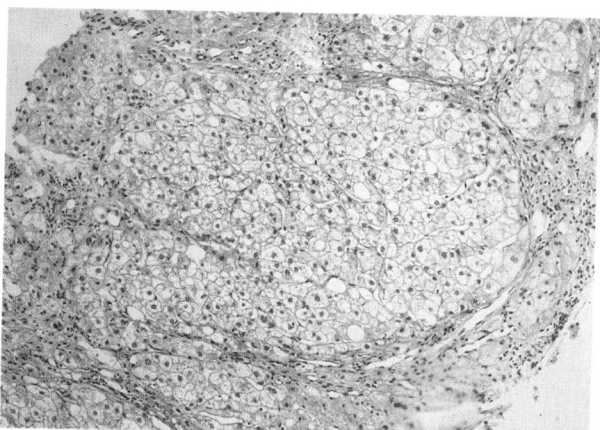

Fig. 18.14. Methotrexate liver injury. Zonal architecture is maintained. The portal zones are expanded with fibrous tissue and mononuclear cells. The hepatocytes show fatty change. (H & E, ×65).

Cytotoxic drugs cause rises in serum transaminases if large amounts are given. Drugs such as methotrexate, azathioprine and cyclophosphamide cause zone 3 necrosis, fibrosis and cirrhosis. Mild sclerosis of some portal zones results in the picture of idiopathic portal hypertension after cytotoxic therapy for leukaemia [179].

Veno-occlusive disease is associated with cyclophosphamide, busulphan and irradiation. *Cholestasis* may be dose-related due to such drugs as cytosine arabinoside, or *hepato-canalicular* due to azathioprine. *Sinusoidal dilatation, peliosis* and *tumours* are associated with sex and anabolic hormone therapy. One drug may enhance the toxicity of another, for instance 6-mercaptopurine effects are worsened by doxorubicin.

Long-term use of cytotoxic agents in recipients of renal transplants or in children with acute lymphatic leukaemia leads to chronic hepatitis, fibrosis and portal hypertension.

Arsenic

The organic, trivalent compounds are particularly poisonous. Arsenic trioxide 1% (Fowler's solution) given for long periods for the treatment of psoriasis has resulted in non-cirrhotic portal hypertension [134]. Acute, probably homicidal, arsenic poisoning can cause peri-sinusoidal fibrosis and veno-occlusive disease [89].

Arsenic in drinking water and native drugs in India may be related to 'idiopathic' portal hypertension. The liver shows portal tract fibrosis and sclerosis of the portal vein branches (fig. 18.15). Angiosarcoma is a complication [160].

Vinyl chloride

Workmen exposed to vinyl chloride monomer over many years develop hepatotoxicity (fig. 18.16). The earliest change is a sclerosis of portal venules in zone 1

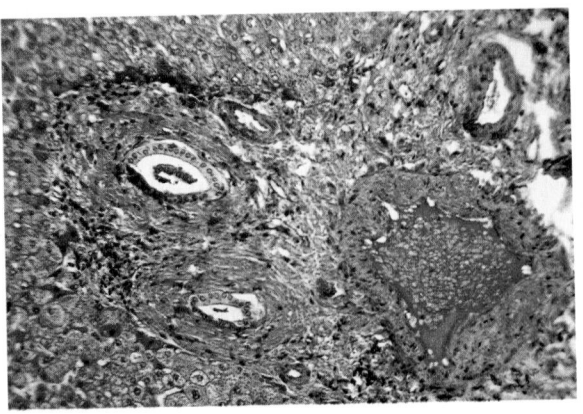

Fig. 18.15. Arsenic hepatotoxicity following treatment of psoriasis. Zone 1 is expanded by fibrosis and sclerosis of portal vein radicles. (Stained Mallory's trichrome.)

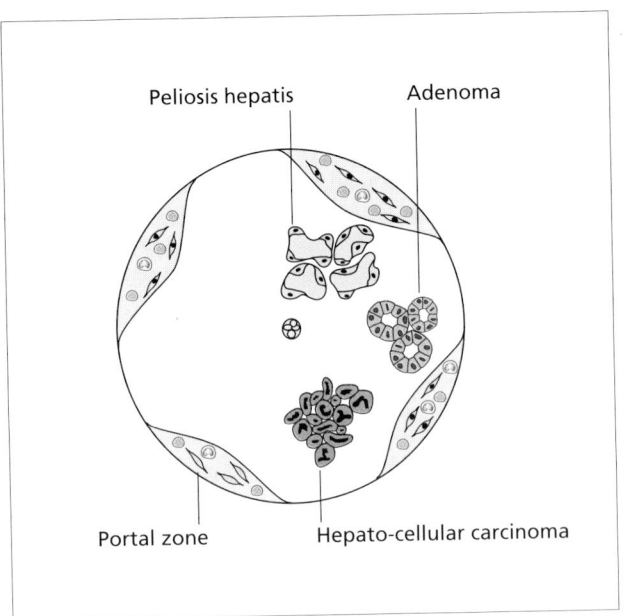

Fig. 18.16. Toxic effects of vinyl chloride, arsenic and thorotrast on the liver.

of the liver with the clinical changes of splenomegaly and portal hypertension. Later associations include angiosarcoma of the liver and peliosis hepatis. Early histological alterations indicative of vinyl monomer exposure are focal hepato-cellular and focal mixed hepatocytes and sinusoidal cells hyperplasia. These are followed by subcapsular portal and peri-sinusoidal fibrosis [196].

Vitamin A

Vitamin A is being increasingly used in dermatology, by food faddists, in cancer prevention and for hypogonadism. Toxicity develops with as little as 25 000 iu over 6 years or 50 000 iu daily for 2 years [51, 123]. It is potentiated by alcohol abuse.

The patient presents with nausea, vomiting, hepatomegaly, abnormal biochemical tests and portal hypertension. Ascites, either exudate or transudate, may develop. Histology shows hyperplasia of fat storing (Ito) cells with vacuoles which fluoresce under ultraviolet light. Fibrosis and cirrhosis may develop [51].

Vitamin A is slowly metabolized from the hepatic stores and may be identified in liver months after stopping treatment.

Retinoids

These vitamin A derivatives are used largely in dermatology. Etretinate, which is structurally similar to retinol, has caused severe hepatic reactions. Hepatotoxicity has also been reported with its metabolite, acitretin [208] and with isotretinoin [113].

Vascular

Sinusoidal dilatation

Focal dilatation of zone 1 sinusoids may complicate contraceptive or anabolic steroid therapy. This can cause hepatomegaly and abdominal pain with rises in serum enzymes. Hepatic arteriography shows stretched, attenuated branches of the hepatic artery with a patchy parenchymal pattern where areas of contrast alternate with areas not well filled.

The condition regresses on stopping the hormone.

A similar change may complicate azathioprine given after renal transplantation and this may be followed 1–3 years later by fibrosis and cirrhosis.

Peliosis hepatis

The large blood-filled cavities may or may not be lined with sinusoidal cells (figs 18.17, 18.27). They are distributed randomly, the diameter varying from 1 mm to several cm [228]. Electron microscopy shows passage of red blood cells through the endothelial barrier and perisinusoidal fibrosis may develop. These alterations might constitute the primary event [227].

Peliosis has been described in patients taking oral contraceptives, in men having androgenic and anabolic steroids, and following tamoxifen for breast cancer [111]. Peliosis has been reported in recipients of renal transplants. It has also complicated danazol therapy [133].

Veno-occlusive disease (VOD)

Small, zone 3 hepatic veins are particularly sensitive to toxic damage, reacting by subendothelial oedema and subsequent collagenization. The disease was originally

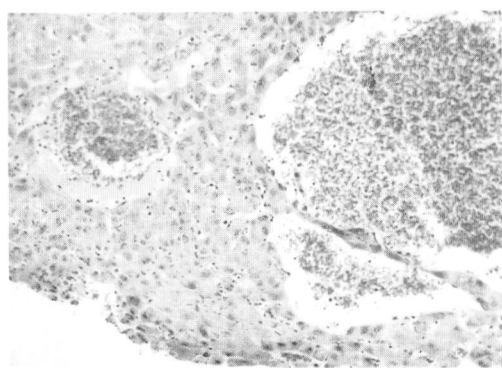

Fig. 18.17. Peliosis hepatis. A dilated blood space is seen with no clear-cut wall.

described from Jamaica due to toxic injury to the minute hepatic veins by pyrrolizidine alkaloids taken as senecio in medicinal bush teas. It has since been described from India [197], Israel, Egypt and even Arizona [162]. It has been related to contamination of wheat [197].

The disease is marked by an acute stage with painful hepatomegaly, ascites and inconspicuous jaundice. The patient may recover, die or pass into a sub-acute stage of hepatomegaly and recurrent ascites. The chronic type resembles any other cirrhosis. Diagnosis is made by liver biopsy.

Azathioprine induces endothelialitis. Its long-term use in kidney and liver transplant recipients is associated with sinusoidal dilatation, peliosis, VOD and nodular regenerative hyperplasia [189].

Cytotoxic therapy especially with cyclophosphamide BNCU, azathioprine, busulphan, VP-16 and total body irradiation exceeding 12 Gy are associated with VOD [79, 101]. VOD follows high-dose cytoreductive therapy in bone marrow recipients [181]. There is widespread damage to zone 3 structures including hepatocytes, sinusoids and particularly small hepatic venules. It is marked by jaundice, painful hepatomegaly and weight gain (ascites). In 25% of patients it is severe with death occurring within 100 days.

Hepatic irradiation. The liver has a low tolerance to radiotherapy. Radiation hepatitis increases when doses reach or exceed 35 Gy to the whole organ delivered as 10 Gy a week. VOD appears 1–3 months after completion of therapy. It may be transient or death may ensue from liver failure. Histologically, zone 3 haemorrhage is seen with hepatic venules showing fibrosis and obliteration.

Hepatic vein occlusion (Budd–Chiari syndrome) has been reported following oral contraceptives, and after azathioprine in a renal transplant patient [154, 206] (see Chapter 11).

Acute hepatitis

Only a very small proportion of patients taking the drug will have the reaction. There is usually no method of selecting who will be susceptible. The reaction is unrelated to dose but is commoner after multiple exposures. The onset is delayed about 1 week after exposure.

The pre-icteric period of gastrointestinal symptoms resembles acute hepatitis and is followed by jaundice associated with pale stools and dark urine and an enlarged tender liver. Biochemical tests indicate hepatocellular damage. Serum γ-globulins are increased.

In those who recover, maximum serum bilirubin levels are reached after 2–3 weeks. The more seriously affected show a shrinking liver and die of hepatic failure. The mortality is high for those that are clinically recognized, higher than for sporadic virus hepatitis. If hepatic precoma or coma is reached the mortality is 70%.

Hepatic histology may be virtually indistinguishable from acute virus hepatitis [74]. Milder cases show spotty necrosis becoming more extensive and reaching a stage of diffuse liver injury and collapse. Bridging is frequent; inflammatory infiltration is variable. Chronic hepatitis may sometimes be a sequel.

The drugs causing this type of reaction may do so by the production of toxic metabolites injurious to the liver *per se* or the metabolite may act as a hapten with cell protein, so inducing immunological liver injury (fig. 18.5).

An enormous number of drugs cause this hepatic reaction. They may emerge only after the drug has been released on the general market. Specialist textbooks should be consulted for individual drugs [43, 194, 229]. Isoniazid, methyl dopa and halothane are described in detail, but any drug should be suspected. An individual drug can cause more than one reaction and there may be overlap between acute hepatitic, cholestatic and hypersensitivity reactions.

The reactions tend to be severe, particularly if the drug is continued after liver damage has started. Patients with acute, fulminant drug-related liver failure must be considered for hepatic transplantation (Chapter 8). Corticosteroids are of doubtful benefit.

Older women are at particular risk, whereas the reactions are unusual in children.

Isoniazid

In one serious outbreak, 19 of 2231 asymptomatic government employers with positive tuberculin skin tests developed clinical signs of liver disease within 6 months of starting isoniazid [48]. Thirteen subjects were jaundiced and two died.

After acetylation the isoniazid is converted to a hydrazine which is changed by drug-metabolizing enzymes to a potent acylating agent which produces liver necrosis (fig. 18.18) [124].

Combination of the isoniazid with an enzyme-inducer such as rifampicin increases the risk [188]. Anaesthetic drugs, paracetamol and alcohol enhance toxicity. Para-amino salicylate, on the other hand, is an enzyme-retarder, and this may account for the relative safety of the para-amino salicylate–isoniazid combination formerly used in the treatment of tuberculosis. The addition of pyrazinamide markedly increases the mortality [38].

The slow acetylator phenotype is caused by decreased or absent *N*-acetyltransferase [57]. The relation of hepatotoxicity to acetylator status remains uncertain, although in Japanese patients fast acetylators are more susceptible [226].

Immunological liver injury is possible. However, 'allergic' manifestations are absent and the incidence of 12–20% developing sub-clinical liver injury is very high.

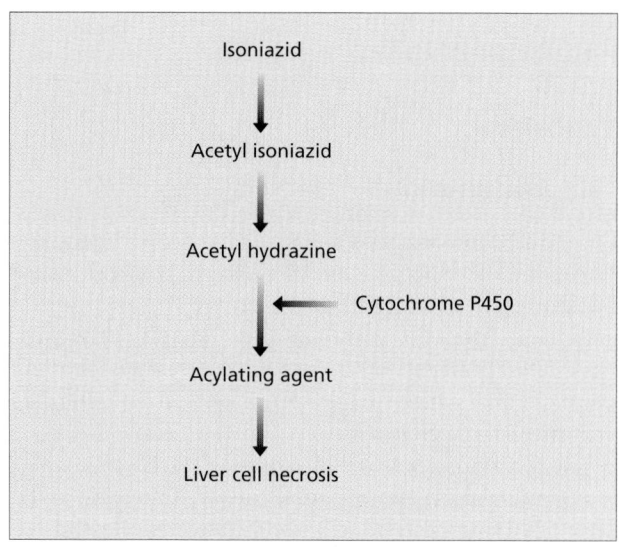

Fig. 18.18. The possible mechanism of isoniazid liver injury.

Elevated serum transaminase values are frequently seen during the first 8 weeks of therapy. There are usually no symptoms and the transaminases subside despite continuing isoniazid. Nevertheless, transaminases should be monitored before treatment is started and 4 weeks later. If increases are found they should be repeated at weekly intervals. Rising levels indicate that treatment must be stopped.

Clinical features

Serious reactions are more frequent in those over 50 years old, usually females. After treatment for 2–3 months, non-specific symptoms include anorexia and weight loss [127]. These continue for 1–4 weeks before the onset of jaundice.

The hepatitis usually resolves rapidly on stopping the drug, but if jaundice develops there is a 10% mortality [13].

Severity is greatly increased if the drug is continued after symptoms develop or serum transaminases rise. The reactions are more serious if the patient presents after more than 2 months on the drug [13]. Malnutrition and alcoholism increase the risk [138].

The *liver biopsy* may show acute hepatitis. Continued administration leads to chronic hepatitis [116]. This is probably non-progressive if the drug is withdrawn.

Rifampicin

This has usually been given with isoniazid. Rifampicin on its own may cause a mild hepatitis, but this is usually in the context of a general hypersensitivity reaction.

Methyl dopa

Increase in serum transaminases, which generally subside despite continued drug administration, are reported in 5%. These may be metabolite related, since human microsomes can convert methyl dopa to a potent arylating agent.

Methyl dopa hepatotoxicity may also be immunologically related to metabolic activation and the production of a drug-associated antigen.

The patient is often post-menopausal and has been on methyl dopa for 1–4 weeks. The reaction usually appears within the first 3 months. Prodromas include pyrexia and are short. Liver biopsy shows bridging and multilobular necrosis. Death may occur in the acute stage, but clinical improvement usually follows stopping the drug.

Other anti-hypertensives

These are subject to the same genetic polymorphism as debrisoquine (P450-II-D6) [96]. Hepatotoxicity has been reported with metoprolol [96], atenolol [175], labetalol [29], acebutalol [198] and hydralazine derivatives [197].

Enalapril, an angiotensin-converting enzyme inhibitor, is a cause of hepatitis with eosinophilia [164]. Verapamil can also cause an acute hepatitis-like reaction [58].

Halothane

Halothane-associated liver damage is very rare. It seems to be of two types: mild, evidenced by raised serum transaminase, and fulminant in a few patients who have usually been exposed previously to halothane.

Mechanisms

Products of reductive metabolism are particularly hepatotoxic in the presence of hypoxaemia. The oxidative metabolites are also reactive. Active metabolites could cause lipid peroxidation and inactivation of drug-metabolizing enzymes.

Halothane is stored in adipose tissue and may be released slowly; obesity is frequently associated with halothane hepatitis.

The association with multiple exposures (fig. 18.19), the pattern of fever and the occasional eosinophilia and skin rash would suggest immunological mechanisms. Patients with halothane hepatitis have specific serum antibodies to liver microsomal proteins bound with halothane metabolites [121].

Lymphocytes show increased cytotoxicity and this is also found in family members. The extreme rarity of the fulminant reaction implies an unusual pathway for drug biotransformation in susceptible patients and/or abnormal tissue responses to electrophilic halothane metabolites.

Clinical features

Halothane hepatitis is much more frequent after multiple anaesthetics. Obese, elderly females seem particularly at risk. Children can be affected [83].

Fever, usually with rigors, develops more than 7 days (range 8–13 days) after the first operation and is usually accompanied by malaise and non-specific gastrointestinal symptoms, including right upper abdominal pain. After several exposures the temperature is noted 1–11 days post-operatively (fig. 18.19). Jaundice appears rapidly after the pyrexia, about 10–28 days after a *single* exposure and 3–17 days after *multiple* anaesthetics. This delay before jaundice, usually of about 1 week, is helpful in excluding other causes of post-operative icterus.

The total white cell count is usually normal, with occasionally eosinophilia. Serum bilirubin levels may be very high, particularly in fatal cases, but are under 170 μmol/litre (10 mg/dl) in 40%. The condition may be anicteric. Serum transaminases are in the range found in viral hepatitis. An occasionally high serum alkaline phosphatase level may be seen. If the patient becomes icteric the mortality is very high. Altogether 139 of 310 patients in one series died (46%). If coma ensues and the one stage prothrombin time rises markedly the condition is virtually hopeless.

Hepatic changes

These may be virtually indistinguishable from those of acute viral hepatitis (fig. 18.20). Leucocytic infiltration in the sinusoids, granulomas and fatty change may suggest

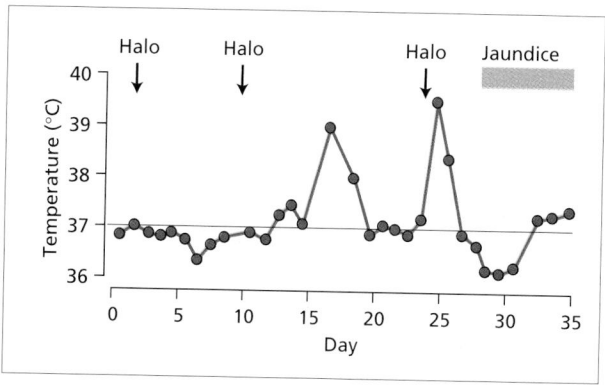

Fig. 18.19. Hepatitis associated with multiple exposures to halothane. Note the febrile response to the halothane anaesthetics. The patient became jaundiced after the third anaesthetic and rapidly became pre-comatose, developing deep coma on the fourth day and dying on the seventh day.

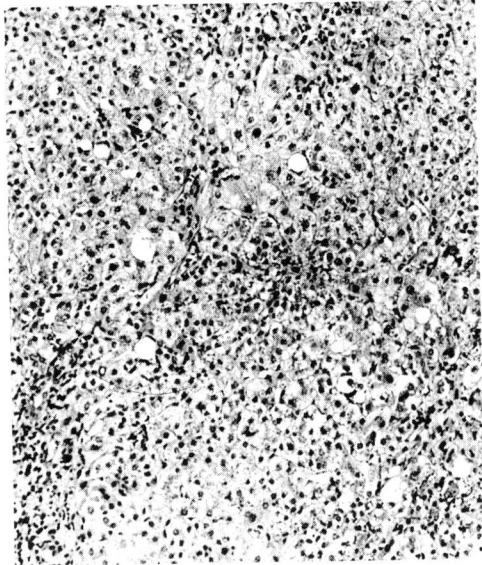

Fig. 18.20. Halothane-associated hepatitis. Hepatic histology shows cellular infiltration largely with mononuclear cells. Centrizonal areas show necrosis and cell swelling. Liver cell columns are disorganized. The appearances are virtually identical to those of acute viral hepatitis. (H & E, × 96.)

a drug aetiology. Necrosis may be sub-massive and confluent or massive [10].

Alternatively, the picture in the first week may be that of direct metabolite-related liver injury with zone 3 massive necrosis involving two-thirds or more of each acinus (fig. 18.21).

Conclusions

Halothane administration should not be repeated if there is the slightest suspicion of even a mild reaction after the first anaesthetic. All case records should be scru-

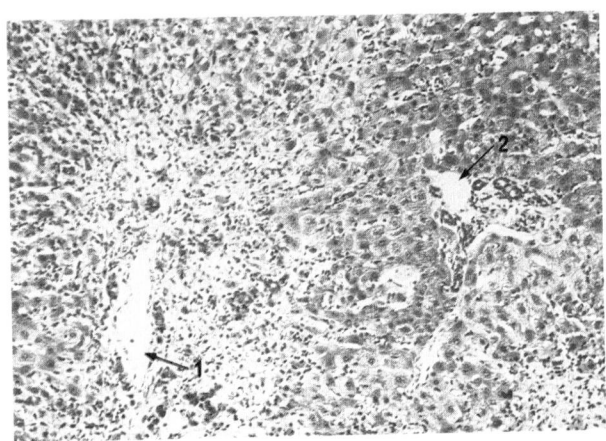

Fig. 18.21. Halothane liver injury. Centrizonal area (1) shows well-defined necrosis without an inflammatory reaction in the portal area (2). (H & E, ×220).

tinized carefully before *any* second anaesthetic is given.

Underlying liver disease is not a risk factor.

Those requiring multiple anaesthetics during a short period should not be given halothane. A second anaesthetic with halothane should not be repeated within 6 months of the first.

Enflurane and *isoflurane* are metabolized much less than halothane and low gas solubilities ensure rapid expiration from the body. Consequently, less toxic metabolites are produced. However, repeated exposures to isoflurane have been followed by fulminant hepatic failure [21, 170]. Although few cases of liver damage have been reported after enflurane [105], these are exceedingly rare. Despite increased cost, enflurane or isoflurane should replace halothane but should probably not be administered at short intervals. Enflurane metabolites are recognized by antibodies from patients with halothane hepatitis. Thus changing from one agent to the other for multiple anaesthetics will not necessarily reduce the risk of liver injury in a susceptible individual.

Ketoconazole

A hepatic reaction causing symptoms is very rare. However, reversible increases in serum transaminases are seen in 5–10% of those taking the drug.

Older people (mean age 57.9 years), and often women, are affected. The patient has usually taken the drug for at least 4 weeks and not for less than 10 days [192]. Cholestasis is often a histological feature [91]. It may be fatal.

The reaction is idiosyncratic but does not seem immunological as fever, rash, eosinophilia and granulomas are rare. Two fatal cases showed massive, predominantly zone 3, hepatic necrosis.

Newer antifungals, fluconazole and itraconazole, may be hepatotoxic.

Cytotoxic drugs

Hepatotoxicity and VOD are discussed above.

Flutamide, an anti-androgen used to treat prostatic cancer, can cause both hepatitis and cholestatic jaundice [37, 166].

Cytoproterone [16] and etoposide can cause acute hepatitis.

Nervous system modifiers

Tacrine, used to treat Alzheimer's disease, causes hepatitis in about 13% of patients receiving it [61]. Half the patients treated will have rises in transaminases usually during the first 3 months of treatment [218]. The patient is usually asymptomatic.

Discontinuation reverses the transaminases increases

and re-challenge in mild cases is usually negative suggesting that the liver may be able to adapt to tacrine. There have been no hepatotoxic deaths but transaminases should be monitored for the first 3 months of therapy with tacrine.

Pemoline is a central nervous system stimulant used in children. It causes acute hepatitis, probably metabolite-related, which can be fatal [132].

Disulfiram, used to treat chronic alcoholism, has been associated with an acute hepatitis picture which is sometimes fatal [26].

Glafenine. This analgesic has been associated with a hepatitic reaction usually between 2 weeks and 4 months of starting. The picture resembles that of cincophen. Five of 12 patients died [191].

Clozapine. This drug, to treat schizophrenia, has caused fulminant liver failure.

Sustained release nicotinic acid (niacin)

Hepatotoxicity is related to the time-release form and not the crystalline form.

The reaction develops 1–4 weeks after 2–4 g per day. It is hepato-cellular and cholestatic and can be fatal [31].

Chronic hepatitis

The picture strikingly resembles 'autoimmune' chronic hepatitis in clinical, biochemical, serological and histological features. The patients recover when the drug is withdrawn. Anti-organelle antibodies have been found in a number of patients [116].

Chronic hepatitis was first described following the laxative oxyphenisatin and this has now been withdrawn from most parts of the world [156]. Chronic active hepatitis can develop insidiously after many years of methyl dopa therapy and without an acute episode. Improvement follows withdrawal of the drug [116].

Nitrofurantoin has been related to chronic hepatitis, usually in women, 4 weeks to 11 years after starting [14].

Other causes include *clometacin, fenofibrate, isoniazid, papaverine, minocyclin* and *dantrolene*. Minocyclin can cause a picture resembling autoimmune chronic hepatitis [55].

General hypersensitivity

A large number of drugs cause hepatic reactions of 'hypersensitivity' type of variable severity and with or without jaundice, rash, arthritis, haemolytic anaemia and eosinophilia. Sometimes the picture resembles infectious mononucleosis. The reaction usually appears within 4 weeks of starting therapy and is most frequent with multiple exposures. Challenge is usually positive. There is considerable overlap with the acute hepatitic

and hepato-canalicular groups. Liver histology shows focal, spotty necrosis of liver cells, with a mononuclear and sometimes eosinophilic reaction in the portal zones. Granulomas are sometimes found (fig. 18.22).

Sulphonamides and derivatives

Sulfasalazine. The hepatic reaction is usually part of a systemic reaction including a serum sickness picture. The patient has usually been taking the drug for less than 1 month. Re-challenge is positive. There is an association with HLA-B8-DR3. The reaction can be fatal [157]. Children can be affected [19].

Co-trimoxazole (Septrin) (see p. 358).

Pyrimethamine–sulfadoxine (Fansidar). This reaction is associated with severe cutaneous reactions and transient liver damage. Occasionally the reaction may be fatal [231]. The sulfadoxine is the likely hepatotoxin.

Non-steroidal anti-inflammatory drugs (NSAIDs)

Most NSAIDs are hepatotoxic, usually through an idiosyncratic or hypersensitivity reaction [149]. The mildest is simply a rise in serum transaminases but fatal liver failure can occur. Acute symptomatic liver disease from NSIADs is not a frequent clinical problem [24], but transaminases should be monitored during the first 6 months of therapy.

Salicylate toxicity is related to dose, duration and age—younger persons are a particular risk.

Sulindac (clinoril) 91 cases (four fatal) have been reported [199]. The reaction may be hepato-cellular, cholestatic or mixed. These are usually hallmarks of hypersensitivity including onset 8 weeks after starting the drug, fever, rash, nausea, vomiting and occasional eosinophilia.

Diclofenac (voltaren) [6, 75]. The patient, usually an elderly osteoarthritic female, presents with jaundice, hepatomegaly, anorexia and nausea. Serum antinuclear antibody may be positive and the patient can be misdiagnosed as having autoimmune liver disease [176]. Liver

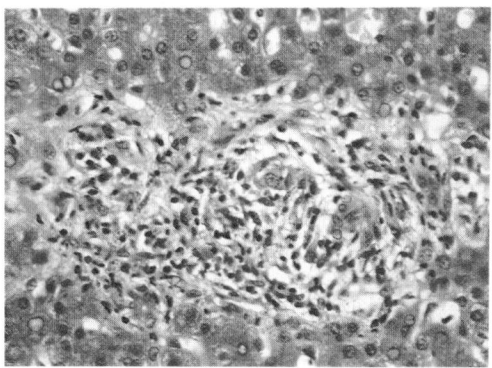

Fig. 18.22. Carbamazepine granulomatous hepatitis.

function should be monitored closely during the first 8 weeks of therapy. The reaction can be fatal. Drug challenge is positive.

Piroxicam hepatotoxicity is being reported after taking this long half-life drug. Onset is 1.5–15 months and the reaction can be fatal [141].

Indomethacin toxicity is exceedingly rare.

Allopurinol can cause a hepatic reaction which can include fibrin ring granulomas [190, 210].

Propafenone can cause an acute hepatic reaction which can be fatal [125].

Hydroxychloroquine has been related to fulminant liver disease.

Feldene and *naprosyn* are rare causes of hepatic dysfunction.

Ibuprofen seems safe.

Anti-thyroid drugs

Propylthiouracil. Elevations in transaminases are common in the first 2 months but are usually transient and asymptomatic. The drug may be continued with caution if there are no symptoms and the serum bilirubin is not increased [106].

Carbimazole has induced cholestasis [137] as has methimazole [135].

Quinidine [85] and quinine

This reaction is marked by rash and fever 6–12 days after starting treatment. Liver biopsy shows inflammatory infiltrates and granulomas. Prompt withdrawal leads to resolution; continued use may cause chronic liver damage.

Diltiazem

This calcium channel blocking agent has been associated with fevers, headache and abnormal transaminases within 18 days of starting. Liver biopsy shows many well-defined granulomas [169].

Benzbromarone, used to treat gout, causes hepatocellular injury [207].

Anti-convulsants

Protracted seizures in children can lead to acute zone 3 ischaemic injury [204]. Serum enzyme levels rise dramatically and fall over the next 2 weeks.

Phenytoin (dilantin). The reaction usually affects adults 2–4 weeks after starting. The picture closely resembles infectious mononucleosis. Eosinophilia is usual.

Mortality is 50% in those who develop jaundice. It is usually due to streptococcal skin infections. Sufferers may have a genetic defect [184] allowing accumu-

lation of a toxic metabolite. Corticosteroids may be of value.

Dantrolene. In one study, 1.8% of patients taking the drug for more than 60 days developed abnormal biochemical tests and a third of these became jaundiced [205]. Seven of 29 jaundiced patients died [205]. Hepatic changes include hepatitis, cholangitis, chronic active hepatitis and cirrhosis. Hepatotoxicity has limited the use of dantrolene as a muscle relaxant.

Carbamazepine. This drug has a wide spectrum of hepatic side-effects, the most usual being hepato-cellular necrosis with granulomas (fig. 18.22). Sometimes, however, itching, fever and right upper quadrant pain may suggest cholangitis and hepatic histology may show marked cholestasis [95].

Herbs and health-store remedies

Vitamin A and arsenic may lead to hepatic fibrosis. Nicotinic acid can cause hepato-cellular necrosis.

Herbs can also be hepatotoxic. VOD may be associated with senecio and comfrey. Herbal medicines used for stress may contain skullcap; valerian can cause acute hepatitis [114]. Chaparral leaf, used for infections, has caused sub-acute hepatic necrosis [17].

Germander causes hepatitis and has resulted in a death from acute hepatic necrosis [98]. A toxic metabolite is produced through P-453A [109].

Chinese herbal remedies for atopic asthma can be hepatotoxic [56].

Jin Bu Huan used for insomnia has caused acute hepatitis [223].

The ingestion of health-store products must be considered in any unexplained case of hepatic disease.

Canalicular cholestasis [211]

Various *androgens* and *oestrogen* steroids can cause canalicular cholestasis. Oestrogens contained in contraceptive pills are good examples but cholestasis is decreasing with reduction in the content of active ingredients. The oestrogen is the important agent, although the progestin may augment the effect.

Bile salt independent bile flow is reduced probably through suppression of $Na^+–K^+–ATPase$ activity. Sinusoidal membranes become less fluid. Peri-cellular permeability (tight junctions) may be increased, Cytoskeleton is affected with failure of the peri-canalicular micro-filaments to contract [145].

The cause is usually, but not always, a C17-alkylated testosterone. The reaction is dose-dependent and reversible even if large doses have been taken over many years [112].

This type of cholestasis is also seen with norethandrolone, methyl testosterone, norandrostenolone, stanozolol [41], megesterol [45] and danazol [182].

Patients with a genetic predisposition to cholestasis of pregnancy are at risk (Chapter 25). An enhanced effect is also seen in those with a tendency to cholestasis such as sufferers from pre-symptomatic primary biliary cirrhosis. Theoretically, patients with acute hepatitis who continue to take oral contraceptives should develop deep jaundice and pruritus. However, this is not so and a woman convalescent from hepatitis may resume use of oral contraceptives as soon as she wishes without causing liver damage.

The patient suffers from itching with variable bilirubinaemia. Serum transaminase values are variable but in about one-third may exceed five times normal. Serum alkaline phosphatase may be disproportionately low [18].

Liver biopsy shows normal architecture and zone 3 cholestasis with surrounding reaction. *Electron microscopy* shows cholestasis and mild hepato-cellular damage.

Prognosis is excellent. Rarely jaundice is severe and prolonged [107] but usually the patient recovers when the drug is stopped. Recurrence is liable to follow resumption.

Cyclosporin A

In rats, cyclosporin inhibits ATP-dependent bile salt transport and may induce cholestasis [76]. Clinical cholestasis in man is rare, but may be treated by ursodeoxycholic acid [148].

Cyclosporin is metabolized by P450-III-A enzymes (fig. 18.4). Enzyme induction and competitive inhibition explains interactions with such drugs as ketoconazole and erythromycin [216].

Hepato-canalicular cholestasis

Here the reaction is predominantly cholestatic but, in addition, hepato-cellular features are present. In many, immunological liver injury is suggested. There is an overlap with hypersensitivity and hepatitic drug reactions.

The cholestatic reaction is usually mild but can be severe and prolonged lasting many months or even years.

Acute cholangitis in the early stages is followed by the chronic phase of ductopenia defined by the absence of interlobular bile ducts in at least 50% of small portal tracts [34]. Recovery is usual, but occasionally, hepatic transplantation is indicated.

Many drugs cause cholestasis. The penicillin derivatives (Augmentin, flucloxacin), sulphonomides (Septrin, Bactrim), the erythromycins, promazines and procarbazine (fig. 18.23) are particularly important.

Chlorpromazine

Only 1–2% of those taking the drug develop cholestasis. The reaction is unrelated to dose and in 80–90% the onset is in the first 4 weeks. There may be associated hypersensitivity. Excess eosinophils may be found in the liver (fig. 18.24). This suggests idiosyncracy.

Chlorpromazine decreases canalicular function and reduces bile flow [80]. Free chlorpromazine radicles may be hepatotoxic.

Genetic differences in the bile transformation of chlorpromazine could theoretically lead to the selective accumulation of cholestatic metabolites [219]. The delay in onset of jaundice and the lack of a dose–response relationship remain unexplained.

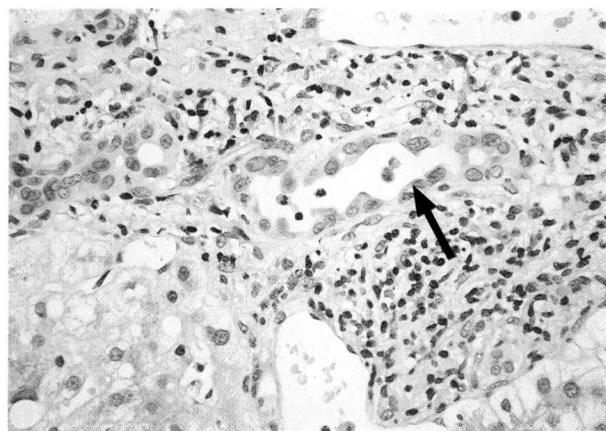

Fig. 18.23. Chronic procarbazine cholestasis: liver biopsy shows a portal area (zone 1) markedly expanded with largely mononuclear cells and some fibrous tissue, and containing a damaged bile duct (arrow). Recovery followed after 6 months jaundice. (H & E, ×100.)

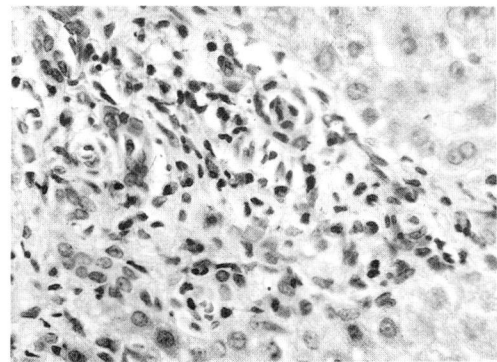

Fig. 18.24. Chlorpromazine hepatitis shows a portal zone reaction with eosinophils prominent.

Clinical picture

The onset may simulate viral hepatitis, prodromas lasting some 4–5 days. Cholestatic jaundice appears concurrently or within a week and lasts 1–4 weeks. Pruritus may precede jaundice. Recovery is usually complete.

Serum biochemistry shows the features of cholestatic jaundice. A sustained rise in alkaline phosphatase values may be the only change. An eosinophilia may be seen in the peripheral blood in the very early stages.

Hepatic changes

Light microscopy shows cholestasis and, in the portal zones, a marked cellular reaction with mononuclear cells and eosinophils prominent (fig. 18.24). Even in the uncomplicated case some damage to liver cells can be noted. Granulomas may be present.

Prognosis and treatment

Jaundice of the chlorpromazine type is rarely fatal.

Occasionally jaundice lasts more than 3 months and even up to 3 years [153]. The picture is of prolonged cholestatic jaundice with steatorrhoea and weight loss. The clinical picture resembles primary biliary cirrhosis. The onset is, however, much more explosive and, in contrast to pimary biliary cirrhosis, which is inevitably progressive, recovery usually ensues. However, the cholestasis can last 6 months or even be permanent with the development of biliary cirrhosis and eventually the need for transplantation.

The mitochondrial antibody test for primary biliary cirrhosis is negative or in low titre.

In the usual case of chlorpromazine jaundice no active treatment is required and recovery is complete. Corticosteroids do not affect the course. Ursodeoxycholic acid may be used to control itching.

Other promazines

An essentially similar picture can complicate therapy with other phenothiazine derivatives such as promazine, prochlorperazine, mepazine or trifluoperazine.

Penicillins

Amoxycillin is an exceedingly rare cause of liver damage [32]. However, in combination with clavulanic acid (*Augmentin*) it can cause cholestasis, predominantly in men and in the elderly, which is usually but not always shortlived [97, 168].

Flucloxacillin causes cholestatic jaundice, usually in older patients taking the drug for more than 2 weeks [42]. Jaundice may appear within 8 weeks, and after the drug has been stopped, making the relationship difficult to establish. Cholestasis can become chronic.

Sulphonomides

Trimethaprim–sulfamethoxazole (*Septrin*, *Bactrim*) can rarely cause cholestatic reactions which usually resolve in 6 months [2, 202]. However, the cholestasis can last 1–2 years [86].

Erythromycin

Hepatic reactions are usually with the estolate, but the proprionate ethylsuccinate and clarithromycin have also been incriminated.

Two patients reacting to the estolate had a further cholestatic reaction when given the ethylsuccinate 12 and 15 years later [81].

The onset is 1–4 weeks after starting therapy with right upper quadrant pain, which may be severe, simulating biliary disease, fever, itching and jaundice. The blood may show eosinophilia and atypical lymphocytes.

Liver biopsy shows cholestasis, hepato-cellular injury and acidophil bodies. Portal zones show the bile duct wall to be infiltrated with leucocytes and eosinophils and the bile duct cells may show mitoses. At autopsy the gallbladder has been shown to be inflamed.

Nitrofurantoin

Nitrofurantoin and its derivative, nifurtoinol, can cause a hepatitis with sometimes cholestasis and even the development of chronic active hepatitis [193]. The reaction is usually in the first 6 weeks and may be accompanied by fever, rash and eosinophilia (fig. 18.25). In chronic cases, circulating autoantibodies can be found. The patients usually improve when the drug is stopped, but may die with progressive liver failure.

Haloperidol

This drug may rarely cause a cholestatic reaction resembling that related to chlorpromazine. It may become chronic [36].

Cimetidine and ranitidine [174, 209]

Very rarely, cimetidine or ranitidine can cause a mild, non-fatal cholestatic jaundice usually developing within 4 weeks of starting the drug.

Oral hypoglycaemics

Cholestasis has been related to chlorpropamide [172], glyburide and acetohexamide [151].

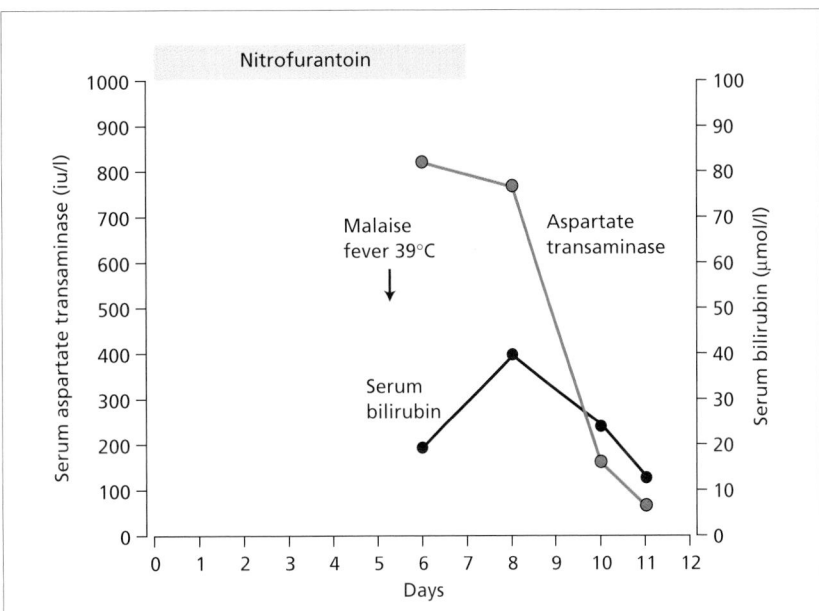

Fig. 18.25. Nitrofurantoin therapy for a urinary tract infection was followed 5 days later by a systemic reaction with jaundice. On stopping the drug the patient recovered rapidly.

Other causes

Prolonged cholestasis can follow cyproheptadine (an appetite suppressant) [94] and thiabendazole (fig. 18.23).

Cholestasis has also been associated with gold, tamoxifen [15], azathioprine, hydralazine [131], captopril [150], propafenone [125] and the quinoline enoxacin [4].

Dextropropoxyphene

This analgesic can induce a reaction with recurrent jaundice, upper abdominal pain and rigors, mimicking biliary tract disease [165].

Ductular cholestasis

The bile ducts and canaliculi are filled with dense, inspissated bile casts without any surrounding inflammatory reaction. The plugs contain bilirubin, probably in combination with a drug metabolite. The picture has been particularly associated with *benoxyprofen*, which has a half-life of 30 hours in the young, but 111 hours in the elderly [195]. Five elderly patients died with jaundice and renal failure. Generalized poisoning by the drug and its metabolites seems likely. Benoxyprofen has now been withdrawn.

Biliary sludge

This complicates treatment with the antibiotic, *ceftriaxone*. The patient may be symptom-free or suffer reversible biliary colic [139]. It is dose dependent [180]. Sludging is related to sharing a common pathway with bile acids for hepatic transport and also to an interaction with biliary lipid excretion. The sludge consists of a small amount of cholesterol and bilirubin but the major component is the calcium salt of ceftriaxone.

Sclerosing cholangitis (Chapter 15)

Causes include hepatic arterial infusion of cytotoxic drugs such as 5-fluorouridine [90], thiabendazole [119], caustics introduced into hydatid cysts [9] and the Spanish toxic oil syndrome [186].

Bile duct stricture can follow 10 years after upper abdominal *radiotherapy* [27, 50].

Hepatic tumours

The association of hepatic adenoma, a hitherto very rare benign tumour, with oral contraceptives was first suggested in 1973 [7]. It is rare but the risk increases dramatically with duration of use, particularly after 48 months [39]. Pills with a high hormone content and use in women over the age of 30 may increase the risk of adenoma [163]. The incidence is falling with the use of pills containing smaller amounts of hormone.

Familial adenomas have been described, where sufferers have never taken oral contraceptives [46].

Adenomas have been induced by norethisterone in patients on renal dialysis [77].

Mechanisms

The mechanism of tumour formation is complex (fig. 18.26). Oestrogens promote hepatic neoplasia [215].

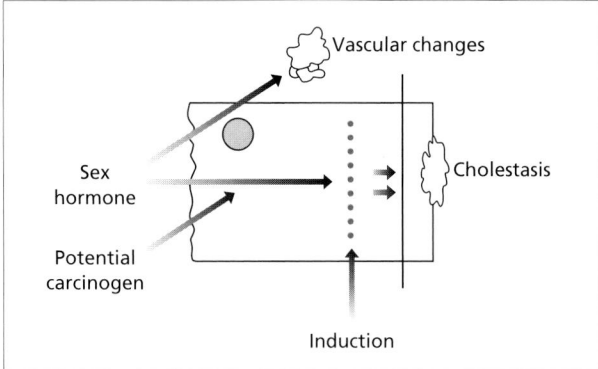

Fig. 18.26. Possible mechanisms of hepatic tumour production by sex hormones.

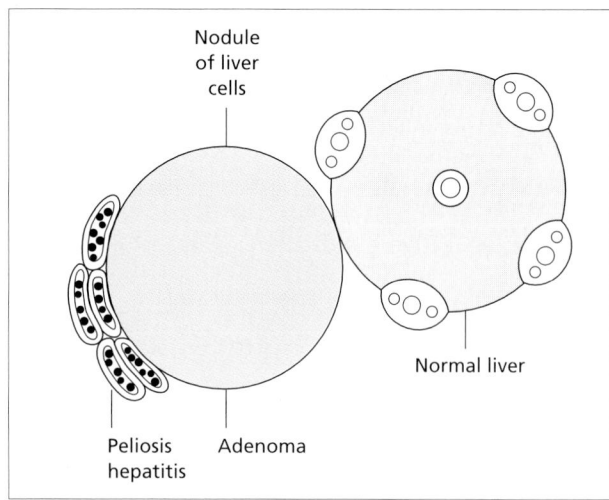

Fig. 18.27. Structure of hepatic adenoma and peliosis hepatis compared with normal liver.

Hepatic adenoma lacks oestrogen receptors. Oral contraceptives, as enzyme-inducers, might potentiate the carcinogenesis of certain compounds by increasing their rate of conversion to toxic (?carcinogenic) metabolites. Cholestatic properties of steroids might enhance the potentially carcinogenic action of substances normally excreted in the bile. Concomitant drugs might act as additional enzyme-inducers. The vascular changes probably represent part of the general vasodilatation associated with sex hormones and are analogous both to vascular spiders and to the endometrial arterial hypertrophy found in pregnancy.

Adenoma

These smooth, encapsulated tumours are usually single but may be multiple. They are about 8–10 cm in diameter, usually subcapsular and sometimes pedunculated. They are most frequent in the right lobe. Microscopically the tumour consists of sheets of near-normal liver cells without portal tracts or central veins (figs 18.27, 18.28). Bile ducts are conspicuously absent.

Hepato-cellular carcinoma

There is a low, although probably increased, risk of hepato-cellular carcinoma in women receiving oral contraceptives for 8 years or more. The tumour develops in a non-cirrhotic liver, metastasizes rarely, and does not infiltrate [69].

Young women with oral contraceptive exposure tend to survive longer, have fewer symptoms and lower serum α-fetoprotein levels than those with hepato-cellular carcinoma without exposure to oral contraceptives. Tumours are more vascular and haemoperitoneum commoner.

Hepatic adenoma rarely transforms into hepato-cellular carcinoma but hepato-cellular carcinoma has developed in a site where a contraceptive steroid-induced adenoma had previously regressed.

Hepato-cellular adenoma and carcinoma have been associated with *danazol* [44]. Multiple adenomas have been associated with *type 1b glycogen storage disease*. These can proceed to carcinoma.

Vascular lesions may accompany adenoma or focal nodular hyperplasia. Large arteries and veins are present in excess, sinusoids may be focally dilated and peliosis may be present. Hepatic haemangiomas are sometimes seen.

Clinical features [84]

The tumour may be symptomless and discovered incidentally at autopsy or at the time of surgery or hepatic scanning for another condition.

The patient may present with a right upper-quadrant mass.

Haemorrhage into the tumour, or infarction, leads to abdominal pain and the tumour is tender.

Rupture is associated with the symptoms and signs of acute intra-peritoneal bleeding.

Serum biochemical tests may be normal. Necrosis and rupture are associated with increase in transaminases and alkaline phosphatase. Serum α-fetoprotein is not increased.

Needle liver biopsy is relatively contraindicated because of the vascular nature of the tumour.

Localization

Ultrasound is useful. *Isotope scans* usually demonstrate the filling defect. However, both this method and an

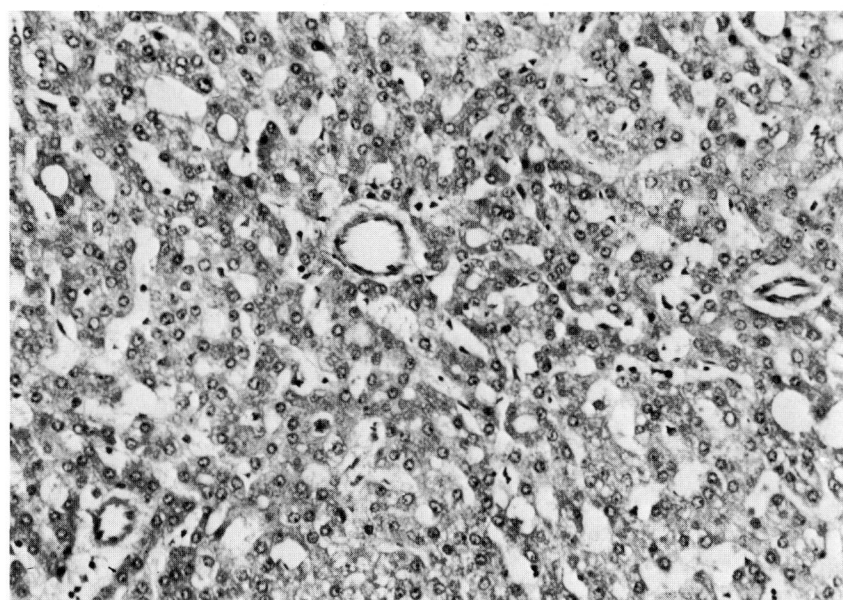

Fig. 18.28. Hepatic adenoma. The appearance is of sheets of near-normal liver cells without portal tracts. (H & E, ×185.)

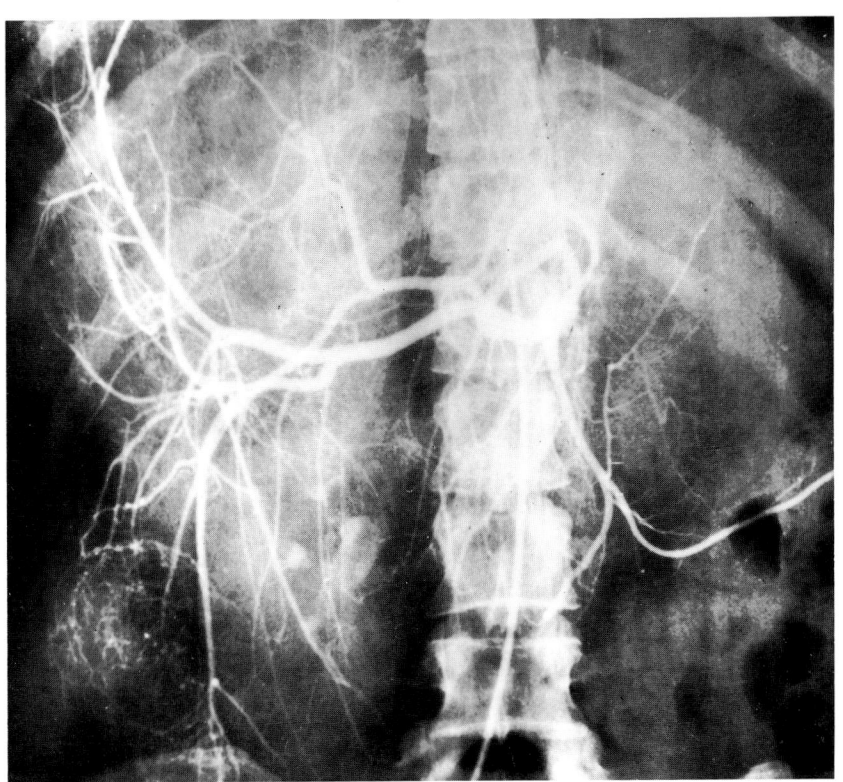

Fig. 18.29. Hepatic adenoma related to oral contraceptives. Coeliac angiogram shows stretching of branches of the hepatic artery around a relatively avascular lesion in the upper part of the right lobe of the liver.

enhanced *CT scan* may fail to demonstrate the tumour when it closely resembles normal liver.

MR imaging. Adenomas have a variable MRI appearance usually hyperintense on T_1- and T_2-weighted images. High signal intensity may be related to increased fat content [142].

Arteriography (figs 18.29, 18.30) shows stretching of the feeding arteries around the mass with branches pene-trating the tumour from the periphery. Irregular vessels course through the lesion. Areas of haemorrhage may be demonstrated. There is a marked capillary blush.

Management

Women who take oral contraceptives, particularly for many years, should be warned of the possibility of

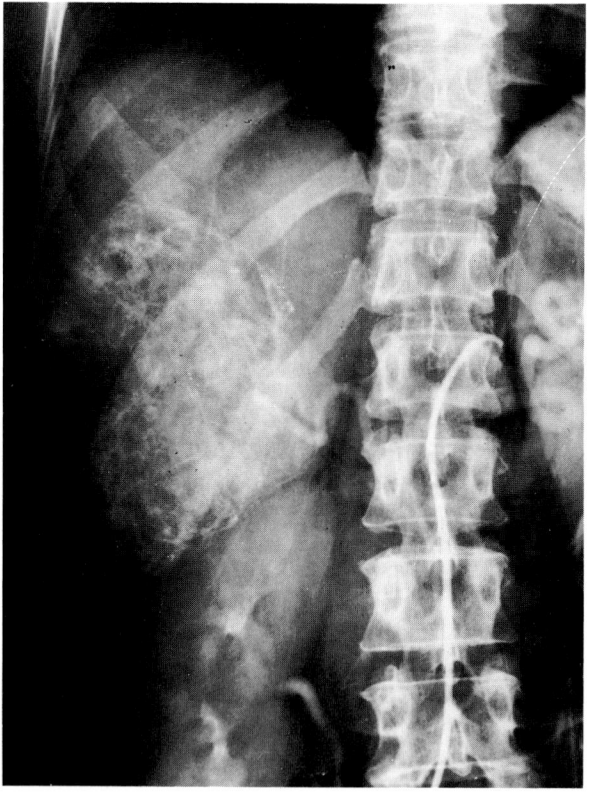

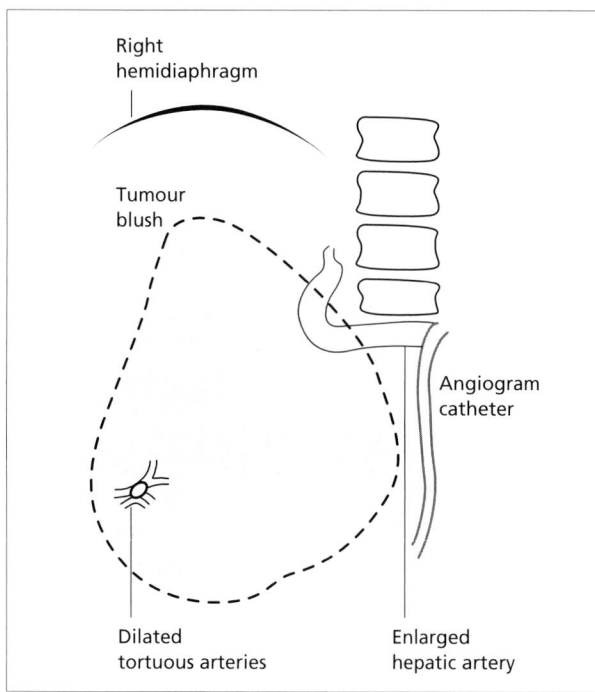

Right
hemidiaphragm

Tumour
blush

Angiogram
catheter

Dilated
tortuous arteries

Enlarged
hepatic artery

Fig. 18.30. Hepatic adenoma related to oral contraceptives. Late stage of coeliac angiogram shows abnormal vascularity in the tumour in the lower part of the right lobe of the liver.

tumours developing. The risk of hepato-cellular carcinoma persists for more than 10 years after discontinuing oral contraceptives [200].

The surgeon is tempted to operate. However, in most uncomplicated cases it is advisable to be conservative. Tumours are often multiple. If the tumour is diagnosed but there are no complications, it should be left *in situ* and sex hormones stopped. Tumours may regress [22] although this is not always the case [120]. Women must be warned of the possibility of rupture and the significance of any unexplained right upper-quadrant pain or swelling in the abdomen. Rupture becomes more likely in pregnancy. Liver ultrasound or scans should be repeated initially every 6 months and then yearly.

Surgery may be needed for complications, particularly intra-peritoneal or intra-tumour bleeding, with severe abdominal pain and anaemia. Excision has virtually no mortality or serious morbidity [100]. In inoperable cases, embolization leads to shrinkage of the tumour and relief of vena-caval obstruction [122].

Even if present, lymph node metastases may regress [201].

Focal nodular hyperplasia

This does not have such a strong association with oral contraceptives as adenoma. It affects both sexes, including children, but especially women in their reproductive years, some of whom may never have taken oral contraceptives.

The well-circumscribed unencapsulated lesion presents in an otherwise normal liver [212]. It is commonly subcapsular but can be pedunculated and can occur in either lobe. The lesions vary in size between 1 and 15 cm and may be multiple. On cut section, a stellate, central scar containing an artery is seen from which septa radiate, subdividing the mass into nodules which simulate cirrhosis (figs 18.31, 18.32). The lesion is supplied by a central artery and may represent a vascular anomaly. This is supported by the association with other vascular lesions such as haemangioma [214]. The lesion is larger and more vascular than adenoma. This would explain regression when oral contraceptives are stopped. Histologically the lesion consists of normal hepatocytes and Kupffer cells. The central core is composed of fibrous tissue and proliferating bile ducts.

The patient may be asymptomatic or may present with pain or an abdominal mass. Serum biochemical tests are normal in the uncomplicated case.

The lesion is identified by ultrasound and CT. Arteriography shows a 'spokes-of-a-wheel' appearance.

Combined angiography and liver scan may be useful in distinguishing between focal nodular hyperplasia (which is hypervascular and exhibits normal uptake)

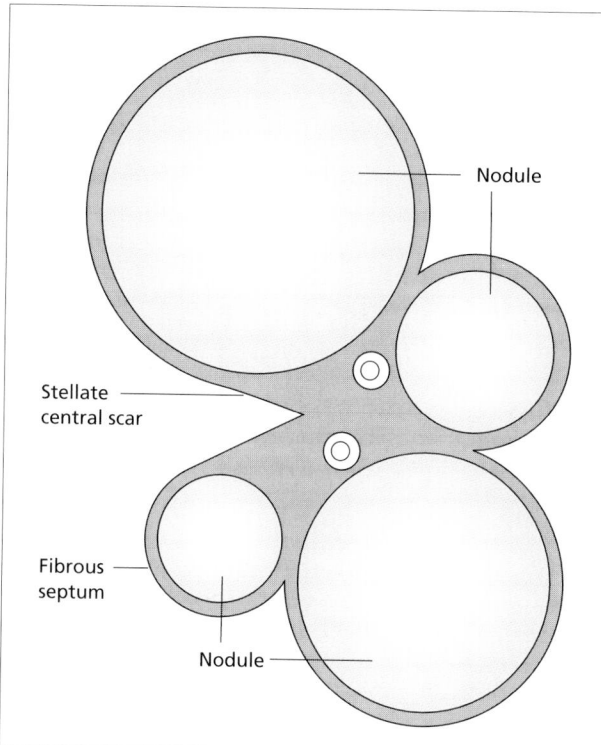

Fig. 18.31. The structure of focal nodular hyperplasia.

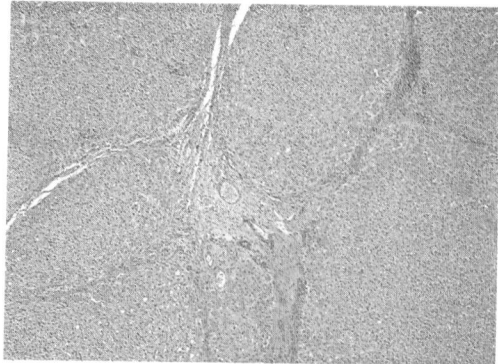

Fig. 18.32. Focal nodular hyperplasia. Note stellate central scar containing an artery.

and liver cell adenoma (which is hypovascular and cold). Enhanced MRI is diagnostic in 70% [28].

Treatment should be flexible [138]. The asymptomatic should be observed regularly with ultrasound examinations. In the symptomatic, stopping the oral contraceptive may lead to the lesion regressing. In others and, in particular, those with complications, surgical resection is indicated.

Androgenic hormones and anabolic steroids

Adenoma, peliosis, nodular regenerative hyperplasia

and particularly hepato-cellular carcinoma may complicate long-term use of C17 substituted testosterones and anabolic steroids. Angiosarcoma may be associated. The drugs may be given for aplastic anaemia, hypopituitarism, eunuchoidism, impotency, in female transsexuals [221] and in athletes to increase muscle mass [30].

Hepato-cellular cancer of a rather benign type is much more frequent with male than with female hormone therapy, perhaps due to the much larger doses given. The incidence of hepatic abnormality is particularly high; in one series, 19 of 60 patients given methyl testosterone showed abnormal liver function tests [221].

Other tumours

Angiosarcoma may follow androgenic–anabolic steroids, vinyl chloride [196], thorotrast and inorganic arsenic [160].

Epithelioid haemangioendothelioma. This rare malignant vascular tumour has been related to oral contraceptive use [33, 47] and to vinyl chloride [49] (see Chapter 35).

Conclusions

Before marketing a new drug, testing must be done on both an acute and chronic basis and on more than one species or strain. Both the drug and its known metabolites must be used. The albumin-binding properties of the drug must be noted. The role of the drug as a hepatic enzyme-inducer must be studied. Clinical trials must include regular pre- and post-treatment estimations of serum bilirubin and transaminase levels. A needle liver biopsy, after informed consent, is particularly helpful in establishing the relation between a drug and liver injury and in determining the type of injury.

The serum transaminases may rise during the first 4 weeks of therapy only to subside despite the drug being continued. When a hepatic reaction is possible, as with isoniazid, it is wise to check serum transaminases 3 and 4 weeks after commencing treatment. If more than three times increased, the drug should be stopped. If less, a further value is taken 1 week later when an increase is an indication for stopping the drug. Continuance of therapy once a hepatic reaction has commenced is the commonest cause of a fatal outcome.

The safety of a drug which causes transient rises in transaminases and apparently no other hepatic effects remains obscure. Many valuable drugs in widespread use fall into this category. In many instances, challenge is the only method of linking a drug with a hepatic reaction, but if its consequence is likely to be serious, this is ethically impossible. However, reporting agencies and drug manufacturers should pay particular attention to the results of inadvertent challenge and to the effects of withdrawing the drug (de-challenge).

Intake of a drug, such as paracetamol, within the therapeutic range, may cause liver injury if the patient is ingesting another drug such as alcohol which by enzyme induction increases the production of hepatotoxic metabolites.

An iatrogenic cause must be considered in any patient presenting with any clinical pattern of hepato-biliary disease. This is particularly so with a picture suggesting viral hepatitis in a middle-aged or elderly patient, especially a woman. In the absence of evidence supporting genuine viral hepatitis, the cause is very frequently drug-related.

Widespread recognition of the relation between a drug and a hepatic reaction would follow increased reporting to agencies such as the Committee for Safety of Medicines in the UK, or MEDWATCH in the USA.

Some catastrophies would be avoided if clinical trials included subjects of all ages from children to old people and those with liver disease.

References

1 Alderman S, Kailas S, Goldfarb S *et al.* Cholestatic hepatitis after ingestion of chaparral leaf: confirmation by endoscopic cholangiopancreatography and liver biopsy. *J. Clin. Gastroenterol.* 1994; **19**: 242.

2 Altraif I, Lilly L, Wanless IR *et al.* Cholestatic liver disease with ductopenia (vanishing bile duct syndrome) after administration of clindamycin and trimethoprim-sulfamethoxazole. *Am. J. Gastroenterol.* 1994; **89**: 1230.

3 Alison MR, Sarraf CE. Liver cell death: patterns and mechanisms. *Gut* 1994; **35**: 577.

4 Amitrano L, Gigliotti T, Guardascione MA *et al.* Enoxacin acute liver injury. *J. Hepatol.* 1992; **15**: 270.

5 Babany G, Uzzan F, Larrey D *et al.* Alcohol-like liver lesions induced by nifedipine. *J. Hepatol.* 1989; **9**: 252.

6 Banks AT, Zimmerman HJ, Ishak KG *et al.* Diclofenac-associated hepatotoxicity: analysis of 180 cases reported to the Food and Drug Administration as adverse reactions. *Hepatology* 1995; **22**: 820.

7 Baum JK, Bookstein JJ, Holtz F *et al.* Possible association between benign hepatomas and oral contraceptives. *Lancet* 1973; **ii**: 926.

8 Beaune P, Dansette PM, Mansuy D *et al.* Human anti-endoplasmic reticulum autoantibodies appearing in a drug-induced hepatitis are directed against a human liver cytochrome P-450 that hydroxylates the drug. *Proc. Natl. Acad. Sci. USA* 1987; **84**: 551.

9 Belghiti J, Benhamou J-P, Houry S *et al.* Caustic sclerosing cholangitis. A complication of the surgical treatment of hydatid disease of the liver. *Arch. Surg.* 1986; **121**: 1162.

10 Benjamin SB, Goodman ZD, Ishak KG *et al.* The morphologic spectrum of halothane-induced hepatic injury. Analysis of 77 cases. *Hepatology* 1985; **5**: 1163.

11 Bernuau J, Larrey D, Campillo B *et al.* Amodiaquine-induced fulminant hepatitis. *J. Hepatol.* 1988; **6**: 109.

12 Bissuel F, Bruneel F, Harbersetzer F *et al.* Fulminant hepatitis with severe lactate acidosis in HIV-infected patients on didanosine therapy. *J. Intern. Med.* 1994; **235**: 367.

13 Black M, Mitchell JR, Zimmerman HJ *et al.* Isoniazid-associated hepatitis in 114 patients. *Gastroenterology* 1975; **69**: 289.

14 Black M, Rabin L, Schatz N. Nitrofurantoin-induced chronic active hepatitis. *Ann. Intern. Med.* 1980; **92**: 62.

15 Blackburn AM, Amiel SA, Millis RR *et al.* Tamoxifen and liver damage. *Br. Med. J.* 1984; **289**: 288.

16 Blake JC, Sawyerr AM, Dooley JS *et al.* Severe hepatitis caused by cyproterone acetate. *Gut* 1990; **31**: 556.

17 Bonkovsky HL, Kane RE, Jones DP *et al.* Acute hepatitis and renal toxicity from low doses of acetaminophen in the absence of alcohol abuse or malnutrition: evidence for increased susceptibility to drug toxicity due to cardiopulmonary and renal insufficiency. *Hepatology* 1994; **19**: 1141.

18 Borhan-Manesh F, Farnum JB. Methyltestosterone-induced cholestasis. The importance of disproportionately low serum alkaline phosphatase level. *Arch. Intern. Med.* 1989; **149**: 2127.

19 Boyer DL, Li BU, Fyda JN *et al.* Sulfasalazine-induced hepatotoxicity in children with inflammatory bowel disease. *J. Pediatr. Gastroenterol. Nutr.* 1989; **8**: 528.

20 Brotodihardjo AE, Batey RG, Farrell GC *et al.* Hepatotoxicity from paracetamol self-poisoning in Western Sydney: a continuing challenge. *Med. J. Aust.* 1992; **157**: 328.

21 Brunt EM, White H, Marsh JW *et al.* Fulminant hepatic failure after repeated exposure to isoflurane anesthesia: a case report. *Hepatology* 1991; **13**: 1017.

22 Buhler H, Pirovino M, Akovbiantz A *et al.* Regression of liver cell adenoma: a follow-up study of three consecutive patients after discontinuation oral contraceptive use. *Gastroenterology* 1982; **82**: 775.

23 Callaghan R, Desmond PV, Paull P *et al.* Hepatic enzyme activity is the major factor determining elimination rate of high-clearance drugs in cirrhosis. *Hepatology* 1993; **18**: 54.

24 Carson JL, Strom BL, Duff A *et al.* Safety of non-steroidal anti-inflammatory drugs with respect to acute liver disease. *Arch. Intern. Med.* 1993; **153**: 1331.

25 Castiella A, Lopez Dominguez L, Txoperena G *et al.* Indication for liver transplantation in *Amanita phalloides* poisoning. *Presse Med.* 1993; **22**: 117 (letter).

26 Cereda J-M, Bernuau J, Degott C *et al.* Fatal liver failure due to disulfiram. *J. Clin. Gastroenterol.* 1989; **11**: 98.

27 Cherqui D, Palazzo L, Piedbois P *et al.* Common bile duct stricture as a late complication of upper abdominal radiotherapy. *J. Hepatol.* 1994; **20**: 693.

28 Cherqui D, Rahnoumi A, Charlotte F *et al.* Management of focal nodular hyperplasia and hepatocellular adenoma in young women: a series of 41 patients with clinical, radiological and pathological correlations. *Hepatology* 1995; **22**: 1674.

29 Clark JA, Zimmerman HJ, Tanner LA. Labetalol hepatotoxicity. *Ann. Intern. Med.* 1990; **113**: 210.

30 Creagh TM, Rubin A, Evans DJ. Hepatic tumours induced by anabolic steroids in an athlete. *J. Clin. Pathol.* 1988; **41**: 441.

31 Dalton TA, Perry RS. Hepatotoxicity associated with sustained-release niacin. *Am. J. Med.* 1992; **93**: 102.

32 Davies MH, Harrison RF, Elias E *et al.* Antibiotic-associated acute vanishing bile duct syndrome: a pattern associated with severe, prolonged, intrahepatic cholestasis. *J. Hepatol.* 1994; **20**: 112.

33 Dean PJ, Haggitt RC, O'Hara CJ. Malignant epithelioid hemangioendothelioma of the liver in young women: rela-

tionship to oral contraceptive use. *Am. J. Surg. Pathol.* 1985; **9**: 695.

34 Degott C, Feldmann G, Larrey D *et al.* Drug-induced prolonged cholestasis in adults: a histological semiquantitative study demonstrating progressive ductopenia. *Hepatology* 1992; **15**: 244.

35 Diaz D, Febre I, Daujat M *et al.* Omeprazole is an aryl hydrocarbon-like inducer of human hepatic cytochrome P-450. *Gastroenterology* 1990; **99**: 737.

36 Dincsoy HP, Saelinger DA. Haloperidol-induced chronic cholestatic liver disease. *Gastroenterology* 1982; **83**: 694.

37 Dourakis SP, Alexopoulou AA, Hadziyannis SJ. Fulminant hepatitis after flutamide treatment. *J. Hepatol.* 1994; **20**: 350.

38 Durand F, Bernuau J, Pessayre D *et al.* Deleterious influence of pyrazinamide on the outcome of patients with fulminant or subfulminant liver failure during antituberculous treatment including isoniazid. *Hepatology* 1995; **21**: 929.

39 Edmondson HA, Henderson B, Benton B. Liver-cell adenomas associated with the use of oral contraceptives. *N. Engl. J. Med.* 1976; **294**: 470.

40 Ellis AJ, Wendon JA, Portmann B *et al.* Acute liver damage and ecstasy ingestion. *Gut* 1996; **38**: 454.

41 Evely RS, Triger DR, Milnes JP *et al.* Severe cholestasis associated with stanozolol. *Br. Med. J.* 1987; **294**: 612.

42 Fairley CK, McNeil JJ, Desmond P *et al.* Risk factors for development of flucloxacillin associated jaundice. *Br. Med. J.* 1993; **306**: 233.

43 Farrell GC. *Drug-induced Liver Disease.* Churchill Livingstone, Edinburgh, 1994.

44 Fermand JP, Levy Y, Bouscary D *et al.* Danazol-induced hepatocellular adenoma. *Am. J. Med.* 1990; **88**: 529.

45 Foitl DR, Hyman G, Lefkowitch JH. Jaundice and intrahepatic cholestasis following high-dose megestrol acetate for breast cancer. *Cancer* 1989; **63**: 438.

46 Foster JH, Donohue TA, Berman MM. Familial liver-cell adenoma and diabetes mellitus. *N. Engl. J. Med.* 1978; **299**: 239.

47 Fries JF, Gurkirpal S, Lenert L *et al.* Aspirin, hydroxychloroquine, and hepatic enzyme abnormalities with methotrexate in rheumatoid arthritis. *Arthritis Rheum.* 1990; **33**: 1611.

48 Garibaldi RA, Drusin RE, Ferebee SH *et al.* Isoniazid-associated hepatitis: report of an outbreak. *Am. Rev. Respir. Dis.* 1972; **106**: 357.

49 Gelin M, Van de Stadt J, Rickaert F *et al.* Epithelioid hemangioendothelioma of the liver following contact with vinyl chloride. *J. Hepatol.* 1989; **8**: 99.

50 Geubel AP. Radiation-induced bile duct injury: a vanishing cause of obstructive jaundice? *J. Hepatol.* 1994; **20**: 687.

51 Geubel AP, De Galocsy C, Alves N *et al.* Liver damage caused by therapeutic vitamin A administration: estimate of dose-related toxicity in 41 cases. *Gastroenterology* 1991; **100**: 1701.

52 Gilbert SC, Klintmalm G, Menter A *et al.* Methotrexate-induced cirrhosis requiring liver transplantation in three patients with psoriasis. A word of caution in the light of the expanding use of this 'steroid-sparing' agent. *Arch. Intern. Med.* 1990; **150**: 889.

53 Goldman IS, Winkler ML, Raper SE *et al.* Increased hepatic density and phospholipidosis due to amiodarone. *Am. J. Roentgenol.* 1985; **144**: 541.

54 Gonzalez FJ, Skoda RC, Kimura S *et al.* Characterization of

the common genetic defect in humans deficient in debrisoquine metabolism. *Nature* 1988; **331**: 442.

55 Gough A, Chapman S, Wagstaff K *et al.* Minocycline induced autoimmune hepatitis and systemic lupus erythematosus-like syndrome. *Br. Med. J.* 1996; **312**: 169.

56 Graham-Brown R. Toxicity of Chinese herbal remedies. *Lancet* 1992; **340**: 673 (letter).

57 Grant DM, Morike K, Eichelbaum M *et al.* Acetylation pharmacogenetics. The slow acetylator phenotype is caused by decreased or absent arylamine N-acetyl transferase in human liver. *J. Clin. Invest.* 1990; **85**: 968.

58 Guarascio P, D'Amato C, Sette P *et al.* Liver damage from verapamil. *Br. Med. J.* 1984; **288**: 362.

59 Gugler R, Jensen JC. Omeprazole inhibits oxidative drug metabolism. Studies with diazepam and phenytoin *in vivo* and 7-ethoxycoumarin *in vitro. Gastroenterology* 1985; **89**: 1235.

60 Guigui B, Perrot S, Berry JP *et al.* Amiodarone-induced hepatic phospholipidosis: a morphological alteration independent of pseudo-alcoholic liver disease. *Hepatology* 1988; **8**: 1063.

61 Hammel P, Larrey D, Bernuau J *et al.* Acute hepatitis after tetrahydroaminoacridine administration for Alzheimer's disease. *J. Clin. Gastroenterol.* 1990; **12**: 329.

62 Harrison PM, Keays R, Bray GP *et al.* Improved outcome of paracetamol-induced fulminant hepatic failure by late administration of acetylcysteine. *Lancet* 1990; **335**: 1572.

63 Harrison PM, Wendon JA, Gimson AES *et al.* Improvement by acetylcysteine of hemodynamics and oxygen transport in fulminant hepatic failure. *N. Engl. J. Med.* 1991; **324**: 1852.

64 Harrison R, Letz G, Pasternak G *et al.* Fulminant hepatic failure after occupational exposure to 2-nitropropane. *Ann. Intern. Med.* 1987; **107**: 466.

65 Hassanein T, Razack A, Gavaler JS *et al.* Heatstroke: its clinical and pathological presentation, with particular attention to the liver. *Am. J. Gastroenterol.* 1992; **87**: 1382.

66 Heier PJ, Mueller HK, Dick B *et al.* Hepatic monooxygenase activities in subjects with a genetic defect in drug oxidation. *Gastroenterology* 1983; **85**: 682.

67 Heim M, Meyer UA. Genotyping of poor metabolisers of debrisoquine by allele-specific PCR amplification. *Lancet* 1990; **336**: 529.

68 Helfgott SM, Sandberg-Cook J, Zakim D *et al.* Diclofenac-associated hepatotoxicity. *JAMA* 1990; **264**: 2660.

69 Henderson BE, Preston-Martin S, Edmondson HA *et al.* Hepatocellular carcinoma and oral contraceptives. *Br. J. Cancer* 1983; **48**: 437.

70 Henry JA, Jeffreys KJ, Dawling S. Toxicity and deaths from 3,4-methylenedioxymethamphetamine ('ecstasy'). *Lancet* 1992; **340**: 384.

71 Hjelm M, de Silva LVK, Seakins JWT *et al.* Evidence of inherited urea cycle defect in a case of fatal valproate toxicity. *Br. Med. J.* 1986; **292**: 23.

72 Hodgson MJ, Heyl AE, Van Thiel DH. Liver disease associated with exposure to 1,1,1-trichloroethane. *Arch. Intern. Med.* 1989; **149**: 1793.

73 Hoyumpa AM, Schenker S. Is glucuronidation truly preserved in patients with liver disease? *Hepatology* 1991; **13**: 786.

74 International Group. Guidelines for diagnosis of therapeutic drug-induced liver injury in liver biopsies. *Lancet* 1974; **i**: 854.

75 Iveson TJ, Ryley NG, Kelly PMA *et al.* Diclofenac-associated hepatitis. *J. Hepatol.* 1990; **10**: 85.

76 Kadmon M, Klünemann C, Böhme M *et al.* Inhibition by cyclosporin A of adenosine triphosphate-dependent transport from the hepatocyte into bile. *Gastroenterology* 1993; **104**: 1507.

77 Kalra PA, Guthrie JA, Dibble JB *et al.* Hepatic adenomas induced by norethisterone in patients receiving renal dialysis. *Br. Med. J.* 1987; **294**: 808.

78 Kanel GC, Cassidy W, Shuster L *et al.* Cocaine-induced liver cell injury: comparison of morphological features in man and in experimental models. *Hepatology* 1990; **11**: 646.

79 Katzka DA, Saul SH, Jorkasky D *et al.* Azathioprine and hepatic venoocclusive disease in renal transplant patients. *Gastroenterology* 1986; **90**: 446.

80 Kawahara H, Marceau N, French SW. Effects of chlorpromazine and low calcium on the cytoskeleton and the secretory function of hepatocytes *in vitro*. *J. Hepatol.* 1990; **10**: 8.

81 Keeffe EB, Reis TC, Berland JE. Hepatotoxicity to both erythromycin estolate and erythromycin ethylsuccinate. *Dig. Dis. Sci.* 1982; **27**: 701.

82 Keeffe EB, Sunderland M, Gabourel JD. Serum gamma-glutamyl transpeptidase activity in patients receiving chronic phenytoin therapy. *Dig. Dis. Sci.* 1986; **31**: 1056.

83 Kenna JG, Neuberger J, Mieli-Vergani G *et al.* Halothane hepatitis in children. *Br. Med. J.* 1987; **294**: 1209.

84 Kerlin P, Davis GL, McGill DB *et al.* Hepatic adenoma and focal nodular hyperplasia: clinical, pathologic, and radiologic features. *Gastroenterology* 1983; **84**: 994.

85 Knobler H, Levij IS, Gavish D *et al.* Quinidine-induced hepatitis. A common and reversible hypersensitivity reaction. *Arch. Intern. Med.* 1986; **146**: 526.

86 Kowdley KV, Keeffe EB, Fawaz KA. Prolonged cholestasis due to trimethoprim sulfamethoxazole. *Gastroenterology* 1992; **102**: 2148.

87 Kremer JM. Liver biopsies in patients with rheumatoid arthritis receiving methotrexate: where are we going? *J. Rheumatol.* 1992; **19**: 189.

88 Kremer JM, Lee RG, Tolman KG. Liver histology in rheumatoid arthritis patients receiving long-term methotrexate therapy. A prospective study with baseline and sequential biopsy samples. *Arthritis Rheum.* 1989; **32**: 121.

89 Labadie H, Stoessel P, Callard P *et al.* Hepatic veno-occlusive disease and perisinusoidal fibrosis secondary to arsenic poisoning. *Gastroenterology* 1990; **99**: 1140.

90 Lafon PC, Reed K, Rosenthal D. Acute cholecystitis associated with hepatic arterial infusion of floxuridine. *Am. J. Surg.* 1985; **150**: 687.

91 Lake-Bakkaar G, Scheuer PJ, Sherlock S. Hepatic reactions associated with ketoconazole in the United Kingdom. *Br. Med. J.* 1987; **294**: 419.

92 Lanse SB, Arnold GL, Gowans JDC *et al.* Low incidence of hepatotoxicity associated with long-term, low-dose oral methotrexate in treatment of refractory psoriasis, psoriatic arthritis and rheumatoid arthritis. An acceptable risk/benefit ratio. *Dig. Dis. Sci.* 1985; **30**: 104.

93 Larrey D, Branch RA. Clearance by the liver: current concepts in understanding the hepatic disposition of drugs. *Semin. Liver Dis.* 1983; **3**: 285.

94 Larrey D, Geneve J, Pessayre D *et al.* Prolonged cholestasis after cyproheptadine-induced acute hepatitis. *J. Clin. Gastroenterol.* 1987; **9**: 102.

95 Larrey D, Hadengue A, Pessayre D *et al.* Carbamazepine-induced acute cholangitis. *Dig. Dis. Sci.* 1987; **32**: 554.

96 Larrey D, Henrion J, Heller F *et al.* Metoprolol-induced hepatitis: rechallenge and drug oxidation phenotyping. *Ann. Intern. Med.* 1988; **108**: 67.

97 Larrey D, Vial T, Micaleff A *et al.* Hepatitis associated with amoxycillin-clavulanic acid combination report of 15 cases. *Gut* 1992; **33**: 368.

98 Larrey D, Vial T, Pauwels A *et al.* Hepatitis after germander (*Teucrium chamaedrys*) administration: another instance of herbal medicine hepatotoxicity. *Ann. Intern. Med.* 1992; **117**: 129.

99 Lee WM. Drug-induced hepatotoxicity. *N. Engl. J. Med.* 1995; **333**: 1118.

100 Leese T, Farges O, Bismuth H. Liver cell adenomas. A 12-year surgical experience from a specialist hepato-biliary unit. *Ann. Surg.* 1988; **208**: 558.

101 Lemley DE, DeLacy LM, Seeff LB *et al.* Azathioprine induced hepatic veno-occlusive disease in rheumatoid arthritis. *Ann. Rheum. Dis.* 1989; **48**: 342.

102 Leonard TB, Morgan DG, Dent JG. Ranitidine: acetaminophen interaction effects on acetaminophen-induced hepatotoxicity in Fischer 344 rats. *Hepatology* 1985; **5**: 480.

103 Lewis JH, Ranard RC, Caruso A *et al.* Amiodarone hepatotoxicity: prevalence and clinicopathologic correlations among 104 patients. *Hepatology* 1989; **9**: 679.

104 Lewis JH, Schiff E. Methotrexate-induced chronic liver injury: guidelines for detection and prevention. *Am. J. Gastroenterol.* 1988; **83**: 1337.

105 Lewis JH, Zimmerman HJ, Ishak KG *et al.* Enflurane hepatotoxicity: a clinicopathologic study of 24 cases. *Ann. Intern. Med.* 1983; **98**: 984.

106 Liaw Y-F, Huang M-J, Fan K-D *et al.* Hepatic injury during propylthiouracil therapy in patients with hyperthyroidism. A cohort study. *Ann. Intern. Med.* 1993; **118**: 424.

107 Lieberman DA, Keeffe EB, Stenzel P. Severe and prolonged oral contraceptive jaundice. *J. Clin. Gastroenterol.* 1984; **6**: 145.

108 Lieh-Lai MW, Sarnaik AP, Newton JF *et al.* Metabolism and pharmacokinetics of acetaminophen in a severely poisoned young child. *J. Pediat.* 1984; **105**: 125.

109 Loeper J, Descatoire V, Letteron P *et al.* Hepatotoxicity of germander in mice. *Gastroenterology* 1994; **106**: 464.

110 Loeper J, Descatoire V, Maurice M *et al.* Presence of functional cytochrome P-450 on isolated rat hepatocyte plasma membrane. *Hepatology* 1990; **11**: 850.

111 Loomus GN, Aneja P, Bota RA. A case of peliosis hepatitis in association with tamoxifen therapy. *Am. J. Clin. Pathol.* 1983; **80**: 881.

112 Lowdell CP, Murray-Lyon IM. Reversal of liver damage due to long term methyltestosterone and safety of non 17α alkylated androgens. *Br. Med. J.* 1985; **291**: 637.

113 McElwee NE, Schumacher MC, Johnson SC *et al.* An observational study of isotretinoin recipients treated for acne in a health maintenance organisation. *Arch. Dermatol.* 1991; **127**: 341.

114 MacGregor FB, Abernethy VE, Dahabra S *et al.* Hepatotoxicity of herbal remedies. *Br. Med. J.* 1989; **299**: 1156.

115 Macilwain C. NIH, FDA seek lessons from hepatitis B drug trial deaths. *Nature* 1993; **364**: 275.

116 Maddrey WC, Boitnott JK. Drug-induced chronic liver disease. *Gastroenterology* 1977; **72**: 1348.

117 Maganto P, Traber PG, Rusnell C *et al.* Long-term maintenance of the adult pattern of liver-specific expression for P-450b, P450e, albumin and α-fetoprotein genes in intrasplenically transplanted hepatocytes. *Hepatology* 1990; **11**: 585.

118 Makin AJ, Wendon J, Williams R. A 7-year experience of severe acetaminophen-induced hepatotoxicity (1987–1993). *Gastroenterology* 1995; **109**: 1907.

119 Manivel JC, Bloomer JR, Snover DC. Progressive bile duct injury after thiabendazole administration. *Gastroenterology* 1987; **93**: 245.

120 Marks WH, Thompson N, Appleman H. Failure of hepatic adenomas (HCA) to regress after discontinuance of oral contraceptives. *Ann. Surg.* 1988; **208**: 190.

121 Martin JL, Kenna JG, Martin BM *et al.* Halothane hepatitis patients have serum antibodies that react with protein disulfide isomerase. *Hepatology* 1993; **18**: 858.

122 Meirowitz RF, Tobin KD, Elias EG *et al.* Resolution of inferior vena cava syndrome after embolization of a hepatic adenoma. *Gastroenterology* 1990; **99**: 1502.

123 Minuk GY, Kelly JK, Hwang W-S. Vitamin A hepatotoxicity in multiple family members. *Hepatology* 1988; **8**: 272.

124 Mitchell JR *et al.* Isoniazid liver injury: clinical spectrum, pathology and probable pathogenesis. *Ann. Intern. Med.* 1976; **84**: 181.

125 Mondardini A, Pasquino P, Bernardi P *et al.* Propafenone-induced liver injury: report of a case and review of the literature. *Gastroenterology* 1993; **104**: 1524.

126 Morse RM, Valenzuela GA, Greenwald TP *et al.* Amiodarone-induced liver toxicity. *Ann. Intern. Med.* 1988; **109**: 838.

127 Moulding TS, Redeker AG, Kanel GC. Twenty isoniazid-associated deaths in one State. *Am. Rev. Respir. Dis.* 1989; **140**: 700.

128 Muñoz SJ, Martinez-Hernandez A, Maddrey WC. Intrahepatic cholestasis and phospholipidosis associated with the use of trimethoprim-sulfamethoxazole. *Hepatology* 1990; **12**: 342.

129 Murphy R, Swartz R, Watkins PB. Severe acetaminophen toxicity in a patient receiving isoniazid. *Ann. Intern. Med.* 1990; **113**: 799.

130 Mutimer DJ, Ayres RCS, Neuberger JM *et al.* Serious paracetamol poisoning and the results of liver transplantation. *Gut* 1994; **35**: 809.

131 Myers JL, Augur NA Jr. Hydralazine-induced cholangitis. *Gastroenterology* 1984; **87**: 1185.

132 Nehra A, Mullick F, Ishak KG *et al.* Pemoline-associated hepatic injury. *Gastroenterology* 1990; **99**: 1517.

133 Nesher G, Dollberg L, Zimran A *et al.* Hepatosplenic peliosis after danazol and glucocorticoids for ITP. *N. Engl. J. Med.* 1985; **312**: 242.

134 Nevens F, Fevery J, Van Steenbergen W *et al.* Arsenic and non-cirrhotic portal hypertension. A report of eight cases. *J. Hepatol.* 1990; **11**: 80.

135 Noseda A, Borsch G, Muller K-M *et al.* Methimazole-associated cholestatic liver injury: case report and brief literative review. *Hepato-Gastroenterol.* 1986; **33**: 244.

136 O'Brien ET, Yeoman WB, Hobby JAE. Hepato-renal damage from toluene in a 'glue sniffer'. *Br. Med. J.* 1971; **ii**: 29.

137 Ozenne G, Manchon ND, Doucet J *et al.* Carbimazole-induced acute cholestatic hepatitis. *J. Clin. Gastroenterol.* 1989; **11**: 95.

138 Pande JN, Singh SPN, Khilnani GC *et al.* Risk factors for hepatotoxicity from antituberculosis drugs: a case-control study. *Thorax* 1996; **51**: 132.

139 Park HZ, Lee SP, Schy AL. Ceftriaxone-associated gallbladder sludge. Indentification of calcium-ceftriaxone salt as a major component of gallbladder precipitate. *Gastroenterology* 1991; **100**: 1665.

140 Parker WB, Cheng YC. Mitochondrial toxicity of antiviral nucleoside analogs. *J. NIH Res.* 1994; **6**: 57.

141 Paterson D, Kerlin P, Walker N *et al.* Piroxicam-induced submassive necrosis of the liver. *Gut* 1992; **33**: 1436.

142 Paulson EK, McClellan JS, Washington K *et al.* Hepatic adenoma: MR characteristics and correlation with pathologic findings. *Am. J. Roenterol.* 1994; **163**: 113.

143 Perry MC. Chemotherapeutic agents and hepatotoxicity. *Semin. Oncol.* 1992; **19**: 551.

144 Phillips CA, Cera PJ, Mangan TF *et al.* Clinical liver disease in patients with rheumatoid arthritis taking methotrexate. *J. Rheumatol.* 1992; **19**: 229.

145 Phillips MJ, Oda M, Mak E *et al.* Microfilament dysfunction as a possible cause of intrahepatic cholestasis. *Gastroenterology* 1975; **69**: 48.

146 Powell-Jackson PR, Tredger JM, Williams R. Progress report, hepatotoxicity to valproate: a review. *Gut* 1984; **25**: 673.

147 Prescott LF, Illingworth RN, Critchley JAJH *et al.* Intravenous *N*-acetylcysteine: the treatment of choice for paracetamol poisoning. *Br. Med. J.* 1979; **ii**: 1097.

148 Queneau PE, Bertault-Peres P, Guitaoui M *et al.* Improvement of cyclosporin A-induced cholestasis by tauroursodeoxycholate in a long-term study in the rat. *Dig. Dis. Sci.* 1994; **39**: 1581.

149 Rabinovitz M, Van Thiel DH. Hepatotoxicity of non-steroidal anti-inflammatory drugs. *Am. J. Gastroenterol.* 1992; **87**: 1696.

150 Rahmat J, Gelfand RL, Gelfand MC *et al.* Captopril-associated cholestatic jaundice. *Ann. Intern. Med.* 1985; **102**: 56.

151 Rank JM, Olson RC. Reversible cholestatic hepatitis caused by acetohexamide. *Gastroenterology* 1989; **96**: 1607.

152 Ratanasavanh D, Beaune P, Morel F *et al.* Intralobular distribution and quantitation of cytochrome P-450 enzymes in human liver as a function of age. *Hepatology* 1991; **13**: 1142.

153 Read AE, Harrison CV, Sherlock S. Chronic chlorpromazine jaundice: with particular reference to its relationship to primary biliary cirrhosis. *Am. J. Med.* 1961; **31**: 249.

154 Read AE, Wiesner RH, LaBreque DR. Hepatic veno-occlusive disease associated with renal transplantation and azathioprine therapy. *Ann. Intern. Med.* 1986; **104**: 651.

155 Redlich CA, West AB, Fleming L *et al.* Clinical and pathological characteristics of hepatotoxicity associated with occupational exposure to dimethylformamide. *Gastroenterology* 1990; **99**: 748.

156 Reynolds TB, Lapin AC, Peters RL *et al.* Puzzling jaundice. Probable relationship to laxative ingestion. *JAMA* 1970; **211**: 86.

157 Ribe J, Benkov KJ, Thung SN *et al.* Fatal massive hepatic necrosis: a probable hypersensitivity reaction to sulfasalazine. *Am. J. Gastroenterol.* 1986; **81**: 205.

158 Rigas B, Rosenfeld LE, Barwick KW. Amiodarone hepatotoxicity: a clinicopathologic study of five patients. *Ann. Intern. Med.* 1986; **104**: 348.

159 Rinder HM, Love JC, Wexler R. Amiodarone hepatotoxicity. *N. Engl. J. Med.* 1986; **314**: 318.

160 Roat JW, Wald A, Mendelow H *et al.* Hepatic angiosarcoma associated with short-term arsenic ingestion. *Am. J. Med.* 1982; **73**: 933.

161 Roenigk HH Jr, Auerbach R, Maibach HI *et al.* Methotrexate in psoriasis: revised guidelines. *J. Am. Acad. Dermatol.* 1988; **19**: 145.

162 Rollins BJ. Hepatic veno-occlusive disease. *Am. J. Med.* 1986; **81**: 297.

163 Rooks JB, Ory HW, Ishak KG *et al.* Epidemiology of hepatocellular adenoma. The role of oral contraceptive use. *JAMA* 1979; **242**: 644.

164 Rosellini SR, Costa PL, Gaudio M *et al.* Hepatic injury related to enalapril. *Gastroenterology* 1989; **97**: 810.

165 Rosenberg WMC, Ryley NG, Trowell JM *et al.* Dextropropoxyphene-induced hepatotoxicity: a report of nine cases. *J. Hepatol.* 1993; **19**: 470.

166 Rosman AS, Frissora-Rodeo C, Marshall AT *et al.* Cholestatic hepatitis following flutamide. *Dig. Dis. Sci.* 1993; **38**: 1756.

167 Ruprah M, Mant TGK, Flanagan RJ. Acute carbon tetrachloride poisoning in 19 patients: implications for diagnosis and treatment. *Lancet* 1985; **i**: 1027.

168 Ryley NG, Fleming KA, Chapman RWG. Focal destructive cholangiopathy associated with amoxycillin clavulanic acid (augmentin). *J. Hepatol.* 1995; **23**: 278.

169 Sarachek NS, London RL, Matulewicz TJ. Diltiazem and granulomatous hepatitis. *Gastroenterology* 1985; **88**: 1260.

170 Scheider DM, Klygis LM, Tsang T-K *et al.* Hepatic dysfunction after repeated isoflurane administration. *J. Clin. Gastroenterol.* 1993; **17**: 168.

171 Schenker S, Bay M. Drug disposition and hepatotoxicity in the elderly. *J. Clin. Gastroenterol.* 1994; **18**: 232.

172 Schneider HL, Horbach KD, Kniaz JL *et al.* Chlorpropamide hepatotoxicity: a report of a case and review of the literature. *Am. J. Gastroenterol.* 1984; **79**: 721.

173 Schultz JC, Adamson JS Jr, Workman WW *et al.* Fatal liver disease after intravenous administration of tetracycline in high dosage. *N. Engl. J. Med.* 1963; **269**: 999.

174 Schwarts JT, Gyorkey F, Graham DY. Cimetidine hepatitis. *J. Clin. Gastroenterol.* 1986; **8**: 681.

175 Schwartz MS, Frank MS, Yanoff A *et al.* Atenolol-associated cholestasis. *Am. J. Gastroenterol.* 1989; **84**: 1084.

176 Scully LJ, Clarke D, Barr RJ. Diclofenac-induced hepatitis: three cases with features of autoimmune chronic active hepatitis. *Dig. Dis. Sci.* 1993; **38**: 744.

177 Seeff LB, Cuccherini BA, Zimmerman HJ *et al.* Acetaminophen hepatotoxicity in alcoholics: a therapeutic misadventure. *Ann. Intern. Med.* 1986; **104**: 399.

178 Seki K, Minami Y, Nishikawa M *et al.* 'Non-alcoholic steatohepatitis' induced by massive doses of synthetic estrogen. *Gastroenterol. Jpn.* 1983; **18**: 197.

179 Shepherd P, Harrison DJ. Idiopathic portal hypertension associated with cytotoxic drugs. *J. Clin. Pathol.* 1990; **43**: 206.

180 Shiffman ML, Keith FB, Moore EW. Pathogenesis of ceftriaxone-associated biliary sludge. *In vitro* studies of calcium-ceftriaxone binding and solubility. *Gastroenterology* 1990; **99**: 1772.

181 Shulman HM, Fisher LB, Schoch G *et al.* Venoocclusive disease of the liver after marrow transplantation: histological correlates of clinical signs and symptoms. *Hepatology* 1994; **19**: 1171.

182 Silva MO, Reddy KR, McDonald T *et al.* Danazol-induced cholestasis. *Am. J. Gastroenterol.* 1989; **84**: 426.

183 Silva MO, Roth D, Reddy KR *et al.* Hepatic dysfunction accompanying acute cocaine intoxication. *J. Hepatol.* 1991; **12**: 312.

184 Spielberg SP, Gordon GB, Blake DA *et al.* Predisposition to phenytoin hepatotoxicity assessed *in vitro*. *N. Engl. J. Med.* 1981; **305**: 722.

185 Simon JB, Manley PN, Brien JF *et al.* Amiodarone hepatotoxicity simulating alcoholic liver disease. *N. Engl. J. Med.* 1984; **311**: 167.

186 Solis-Herruzo JA, Castellano G, Colina F *et al.* Hepatic injury in the toxic epidemic syndrome caused by ingestion of adulterated cooking oil (Spain 1981). *Hepatology* 1984; **4**: 131.

187 Somani P, Bandyopadhyay S, Klaunig JE *et al.* Amiodarone- and desethylamiodarone-induced myelinoid inclusion bodies and toxicity in cultured rat hepatocytes. *Hepatology* 1990; **11**: 81.

188 Steele MA, Burk RF, DesPrez RM. Toxic hepatitis with isoniazid and rifampicin. A meta-analysis. *Chest* 1991; **99**: 465.

189 Sterneck M, Wiesner R, Ascher N *et al.* Azathioprine hepatotoxicity after liver transplantation. *Hepatology* 1991; **14**: 806.

190 Stricker BHCh, Blok APR, Babany G *et al.* Fibrin ring granulomas and allopurinol. *Gastroenterology* 1989; **96**: 1199.

191 Stricker BHC, Blok APR, Bronkhorst FB. Glafenine-associated hepatic injury. Analysis of 38 cases and review of the literature. *Liver* 1986; **6**: 63.

192 Stricker BHC, Blok APR, Bronkhorst FB *et al.* Ketoconazole-associated hepatic injury: a clinicopathological study of 55 cases. *J. Hepatol.* 1986; **3**: 399.

193 Stricker BHCh, Blok APR, Claas FHJ *et al.* Hepatic injury associated with the use of nitrofurans: a clinicopathological study of 52 reported cases. *Hepatology* 1988; **8**: 599.

194 Stricker BHC, Spoelstra P. *Drug-induced Hepatic Injury.* Amsterdam, Elsevier, 1985.

195 Taggart HMcA, Alderdice JM. Fatal cholestatic jaundice in elderly persons taking benoxaprofen. *Br. Med. J.* 1982; **284**: 1372.

196 Tamburro CH, Makk L, Popper H. Early hepatic histologic alterations among chemical (vinyl monomer) workers. *Hepatology* 1984; **4**: 413.

197 Tameda Y, Hamada M, Takase K *et al.* Fulminant hepatic failure caused by ecarazine hydrochloride (a hydralazine) derivative. *Hepatology* 1996; **23**: 465.

198 Tanner LA, Bosco LA, Zimmerman HJ. Hepatic toxicity after acebutolol therapy. *Ann. Intern. Med.* 1989; **111**: 533.

199 Tarazi EM, Harter JG, Zimmerman HJ *et al.* Sulindac-associated hepatic injury: analysis of 91 cases reported to the Food and Drug Administration. *Gastroenterology* 1993; **104**: 569.

200 Tavani A, Negri E, Parazzini F *et al.* Female hormone utilisation and risk of hepatocellular carcinoma. *Br. J. Cancer* 1993; **67**: 635.

201 Terpstra OT, Ten Kate FJW, Van Urk H. Long-term survival after resection of a hepatocellular carcinoma with lymph node metastasis and discontinuation of oral contraceptives. *Am. J. Gastroenterol.* 1984; **79**: 474.

202 Thies PW, Duil WL. Trimethoprin-sulfamethoxazole-induced cholestatic hepatitis — inadvertent rechallenge. *Arch. Intern. Med.* 1984; **144**: 1691.

203 Tyrrell DLJ, Mitchell MC, De Man RA *et al.* Phase II trial of lamivudine for chronic hepatitis B. *Hepatology* 1993; **18**: 112A.

204 Ussery XT, Henar EL, Black DD *et al.* Acute liver injury after protracted seizures in children. *J. Pediatr. Gastroenterol. Nutr.* 1989; **9**: 421.

205 Utili R, Boitnott JK, Zimmerman HJ. Dantrolene-associated hepatic injury. *Gastroenterology* 1977; **72**: 610.

206 Valla D, Le MG, Poynard T *et al.* Risk of hepatic vein thrombosis in relation to recent use of oral contraceptives: a case-control study. *Gastroenterology* 1986; **90**: 807

207 Van der Klauw MM, Houtman PM, Stricker BHC *et al.* Hepatic injury caused by benzbromarone. *J. Hepatol.* 1994; **20**: 376.

208 Van Ditzhuijsen TJM, van Haelst UJGM, van Dooren-Greebe RJ. Severe hepatotoxic reaction with progression to cirrhosis after use of a novel retinoid (acitretin). *J. Hepatol.* 1990; **11**: 185.

209 Van Steenbergen W, Vanstapel MJ, Desmet V *et al.* Cimetidine-induced liver injury. Report of three cases. *J. Hepatol.* 1985; **1**: 359.

210 Vanderstigel M, Zafrani ES, Lajonc JL *et al.* Allopurinol hypersensitivity syndrome as a cause of hepatic fibrin-ring granulomas. *Gastroenterology* 1986; **90**: 188.

211 Vore M. Estrogen cholestasis. Membranes, metabolites, or receptors? *Gastroenterology* 1987; **93**: 643.

212 Wanless IR and the International Working Party. Terminology of nodular hepato-cellular lesions. *Hepatology* 1995; **22**: 983.

213 Wanless IR, Dore S, Gopinath N *et al.* Histopathology of cocaine hepatotoxicity. Report of four patients. *Gastroenterology* 1990; **98**: 497.

214 Wanless IR, Mawdsley C, Adams R. On the pathogenesis of focal nodular hyperplasia of the liver. *Hepatology* 1985; **5**: 1194.

215 Wanless IR, Medline A. Role of estrogens as promoters of hepatic neoplasia. *Lab. Invest.* 1982; **46**: 313.

216 Watkins PB. The role of cytochromes P-450 in cyclosporine metabolism. *J. Am. Acad. Dermatol.* 1990; **23**: 1301.

217 Watkins PB. Role of cytochromes P-450 in drug metabolism and hepatotoxicity. *Semin. Liver Dis.* 1990; **10**: 235.

218 Watkins PB, Zimmerman HJ, Knapp MJ *et al.* Hepatotoxic effects of tacrine administration in patients with Alzheimer's disease. *JAMA* 1994; **271**: 992.

219 Watson RGP, Olomu A, Clements D *et al.* A proposed mechanism for chlorpromazine jaundice-defective hepatic sulphoxidation combined with rapid hydroxylation. *J. Hepatol.* 1988; **7**: 72.

220 Wepler W, Optiz K. Histologic changes in the liver biopsy in *Amanita phalloides* intoxication. *Hum. Pathol.* 1972; **3**: 249.

221 Westaby D. Ogle SJ, Paradinas FJ *et al.* Liver damage from long term methyltestosterone. *Lancet* 1977; **ii**: 261.

222 Whiting-O'Keefe QE, Fye KH, Sack KD. Methotrexate and histologic hepatic abnormalities: a meta-analysis. *Am. J. Med.* 1991; **90**: 711.

223 Woolf GM, Petrovic LM, Rojter SE *et al.* Acute hepatitis associated with the Chinese herbal product Jin Bu Huan. *Ann. Intern. Med.* 1994; **121**: 729.

224 Wynne HA, Lope LH, Mutch E *et al.* The effect of age upon liver volume and apparent liver blood flow in healthy men. *Hepatology* 1989; **9**: 297.

225 Yagupsky P, Gazala E, Sofer S *et al.* Fatal hepatic failure and encephalopathy associated with amiodarone therapy. *J. Pediat.* 1985; **107**: 967.

226 Yamamoto T, Suou T, Hirayama C. Elevated serum aminotransferase induced by isoniazid in relation to isoniazid acetylator phenotype. *Hepatology* 1986; **6**: 295.

227 Zafrani ES, Cazier A, Baudelot A-M *et al.* Ultra-structural lesions of the liver in human peliosis: a report of 12 cases. *Am. J. Pathol.* 1984; **114**: 349.

228 Zafrani ES, Pinaudeau Y, Dhumeaux D. Drug-induced vascular lesions of the liver. *Arch. Intern. Med.* 1983; **143**: 495.

229 Zimmerman HJ. *The Adverse Effects of Drugs and Other Chemicals on the Liver*, 2nd edn. Raven Press, New York, in press.

230 Zimmerman HJ, Maddrey WC. Acetaminophen (paracetamol) hepatotoxicity with regular intake of alcohol: analysis of instances of therapeutic misadventure. *Hepatology* 1995; **22**: 767.

231 Zitelli BJ, Alexander J, Taylor S *et al.* Fatal hepatic necrosis due to pyrimethamine-sulfadoxine (fansidar). *Ann. Intern. Med.* 1987; **106**: 393.

Chapter 19
Hepatic Cirrhosis

Definition

Cirrhosis is defined anatomically as a diffuse process with fibrosis and nodule formation. It has followed hepato-cellular necrosis. Although the causes are many, the end result is the same.

Fibrosis is not synonymous with cirrhosis. Fibrosis may be in acinar zone 3 in heart failure, or in zone 1 in bile duct obstruction and congenital hepatic fibrosis (fig. 19.1) or interlobular in granulomatous liver disease, but without a true cirrhosis.

Nodule formation without fibrosis, as in partial nodular transformation (fig. 19.1), is not cirrhosis.

The relation of chronic hepatitis to cirrhosis is discussed in Chapter 17.

Production of cirrhosis

The responses of the liver to necrosis are limited; the most important are collapse of hepatic lobules, formation of diffuse fibrous septa and nodular regrowth of liver cells. Thus, irrespective of the aetiology, the ultimate histological pattern of the liver is the same, or nearly the same. Necrosis may no longer be apparent at autopsy.

Fibrosis follows hepato-cellular necrosis (fig. 19.2). This may follow interface hepatitis in zone 1 leading to portal–portal fibrous bridges. Confluent necrosis in zone 3 leads to central–portal bridging and fibrosis. Focal necrosis is followed by focal fibrosis. The cell death is fol-

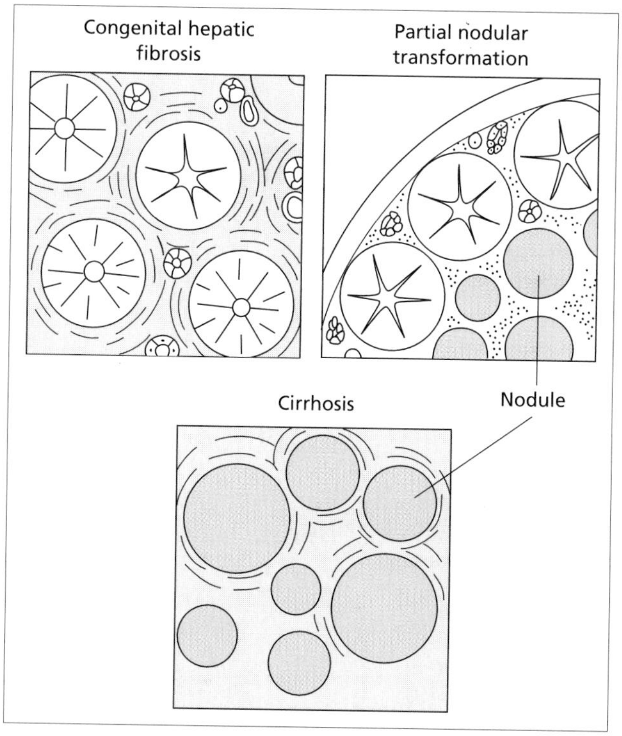

Fig. 19.1. Cirrhosis is defined as widespread fibrosis and nodule formation. Congenital hepatic fibrosis consists of fibrosis without nodules. Partial nodular transformation consists of nodules without fibrosis.

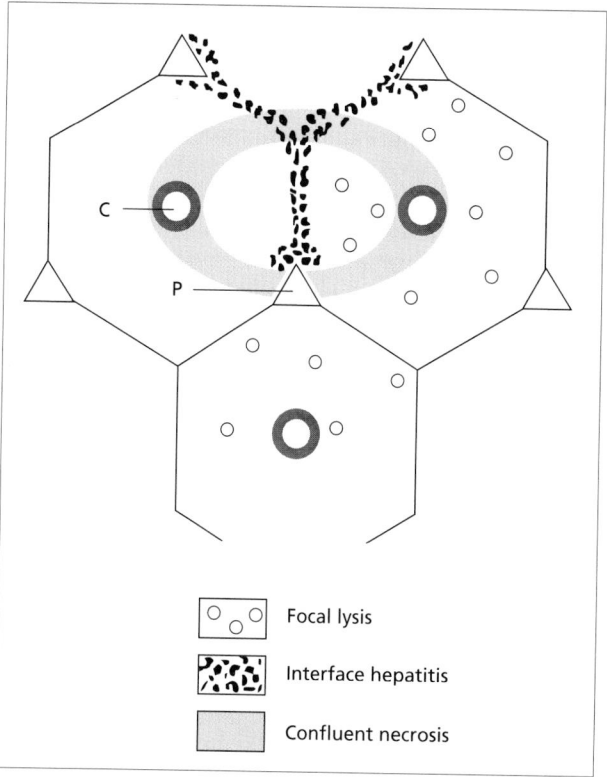

Fig. 19.2. Focal necrosis, interface hepatitis and confluent necrosis and their relationship to portal–portal and portal–central fibrosis (C = central vein; P = portal tract). (Courtesy L. Bianchi.)

lowed by nodules which disturb the hepatic architecture and a full cirrhosis develops.

Sinusoids persist at the periphery of the regenerating nodules at the site of the portal–central bridges. Portal blood is diverted past functioning liver tissue leading to vascular insufficiency at the centre of the nodules (zone 3) and even to persistence of the cirrhosis after the cause has been controlled. Abnormal connective tissue matrix is laid down in the space of Disse, so impeding metabolic exchange with the liver cells.

New fibroblasts form around necrotic liver cells and proliferated ductules. The fibrosis (collagen) progresses from a reversible to an irreversible state where acellular permanent septa have developed in zone 1 and in the lobule. The distribution of the fibrous septa varies with the causative agent. In haemochromatosis, the iron excites portal zone fibrosis. In alcoholism, the fibrosis is predominantly in zone 3.

Fibrogenesis [5, 20, 25]

Normal liver has a connective tissue matrix including type IV collagen, laminin, heparan sulphate, protoglycan and fibronectin. These are in basement membrane. Following hepatic injury there is an increase in extracellular matrix which contains fibril-formin collagens (types I and III) as well as proteoglycans, fibronectin, hyaluronic acid and other matrix glycoconjugates.

The formation of fibrous scar is the net result of increased formation and reduced degradation of extracellular matrix (fig. 19.3). Both processes are complex with many components. Greater understanding will allow trials of new therapies. Early fibrosis is reversible; cirrhosis with cross-linked collagen and regenerative nodules is not.

The *hepatic stellate cell* (also called lipocyte, fat-storing cell, Ito cell, pericyte) is the principle cell involved in fibrogenesis. It lies in the space of Disse, between endothelial cell and sinusoidal surface of the hepatocyte

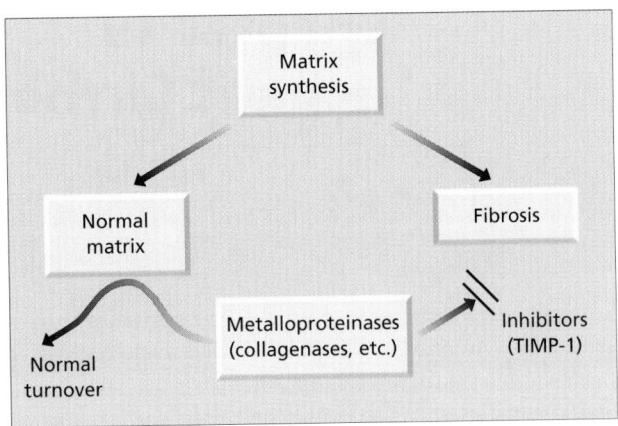

Fig. 19.3. Mechanism of normal and abnormal connective tissue production.

(figs 1.14, 1.17). There are equivalent peri-vascular cells in the kidney and other tissues. In the resting state the hepatic stellate cells have intra-cellular droplets containing vitamin A, and are the primary storage site for retinoids. They express desmin, a filament protein seen in muscle.

Following hepatic injury, these cells are activated (fig. 19.4). There is loss of retinoid droplets, proliferation and enlargement of cells, increased rough endoplasmic reticulum, and expression of smooth muscle specific α-actin [20]. Receptors for proliferative and fibrogenic cytokines appear or are upregulated. The triggers for stellate cell activation are not well understood. Transforming growth factor-β (TGF-β) derived from Kupffer cells may play a role. Initiating factors may also come from hepatocytes, platelets and lymphocytes.

Activated cells are influenced by cytokines some of which have proliferative effects, such as platelet-derived growth factor (PDGF), while others stimulate fibrogenesis, for example TGF-β. Numerous other growth factors and cytokines effect stellate cells including fibroblast

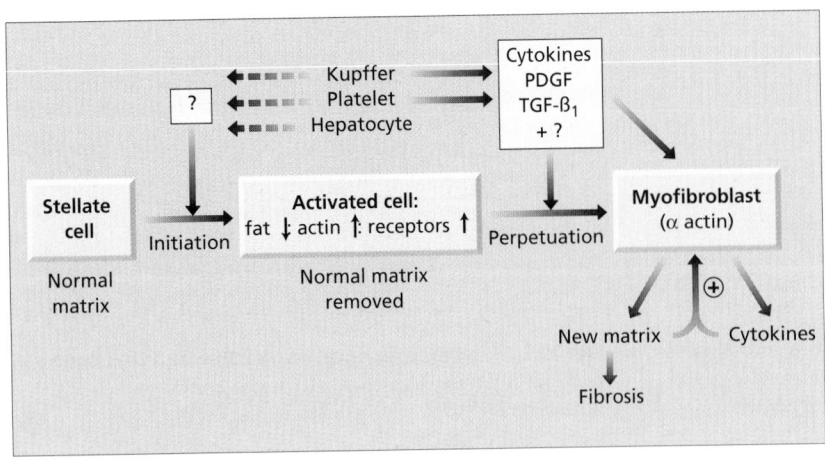

Fig. 19.4. Activation of hepatic stellate cells in fibrogenesis. Myofibroblasts probably also produce inhibitors of collagenases, enhancing fibrogenesis.

growth factor, interleukin-1, epidermal growth factor and tumour necrosis factor-α [53]. Some of these are derived from Kupffer cells and also the stellate cell itself, thereby having an autocrine effect. Acetaldehyde from alcohol metabolism, and products of lipid peroxidation due to damage from alcohol or excess iron, may also be involved. Thrombin stimulates stellate cell proliferation [42]. Alterations in the extra-cellular matrix produced by stellate cells sustain activation.

Activated stellate cells (myofibroblasts) show features of smooth muscle and are contractile. Endothelin-1 is synthesized by these cells and can stimulate reversible cell contraction [54]. Thus these cells may also have a role in blood flow regulation.

The other major factor in the formation of fibrous tissue is the degradation of matrix proteins (fig. 19.3). This is regulated by a family of enzymes called metalloproteinases [5]. There are three main groups: collagenases, gelatinases (type IV collagenases) and stromelysins. Collagenases degrade interstitial collagens (types I, II and III). Gelatinases act on basement membrane (type IV) collagen and gelatins. Stromelysins degrade many substrates including proteoglycans, laminin, gelatins and fibronectin. These enzymes are synthesized primarily by Kupffer cells and activated stellate cells. The metalloproteinases are inhibited by tissue inhibitors of metalloproteinases (TIMPs). The activated stellate cell secretes TIMP-1 [31], and therefore occupies a prime position in both the regulation of degradation of matrix, as well as the production of fibrous tissue. TIMP is increased in the serum of pre-cirrhotic and cirrhotic alcoholic patients [39].

Following hepatic injury, the early changes in matrix in the space of Disse are important with laying down of fibril-forming collagens (types I, III and V) and fibronectin. Sinusoids are converted to capillaries ('capillarization') and there is loss of endothelial fenestrae (fig. 1.16) so impeding metabolic exchange between blood and liver cells. Experimentally, sinusoidal stenoses lead to an increase in hepatic vascular resistance and to portal hypertension [60]. Progression of fibrosis disrupts hepatic architecture and leads to cirrhosis and portal hypertension.

Cytokines and hepatic growth factors

Apart from their role in fibrogenesis, cytokines have a wide range of other effects. They are hormone-like proteins which co-ordinate differentiating cells, and maintain or restore physiological homeostasis [3]. They are essential for communication not only within the liver itself but also between the liver and extra-hepatic sites. Cytokines regulate the intermediate metabolism of amino acids, proteins, carbohydrates, lipids and minerals. They interact with classical hormones such as gluco-corticoids. Since many cytokines exert growth factor like activity, in addition to their specific pro-inflammatory effects, the distinction between cytokines and growth factors is somewhat artificial.

The liver, predominantly the Kupffer cells, produces pro-inflammatory cytokines such as tumour necrosis factor-α (TNF-α), interleukin-1 (IL1) and interleukin-6 (IL6) (fig. 6.9). The liver also clears circulating cytokines, so limiting their systemic action. Failure of clearance may account for some of the immunological changes in cirrhosis.

Cytokine production is mediated through activation of monocytes and macrophages by endotoxin of gut origin. In cirrhosis, endotoxaemia is enhanced by increased gut permeability and depressed Kupffer cells which prevent uptake by the hepatocyte for detoxification and elimination. There is monokine overproduction [15]. Some of the systemic changes of cirrhosis, such as fever and anorexia, are mediated by cytokines [15]. Fatty acid synthesis is increased by TNF-α, IL1, and interferon alpha (IFN-α) with resultant fatty liver.

Cytokines inhibit hepatic regeneration. IL6, IL1 and TNF-α induce hepatic acute-phase protein synthesis with production, amongst others, of C-reactive protein, amyloid-A, haptoglobin, complement B and α_1-antitrypsin.

The remarkable hepatocyte regenerative capacity after such insults as viral hepatitis or hepatic resection might be initiated by growth factors interacting with specific receptors on cell surfaces [37].

Hepatocyte growth factor (HGF) is the most potent stimulator of DNA synthesis in mature hepatocytes, and triggers liver regeneration after injury. However, it is produced not only by liver cells (including stellate cells) but also in other tissues and by tumours [8]. Production is regulated by several factors including IL1α and IL1β, as well as TGF-β_1 and glucocorticoids. It stimulates growth of other cell types including melanocytes and haemopoietic cells.

Epidermal growth factor (EGF) is formed in regenerating hepatocytes. EGF receptors have a high density on hepatocyte membranes and are also found in the nucleus. Uptake is greatest in zone 1 (periportal) where regeneration is most active.

Transforming growth factor-α (TGF-α) has a 30–40% sequence homology with EGF and can bind to EGF receptors so initiating hepatocyte replication.

Transforming growth factor-β_1 (TGF-β_1) is probably the major inhibitor of hepatocyte proliferation and is strongly expressed in non-parenchymal cells during liver regeneration. Experimentally TGF-β_1 exerts both positive and negative effects, depending on the cell type and culture conditions.

TGF-β inhibits and EGF stimulates amino-acid uptake by cultured hepatocytes.

No growth factor or cytokine acts independently and the whole field is complex and growing rapidly.

Monitoring fibrogenesis

The proteins and metabolites of connective tissue metabolism spill-over into the plasma where they can be measured. Unfortunately, results reflect fibrosis generally and do not give information specifically about hepatic fibrosis.

Aminoterminal *procollagen type III peptide* (P-III-P) is cleaved off the procollagen molecule in the synthesis of a collagen type III fibril. Values in serum are not of practical *diagnostic* value. They are useful in *monitoring* liver fibrosis, particularly in the alcoholic [50]. However, increased levels may reflect inflammation and necrosis rather than fibrosis in chronic liver disease [40], primary biliary cirrhosis [6] and haemochromatosis [56]. Increased values are found in children, pregnant women and patients with renal failure.

Other assays that have been studied include procollagen IV propeptide, laminin, undulin, hyaluronan [27], TIMP-1 and integrin-β_1 [58]. In general, however, these estimations are largely of experimental interest and have not gained widespread clinical acceptance. Liver biopsy cannot be replaced by serum markers for individual diagnosis of liver injury.

Classification of cirrhosis

Morphological classification

Three anatomical types of cirrhosis are recognized: micronodular, macronodular and mixed.

Micronodular cirrhosis is characterized by thick, regular septa, by regenerating small nodules varying little in size, and by involvement of every lobule (figs 19.5, 19.6). The micronodular liver may represent impaired capacity for regrowth as in alcoholism, malnutrition, old age or anaemia.

Macronodular cirrhosis is characterized by septa and nodules of variable sizes and by normal lobules in larger nodules (figs 19.7, 19.8). Previous collapse is shown by juxtaposition in the fibrous scars of three or more portal tracts. Regeneration is reflected by large cells with large nuclei and by cell plates of varying thickness.

Regeneration in a micronodular cirrhosis results in a macronodular or *mixed* appearance. With time, micronodular cirrhosis often converts to macronodular [18].

Aetiology (table 19.1)

1 Viral hepatitis types B; ±delta; C.
2 Alcohol.

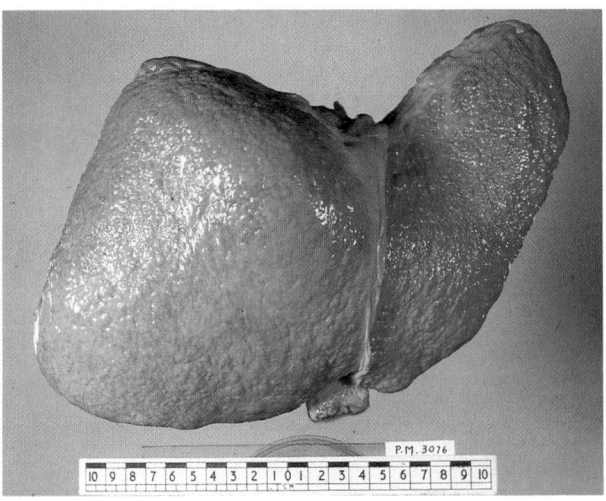

Fig. 19.5. The small finely nodular liver of micronodular cirrhosis.

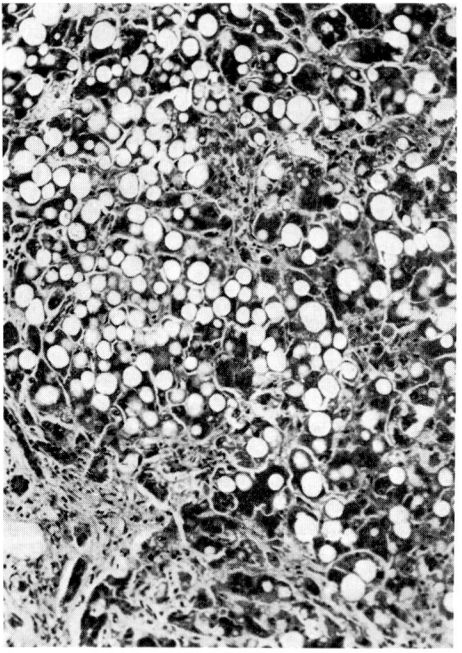

Fig. 19.6. Micronodular cirrhosis. Gross fatty change. The liver cells are often necrotic. Fibrous septa dissect the liver. (H & E, × 135.)

3 Metabolic, e.g. haemochromatosis, Wilson's disease, α_1-antitrypsin deficiency, type IV glycogenosis, galactosaemia, congenital tyrosinosis.
4 Prolonged cholestasis, intra- and extra-hepatic.
5 Hepatic-venous outflow obstruction, e.g. venoocclusive disease, Budd–Chiari syndrome, constrictive pericarditis.
6 Disturbed immunity ('lupoid' hepatitis).
7 Toxins and therapeutic agents, e.g. methotrexate, amiodarone.

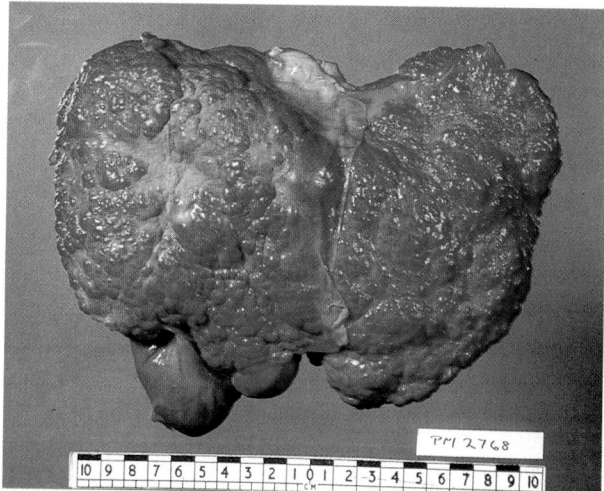

Fig. 19.7. The grossly distorted coarsely nodular liver of macronodular cirrhosis.

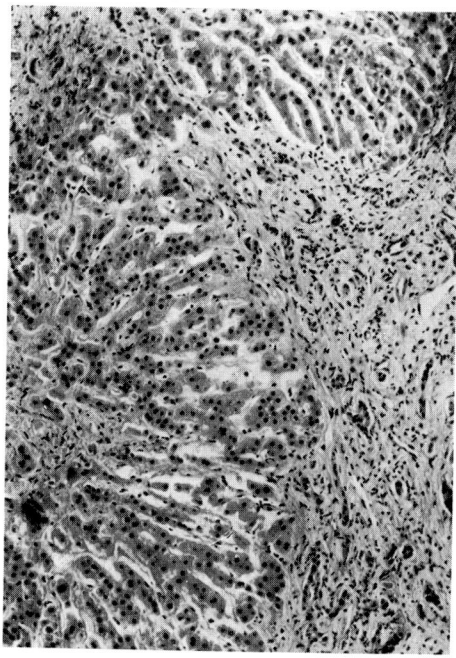

Fig. 19.8. Macronodular cirrhosis. Nodules of regenerating liver cells of different sizes are intersected by fibrous bands of various widths containing proliferating bile ducts. Fatty change is not seen. (H & E, ×135.)

8 Intestinal bypass.

9 Indian childhood cirrhosis.

Other possible factors to be considered include:

Malnutrition (Chapter 23).

Infections. Malarial parasites do not cause cirrhosis. The coexistence of malaria and cirrhosis probably reflects malnutrition and viral hepatitis in the community.

Syphilis causes cirrhosis in neonates but not in adults.

In schistosomiasis, the ova excite a fibrous tissue reaction in the portal zones. The association with cirrhosis in certain countries is probably related to other aetiological factors for example hepatitis C.

Granulomatous lesions. Focal granuloma in such conditions as brucellosis, tuberculosis and sarcoidosis heal with fibrosis, but the liver does not show nodular regrowth.

Cryptogenic cirrhosis. The aetiology is unknown and this is clearly a heterogeneous group. Frequency varies in different parts of the world; in the UK it is about 5–10%, whereas in other areas such as France or in urban parts of the USA where alcoholism is prevalent the pro-

Table 19.1. Aetiology and definitive treatment of cirrhosis

Aetiology	Treatment
Viral hepatitis (B, C and D)	?Antivirals
Alcohol	Abstention
Metabolic	
Iron overload	Venesection. Desferrioxamine
Copper overload (Wilson's disease)	Penicillamine
α_1-antitrypsin deficiency	?Transplant
Type IV glycogenesis	?Transplant
Galactosaemia	Withdraw milk and milk products
Tyrosinaemia	Withdraw dietary tyrosine. ?Transplant
Cholestasis (biliary)	Relieve biliary obstruction
Hepatic venous outflow block	
Budd–Chiari syndrome	Relieve main vein block. ?Transplant
Heart failure	Treat cardiac cause
Immunological ('lupoid' hepatitis)	Prednisolone
Toxins and drugs, e.g. methotrexate, amiodarone	Identify and stop
Indian childhood	?Penicillamine
Cryptogenic	—

portion is lower. As specific diagnostic criteria appear, so the percentage falls. The advent of HBsAg and anti-HCV transferred many previously designated cryptogenic cirrhotics to the post-hepatitic group. Estimations of serum smooth muscle and mitochondrial antibodies and better interpretation of liver histology separate others into the autoimmune chronic hepatitis — primary biliary cirrhosis category. Some of the remainder may be alcoholics who deny alcoholism or have forgotten that they ever consumed alcohol. There remains a hard core of patients in whom the cirrhosis remains cryptogenic. Aetiological diagnosis in these awaits further specific criteria.

Mechanisms are discussed in individual chapters. The clinical and pathological picture may be that of 'chronic hepatitis' which has proceeded to cirrhosis (Chapter 17).

Anatomical diagnosis

The diagnosis of cirrhosis depends on demonstrating widespread nodules in the liver combined with fibrosis. This may be done by *direct visualization*, for instance at laparotomy or laparoscopy. However, laparotomy should never be used to diagnose cirrhosis because it may precipitate liver failure even in those with very well-compensated disease.

Laparoscopy visualizes the nodular liver and allows directed liver biopsy (fig. 19.9).

Radioisotope scanning may show decreased uptake, an irregular pattern and uptake by spleen and bone marrow. Nodules are not identified.

Using *ultrasound*, cirrhosis is suggested by dense reflective areas of irregular distribution and increased echogenicity (fig. 5.5). The caudate lobe is enlarged relative to the right lobe [21]. However, ultrasound is not reliable for the diagnosis of cirrhosis unless ascites is present. Regenerating nodules may be shown as focal lesions [36]. These should be considered malignant unless proved otherwise by serial imaging and α-fetoprotein levels.

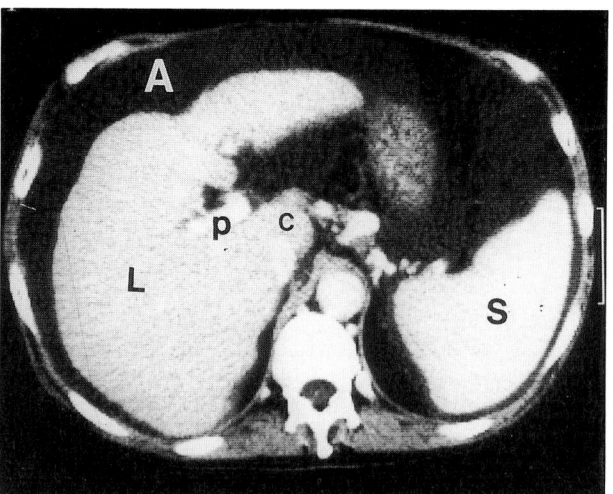

Fig. 19.10. CT scan, after intravenous contrast, in cirrhosis shows ascites (A), small liver with irregular surface (L), enlarged caudate lobe (c), splenomegaly (S) and patent portal vein (p).

CT scan is cost-effective for the diagnosis of cirrhosis and its complications (fig. 19.10). Liver size can be assessed and the irregular nodular surface seen. Benign regenerative nodules are not visualized by CT. Fatty change, increased density due to iron and a space-occupying lesion can be recognized. After intravenous contrast, the portal vein and hepatic veins can be identified in the liver, and a collateral circulation with splenomegaly may give confirmation to the diagnosis of portal hypertension. Large collateral vessels, usually perisplenic or paraoesophageal, may add confirmation to a clinical diagnosis of chronic porto-systemic encephalopathy. Ascites can be seen. Gallstones may be noted in the gallbladder or common bile duct. The CT scan provides an objective record useful for following the course. Directed biopsy of a selected area can be performed safely.

Biopsy diagnosis of cirrhosis may be difficult. Reticulin and collagen stains are essential for the demonstration of a rim of fibrosis around the nodule (table 19.2) (fig. 19.11).

Helpful diagnostic points include absence of portal tracts, abnormal vascular arrangements, hepatic arteri-

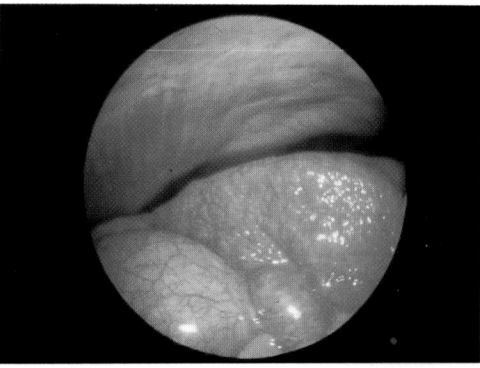

Fig. 19.9. Laparoscopy shows the nodular liver of cirrhosis. Note gallbladder to the left.

Table 19.2. Staining of connective tissue collagen in biopsies

Type	Site	Stained by
I	Portal zones, central zones, broad scars	Van Giesen
II	Sinusoids (elastic tissue)	Elastin
III	Reticulin fibres (sinusoids, portal zones)	Silver
IV	Basement membranes	Periodic–acid Schiff (PAS)

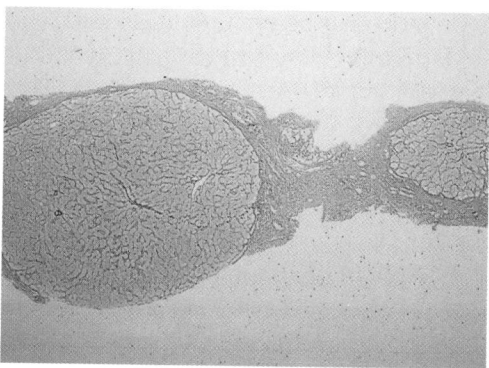

Fig. 19.11. Liver biopsy in cirrhosis: the specimen is small but nodules are shown outlined by reticulin. (Stained reticulin, ×40.)

oles not accompanied by portal veins, the presence of nodules with fibrous septa, variability in liver cell size and appearance in different areas, and thickened liver cell plates [57].

Functional assessment

Liver failure is assessed by such features as jaundice, ascites (Chapter 9), encephalopathy (Chapter 7), low serum albumin, and a prothrombin deficiency not corrected by vitamin K.

Portal hypertension (Chapter 10) is shown by splenomegaly, oesophageal varices and by the newer methods of measuring portal pressure.

Evolution is monitored by serial clinical, biochemical and histological observations, and classified as progressing, regressing or stationary.

Examples of classification

In every patient, diagnosis must be in terms of aetiology, morphology and hepatic function. Examples of such complete diagnoses are as follows.

1 Macronodular cirrhosis following type B hepatitis with liver cell failure and portal hypertension. Progressing.

2 Micronodular cirrhosis in an alcoholic with liver cell failure and minimal portal hypertension. Regressing.

3 Mixed micronodular and macronodular cirrhosis following bile duct stricture with minimal liver cell failure and portal hypertension. Progressing.

Clinical cirrhosis (table 19.3)

Cirrhosis, apart from other features peculiar to the cause, results in two major events: hepato-cellular failure (Chapters 6, 7, 9) and portal hypertension (Chapter 10). Prognosis and treatment depend on the magnitude of

Table 19.3. General investigations in the patient with cirrhosis (see also table 10.1)

Occupation, age, sex, domicile

Clinical history
Fatigue and weight loss
Anorexia and flatulent dyspepsia
Abdominal pain
Jaundice. Colour of urine and faeces
Swelling of legs or abdomen
Haemorrhage—nose, gums, skin, alimentary tract
Loss of libido
Past health: jaundice, hepatitis, drugs ingested, blood transfusion
Social. Alcohol consumption
Hereditary

Examination
Nutrition, fever, fetor hepaticus, jaundice, pigmentation, purpura, finger clubbing, white nails, vascular spiders, palmar erythema, gynaecomastia, testicular atrophy, distribution of body hair. Parotid enlargement. Dupuytren's contracture. Blood pressure
Abdomen: ascites, abdominal wall veins, liver, spleen
Peripheral oedema
Neurological changes: mental functions, stupor, tremor

Investigations
Haematology:
   Haemoglobin, absolute values, leucocyte and platelet count, prothrombin time
Biochemical:
   Serum—bilirubin
            transaminase
            alkaline phosphatase
            albumin and globulin
            immunoglobulins
If ascites present:
   serum sodium, potassium, bicarbonate, chloride, urea and creatinine levels
   weigh daily
   24-hour urine volume and sodium excretion
Serum immunological:
   smooth muscle, mitochondrial and nuclear antibodies
   hepatitis B antigen (HBsAg), anti-HCV (other markers of hepatitis, see Chapter 16)
   α-fetoprotein
Endoscopy
Hepatic CT scan or ultrasound
Needle liver biopsy if blood coagulation permits
EEG if neuropsychiatric changes

these two factors. In clinical terms, the types are either 'compensated' or 'decompensated'. In addition, cirrhosis, whatever its type, has certain clinicopathological associations.

It is difficult to relate the clinical picture with the underlying pathology although there are certain similarities. In Europe and the USA, cirrhosis of the alcoholic, chronic hepatitis B and C and cryptogenic cirrhosis account for the majority. In developing countries, the predominant causes are hepatitis viruses B and C. The age and sex distribution of the various types differ.

The terminal stages of the various types may be identical. The aetiological distinction is important both for prognosis and for specific treatment, such as alcohol withdrawal, venesection in haemochromatosis or prednisolone in autoimmune chronic hepatitis (table 19.1). Finally, comparison of cirrhosis in different parts of the world must allow for different aetiologies, although the basic pattern of liver cell failure and portal hypertension may be similar.

Clinical and pathological associations

1 *Nutrition.* Fat stores and muscle mass are reduced in many cirrhotic patients, with a greater reduction in the alcoholic and those who are Child's grade C (table 10.4) [13, 32]. Muscle wasting is related to reduced muscle protein synthesis with an overall fall in whole body protein turnover [47]. Resting energy expenditure is increased in cirrhotic patients with more advanced disease. This persists after transplantation with associated poor nutrition [48].

Taste and smell may be impaired [9]. Cirrhosis does not predispose to dental and peridontal disease. Poor oral hygiene and dental care appear to be responsible especially in alcoholics [52].

2 *Eye signs.* Lid retraction and lid lag is significantly increased in patients with cirrhosis compared with a control population [62].

There is no evidence of thyroid disease. Serum-free thyroxin is not increased.

3 *Parotid gland enlargement* and *Dupuytren's contracture* are seen in some alcoholic patients with cirrhosis.

4 *Digital clubbing* and *hypertrophic osteoarthropathy* may complicate cirrhosis, especially biliary cirrhosis [17]. These changes may be due to aggregated platelets, passing peripherally through pulmonary arteriovenous shunts, plugging capillaries and releasing PDGF [16].

5 *Muscle cramps* occur significantly more frequently in cirrhotic patients than in patients without liver disease, and correlate with the presence of ascites, low mean arterial pressure and plasma renin activity [4]. Cramps often respond to oral quinine sulphate. Weekly infusion of human albumin is beneficial by improving effective circulating volume [4].

6 *Steatorrhoea* is frequent even in the absence of pancreatitis or alcoholism. It can be related to reduced hepatic bile salt secretion.

7 *Splenomegaly* and *abdominal wall venous collaterals* usually indicate portal hypertension.

8 *Abdominal herniae* are common with ascites. They should not be repaired unless endangering life or unless the cirrhosis is very well compensated.

9 *Gastrointestinal.* Varices are visualized by endoscopy.

Peptic ulceration has been found in 11% of 324 patients with cirrhosis [61], more frequently those HBsAg positive. Seventy per cent were asymptomatic. Duodenal ulcers were more frequent than gastric ulcers, which healed more slowly and recurred more frequently than in non-cirrhotics.

Small bowel bacterial overgrowth occurs in 30% of patients with alcoholic cirrhosis, being more frequent in those with than without ascites (37 versus 5%) [46].

10 *Primary liver cancer* is frequent with all forms of cirrhosis except the biliary and cardiac types. *Metastatic cancer* is said to be rare, due to the reduced frequency of extra-hepatic carcinoma in cirrhosis [22]. However, when groups of patients with cancer and with or without cirrhosis were compared, the incidence of hepatic metastases was the same in each group.

11 *Gallstones.* Ultrasound shows that 18.5% of males and 31.2% of females with chronic liver disease have gallstones, usually of pigment type [59]. This is 4–5 times higher than the general population. The gallstones do not affect survival [19]. The low bile salt/unconjugated bilirubin ratio with very high biliary monoconjugated bilirubin predisposes to pigment gallstones [2]. Surgery should be avoided unless life saving, for the patient is a poor operative risk.

12 Chronic relapsing *pancreatitis* and pancreatic calcification are often associated with alcoholic liver disease.

13 *Cardiovascular.* Cirrhotics are less liable to coronary and aortic atheroma than the rest of the population [55]. At autopsy, the incidence of myocardial infarction is about a quarter of that among total cases examined without cirrhosis [29]. Cirrhosis is associated with an increased cardiac output and heart rate, as well as decreased systemic peripheral vascular resistance and blood pressure. There is an impaired cardiovascular response to exercise, with lower than expected peak heart rate and cardiac output, and autonomic dysfunction [26]. Vascular tone is reduced accounting for blunted systemic and renal effects of volume expansion [28]. Impaired response to catecholamines plays a part, as well as increased vascular synthesis of *nitric oxide* [11, 45]. Nitric oxide output in the breath of patients with Child's grade C decompensated cirrhosis is double that in control patients [43].

14 *Renal.* Changes in intra-renal circulation, and particularly a redistribution of blood flow away from the cortex, are found in all forms of cirrhosis. This predisposes to the *hepato-renal syndrome.* Intrinsic renal failure follows periods of hypotension and shock.

Glomerular changes include a thickening of the mesangial stalk and to a lesser degree of the capillary walls (*cirrhotic glomerular sclerosis*). Deposits of IgA are most frequent (fig. 19.12) [49, 51]. These are particularly found with alcoholic liver disease. The changes are usually latent, but occasionally are associated with pro-

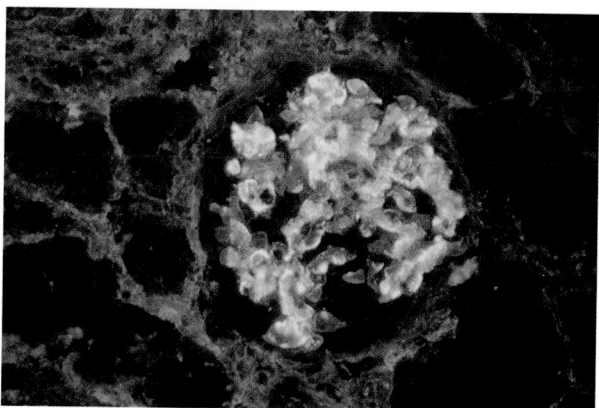

Fig. 19.12. IgA nephropathy: renal biopsy showing IgA deposition in glomerulus of cirrhotic patient (alcohol-related) with creatinine clearance of 20 ml/min and proteinuria (immunostaining with FITC rabbit anti-human IgA).

liferative changes and the clinical manifestations of glomerular involvement. Chronic hepatitis C infection is associated with cryoglobulinaemia and membranoproliferative glomerulonephritis [33].

15 *Infections.* Reticulo-endothelial system phagocytic activity is impaired [23], in part related to intra-hepatic portal-systemic shunting. Bacterial infections, often of intestinal origin, are common, affecting 4.5% of cirrhotic patients per year [24].

Septicaemias are frequent in end-stage cirrhosis and should always be suspected in patients with unexplained pyrexia or deterioration. The diagnosis is often missed. Spontaneous bacterial peritonitis must always be considered (Chapter 9). In patients with decompensated cirrhosis the plasma level of IL6 (>200 pg/ml) on admission to hospital is a sensitive measure of infection [38].

Tuberculosis has decreased, but tuberculous peritonitis is still encountered and often unsuspected. Respiratory infections have also lessened in severity.

16 *Drug metabolism.* Intrinsic drug metabolism is reduced in cirrhotic liver biopsies due to loss of hepatocytes. The metabolic activity of the remaining hepatocytes is preserved [44].

Histocompatibility antigens (HLA)

Sixty per cent of patients with HBsAg-negative chronic hepatitis are HLA-B8 positive. The patients who are positive tend to be female, less than 40 years old, have a remission with corticosteroid therapy and show positive non-specific serum antibody tests and high serum gamma-globulins. This association does not apply to HBsAg-positive chronic hepatitis. The HLA class II antigen Dw3 may show an even stronger association with non-B chronic hepatitis than does serotype B8.

In alcoholic liver disease there are geographic differences in the HLA association with no consistent pattern (Chapter 20).

In idiopathic haemochromatosis there is an association with HLA-A3, -B7 and -14 (Chapter 21). Genetic linkage to HLA-A and -B has been useful in detecting siblings at risk of developing the disease.

In primary biliary cirrhosis the data on HLA class II association have been conflicting.

Hyperglobulinaemia

Elevation of the total serum globulin, and particularly gamma level, is a well-known accompaniment of chronic liver disease. Electrophoresis shows a polyclonal gamma response, but rarely a monoclonal picture may be seen. The increased gamma-globulin values may be related in part to increased tissue autoantibodies, such as smooth muscle antibody. However, the major factor seems to be failure of the damaged liver to clear intestinal antigens (fig. 19.13). Patients with cirrhosis show increased serum antibodies to gastrointestinal tract antigens, particularly *Escherichia coli* [63]. Such antigens bypass the liver through portal-systemic channels or through the internal shunts developing around the cirrhotic nodule. Once in the systemic circulation they provoke an increased antibody response from such organs as the spleen. Systemic endotoxaemia may arise similarly. Polymeric IgA and IgA-antigen complexes of gut origin can also reach the systemic circulation [35]. Suppressor T-lymphocyte function is depressed in chronic liver disease and this would reduce the suppression of B-lymphocytes and so favour antibody production.

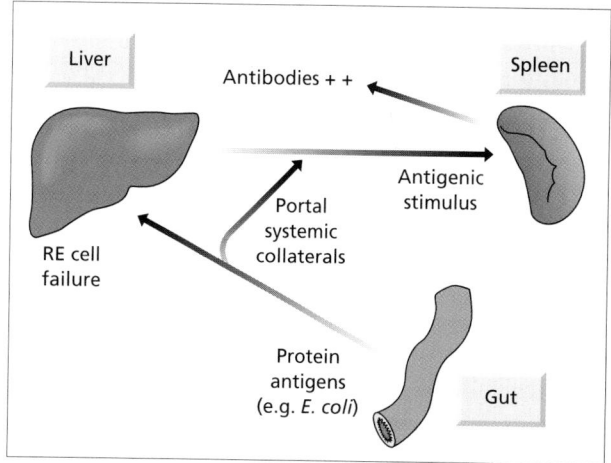

Fig. 19.13. A possible mechanism for the increased serum antibody (and globulin) levels in cirrhosis. Protein antigens from the gut bypass reticulo-endothelial (RE) Kupffer cells in the liver and present an antigenic stimulus to other organs, particularly the spleen, so increasing serum antibodies.

Compensated cirrhosis

The disease may be discovered at a routine examination or biochemical screen, or at operation undertaken for some other condition (fig. 19.14). Cirrhosis may be suspected if the patient has mild pyrexia, vascular spiders, palmar erythema, or unexplained epistaxis or oedema of the ankles. Firm enlargement of the liver and splenomegaly are helpful diagnostic signs. Vague morning indigestion and flatulent dyspepsia may be early features in the alcoholic cirrhotic. Confirmation should be sought by biochemical tests, scanning and, if necessary, by liver biopsy.

Biochemical tests may be quite normal in this group. The most frequent changes are a slight increase in the serum transaminase or gamma-GT level.

Diagnosis is confirmed by *needle liver biopsy*.

These patients may remain compensated until they die from another cause. Some proceed, in a period from months to years, to the stage of hepato-cellular failure. In others the problem is of portal hypertension with oesophageal bleeding. Portal hypertension may be present even with normal liver function tests. The course in the individual patient is very difficult to predict.

Decompensated cirrhosis

The patient usually seeks medical advice because of ascites and/or jaundice. General health fails with weakness, muscle wasting and weight loss. Continuous mild fever (37.5–38°C) is often due to Gram-negative bacteraemia, to continuing hepatic cell necrosis or to a complicating liver cell carcinoma. Fetor hepaticus may be present. Cirrhosis is the commonest cause of hepatic encephalopathy.

Jaundice implies that liver cell destruction exceeds the capacity for regeneration and is always serious. The deeper the jaundice the greater the inadequacy of liver cell function.

The skin may be pigmented. Clubbing of the fingers is occasionally seen. Purpura over the arms, shoulders and shins may be associated with a low platelet count. Spontaneous bruising and epistaxes reflect a prothrombin deficiency. The circulation is over-active. The blood pressure is low. Sparse body hair, vascular spiders, palmar erythema, white nails and gonadal atrophy are common.

Ascites is usually preceded by abdominal distension. Oedema of the legs is frequently associated.

The liver may be enlarged, with a firm regular edge, or contracted and impalpable. The spleen may be palpable.

The differential diagnosis of ascites, hepatic encephalopathy and jaundice are described in Chapters 7, 9, 12.

Laboratory findings

Haematology. There is usually a mild normocytic, normochromic anaemia; it is occasionally macrocytic. Gastrointestinal bleeding leads to hypochromic anaemia. The leucocyte and platelet counts are reduced ('hypersplenism'). The prothrombin time is prolonged and does not return to normal with vitamin K therapy. The bone marrow is macronormoblastic. Plasma cells are increased in proportion to the hyperglobulinaemia.

Serum biochemical changes. In addition to the raised serum bilirubin level, albumin is depressed and gamma-globulin raised. The serum alkaline phosphatase is usually raised to about twice normal; very high readings are occasionally found, particularly with alcoholic cirrhosis. Serum transaminase values may be increased.

Urine. Urobilinogen is present in excess; bilirubin is also present if the patient is jaundiced. The urinary sodium excretion is diminished in the presence of ascites, and in a severe case less than 4 mmol/l is passed daily.

Needle biopsy diagnosis (table 19.4) [57]

This may give a clue to the aetiology and activity. If there are contraindications, such as ascites or a coagulation defect, the transjugular approach should be used. Serial biopsies are valuable in assessing progress.

In cirrhosis, directed biopsies, using ultrasound or CT and a trucut needle, are particularly helpful in obtaining adequate samples and avoiding other viscera, especially the gallbladder.

Prognosis

Cirrhosis is usually believed to be irreversible, but fibrosis may regress as seen in treated haemochromatosis or Wilson's disease and the concept of irreversibility is not proven.

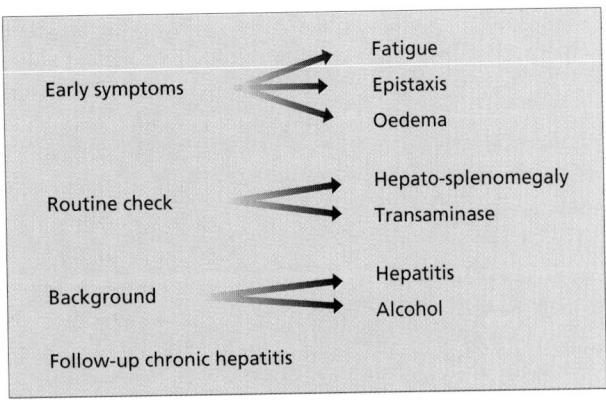

Fig. 19.14. Presentation of 'compensated' hepatic cirrhosis.

Table 19.4. Histopathology and aetiology of cirrhosis

Aetiology	Morphological pattern	Fat	Cholestasis	Iron	Copper	Acidophilic bodies	PAS-positive globules	Mallory's hyalin	Ground-glass hepatocytes
Viral hepatitis B	Macro- or micronodular	−	−	−	−	+	−	−	+
Viral hepatitis C	Macro- or micronodular	+	−	±	−	+	−	−	−
Alcohol	Micro- or macronodular	+	±	±	−	±	−	+	−
Haemochromatosis	Micronodular	±	−	+	−	−	−	−	−
Wilson's disease	Macronodular	±	±	−	±	+	−	+	−
α_1-antitrypsin deficiency	Micro- or macronodular	±	±	−	±	±	+	±	−
Primary biliary	Biliary	−	+	−	+	−	−	±	−
Venous outflow obstruction	Reversed	−	−	−	−	−	−	−	−
Intestinal bypass operation	Micronodular	+	−	−	−	±	−	±	−
Indian childhood	Micronodular	−	±	−	+	−	−	+	−

− usually absent; ± may be present; + usually present.

Cirrhosis need not be a progressive disease. With therapy the downhill progress may be checked.

The advent of liver transplantation has emphasized the need for an accurate prognosis so that surgery may be performed at the right time.

Child's classification (grades A–C)—which depends on jaundice, ascites, encephalopathy, serum albumin concentration and nutrition (see table 10.4)—gives a good short-term prognostic guide. Prothrombin time can be used rather than nutritional status (Child–Pugh modification) and individual features scored by severity. The total score classifies patients into grade A, B or C [30], although published studies often differ in their choice of numerical boundary between one grade and another [41].

Cox's regression model using proportional hazards has been applied to cirrhosis and a prognostic index formulated [12]. Poor prognosis is associated with a prolonged prothrombin time, marked ascites, gastrointestinal bleeding, advanced age, high daily alcohol consumption, high serum bilirubin and alkaline phosphatase, low albumin values, and poor nutrition.

In a very large series of cirrhotic patients from Southern Italy, those originally compensated became decompensated at the rate of 10% per year. Ascites was the usual first sign. Decompensated patients had a 21% 6-year survival. Significant indicators of death risk were advanced age, male sex, encephalopathy, haemorrhage, varices, prothrombin time, HBsAg positivity and, of course, hepato-cellular carcinoma [14].

The 1-year survival rate of cirrhotic patients following the first episode of spontaneous bacterial peritonitis is 30–45% [1]. Studies of functional liver function tests generally add little to Child's grading, although the aminopyrine breath test has been reported to add prognostic information in Child's grade A and B but not grade C alcoholic cirrhotics [64].

The following points are useful prognostically:

1 *Aetiology*. Alcoholic cirrhotics, if they abstain, respond better than those with 'cryptogenic' cirrhosis.

2 If decompensation has followed haemorrhage, infection or alcoholism, the prognosis is better than if it is spontaneous, because the *precipitating factor* is correctable.

3 The *response to therapy*. If the patient has failed to improve within 1 month of starting hospital treatment, the outlook is poor.

4 *Jaundice*, especially if persistent, is a serious sign.

5 *Neurological complications*. The significance depends on their mode of production. Those developing in the course of progressive hepato-cellular failure carry a bad prognosis, whereas those developing chronically and associated with an extensive portal-systemic collateral circulation respond well to dietary protein restriction.

6 *Ascites* worsens the prognosis, particularly if large doses of diuretics are needed for control.

7 *Liver size.* A large liver carries a better prognosis than a small one because it is likely to contain more functioning cells.

8 *Haemorrhage from oesophageal varices.* Portal hypertension must be considered together with the state of the liver cells. If function is good, haemorrhage may be tolerated; if poor, hepatic coma and death are probable.

9 *Biochemical tests.* If the serum albumin is less than 2.5 g the outlook is poor. Hyponatraemia (serum sodium <120 mmol/l), if unrelated to diuretic therapy, is grave. Serum transaminase and globulin levels give no guide to prognosis.

10 Persistent *hypoprothrombinaemia* with spontaneous bruising is serious.

11 Persistent *hypotension* (systolic BP <100 mmHg) is serious.

12 *Hepatic histological changes.* Sections are useful in evaluating the extent of necrosis and of inflammatory infiltration. A fatty liver responds well to treatment.

Conclusions

The prognosis is determined by the extent of hepatocellular failure. Jaundice, spontaneous bruising and ascites resistant to treatment are grave signs. If specific treatment is available the outlook is better.

Treatment

The management of the *well-compensated* cirrhotic is directed towards the early detection of hepato-cellular failure. An adequate balanced diet and avoidance of alcohol are essential.

A diet of 1 g of protein per kilogram of body weight is adequate unless the patient is obviously malnourished. Additional methionine or various 'hepato-protectives' are unnecessary. Avoidance of butter and other fats, eggs, coffee or chocolate is not of any therapeutic value.

Additional branched-chain amino acids are not indicated in stable cirrhotic patients [65]. In the severely malnourished, sip-feed supplements to a standard kitchen diet are useful. Total enteral nutrition for about three weeks improves serum albumin and Child's score [10].

The onset of hepato-cellular failure with oedema and ascites demands sodium restriction and diuretics (Chapter 9); complicating encephalopathy is an indication for a lowered protein intake and lactulose or lactitol (Chapter 7).

Portal hypertension may demand special treatment (Chapter 10).

Anti-fibrotic drugs [20, 66]

The treatment of cirrhosis may lie in switching off collagen synthesis.

Procollagen secretion requires the polymerization of microtubules, a process which can be inhibited by microtubular disruptive drugs such as *colchicine*. A controlled trial of colchicine (1 mg daily for 5 days per week) showed improved survival over the placebo treated [34]. However, the initial serum albumin level was higher in the treated, and compliance was poor, many patients being lost to follow-up. Evidence is not sufficiently strong to recommend the use of colchicine long-term for patients with cirrhosis. It is, however, relatively harmless —the only side-effect being diarrhoea.

Corticosteroids are anti-inflammatory and inhibit the activity of prolyl hydroxylase. They inhibit collagen synthesis but also inhibit pro-collagenase. They are used in autoimmune chronic hepatitis.

Other promising drugs for the treatment of hepatic fibrosis exist, such as γ-interferon and other inhibitors of prolylhydroxylase such as HOE 077 [20]. They have not been subjected to clinical trial.

Other therapeutic strategies for the future include the augmentation of the activity of extra-cellular proteases responsible for degrading collagen. The possibility of directly blocking the synthesis of connective tissue proteins by somatic gene therapy remains for the future.

Therapeutic strategies for the alcoholic cirrhotic are described in Chapter 20.

Surgical procedures

All operations in cirrhotic patients carry a high risk and a high mortality. Surgery in non-bleeding cirrhotic patients has an operative mortality of 30% and an additional morbidity rate of 30%. These are related to Child's grade—mortality being 10% in grade A, 31% in grade B, and 76% in grade C patients. Operations on the biliary tract, for peptic ulcer disease or for colon resection have a particularly bad prognosis. Poor predictive features include a low serum albumin, the presence of infection and a prolonged prothrombin time.

Upper abdominal surgery increases the difficulty, and should be avoided, in possible candidates for liver transplantation (Chapter 35).

Using segmental surgery, small hepato-cellular carcinomas arising in a cirrhotic liver can be successfully resected [7].

References

1 Altman C, Grange J-D, Amiot X *et al.* Survival after a first episode of spontaneous bacterial peritonitis. Prognosis of potential candidates for orthotopic liver transplantation. *J. Gastroenterol. Hepatol.* 1995; **10**: 47.

2 Alvaro D, Angelico M, Gandin C *et al.* Physico-chemical factors predisposing to pigment gallstone formation in liver cirrhosis. *J. Hepatol.* 1990; **10**: 228.

3 Andus T, Bauer J, Gerok W. Effects of cytokines on the liver.

Hepatology 1991; **13**: 364.

4 Angeli P, Albino G, Carraro P *et al.* Cirrhosis and muscle cramps: evidence of a causal relationship. *Hepatology* 1996; **23**: 264.

5 Arthur MJP, Iredale JP. Hepatic lipocytes, TIMP-1 and liver fibrosis. *J. Roy. Coll. Phys. London* 1994; **28**: 200.

6 Babbs C, Smith A, Hunt LP *et al.* Type III procollagen peptide: a marker of disease activity and prognosis in primary biliary cirrhosis. *Lancet* 1988; **i**: 1021.

7 Bismuth H, Houssin D, Ornowski J *et al.* Liver resections in cirrhotic patients: a Western experience. *World J. Surg.* 1986; **10**: 311.

8 Boros P, Miller CM. Hepatocyte growth factor: a multifunctional cytokine. *Lancet* 1995; **345**: 293.

9 Burch RE, Sackin DA, Ursick JA *et al.* Decreased taste and smell acuity in cirrhosis. *Arch. Intern. Med.* 1978; **138**: 743.

10 Cabre E, Gonzalez-Huix F, Abad-Lacruz A *et al.* Effect of total enteral nutrition on the short-term outcome of severely malnourished cirrhotics. A randomized controlled trial. *Gastroenterology* 1990; **98**: 715.

11 Campillo B, Chabrier P-E, Pelle G *et al.* Inhibition of nitric oxide synthesis in the forearm arterial bed of patients with advanced cirrhosis. *Hepatology* 1995; **22**: 1423.

12 Christensen E, Schlichting P, Anderson PK *et al.* Updating prognosis and therapeutic evaluation in cirrhosis with Cox's multiple regression model for time-dependent variables. *Scand. J. Gastroenterol.* 1986; **21**: 163.

13 Crawford DHG, Shepherd RW, Halliday JW *et al.* Body composition in non-alcoholic cirrhosis: the effect of disease etiology and severity on nutritional compartments. *Gastroenterology* 1994; **106**: 1611.

14 D'Amico G, Morabito A, Pagliaro L *et al.* Survival and prognostic indicators in compensated and decompensated cirrhosis. *Dig. Dis. Sci.* 1986; **31**: 468.

15 Devière J, Content J, Denys C *et al.* Excessive *in vitro* bacterial lipopolysaccharide-induced production of monokines in cirrhosis. *Hepatology* 1990; **11**: 628.

16 Dickinson CJ. The aetiology of clubbing and hypertrophic osteoarthropathy. *Eur. J. Clin. Invest.* 1993; **23**: 330.

17 Epstein O, Ajdukiewicz AB, Dick R *et al.* Hypertrophic hepatic osteoarthropathy. *Am. J. Med.* 1979; **67**: 88.

18 Fauerholdt L, Schlichting P, Christensen E *et al.* Conversion of micronodular cirrhosis into macronodular cirrhosis. *Hepatology* 1983; **3**: 928.

19 Finucci G, Tirelli M, Bellon S *et al.* Clinical significance of cholelithiasis in patients with decompensated cirrhosis. *J. Clin. Gastroenterol.* 1990; **12**: 538.

20 Friedman SL. The cellular basis of hepatic fibrosis: mechanisms and treatment strategies. *N. Engl. J. Med.* 1993; **328**: 1828.

21 Giorgio A, Amoroso P, Lettieri G *et al.* Cirrhosis: value of caudate to right lobe ratio in diagnosis with US. *Radiology* 1986; **161**: 443.

22 Goldstein MJ, Franle WJ, Sherlock P. Hepatic metastases and portal cirrhosis. *Am. J. Med. Sci.* 1966; **252**: 26.

23 Gomez F, Ruiz P, Schreiber AD. Impaired function of macrophage Fc-gamma receptors and bacterial infection in alcoholic cirrhosis. *N. Engl. J. Med.* 1994; **331**: 1122.

24 Graudal N, Milman N, Kirkegaard E *et al.* Bacteremia in cirrhosis of the liver. *Liver* 1986; **6**: 297.

25 Gressner AM. Cytokines and cellular crosstalk involved in the activation of fat-storing cells. *J. Hepatol.* 1995; **22** (Suppl. 2): 28.

26 Grose RD, Nolan J, Dillon JF *et al.* Exercise-induced left ventricular dysfunction in alcoholic and non-alcoholic cirrhosis. *J. Hepatol.* 1995; **22**: 326.

27 Guechot J, Loria A, Serfaty L *et al.* Serum hyaluronan as a marker of liver fibrosis in chronic viral hepatitis C: effect of α-interferon therapy. *J. Hepatol.* 1995; **22**: 22.

28 Hadengue A, Moreau R, Gaudin C *et al.* Total effective vascular compliance in patients with cirrhosis: a study of the response to acute blood volume expansion. *Hepatology* 1992; **15**: 809.

29 Howel WL, Manion WC. The low incidence of myocardial infarction in patients with portal cirrhosis of the liver: a review of 639 cases of cirrhosis of the liver from 17,731 autopsies. *Am. Heart J.* 1960; **60**: 341.

30 Infante-Rivard C, Esnaola S, Villeneuve J-P *et al.* Clinical and statistical validity of conventional prognostic factors in predicting short-term survival among cirrhotics. *Hepatology* 1987; **7**: 660.

31 Iredale JP, Murphy G, Hembry RM *et al.* Human hepatic lipocytes synthesise tissue inhibitor of metalloproteinases-1 (TIMP-1): implications for regulation of matrix degradation in liver. *J. Clin. Invest.* 1992; **90**: 282.

32 Italian Multicentre Cooperative Project. Nutritional status in cirrhosis. *J. Hepatol.* 1994; **21**: 317.

33 Johnson RJ, Gretch DR, Yamabe H *et al.* Membranoproliferative glomerulonephritis associated with hepatitis C virus infection. *N. Engl. J. Med.* 1993; **328**: 465.

34 Kershenobich D, Vargas F, Garcia-Tsao G *et al.* Colchicine in the treatment of cirrhosis of the liver. *N. Engl. J. Med.* 1988; **318**: 1709.

35 Kleinman RE, Harmatz PR, Walker WA. The liver: an integral part of the enteric mucosal immune system. *Hepatology* 1982; **2**: 379.

36 Kondo F, Ebara M, Sugiura N *et al.* Histological features and clinical course of large regenerative nodules: evaluation of their precancerous potential. *Hepatology* 1990; **12**: 592.

37 LaBrecque D. Liver regeneration: a picture emerges from the puzzle. *Am. J. Gastroenterol.* 1994; **89**: 586.

38 Le Moine O, Deviere J, Devaster J-M *et al.* Interleukin-6: an early marker of bacterial infection in decompensated cirrhosis. *J. Hepatol.* 1994; **20**: 819.

39 Li J, Rosman AS, Leo MA *et al.* Tissue inhibitor of metalloproteinase is increased in the serum of precirrhotic and cirrhotic alcoholic patients and can serve as a marker of fibrosis. *Hepatology* 1994; **19**: 1418.

40 McCullough AJ, Stassen WN, Wiesner RH *et al.* Serum type III procollagen peptide concentrations in severe chronic active hepatitis: relationship to cirrhosis and disease activity. *Hepatology* 1987; **7**: 49.

41 McIntyre N. The Child–Turcotte and Child–Pugh classification. In Reichen J, Poupon RE. *Surrogate Markers to Assess Efficacy of Treatment in Chronic Liver Disease.* Kluwer Academic Publishers, London, 1996, p. 69.

42 Marra F, Grandaliano G, Valente AJ *et al.* Thrombin stimulates proliferation of liver fat-storing cells and expression of monocyte chemotactic protein-1: potential role in liver injury. *Hepatology* 1995; **22**: 780.

43 Matsumoto A, Ogura K, Hirata Y *et al.* Increased nitric oxide in the exhaled air of patients with decompensated cirrhosis. *Ann. Intern. Med.* 1995; **123**: 110.

44 Meyer B, Luo H, Bargetzi M *et al.* Quantitation of intrinsic drug-metabolizing capacity in human liver biopsy specimens: support for the intact-hepatocyte theory. *Hepatology*

1991; **13**: 475.

45 Moreau R, Lebrec D. Endogenous factors involved in the control of arterial tone in cirrhosis. *J. Hepatol.* 1995; **22**: 370.

46 Morencos FC, De Las Heras Castano G, Ramos LM *et al.* Small bowel bacterial overgrowth in patients with alcoholic cirrhosis. *Dig. Dis. Sci.* 1996: **41**: 552.

47 Morrison WL, Bouchier IAD, Gibson JNA *et al.* Skeletal muscle and whole-body protein turnover in cirrhosis. *Clin. Sci.* 1990; **78**: 613.

48 Muller MJ, Boker KHW, Selberg O. Are patients with liver cirrhosis hypermetabolic? *Clin. Nutr.* 1994; **13**: 131.

49 Newell GC. Cirrhotic glomerulonephritis: incidence, morphology, clinical features, and pathogenesis. *Am. J. Kidney Dis.* 1987; **9**: 183.

50 Niemela O, Risteli L, Sotaniemi EA *et al.* Aminoterminal propeptide of type III procollagen in serum in alcoholic liver disease. *Gastroenterology* 1983; **85**: 254.

51 Noble-Jamieson G, Thiru S, Johnston P *et al.* Glomerulonephritis with end-stage liver disease in childhood. *Lancet* 1992; **339**: 706.

52 Novacek G, Plachetzky U, Potzi R *et al.* Dental and periodontal disease in patients with cirrhosis—role of etiology of liver disease. *J. Hepatol.* 1995; **22**: 576.

53 Pinzani M. Hepatic stellate (Ito) cells: expanding roles for a liver-specific pericyte. *J. Hepatol.* 1995; **22**: 700.

54 Pinzani M, Milani S, De Franco R *et al.* Endothelin 1 is over-expressed in human cirrhotic liver and exerts multiple effects on activated hepatic stellate cells. *Gastroenterology* 1996; **110**: 534.

55 Platt D, Kie FE, Luboeinski HP. Der Einflüss des Atters auf die negative Syntropie zwischen malignen Tumören, Lebercirrhöse und arterioskleorischen Umbaurorgangen der Aortawand Coronar und Cerebral. *Arterien Klin. Wschr.* 1973; **51**: 176.

56 Roberts FD, Sandford NL, Bradbear RA *et al.* Serum procollagen-III-peptide: failure to reflect the extent of hepatic fibrosis. *J. Gastroenterol. Hepatol.* 1986; **1**: 27.

57 Scheuer PJ, Lefkowitch JH. *Liver Biopsy Interpretation*, 5th edn. London: WB Saunders, 1994; 135.

58 Scuppan D, Stolzel U, Oesterling C *et al.* Serum assays for liver fibrosis. *J. Hepatol.* 1995; **22** (Suppl. 2): 82.

59 Sheen I-S, Liaw Y-F. The prevalence and incidence of cholecystolithiasis in patients with chronic liver diseases: a prospective study. *Hepatology* 1989; **9**: 538.

60 Shibayama Y, Nakata K. The role of sinusoidal stenoses in portal hypertension of liver cirrhosis. *J. Hepatol.* 1989; **8**: 60.

61 Siringo S, Burroughs AK, Bolondi L *et al.* Peptic ulcer and its course in cirrhosis: an endoscopic and clinical prospective study. *J. Hepatol.* 1995; **22**: 633.

62 Summerskill WHJ, Molnar GD. Eye signs in hepatic cirrhosis. *N. Engl. J. Med.* 1962; **266**: 1244.

63 Triger DR, Wright R. Hyperglobulinaemia in liver disease. *Lancet* 1973; **i**: 1494.

64 Urbain D, Muls V, Thys O *et al.* Aminopyrine breath test improves long-term prognostic evaluation in patients with alcoholic cirrhosis in Child classes A and B. *J. Hepatol.* 1995; **22**: 179.

65 Weber FL Jr, Bagby BS, Licate L *et al.* Effects of branched-chain amino acids on nitrogen metabolism in patients with cirrhosis. *Hepatology* 1990; **11**: 942.

66 Wu J, Danielsson A. Inhibition of hepatic fibrogenesis: a review of pharmacologic candidates. *Scand. J. Gastroenterol.* 1994; **29**: 385.

Chapter 20
Alcohol and the Liver

The association of alcohol with cirrhosis was recognized by Matthew Baillie in 1793. Over the last 20 years alcohol consumption has correlated with deaths from cirrhosis. In the USA, cirrhosis is the fourth commonest cause of death in adult males. The prevalence of alcoholic liver disease depends largely on religious and other customs and on the relation between the cost of alcohol and earnings — the lower the cost of alcohol, the more are lower socioeconomic groups affected.

World-wide, alcohol consumption is increasing. In France, however, the past 20 years has seen a decrease, perhaps due to Government propaganda. In the USA, alcohol consumption, particularly of spirits, has fallen, perhaps due to changing lifestyles (table 20.1).

Table 20.1. Alcohol consumption in the USA. Note the fall, particularly in the consumption of spirits

	Gallons/person/yr		
	1980	1987	% fall
Beer	37	34	7
Wine	3.2	2.7	14
Spirits	3.0	2.3	23

Risk factors for alcoholic liver diseases

Not all those who abuse alcohol develop liver damage; the incidence of cirrhosis among alcoholics at autopsy is about 10–15% (fig. 20.1) [81]. The explanation of the apparent predisposition of certain people to develop alcoholic cirrhosis is unknown.

Drinking patterns

The average intake of alcohol in a large group of male alcoholic cirrhotics was 160 g/day for 8 years [46]. Alcoholic hepatitis, a pre-cirrhotic lesion, was noted in 40% of those who drank less than 160 g/day. For most individuals the danger dose is greater than 80 g alcohol daily (table 20.2). Duration is important. Neither cirrhosis nor alcoholic hepatitis was seen in patients who consumed an average of 160 g of ethanol per day for less than 5

Table 20.2. Alcohol equivalents

Whisky	30 ml	10 g
Wine	100 ml	10 g
Beer	250 ml	10 g

?80 g/day safe.

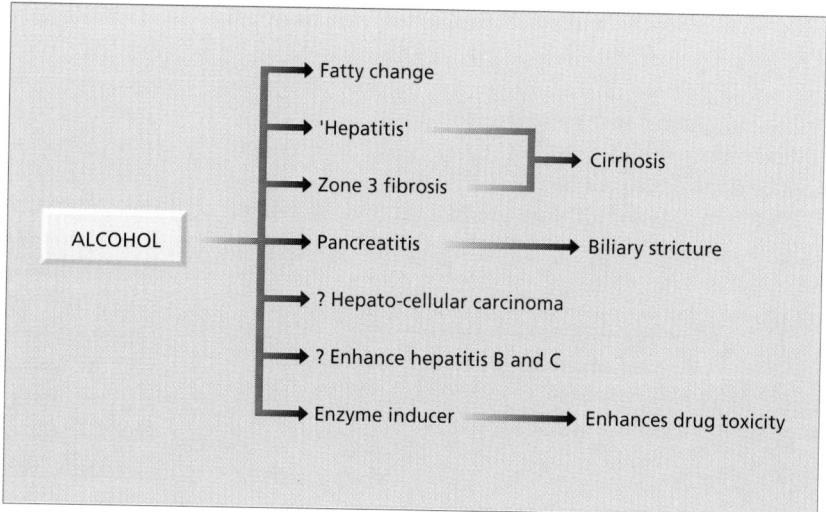

Fig. 20.1. The hepato-biliary effects of alcohol abuse. 80–90% of abusers have no liver disease.

years, whereas 50% of 50 patients consuming high levels of alcohol for an average of 21 years developed cirrhosis.

The liver injury is unrelated to the type of beverage; it is related only to its alcohol content. The non-alcoholic constituents of the drink—congeners—are not particularly hepato-toxic.

Continued daily imbibing is more dangerous than intermittent consumption when the liver is given a chance to recover. For at least 2 days in the week a person should not drink alcohol.

Those who develop alcoholic liver damage are only mildly dependent on alcohol [97]. They escape florid withdrawal symptoms, and are at greater risk of developing liver damage because they are able to maintain a high consumption over many years.

Sex

Alcoholism is increasing among women, owing to a decline in the social stigmas attached to drinking and to the ready availability of alcohol in supermarkets. Women are less likely to be suspected of alcohol abuse; they present at a later stage, are more susceptible to hepatic damage and are more likely to relapse after treatment (table 20.3) [64]. Women develop higher blood ethanol values following a standard dose of ethanol, possibly because of a smaller mean apparent volume of distribution of alcohol [58]. Women are more likely to progress from alcoholic hepatitis to cirrhosis even if they stop drinking.

Alcohol dehydrogenase in the gastric mucosa contributes to alcohol metabolism and this is reduced in women [28].

Genetics

Patterns of alcohol drinking behaviour are inherited, but no single genetic marker has been shown to be associated with susceptibility to alcoholic liver damage. However, the rates of alcohol elimination vary as much as three-fold among individuals. Prevalence of alcoholism is greater among monozygotic than dizygotic twins suggesting an inherited defect.

Histocompatibility studies have given inconsistent associations with alcoholic liver disease.

Different rates of alcohol elimination may be related to genetic polymorphism of enzyme systems [11, 20]. Alcohol dehydrogenase (ADH) is encoded at five different gene loci on chromosome 4. Individuals with different ADH isoenzymes have different alcoholic elimination rates. Polymorphism of ADH2 and ADH3, more active forms, may be protective as faster acetaldehyde accumulation leads to lower tolerance to alcohol. However, if such persons do imbibe more acetaldehyde is produced so increasing the risk of liver disease.

Alcohol is also metabolized by microsomal cytochrome P450-II-E1 and the gene encoding it has been cloned and sequenced but so far no studies on variants in alcoholic liver disease have been described.

Acetaldehyde is metabolized to acetate by aldehyde dehydrogenase (ALD). This is encoded at four different loci on four different chromosomes. ALDH2, the main mitochondrial enzyme, is responsible for the majority of aldehyde oxidation. Inactive ALDH2 is found in 50% of Japanese and Chinese and this explains the embarrassing acetaldehyde flush reaction seen when they consume alcohol. This inhibits Orientals from taking alcohol and is a negative risk for the development of alcoholic liver damage. However, heterozygotes for the ALDH2 genes have impaired metabolism of acetaldehyde and may be at high risk of alcoholic liver disease [23].

Polymorphism in genes encoding enzymes involved in fibrogenesis may prove important in determining individual susceptibility to the fibrotic effect of alcohol.

Susceptibility to liver damage from alcohol is probably not caused by a single gene defect but cumulative interaction of a number of genes [53]. Alcoholism and alcoholic liver damage are polygenic disorders.

Nutrition

Body composition analysis has shown protein depletion in chronic, stable, alcoholic cirrhotics related to the severity of the liver disease [85]. The extent of the nutritional defect depends on the type of alcoholic, whether of low socioeconomic status where protein-calorie malnutrition often precedes liver injury or in the socially adequate where diet is good and liver damage seems unrelated to nutrition [89]. Animals show species variation [73]. The rat given alcohol develops liver damage only if the diet is deficient, whereas baboons develop cirrhosis with a good diet. In rhesus monkeys, alcoholic liver damage is prevented by increasing dietary protein and choline [88]. Certainly, patients with decompensated liver disease, given a third of their calories as alcohol together with a nutritious diet, improve steadily [87], whereas liver function does not improve with alcohol abstinence if dietary protein remains low [83]. Nutrition and hepatotoxicity may act synergistically.

Alcohol may increase minimum daily requirements of choline, folic acid and other nutrients. Nutritional defi-

Table 20.3. Alcoholic liver disease—males:females [64]

Females suspected	38%
Males suspected	77%
Continued to abuse alcohol	
males	71%
females	91%

ciencies, particularly of protein, may promote the toxic effects of alcohol by depleting hepatic amino acids and enzymes.

It seems likely that both alcohol and nutrition play a part in alcohol hepato-toxicity, alcohol being the more important. There may be a range of alcohol intake that is tolerated without liver damage under optimal dietary conditions. However, it is also likely that there is a threshold of alcohol toxicity beyond which no protection is afforded by dietary manipulation [80].

Metabolism of alcohol (figs 20.2, 20.3)

Alcohol cannot be stored and obligatory oxidation must take place, predominantly in the liver. The healthy individual cannot metabolize more than 160–180 g/day. Alcohol induces enzymes used in its catabolism, and the alcoholic, at least while his liver is relatively unaffected, may be able to metabolize more.

One gram of alcohol gives seven calories and alcoholics literally run on spirit. The empty calories provide only energy with no contribution to nutrition (table 20.4).

Eighty to 85% ethanol oxidation is by initial conversion to acetaldehyde catabolized by ADH (fig. 20.3). This takes place in the cytosol. Acetaldehyde in mitochondria and cytosol may be injurious, causing membrane damage and cell necrosis. The acetaldehyde is converted to acetyl CoA with ALD acting as a co-enzyme (fig. 20.3). This can be further broken down to acetate, which may be oxidized to carbon dioxide and water, or converted by the citric acid cycle to other biochemically important compounds including fatty acids. NAD is a co-factor and hydrogen acceptor when alcohol is converted to acetaldehyde and further to acetyl CoA. The NADH

Table 20.4. The 'empty' (i.e. nutritionally valueless) calories supplied by alcohol

1 g alcohol = 7 calories
200 g (500 ml proof spirits) = approx. 1400 calories

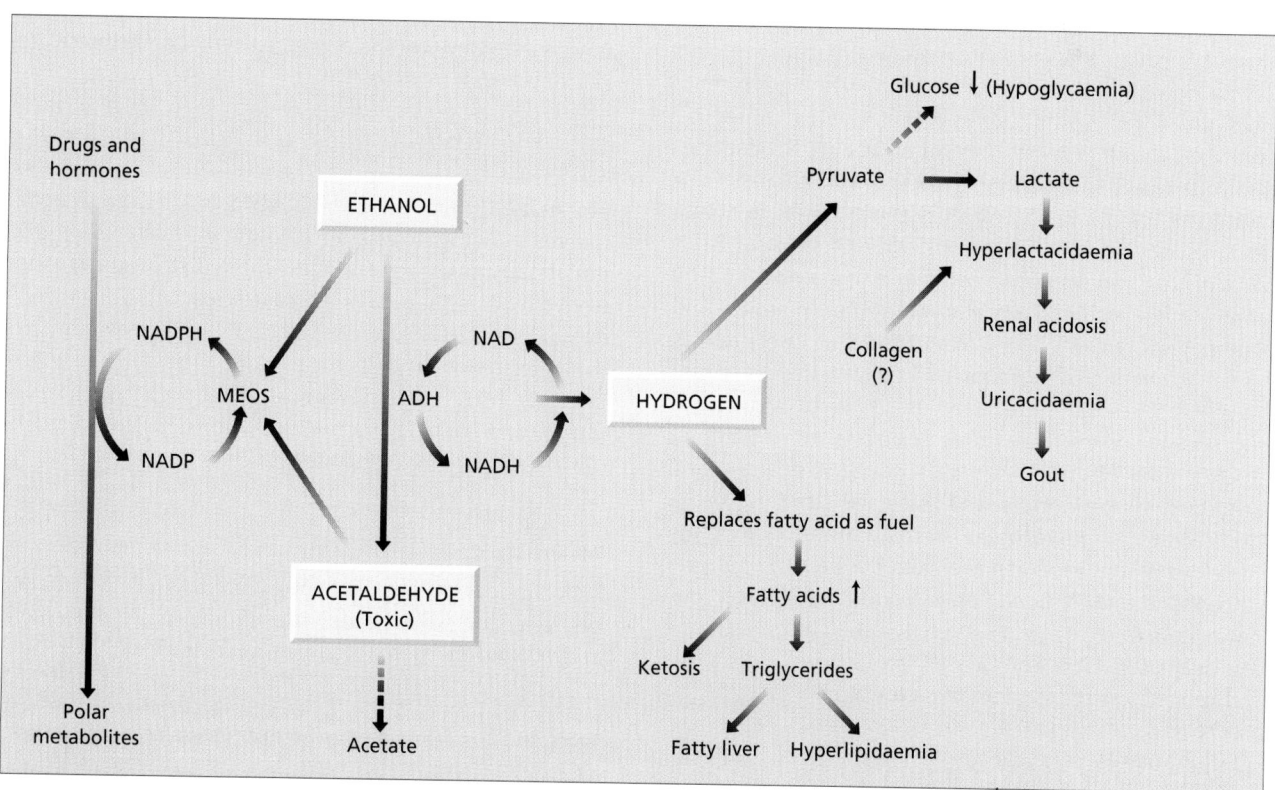

Fig. 20.2. Oxidation of alcohol in the hepatocyte. The production of acetaldehyde (toxic) is enhanced and conversion to acetate reduced. The hydrogen produced replaces fatty acid as a fuel so that fatty acids accumulate with consequent ketosis, triglyceridaemia, fatty liver and hyperlipidaemia. Unwanted hydrogen is used to convert pyruvate to lactate, which is produced in excess. Hyperlactacidaemia leads to renal acidosis, a rise in serum uric acid and gout. Collagen synthesis may be stimulated. Reduction of the pyruvate to glucose pathway results in hypoglycaemia.

Stimulation of the MEOS drug-metabolizing system leads to drug and alcohol tolerance, and increased testosterone metabolism may be related to feminization and to infertility.

Broken lines indicate depressed pathways.

ADH = alcohol dehydrogenase; MEOS = microsomal ethanol oxidizing system; NAD = nicotinamide adenine dinucleotide; NADP = nicotinamide adenine dinucleotide phosphate (after [49]).

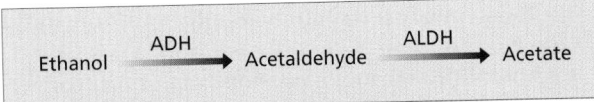

Fig. 20.3. Alcohol metabolism in the liver. ADH = alcohol dehydrogenase; ALDH = aldehyde dehydrogenase.

generated shuttles into the mitochondria and changes the NADH:NAD ratio and the redox state of the liver. The hydrogen generated replaces fatty acid as a fuel and is followed by triglyceride accumulation and fatty liver. The redox state of the liver changes, protein synthesis is inhibited and lipid peroxidation increases [90].

Diminished hepatic ADH and ALD are secondary to zone 3 necrosis.

Gastric ADH may metabolize some alcohol and the gastric atrophy of the alcoholic would reduce this process.

The activity of the citric acid cycle is reduced, and this may be responsible for decreased fatty acid oxidation. Lipoprotein synthesis is increased by alcohol. The NADH may serve as the hydrogen carrier for the conversion of pyruvate to lactate and blood lactate and uric acid levels rise after alcohol. Post-alcoholic hypoglycaemia and gout after alcohol ingestion may be explained by this mechanism. The conversion of alcohol to acetaldehyde also leads to inhibition of protein synthesis.

10–15% of alcohol is metabolized by a microsomal P450 ethanol oxidizing system (MEOS). P450-II-E1 is part of this system and is inducible by alcohol and by some drugs such as paracetamol (acetaminophen) and carcinogens [48, 49]. This accounts for the susceptibility of the alcoholic to drugs that are hepatotoxic on account of metabolites and which, when given in recognized therapeutic doses, can cause serious liver injury. Induction of P450-II-E1 increases oxygen consumption, acetaldehyde production and promotes lipid peroxidation. During microsomal peroxidation, potentially injurious reactive oxygen radicals (*free radicals*) are produced and may initiate lipid peroxidation [16]. The endogenous free radical scavengers such as glutathione are decreased [25]. The lack of protection against free radicals may partly explain mitochondrial injury.

Mechanisms of liver injury [27, 49]

Relation to alcohol and its metabolites

Rodents given alcohol develop only a fatty liver. However, they cannot match the quantities of alcohol consumed by the human who may take 50% of total calories as alcohol. This level can be achieved in the baboon who, after 2–5 years of alcoholism, develops cirrhosis. Evidence for the direct hepato-toxic effect of alcohol,

apart from nutritional changes, comes from human volunteers, both normal and alcoholic who, after 10–20 ounces (300–600 ml) of 86% proof alcohol daily for 8–10 days, develop fatty change and electron microscopic abnormalities on liver biopsy [48].

Acetaldehyde

Acetaldehyde is generated by both ADH and the MEOS systems. Blood acetaldehyde levels in alcoholics increase after chronic alcohol consumption but only very small amounts leave the liver.

Acetaldehyde is a toxic substance held responsible for many of the features of acute alcoholic hepatitis (table 20.5). Acetaldehyde is extremely reactive and toxic; it binds to phospholipids, amino acid residues and sulphydryl groups. It affects the plasma membranes by depolymerizing proteins and producing altered surface antigens. Lipid peroxidation is favoured. Acetaldehyde binds to tubulin, so impairing the microtubules of the cytoskeleton [40].

Acetaldehyde reacts with serotonin, dopamine and noradrenaline, yielding pharmacologically active compounds. It stimulates procollagen type I and fibronectin synthesis from Ito cells [15].

Changes in the intracellular redox potential

The marked increase in the NADH:NAD ratio in hepatocytes actively oxidizing alcohol produces profound metabolic consequences. Thus the redox ratio of lactate to pyruvate is markedly increased, leading to lactic acidosis. This acidosis, in conjunction with ketosis, impairs urate excretion and leads to gout. The altered redox potential has also been implicated in the pathogenesis of fatty liver, collagen formation, altered steroid metabolism and impaired gluconeogenesis.

Mitochondria

Mitochondria show swelling and abnormal cristae, perhaps due to acetaldehyde. Functionally, fatty acid and acetaldehyde oxidation is decreased with a reduc-

Table 20.5. The possible hepato-toxic effects of acetaldehyde

Increases lipid peroxidation
Binds plasma membranes
Interferes with mitochondrial electron-transport chain
Inhibits nuclear repair
Interferes with microtubule function
Forms adducts with proteins
Activates complement
Stimulates superoxide formation by neutrophils
Increases collagen synthesis

tion in cytochrome oxidase activities, respiratory capacity and oxidative phosphorylation.

Liver cell water and protein retention

In rat liver slices, alcohol inhibits secretion of newly synthesized glycoprotein and albumin by the hepatocyte [47]. This may be due to acetaldehyde binding to tubulin so impairing the microtubules on which protein secretion from the cell depends. In rats fed alcohol, fatty acid binding protein increases and this accounts for some of the total rise in cytosolic protein.

Water is retained in proportion to the protein and the resultant hepatocyte swelling is the major cause of hepatomegaly in alcoholics.

Hypermetabolic state

Chronic alcohol ingestion results in an increased consumption of oxygen largely due to increased re-oxidation of NADH. The increased hepatic oxygen requirement results in a steeper oxygen gradient along the sinusoidal length so that cell necrosis is in zone 3 (centrizonal) (fig. 20.4). Necrosis in this area may be hypoxic. P450-II-E1 is found in greatest concentration in zone 3 where the redox changes are also most marked.

Increased liver fat

Increased amounts of fat can be of exogenous (dietary) origin, can come from adipose tissue being transported to the liver as free fatty acids, or come from lipids synthesized in the liver itself. The origin depends upon the dose of ethanol ingested and the lipid content of the diet. After an acute, isolated ingestion of a large dose of ethanol the fatty acids found in the liver originate from adipose

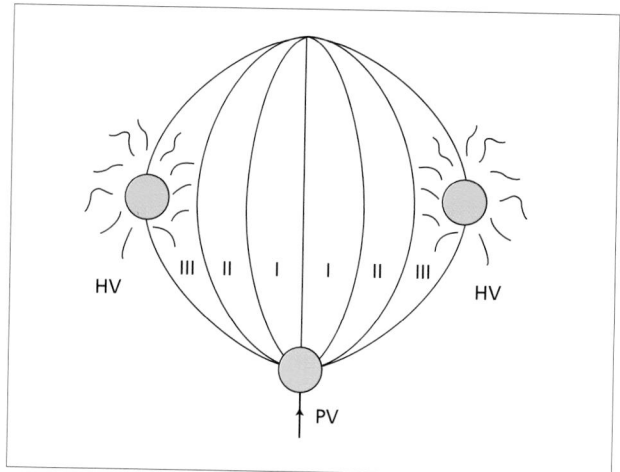

Fig. 20.4. Zone 3 collagenosis. HV = hepatic venule; PV = portal venule.

tissue, whereas following chronic ingestion, there is increased synthesis and decreased degradation of fatty acids in the liver.

Immunological liver damage

Immunological mechanisms might explain the occasional progression of the liver disease despite cessation of alcohol intake [45]. However, the histological picture of an immunological chronic active hepatitis is a rare sequel of alcohol excess [94]. Viral markers for hepatitis B and C must be absent.

Impaired humoral immunity in alcoholic liver disease is shown by elevations of serum immunoglobulin levels and deposition of IgA along hepatic sinusoidal walls.

Impaired cell-mediated hepatic injury is shown by antibodies reacting with ethanol-altered rabbit liver cell membrane antigens [69]. Circulating lymphocytes from patients with alcoholic hepatitis are directly cytotoxic to different target cells. In the active stage of alcoholic hepatitis, the infiltrate is largely neutrophilic, soon becoming lymphocytic. The distribution and persistence of CD4- and CD8-expressing lymphocytes in actively advancing alcoholic hepatitis with enhanced major histocompatibility complex expression on hepatocytes and their relationship to alcoholic hyalin and necrosis would support the hypothesis that a cytotoxic T-lymphocyte–hepatocyte interaction plays a role in the genesis or perpetuation of alcoholic liver disease [18].

The nature of the antigenic stimulant is uncertain. Mallory's alcoholic hyaline has been suggested but not confirmed. The antigen is unlikely to be alcohol or its metabolites because of their small molecular size although they might act as haptens. Acetaldehyde–collagen adducts are found in liver biopsies from subjects with alcoholic liver disease. They correlate with parameters of disease activity [93]. It remains possible that the impaired cell-mediated immunity reflects no more than a secondary response to systemic disease.

Fibrosis

In the alcoholic, cirrhosis can develop from fibrosis without an intervening acute alcoholic hepatitis. The mechanism of the fibrosis is uncertain. Lactic acid, which increases fibrogenesis, seems to be related to any type of severe liver disease.

The fibrosis is due to transformation of fat-storing Ito cells to fibroblasts and myofibroblasts [63]. Type III procollagen is found in the peri-sinusoidal collagen deposits (fig. 20.5) [59]. Alcohol dehydrogenase (ADH) can be found in the Ito cells of rat liver.

Although cell necrosis is the major stimulus to collagen formation there are other possibilities. Centrizonal (zone 3) hypoxia might be the stimulus. Increased intra-

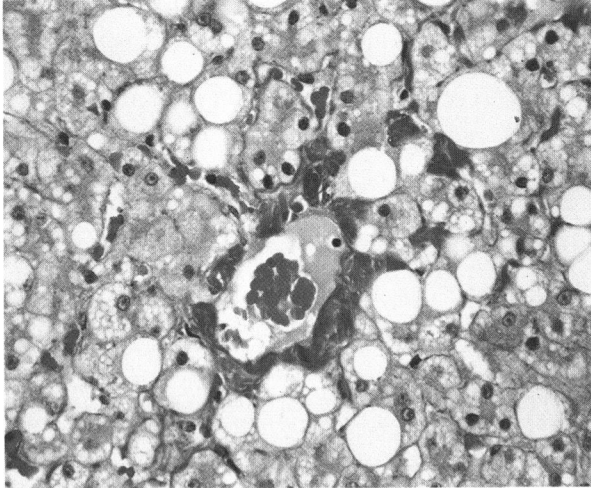

Fig. 20.5. Perivenular (zone 3) and phlebosclerosis fibrosis with adjacent fatty change. (Chromophobe aniline blue, ×100.)

cellular pressure due to hepatocyte enlargement is another possible fibrogenic stimulus.

Degradation products from lipid peroxidation activate Ito cells to stimulate collagen synthesis.

Cytokines

In the severely ill, cirrhotic patient, endotoxin frequently appears in the peripheral blood and ascitic fluid [8]. This is of intestinal origin related to impairment of endotoxin detoxification by the reticulo-endothelial system and to increased gut permeability. Endotoxin releases cytochromes IL1, IL2 and TNF from non-parenchymal cells. Circulating TNF, IL1 and IL6 concentrations are increased in chronic alcoholic patients [44]. In alcoholic hepatitis, TNF produced by monocytes in increased [54]. IL8, the neutrophilic chemotactic factor, is increased in plasma in alcoholic hepatitis [36]. It might be related to the neutrophilia and hepatic polymorph infiltration. It is also possible that the stimulus for cytokine production comes from alcohol-induced or alcohol-injured hepatocytes.

There is a striking similarity between the biological effects of certain cytokines and the clinical manifestations of acute alcoholic liver disease (table 20.6). These are shown by anorexia, muscle wasting, fever, neutrophilia and reduced albumin synthesis. Cytokines stimulate fibroblast proliferation. TGF-β activates collagen production from lipocytes [59]. TNF-α can depress P450 drug metabolism, induce cell surface expression of mixed HLA antigens and cause hepato-toxicity. Plasma levels correlate with the severity of liver injury [10].

Table 20.6. The biological effects of cytokine inducers of the acute phase response compared with the changes seen in acute alcoholic liver disease (ALD)

Change	ALD	Cytokines
Fever	+	+
Anorexia	+	+
Muscle wasting	+	+
Hypermetabolism	+	+
Neutrophilia	+	+
Decreased albumin	+	+
Collagen disposition	+	+
Increased triglycerides	+	+
Decreased bile flow	+	+
Shock	+	+

Morphological changes [27]

The changes are usually classified into fatty liver, alcoholic hepatitis and cirrhosis.

Fatty liver (steatosis) (figs 20.6, 20.7)

The fat accumulates in zones 3 and 2 (centrizonal and mid-zonal). In the more severely affected, the fatty change is diffuse. The fat may be in macrovesicular (large droplet) form. Less often it is in microvesicular (small droplet) form.

Large fat droplets appear in hepatocytes within 3–7 days of excess alcohol ingestion. Microvesicular fat represents mitochondrial damage and more active lipid synthesis by the hepatocyte. Hepatic mitochondrial DNA deletion is associated [29].

The fatty change can be quantitated:

+   less than 25% of liver cells contain fat
++   25–50% of liver cells contain fat
+++   50–75% of liver cells contain fat
++++ more than 75% of liver cells contain fat.

Alcoholic hepatitis

The full picture of a florid, acute alcoholic hepatitis is relatively rare. There are all gradations of severity. The hepatitis may be separate or can be combined with an established cirrhosis.

Balloon degeneration. Hepatocytes are swollen with granular cytoplasm often dispersed into fine strands. The nucleus is small and hyperchromatic. Steatosis, usually macrovesicular, but with some microvesicular change is usual. The ballooning is due to retention of water and to failure of the microtubules to support excretion of protein from the hepatocyte.

Acidophilic bodies represent apoptosis.

Mallory bodies are seen by haematoxylin and eosin as

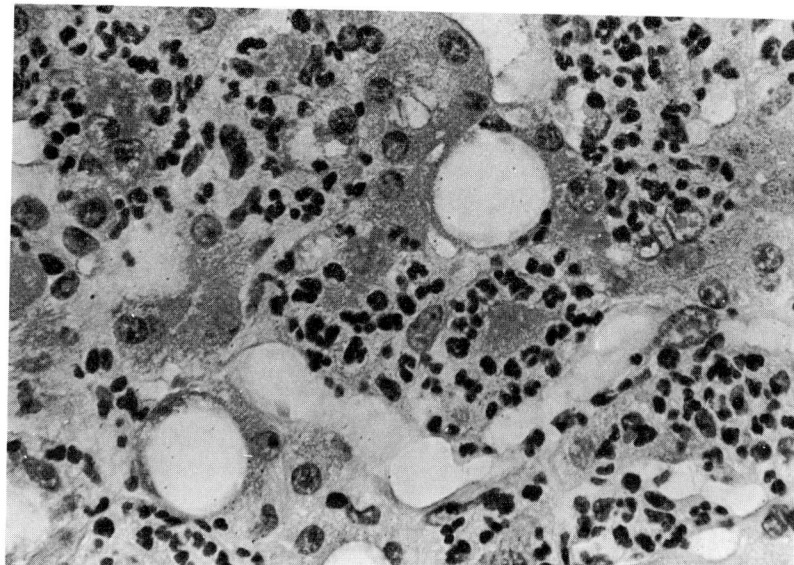

Fig. 20.6. Acute alcoholic hepatitis. Liver cells undergoing necrosis and containing clumps of Mallory's hyaline are surrounded by cuffs of polymorphonuclear cells. There is fatty change. (H & E, ×120.)

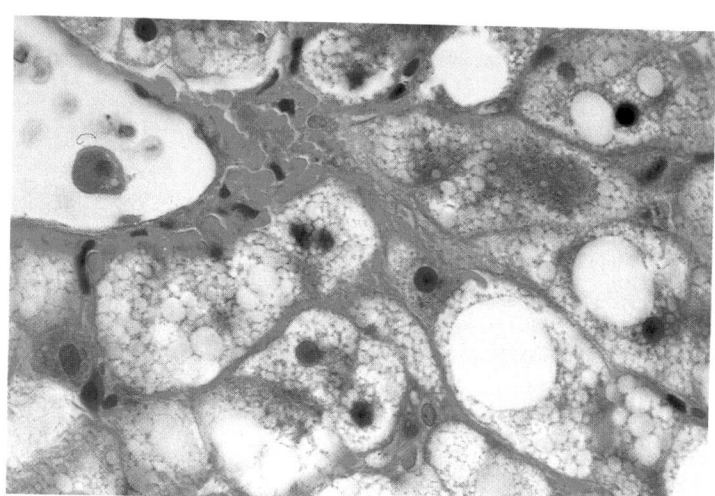

Fig. 20.7. Acute alcoholic hepatitis. Hepatocytes are ballooned and contain micro- and macrovesicular fat and clumps of purplish-red Mallory's alcoholic hyaline. (Chromophobe aniline blue, ×100).

purplish-red intra-cytoplasmic inclusions [41, 42]. They may be more obvious with Masson's trichrome or chromophobe aniline blue stains (fig. 20.7). They consist of clumped organelles, largely intermediate filaments and are composed of cytokeratin proteins cross-linked by transglutaminase [98]. They target the hepatocyte for destruction. The Mallory-containing cell is surrounded by a satellite of polymorphs which can also be seen within the injured hepatocytes (see fig. 20.6).

Giant mitochondria form globular intra-cytoplasmic inclusion seen by light microscopy using a Masson trichrome stain.

Sclerosing hyaline necrosis. Collagen deposition is maximal in zone 3. The fibres are peri-sinusoidal and enclose normal or ballooned hepatocytes. The pericellular fibrosis is like lattice or chicken wire and has been termed 'creeping collagenosis' [22] (fig. 20.8).

Collagenization of the space of Disse can be shown by electron microscopy (fig. 20.9). This shows that the number and porosity of the sinusoidal lining cells are reduced [37]. All these changes interfere with the exchange of substances between plasma and hepatocyte cell membrane and also contribute to portal hypertension [70].

Venous lesions include lymphocytic phlebitis in terminal hepatic venules and sublobular veins, peri-venular scarring with gradual obliteration of the lumen of terminal hepatic venules and veno-occlusive lesions of terminal hepatic venules and occasionally portal veins [35].

Portal zone changes are inconspicuous with mild to moderate chronic inflammatory infiltrate in the advanced case. Marked portal zone fibrosis suggests a complicating chronic pancreatitis (fig. 20.10) [66].

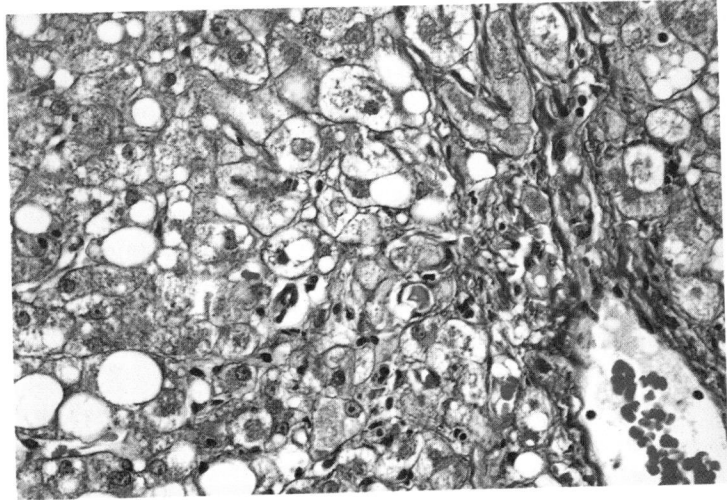

Fig. 20.8. Advanced zone 3 collagenosis with fatty change. A thickened hepatic vein is bottom right. (Chromophobe aniline blue, ×100.)

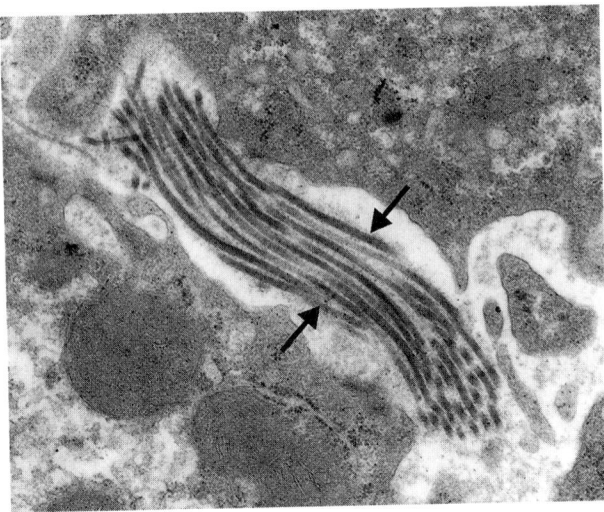

Fig. 20.9. Electron micrograph of liver in a patient with alcoholic liver disease. Note deposition of collagen fibrils in Disse's space (arrowed). This could interfere with oxygen and metabolite exchange between blood and hepatocyte.

Cholestasis in bile canaliculi is a feature of all types of alcoholic liver disease. It is strongly associated with decreased survival [72].

The *histological patterns* form a spectrum from minimal alcoholic hepatitis to an advanced, probably irreversible, picture, where necrosis is more extensive and fibrotic scars form. Alcoholic hepatitis can be regarded as a precursor of cirrhosis.

Hyperplastic nodules develop in those who reduce their alcohol consumption [32].

Cirrhosis

Classically, cirrhosis of the alcoholic is micronodular (fig. 20.11). No normal zonal architecture can be identified, and zone 3 venules are difficult to find. The formation of

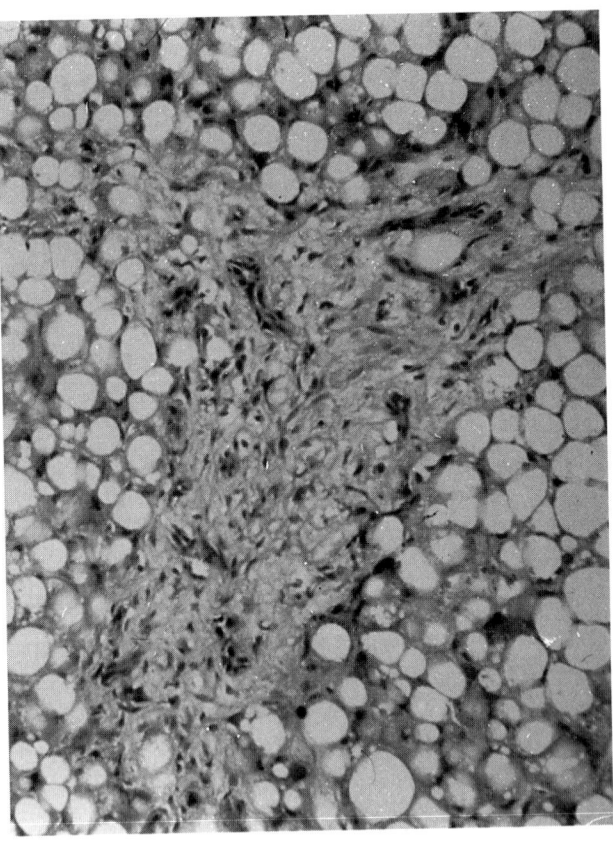

Fig. 20.10. Portal zone (zone 1) with marked fibrosis and fatty change in the hepatocytes. This patient suffered from chronic alcoholic pancreatitis with partial biliary obstruction. (H & E, ×120.)

nodules is often slow because of a presumed inhibitory effect of alcohol on hepatic regeneration. The amount of fat is variable and acute alcoholic hepatitis may or may not coexist. With continuing necrosis and replacement fibrosis, the cirrhosis may progress from a micro- to a

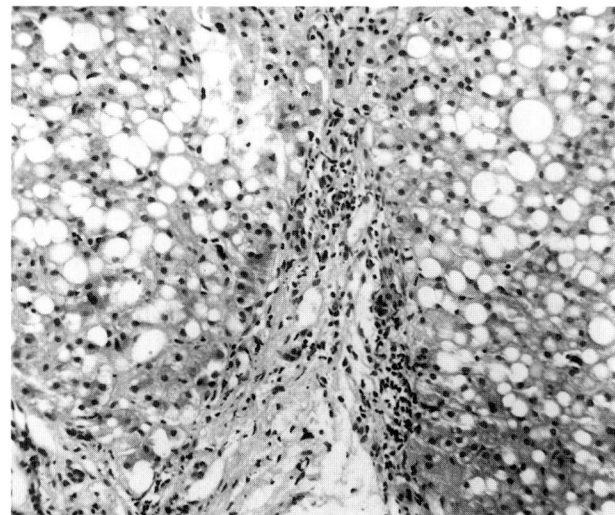

Fig. 20.11. Cirrhosis of the alcoholic. Fibrous bands divide the liver into small regular nodules. Fatty change is conspicuous. (H & E, ×120.)

macronodular pattern, but this is usually accompanied by a reduction in steatosis. When this end-stage picture is reached, an alcoholic aetiology is difficult to confirm on histological grounds.

Cirrhosis may follow peri-cellular fibrosis without apparent hepatic necrosis and inflammation. Zone 3 myofibroblastic proliferation and collagen deposition may be the first apparent lesions in the sequence of events leading to alcoholic cirrhosis.

Increased hepatic iron can be related to increased iron absorption, to the iron content of beverages (especially wines), to haemolysis and to porta-caval shunting. Body iron stores are only moderately increased [39].

Early recognition

This depends on a high index of suspicion by the physician. If alcoholism is suspected, the CAGE questionnaire should be used (table 20.7). Score 1 point for each positive response. Scores of 2 or more suggest alcohol-related problems. A patient may present with non-specific digestive symptoms such as anorexia, morning nausea with dry retching, diarrhoea, vague right upper abdominal pain and tenderness or pyrexia.

The patient may seek medical advice because of the effects of alcoholism such as social disruption, poor

Table 20.7. Alcoholism — the CAGE questionaire

C	Have you felt the need to cut down?
A	Annoyed at the suggestion of a drinking problem
G	Guilty of excess drinking
E	Drink (eye opener) in the morning

work performance, accidents, violent behaviour, fits, tremulousness or depression.

The diagnosis may be made when hepatomegaly, a raised serum transaminase or γ-glutamyl transpeptidase level or macrocytosis are discovered at a routine examination, for instance at a life insurance check-up or during investigation of another condition.

Physical signs may be non-contributory, although tender hepatomegaly, prominent vascular spiders and associated features of alcoholism may be helpful. The clinical features do not reflect the hepatic histology and biochemical tests of liver function may be normal.

BIOCHEMICAL TESTS [61]

Serum transaminase levels rarely exceed 300 iu/dl. SGOT (AST), which is derived from alcoholic damage to mitochondria or smooth muscle, is more increased than the SGPT (ALT) which is confined to the liver. In alcoholic liver disease, the SGOT : SGPT ratio usually exceeds 2. This is partially explained by the depletion in alcoholics of pyridoxal 5-phosphate, the biologically active form of vitamin B_6 which is necessary for the activity of both enzymes and is depleted in alcoholics.

The serum γ-glutamyl transpeptidase (γ-GTP) is a widely used screening test for alcohol abuse. The rise results mainly from enzyme induction, although hepatocellular damage and cholestasis may contribute. There are many false positives due to other factors, such as drugs, other diseases and the patient having a value at the upper limit of the normal range.

Serum alkaline phosphatase may be markedly increased (greater than four times normal) especially in those with severe cholestasis and alcoholic hepatitis [82]. Serum IgA values may be very high.

Blood and urinary alcohol levels can be used in the clinic to refute the individual who has a high blood alcohol level but denies imbibing.

Non-specific serum changes in acute and chronic alcoholism include elevations in uric acid, lactate and triglyceride, and reductions in glucose and magnesium. Hypophosphataemia is related to a renal tubular defect, independent of liver function impairment [2]. Low serum tri-iodothyronine (T3) levels presumably reflect decreased hepatic conversion of T4 to T3. Levels correlate inversely with the severity of alcoholic liver disease.

Type III collagen can be estimated by the serum procollagen type III peptides. Serum type IV collagen and laminin estimate components of basement membranes. Results of these three tests correlate with disease severity, degree of alcoholic hepatitis and alcohol intake [3, 70].

Other serum tests are markers of alcohol abuse rather than alcoholic liver damage. They include serum glutamate dehydrogenase, the mitochondrial isoenzyme of aspartate transaminase [52, 68]. Serum carbohydrate-deficient (desialylated) transferrin levels may be a useful marker of excessive alcohol intake irrespective of liver disease but this test is not generally available [6].

Even sensitive biochemical methods may fail to reveal alcoholic liver damage and liver biopsy is necessary in cases of doubt.

HAEMATOLOGICAL CHANGES

Macrocytosis (MCV) greater than 95 fl is presumably due to a direct effect of alcohol on bone marrow. Deficiencies of folate and vitamin B_{12} contribute in the malnourished. The combination of a raised MCV and serum γ-GTP will identify 90% of alcohol-dependent patients.

LIVER BIOPSY

This confirms liver disease and identifies alcohol abuse as the likely cause. The dangers of the liver damage can be emphasized more forcibly to the patient.

Liver biopsy is important prognostically. Fatty change alone is not nearly so serious as peri-venular sclerosis, which is a precursor of cirrhosis [91]. An established cirrhosis can be confirmed.

Non-alcoholic steato-hepatitis (NASH) may be due to various causes (table 20.8) [4]. In contrast to the alcoholic, the lesion is largely peri-portal.

PORTAL HYPERTENSION

Splenomegaly is not prominent. Portal hypertension and gastrointestinal bleeding, however, are frequent at all stages. Bleeding comes not only from oesophageal varices but from duodenal ulcers, gastritis and Mallory–Weiss lower oesophageal tears following repeated vomiting.

The portal hypertension may be related to cirrhosis.

Table 20.8. Differential diagnosis of NASH

Condition	Diagnostic points
Diabetes and pre-diabetes	Fasting blood glucose
Obesity	Body weight
Jejuno-ileal bypass	History
Parenteral nutrition	History—cholestasis
Wilson's disease	Kayser–Fleischer ring
	Copper metabolism
Abetalipoproteinaemia	Lipid profile
Drugs	History
amiodarone	
nifedipine	
oestrogens	
Indian childhood cirrhosis	Excess liver copper

Fatty change and zone 3 collagenosis (perivenular sclerosis) lead to a pre-sinusoidal portal hypertension [35]. Collagenization of the space of Disse decreases sinusoidal diameter, increases resistance to sinusoidal blood flow and raises portal pressure. Enlargement of hepatocytes probably plays little part.

Scanning

With severe acute alcoholic hepatitis or advanced cirrhosis, isotopes, such as technetium labelled colloid, are hardly taken up by the liver because the blood shunts past the reticulo-endothelial cells.

Ultrasound will not detect minimal change, fat or fibrosis. However, in more advanced alcoholic liver disease, the liver is diffusely abnormal and the changes correlate with those seen on liver biopsy.

CT scanning is very useful in demonstrating fatty liver (low attenuation), irregular liver surface, splenomegaly, portal collateral circulation, ascites and pancreatitis. It may demonstrate alcoholic pseudo-tumour (fig. 20.12).

Clinical syndromes

FATTY LIVER

The patients are usually asymptomatic, diagnosis being made when an enlarged, smooth, firm liver is discovered. Liver function tests may be normal or the transaminases and alkaline phosphatase slightly

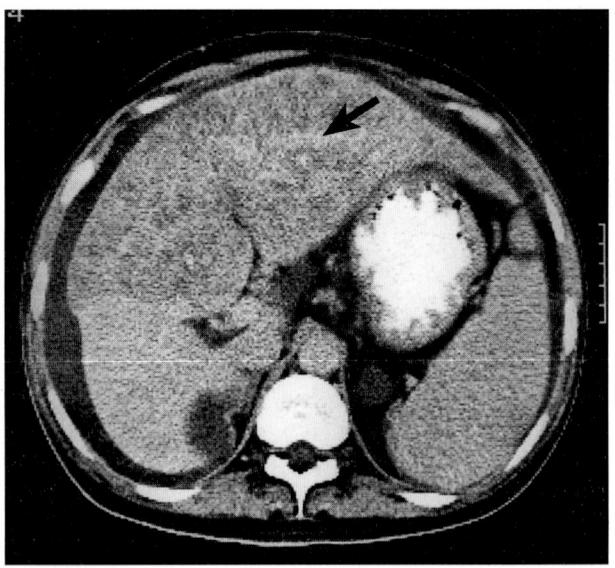

Fig. 20.12. Alcoholic pseudo-tumour. A mass was felt in the upper abdomen and a liver tumour was suspected. CT scan (enhanced oral contrast) showed features suggestive of hepato-cellular carcinoma (arrowed). Directed needle biopsy showed only acute alcoholic hepatitis. This is a rare type of alcoholic hepatitis, affecting particularly one part of the liver.

increased. If the alcoholic fatty liver is sufficiently severe to merit admission to hospital the patient has usually been drinking heavily for some time and is anorexic. There may be nausea and vomiting with peri-umbilical, epigastric or right upper-quadrant pain. Clinically, the fatty liver patient cannot be separated from one with mild alcoholic hepatitis. Needle liver biopsy is essential to diagnose alcoholic hepatitis.

ACUTE ALCOHOLIC HEPATITIS

In the very mildest case, the diagnosis may be made only by a liver biopsy in an asymptomatic patient who is mis-using alcohol and has shown abnormal serum enzyme tests and macrocytosis.

Patients in the next category complain only of fatigue, anorexia and weight loss. There is tender hepatomegaly and usually pyrexia. The patient may be obese, but some features of malnutrition are present in 90% of patients.

In the more severe case, the patient has usually been drinking particularly heavily and not eating. The severe hepatic decompensation may be precipitated by vomiting, diarrhoea or an intercurrent infection, such as pneumonia or urinary tract infection, or by prolonged anorexia.

Intake of quite modest doses of paracetamol may precipitate the alcoholic into severe hepatitis (fig. 20.13) [55]. Transaminase levels are enormous [101].

Severe alcoholic hepatitis is marked by pyrexia, anorexia, jaundice and repeated vomiting. The patient may experience pain over a very enlarged tender liver. In about half, an arterial murmur may be heard over the liver. Florid vascular spiders are usual on the skin. There may be associated signs of liver failure such as ascites, hepatic encephalopathy and a bleeding diathesis. The blood pressure is usually low with a hyperdynamic circulation. Signs of associated vitamin deficiencies, such as beri beri or scurvy, are usual in the malnourished.

Diarrhoea with steatorrhoea can be related to decreased biliary excretion of bile salts, to pancreatic insufficiency and to a direct, toxic effect of alcohol on the intestinal mucosa.

Patients with acute fatty liver may die suddenly in shock, attributable to pulmonary fat emboli. Sudden deaths have also been reported in hypoglycaemia.

Gastrointestinal haemorrhage is frequently from a local gastric or duodenal lesion, and is secondary to the general bleeding tendency, rather than related to portal hypertension.

Acute alcoholic hepatitis may be confused with acute virus hepatitis. Helpful diagnostic points are the history, the florid vascular spiders, the very large liver and the leucocytosis.

Laboratory tests

Serum transaminases are increased, but rarely to greater than 300 iu/litre. Very high values suggest complicating ingestion of paracetamol (fig. 20.13). The AST:ALT ratio exceeds 2. Serum alkaline phosphatase is usually increased.

The severity is best correlated with the serum bilirubin level and prothrombin time after vitamin K administration [56]. Serum IgA is markedly increased with IgG and IgM raised to a much lesser extent, and serum IgG falls with improvement. The serum albumin level is decreased, increasing as the patient improves. Serum cholesterol levels are usually increased.

The serum potassium value is low, largely due to the low dietary protein intake, to diarrhoea, and to secondary hyperaldosteronism if fluid retention is present. Albumin-bound serum zinc is decreased, and this is related to a low liver zinc concentration, not found in patients with non-alcoholic liver disease. The blood urea and creatinine values increase and these reflect severity. They predict the development of the hepato-renal syndrome.

A polymorph leucocytosis of about $15–20 \times 10^9$/litre is found in proportion to the severity of the alcoholic hepatitis.

Platelet function is depressed even in the absence of thrombocytopenia or of alcohol in the blood.

HEPATIC CIRRHOSIS

Established cirrhosis can present without a stage of acute alcoholic hepatitis having been recognized clinically or histologically and the picture can resemble any end-stage liver disease. The points suggesting an alcoholic aetiology include the history of alcohol abuse (which may be forgotten), the hepatomegaly and the associated features of alcoholism. Splenomegaly is a late feature.

Liver biopsy findings supporting an alcoholic aetiology include a micronodular cirrhosis, perivenular scler-

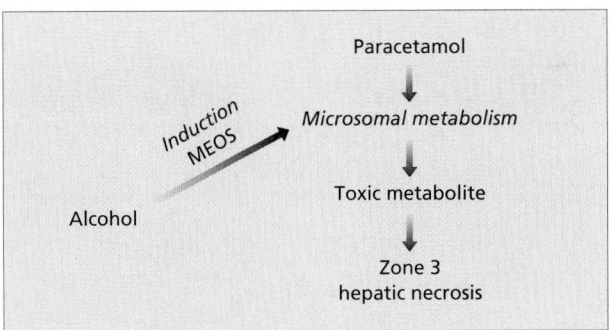

Fig. 20.13. Alcohol, by inducing microsomal metabolism, enhances the effects of toxic metabolites of drugs such as paracetamol (acetaminophen) on the liver.

osis and paucity of hepatic veins. It may be impossible on histological grounds to determine an alcoholic cause.

CHOLESTATIC SYNDROMES

Occasionally, the patient presents with deep jaundice, hepatomegaly and an increase in serum alkaline phosphatase, transaminases, triglycerides and cholesterol [95]. Functional renal failure is usual. This is usually the first episode of decompensation.

Liver biopsy shows massive accumulation of microvesicular fat (fig. 20.7) with cholestasis in centrizonal areas. Inflammation is inconspicuous and there is little or no hyaline [65]. Electron microscopy shows extensive disorganization of the organelles in affected hepatocytes. The condition has been termed *alcoholic foamy degeneration* [95]. Prognosis is very variable and foamy degeneration can be found in the asymptomatic.

Cholestasis may also be due to compression of the intra-pancreatic portion of the common bile duct by chronic pancreatitis. ERCP confirms the diagnosis (figs 20.14, 20.15).

RELATIONSHIP TO HEPATITIS B AND C

Markers of past or current hepatitis B or C are commoner in patients with alcoholic liver disease than in the general population [71]. It may be difficult to distinguish the viral from the alcoholic aetiology. The identification of risk factors is helpful. The effect of abstinence in the alcoholic is a fall in transaminases but in the viral patient these continue their fluctuant course. Liver biopsy appearances may be helpful although there may be considerable difficulty in interpretation. Serological HBsAg may be absent and serum hepatitis B virus DNA testing may be necessary to diagnose hepatitis B infection [100]. Positive second-generation ELISA tests usually correlate with a positive hepatitis C virus RNA and allow diagnosis of complicating hepatitis C disease [26]. Coexistence of viral infection is believed to increase the severity of the alcoholic liver disease.

HEPATOCELLULAR CANCER

This occasionally develops in the alcoholic cirrhotic liver,

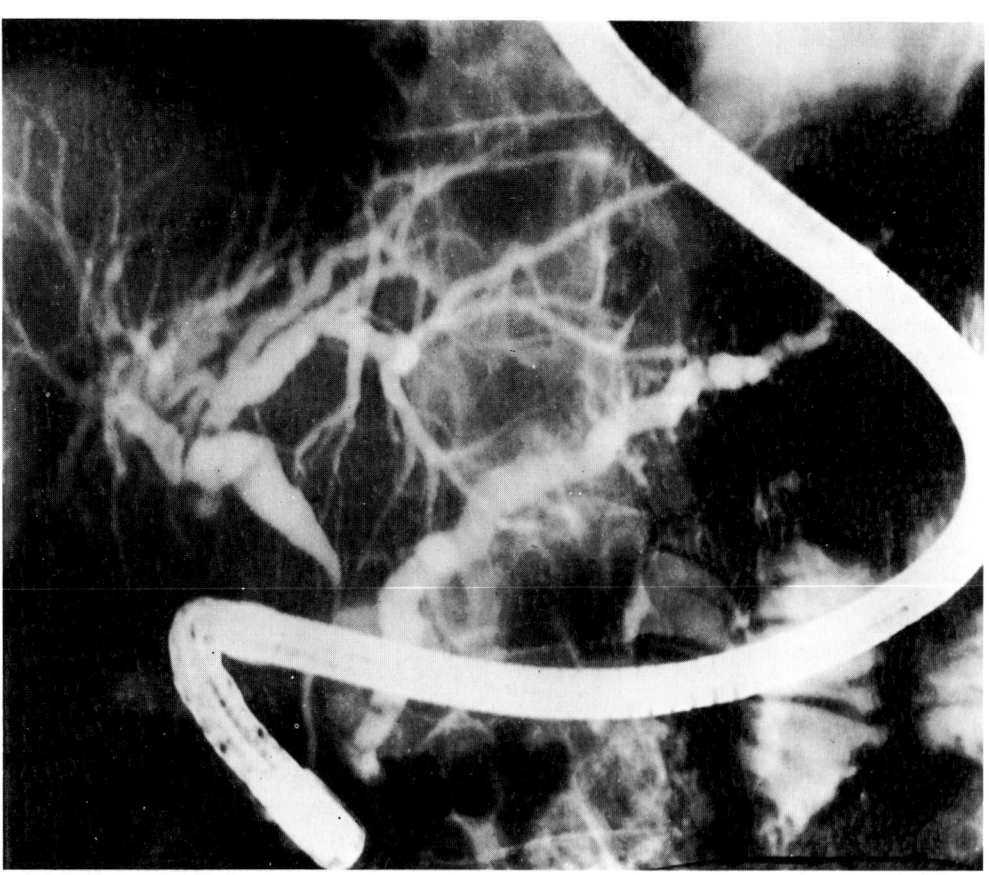

Fig. 20.14. ERCP in an alcoholic patient with chronic pancreatitis and cholestasis. It shows dilatation and irregularity of the pancreatic duct and smooth constriction of the common bile duct as it passes behind the inflamed pancreas.

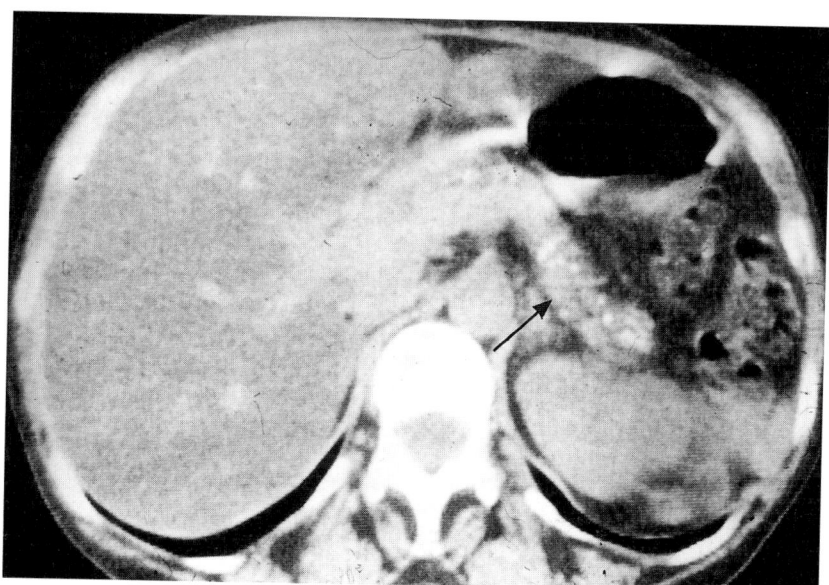

Fig. 20.15. CT scan showing an enlarged fatty liver with a chronic calcific pancreatitis (arrowed).

usually after a period of abstention when a macronodular cirrhosis has developed.

There is a strong association between hepatitis B and cancer developing in an alcoholic. Integrated hepatitis B sequences are found in the livers of alcoholic patients with primary liver cancer.

Associated features

The occasional, bilaterally enlarged parotids may be analogous to those seen with other types of malnutrition. Gynaecomastia often appears after treatment and is a frequent complication of spironolactone therapy. The testes atrophy and sexual performance in men declines [30]. Muscle mass wastes.

Dupuytren's contracture of the palmar fascia is related to the alcoholism and not to the cirrhosis [12].

Loss of memory and concentration, insomnia, irritability, hallucinations, convulsions, 'rum-fits' and tremor may be the stigmas of alcoholism. These must be distinguished from early hepatic pre-coma.

Hepato-renal syndrome seems particularly common in alcoholics.

Serum IgA is increased and deposits are found along the sinusoids. They are probably related to local stimulation of the secretory immune system [96]. It may trigger TNF-α secretion by monocytes [21].

Renal glomerular abnormalities, in particular mesangial expansion are probably related to immune complex deposition [7]. These contain IgA, Mallory body antigen and complement.

Impaired renal acidification in alcoholic liver disease may be a sign of liver cell failure [79].

Prognosis

The prognosis in alcoholics is much better than with other forms of cirrhosis. Everything depends on whether the alcoholic can overcome his addiction. This in turn is related to family support, financial resources and socio-economic state. In a large group of working-class, often 'skid row' type, alcoholic cirrhotics studied in Boston, the mean life expectancy for men was 33 months, compared with 16 months for a non-alcoholic group of cirrhotics. In a study at Yale, patients from a higher socioeconomic class, with cirrhosis complicated by ascites, jaundice and haematemesis, showed an overall 5-year survival of 50%. If they persisted in alcoholism this fell to 40%, whereas if they abstained it was 60% [84]. Very similar figures come from the UK (fig. 20.16) [13]. Continued heavy drinking is associated with poor survival.

Women with alcoholic cirrhosis survive a shorter time than men (fig. 20.17).

Liver biopsy gives the best indication of prognosis. Zone 3 fibrosis and peri-venular sclerosis are very unfavourable features [57, 99]. At present this lesion can only be detected by liver biopsy with appropriate connective tissue staining.

Histological cholestasis is a bad prognostic indicator in alcoholic hepatitis [72]. Hepatocyte proliferation factors, TGF-α and HGF, in liver biopsy specimens show greater expression in patients who survive acute alcoholic hepatitis [24].

In one study, 50% of patients with alcoholic hepatitis developed cirrhosis after 10–13 years [91]. In another study, 23% of patients with alcoholic liver disease but without cirrhosis developed cirrhosis after an average of 8.1 years [57]. Fatty change is probably not a risk factor.

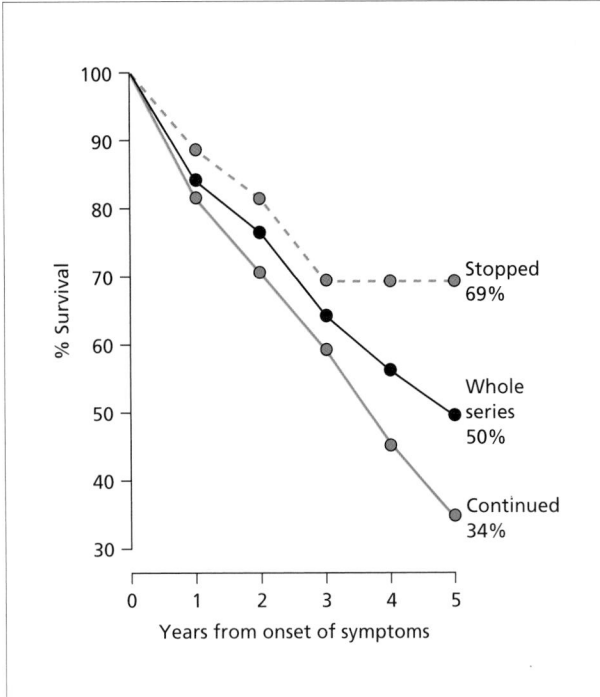

Fig. 20.16. The probability of survival of patients with established alcoholic liver disease: 50% survived 5 years. 69% of those who abstained from alcohol were alive at 5 years, but only 34% of those who continued to imbibe [13].

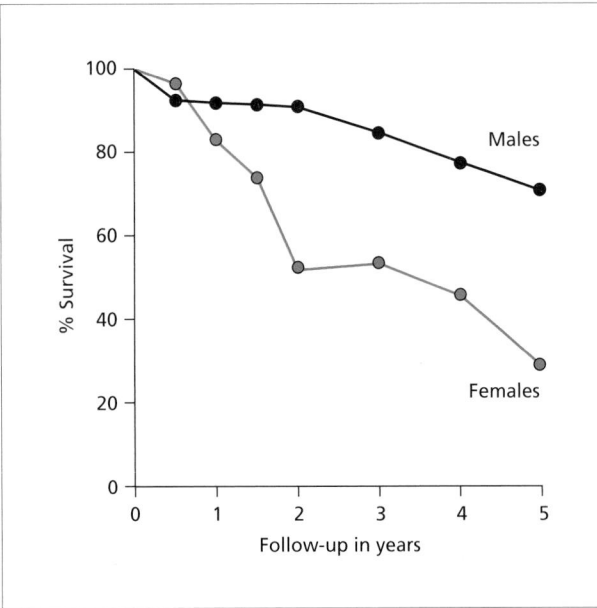

Fig. 20.17. The percentage survival of males and females with alcoholic cirrhosis.

Patients with fibrosis and nodules only, and without hepatitis, have the same prognosis as those with non-cirrhotic liver disease without hepatitis who usually have a fatty liver [76].

Symptoms with independent but bad prognostic significance seem to be encephalopathy, low serum albumin, increased prothrombin time and low haemoglobin level [33, 77]. Patients with pre-coma, persistent jaundice and azotaemia are very liable to develop the hepato-renal syndrome.

The patient with decompensated disease improves slowly. Overt jaundice and ascites after 3 months carry a grave prognosis. In the very late, irreversible stage, abstinence from alcohol cannot be expected to affect the prognosis. The damage has been done and there is no turning back. The highest mortality for patients with either cirrhosis or alcoholic hepatitis or both is in the first year of follow-up [76].

Megamitochondria on liver biopsy categorize a mild illness with a good long-term survival [19].

Patients with acute alcoholic hepatits often deteriorate during the first few weeks in hospital. It may take 1–6 months for resolution, and 20–50% die. Those with a markedly prolonged prothrombin time, unresponsive to intramuscular vitamin K, and with a serum bilirubin level greater than 20 mg, have a particularly bad outlook [56]. Alcoholic hepatitis is slow to resolve even in those who abstain.

In a multi-centre Veterans Hospital study, the combination of cirrhosis and alcoholic hepatitis had the worst prognosis [17]. Predictors of survival were age, grams of alcohol consumed, ratio of AST : ALT and the histological and clinical severity of the disease. Those with poor nutrition who had been starving recently were particularly liable to die [60]. Levels of prothrombin time and bilirubin can be used to determine a *discriminant function* which estimates prognosis in alcoholic hepatitis (fig. 20.18) [14].

Treatment

The most important measure is to ensure total and immediate abstinence from alcohol. Patients with severe physical ailments are more likely to abstain than those who present psychological problems. In a long-term follow-up of men attending a liver clinic, severe medical illness was critical in the decision to stop drinking [80].

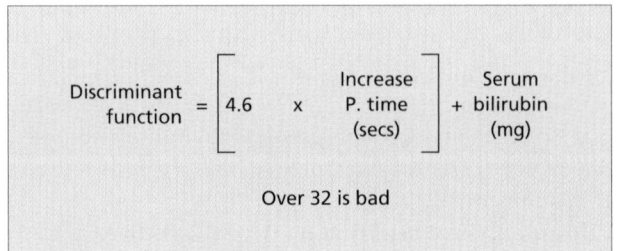

Fig. 20.18. Discriminant function for prognosis in alcoholic hepatitis [14]. P = prothrombin.

Continued medical care is also essential. Follow-up of patients with alcoholic liver disease treated at the Royal Free Hospital between 1975 and 1990 showed 50% remained abstinent, 25% took alcohol but were not abusing it and 25% continued alcohol abuse regardless of therapy. Less severely affected can receive *'brief interventional counselling'* from doctor, nurse or similar person. This results in a 38% treatment benefit albeit often temporary [9]. The more severely affected will need psychiatric referral.

The development of a withdrawal syndrome (*delirium tremens*) should be anticipated by the administration of chlormethiazole or chlordiazepoxide.

Improvement following abstinence and bed rest may be so striking that it is virtually diagnostic of previous alcoholism.

During 'drying out' or recovery from hepatic decompensation, the alcoholic requires dietary supplements of protein and vitamins. Dietary protein should be 0.5 g/kg initially, increasing to 1 g/kg as soon as possible. Encephalopathy may restrict protein intake. Potassium stores are usually low and supplements of potassium chloride together with magnesium and zinc are usually given. Vitamins, especially the B complex, C and K are given in large doses, if necessary intravenously.

Stable middle-class alcoholics should, of course, be advised to abstain completely, particularly if the liver biopsy shows zone 3 fibrosis. If they fail to do so they should be encouraged to take at least 2000 calories daily of a well-balanced diet containing 1 g protein per kg body weight. Modest vitamin supplements are advisable (table 20.9) [89].

Acute alcoholic hepatitis

Ascites is treated cautiously as functional renal failure is a likely development (table 20.10).

The results of *corticosteroid therapy* have been

Table 20.9. Minimum daily requirements for an alcoholic [89]

Item	Amounts	Remarks
Protein	1 g/kg body weight	Eggs, lean meat, cheese, chicken, liver
Calories	2000	Mixed foods with fruit and vegetables
Vitamins		
A	One	or one carrot
B complex	multivitamin	or yeast
C	tablet	or one orange
D		Sunlight
Folate		Good mixed diet
K_1		Good mixed diet

Table 20.10. Treatment of acute alcoholic hepatitis

Stop alcohol
Search precipitant (infections, bleeding, etc.)
Anticipate acute alcohol withdrawal
Intramuscular multivitamins
Treat ascites and encephalopathy
Potassium and zinc supplements
Maintain nitrogen intake—oral or enteral
Consider corticosteroids in severe disease with encephalopathy, without GI bleeding

extremely conflicting. Seven clinical trials in mild or moderately ill patients with acute alcoholic hepatitis seemed to show no effect on clinical recovery, biochemical tests or rate of histological progression. However, more favourable results were reported from a randomized, multi-centre trial. Patients were included with either spontaneous hepatic encephalopathy or a discriminant function value exceeding 32 (fig. 20.18) [14]. Methyl prednisolone (30 mg daily) or placebo were given within 7 days of admission and continued for 28 days when they were tapered over 2 weeks and discontinued. The mortality rate was 35% of 31 receiving placebo, compared with 6% of 35 given prednisolone (*P* = 0.006). The prednisolone therefore decreased short-term mortality. It seemed particularly valuable in those with encephalopathy. The fall in serum bilirubin and prothrombin time was greater in the treated group. A randomized trial [86] and meta-analysis of all trials [38] confirmed initial survival benefit. It is difficult to reconcile these results with the negative ones reported with 12 previous trials, many of which, however, contained only small numbers of patients. A type I error (the control and corticosteroid group not being comparable) or type II error (too many patients included not at risk of death) is possible. Perhaps the patients included in the recent trial were less sick than those in the previous ones. Corticosteroids are probably useful in those with encephalopathy but without bleeding, systemic infections or renal failure. Only about 25% of hospitalized patients with alcoholic hepatitis fulfil all the above criteria for the use of corticosteroids.

Testosterone is of little benefit [34]. Oxandrolone (an anabolic steroid) is useful in those with moderately severe disease but ineffective in those with severe malnutrition and inadequate caloric intake [60].

Severe *protein malnutrition* can favour immuno-incompetence and infections and exacerbate hypoalbuminaemia and ascites. It is clearly important to maintain and improve nutrition particularly during the first few days in hospital. Most patients can take adequate natural protein by mouth. Accelerated improvement may follow the use of casein-based naso-duodenal tube-feeding supplements (1.5 g protein per kg body weight) [43]. There is however only a trend towards increased survival.

Controlled trials of intravenous *amino acid supplementation* have given conflicting results. In one, 70–85 g daily lowered mortality and improved serum bilirubin and albumin concentrations. In another, benefit was transient and not significant. In yet another, sepsis and fluid retention were enhanced in the treated group, although serum bilirubin level was reduced. Trials of branched-chain amino acid enriched enteral diets have shown no effect on mortality. Oral or intravenous amino-acid supplementation should be reserved for a very few jaundiced and severely malnourished patients [73].

Colchicine has failed to improve short-term survival in patients with alcoholic hepatitis [1].

Propylthiouracil. Alcohol induces a hypermetabolic state, potentiating anoxic liver injury in zone 3. Propylthiouracil reduces hypoxic liver injury in hypermetabolic animals and has been used to treat patients with alcoholic liver disease, largely in the cirrhotic stage. A controlled trial confirmed the benefit particularly long-term in those who continued to drink at lower levels [75]. Nevertheless, propylthiouracil has never gained acceptance for the treatment of alcoholic liver disease.

Cirrhosis

Cirrhosis is irreversible and therapy has to be directed at the complications. These include portal hypertension, encephalopathy and ascites. Drug metabolism is impaired and particular care must be taken, especially with sedatives. Diazepam seems to be the safest.

Oral supplementation with a purified soya bean, polyunsaturated, lecithin extract containing 94–98% phosphatidyl choline prevents the development of septal fibrosis and cirrhosis in baboons fed alcohol long term [47]. The mechanism is unknown, but is possibly by stimulating lipocyte collagenase.

Porta-caval shunting, including trans-jugular intra-hepatic portal-systemic stent shunt (TIPPS), in alcoholics is associated with a reduction of bleeding from varices but a 30% incidence of hepatic encephalopathy and only a marginal increase in survival. Results with the selective spleno-renal shunt are less good in alcoholic than in non-alcoholic patients. In general, alcoholics are not good candidates for any surgical procedure, especially if they continue to imbibe.

Hepatic transplantation

End-stage alcoholic liver disease accounts for 20 000 deaths from liver failure per year in the USA. Early mortality results for transplantation are similar to those for other subjects suffering from other types of liver disease. The selection for transplant is difficult (table 20.11) [89].

Table 20.11. Selection of patients with alcoholic liver disease for liver transplantation

Abstinent for 6 months
Child's grade C
Socioeconomically stable
Job to return to
No extra-hepatic organ alcoholic damage

Table 20.12. Liver biopsy follow-up 177–711 days post-transplant of 330 patients having a liver transplant for alcoholic liver disease. 23 definitely resumed alcohol abuse [5]

Definitely resumed alcohol	23
alcoholic hepatitis	22
cirrhosis	4

The cirrhosis is self-inflicted. The patient may return to alcoholism and compliance with immunosuppressive regimes may be poor. Should alcoholics compete with other patients when donor livers are in short supply? Those selected should have a stable psychiatric and socioeconomic background, a job to return to after the transplant and no extra-hepatic, for instance cerebral, alcoholic damage. They should have been abstinent for at least 6 months, indeed this proves the most important predictor of post-transfusion recidivism [78]. Psychiatric advice should be obtained and the candidate should sign an alcohol contract which includes a commitment to abstinence and to alcoholic rehabilitation before and after the operation [31]. The longer the follow-up the worse the recidivism. Alcoholic hepatitis may develop rapidly in the new liver. 23 patients surviving transplant returned to alcohol abuse and within 177–711 days 22 had liver biopsy evidences of alcoholic hepatitis and four of these showed cirrhosis [5] (table 20.12).

Selection is all important [51]. Those patients who are rejected for transplantation because they are too well need continued surveillance as their condition can deteriorate. Those omitted because they are too sick or psychiatrically unsuitable have a significantly lower survival than those transplanted. Hepatic transplantation for acute alcoholic hepatitis, where a period of pre-transplant sobriety is unlikely, is even more difficult to justify than for end-stage alcoholic cirrhosis in a person who has a proven record of compliance. Hepatic transplants should not be performed for acute alcoholic hepatitis until we have reliable techniques to predict recidivism and especially the potential to return to problem drinking [92]. Well-designed controlled trials must be performed [62].

References

1 Akriviadis EA, Steindel H, Pinto PC *et al.* Failure of colchicine to improve short-term survival in patients with alcoholic hepatitis. *Gastroenterology* 1990; **99**: 811.

2 Angeli P, Gatta A, Caregaro L *et al.* Hypophosphatemia and renal tubular dysfunction in alcoholics: are they related to liver function impairment? *Gastroenterology* 1991; **100**: 502.

3 Annoni G, Colombo M, Cantaluppi MC *et al.* Serum type III procollagen peptide and laminin (Lam-P1) detect alcoholic hepatitis in chronic alcohol abusers. *Hepatology* 1989; **9**: 693.

4 Bacon BR, Farahvash MJ, Janney CG *et al.* Non-alcoholic steatohepatitis: an expanded clinical entity. *Gastroenterology* 1994; **107**: 1103.

5 Baddour N, Demetris AJ, Shah G *et al.* The prevalence, rate of onset and spectrum of histologic liver disease in alcohol abusing liver allograft recipients. *Gastroenterology* 1992; **102**: A777.

6 Bell H, Tallaksen C, Sjahel M *et al.* Serum carbohydrate-deficient transferrin as a marker of alcohol consumption in patients with chronic liver disease. *Alcohol Clin. Exp. Res.* 1993; **17**: 246.

7 Bene MC, De Korwin JD, De Ligny BH *et al.* IgA nephropathy and alcoholic liver disease. A prospective necropsy study. *Am. J. Clin. Path.* 1988; **89**: 769.

8 Bigatello LM, Broitman SA, Fattori L *et al.* Endotoxemia, encephalopathy, and mortality in cirrhotic patients. *Am. J. Gastroenterol.* 1987; **82**: 11.

9 Bien TH, Miller WR, Tonigan JS. Brief interventions for alcohol problems: a review. *Addiction* 1993; **88**: 315.

10 Bird GLA, Sheron N, Goka AKJ *et al.* Increased plasma tumor necrosis factor in severe alcoholic hepatitis. *Ann. Intern. Med.* 1990; **112**: 917.

11 Bosron WF, Ehrig T, Li TK. Genetic factors in alcohol metabolism and alcoholism. *Sem. Liver Dis.* 1993; **13**: 126.

12 Bradlow A, Mowat AG. Dupuytren's contracture and alcohol. *Ann. Rheum. Dis.* 1986; **45**: 304.

13 Brunt PW, Kew MC, Scheuer PJ *et al.* Studies in alcoholic liver disease in Britain. I. Clinical and pathological patterns related to natural history. *Gut* 1974; **15**: 52.

14 Carithers RL, Herlong HF, Diehl AM *et al.* Methyl-prednisolone therapy in patients with severe alcoholic hepatitis. A randomized multicenter trial. *Ann. Intern. Med.* 1989; **110**: 685.

15 Casini A, Cunningham M, Rojkind M *et al.* Acetaldehyde increases procollagen type I and fibronectin gene transcription in cultured rat fat-storing cells through a protein synthesis-dependent mechanism. *Hepatology* 1991; **13**: 758.

16 Castillo T, Koop DR, Karmimura S *et al.* Role of cytochrome P-450 2E1 in ethanol-carbon tetrachloride and iron-dependent microsomal lipid peroxidation. *Hepatology* 1992; **16**: 992.

17 Chedid A, Mendenhall CL, Gartside P *et al.* Prognostic factors in alcoholic liver disease. *Am. J. Gastroenterol.* 1991; **86**: 210.

18 Chedid A, Mendenhall CL, Moritz TE *et al.* Cell-mediated hepatic injury in alcoholic liver disease. *Gastroenterology* 1993; **105**: 254.

19 Chedid A, Mendenhall CL, Tosch T *et al.* Significance of megamitochondria in alcoholic liver disease. *Gastroenterology* 1986; **90**: 1858.

20 Day CP, Bassendine MF. Genetic pre-disposition to alcoholic liver disease. *Gut* 1992; **33**: 1444.

21 Deviere J, Vaerman J-P, Content J *et al.* IgA triggers tumour necrosis factor α secretion by monocytes: a study in normal subjects and patients with alcoholic cirrhosis. *Hepatology* 1991; **13**: 670.

22 Edmondson HA, Peters RL, Reynolds TB *et al.* Sclerosing hyaline necrosis of the liver in the chronic alcoholic. A recognizable clinical syndrome. *Ann. Intern. Med.* 1963; **59**: 646.

23 Enomoto N, Takase S, Takada N *et al.* Alcoholic liver disease in heterozygotes of mutant and normal aldehyde dehydrogenase-2 genes. *Hepatology* 1991; **13**: 1071.

24 Fang JWS, Bird GLA, Nakamura T *et al.* Hepatocyte proliferation as an indicator of outcome in acute alcoholic hepatitis. *Lancet* 1994; **343**: 820.

25 Fernández-Checa JC, García-Ruiz C, Ookhtens M *et al.* Impaired uptake of glutathione by hepatic mitochondria from chronic ethanol-fed rats. *J. Clin. Invest.* 1991; **87**: 397.

26 Fong T-L, Kanel GC, Conrad A *et al.* Clinical significance of concomitant hepatitis C infection in patients with alcoholic liver disease. *Hepatology* 1994; **19**: 554.

27 French SW, Nash J, Shitabata P *et al.* Pathology of alcoholic liver disease. *Sem. Liver Dis.* 1993; **13**: 154.

28 Frezza M, Di Padova C, Pozzato G *et al.* High blood alcohol levels in women: the role of decreased gastric alcohol dehydrogenase activity and first-pass metabolism. *N. Engl. J. Med.* 1990; **322**: 95.

29 Fromerty B, Grimbert S, Yensouri A *et al.* Hepatic mitochondrial DNA detection in alcoholics: association with microvesicular steatosis. *Gastroenterology* 1995; **108**: 193.

30 Gavaler JS, Van Thiel DH. Gonadal dysfunction and inadequate sexual performance in alcoholic cirrhotic men (editorial). *Gastroenterology* 1988; **95**: 1680.

31 Gish RG, Lee AH, Keeffe EB *et al.* Liver transplantation for patients with alcoholism and end-stage liver disease. *Am. J. Gastroenterol.* 1993; **88**: 1337.

32 Gluud C, Christoffersen P, Eriksen J *et al.* Influence of ethanol on development of hyperplastic nodules in alcoholic men with micronodular cirrhosis. *Gastroenterology* 1987; **93**: 256.

33 Gluud C, Henriksen JH, Nielsen G. Prognostic indicators in alcoholic cirrhotic men. *Hepatology* 1988; **8**: 222.

34 Gluud C, Wantzin P, Eriksen J. No effect of oral testosterone treatment on sexual dysfunction in alcoholic cirrhotic men. *Gastroenterology* 1988; **95**: 1582.

35 Goodman ZD, Ishak KG. Occlusive venous lesions in alcoholic liver disease. *Gastroenterology* 1982; **83**: 786.

36 Hill DB, Marsano LS, McClain CJ. Increased plasma interleukin-8 concentrations in alcoholic hepatitis. *Hepatology* 1993; **18**: 576.

37 Horn T, Christoffersen P, Henriksen JH. Alcoholic liver injury: defenestration in non-cirrhotic livers — a scanning electron microscopic study. *Hepatology* 1987; **7**: 77.

38 Imperiale TF, McCullough AJ. Do corticosteroids reduce mortality from alcoholic hepatitis? A meta-analysis of the randomized trials. *Ann. Intern. Med.* 1990; **113**: 299.

39 Jakobovits AW, Morgan MY, Sherlock S. Hepatic siderosis in alcoholics. *Dig. Dis. Sci.* 1979; **24**: 305.

40 Jennett RB, Sorrell MF, Saffari-Fard A *et al.* Preferential covalent biding of acetaldehyde to the α-chain of purified rat liver tubulin. *Hepatology* 1989; **9**: 57.

41 Jensen K, Gluud C. The Mallory body: morphological, clinical and experimental studies (part 1 of a literature survey). *Hepatology* 1994; **20**: 1061.

42 Jensen K, Gluud C. The Mallory body: theories on development and pathological significance (part 2 of a literature survey). *Hepatology* 1994; **20**: 1330.

43 Kearns PJ, Youno H, Garcia G *et al.* Accelerated improvement of alcoholic liver disease with enteral nutrition. *Gastroenterology* 1992; **100**: 200.

44 Khoruts A, Stahnke L, McClain CJ *et al.* Circulating tumor necrosis factor, interleukin-1 and interleukin-6 concentrations in chronic alcoholic patients. *Hepatology* 1991; **13**: 267.

45 Klassen LW, Tuma D, Sorrell MF. Immune mechanisms of alcohol-induced liver disease. *Hepatology* 1995; **22**: 355.

46 Lelbach WK. Cirrhosis in the alcoholic and the relation to the volume of alcohol abuse. *Ann. NY Acad. Sci.* 1975; **252**: 85.

47 Lieber CS. Alcohol and the liver: 1994 update. *Gastroenterology* 1994; **106**: 1085.

48 Lieber CS (ed). Alcoholic liver disease. *Sem. Liver Dis.* 1993; **13**: 109.

49 Lieber CS. Medical disorders of alcoholism. *N. Engl. J. Med.* 1995; **333**: 1058.

50 Lieber CS, Robin SJ, Li J *et al.* Phosphatidylcholine protects against fibrosis and cirrhosis in the baboon. *Gastroenterology* 1994; **106**: 152.

51 Lucey MR, Merion RM, Henley KS *et al.* Selection for and outcome of liver transplantation in alcoholic liver disease. *Gastroenterology* 1992; **102**: 1736.

52 Lumeng L. New diagnostic markers of alcohol abuse. *Hepatology* 1986; **4**: 742.

53 Lumeng L, Crabb DW. Genetic aspects and risk factors in alcoholism and alcoholic liver disease. *Gastroenterology* 1994; **107**: 572.

54 McLain CJ, Cohen DA. Increased tumor necrosis factor production by monocytes in alcoholic hepatitis. *Hepatology* 1989; **9**: 349.

55 Maddrey WC. Hepatic effects of acetaminophen. Enhanced toxicity in alcoholics. *J. Clin. Gastroenterol.* 1987; **9**: 180.

56 Maddrey WC, Boitnott JK, Bedine MS *et al.* Corticosteroid therapy of alcoholic hepatitis. *Gastroenterology* 1978; **75**: 193.

57 Marbet UA, Bianchi L, Meury U *et al.* Long-term histological evaluation of the natural history and prognostic factors of alcoholic liver disease. *J. Hepatol.* 1987; **4**: 364.

58 Marshall AW, Kingstone D, Boss M *et al.* Ethanol elimination in males and females: relationship to menstrual cycle and body composition. *Hepatology* 1983; **3**: 701.

59 Matsuoka M, Tsukamoto H. Stimulation of hepatic lipocyte collagen production by Kupffer cell-derived transforming growth factor β: implication for a pathogenetic role in alcoholic liver fibrogenesis. *Hepatology* 1990; **11**: 599.

60 Mendenhall CL, Moritz TE, Roselle GA *et al.* A study of oral nutritional support with oxandrolone in malnourished patients with alcoholic liver hepatitis: results of a Department of Veterans Affairs Cooperative Study. *Hepatology* 1993; **17**: 564.

61 Mihas AA, Tavassoli M. Laboratory markers of ethanol intake and abuse: a critical appraisal. *Am. J. Med. Sci.* 1992; **303**: 415.

62 Miller C, Kamean J, Berk PD. Liver transplantation for alcoholic hepatitis? An unanswered question. *Alcohol Clin. Exp. Res.* 1994; **18**: 224.

63 Minato Y, Hasumura Y, Takeuchi J. The role of fat-storing cells in Dissë space fibrogenesis in alcoholic liver disease. *Hepatology* 1983; **3**: 559.

64 Morgan MY, Sherlock S. Sex-related differences among 100 patients with alcoholic liver disease. *Br. Med. J.* 1977; **i**: 939.

65 Morgan MY, Sherlock S, Scheuer PJ. Acute cholestasis, hepatic failure and fatty liver in the alcoholic. *Scand. J. Gastroenterol.* 1978; **13**: 299.

66 Morgan MY, Sherlock S, Scheuer PJ. Portal fibrosis in the livers of alcoholic patients. *Gut* 1978; **19**: 1015.

67 Moss AH, Siegler M. Should alcoholics compete equally for liver transplantation? *JAMA* 1991; **265**: 1295.

68 Nalpas B, Vassault A, Charpin S *et al.* Serum mitochondrial aspartate aminotransferase as a marker of chronic alcoholism: diagnostic value and interpretation in a Liver Unit. *Hepatology* 1986; **4**: 608.

69 Neuberger J, Crossley IR, Saunders JB *et al.* Antibodies to alcohol-altered liver cell determinants in patients with alcoholic liver disease. *Gut* 1984; **25**: 300.

70 Niemela O, Risteli J, Blake JE *et al.* Markers of fibrogenesis and basement membrane formation in alcoholic liver disease. Relation to severity, presence of hepatitis, and alcohol intake. *Gastroenterology* 1990; **98**: 1612.

71 Nishiguchi S, Kuroki T, Yabusako T *et al.* Detection of hepatitis C virus antibodies and hepatitis C virus RNA in patients with alcoholic liver disease. *Hepatology* 1991; **14**: 985.

72 Nissenbaum M, Chedid A, Mendenhall C *et al.* Prognostic significance of cholestatic alcoholic hepatitis. *Dig. Dis. Sci.* 1990; **35**: 891.

73 Nompleggi DJ, Bonkovsky HL. Nutritional supplementation in chronic liver disease: an analytical review. *Hepatology* 1994; **19**: 518.

74 Orrego H, Blake JE, Blendis LM *et al.* Long-term treatment of alcoholic liver disease with propylthiouracil. *N. Engl. J. Med.* 1987; **317**: 1421.

75 Orrego H, Blake JE, Blendis LM *et al.* Long-term treatment of alcoholic liver disease with propylthiouracil. Part 2: Influence of drop-out rates and of continued alcohol consumption in a clinical trial. *J. Hepatol.* 1994; **20**: 343.

76 Orrego H, Blake JE, Blendis LM *et al.* Prognosis of alcoholic cirrhosis in the presence and absence of alcoholic hepatitis. *Gastroenterology* 1987; **92**: 208.

77 Orrego H, Israel Y, Blake JE *et al.* Assessment of prognostic factors in alcoholic liver disease: toward a global quantitative expression of severity. *Hepatology* 1983; **3**: 896.

78 Osorio RW, Ascher NL, Avery M *et al.* Predicting recidivism after orthotopic liver transplantation for alcoholic liver disease. *Hepatology* 1994; **20**: 105.

79 Pare P, Reynolds TB. Impaired renal acidification in alcoholic liver disease. *Arch. Intern. Med.* 1984; **144**: 941.

80 Patek AJ Jr, Hermos JA. Recovery from alcoholism in cirrhotic patients: a study of 45 cases. *Am. J. Med.* 1981; **70**: 782.

81 Pequignot G, Cyrulnik F. Chronic disease due to overconsumption of alcoholic drinks (excepting neuropsychiatric pathology). In *International Encyclopaedia of Pharmacology and Therapeutics*, vol. II, Chapter 14. Pergamon Press, Oxford, 1970; 375–412.

82 Perrillo RP, Griffin R, De Schryver-Kecskemeti K *et al.* Alcoholic liver disease presenting with marked elevation

of serum alkaline phosphatase. A combined clinical and pathological study. *Am. J. Dig. Dis.* 1978; **23**: 1061.

83 Phillips GB, Gabuzda GJ Jr, Davidson CS. Comparative effects of a purified and an adequate diet on the course of fatty cirrhosis in the alcoholic. *J. Clin. Invest.* 1952; **31**: 351.

84 Powell WJ Jr, Klatskin G. Duration of survival in patients with Laennec's cirrhosis. *Am. J. Med.* 1968; **44**: 406.

85 Prijatmoko D, Strauss PJG, Lambert JR *et al.* Early detection of protein depletion in alcoholic cirrhosis: role of body composition analysis. *Gastroenterology* 1993; **105**: 1839.

86 Ramond M, Poynard T, Rueff B *et al.* A randomized trial of prednisolone in patients with severe alcoholic hepatitis. *N. Engl. J. Med.* 1992; **326**: 507.

87 Reynolds TB, Redeker AG, Kuzma OT. Role of alcohol in pathogenesis of alcoholic cirrhosis. In McIntyre N & Sherlock S, eds. *Therapeutic Agents and the Liver.* Blackwell Scientific Publications, Oxford, 1965; 131.

88 Rogers AE, Fox JG, Whitney K *et al.* Acute and chronic effects of ethanol in non-human primates. In Hayes KC, ed. *Primates in Nutritional Research.* Academic Press, New York, 1979; 249.

89 Sherlock S. Alcoholic liver disease. *Lancet* 1995; **345**: 227.

90 Situnayake RD, Crump BJ, Thurnham DI *et al.* Lipid peroxidation and hepatic antioxidants in alcoholic liver disease. *Gut* 1990; **31**: 1311.

91 Sorensen TIA, Orholm M, Bentsen KD *et al.* Prospective evaluation of alcohol abuse and alcoholic liver injury in men as predictors of development of cirrhosis. *Lancet* 1984; **ii**: 241.

92 Sorrell MF, Zetterman RK, Donovan JP. Alcoholic hepatitis

93 Svegliati-Baroni G, Baraona E, Rosman AS *et al.* Collagen-acetaldehyde adducts in alcoholic and nonalcoholic liver diseases. *Hepatology* 1994; **20**: 111.

94 Takase S, Takada N, Enomoto N *et al.* Different types of chronic hepatitis in alcoholic patients: does chronic hepatitis induced by alcohol exist? *Hepatology* 1991; **13**: 876.

95 Uchida T, Kao H, Quispe-Sjogren M *et al.* Alcoholic foamy degeneration — a pattern of acute alcoholic injury of the liver. *Gastroenterology* 1983; **84**: 683.

96 Van de Weil A, Delacroix DL, van Hattum J *et al.* Characteristics of serum IgA and liver IgA deposits in alcoholic liver disease. *Hepatology* 1987; **7**: 95.

97 Wodak AD, Saunders JB, Ewuis-Mensah I *et al.* Severity of alcohol dependence in patients with alcoholic liver disease. *Br. Med. J.* 1983; **287**: 1420.

98 Worman HJ. Cellular intermediate filament networks and their derangement in alcoholic hepatitis. *Alcohol Clin. Exp. Res.* 1990; **14**: 789.

99 Worner TM, Lieber CS. Perivenular fibrosis as precursor lesion of cirrhosis. *JAMA* 1985; **253**: 627.

100 Zignego AL, Forschi M, Laffi G *et al.* 'Inapparent' hepatitis B virus infection and hepatitis C virus replication in alcoholic subjects with and without liver disease. *Hepatology* 1994; **19**: 577.

101 Zimmerman HJ, Maddrey WC. Acetaminophen (paracetamol) hepatotoxicity with regular intake of alcohol: analysis of instances of therapeutic misadventure. *Hepatology* 1995; **22**: 767.

and liver transplantation: the controversy continues. *Alcohol Clin. Exp. Res.* 1994; **18**: 222.

Chapter 21
Iron Overload States

Normal iron metabolism

The normal daily diet contains about 10–20 mg of iron (90% free; 10% bound in haem). Of this 1–1.5 mg is absorbed. This amount depends on body stores, more being absorbed the greater the need. The absorption process, sited in the upper small intestine, is active and capable of transporting iron against a gradient. The mechanisms involved, however, are not understood. Transport proteins have been identified but await confirmation.

In the mucosal cell iron enters a cytosolic pool. Some passes to be stored in ferritin, and thence either mobilized or lost with exfoliation of mucosal cells. That destined for cellular metabolism in other tissues passes to, and crosses, the basolateral surface of the cell (by an unknown mechanism), and is bound to transferrin, the major transport protein in the blood.

Transferrin (mol. wt 77 000 Da) is a glycoprotein largely synthesized in the liver. It can bind two ferric iron molecules, and is responsible for the 'total iron binding capacity' of serum of 250–370 µg/dl. This is normally about one-third saturated with iron. Physiological entry of iron into reticulocytes and hepatocytes depends upon transferrin receptors at the cell surface which preferentially bind transferrin carrying iron. The receptor/iron complex is internalized and the iron released. This process is saturable. Transferrin receptors are downregulated as the cell becomes replete with iron. When transferrin is fully saturated, as in overt haemochromatosis, iron circulates in 'non-transferrin bound' forms, associated with low molecular weight chelators. Iron in this form readily enters cells by a non-saturable process.

Iron is stored in cells as ferritin (mol. wt 480 000 Da), the combination of the protein apoferritin (H and L subunits) and iron, which appears under electron microscopy as particles 50 Å in diameter lying free in the cytoplasm. Up to 4500 atoms of iron can be stored within a single ferritin molecule. High concentrations of iron stimulate apoferritin synthesis.

Aggregates of degraded ferritin molecules make up haemosiderin which stains as blue granules with ferrocyanide. Approximately one-third of iron is stored in this form, increasing in iron storage disorders.

Lipofuscin, or wear and tear pigment, accumulates in association with iron overload. It is yellow–brown in colour and does not contain iron.

Iron contained in depots as ferritin or haemosiderin is available for mobilization and haemoglobin formation should the demand arise.

The normal total body content of iron is about 4 g, of which 3 g are present in haemoglobin, myoglobin, catalase and other respiratory pigments or enzymes. Storage iron comprises 0.5 g; of this 0.3 g is in the liver but is not revealed by the usual histological stains for iron. The liver is the predominant site for storage of iron absorbed from the gut. When its capacity is exceeded, iron is deposited in other parenchymal tissues, including the acinar cells of the pancreas, and the cells of the anterior pituitary gland. The reticulo-endothelial system plays only a limited part in iron storage unless the iron is given intravenously, when it becomes the preferential site for deposition. Iron from erythrocyte breakdown is concentrated in the spleen.

Iron overload and liver damage

Fibrosis and hepato-cellular damage are directly related to the iron content of the liver cell. The pattern of damage is similar irrespective of whether the overload is due to genetic haemochromatosis or to multiple transfusions. The severity of fibrosis is maximal in peri-portal areas where iron is particularly deposited. Chronic liver damage with fibrosis has been produced in rats by dietary carbonyl iron overload [46].

When iron deposition is low it is stored as ferritin. As the load increases more is present as haemosiderin.

Removal of iron by venesections or chelation leads to clinical and biochemical improvement with reduction or prevention of hepatic fibrosis [14].

There are several processes by which iron can damage the liver. Iron causes lipid peroxidation of membranes of organelles leading to functional defects of lysosomes, mitochondria and microsomes [4]. Mitochondrial cytochrome C oxidase activity is reduced [5]. There is lysosomal membrane fragility and release of hydrolytic enzymes into the cytosol. Hepatic stellate cells (lipocytes) are activated in animal models of iron overload [60] and collagen type 1 synthesis is stimulated [51]. The precise events leading to stellate cell activation are under study. Anti-oxidant treatment protects against hepatic fibrosis in an animal model of iron overload [52].

Genetic haemochromatosis

Described in 1886 as *bronze diabetes* [29], this is an autosomal recessive metabolic disorder in which there is increased iron absorption over many years [27]. The tissues contain enormous quantities of iron, of the order of 20–60g. If 5mg dietary iron were retained by the tissues daily it would take about 28 years for 50g to accumulate.

Molecular genetics

Sheldon [65] in his classical monograph described idiopathic haemochromatosis as an inborn error of metabolism. The discovery of genetic linkage of haemochromatosis to the HLA-serotype allowed the inheritance to be defined as autosomal recessive, and placed the gene on chromosome 6 [66]. Studies of Caucasian populations show 0.3% to be homozygote (affected) and 8–10% heterozygote (carriers) [66].

Genetic linkage to HLA-A was tight with a recombination fraction of 0.01 (1% recombination) [66]. The area around HLA-A (fig. 21.1) was therefore the first area to be searched for a candidate gene for haemochromatosis but none was found. Molecular techniques allowed the assembling of genomic DNA resources telomeric to HLA-A and the identification of new polymorphic markers. Linkage disequilibrium studies using these showed closer association of haemochromatosis with D_6S_{105} [33, 74], and subsequently D_6S_{1260} [59] (fig. 21.1). Further fine-linkage and haplotype analysis suggested that the gene lay between D_6S_{2238} and D_6S_{2241} [26], 3–4 Mb telomeric to HLA-A. A comprehensive search for new genes in the 250kb between these markers showed

one, designated 'HLA-H', in which a mutation (Cys282Tyr) was present in approximately 85% of haemochromatotic chromosomes compared with 3% of control chromosomes [26]. Eighty-three per cent of patients with haemochromatosis were homozygous for this mutation.

This candidate gene has homology to HLA, and the mutation seems to be in a region critical for normal function. However, studies of the protein product and its role in iron metabolism are awaited to confirm whether this is the haemochromatosis gene. The only previous link between HLA and iron metabolism is the β_2-microglobulin knock-out mouse [62] in which iron accumulates by an unknown mechanism.

In previous studies approximately 50% of chromosomes carrying the haemochromatosis defect were found to have a common set of marker alleles between HLA-A and D_6S_{1260}, rarely found among non-haemochromatotic individuals. This has been termed the ancestral or founder haplotype [34, 59]. It is thought to be· the haplotype of the first individual with haemochromatosis and now includes the recently described mutated candidate gene. Comparison of the haplotype with the degree of iron overload has shown that the founder haplotype correlates with more severe overload [17, 53]. Based on iron studies, it has also been suggested that the heterozygote state may protect against iron deficiency [17], which might give a survival advantage and explain why haemochromatosis is one of the most frequent single gene disorders.

Because of the tight linkage of haemochromatosis to HLA, serotyping is of value in identifying affected siblings of a proband before iron accumulation has occurred [11]. Mutation analysis of the haemochromatosis gene should replace this in the future.

Heterozygotes

One-quarter of heterozygotes have mild elevation of serum iron indices, but these patients do not develop

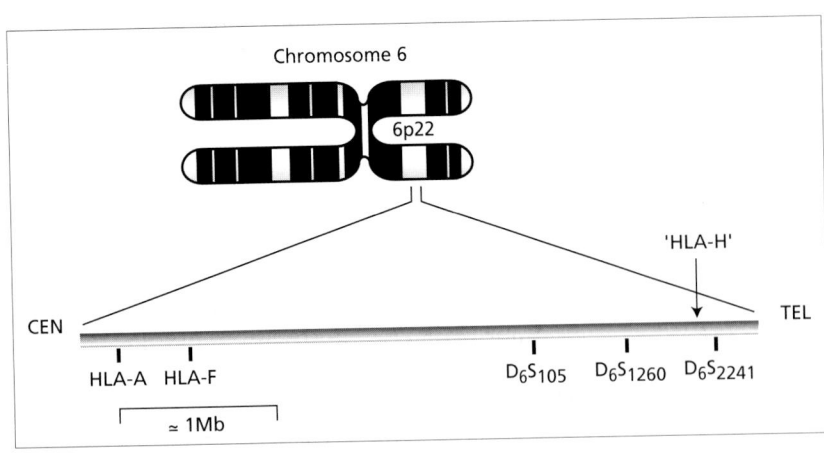

Fig. 21.1. Region of the haemochromatosis gene on the short arm of chromosome 6 implicated by linkage and haplotype analysis. Positional cloning has identified a possible candidate gene, 'HLA-H' [26]. CEN = centromeric; TEL = telomeric.

iron overload or tissue damage [11]. However, it is possible that heterozygotes accumulate iron if they suffer from another disturbance in iron metabolism such as haemolytic anaemia [41].

Pathogenesis

At present this is not known. Intestinal absorption of iron, greater than normal and inappropriate for the accumulating body iron stores, dates from birth. Absorption only becomes 'normal' (but still excessive for the iron replete state) when storage iron reaches injurious levels and then increases again after iron stores have been reduced by venesection [72].

The mechanism controlling iron absorption is unknown as is the defect leading to genetic haemochromatosis. The presence and role of a specific microvillous-membrane iron transporter remains to be confirmed. Whether the intestinal mucosal cell itself regulates absorption by an unknown mechanism, or whether a signal from liver, bone marrow or reticulo-endothelial cell is the controlling influence remains speculation. However, duodenal ferritin mRNA and protein expression are reduced in genetic haemochromatosis [50] suggesting that the cell may be reacting as if iron deficient [40].

To date, no abnormality of ferritin or transferrin structure has been found in genetic haemochromatosis. There is, however, a failure to downregulate duodenal, but not hepatic, transferrin receptors [40, 64]. The genetic defect is on chromosome 6, ruling out the primary involvement of ferritin subunits (expressed from chromosomes 11 (H subunit) and 19 (L subunit)), transferrin (chromosome 3), transferrin receptor (chromosome 3) or the protein interacting with iron response elements (chromosome 9). Characterization of the protein expressed by the candidate gene on chromosome 6, if confirmed as the haemochromatosis gene, will provide new insights into the control of iron metabolism.

Pathology

A fibrous tissue reaction is found wherever the iron is deposited.

The *liver* in the early stages may show only portal zone fibrosis with deposition of iron in the peri-portal liver cells and, to a lesser extent, in the Kupffer cells. Fibrous septa then surround groups of lobules and irregularly shaped nodules (*holly-leaf* appearance). There is partial preservation of the architecture, although ultimately a macronodular cirrhosis develops (fig. 21.2). Fatty change is unusual and the glycogen content of the liver cells is normal.

Cirrhotic patients with iron-free foci have a higher risk of developing hepatocellular carcinoma [20].

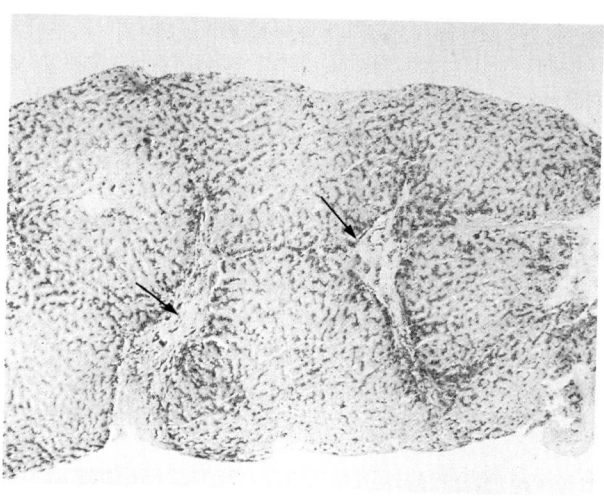

Fig. 21.2. The liver in genetic haemochromatosis. Cirrhosis is seen, the liver cells being filled with blue-staining iron pigment. Fibrous tissue is also infiltrated with iron. The arrows indicate portal tracts. (Stained Perls, ×13.)

The *pancreas* shows fibrosis and parenchymal degeneration with iron deposition in acinar cells, macrophages, islets of Langerhans and fibrous tissue.

Heart muscle is heavily involved, muscle fibres being replaced by a mass of iron pigment within the sheath. Degeneration of the fibres is rare. Coronary sclerosis, however, is common.

Spleen, bone marrow and duodenal epithelium do not show the iron overload seen elsewhere. *Brain* and *nervous tissue* are also usually free of iron.

Epidermal atrophy may reduce the *skin* to a flattened sheet. Hair follicles and sebaceous glands are inconspicuous. Characteristically the melanin content of the basal layer is increased. Iron is usually absent from the epidermis but can often be seen deeper, especially in the basal layer.

Endocrine glands, including adrenal cortex, anterior lobe of pituitary, and thyroid show varying amounts of iron and fibrosis.

The testes are small and soft with atrophy of the germinal epithelium without iron overload. There is interstitial fibrosis and iron is found in the walls of capillaries.

Relation to alcoholism

Alcoholism is frequent in patients with clinical haemochromatosis, but low among asymptomatic relatives with disordered iron metabolism [71]. Abuse of alcohol may accelerate the accumulation of iron in a subject genetically disposed to the disease. In patients, the combination of haemochromatosis and excess alcohol intake results in more advanced liver disease [2]. In an experimental model of alcoholic liver disease, the addition of iron to the diet results in cirrhosis [69].

Clinical features

The classical picture (fig. 21.3) is of a lethargic, middle-aged man with pigmentation, hepatomegaly, diminished sexual activity and loss of body hair; diabetes is common.

Diagnosis depends on a high degree of suspicion and should be considered in any male with symptomless hepatomegaly and virtually normal biochemical tests of liver function. In view of the high heterozygote frequency in the community, the condition must be considerably more frequent than is recognized. There is a mean delay of 5–8 years between presentation and diagnosis [1].

Overt haemochromatosis is 10 times more frequent in males than females [27, 65]. Women are spared by iron loss with menstruation and pregnancy. Female patients with haemochromatosis usually, but not always [39], have absent or scanty menstruation, have had a hysterectomy, or are many years post-menopausal. Families have been reported which included two generatons of women, two of whom were menstruating [39]. Familial juvenile haemochromatosis is described [37, 47]. The symptoms appear earlier in males than in females.

Haemochromatosis is rarely diagnosed before the age of 20, and the peak incidence is between 40 and 60. Chil-

dren developing the disease show a more acute course, presenting with skin pigmentation, endocrine changes and cardiac disease [47].

The grey-slaty pigmentation is maximal in the axillae, groins, genitalia, old scars and exposed parts. It can occur in the mouth. The colour, due to increased melanin in the basal layer, appears through the atrophied, superficial epidermis. The skin is shiny, thin and dry, like that of eunuchs.

Hepatic changes

The liver is enlarged and firm. Abdominal pain, usually a dull ache with hepatic tenderness, is noted in 37% of cases [27]. The pain may be so severe that an acute abdominal emergency is simulated. Circulatory collapse and sudden death can occur. The mechanism is obscure, although release of ferritin, a vasoactive substance, from the liver has been postulated.

Signs of hepato-cellular failure are usually absent and ascites rare. The spleen is palpable but rarely large. Bleeding from oesophageal varices is unusual.

Primary liver cancer develops in 15–30% of cirrhotic patients [21, 27, 42]. It may be the mode of presentation, particularly in the elderly. It should be suspected if the patient shows clinical deterioration with rapid liver enlargement, abdominal pain and ascites. Serum α-fetoprotein may be increased.

Endocrine changes

Clinical diabetes is present in about two-thirds [23]. This may be complicated by nephropathy, neuropathy, peripheral vascular disease and proliferative retinopathy [23]. The diabetes may be easy to control or may be resistant to large doses of insulin. It could be related to a family history of diabetes, to cirrhosis of the liver which impairs glucose tolerance, or to direct damage to the pancreas by iron deposition.

Pituitary function is impaired to a variable extent in about two-thirds of patients. This can be related to iron deposition in the anterior pituitary, and not to the severity of liver disease or to the degree of abnormality of iron metabolism. Gonadotrophin producing cells are selectively affected. Basal serum prolactin and luteinizing hormone levels are low with impaired response to thyroid or luteinizing releasing hormones [70] or to clomiphene. Hypogonadotrophic testicular failure is shown by impotence, loss of libido, testicular atrophy, skin atrophy and loss of secondary sexual hair. Plasma testosterone levels are subnormal. Testosterone levels increase following administration of gonadotrophins suggesting that the testes are capable of responding.

Pan-hypopituitarism with hypothyroidism and adrenal cortico-deficiency are rarer.

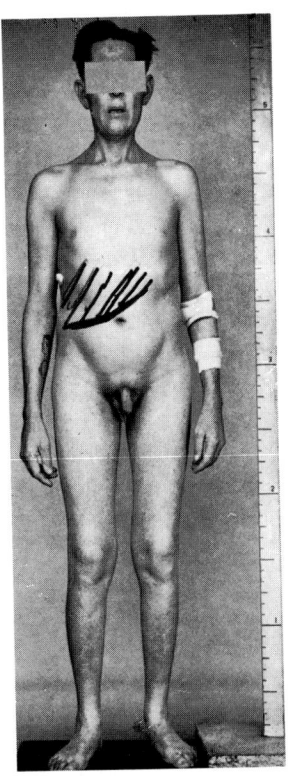

Fig. 21.3. Pigmented man showing loss of secondary sexual hair, gonadal atrophy and hepatomegaly.

Cardiac changes

Changes on ECG are reported in 88% of patients presenting with haemochromatosis [42]. Presentation with heart failure particularly in younger subjects is seen but is unusual. The picture is of progressive right-sided heart failure sometimes with sudden death. Constrictive pericarditis or cardiomyopathy may be simulated. The 'iron heart' is a weak one. The heart is globular in shape. Arrhythmias are also seen.

Cardiac complications are presumably related to iron deposits in the myocardium and conducting system.

Arthropathy

In about two-thirds of patients a specific arthropathy starts in the metacarpophalangeal joints. Wrists and hips may also be affected [24]. It may be a presenting feature. It is related to an acute crystal synovitis with calcium pyrophosphate. Radiologically there is a hypertrophic osteoarthritis [3]. Chondrocalcinosis is seen in menisci and articular cartilage (fig. 21.4).

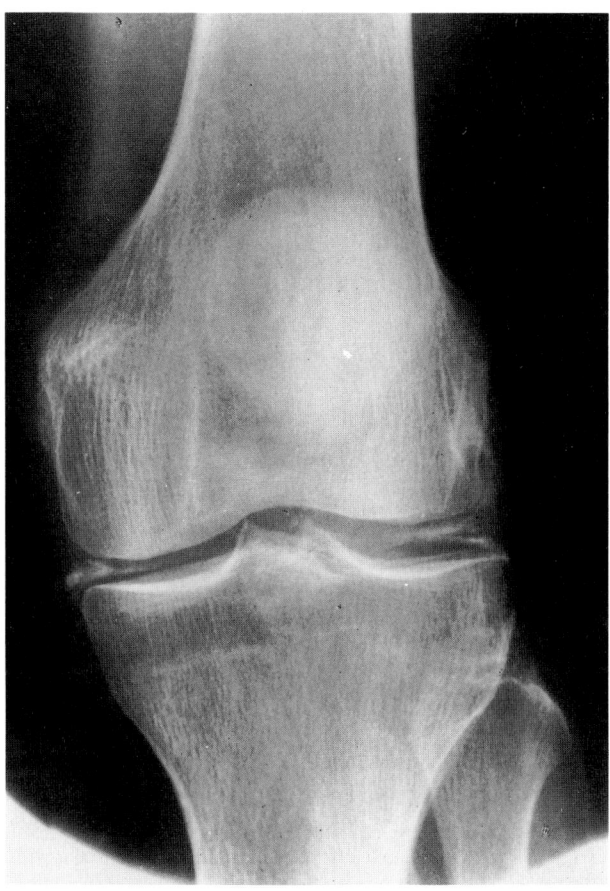

Fig. 21.4. Genetic haemochromatosis. Radiograph of the knee joint shows chondrocalcinosis in menisci and articular cartilage. (Courtesy M. Barry.)

Special investigations

Biochemical tests show surprisingly little disturbance. Later the changes are those of cirrhosis.

The *serum iron* is raised to about 220 µg/dl compared with the normal of about 125 µg/dl. The *serum transferrin* is about 90% saturated compared with 30% in the normal.

Serum ferritin

Ferritin is the major cellular iron-storage protein. The form present in normal serum contains little iron. Its function there is uncertain. The concentration is proportional to body iron stores (fig. 21.5). It is of value in assessing uncomplicated iron overload [56], but can be unreliable in early diagnosis of the pre-cirrhotic stage. A normal value does not exclude iron storage disease [13, 56]. It is useful in following treatment.

With severe hepato-cellular necrosis, serum ferritin levels increase as it is released from liver cells [56]. High serum ferritin levels are also seen with some cancers.

Needle liver biopsy

This is the best method of confirming the diagnosis and will show the degree of hepatic fibrosis/cirrhosis and of iron loading. The amount of iron in the specimen correlates well with total body iron [9]. A tough, fibrous liver may cause technical difficulties, but if a sample is obtained, this shows the characteristic pigmentary cirrhosis (fig. 21.2).

The liver section is stained with Perls' reagent. Visual scoring of the iron load (0–4+) depends upon the percentage of parenchymal cells with positive staining (0–100%). Chemical measurement of iron should be made. This can be done on tissue extracted from the paraffin block if fresh tissue was not provided [44]. From the iron content (µg or µmol/g dry weight) the hepatic iron index is calculated (µmol/g dry weight divided by age in years). In the homozygote haemochromatosis patient, hepatic iron is related to age [12], and the hepatic iron index has been validated as a method of differentiating homozygotes (index greater than 1.9) from heterozygotes (less than 1.5) (fig. 21.6) [67] and patients with alcoholic liver disease [12], both of whom may have a raised ferritin and/or percent saturation.

In the absence of other pathology (for example transfusion iron overload, alcohol, hepatitis C, haematological diseases) moderate to heavy (3+ to 4+) siderosis will be due to genetic haemochromatosis. Chemical measurement of iron and calculation of the hepatic iron index will confirm this. If siderosis is mild to moderate (1+ to 2+), and/or another confusing pathology is present (alcohol, hepatitis C), then measurement of the liver

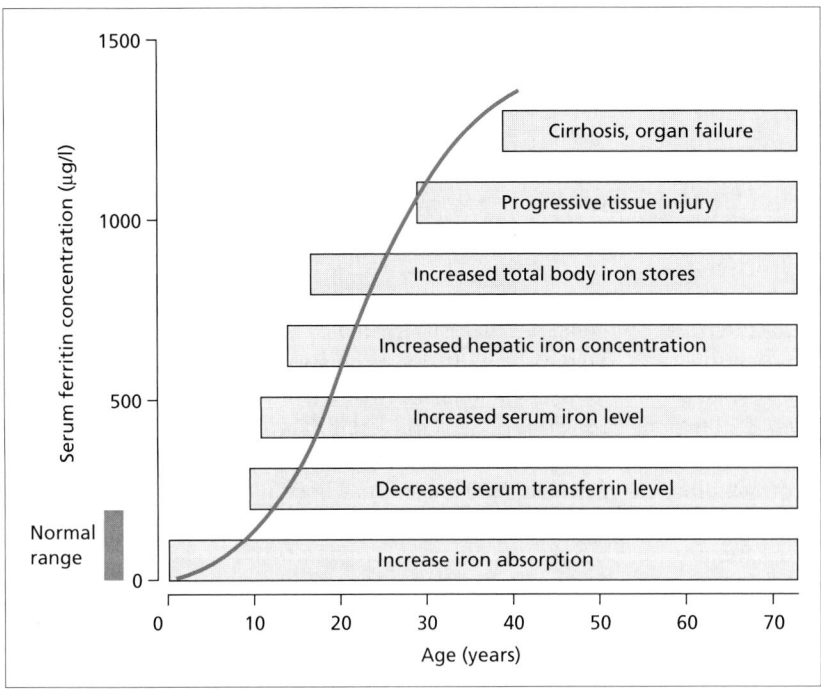

Fig. 21.5. Natural history of genetic haemochromatosis. Progression of events leading to the clinical syndrome [56].

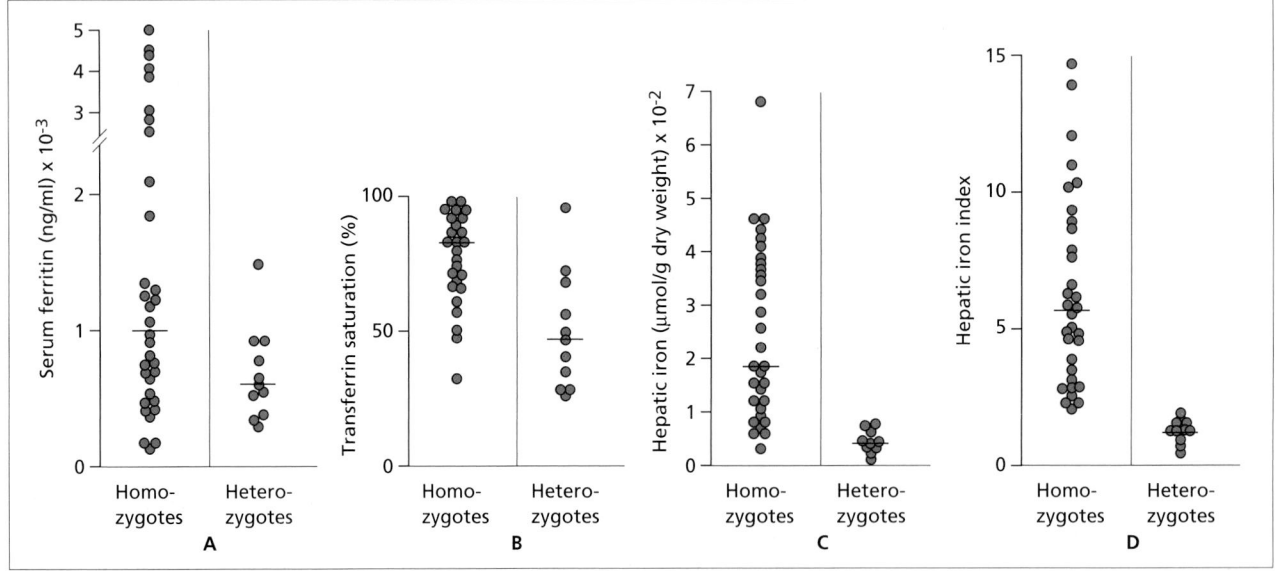

Fig. 21.6. Iron indices in men with haemochromatosis. Note that only the hepatic iron index (D) clearly separates homozygotes (left-hand panels) from heterozygotes (right-hand panels). There is overlap for serum ferritin (A), transferrin saturation (B) and hepatic iron concentration (C). The same was found for women with haemochromatosis. Horizontal lines are mean values (modified from [67]).

iron index is essential to distinguish patients with genetic haemochromatosis.

The index has no place, however, in the evaluation of patients with transfusion iron overload.

Liver biopsy is not necessary to follow de-ironing during treatment. Serum iron indices are sufficient.

Imaging

Using single energy *CT scanning*, hepatic attenuation correlates with serum ferritin, but it is unable to detect hepatic iron overload less than five times the normal limit (40% of patients) [15].

The accuracy is greatly improved if dual-energy CT scanning is available.

MRI detects iron which is a naturally occurring paramagnetic contrast agent. In overload states, marked decreases in T2 relaxation time are shown.

Although both CT and MRI detect heavy iron overload, they are not yet sufficiently precise to predict hepatic iron concentrations with accuracy.

Differential diagnosis

Serum iron and per cent saturation, as well as serum ferritin, are sometimes increased in cirrhosis due to causes other than genetic haemochromatosis. These include alcohol and hepatitis C. The clinical picture may confuse, since the association of diabetes mellitus and cirrhosis is not uncommon, and patients with cirrhosis may become impotent, hairless and develop skin pigmentation. Hepato-cellular failure, however, is usually minimal in haemochromatosis. Liver biopsy resolves any doubt. Although hepatic siderosis is frequent in alcoholics (57%), significant siderosis is rare (7%). Calculation of the hepatic iron index differentiates genetic haemochromatosis (index greater than 1.9) from other causes of increased liver iron.

The distinction from other forms of secondary iron overload is discussed later.

Prognosis

Much depends upon the amount and duration of iron overload. Early diagnosis and treatment is central to improving prognosis. Those treated in the pre-cirrhotic stage and before diabetes mellitus has developed, and who subsequently have normal iron levels maintained by phlebotomy, have a normal life expectancy [42]. This is important for patients applying for life insurance [55].

Cardiac failure worsens the outlook and such patients rarely survive longer than 1 year without treatment. Hepatic failure or bleeding oesophageal varices are rare terminal features.

The outlook is better than for cirrhosis in alcoholics who stop drinking. However, the patient with haemochromatosis who also abuses alcohol does worse than the abstinent patient.

The risk of developing hepato-cellular carcinoma in haemochromatotic patients with cirrhosis is increased about 200 times [42] and is not reduced by de-ironing [14]. A minority (approx. 15%) of hepato-cellular carcinoma develop in non-cirrhotic haemochromatotic liver [21]—as is found for hepato-cellular carcinoma related to other aetiologies.

Treatment

Iron can be removed by venesection and can be mobilized from tissue stores at rates as high as 130 mg/day [18]. Blood regeneration is extraordinarily rapid, haemo-

globin production increasing to six or seven times normal. Large quantities of blood must be removed, for 500 ml removes only 250 mg of iron, whereas the tissues contain up to 200 times this amount. Depending on the initial iron stores, the amount necessary to reduce them effectively varies from 7 to 45 g. Venesections of 500 ml are carried out weekly, or even twice weekly in particularly co-operative patients, and continued until serum iron, percentage saturation, and ferritin levels fall into the low normal range. Comparison of a venesection-treated with an untreated group showed a survival of 8.2 compared with 4.9 years and a 5-year mortality of 11% compared with 67% [57, 72]. Venesection treatment results in increased well-being and gain in weight. Pigmentation and hepatosplenomegaly decrease. Liver function tests improve. Control of diabetes improves in some patients [14]. The arthropathy is unaffected. Cardiac failure may decrease [61]. Hypogonadism may lessen in men aged less than 40 years at diagnosis [19]. In two patients, serial hepatic biopsies showed apparent reversal of established cirrhosis [57]. This would agree with the type of fibrosis seen in haemochromatosis; architecture is preserved so making reversibility possible.

Rates of iron accumulation vary between 1.4 and 4.8 mg daily [14] and after de-ironing a 500 ml venesection every 3 months should prevent iron accumulation. A low iron diet is impossible to achieve.

Gonadal atrophy may be treated by replacement therapy with an intramuscular, depot testosterone. Human chorionic gonadotrophin (HCG) injections will increase testicular volume and sperm counts.

Diabetes should be treated by diet and, if necessary, insulin. Resistant cases may be encountered.

The *cardiac complications* respond poorly to the usual measures but can be reversible with venesection [61].

Transplantation

The survival of patients with genetic haemochromatosis after liver transplant is less than for other recipients (53% versus 81% survival at 25 months) [25]. The lower survival is related to cardiac complications and sepsis, emphasizing the need for early diagnosis and treatment [55].

Follow-up of haemochromatotic patients receiving a normal liver, and non-haemochromatotics inadvertently transplanted with a haemochromatotic liver, has not resolved whether or not the liver is the site of the metabolic defect [54].

Screening for early haemochromatosis in relatives

First-degree relatives, particularly siblings, should be screened so that treatment may be started before tissue damage occurs. If serum iron, percentage transferrin saturation and serum ferritin are within the normal range, iron stores are normal. The combination of an increased transferrin saturation (greater than 50%) with an elevated serum ferritin concentration (greater than 200 µg/litre in men or 150 µg/litre in women) is 94% sensitive and 86% specific for genetic haemochromatosis in younger homozygotes [10]. If any one of the tests is persistently abnormal, liver biopsy, with measurement of hepatic iron and iron index, is indicated. If homozygous haemochromatosis is confirmed, the relative, even if symptom free, should be venesected.

Affected siblings may also be identified by comparing their HLA-A serotype with that of the proband. Any sibling whose serotype is the same as the proband is at risk of developing homozygous haemochromatosis. Mutation analysis will soon replace HLA typing. Progressive iron overload does not develop in heterozygotes [11].

The risk of children of an affected individual developing haemochromatosis is low since the affected parent would have to marry a heterozygote (carrier)—a risk of approximately 1 in 10. However, serum iron, percent saturation and ferritin should be measured in all children in their teenage years so that early iron overload can be detected. When the haemochromatosis gene is securely identified, mutation analysis should simplify the diagnosis in affected individuals.

Population screening

Screening the Caucasian population for genetic haemochromatosis using transferrin saturation is cost-effective [7, 49]. Screening of selected groups is also valuable. Genetic haemochromatosis was found in 1.5% of patients attending a rheumatology clinic [43]. There was an additional benefit detecting iron deficiency in 15% of patients.

Other iron storage diseases

Transferrin deficiency

Absence of this binding protein has been found in a child with iron overload [31]. The haematological picture was of severe iron deficiency although the tissues were loaded with iron. The parents were heterozygotes and the patient a homozygote.

Cancer inducing iron overload

A primary bronchial carcinoma produced an abnormal ferritin that was thought to cause excess iron deposition in the liver and spleen [38].

Porphyria cutanea tarda (Chapter 23)

Increased hepatic iron has been related to additional heterozygosity for the haemochromatosis gene [36].

Erythropoietic siderosis

Siderosis is associated with extremely high rates of erythropoiesis. The hyperplastic bone marrow may in some way direct the intestinal mucosa to take in excessive quantities of iron. This continues even in the presence of large iron stores. The iron is deposited first in the macrophages of the reticulo-endothelial system and later in parenchymal cells of liver, pancreas and other organs.

Siderosis can therefore be expected in chronic haemolytic states, especially β-thalassaemia, sickle cell disease, congenital spherocytosis [8] and hereditary dyserythropoietic anaemia. Patients with chronic aplastic anaemia may also be at risk. Iron overload may develop in mild sideroblastic anaemia without severe anaemia or transfusions [48].

The siderosis is enhanced by *blood transfusions* as the iron given with the blood cannot be lost from the body. More than 100 units must have been transfused before siderosis is clinically recognizable. Misdirected iron therapy enhances the siderosis.

The siderosis is recognized clinically by increasing skin pigmentation and by hepatomegaly. Children fail to grow and to develop secondary sexual characteristics. Liver failure and frank portal hypertension are rare. The fasting blood glucose is raised, but clinical diabetes is excessively rare.

Although the amount of iron deposited in the heart is relatively small, myocardial damage is a major factor determining prognosis, especially in younger children [63]. In children, symptoms arise when body iron reaches 20 g (100 units blood transfused); death from heart failure is likely when 60 g is reached.

Treatment is difficult. Splenectomy may reduce transfusion needs. A well-balanced, low-iron diet is virtually impossible. 12-hour overnight subcutaneous infusion of 2–4 g desferrioxamine given with a small syringe pump into the anterior abdominal wall is effective [32]. Such measures can only be available to a very few children with haemoglobinopathies: the cost is prohibitive. Oral iron chelators remain at an experimental stage.

Bantu siderosis

This condition is seen in South African Black people whose diet consists of porridge fermented in iron pots at an acid pH. Absorption is facilitated by the acid diet and by malnutrition. Traditional beer brewed in steel drums continues to cause iron overload in rural sub-Saharan

Africa. Studies suggest that genetic (non-HLA linked) as well as environmental factors effect the degree of iron overload [28].

Cirrhosis of the alcoholic

Multiple factors contribute to increased hepatic iron deposition. Protein deficiency is frequent. Increased iron absorption is found in cirrhotic patients irrespective of aetiology [73]. Cirrhotic patients with a large portal–systemic collateral circulation may absorb somewhat more.

Alcoholic beverages, particularly wine, have a high iron content. Chronic pancreatitis seems to increase iron absorption. Iron medications and haemolysis add to the load of iron, whereas intestinal blood loss diminishes it.

Iron deposition is rarely as great as in genetic haemochromatosis. Iron deficiency soon follows multiple venesections showing that body iron stores are only moderately increased. Hepatic histology shows the features of alcoholism as well as iron deposition. Calculation of the hepatic iron index will distinguish early haemochromatosis from alcoholic siderosis [12]. Some alcoholic patients with hepatic siderosis may turn out to be heterozygotes for genetic haemochromatosis when a genetic test becomes available.

Siderosis after portal–caval shunting

Iron may accumulate rapidly in the liver with surgical or spontaneous portal–systemic shunts [16, 73]. In general, siderosis is slight and clinically insignificant. It is probably an exaggeration of that frequently observed in cirrhosis.

Haemodialysis

Massive overload in liver and spleen reflect transfusion and haemolysis.

Relation of the pancreas to iron metabolism

Increased iron absorption and storage have been found in experimental pancreatic damage and also in patients with calcific pancreatitis and with cystic fibrosis where absorption of inorganic iron but not haemoglobin iron was increased [68]. This suggests that some factor in the exocrine secretion of the pancreas can decrease iron absorption.

Neonatal haemochromatosis

This very rare and fatal disorder is characterized by liver failure which starts *in utero*, together with hepatic and extra-hepatic parenchymal iron overload which spares the reticulo-endothelial system. Whether it represents a primary iron storage disorder or the effect of liver disease of another cause superimposed on a liver already physiologically replete with iron, is not certain [35]. It is not related to genetic haemochromatosis [30].

Chronic viral hepatitis

Nearly half of patients with chronic viral hepatitis (B and C) have an abnormal percentage saturation and/or serum ferritin [22]. Liver biopsy, with iron estimation and calculation of the hepatic iron index is currently the only way to evaluate the possibility of genetic haemochromatosis. A high liver iron reduces the response rate to α-interferon in chronic hepatitis C [45]. Whether removal of iron by venesection increases the response rate awaits prospective study.

Non-alcoholic steato-hepatitis

Serum iron indices were abnormal in 58% of 33 patients with non-alcoholic steato-hepatitis. None had haemochromatosis based on the hepatic iron index [6].

Iron overload related to acaeruloplasminaemia

In this very rare syndrome, acaeruloplasminaemia, due to a mutation in the caeruloplasmin gene, is associated with excessive iron deposition mainly in the brain, liver and pancreas. Patients show extra-pyramidal disorders, cerebellar ataxia and diabetes mellitus [75].

References

1 Adams PC, Kertesz AE, Valberg LS. Clinical presentation of hemochromatosis: a changing scene. *Am. J. Med.* 1991; **90**: 445.

2 Adams PC, Agnew S. Alcoholism in hereditary hemochromatosis revisited: prevalence and clinical consequences among homozygous siblings. *Hepatology* 1996; **23**: 724.

3 Axford JS. Rheumatic manifestations of haemochromatosis. *Baillières Clin. Rheumatol.* 1991; **5**: 351.

4 Bacon BR, Britton RS. The pathology of hepatic iron overload: a free radical-mediated process? *Hepatology* 1990; **11**: 127.

5 Bacon B, O'Neill R, Britton R. Hepatic mitochondrial energy production in rats with chronic iron overload. *Gastroenterology* 1993; **105**: 1134.

6 Bacon BR, Farakvash L, Faginoli S *et al*. Nonalcoholic steatohepatitis: an expanded clinical entity. *Gastroenterology* 1994; **107**: 1103.

7 Baer DM, Simons JL, Staples RL *et al*. Hemochromatosis screening in asymptomatic ambulatory men 30 years of age and older. *Am. J. Med.* 1995; **98**: 464.

8 Barry M, Scheuer PJ, Sherlock S *et al*. Hereditary spherocytosis with secondary haemochromatosis. *Lancet* 1968; **ii**: 481.

9 Barry M, Sherlock S. Measurement of liver iron concentration in needle biopsy specimens. *Lancet* 1971; **i**: 100.

10 Bassett ML, Halliday JW, Ferris RA *et al*. Diagnosis of haemochromatosis in young subjects: predictive accuracy of biochemical screening tests. *Gastroenterology* 1984; **87**: 628.

11 Bassett ML, Halliday JW, Powell LW. HLA typing in idiopathic haemochromatosis: distinction between homozygotes and heterozygotes with biochemical expression. *Hepatology* 1981; **1**: 120.

12 Bassett ML, Halliday JW, Powell LW. Value of hepatic iron measurements in early haemochromatosis and determination of the critical iron level associated with fibrosis. *Hepatology* 1986; **6**: 24.

13 Batey RG, Hussein S, Sherlock S *et al*. The role of serum ferritin in the management of idiopathic haemochromatosis. *Scand. J. Gastroenterol.* 1978; **13**: 953.

14 Bomford A, Williams R. Long term results of venesection therapy in idiopathic haemochromatosis. *Q. J. Med.* 1976; **45**: 611.

15 Bonkovsky HL, Slaker DP, Bills EB *et al*. Usefulness and limitations of laboratory and hepatic imaging studies in iron-storage disease. *Gastroenterology* 1990; **99**: 1079.

16 Conn HO. Portacaval anastomosis and hepatic haemosiderin disposition: a prospective controlled investigation. *Gastroenterology* 1972; **62**: 61.

17 Crawford DHG, Powell LW, Leggett BA *et al*. Evidence that the ancestral haplotype in Australian hemochromatosis patients may be associated with a common mutation in the gene. *Am. J. Hum. Genet.* 1995; **57**: 362.

18 Crosby WH. Treatment of haemochromatosis by energetic phlebotomy. One patient's response to the letting of 55 litres of blood in 11 months. *Br. J. Haematol.* 1958; **4**: 82.

19 Cundy T, Butler J, Bomford A *et al*. Reversibility of hypogonadotrophic hypogonadism associated with genetic haemochromatosis. *Clin. Endocrinol.* 1993; **38**: 617.

20 Deugnier Y, Charalambous P, Quilleuc D *et al*. Preneoplastic significance of hepatic iron-free foci in genetic hemochromatosis: a study of 185 patients. *Hepatology* 1993; **18**: 1363.

21 Deugnier Y, Guyader D, Crantock L *et al*. Primary liver cancer in genetic hemochromatosis: a clinical, pathological, and pathogenetic study of 54 cases. *Gastroenterology* 1993; **104**: 228.

22 Di Bisceglie AM, Axiotis CA, Hoofnagle JH *et al*. Measurement of iron status in patients with chronic hepatitis. *Gastroenterology* 1992; **102**: 2108.

23 Dymock IW, Cassar J, Pyke DA *et al*. Observations on the pathogenesis, complications and treatment of diabetes in 115 cases of haemochromatosis. *Am. J. Med.* 1972; **52**: 203.

24 Faraawi R, Harth M, Kertesz A *et al*. Arthritis in hemochromatosis. *J. Rheumatol.* 1993; **20**: 448.

25 Farrell FJ, Nguyen M, Woodley S *et al*. Outcome of liver transplantation in patients with haemochromatosis. *Hepatology* 1994; **20**: 404.

26 Feder JN, Gnirke A, Thomas W *et al*. A novel MHC class I-like gene is mutated in patients with hereditary haemochromatosis. *Nature Genet.* 1996; **13**: 399.

27 Finch SC, Finch CA. Idiopathic haemochromatosis. *Medicine (Baltimore)* 1955; **34**: 381.

28 Gordeuk V, Mukiibi J, Hasstedt SJ *et al*. Iron overload in Africa: interaction between a gene and dietary iron content. *N. Engl. J. Med.* 1992; **326**: 95.

29 Hanot V, Schachmann M. Sur le cirrhose pigmentaire dans le diabète sucré. *Arch. Physiol. Norm. Path.* 1886; **7**: 50.

30 Hardy L, Hansen JL, Kushner JP *et al*. Neonatal haemochromatosis: genetic analysis of transferrin-receptor, H-apoferritin, and L-apoferritin loci and of the human leukocyte antigen class I region. *Am. J. Pathol.* 1990; **137**: 149.

31 Heilmeyer L, Keller W, Vivell O *et al*. Congenital transferrin deficiency in a seven-year-old girl. *Germ. Med. Mth.* 1961; **6**: 385.

32 Hoffbrand AV, Gorman A, Laulicht M *et al*. Improvement in iron status and liver function in patients with transfusional iron overload with long-term subcutaneous desferrioxamine. *Lancet* 1979; **i**: 947.

33 Jazwinska EC, Lee SC, Webb SI *et al*. Localization of the haemochromatosis gene close to D6S105. *Am. J. Hum. Genet.* 1993; **53**: 347.

34 Jazwinska EC, Pyper W, Burt M *et al*. Haplotype analysis in Australian hemochromatosis patients: evidence for a predominant ancestral haplotype exclusively associated with hemochromatosis. *Am. J. Hum. Genet.* 1995; **56**: 428.

35 Knisely AS. Neonatal hemochromatosis. *Adv. Pediatr.* 1992; **39**: 383.

36 Kushner JP, Edwards CQ, Dadone MM *et al*. Heterozygosity for HLA-linked haemochromatosis as a likely cause of the hepatic siderosis associated with sporadic porphyria cutanea tarda. *Gastroenterology* 1985; **88**: 1232.

37 Lamon JM, Marynick SP, Rosenblatt R *et al*. Idiopathic haemochromatosis in a young female. A case study and review of the syndrome in young people. *Gastroenterology* 1979; **76**: 178.

38 Li AKC, Batey RG. A tumour inducing iron overload. *Br. Med. J.* 1977; **ii**: 1327.

39 Lloyd HM, Powell LW, Thomas MJ. Idiopathic haemochromatosis in menstruating women. *Lancet* 1964; **ii**: 555.

40 Lombard M, Bomford A, Polson RJ *et al*. Differential expression of transferrin receptor in duodenal mucosa in iron overload. *Gastroenterology* 1990; **98**: 976.

41 Mohler DN, Wheby MS. Case report: haemochromatosis heterozygotes may have significant iron overload when they also have hereditary spherocytosis. *Am. J. Med. Sci.* 1986; **29**: 320.

42 Niederau C, Fischer R, Purschel A *et al*. Long-term survival in patients with hereditary hemochromatosis. *Gastroenterology* 1996; **110**: 1107.

43 Olynyk J, Hall P, Ahern M *et al*. Screening for genetic haemochromatosis in a rheumatology clinic. *Austr. NZ J. Med.* 1994; **24**: 22.

44 Olynyk JK, O'Neill R, Britton RS, Bacon BR. Determination of hepatic iron concentration in fresh and paraffin-embedded tissue: diagnostic implications. *Gastroenterology* 1994; **106**: 674.

45 Olynyk JK, Reddy RK, Di Bisceglie AM *et al*. Hepatic iron concentration as a predictor of response to alpha interferon therapy in chronic hepatitis C. *Gastroenterology* 1995; **108**: 1104.

46 Park CH, Bacon BR, Brittenham GM *et al*. Pathology of dietary carbonyl iron overload in rats. *Lab. Invest.* 1987; **57**: 555.

47 Perkins KW, McInnes IWS, Blackburn CRB *et al*. Idiopathic haemochromatosis i n children. *Am. J. Med.* 1965; **39**: 118.

48 Peto TEA, Pippard MJ, Weatherall DJ. Iron overload in mild sideroblastic anaemias. *Lancet* 1983; **i**: 375.

49 Phatak P, Guzman G, Woll J *et al*. Cost-effectiveness of screening for hereditary hemochromatosis. *Arch. Intern. Med.* 1994; **154**: 769.

50 Pietrangelo A, Casalgrandi G, Quaglino D *et al*. Duodenal

ferritin synthesis in genetic haemochromatosis. *Gastroenterology* 1995; **108**: 208.

51 Pietrangelo A, Gualdi R, Casalgrandi G *et al.* Enhanced hepatic collagen type I mRNA expression in fat-storing cells in a rodent model of hemochromatosis. *Hepatology* 1994; **19**: 714.

52 Pietrangelo A, Gualdi R, Casalgrandi G *et al.* Molecular and cellular aspects of iron-induced hepatic cirrhosis in rodents. *J. Clin. Invest.* 1995; **95**: 1824.

53 Piperno A, Arosio C, Fargion S *et al.* The ancestral hemochromatosis haplotype is associated with a severe phenotype expression in Italian patients. *Hepatology* 1996; **24**: 43.

54 Powell LW. Does transplantation of the liver cure haemochromatosis? *J. Hepatol.* 1992; **16**: 259.

55 Powell LW. Hemochromatosis: the impact of early diagnosis and therapy. *Gastroenterology* 1996; **110**: 1304.

56 Powell LW, Halliday JW, Cowlishaw JL. Relationship between serum ferritin and total body iron stores in idiopathic haemochromatosis. *Gut* 1978; **19**: 538.

57 Powell LW, Kerr JFR. Reversal of 'cirrhosis' in idiopathic haemochromatosis following long-term intensive venesection therapy. *Aust. Ann. Med.* 1970; **19**: 54.

58 Prieto J, Barry M, Sherlock S. Serum-ferritin in patients with iron overload and with acute and chronic liver diseases. *Gastroenterology* 1975; **68**: 525.

59 Raha-Chowdhury R, Bowen DJ, Stone C *et al.* New polymorphic microsatellite markers place the haemochromatosis gene telomeric to D6S105. *Hum. Mol. Genet.* 1995; **4**: 1869.

60 Ramm GA, Li SCY, Li L *et al.* Chronic iron overload causes activation of rat lipocytes in vivo. *Am. J. Physiol.* 1995; **268**: G451.

61 Rivers J, Garrahy P, Robinson W *et al.* Reversible cardiac dysfunction in haemochromatosis. *Am. Heart J.* 1987; **113**: 216.

62 Rothenberg BE, Voland JR. β2 knockout mice develop parenchymal iron overload: a putative role for class I genes of the major histocompatibility complex in iron metabolism. *Proc. Natl. Acad. Sci. USA* 1996; **93**: 1529.

63 Schafer AI, Cheron RG, Dluhy R *et al.* Clinical consequences of acquired transfusional iron overload in adults. *N. Engl. J. Med.* 1981; **304**: 319.

64 Sciot R, Paterson AC, Van Den Oord JJ *et al.* Lack of hepatic transferrin receptor expression in haemochromatosis. *Hepatology* 1987; **7**: 831.

65 Sheldon JH. *Haemochromatosis.* Oxford University Press, Oxford, 1935.

66 Simon M, Brissot P. The genetics of haemochromatosis. *J. Hepatol.* 1988; **6**: 116.

67 Summers KM, Halliday JW, Powell LW. Identification of homozygous haemochromatosis subjects by measurement of hepatic iron index. *Hepatology* 1990; **12**: 20.

68 Tonz O, Weiss S, Strahm HW *et al.* Iron absorption in cystic fibrosis. *Lancet* 1965; **ii**: 1096.

69 Tsukamoto H, Horne W, Kamimura S *et al.* Experimental liver cirrhosis induced by alcohol and iron. *J. Clin. Invest.* 1995; **96**: 620.

70 Walton C, Kelly WF, Laing I *et al.* Endocrine abnormalities in idiopathic haemochromatosis. *Q. J. Med.* 1983; **52**: 99.

71 Williams R, Scheuer PJ, Sherlock S. The inheritance of idiopathic haemochromatosis: a clinical and liver biopsy study of 16 families. *Q. J. Med.* 1962; **31**: 249.

72 Williams R, Smith PM, Spicer EJF *et al.* Venesection therapy in idiopathic haemochromatosis. *Q. J. Med.* 1969; **38**: 1.

73 Williams R, Williams HS, Scheuer PJ *et al.* Iron absorption and siderosis in chronic liver disease. *Q. J. Med.* 1967; **36**: 151.

74 Worwood M, Raha-Chowdhury R, Dorak MT *et al.* Alleles at D6S265 and D6S105 define a haemochromatosis-specific genotype. *Br. J. Haematol.* 1994; **86**: 863.

75 Yoshida K, Furihata K, Takeda S *et al.* A mutation in the ceruloplasmin gene is associated with systemic hemosiderosis in humans. *Nature Genet.* 1995; **9**: 267.

Chapter 22
Wilson's Disease

This rare inherited disease, predominantly of young people, is characterized by cirrhosis of the liver, bilateral softening and degeneration of the basal ganglia of the brain, and greenish-brown pigmented rings in the periphery of the cornea (Kayser–Fleischer rings). Kinnier Wilson (1912) [60] was the first to define it in an article entitled 'Progressive lenticular degeneration: a familial nervous disease associated with cirrhosis of the liver'.

Aetiology

Increased amounts of copper, deposited in the tissues, are responsible for the hepatic and neurological changes, the Kayser–Fleischer rings in the cornea and lesions in kidneys and other organs [1].

Biliary copper excretion is low [12]. Urinary copper excretion is increased. The serum copper level, however, is almost invariably reduced (fig. 22.1). Caeruloplasmin, an α_2-globulin responsible for transfer of copper in the plasma, is reduced [1].

The normal daily dietary intake of copper is 4 mg, of which 2 mg is absorbed and excreted in bile so that the patient is in balance. In Wilson's disease, only 0.2–0.4 mg can be excreted in bile with 1 mg in the urine so that a positive copper balance develops.

The disease is worldwide but occurs particularly in Jews of eastern European origin, Arabs, Italians, Japanese, Chinese, Indians and any community having a high inter-marriage rate.

Molecular genetics: pathogenesis

Inheritance is autosomal recessive. The prevalance is about 1 in 30 000 with a carrier frequency of around 1 in 90 [34]. The Wilson's disease gene is on the long arm of chromosome 13 and has been cloned and characterized [6, 26, 62]. The gene product is a copper transporting ATPase [6, 48] which binds six copper atoms (fig. 22.2). It is not clear where in the cell this transporter lies nor its exact function. It may be involved in the biliary excretion of copper or the transfer of copper to caeruloplasmin. To date more than 25 different mutations in the Wilson's disease gene have been identified [49]. Most are in the ATPase functional domain (fig. 22.2) rather than the copper binding regions. In many patients the mutation

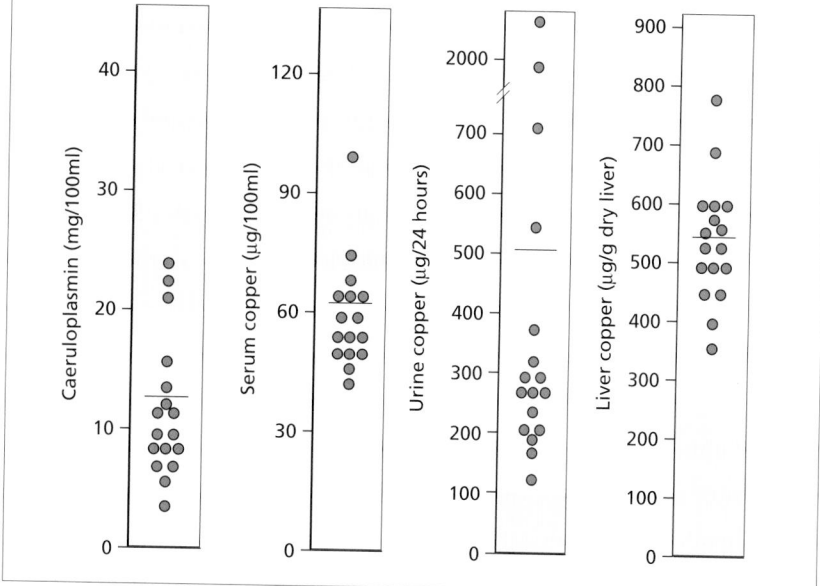

Fig. 22.1. Copper studies in 17 patients with Wilson's disease presenting as chronic hepatitis. Horizontal lines indicate mean values. Tinted areas represent the normal ranges for serum caeruloplasmin and serum copper, and delineate the levels above which urine copper (>100 μg/24 h) and liver copper concentration (>250 μg/g dry weight) are compatible with the diagnosis of Wilson's disease [37].

417

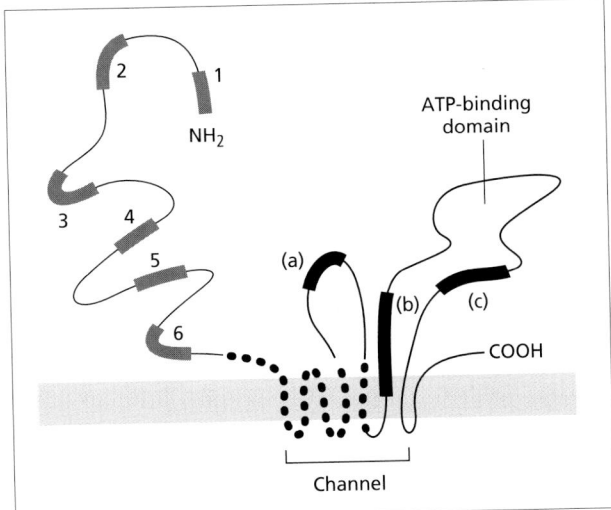

Fig. 22.2. Model of Wilson's disease gene product: a copper-transporting P-type ATPase. 1–6 = copper-binding sequences; dotted regions = transmembrane helices. Conserved regions of P-type ATPases are shown: (a) energy transduction; (b) invariant cytoplasmic motif; and (c) cytoplasmic ATP-binding domain (reproduced with permission from [5]).

has yet to be identified. There is a suggestion that patients with mutations that destroy the function of the gene have an earlier onset of disease [49]. Most patients have a different mutation on each chromosome making phenotype/genotype correlations more difficult. Because of the large number of mutations, mutation analysis is not a practical method of diagnosis in individual patients.

Haplotype analysis — that is analysis of the alleles of microsatellite markers in the area of the gene on chromosome 13 — was important in identifying the area of the gene on chromosome 13 before it was cloned, and remains valuable in determining the disease status in siblings of affected patients (homozygote, heterozygote or normal) [15].

Such a distinction is important since heterozygote carriers do not develop clinical disease. There is a correlation between the haplotype and some mutations [50] and this may aid the search for new mutations.

The Long–Evans Cinnamon (LEC) rat is an animal model for Wilson's disease. There is marked hepatic copper accumulation in the first few months of life, a low serum caeruloplasmin and development of an acute and later chronic hepatitis [23]. D-penicillamine protects against these changes [51]. This inbred rat has a deletion in the copper-transporting ATPase gene homologous to the Wilson's disease gene [61].

Reduced biliary excretion of copper in Wilson's disease and the animal model results in toxic levels of copper in the liver and other tissues. There is oxidant damage to mitochondria with lipid peroxidation [40]

which can be reduced experimentally by vitamin E administration [41].

Normal neonates have greatly elevated hepatic copper concentrations and a reduced serum caeruloplasmin. In the neonatal guinea-pig, copper distribution and plasma binding protein soon revert to the adult form [43]. Whether this relates to the activity of the Wilson's disease gene is unknown.

Pathology

Liver

The liver shows all grades of change from peri-portal fibrosis through submassive necrosis to a coarse, macronodular cirrhosis [47].

Liver cells are ballooned, show multiple nuclei, clumped glycogen and glycogen vacuolation of the nuclei (fig. 22.3). Fatty change is usual. Kupffer cells are large. In some patients a particularly florid picture is seen with Mallory's bodies, simulating acute alcoholic hepatitis. Alternatively the changes are those of a chronic hepatitis (fig. 22.4). Hepatic histology is not diagnostic, but in a young person with cirrhosis such a picture should always suggest Wilson's disease.

Rubeanic acid or rhodanine stains for copper may be unreliable as the metal is patchily distributed, being absent from regenerating nodules. The copper is usually peri-portal in distribution and associated with atypical lipofuscin deposits.

Electron microscopy [33]

Autophagic vacuoles are seen and mitochondria are

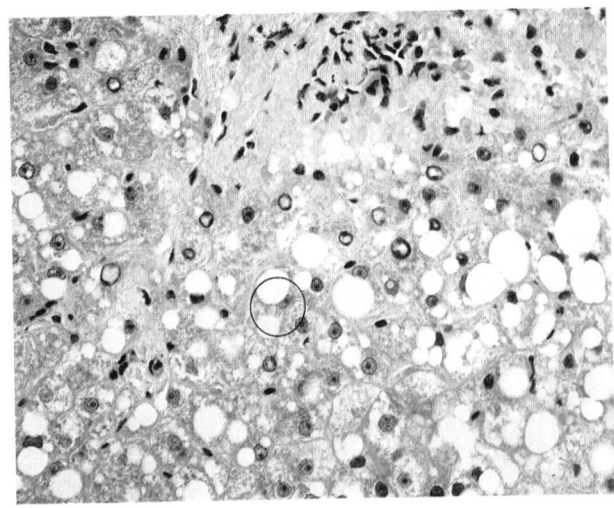

Fig. 22.3. Hepato-lenticular degeneration (Wilson's disease). Liver cells adjoining a fibrous tissue band show gross vacuolation of their nuclei (glycogenic degeneration) and fatty change. (Stained H & E, ×65.)

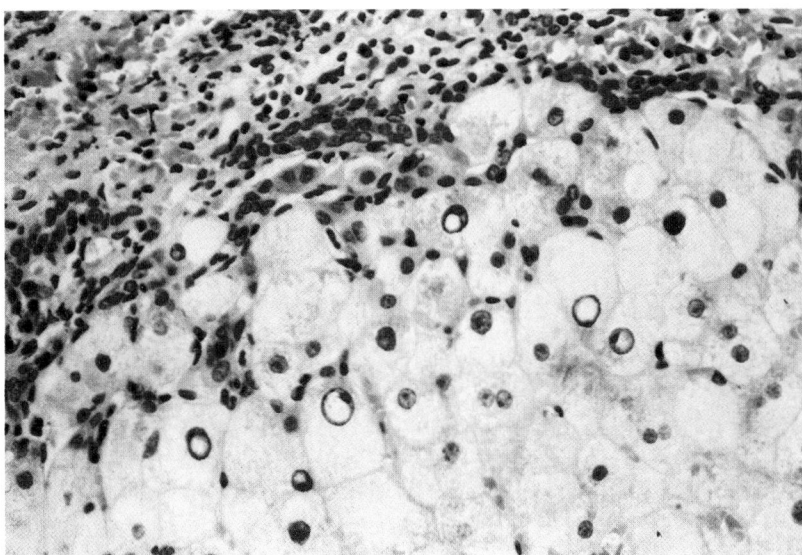

Fig. 22.4. Wilson's disease. In this example there is piecemeal necrosis and lymphocytic infiltration as in chronic hepatitis of other aetiologies. Note hepato-cellular swelling due to finely divided fat, and vacuolization of nuclei. (Stained H & E, ×350.)

large and abnormal even in asymptomatic patients. Fatty change can be related to the mitochondrial alterations. Collagen fibrils infiltrate between cells and light and dark liver cells are seen.

Other organs

The *kidney* shows fatty and hydropic change with copper deposition in the proximal convoluted tubules.

The *Kayser–Fleischer* ring is due to a copper-containing pigment deposited in Descemet's membrane at the periphery of the posterior surface of the cornea.

Clinical picture

The picture is a composite one due to general poisoning of the tissues with copper. The emphasis falls on different tissues at different ages (fig. 22.5). In children the liver is chiefly involved (*hepatic form*). Later neuropsychiatric changes become increasingly important (*neurological form*). Patients presenting after age 20 usually have neurological symptoms [46]. The two types may overlap. Most patients have developed symptoms or been diagnosed between the ages of 5 and 30 [46].

The *Kayser–Fleischer* ring (fig. 22.6) is a greenish-brown ring at the periphery of the cornea. The upper pole is first affected. Slit-lamp examination by an expert is usually necessary to show it. It is usually present with neurological abnormalities. It may be absent in young people with an acute presentation [37]. A rather similar ring may rarely be found with prolonged cholestasis and cryptogenic cirrhosis [11, 13].

Rarely the posterior layer of the capsule of the lens may show greyish-brown 'sunflower' cataracts, similar to those due to copper-containing foreign bodies [7].

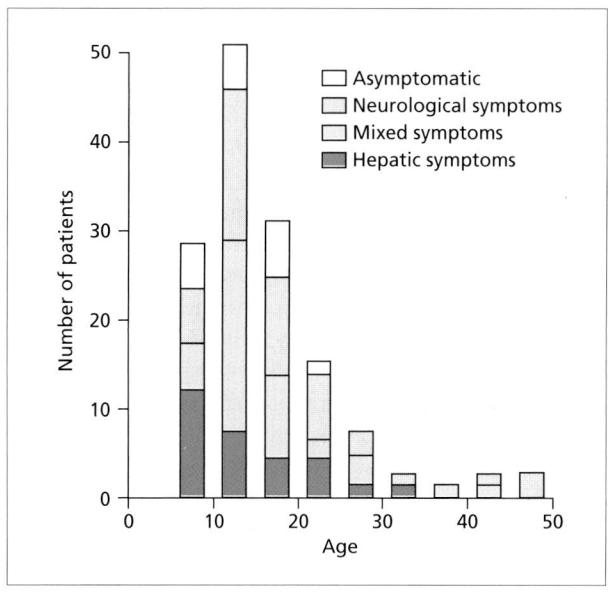

Fig. 22.5. Type of symptom complex at onset by age in 142 British and Chinese patients with Wilson's disease [46].

Hepatic forms

Fulminant hepatitis. This is characterized by progressive jaundice, ascites and hepatic and renal failure, usually in a child or young person [21, 31]. The liver cell necrosis is presumably related to accumulation of copper. Virtually all patients are already cirrhotic [32]. Acute intravascular haemolysis may be due to destruction of erythrocytes by a sudden flux of copper from the necrotic hepatocytes (fig. 22.7) [22]. Haemolysis of similar type is reported in sheep with copper intoxication, and in humans in accidental copper poisoning.

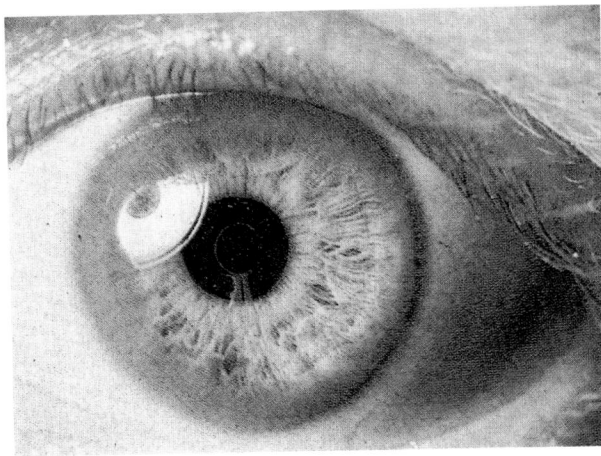

Fig. 22.6. Kayser–Fleischer ring. A brownish deposit is seen at the periphery of the cornea.

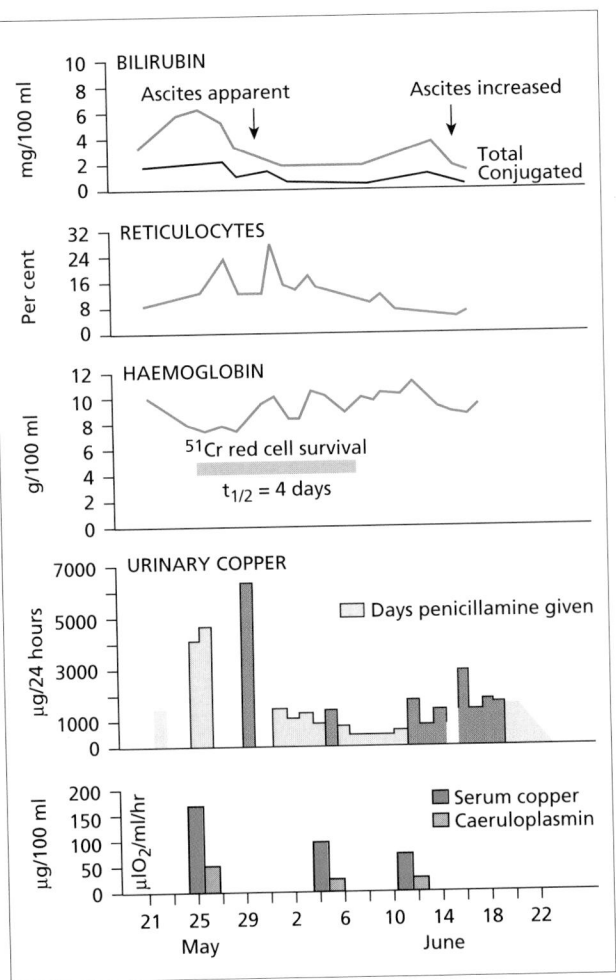

Fig. 22.7. Haemolytic crisis in Wilson's disease, marked by a rise in serum (mainly unconjugated) bilirubin and followed by reticulocytosis. The haemoglobin fell and red cell survival was reduced. Urinary copper was very high even without the administration of penicillamine. Serum copper was higher than that usually found in Wilson's disease. Ascites developed. The second episode of haemolysis, which was noted in June, was marked by a slight rise in serum bilirubin and a fall in haemoglobin [22].

Kayser–Fleischer rings may be absent. Urinary and serum copper levels are very high. Serum caeruloplasmin is usually low. However, it may be normal or raised as caeruloplasmin is an acute phase reactant, increased by underlying active liver disease. Serum transaminases and alkaline phosphatase levels are inappropriately low for fulminant viral hepatitis [21, 38]. A low alkaline phosphatase/bilirubin ratio although not diagnostic of fulminant Wilson's disease is suggestive [32].

Chronic hepatitis. The condition presents at 10–30 years of age as a chronic hepatitis with jaundice, high transaminase values and hypergammaglobulinaemia (fig. 22.8) [37]. Neurological changes appear some 2–5 years later. The picture may resemble other forms of chronic hepatitis very closely. This emphasizes the need to screen all such patients for Wilson's disease.

Cirrhosis. The patient may present with insidiously developing cirrhosis. Clinical features include vascular spiders, splenomegaly, ascites and portal hypertension. The disease can exist without any neurological signs. In some patients the cirrhosis is well compensated. Hepatic biopsy may be necessary for diagnosis. If possible the copper content of the biopsy should be estimated quantitatively.

All young patients with chronic liver disease showing any mental peculiarity, any slurring of the speech, early ascites or haemolysis, and especially with a family history of cirrhosis should be screened for Wilson's disease.

Hepato-cellular carcinoma is very rare and copper may be protective [27].

Neuropsychiatric forms

These broadly form subgroups according to the predominant features, and in order of incidence are: parkin-sonian, pseudosclerotic, dystonic (dyskinetic) and choreic [58]. The neurological presentation may be acute and rapidly progressive. Early changes include a flexion–extension tremor of the wrists, grimacing, difficulty in writing and slurred speech. The limbs show a fluctuating rigidity. The intellect is fairly well preserved although 61% of patients have some psychiatric disturbance usually presenting as a slow deterioration of the personality.

More usually the neurological changes are chronic. Onset is in early adult life with tremor, gross and of a wing-beating type, exaggerated by voluntary movement. Sensory loss and pyramidal tract signs are absent.

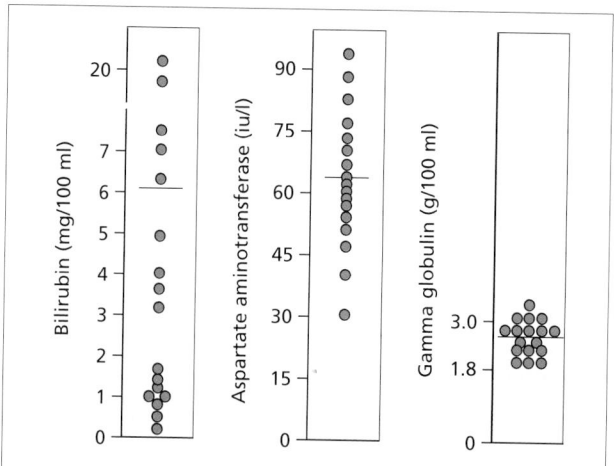

Fig. 22.8. Biochemical tests in 17 patients with Wilson's disease presenting as chronic hepatitis. Horizontal lines indicate mean values. Normal ranges are denoted by hatching (serum bilirubin 0.2–0.8 mg/dl; aspartate aminotransferase 4–15 iu/l; gamma globulin 0.7–1.8 g/dl) [37].

The expression is fatuous. Severely dystonic patients have a worse prognosis than the other groups [57].

The EEG shows generalized non-specific changes which may also be seen in asymptomatic siblings.

Renal changes

Aminoaciduria, glycosuria, phosphaturia, uricosuria and failure to excrete *p*-amino-hippurate (PAH) reflect renal tubular changes. These are presumably due to copper deposition in the proximal renal tubules.

Renal tubular acidosis is frequent and may be related to stone formation [59].

Other changes

Rarely, the lunulae of the nails are blue [2] due to increased copper. Skeletal changes include demineralization, premature osteoarthritis, subarticular cysts and fragmentation of bone about the joints. Changes in the spine are common and due to calcium pyrophosphate dihydrate deposition [20]. Gallstones are related to haemolysis. Hypoparathyroidism is an association, possibly due to copper deposition. Acute rhabdomyolysis has been reported with high skeletal muscle copper levels [29].

Laboratory tests

Serum caeruloplasmin and copper levels are usually reduced [14]. Distinction must be made from acute or chronic hepatitis with reduced serum caeruloplasmin

due to failure of synthesis [42]. Malnutrition also reduces serum caeruloplasmin. The level may be raised by oestrogen administration, oral contraceptive drugs, biliary obstruction or pregnancy.

Twenty-four-hour urinary copper excretion is increased. Results may be difficult to evaluate unless strict precautions are taken. Wide-necked bottles with copper-free disposable polyethylene liners are recommended [52].

In those in whom liver biopsy is contraindicated and where the serum caeruloplasmin level is normal, incorporation of orally administered radio-copper into caeruloplasmin may be diagnostic [34].

Liver biopsy

The copper content must be measured although concentrations vary widely within a cirrhotic liver [10]. The biopsy can be extracted from the paraffin block for copper measurement [19]. The normal is less than 55 μg/g dry liver weight, and concentrations greater than 250 μg are usual in homozygous Wilson's disease [39] (fig. 22.9). High values may even be found in those with normal hepatic histology [17]. High values are also found in all forms of long-standing cholestasis (fig. 22.9).

Scanning

Cranial CT scanning may show changes including ventricular enlargement before neurological changes appear [16]. MRI is more sensitive. Dilatation of the third ventricle, focal lesions in the thalamus, putamen and pallidum are seen and bear a relationship to clinical subgroups [25].

Detection of symptom-free homozygotes

All siblings of sufferers must be screened [17, 34]. A homozygote is suggested by such features as hepatomegaly, splenomegaly, vascular spiders and a slight rise in serum transaminase values. The Kayser–Fleischer rings may or may not be seen. Serum caeruloplasmin will usually be reduced to below 20 mg/100 ml. Liver biopsy with copper analysis is confirmatory.

Some difficulty may arise in distinguishing the homozygote from the heterozygote but the distinction is usually clear-cut. To be certain haplotype analysis, comparing the affected patient with siblings, should be done [15]. The homozygote must be treated with penicillamine, even if symptom-free. The heterozygote does not require treatment. Thirty-nine symptom-free homozygotes remained well with treatment, whereas seven left untreated have all developed the disease and five died of Wilson's disease [44].

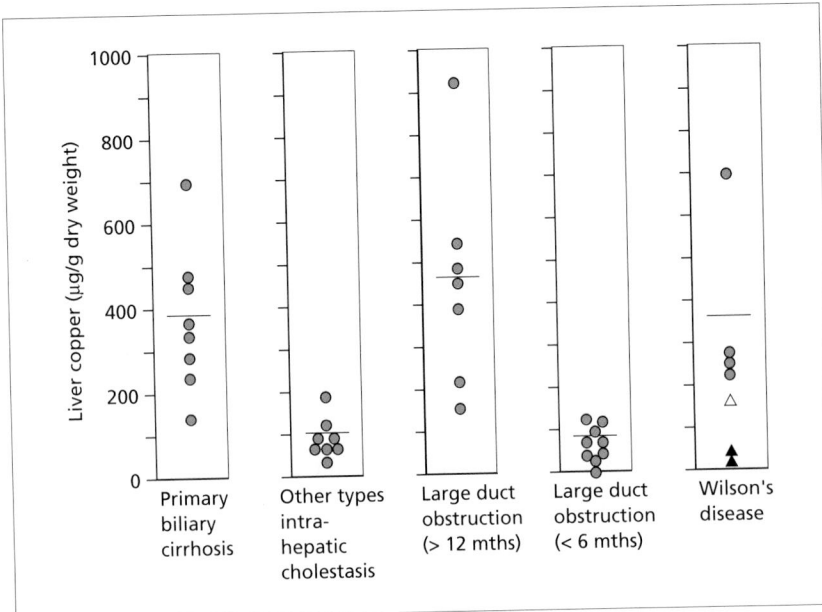

Fig. 22.9. Liver copper levels in patients with Wilson's disease and various types of cholestasis. Wilson's disease: △: heterozygote, ▲: siblings probably homozygous normal (these three patients not included in the calculation of the mean) [39].

Treatment (table 22.1)

Penicillamine is the treatment of choice [53]. This chelates copper and increases urinary excretion to as much as 1000–3000 µg daily. Treatment is started with 1.5 g D-penicillamine hydrochloride daily by mouth in four divided doses taken before meals. Improvement is slow and at least 6 months' continuous therapy should be given at this dose. If there is no improvement, the dose may be increased to 2 g daily. 25% of patients with neurological disease may deteriorate before improvement is seen [57]. Improvement is marked by fading and disappearance of the Kayser–Fleischer rings. Speech is clearer, tremor and rigidity lessen. Mentality is more normal. Hand-writing is a good test of progress. Liver function improves. Hepatic biopsy shows lessening of activity and reversion to an inactive cirrhosis. Failure to improve implies that irreparable tissue damage was present before treatment started or lack of compliance with treatment. Failure should not be admitted until 2 years' optimal therapy has been given. This is the usual period for adequate initial therapy.

Success during this initial period of therapy is judged by clinical improvement, a fall in serum free copper below 10 µg/dl (total serum copper minus caeruloplasmin-bound copper) and de-coppering indicated by a 24-hour urine copper excretion falling to 500 µg or less. There is controversy whether the liver copper level returns to normal [35]—a situation complicated further by the different copper levels found within the same liver [10]—but when it does, it takes many years of treatment (fig. 22.10). After the initial period of treatment, if there is the expected improvement, the dose of D-penicillamine should be reduced to 750–1000 mg/day

Table 22.1. Treatment of Wilson's disease

Penicillamine 1.5 daily initially
Monitor clinical improvement, serum-free copper, urinary copper
Maintenance therapy: reduce to 0.75–1 g daily

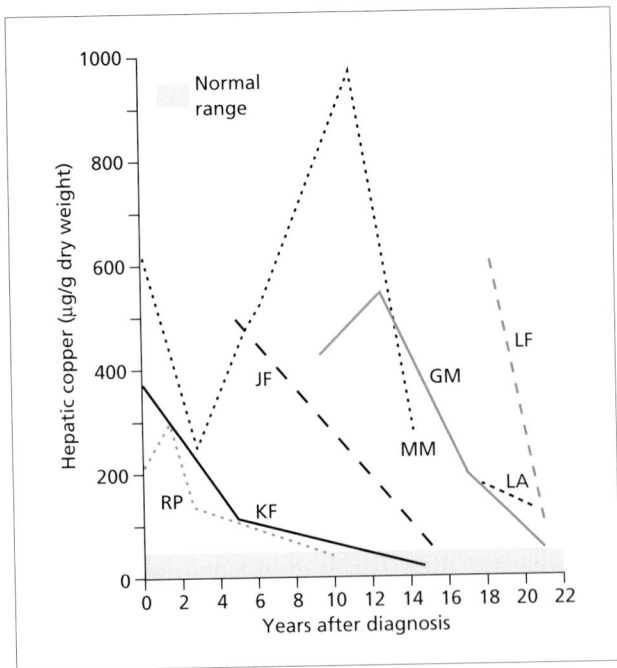

Fig. 22.10. Liver copper levels in seven penicillamine-treated patients with Wilson's disease (some reduced their dose). Many years passed before the liver copper reached the normal range (shaded area).

[45, 63]. Close follow-up is necessary to ensure continued improvement/stability, and to monitor the free serum copper concentration and urinary copper output and thus compliance. A fulminant course may follow non-compliance of penicillamine treatment in a previously well-controlled patient [35, 56].

Reactions to D-penicillamine occur in about 20% of patients with Wilson's disease [57]. These include sensitivity reactions within the first few weeks of treatment with fever and rash, leucopenia, thrombocytopenia and lymphadenopathy. These are usually resolved by stopping D-penicillamine and recommencing with slowly increasing doses of penicillamine in combination with prednisolone [45]. Prednisolone is gradually withdrawn after about 2 weeks. D-penicillamine may also cause proteinuria and an SLE-like syndrome. Skin changes include elastosis perforans serpiginosa and cutis laxa (progeric wrinkling). The latter is dose-related, so that long-term treatment with doses over 1 g/day are not recommended [34]. In the event of serious or unremitting adverse effects of penicillamine, trientine, another copper chelator should be substituted.

During the first 2 months of D-penicillamine treatment, white cell and platelet counts are done twice a week, then monthly up to 6 months and thereafter less frequently. Proteinuria should be checked on these occasions. Clinical pyridoxine deficiency is a theoretical possibility with penicillamine therapy but exceedingly rare. When large doses have been given, pyridoxine supplements can be added.

Trientine (tetraethylene tetramine dihydrochloride) may be tried in those unable to take penicillamine [35, 55]. It has a lower cupriuretic effect than penicillamine but is clinically effective [9].

Elemental zinc (50 mg) as acetate three times a day between meals inhibits gastrointestinal absorption of copper. Despite increasing experience [4, 8] its overall clinical effectiveness and its role over a prolonged period remain to be fully established. Side-effects occur including gastrointestinal symptoms but these are less severe than with penicillamine. It may be tried only in patients who have not responded to a long course of penicillamine or who have had reactions to both penicillamine and triene [18].

Physiotherapy is of value in the re-education of the patient's gait, writing and movement generally.

A low-copper diet is of little value but high copper-containing foods, including chocolate, peanuts, mushrooms, liver and shell fish, should be avoided.

Hepatic transplantation may be indicated for the fulminant form (which is usually fatal) [32], the young cirrhotic in severe hepato-cellular failure who fails to improve after 2–3 months' penicillamine, or the patient who develops severe liver failure with haemolysis after unwisely stopping therapy. Survival at 1 year is 79% [3,

36]. Neurological features show improvement in some but not all cases [28]. The metabolic defect is corrected. Before transplant, renal failure may be treated by post-dilution and continuous arteriovenous haemofiltration which removes large quantities of copper as large molecules of copper/penicillamine complex [30].

Prognosis

Untreated Wilson's disease is progressive and fatal. The great danger is that the patient remains undiagnosed and dies untreated.

In the acute neurological form the prognosis is poor, for cystic changes in the basal ganglia are irreversible. In the more chronic form the outlook depends on early diagnosis, preferably before symptoms have appeared. The final prognosis also depends on the response to 6 months' continuous penicillamine treatment. In one series [46], 16 asymptomatic patients were treated and have remained alive and asymptomatic, and three-quarters of 22 symptomatic patients treated for longer than 2 years are now asymptomatic. Dystonia carries a poor prognosis, being little affected by chelation therapy. Successful pregnancies have been reported in well-treated cases and penicillamine causes little problem to the fetus [54].

In chronic hepatitis, response to treatment can be poor, nine of 17 patients dying in one series [37]. The fulminant cases are frequently fatal despite chelation therapy [31]. Jaundice, ascites, and a high serum bilirubin, asparate transaminase and prothrombin time are ominous signs [24]. Liver transplantation is life saving in such patients.

Otherwise death is from liver failure, bleeding oesophageal varices or intercurrent infections in those bedridden from neurological disability.

Indian childhood cirrhosis

See Chapter 24.

Hereditary acaeruloplasminaemia

See Chapter 21.

References

1 Bearn AG. Wilson's disease. An inborn error of metabolism with multiple manifestations. *Am. J. Med.* 1957; **22**: 747.
2 Bearn AG, McKusick VA. Azure lunulae. An unusual change in the finger nails in two patients with hepatolenticular degeneration (Wilson's disease). *JAMA* 1958; **166**: 904.
3 Bellary S, Hassanein T, Van Thiel D. Liver transplantation for Wilson's disease. *J. Hepatol.* 1995; **23**: 373.
4 Brewer GJ, Dick RD, Yuzbasiyan-Gurkan V *et al.* Treatment

of Wilson's disease with zinc XIII: therapy with zinc in presymptomatic patients from the time of diagnosis. *J. Lab. Clin. Med.* 1994; **123**: 849.

5 Bull PC, Cox DW. Wilson disease and Menkes disease; new handles on heavy-metal transport. *Trends Genet.* 1994; **10**: 246.

6 Bull PC, Thomas GR, Rommens JM *et al.* The Wilson disease gene is a putative copper transporting P-type ATPase similar to the Menkes gene. *Nature Genet.* 1993; **5**: 327.

7 Cairns JE, Williams HP, Walshe JM. 'Sunflower cataract' in Wilson's disease. *Br. Med. J.* 1969; **iii**: 95.

8 Czlonkowska A, Gajda J, Rodo M. Effects of long term treatment in Wilson's disease with D-penicillamine and zinc sulphate. *J. Neurol.* 1996; **243**: 269.

9 Dahlman T, Hartvig P, Löholm M *et al.* Long-term treatment of Wilson's disease with triethylene tetramine dihydrochloride (trientine). *Q. J. Med.* 1995; **88**: 609.

10 Faa G, Nurchi V, Demelia L *et al.* Uneven hepatic copper distribution in Wilson's disease. *J. Hepatol.* 1995; **22**: 303.

11 Flemming CR, Dickson ER, Wahner HW *et al.* Pigmented corneal rings in non-Wilsonian liver disease. *Ann. Intern. Med.* 1977; **86**: 285.

12 Frommer D. The binding of copper by bile and serum. *Clin. Sci.* 1971; **41**: 485.

13 Frommer D, Morris J, Sherlock S *et al.* Kayser–Fleischer-like rings in patients without Wilson's disease. *Gastroenterology* 1977; **72**: 1331.

14 Gibbs K, Walshe JM. A study of the caeruloplasmin concentrations found in 75 patients with Wilson's disease, their kinships and various control groups. *Q. J. Med.* 1979; **48**: 447.

15 Houwen RHJ, Roberts EA, Thomas GR *et al.* DNA markers for the diagnosis of Wilson disease. *J. Hepatol.* 1993; **17**: 269.

16 Kendall BE, Pollock SS, Barr NM *et al.* Wilson's disease: clinical correlation with cranial computed tomography. *Neuroradiology* 1981; **22**: 1.

17 Levi AJ, Sherlock S, Scheuer PJ *et al.* Presymptomatic Wilson's disease. *Lancet* 1967; **ii**: 575.

18 Lipsky MA, Gollan JL. Treatment of Wilson's disease: In D-penicillamine we trust—what about zinc? *Hepatology* 1987; **7**: 593.

19 Ludwig J, Moyer TP, Rakela J. The liver biopsy diagnosis of Wilson's disease: methods in pathology. *Am. J. Clin. Pathol.* 1994; **102**: 443.

20 McClure J, Smith PS. Calcium pyrophosphate dihydrate deposition in the intervertebral discs in a case of Wilson's disease. *J. Clin. Pathol.* 1983; **36**: 764.

21 McCollough AJ, Fleming CR, Thistle JL *et al.* Diagnosis of Wilson's disease presenting as fulminant hepatic failure. *Gastroenterology* 1983; **84**: 161.

22 McIntyre N, Clink HM, Levi AJ *et al.* Hemolytic anemia in Wilson's disease. *N. Engl. J. Med.* 1967; **276**: 439.

23 Mori M, Hattori A, Sawaki M *et al.* The LEC rat: a model for human hepatitis, liver cancer and much more. *Am. J. Pathol.* 1994; **144**: 200.

24 Nazer H, Ede RJ, Mowat AP *et al.* Wilson's disease: clinical presentation and use of prognostic index. *Gut* 1986; **27**: 1377.

25 Oder W, Prayer L, Grimm G *et al.* Wilson's disease: evidence of subgroups derived from clinical findings and brain lesions. *Neurology* 1993; **43**: 120.

26 Petrukhin K, Fischer SG, Pirastu M *et al.* Mapping, cloning and genetic characterization of the region containing the Wilson disease gene. *Nature Genet.* 1993; **5**: 338.

27 Polio J, Enriquez RE, Chow A *et al.* Hepatocellular carcinoma in Wilson's disease: case report and review of the literature. *J. Clin. Gastroenterol.* 1989; **11**: 220.

28 Polson RJ, Rolles K, Calne RY *et al.* Reversal of severe neurological manifestations of Wilson's disease following orthotopic liver transplantation. *Q. J. Med.* 1987; **64**: 685.

29 Propst A, Propst T, Feichtinger H *et al.* Copper-induced acute rhabdomyolysis in Wilson's disease. *Gastroenterology* 1995; **108**: 885.

30 Rakela J, Kurtz SB, McCarthy JT *et al.* Fulminant Wilson's disease treated with post dilution hemofiltration and orthotopic liver transplantation. *Gastroenterology* 1986; **90**: 2004.

31 Roche-Sicot J, Benhamou J-P. Acute intravascular hemolysis and acute liver failure associated as a first manifestation of Wilson's disease. *Ann. Intern. Med.* 1977; **86**: 301.

32 Sallie R, Katsiyiannakis L, Baldwin D *et al.* Failure of simple biochemical indexes to reliably differentiate fulminant Wilson's disease from other causes of fulminant liver failure. *Hepatology* 1992; **16**: 1206.

33 Schaffner F, Sternlieb I, Barka T *et al.* Hepatocellular changes in Wilson's disease: histochemical and electron microscopic studies. *Am. J. Pathol.* 1962; **41**: 315.

34 Scheinberg H, Sternlieb I. *Wilson's Disease.* WB Saunders, Philadelphia, 1984.

35 Scheinberg IH, Jaffe ME, Sternlieb I. The use of trientine in preventing the effects of interrupting penicillamine therapy in Wilson's disease. *N. Engl. J. Med.* 1987; **317**: 209.

36 Schilsky ML, Scheinberg IH, Sternlieb I. Liver transplantation for Wilson's disease: indications and outcome. *Hepatology* 1994; **19**: 583.

37 Scott J, Gollan JL, Samourian S *et al.* Wilson's disease, presenting as chronic active hepatitis. *Gastroenterology* 1978; **74**: 645.

38 Shaver WA, Bhartt H, Combes B. Low serum alkaline phosphatase activity in Wilson's disease. *Hepatology* 1986; **6**: 859.

39 Smallwood RA, Williams HA, Rosenoer VM *et al.* Liver-copper levels in liver disease. Studies using neutron activation analysis. *Lancet* 1968; **ii**: 1310.

40 Sokol RJ, Twedt D, McKim JM *et al.* Oxidant injury to hepatic mitochondria in patients with Wilson's disease and Bedlington terriers with copper toxicosis. *Gastroenterology* 1994; **107**: 1788.

41 Sokol RJ, McKim JM, Devereaux MW. α-Tocopherol ameliorates oxidant injury in isolated copper-overloaded rat hepatocytes. *Pediatr. Res.* 1996; **39**: 259.

42 Spechler SJ, Koff RS. Wilson's disease: diagnostic difficulties in the patient with chronic hepatitis and hypoceruloplasminemia. *Gastroenterology* 1980; **78**: 103.

43 Srai SKS, Burroughs AK, Wood B *et al.* The ontogeny of liver copper metabolism in the guinea pig: clues to the etiology of Wilson's disease. *Hepatology* 1986; **6**: 427.

44 Sternlieb I, Scheinberg IJ. The prevention of clinical Wilson's disease. *J. Clin. Invest.* 1967; **46**: 1121.

45 Sternlieb I, Scheinberg IJ. Wilson's disease. In: *Wright's Liver and Biliary Disease*, Millward-Sadler GH, Wright R, Arthur MJP, eds. WB Saunders, 3rd edn, 1992: 965.

46 Strickland GT, Frommer D, Leu M-L *et al.* Wilson's disease in the United Kingdom and Taiwan. I. General characteristics of 142 cases and prognosis. II. A genetic analysis of 88 cases. *Q. J. Med.* 1973; **42**: 619.

47 Stromeyer FW, Ishak KG. Histology of the liver in Wilson's disease. *Am. J. Clin. Pathol.* 1980; **73**: 12.

48 Tanzi RE, Petrukhin K, Chernov I *et al.* The Wilson disease gene is a copper transporting ATPase with homology to the Menkes disease gene. *Nature Genet.* 1993; **5**: 344.

49 Thomas GR, Forbes JR, Roberts EA *et al.* The Wilson disease gene: spectrum of mutations and their consequences. *Nature Genet.* 1995; **9**: 210.

50 Thomas GR, Roberts EA, Walshe JM *et al.* Haplotypes and mutations in Wilson disease. *Am. J. Hum. Genet.* 1995; **56**: 1315.

51 Togashi Y, Li Y, Kang J-H *et al.* D-Penicillamine prevents the development of hepatitis in Long–Evans Cinnamon rats with abnormal copper metabolism. *Hepatology* 1992; **15**: 82.

52 Walshe JM. Copper: not too little, not too much, but just right. *J. RCP (Lon.)* 1995; **29**: 280.

53 Walshe JM. Treatment of Wilson's disease with penicillamine. *Lancet* 1960; **i**: 188.

54 Walshe JM. Pregnancy in Wilson's disease. *Q. J. Med.* 1977; **46**: 73.

55 Walshe JM. Treatment of Wilson's disease with trientine (triethylene tetramine) dihydrochloride. *Lancet* 1982; **ii**: 643.

56 Walshe JM, Dixon AK. Dangers of non-compliance in Wilson's disease. *Lancet* 1986; **i**: 845.

57 Walshe JM, Yealland M. Chelation treatment of neurological Wilson's disease. *Q. J. Med.* 1993; **86**; 197.

58 Walshe JM, Yealland M. Wilson's disease: the problem of delayed diagnosis. *J. Neurol. Neurosurg. Psych.* 1992; **55**: 692.

59 Wieber DO, Wilson DM, McLeod RA *et al.* Renal stones in Wilson's disease. *Am. J. Med.* 1979; **67**: 249.

60 Wilson AK. Progressive lenticular degeneration: a familial nervous disease associated with cirrhosis of the liver. *Brain* 1912; **34**: 295.

61 Wu J, Forbes JR, Chen HS *et al.* The LEC rat has a deletion in the copper transporting ATPase gene homologous to the Wilson disease gene. *Nature Genet.* 1994; **7**: 541.

62 Yamaguchi Y, Heiny ME, Gitlin JD. Isolation and characterization of a human liver cDNA as a candidate gene for Wilson disease. *Biochem. Biophys. Res. Commun.* 1993; **197**: 271.

63 Yarze JC, Martin P, Munoz SJ *et al.* Wilson's disease: current status. *Am. J. Med.* 1992; **92**: 643.

Chapter 23
Nutritional and Metabolic Liver Diseases

Clinical nutritional liver injury

Hepatic necrosis and fibrosis can be produced in experimental animals by certain diets, particularly those low in protein and essential amino acids [12]. World-wide, protein malnutrition is extremely common [31]. The liver suffers in common with other organs.

The most clearly defined syndrome is *kwashiorkor*, but this represents only one end of the malnutrition spectrum. The liver is involved in *wasting diseases*, especially with chronic diarrhoea such as ulcerative colitis, and the hepatic changes in the *alcoholic* may be, at least in part, nutritional [25].

In *starvation* and hunger oedema, the liver shrinks, increased lipochrome pigment is seen in the liver cells, but there is no fatty change [26]. Liver biopsies from malnourished children show a reduction in liver protein [31]. Liver biopsies from patients with *anorexia nervosa* are essentially normal. Previous malnutrition may 'condition' the liver to toxic and infective agents, but this has

not been proved. Increased mortality from viral hepatitis, particularly in pregnancy, may occur in protein-deficient communities.

Fatty liver

This is defined as fat, largely triglyceride, exceeding 5% of the liver weight. It is caused by failure of normal hepatic fat metabolism either due to a defect within the hepatocyte or to delivery of excess fat, fatty acid or carbohydrate beyond the secretory capacity for lipid of the liver cell. Liver biopsy and imaging procedures, such as ultrasound and CT, are resulting in increasing numbers of patients being identified with excess fat in the liver.

Theoretically fatty liver could accumulate through at least four mechanisms.

1 *Increased delivery of dietary fat or fatty acids to the liver.* Dietary fat is transported in the circulation mainly as chylomicrons (fig. 23.1). Lipolysis in adipose tissue liber-

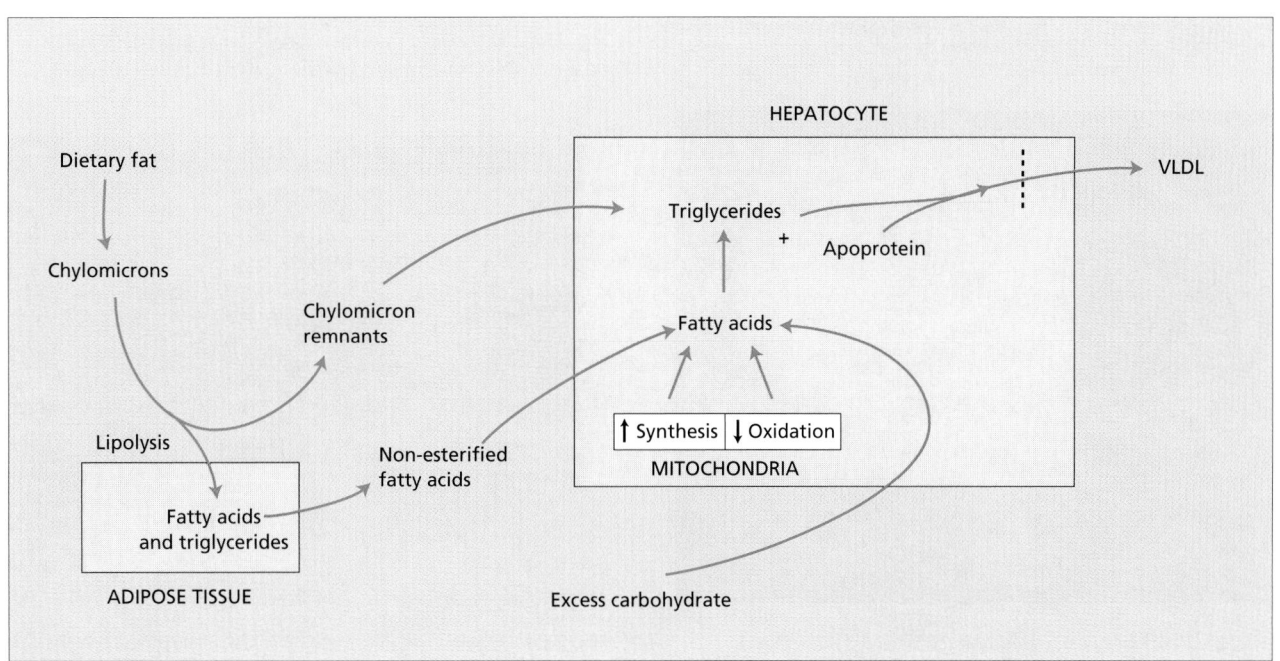

Fig. 23.1. Factors in fatty liver.

ates the fatty acids. These are incorporated into triglyceride within the adipocyte but some fatty acid may be released into the circulation and taken up by the liver. The chylomicron remnants also enter the liver.

2 *Increased mitochondrial synthesis of fatty acids or reduced oxidation.* Both augment triglyceride production.

3 *Impaired export of triglyceride out of the liver cell.* Export of triglycerides from the hepatocyte depends upon packaging with apoprotein, phospholipid and cholesterol to form very low density lipoprotein (VLDL). This process may be inhibited.

4 *Excess carbohydrate* delivered to the liver may be converted to fatty acids.

DIAGNOSIS

Fatty liver may present as diffuse, smooth hepatomegaly in appropriate circumstances such as obesity, diabetes or alcoholism.

Ultrasound may show a bright echo pattern but can be normal. Reflective echoes from fibrosis or cirrhosis are difficult to distinguish. CT shows a reduced attenuation. Portal and hepatic vein radicles appear prominent in a scan unenhanced with contrast. The attenuation is less than that of the spleen or kidneys (fig. 23.2). CT scan is useful to follow the effects of therapy. MRI scanning may also detect fatty infiltration.

Liver biopsy is the best method of diagnosing fatty liver. Appropriate stains such as oil red O on frozen sections are essential to diagnose lesser degrees of fatty change. Liver biopsy appearances are not diagnostic of the cause of the fatty change.

In most instances, the fat is maximal in hepatocytes in zone 3 (central). A zone 1 (peri-portal) distribution is found in protein calorie malnutrition, kwashiorkor, total parenteral nutrition, phosphorus poisoning, methotrexate injury and various other toxic states.

CLASSIFICATION

Increased fat in the liver is divided into two morphological categories: macroscopic and microscopic (figs 23.3, 23.4, 23.5). The two may be combined.

Macroscopic (large droplet)

In haematoxylin and eosin stained liver sections, the hepatocytes contain punched out, empty vacuoles. The nucleus is displaced to the periphery of the cell (fig. 23.4).

Fat in the hepatocyte *per se* is not damaging. The serious association is with steatonecrosis (alcoholic hepatitis) (table 23.1). This is marked by zone 3 (Disse space) pericellular fibrosis (creeping collagenosis) often

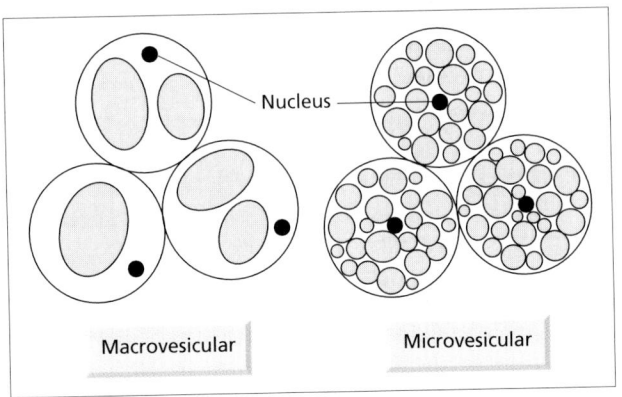

Fig. 23.3. Fatty liver may be classified into macrovesicular (large droplet) and microvesicular (small droplet) types.

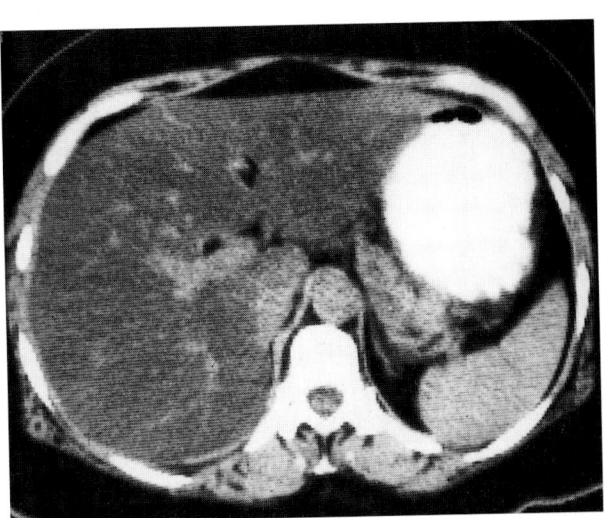

Fig. 23.2. CT fatty liver (unenhanced). Liver is enlarged, smooth and less dense than spleen. The intra-hepatic portal vein radicles are more prominent than normal.

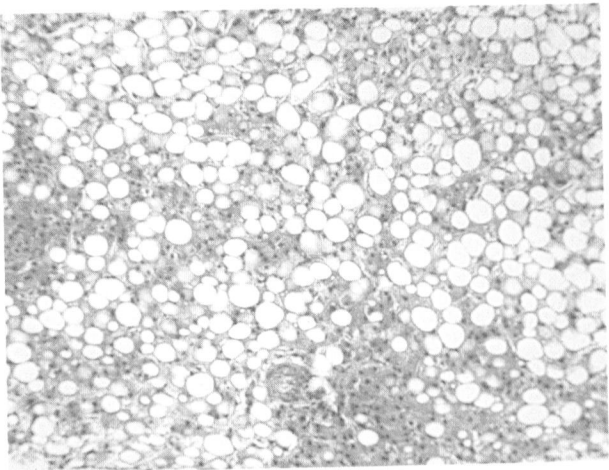

Fig. 23.4. Macrovesicular fat. The liver cells appear empty. The change is maximal in zone 1 ('portal'). (Stained H & E, ×135.)

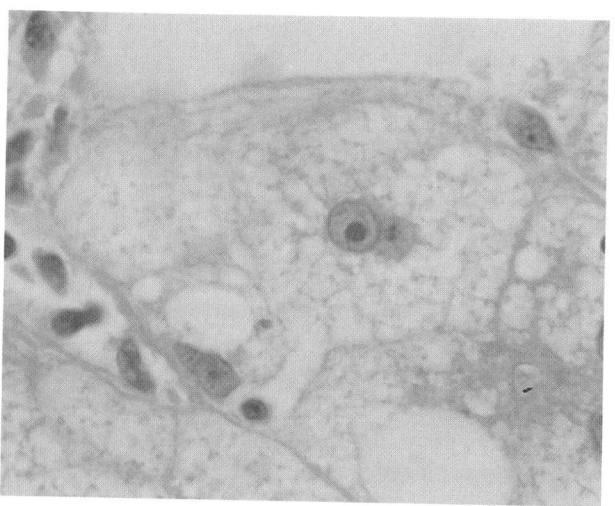

Fig. 23.5. Microvesicular fat. The hepatocyte has a foamy appearance. The nucleus is central with a dense nucleolus.

Table 23.1. The aetiology of large droplet macrovesicular fatty liver

Nutritional
Kwashiorkor
Gastrointestinal disease
Pancreatic disease
Obesity*
Intestinal bypass*
Prolonged parenteral nutrition*

Metabolic diseases
Type II diabetes mellitus*
Galactosaemia
Glycogenoses
Fructose intolerance
Wilson's disease
Tyrosinaemia
Hyperlipidaemias
Abetalipoproteinaemia
Weber–Christian disease
Acylcoenzyme A dehydrogenase deficiency

Drug-related
Alcohol*
Corticosteroids
Direct hepatotoxicity (Chapter 18)
High dose oestrogens*
Amiodarone*

General
Fever
Systemic disease
Viral infections
Cryptogenic

* Steatonecrosis ('alcoholic hepatitis') can develop.

with hepatocyte swelling and deposits of Mallory's hyaline in hepatocytes which are surrounded by neutrophils. This lesion is due to some factor in addition to that which causes fatty liver. It is precirrhotic and can be diagnosed only by liver biopsy.

Clinical features. The patient is usually symptom free. He may complain of right upper quadrant heaviness and discomfort, worse on movement. Pain over the liver is usually related to rapid accumulation of fat associated with alcoholism or with diabetes.

The liver is usually, but not always, smoothly enlarged.

Biochemical tests. These correlate poorly with hepatic histology. Gamma glutamyl transpeptidase is usually elevated. Serum transaminases and alkaline phosphatase show mild increases. Bilirubin and serum albumin are usually normal. Fatty liver is one of the commonest causes of a raised serum transaminase value detected in 'healthy' blood donors.

Cryptogenic fatty liver

When common causes, such as obesity, alcoholism and diabetes, have been excluded a hard core remains with no obvious aetiology. Some may be pre-diabetic [2] or give a family history of diabetes. Patients usually have no symptoms other than anxiety. Serum transaminases may be slightly increased. Treatment is by reassurance and avoiding over-investigation.

Microvesicular fat (fig. 23.5)

Hepatic histology shows zone 3 microvesicular fat. Cell necrosis is variable and minor, although, occasionally, there may be massive zone 3 necrosis. Hepatocytes show central nuclei with prominent nucleoli. Inflammation is minimal, and centrizonal cholestasis is occasionally found. Frozen sections stained for fat are necessary for diagnosis in mild cases. Electron microscopy shows the mitochondria swollen, pleomorphic and varying in shape. The smooth endoplasmic reticulum is increased.

The microvesicular fat diseases can be related to a widespread hepatic metabolic disturbance, particularly involving mitochondria. Perhexiline inhibits both oxidative phosphorylation and the mitochondrial β-oxidation of fatty acids, and is associated with microvesicular steatosis [7]. Experimentally, administration of oestradiol and progesterone (to simulate changes in pregnancy) produce ultrastructural changes in mitochondria and decrease oxidation of fatty acids [10]. Disruption of mitochondrial DNA either due to an inborn error [3], a sporadic deletion [9] or incorporation of a nucleo-side analogue [17] may lead to steatosis, more of the microvesicular than macrovesicular pattern. There are mitochondrial abnormalities on electron microscopy.

Fatty acid oxidation may be depressed. Increases in blood ammonia and low citrulline values can be related to reduction of mitochondrial Krebs' cycle enzymes. Hypoglycaemia is frequent.

Triglyceride accumulation reflects disordered lipoprotein secretion and assembly. Synthesis of the apoprotein of VLDL is depressed with interference with the exit of lipid from the liver.

This group has several members (table 23.2) [11, 24]. Although many show the same clinical pattern, the recognition of this pathology in a wider range of disorders has revealed a heterogeneity of features and outcome.

The onset is often marked by fatigue, nausea, vomiting with variable jaundice, impairment of consciousness, coma and fits (table 23.3). Renal failure and disseminated intravascular coagulation may be complications. The liver is not the only organ involved, and triglyceride accumulations may be found in the renal tubules and occasionally in myocardium, brain and pancreas. Liver failure is not the usual cause of death. Coma may be related to an increase in blood ammonia levels or to cerebral oedema.

Table 23.2. The microvesicular fat diseases

Acute fatty liver of pregnancy
Reye's syndrome
Vomiting disease of Jamaica
Drug toxicity
  sodium valproate
  tetracycline
  salicylate
  fialuridine (FIAU)
Congenital defects of urea cycle enzymes
Genetic defects of mitochondrial fatty acid oxidation
Wolman's disease
Cholesterol ester storage disease
Alcoholic foamy fat syndrome
Delta virus hepatitis in northern South America

Table 23.3. Features of the microvesicular fat diseases [24]

Vomiting
Variable jaundice
Coma
Disseminated intravascular coagulation
Renal failure
Raised blood ammonia values
Hypoglycaemia
Rise in serum fatty acids
Liver biopsy
  microvesicular fat
  necrosis and cellular infiltration not prominent
Electron microscopy
  mitochondrial abnormalities

The mode of initiation of these diseases is diverse and in most instances not fully understood. Viral, toxic and nutritional factors have been implicated.

Focal fatty liver

This condition is recognized by ultrasound, when areas of increased echogenicity are seen. The CT scan shows areas of low attenuation (figs 23.6, 23.7). Dual energy CT helps to differentiate focal fat from other low density lesions [22]. Needle biopsy under CT guidance confirms the diagnosis. The lesions are usually multiple and resolve with time. They may recur. Patients at risk include diabetics, alcoholics, the obese, those on hyperalimentation and sufferers from Cushing's syndrome.

Kwashiorkor syndrome

Children may develop a syndrome of protein malnutri-

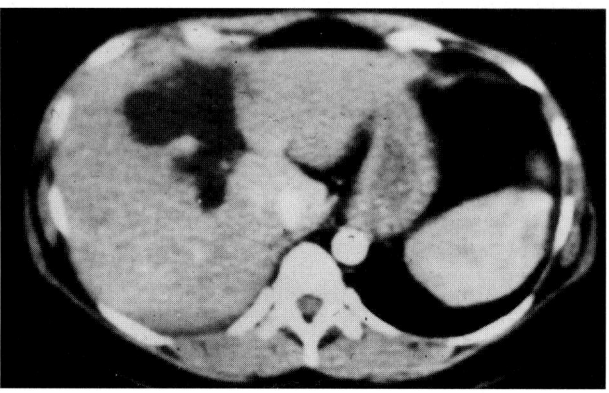

Fig. 23.6. Focal fatty liver. CT scan shows a low attenuation filling defect in the right lobe of liver. This lesion disappeared spontaneously.

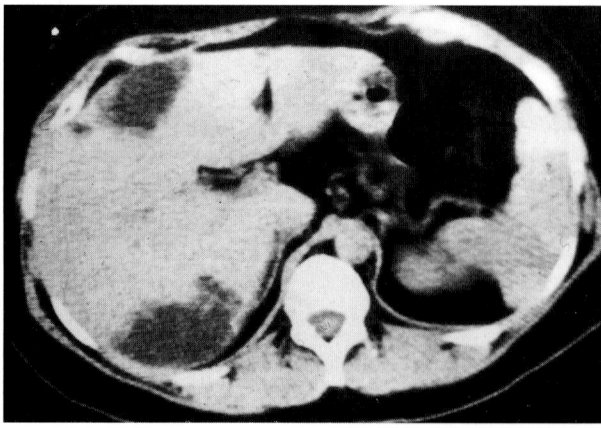

Fig. 23.7. The same patient as in fig. 23.6. A further CT scan performed 6 months later showed two further areas of focal filling defects anteriorly and posteriorly in the right lobe of the liver.

tion called kwashiorkor. It has a worldwide distribution in under-privileged, overpopulated communities, especially tropical and subtropical [31]. It is rare in Europe and indeed in the temperate areas of any continent.

PATHOLOGY

Deficiency of dietary protein affects particularly organs concerned with the elaboration of proteins and protein-containing enzymes.

The acinar cells of the pancreas, salivary and lacrymal glands, and glands of the small intestinal wall are atrophied. There is muscle wasting. The parotid glands may enlarge during recovery.

The liver shows extensive zone 1 fatty change. This might be secondary to the pancreatic damage and analogous to the fatty liver of depancreatized dogs. Alternatively, it may be due to dietary protein deficiency. The liver loses protein and gains water, sharing in the general oedema [31]. The very fatty liver may be related to mobilization of fat from adipose tissue. The hepatic glucose-6-phosphatase level is reduced. Although hepatic glycogen is increased, this suggests failure to handle dietary carbohydrate which may then be converted into fat. Electron microscopy shows surprisingly mild changes [32].

The hepatic change is not specific. It might be an epiphenomenon: the fatty infiltration bears very little relation to clinical severity and causes little disturbance of liver function [31]. There is no progressive fibrosis or cirrhosis [6].

CLINICAL FEATURES

Children are most commonly affected 6–18 months after weaning when they are fed on an almost pure carbohydrate diet. Even before weaning, the milk of the undernourished mother may have been poor in protein, and this lack is emphasized by the demands of growth. Malaria and hookworm disease or an additional insult such as aflatoxin may contribute.

The acute breakdown is often initiated by a diminished food intake due to deprivation of mother love, the birth of another child or to an infection [30]. The child is extremely miserable with arrested growth, generalized oedema and cold extremities. The hair shows characteristic depigmentation, becoming pale and losing its crisp black curliness, thin, straight and soft. The characteristic dermatosis starts in the inguinal region and napkin area and spreads to sites of pressure and irritation. The dusky red patches have been likened to crazy paving. The skin desquamates and becomes pallid.

Appetite is decreased and diarrhoea is prominent, especially in the severe case, the stools showing undigested food. The liver may be enlarged or of normal size.

Severe protein malnutrition in *adults*, resembling kwashiorkor, can be related to ineffective utilization of dietary protein due to pancreatic exocrine deficiency or enteric bacterial colonization [13, 19].

Laboratory findings include reduced haemoglobin and plasma protein concentrations. Pancreatic enzymes are diminished.

Analysis of liver biopsy material shows reduction of pseudo-cholinesterase, D-amino acid oxidase and xanthine oxidase [24]. Enzymes subserving respiration and oxidative phosphorylation are well preserved.

Serum enzymes are depressed in keeping with all protein production [24]. Serum transaminase and plasma-free fatty acid levels are increased [15].

The liver in obesity

Fatty liver is associated with obesity. The degree of steatosis correlates with the increase in body weight in both adults and children [28, 29].

Lipolysis from expanded fat depots is markedly increased and more fatty acids are supplied to the liver. This leads to an imbalance of triglyceride synthesis and secretion. There is also an imbalance between protein and calorie intake.

The fatty change is macrovesicular and in zone 3.

Weight loss by low-calorie dieting or starvation is accompanied by improvement in fatty change and return of liver function tests to normal [8].

In the absence of pre-existing fibrosis or inflammation, the fatty liver of non-alcoholic origin appears to be non-progressive and benign [27]. In some patients, however, inflammation and other changes are associated with steatosis (*steato-hepatitis*) and this may have a less benign course.

NON-ALCOHOLIC STEATO-HEPATITIS [1, 20]

Occasionally the liver shows the changes of acute alcoholic hepatitis (steatonecrosis) in the non-alcoholic. The most common risk factors are obesity and diabetes mellitus [29]. These changes are also seen in patients with jejuno-ileal bypass and drug toxicity, for example amiodarone, but there may be no recognizable risk factor. Symptoms are minor or absent. The diagnosis is made on liver biopsy when investigating a patient with raised transaminases and an otherwise negative biochemical and serological work-up. There is steatosis (macrovesicular or microvesicular) and inflammation; Mallory bodies, fibrosis and cirrhosis may be present. The hepatic damage may relate to lipid peroxidation due to oxidizable fat [14]. Serum transferrin saturation and ferritin may be raised.

Fibrosis and cirrhosis can be present on the initial biopsy. Progression occurs but the speed and severity varies between reports [1, 20]. This may relate to the patient population studied and the morphological definition of the syndrome. However, progression has been seen in 40% of patients, more frequently in obese women [1].

This entity should be considered in the individual with otherwise unexplained raised transaminases whether or not they are diabetic or obese.

EFFECTS OF JEJUNO-ILEAL BYPASS

The hepatic changes of obesity are enhanced. Hepatic lipid concentration increases, and the morphological changes of alcoholic liver disease may be present. Progressive inflammation, fibrosis, zone 3 sclerosis and cirrhosis can develop. Liver disease including the development of cirrhosis is seen in 10% of patients at 15 years after operation [23]. The patient may die in hepatic failure. Reversal of the bypass may not be effective treatment although liver fat decreases.

The liver changes are probably related to rapid weight loss, protein-calorie malnutrition, bacterial overgrowth in the blind loop of intestine, malabsorption and other complex nutritional deficiencies. They can also follow gastric partitioning operations, and are found associated with small intestinal diverticulosis [18] and coeliac disease [16].

Parenteral nutrition [21]

Cholestasis has developed in infants given long-term parenteral nutrition for neonatal intestinal obstruction. In adults, increases in serum transaminase, alkaline phosphatase and bilirubin values follow fat-free total parenteral nutrition for 2 weeks or longer. Liver biopsies show fatty change and mild peri-portal cholestasis. Abnormal biochemical tests also complicate enteral elemental diets in adults [4].

Hepatic fatty change occurs particularly with high glucose feeding and when the rate of infusion exceeds the hepatic oxidative capacity so that fat is synthesized. Similar effects follow intravenous fat emulsions. These changes do not develop if the infusion is balanced in terms of carbohydrate and fat. Choline deficiency may play a part and steatosis reversed by choline supplementation [5].

Gallbladder biliary sludge and pigment gallstones may follow prolonged total parenteral nutrition, especially in infants. It is detected by ultrasound.

Vitamins

The fat-soluble vitamins A, D, E and K are not absorbed if biliary bile acid excretion is inadequate. Deficiencies therefore complicate cholestasis (Chapter 13).

Hypervitaminosis A leads to perisinusoidal fibrosis, central vein sclerosis and focal congestion with perisinusoidal lipid storage cells. Vitamin A fluorescence may be shown in frozen sections. Portal hypertension and ascites are consequences. Similar changes can complicate *retinoid* treatment for psoriasis or acne.

Vitamin E deficiency causes a neuromuscular syndrome in cholestatic children, but rarely in adults.

Alcoholics may show thiamine deficiency. Clinical evidence of this in non-alcoholic patients with liver disease is very rare. Similarly folic acid may be reduced in alcoholics.

Low circulating levels of pyridoxal phosphate, the active form of vitamin B_6 compounds, in cirrhosis is probably due to increased degradation.

References

1 Bacon BR, Farahvash MJ, Janney CG *et al.* Non-alcoholic steatohepatitis: an expanded clinical entity. *Gastroenterology* 1994; **107**: 1103.

2 Batman PA, Scheuer PJ. Diabetic hepatitis preceding the onset of glucose intolerance. *Histopathology* 1985; **9**: 237.

3 Bioulac-Sage P, Parrot-Roulaud F, Mazat JP *et al.* Fatal neonatal liver failure and mitochondrial cytopathy (oxidative phosphorylation deficiency): a light and electron microscopic study of the liver. *Hepatology* 1993; **18**: 839.

4 Bower RH. Hepatic complications of parenteral nutrition. *Semin. Liver Dis.* 1983; **3**: 216.

5 Buchman AL, Dubin MD, Moukarzel AA *et al.* Choline deficiency: a cause of hepatic steatosis during parenteral nutrition that can be reversed with intravenous choline supplementation. *Hepatology* 1995; **22**: 1399.

6 Cook GC, Hutt MSR. The liver after kwashiorkor. *Br. Med. J.* 1967; **iii**: 454.

7 Deschamps D, DeBeco V, Fisch C *et al.* Inhibition by perhexiline of oxidative phosphorylation and the β-oxidation of fatty acids: possible role in pseudoalcoholic liver lesions. *Hepatology* 1994; **19**: 948.

8 Drenick EJ, Simmons F, Murphy JF. Effect on hepatic morphology of treatment of obesity by fasting, reducing diets and small bowel bypass. *N. Engl. J. Med.* 1970; **282**: 829.

9 Fromenty B, Grimbert S, Mansouri A *et al.* Hepatic mitochondrial DNA deletion in alcoholics: association with microvesicular steatosis. *Gastroenterology* 1995; **108**: 193.

10 Grimbert S, Fisch C, Deschamps D *et al.* Effects of female sex hormones on mitochondria: possible role in acute fatty liver of pregnancy. *Am. J. Physiol.* 1995; **268**: G107.

11 Hautekeete ML, Degott C, Benhamou J-P. Microvesicular steatosis of the liver. *Acta Clin. Belgica* 1990; **45**: 311.

12 Himsworth HP, Glynn LE. Massive hepatic necrosis and diffuse hepatic fibrosis (acute yellow atrophy and portal cirrhosis): their production by means of diet. *Clin. Sci.* 1994; **5**: 93.

13 Jones EA, Craigie A, Tavill AS *et al.* Protein metabolism in the intestinal stagnant loop syndrome. *Gut* 1968; **9**: 466.

14 Letteron P, Fromenty B, Terris B *et al.* Acute and chronic hepatic steatosis lead to *in vivo* lipid peroxidation in mice. *J. Hepatol.* 1996; **24**: 200.

15 Lewis B, Hansen JDL, Wittman W *et al.* Plasma free fatty

acids in kwashiorkor and the pathogenesis of the fatty liver. *Am. J. Clin. Nutr.* 1964; **15**: 161.

16 Lynch DA, Thornton JR, Axon AT. Acute fatty liver complicating coeliac disease. *Eur. J. Gastroenterol. Hepatol.* 1994; **6**: 745.

17 McKenzie R, Fried MW, Sallie R *et al.* Hepatic failure and lactic acidosis due to fialuridine (FIAU), an investigational nucleoside analogue for chronic hepatitis B. *N. Engl. J. Med.* 1995; **333**: 1099.

18 Nazim M, Stamp G, Hodgson HJF. Non-alcoholic steatohepatitis associated with small intestinal diverticulosis and bacterial overgrowth. *Hepato-gastroenterology* 1989; **36**: 349.

19 Neale G, Antcliff AC, Welbourn RB *et al.* Protein malnutrition after partial gastrectomy. *Q. J. Med.* 1967; **36**: 469.

20 Powell EE, Cooksley WGE, Hanson R *et al.* The natural history of nonalcoholic steatohepatitis: a follow-up study of forty-two patients for up to 21 years. *Hepatology* 1990; **11**: 74.

21 Quigley EMM, Marsh MN, Shaffer JL *et al.* Hepatobiliary complications of total parenteral nutrition. *Gastroenterology* 1993; **104**: 286.

22 Raptopoulos V, Karellas A, Bernstein J *et al.* Value of dual-energy CT in differentiating focal fatty infiltration of the liver from low-density masses. *Am. J. Roentgenol.* 1991; **157**: 721.

23 Requarth JA, Burchard KW, Colacchio TA *et al.* Long-term morbidity following jejunoileal bypass. The continuing potential need for surgical reversal. *Arch. Surg.* 1995; **130**: 318.

24 Sherlock S. Acute fatty liver of pregnancy and the microvesicular fat diseases. *Gut* 1983; **24**: 265.

25 Sherlock S. Nutrition and the alcoholic. *Lancet* 1984; **i**: 436.

26 Sherlock S, Walshe VM. Hepatic structure and function. In: *Studies of Undernutrition, Wuppertal, 1946 9.* Medical Research Council Special Report, 1951 Series No. 275, p. 111.

27 Teli MR, James OFW, Burt AD *et al.* The natural history of non-alcoholic fatty liver: a follow-up study. *Hepatology* 1995; **22**: 1714.

28 Tominaga K, Kurata JH, Chen YK *et al.* Prevalence of fatty liver in Japanese children and relationship to obesity. An epidemiological ultrasonographic study. *Dig. Dis. Sci.* 1995; **40**: 2002.

29 Wanless IR, Lentz JS. Fatty liver hepatitis (steatohepatitis) and obesity: an autopsy study with analysis of risk factors. *Hepatology* 1990; **12**: 1106.

30 Waterlow JC. Kwashiorkor revisited: the pathogenesis of oedema in Kwashiorkor and its significance. *Trans. R. Soc. Trop. Med. Hyg.* 1984; **78**: 436.

31 Waterlow JC, Cravioto J, Stephen JML. Protein malnutrition in man. *Adv. Protein Chem.* 1960; **15**: 131.

32 Webber BL, Freiman I. The liver in kwashiorkor. *Arch. Pathol.* 1974; **98**: 400.

Carbohydrate metabolism in liver disease

HYPOGLYCAEMIA

This is usually due to reduction in hepatic glucose release. The hepatectomized dog rapidly develops hypoglycaemia [1] and this is seen in acute liver failure (Chapter 8). In fulminant hepatitis it may be intractable [2]. Hypoglycaemia is rare in chronic liver disease, even terminally. Very rarely it is found in cirrhotic patients after a porta-caval anastomosis. Reactive hypoglycaemia, 1.5–2 hours after glucose, has been seen in two patients with chronic hepatitis; blood insulin levels were high. Alcohol can also induce hypoglycaemia, especially in cirrhotic patients.

Hypoglycaemia may complicate Reye's syndrome in children and primary hepatic carcinoma.

HYPERGLYCAEMIA

See page 435.

References

1 Mann FC, Magath TB. Studies on the physiology of the liver. II. The effect of the removal of the liver on the blood sugar level. *Arch. Intern. Med.* 1992; **30**: 73.

2 Samson RI, Trey G, Timme AH *et al.* Fulminating hepatitis with recurrent hypoglycaemia and hemorrhage. *Gastroenterology* 1967; **53**: 291.

The liver in diabetes mellitus

Insulin and the liver

The liver is the principal organ for the degradation of insulin. Peripheral tissues take up insulin to a lesser extent and also remove glucagon. Hyperinsulinaemia is a characteristic association of cirrhosis and is due to failure of degradation and clearance, and not to portal-systemic shunting [12].

In diabetes, glucose-6-phosphatase increases in the liver, facilitating glucose release into the blood. The opposing enzymes which phosphorylate glucose are hexokinase, which is unaffected by insulin, and glucokinase, which decreases in diabetes. As a result, the liver continues to produce glucose even with severe hyperglycaemia. Under these circumstances the normal liver would shut off and deposit glycogen. Fructose-1-6-phosphate activity is also increased in diabetes. Gluconeogenesis is thus favoured.

Substances released from the pancreas into the portal blood are known to increase hepatic regeneration (*hepatotrophic substances*). Insulin is the main hepatotrophic substance although glucagon may also be important. Blood glucagon is increased in liver disease, probably due to pancreatic over-secretion.

Liver changes

Needle biopsy shows normal or increased amounts of glycogen in the livers of severe untreated diabetes [5]. Even higher values follow the administration of insulin, provided hypoglycaemia is prevented.

Histologically the zonal structure is normal. In sections stained with haematoxylin and eosin, the glycogen-filled cells appear pale and fluffy. Zone 1 cells always contain less than zone 3 and this is accentuated by glycogenolysis. In type 1 diabetes, the liver cells appear bloated and oedematous: glycogen is maintained or even increased [5].

Glycogenic infiltration of the liver cell nuclei (fig. 23.8) is shown as vacuolization, the nature of which is confirmed by glycogen stains. It is not specific but is found in about two-thirds of diabetics.

Fatty change of large droplet type is common in the obese type 2 diabetic, but is minimal in type 1 (fig. 23.9). It is mainly in zone 1.

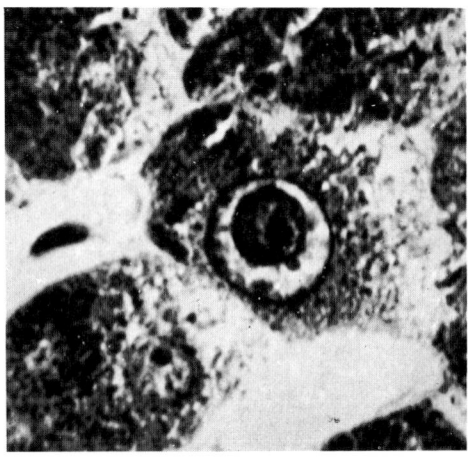

Fig. 23.8. Glycogen infiltration of a hepatic nucleus. Cells contain much glycogen. (Best's carmine for glycogen, ×1150).

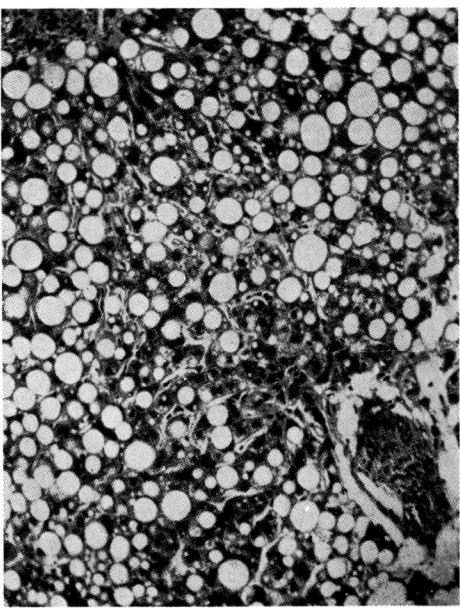

Fig. 23.9. Diabetes mellitus. Liver biopsy sections show great increase in fat in the liver cells. (H & E, ×145) (Sherlock et al. 1951).

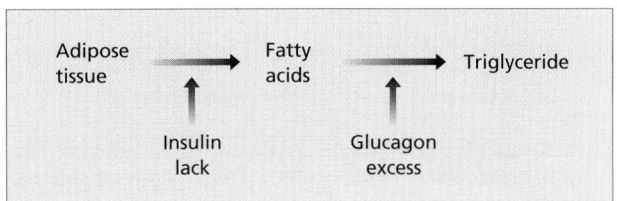

Fig. 23.10. The mechanism of macrovesicular fatty change in type 2 diabetes.

Mechanisms. Diabetes is marked by insulin deficiency and glucagon excess (fig. 23.10). This enhances lipolysis and inhibits glucose uptake so increasing triglyceride formation by adipose tissue. Hepatic uptake of free fatty acids increases. In the liver, glycogen degradation and gluconeogenesis are increased while glucose utilization is inhibited. Ketoacidosis enhances the lipolysis. These factors are responsible for the fatty liver of diabetics.

Steatonecrosis resembling alcoholic hepatitis, but without polymorph infiltration, can be seen particularly in type 2 diabetes [3], even preceding glucose intolerance [1]. This collagenosis of Disse's space can develop in both types of diabetes and may be aetiologically similar to that seen in systemic capillaries in diabetes [8]. Cirrhosis can develop.

At autospy cirrhosis is seen twice as commonly in 'diabetics' as in the general population, but this excess incidence may be flawed because the hyperglycaemia recorded in life might be secondary to unrecognized cirrhosis.

Liver changes in various types of diabetes mellitus

JUVENILE TYPE 1 OR INSULIN-DEPENDENT

There are usually no clinical features referable to the liver. Occasionally, however, the liver is greatly enlarged, firm and with a smooth, tender edge. Some of the nausea, abdominal pain and vomiting of diabetic ketosis may be due to hepatomegaly [4]. Hepatic enlargement is found particularly in young people and children with severe, uncontrolled diabetes. In adults, hepatomegaly occurs with prolonged acidosis. In one large series, hepatomegaly was noted in only 9% of well-controlled diabetics, in 60% of uncontrolled diabetics and in 100% of patients in ketosis [4]. The liver returns to a normal size when the diabetes is brought under complete control. The enlargement is due to increased glycogen. Insulin therapy in the presence of a very high blood sugar level augments still further the glycogen content of the liver and, in the initial stages of treatment, hepatomegaly may increase. The liver cells in severe acidosis may contain more water than usual; it is probably retained to keep the glycogen in solution.

The blood glucose levels and hepatic glucose output fall promptly with insulin [2]. In ketosis, hepatic insulin sensitivity is lost.

TYPE 2 OR NON-INSULIN-DEPENDENT

The liver may be enlarged with a firm, smooth, non-tender edge. Enlargement is due to increased deposition of liver fat largely related to the obesity.

The blood glucose level and the hepatic glucose output respond poorly to a small dose of insulin [1, 2].

Diabetes in childhood

The liver may be enlarged and this enlargement has been attributed both to fatty infiltration and to increased amounts of glycogen. Aspiration biopsy studies show that the fatty change is slight but that the liver does contain an excess of glycogen. The hepatic changes are similar to those already described in the type 1, insulin-sensitive diabetic.

Sometimes a huge liver is associated with retarded growth, obesity, florid facies and hypercholesterolaemia (*Mauriac syndrome*) [9]. Splenomegaly, portal hypertension and hepato-cellular failure do not occur.

Liver function tests

In well-controlled diabetics, routine tests are usually normal and any change is due to a cause other than diabetes. Acidosis may produce mild changes including hyperglobulinaemia and a slightly raised serum bilirubin level. These return to normal with diabetic control.

Eighty per cent of diabetics with a fatty liver have abnormal results for one or more serum biochemical test such as transaminases, alkaline phosphatase and gamma-glutamyl transpeptidase.

Hepatomegaly, whether due to increased amounts of glycogen in type 1 diabetes or to fatty change in type 2, does not correlate with the results of the liver function tests.

Hepato-biliary disease and diabetes

Any real increase of cirrhosis in diabetics seems unlikely. In most instances, the cirrhosis is diagnosed first before impaired glucose tolerance is recognized.

Diabetes mellitus is associated with genetic haemochromatosis. It is also associated with autoimmune chronic hepatitis and with the histocompatibility antigens HLA-B8 and DR3, which are common to both.

Gallstones are frequent in non-insulin-dependent diabetics. This is probably more related to the biliary changes of obesity than a direct effect of diabetes. The same applies to the finding of a reduced gallbladder contractility in these patients.

Elective surgery for gallbladder disease is not dangerous but emergency biliary surgery in diabetics is associated with an increased mortality and a high risk of wound infections.

Sulfonylurea therapy can be complicated by cholestatic or granulomatous liver disease.

Glucose intolerance of cirrhosis

Cirrhotic patients often become hyperglycaemic following an oral glucose load [10] (fig. 23.11). The underlying mechanism is complex and not fully understood [6]. There is peripheral insulin resistance [13] and reduced insulin clearance in most cirrhotics. Adipocytes show defects in insulin sensitivity [13]. The first pass hepatic extraction of insulin is reduced compared with controls [7]. Most patients compensate for the peripheral insulin resistance with increased pancreatic insulin secretion. The result is high circulating insulin levels, a normal fasting blood glucose and minimal glucose intolerance.

In some patients there is a blunted or subnormal pancreatic secretion of insulin after oral glucose, shown by the delayed appearance of C-peptide [7] (fig. 23.11). This leads to delayed peripheral utilization of glucose. The fasting glucose remains normal. With more severe hyposecretion of insulin, there is also continued hepatic glucose production due to lack of inhibition by insulin [11]. The net result of these changes is fasting hyperglycaemia and marked hyperglycaemia after oral glucose. The patient is diabetic.

The glucose intolerance of cirrhotic patients can be distinguished from genuine diabetes mellitus as the fasting blood glucose is usually normal. Clinical features of diabetes are not seen.

Diagnosis of cirrhosis in the presence of diabetes is usually easy, for diabetes alone does not cause vascular spiders, jaundice, hepato-splenomegaly and ascites. If necessary liver biopsy is diagnostic.

High carbohydrate feeding may be necessary in the management of cirrhosis, especially if there is encephalopathy. This always takes precedence over any impairment of glucose tolerance whether from genuine diabetes or secondary to the liver disease.

Treatment of diabetes in cirrhotic patients

There are few data on treatment of diabetes in patients with cirrhosis [6]. Decisions depend upon the degree of hyperglycaemia and the severity and prognosis of the liver disease. Diet is appropriate for mild hyperglycaemia. Sulphonylureas can be used if diet is unsuccessful or the blood glucose is higher, but because these agents are metabolized by the liver, the shorter acting

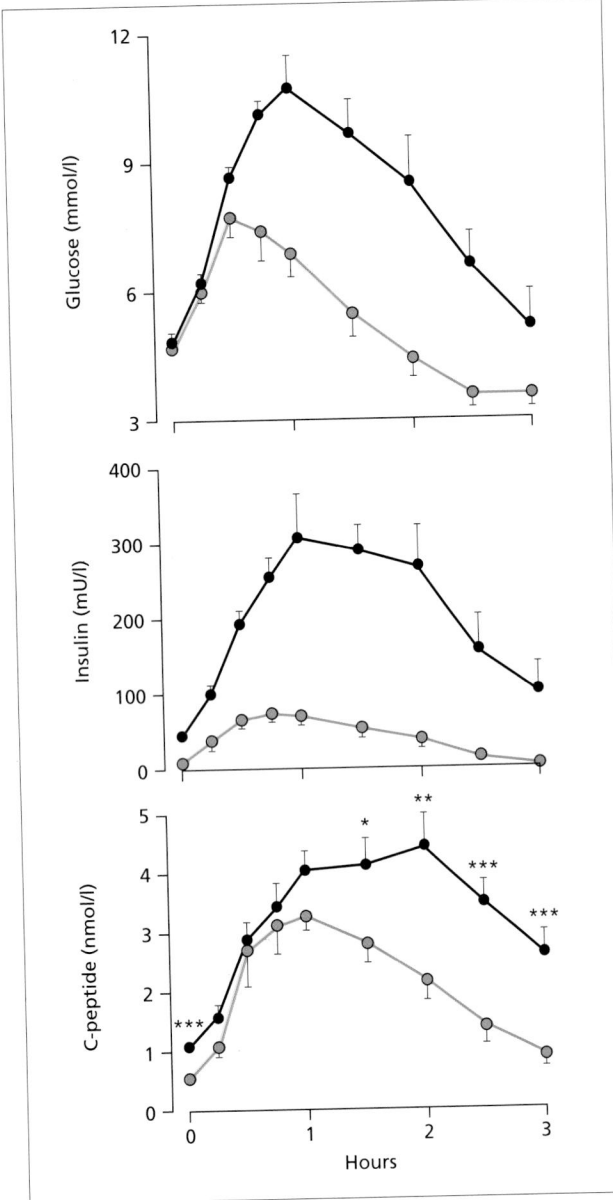

Fig. 23.11. Blood glucose, serum insulin and C-peptide responses to 75 g of oral glucose in cirrhotics (*n* = 10) (black circles) and normal controls (*n* = 9) (green dots). Note the normal fasting glucose followed by hyperglycaemia in the cirrhotics, despite greater insulin levels. The C-peptide response is blunted and only becomes significantly greater than controls at 90 minutes (*$P < 0.05$; **$P < 0.01$; ***$P < 0.001$) [7].

agents such as tolbutamide are preferred to reduce the risk of hypoglycaemia [6]. Because of the risk of lactic acidosis, biguanides such as metformin should be avoided. Insulin may be necessary but, as with other diabetics, regular self-monitoring of blood glucose is necessary. Short-acting insulin before meals, and intermediate acting insulin in the evening, may be used. Strict guidelines do not exist and good control in this group of patients is often difficult and unsatisfactory. Steroid administration, necessary for example in autoimmune chronic liver disease, further complicates diabetic control.

References

1 Batman PA, Scheuer PJ. Diabetic hepatitis preceeding the onset of glucose intolerance. *Histopathology* 1985; **9**: 237.
2 Bearn AG, Billing BH, Sherlock S. Hepatic glucose output and hepatic insulin sensitivity in diabetes mellitus. *Lancet* 1951; **ii**: 698.
3 Falchuk KR, Fiske SC, Haggitt RC *et al*. Pericentral hepatic fibrosis and intracellular hyalin in diabetes mellitus. *Gastroenterology* 1980; **78**: 535.
4 Goodman JI. Hepatomegaly and diabetes mellitus. *Ann. Intern. Med.* 1953; **39**: 1077.
5 Hildes JA, Sherlock S, Walsh V. Liver and muscle glycogen in normal subjects, in diabetes mellitus and in acute hepatitis. *Clin. Sci.* 1949; **7**: 287.
6 Kruszynska YT. Glucose control in liver disease. *Curr. Med. Lit. Gastroenterol.* 1992; **11**: 9.
7 Kruszynska YT, Home PD, McIntyre N. Relationship between insulin sensitivity, insulin secretion and glucose tolerance in cirrhosis. *Hepatology* 1991; **14**: 103.
8 Latry P, Bioulac-Sage P, Echinard E *et al*. Peri-sinusoidal fibrosis and basement membrane-like material in the livers of diabetic patients. *Hum. Path.* 1987; **18**: 775.
9 Mauriac P. Hepatomégalie, nanismé, obesité dans le diabète infantile: pathogenie du syndrome. *Presse Med.* 1946; **54**: 826.
10 Megyesi C, Samols E, Marks V. Glucose tolerance and diabetes in chronic liver disease. *Lancet* 1967; **ii**; 1051.
11 Petrides AS, Vogt C, Schulze-Berge D *et al*. The pathogenesis of glucose intolerance and diabetes mellitus in cirrhosis. *Hepatology* 1994; **19**: 616.
12 Smith-Laing G, Sherlock S, Faber OK. Effects of spontaneous portal-systemic shunting on insulin metabolism. *Gastroenterology* 1979; **76**: 685.
13 Taylor R, Heine RJ, Collins J *et al*. Insulin action in cirrhosis. *Hepatology* 1985; **5**: 64.

The glycogenoses

These are diseases with excessive and/or abnormal glycogen in the tissues. Various forms have different enzymatic or structural defects. Most affect the liver (table 23.4). In the hepatic forms diagnosis is usually in infancy or early childhood with hypoglycaemia, massive hepatomegaly, poor physical growth, a tendency to increased fat deposition particularly in the cheeks, and biochemical abnormalities. Type V (muscle phosphorylase) and VII (phosphofructokinase) involve only muscle, or muscle and erythrocyte, respectively.

For those involving the liver, needle biopsy specimens should be examined histologically, quantitative glycogen analysis is helpful and a portion should be sent, appropriately preserved, to a centre where *in vitro* study

Table 23.4. The hepatic glycogen storage diseases

Type	Enzyme defect	Tissues involved
0	Glycogen synthetase	Liver
I	Glucose-6-phosphatase	Liver, kidney, intestines
II	Lysosomal α-1,4 glucosidase (acid maltase)	Generalized
III	Amylo-1,6 glucosidase (debranching enzyme)	Liver, muscle, WBC
IV	Amylo-1,4,1,6 transglucosidase (branching enzyme)	Generalized
VI	Liver phosphorylase	Liver, WBC
VIII	Phosphorylase activation	Liver
IXa, IXb	Phosphorylase kinase	Liver, WBC, RBC

of the enzymes present and of glycogen structure can be made (table 23.4). The diagnosis cannot be made on hepatic histology alone. All forms seem to be inherited, usually as an autosomal recessive except type VI which

is sex-linked. The types vary greatly in their severity and in their clinical picture. The critical abnormality is usually insufficient glucose production by the liver, which results in hypoglycaemia when the blood glucose level is not supported by an inflow of glucose from the intestinal tract. The other abnormalities follow this defect and from the metabolic reactions to hypoglycaemia (fig. 23.12).

Type I (Von Gierke's disease)

This type involves liver and kidney but not muscle and heart. The inheritance is autosomal recessive. Siblings may be involved, but transmission through successive generations has not been shown.

Type Ia is due to deficiency in the liver of glucose-6-phosphatase. In *type Ib*, the defect is in the translocase for glucose-6-phosphatase at the membrane of the endoplasmic reticulum [14]. The clinical features of Ia and Ib are generally similar. Type Ib may affect adults.

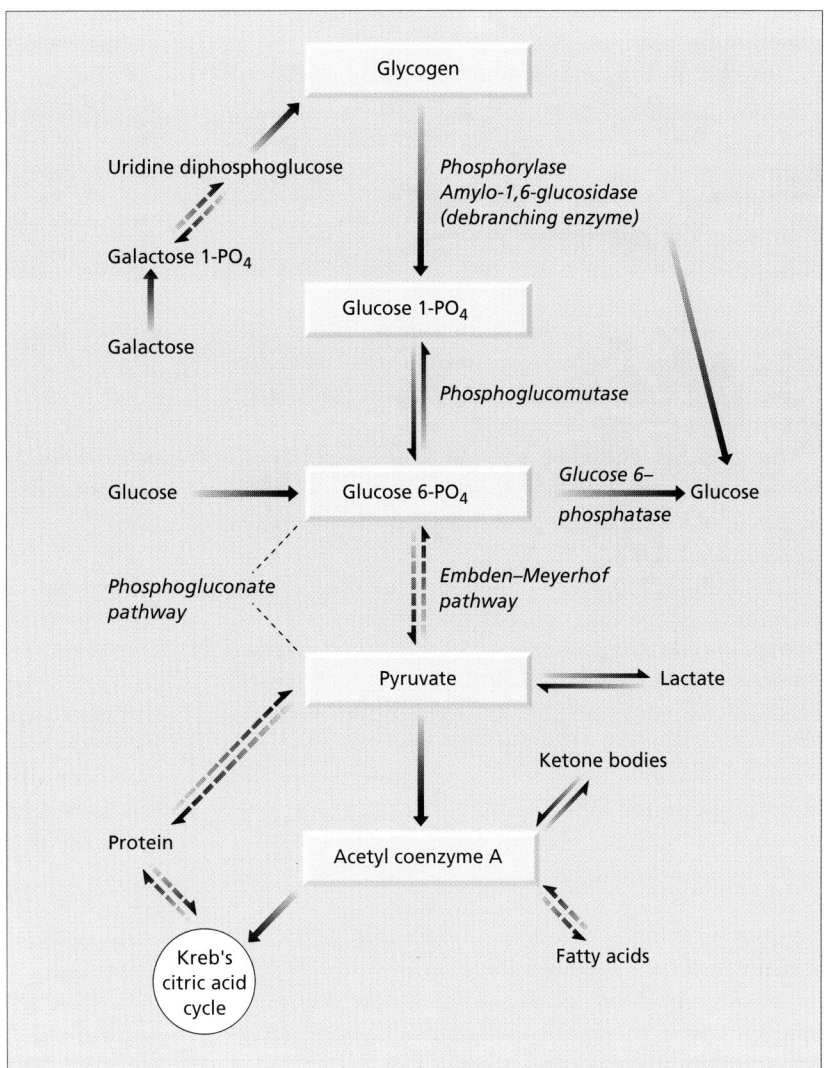

Fig. 23.12. Metabolic pathways in glycogen breakdown (Sokal 1962).

Pericellular zone 3 fibrosis and Mallory bodies have been described in type Ia glycogenesis [12].

Type Ic is due to a defect in hepatic microsomal phosphate/pyrophosphate translocase T_2 [5].

HEPATIC CHANGES

The liver is enlarged, smooth and brown. The liver cells and their nuclei are laden with glycogen, but this is not diagnostic. In formol-fixed material, glycogen is washed out leaving an appearance of clear, plant-like cells. Excess fat is usually present. The glycogen is usually stable, persisting many days *post-mortem* and despite severe ketosis or prolonged anaesthesia. Cirrhosis does not develop. Hepato-cellular adenomas and, rarely carcinomas are late developments [3].

CLINICAL FEATURES

In early infancy the symptoms include irritability, pallor, cyanosis, feeding difficulties and seizures usually associated with hypoglycaemia. Episodes of diarrhoea and vomiting are frequent.

Presentation is as massive hepatomegaly at about 2 years old. The spleen is not enlarged—a point of distinction from the lipoidoses, the cirrhoses and congenital hepatic fibrosis.

The child is short and fat with particularly fat cheeks. Mental development is usually normal.

Hypoglycaemic episodes and fasting ketosis are usual.

Excessive bleeding is due to abnormal platelet function. In type Ib, infectious complications are due to neutropenia and neutrophil dysfunction related to abnormal glucose-6-phosphatase transport [1].

Untreated patients have a doll-like facies and hypotonia with delayed motor milestones. Chronic renal failure occurs in older patients whose disease has been ineffectively treated [20].

Type I glycogenosis can present in adults as hypoglycaemic symptoms and/or hepatomegaly [5].

Hepato-cellular adenomas develop. At least one was found on ultrasound in 75% of 37 patients with type 1a aged 18 years or more [20]; 41% had multiple lesions. There may be pain. Haemorrhage into the tumour is reported. Malignant transition to hepato-cellular carcinoma is recognized [3].

INVESTIGATIONS

Routine liver function tests are usually normal. Occasionally transaminases are raised.

The fasting blood glucose level is low. Ketosis is related to defective glucose metabolism. Hyperlipaemia, hypercholesterolaemia and a fatty liver are common.

Plasma uric acid levels are raised and gout develops after puberty. There is chronic lactic acidosis.

Diagnosis depends on showing that the blood glucose fails to rise adequately when hepatic glycogenolysis is stimulated. *Glucagon* (20 µg/kg body weight) is given intramuscularly after a fast of 10–12 hours, or 3–4 hours if hypoglycaemia is severe. Results are classified according to the blood glucose response. Normals show a rise of 35 mg/100 ml (2 mmol/l), subnormals 15–35 mg/100 ml, and absent or minimal less than 15 mg/100 ml. Lactic acid changes are classified as normal with increases of less than 10 mg/100 ml or abnormal with increases of more than 10 mg/100 ml.

These patients cannot utilize galactose or fructose as a source of blood glucose and intravenous lactose and fructose tests may also be performed.

The erythrocyte glycogen level is increased.

If a test is positive, liver biopsy should be taken for histology, including histochemistry, quantitative glycogen analysis and enzyme analysis.

Classification into the actual type can then be attempted. Mutation analysis as a diagnostic method is being developed [16].

Ultrasound shows marked parenchymal changes in 40% of patients due to fat, and will identify tumours, usually adenoma [15].

TREATMENT

Repeated enteral glucose feeds, often given as a continual nocturnal infusion, are needed to prevent hypoglycaemia [17]. Uncooked corn starch, a slow release source of glucose, is an alternative regime [7] and can be given with milk feeds every 4 hours [21]. Parenteral hyperalimentation may be useful [6]. Allopurinol may be given for the high serum uric acid.

Haemorrhage into an adenoma may necessitate resection [10].

Hepatic transplantation has been successfully performed both because of poor control of blood glucose with usual therapeutic measures and for hepatic adenomas [8]. With longer survival through improved dietary regimens, adenoma-related complications (haemorrhage, malignant transformation) are clinical problems. Ideally transplantation should predate malignant transformation but data are needed to show when this intervention is most appropriate.

PROGNOSIS

Many patients die in early childhood, often with infections. There are great variations in severity and some patients seem to recover completely. The disease tends to become milder after puberty. Later deaths are due to gouty nephropathy or to hepato-cellular tumours.

Type II (Pompe's disease)

This primary lysosomal disease is due to deficiency of lysosomal acid α-1,4 glucosidase which normally degrades glycogen within lysosomes.

There is weakness of skeletal muscle, cardiomegaly, hepatomegaly and macroglossia. Mental development is normal. Infantile, childhood and adult onset forms exist. The infantile form is the most severe. Glucagon and adrenaline tests are normal and hypoglycaemia does not occur. Hyperlipidaemia is conspicuous.

All organs show vacuolated cells due to the enlarged lysosomes which contain the glycogen. Vacuolated lymphocytes are found in peripheral blood and marrow. The liver cells at autopsy show particularly prominent vacuoles.

Type III (Cori's disease) (fig. 23.13)

Clinically this resembles type I glycogenosis. Acidosis, hypoglycaemia and hyperlipidaemia may be present.

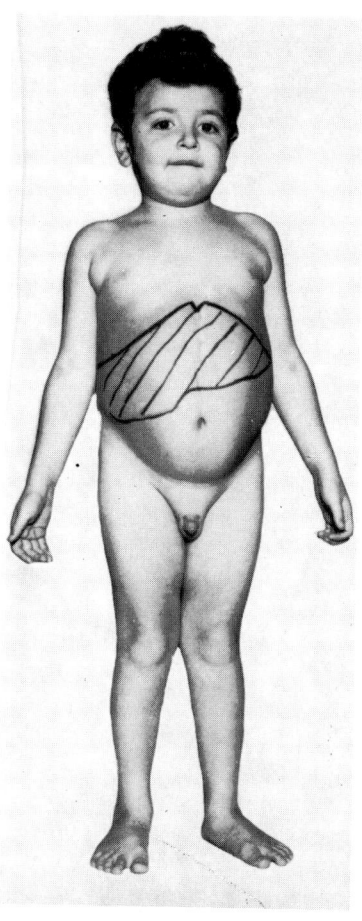

Fig. 23.13. Type III glycogen storage disease (Cori's disease). A boy of 4 years with enormous hepatomegaly but without splenomegaly. At the age of 30, this young man is well and has finished his military service.

Blood glucose does not rise after glucagon, but galactose and fructose tolerance are normal. Serum transaminases are usually increased. Symptoms may be mild and by adult life only the hepatomegaly may remain. The prognosis is fair to good.

Peri-portal fibrosis occurs but cirrhosis is rare. Liver biopsy is rarely necessary for diagnosis which is made by measuring debrancher activity in a mixed white blood cell pellet.

Glycogen is increased in muscle and liver and the debranching enzyme, amylo-1,6 glucosidase, is absent.

Corn starch therapy may improve growth and liver function [4]. Ultrasound shows hepatic changes and tumour less often than in type 1 [15].

Type IV (Andersen's disease)

This very rare form of generalized glycogenosis is associated with low normal tissue levels of glycogen. The glycogen structure is abnormal due to deficiency of the branching enzyme amylo-1,4,1,6 transglucosidase.

A cirrhosis develops which may be associated with many giant cells. It can resemble that of the alcoholic. The chief distinction is the presence of intra-cellular deposits of abnormal glycogen partially removed by diastase digestion. This may show abnormal staining properties turning purplish with iodine instead of the usual reddish-brown. It stains strongly with PAS. The cirrhosis is presumably due to a reaction to this abnormal glycogen which is found in every organ examined.

The child develops hepatosplenomegaly, ascites and finally liver failure. Enzyme deficiency in skin fibroblasts has been shown and may allow diagnosis and detection of heterozygotes. The features of cirrhosis are present. Hepato-cellular adenoma is reported [2]. Death is in early childhood. Hepatic transplantation has been successful. Because of the persistent metabolic abnormality in extra-hepatic sites, there may be progressive extra-hepatic disease [19] but it is not known why this does not occur in all patients [18].

Type VI (Hers' disease)

This involves only the liver and is marked by deficiency of phosphorylase. Growth retardation and hepatomegaly are marked. Hypoglycaemia and acidosis are usually found. Mental function is normal. Liver ultrasound shows less frequent and less severe changes than in types I and III [15]. Survival into adult life is usual.

Variants have been described where, although phosphorylase is reduced, it can be increased to normal by glucagon or adrenaline, or *in vitro* by substitution of an activation system [11]. In these patients the low hepatic phosphorylase activity is not the result of deficiency of the enzymes.

Type IXa and IXb

This benign condition is due to phosphorylase kinase deficiency. It presents with short stature and hepatomegaly. The outlook is excellent and in time the patient catches up growth and hepatomegaly becomes less. It is diagnosed by measuring phosphorylase kinase in red blood cells. Autosomal and X-linked forms exist.

Low molecular weight glycogen

This very rare condition is associated with cirrhosis, early death and a widespread deposition in tissues, including the liver, of a polysaccharide material of low molecular weight [13].

Hepatic glycogen synthetase deficiency (type 0) [9]

This very rare condition is associated with glucose intolerance, hypoglycaemia and mental retardation. Analysis of liver biopsy material shows complete absence of the enzyme glycogen synthetase.

References

1 Ambruso DR, McCabe ERB, Anderson D *et al.* Infectious and bleeding complications in patients with glycogenosis 1b. *Am. J. Dis. Child.* 1985; **139**: 691.

2 Alshak NS, Cocjin J, Podesta L *et al.* Hepatocellular adenoma in glycogen storage disease type IV. *Arch. Path. Lab. Med.* 1994; **118**: 88.

3 Bianchi L. Glycogen storage disease I and hepatocellular tumours. *Eur. J. Pediatr.* 1993; **152** (Suppl. 1): S63.

4 Borowitz SM, Greene HL. Cornstarch therapy in a patient with type III glycogen storage disease. *J. Pediatr. Gastroenterol. Nutr.* 1987; **6**: 631.

5 Burchell A, Jung RT, Lang CC *et al.* Diagnosis of type 1a and type 1c glycogen storage diseases in adults. *Lancet* 1987; **i**: 1059.

6 Burr IM, O'Neill JA, Karson DT *et al.* Comparison of the effects of total parenteral nutrition, continuous intragastric feeding and portacaval shunt on a patient with type 1 glycogen storage disease. *J. Pediatr.* 1974; **85**: 792.

7 Chen Y-T, Cornblath M, Sidbury JB. Corn starch therapy in type 1 glycogen-storage disease. *N. Engl. J. Med.* 1984; **310**: 171.

8 Coire CI, Qizilbash AH, Castelli MF. Hepatic adenomata in type 1a glycogen storage disease. *Arch. Pathol. Lab. Med.* 1987; **111**: 166.

9 Dykes JRW, Spencer-Peet J. Hepatic glycogen synthetase deficiency. Further studies on a family. *Arch. Dis. Child.* 1972; **47**: 558.

10 Fink AS, Appleman HD. Hemorrhage into a hepatic adenoma and type 1a glycogen storage disease: a case report and review of the literature. *Surgery* 1985; **97**: 117.

11 Hug G, Schubert WK, Chuck G *et al.* Liver phosphorylase. Deactivation in a child with progressive brain disease, elevated hepatic glycogen and increased urinary catecholamines. *Am. J. Med.* 1967; **42**: 139.

12 Itoh S, Ishida Y, Matsuo S. Mallory bodies in a patient with type 1a glycogen storage disease. *Gastroenterology* 1987; **92**: 520.

13 Krivit W, Sharp HL, Lee JC. Low molecular weight glycogen as a cause of generalised glycogen storage disease. *Am. J. Med.* 1973; **54**: 88.

14 Kuzuya T, Matsuda A, Yoshida S *et al.* An adult case of type 1b glycogen-storage disease. *N. Engl. J. Med.* 1983; **308**: 566.

15 Lee P, Mather S, Owens C *et al.* Hepatic ultrasound findings in the glycogen storage diseases. *Br. J. Radiol.* 1994; **67**: 1062.

16 Lei KJ, Chen YT, Chen H *et al.* Genetic basis of glycogen storage disease type 1a: prevalent mutations at the glucose-6-phosphatase locus. *Am. J. Hum. Genet.* 1995; **57**: 766.

17 Schwenk WF, Haymond MW. Optimal rate of enteral glucose administration in children with glycogen storage disease type 1. *N. Engl. J. Med.* 1986; **314**: 680.

18 Selby R, Starzl TE, Yunis E *et al.* Liver transplantation for type I and type IV glycogen storage disease. *Eur. J. Pediatr.* 1993; **152** (Suppl. 1): S71.

19 Sokal EM, Van Hoof F, Alberti D *et al.* Progressive cardiac failure following orthotopic liver transplantation for type IV glycogenosis. *Eur. J. Pediatr.* 1992; **151**: 200.

20 Talente GM, Coleman RA, Alter C *et al.* Glycogen storage disease in adults. *Ann. Intern. Med.* 1994; **120**: 218.

21 Wolfsdorf JI, Keller RJ, Landy H *et al.* Glucose therapy for glycogenosis type 1 in infants: comparison of intermittent uncooked cornstarch and continuous overnight glucose feedings. *J. Pediatr.* 1990; **117**: 384.

Hereditary fructose intolerance

This autosomal recessive condition is caused by mutations in the gene for aldolase B on chromosome 9 [1]. Deficiency of this enzyme impairs the cleavage of fructose-1-phosphate in liver, renal cortex and intestinal epithelium. Exposure to fructose induces cytoplasmic accumulation of fructose-1-phosphate and hence fructose intoxication [2].

The acute syndrome is marked by abdominal pain, vomiting and hypoglycaemia. The chronic syndrome is one of severe metabolic derangement with failure to thrive, vomiting, hepatomegaly and liver and renal tubular dysfunction. Fructosaemia, fructosuria and hypophosphataemia are features. Diagnosis is confirmed by the intravenous fructose tolerance test or by direct assay of fructaldolase activity in tissue biopsy samples. Hepatic histology shows similar findings to galactosaemia with the ultimate development of cirrhosis.

Older children learn to avoid fructose and sucrose and isolated hepatomegaly may be the only abnormality.

Treatment is by a diet without sucrose and fructose. Sometimes the symptoms persist in older children and are marked by growth retardation when even more strict fructose restriction may be necessary [3].

References

1 Cross NCP, De Franchis R, Sebastio G *et al.* Molecular analysis of aldolase B genes in hereditary fructose intolerance.

Lancet 1990; **335**: 306.

2 Froesch ER, Wolf HP, Baitsch H *et al.* Hereditary fructose intolerance: inborn defect of hepatic fructose-1-phosphate splitting aldolase. *Am. J. Med.* 1963; **34**: 151.

3 Mock DM, Perman JA, Thaler MM *et al.* Chronic fructose intoxication after infancy in children with hereditary fructose intolerance: a cause of growth retardation. *N. Engl. J. Med.* 1983; **309**: 764.

Glutaric aciduria type II

This disturbance of organic acid metabolism presents in infants or adults as recurrent hypoglycaemia with elevated serum free fatty acid. There may be hepatomegaly. The liver often shows fatty change. Peri-portal fibrosis and hypoplastic extra-hepatic ducts are reported [1]

Reference

1 Wilson GN, De Chadarevian J-P, Kaplan P *et al.* Glutaric aciduria type II: review of the phenotype and report of an unusual glomerulopathy. *Am. J. Med. Genet.* 1989; **32**: 395.

Galactosaemia

The liver and red blood cells lack the specific enzyme, galactose-1-phosphate-uridyl transferase, essential for galactose metabolism. Toxic effects are related to the accumulation in the tissues of galactose-1-phosphate. The mechanism of toxicity is uncertain [3].

Transferase deficiency is inherited as an autosomal recessive with a frequency of between 1 in 10 000 and 1 in 60 000. There are several mutations [6]. These would explain the clinical variability seen. A significant reduction of the transferase is found in heterozygotes.

CLINICAL PICTURE

The disease starts *in utero*. The infant presents with feeding difficulties, with sepsis, and with vomiting, diarrhoea and malnutrition, often with jaundice. Ascites and hepatosplenomegaly are noted. Cataracts develop. Death may result in the first few weeks, but survivors become mentally retarded and finally show the features of cirrhosis, portal hypertension and, later, ascites.

HEPATIC CHANGES

Those dying in the first few weeks show diffuse hepatocellular fatty change. In the next few months the liver shows pseudoglandular or ductular structures around the canaliculi which may contain bile. Regeneration is conspicuous, necrosis scanty and a macronodular cirrhosis results. Giant cells may be numerous.

DIAGNOSIS [5]

The biochemical changes include galactosaemia, galactosuria, hyperchloraemic acidosis, albuminuria and aminoaciduria. Diagnosis is made by finding a urinary reducing substance which is glucose oxidase negative. Definite diagnosis comes from determining galactose-1-phosphate uridyl transferase levels in the erythrocytes.

The condition should be considered in all young patients with cirrhosis and even in the adult if there are suggestive features such as cataract. Galactosaemia has been diagnosed as late as 63 years [4]. A survey of a group of juvenile cirrhotics for this disease, however, failed to reveal a single case and this must be a rare cause of adult cirrhosis [2].

PROGNOSIS AND TREATMENT

Great improvement results from withdrawal of dietary milk and milk products from the diet. If the child survives to 5 years of age, recovery may be complete apart from persistent cataracts or cirrhosis. Delayed puberty, speech abnormalities and reduced intelligence are seen in the longer term [7]. There is endogenous production of galactose explaining the persistence of galactose metabolites despite compliance with dietary restriction [1]. Those living into childhood and adult life without treatment may be only partially enzyme deficient. Alternatively, they may have developed another pathway for handling galactose. The consumption of galactose-containing foods also decreases with age.

References

1 Berry GT, Nissim I, Lin Z *et al.* Endogenous synthesis of galactose in normal men and patients with hereditary galactosemia. *Lancet* 1995; **346**: 1073.

2 Fisher MM, Spear S, Samols E *et al.* Erythrocytic galactose-1-phosphate uridyl transferase levels in hepatic cirrhosis. *Gut* 1964; **5**: 170.

3 Gitzelmann R. Galactose-1-phosphate in the pathogenesis of galactosemia. *Eur. J. Pediatr* 1995; **154** (Suppl. 2): S45.

4 Hsia DY-Y, Walker FA. Variability in the clinical manifestations of galactosaemia. *J. Pediatr.* 1961; **59**: 872.

5 Monk AM, Mitchell AJH, Milligan DWA *et al.* The diagnosis of classical galactosaemia. *Arch. Dis. Child.* 1977; **52**: 943.

6 Reichardt JK. Mutations in galactosemia. *Am. J. Hum. Genet.* 1995; **57**: 978.

7 Schweitzer S, Shin Y, Jakobs C *et al.* Long-term outcome in 134 patients with galactosaemia. *Eur. J. Pediatr* 1993; **152**: 36.

Mucopolysaccharidoses [2]

These are a group of lysosomal storage diseases, each of which is due to a deficiency of a specific lysosomal enzyme involved in the degradation of dermatin sulphate, heparin sulphate, chondroitin sulphate or keratin sulphate. Hepatosplenomegaly is a feature.

Hepatocyte and Kupffer cell swelling and vacuolization are due to storage of poorly degraded mucopolysaccharide.

In addition, hepatic fibrosis outlining the hepatic lobule (zone 1) may be seen. The mechanism is unknown, but is possibly due to abnormal accumulation of a hepatotoxic metabolite of mucopolysaccharide.

Hurler's syndrome (gargoylism) is inherited as an autosomal recessive and is characterized by deficiency of the lysosomal degrading enzyme, alpha-L-iduronidase, in liver, cultured skin fibroblasts and leucocytes. It is characterized by coarse facial features, dwarfism, limitation of joint movement, deafness, abdominal hernias, hepatosplenomegaly, cardiac abnormalities and mental retardation.

The liver in the mucopolysaccharidoses is large and firm. Microscopically liver cells are swollen and together with Kupffer cells accumulate glycosaminoglycan, demonstrated by colloidal iron stain. Electron microscopy shows characteristic membrane-bound inclusions in hepatocytes and Kupffer cells. This lysosomal storage material disappears in the majority of patients after bone marrow transplantation [1].

Diagnosis may be made by finding increased urinary or leucocyte mucopolysaccharides. Culture of skin biopsies shows fibroblasts containing mucopolysaccharides.

References

1 Resnick JM, Krivit W, Snover DC *et al*. Pathology of the liver in mucopolysaccharidosis: light and electron microscopic assessment before and after bone marrow transplantation. *Bone Marrow Transplant* 1992; **10**: 273.
2 Wraith JE. The mucopolysaccharidoses: a clinical review and guide to management. *Arch. Dis. Child.* 1995; **72**: 263.

Familial hypercholesterolaemia

This is an autosomal dominant disease due to absence of a gene which codes for the LDL receptor on cell membranes [2]. The liver contains 60% of such receptors. Sufferers have increased plasma total cholesterol and LDL from birth, cutaneous xanthomas develop and most homozygotes die from coronary artery disease before the age of 30.

Hypercholesterolaemia is controlled by reduction in dietary saturated fats and administration of bile acid sequestrants such as cholestyramine. One child has been successfully treated by simultaneous heart transplant for the coronary disease and liver transplant to provide low-density lipoprotein receptors [1, 4]. Follow-up showed decreases in LDL and plasma cholesterol [5].

Gene therapy, using 'transplant' of autologous hepatocytes genetically corrected with recombinant retroviruses carrying the LDL receptor, was successful with 18 months follow-up [3].

References

1 Bilheimer DW, Goldstein JL, Grundy SM *et al*. Liver transplantation to provide low-density-lipoprotein receptors and lower plasma cholesterol in a child with homozygous familial hypercholesterolemia. *N. Engl. J. Med.* 1984; **311**: 1658.
2 Brown MS, Goldstein JL. Lipoprotein receptors in the liver: control signals for plasma cholesterol traffic. *J. Clin. Invest.* 1983; **72**: 743.
3 Grossman M, Raper SE, Kozarsky K *et al*. Successful *ex vivo* gene therapy directed to liver in a patient with familial hypercholesterolaemia. *Nature Genet.* 1994; **6**: 335.
4 Starzl TE, Bilheimer DW, Bahnson HT *et al*. Heart–liver transplantation in a patient with familial hypercholesterolaemia. *Lancet* 1984; **i**: 1382.
5 Valdivielso P, Escolar JL, Cuervas-Mons V *et al*. Lipids and lipoprotein changes after heart and liver transplantation in a patient with homozygous familial hypercholesterolemia. *Ann. Intern. Med.* 1988; **108**: 204.

Hepatic amyloidosis

This waxy infiltration of the organs was termed amyloidosis because it resembled starch in its staining [17].

The diseases have in common extra-cellular deposition of a number of relatively insoluble proteins as fibrils with typical staining properties. All forms are related to overproduction of a protein which can assume a fibrillar form [16]. The amyloid is deposited in association with glycoprotein composed of globular subunits. At least 12 different proteins can be involved.

The amyloidoses may be classified according to the protein deposited (table 23.5). AL and AA account for the majority. Other amyloid proteins are implicated in hereditary, renal and cardiac amyloidoses and the amyloid associated with chronic dialysis.

In the case of AA amyloidosis (also called 'secondary') the protein shares antigenicity and structure with the acute phase protein of human serum. AA amyloidosis complicates chronic inflammation, either

Table 23.5. Classification of amyloidosis

Type	Fibril	Syndrome
AA	Serum amyloid A	Reactive (secondary) amyloid — acquired (e.g. rheumatoid) — hereditary (FMF)
AL	Monoclonal immunoglobulin light chain	Primary amyloid — myeloma associated — no association
ATTR	Transthyretin	Familial amyloidotic polyneuropathy

Other types: $A\beta_2M$ (renal failure dialysis), $A\beta$ (Alzheimer), A1APP (diabetes/insulinoma).

acquired as in rheumatoid arthritis, or hereditary as in familial Mediterranean fever (FMF).

During the acute phase response, interleukin 1 is produced through activated macrophages. This causes reduced hepatic albumin synthesis, with production of acute phase proteins including serum amyloid A protein (SAA) [3]. A persistently high SAA level is a prerequisite for AA amyloidosis, but not every patient with such levels will develop the disease. Predisposing factors include failure of AA degradation, a low serum albumin level, the activity of proteolytic enzymes from macrophages and genetics [2].

In the case of AL amyloidosis (also called 'primary') the protein consists of immunoglobulin light chains of kappa or lambda types [10]. The classical association of AL amyloidosis is with multiple myeloma.

Amyloid fibrils may resolve. This emphasizes the importance of searching for precipitating chronic diseases in patients with amyloidosis.

Hepatic involvement is constant. The pattern (sinusoidal vs. portal) is not diagnostically valuable. The sinusoidal ('space of Disse'; 'parenchymal') pattern is statistically more common in AL type than AA, but does not exclude AA. Modern histochemical techniques are essential for accurate identification of the amyloid type. Both AA and AL can be deposited under the lining epithelium of intra-hepatic large bile ducts.

Globular amyloid. Eosinophilic globules 5–40 μm in diameter are found in the space of Disse and aggregated within the portal tracts. There are no distinctive clinical or laboratory features distinguishing this type from classical hepatic amyloidosis. It is, however, not associated with multiple myeloma [9]. Globular amyloid usually coexists with classical (AA) systemic amyloidosis.

CLINICAL TYPES

Reactive amyloidosis (acquired, secondary) (AA). Acquired reactive amyloid is the most common form involving spleen, kidneys, liver and adrenal glands, in that order of frequency. It follows chronic diseases such as tuberculosis, pleuropulmonary suppuration, long-standing rheumatoid arthritis, ulcerative colitis, Crohn's disease, leprosy, some neoplasms and Hodgkin's disease. Affected organs have a firm waxy consistency and develop a deep red–brown colour on the addition of dilute iodine.

Familial Mediterranean fever (FMF) (AA) is an autosomal recessive disease which is characterized by acute attacks of fever with sterile peritonitis, pleurisy or synovitis. The amyloid deposited is AA but the mechanism is unknown. FMF primarily affects non-Ashkenazi Jewish, Armenian, Turkish and Middle-Eastern Arab populations. The gene has been mapped to chromosome 16 [13]. The hepatic sinusoids are spared. Hepatic involvement is seen only in the arterioles. The glomeruli, spleen and pulmonary alveoli bear the brunt of the disease. Renal failure may be fatal.

Primary systemic amyloidosis ('atypical') (AL). This is rare and occurs without pre-existing disease. The liver is sometimes involved by deposits in the walls of the small hepatic arterioles in the portal tracts. The deposits may stain poorly with Congo red. Parenchymal deposits are also seen.

Amyloidosis complicating myeloma (AL). This occurs in about 15% of patients. The deposits are usually in the atypical ('primary') distribution.

CLINICAL FEATURES OF HEPATIC INVOLVEMENT

Amyloidosis is suspected when an enlarged, smooth, non-tender liver is detected in a patient with a predisposing cause; however, occasionally the liver may not be enlarged. An enlarged spleen, infiltrated with amyloid, may be found. Hepato-cellular failure is rare as is portal hypertension which is of the sinusoidal type and has a poor prognosis [1]. Jaundice is present in about 5%. Biochemical tests are usually normal apart from a slight rise in alkaline phosphatase.

Severe intra-hepatic cholestasis may rarely complicate kappa and lambda AL amyloidosis [12]. It is presumably due to the intense amyloid deposition interfering with bile passage into canaliculi and small bile ducts. The prognosis is very poor for the cholestatic type. Light-chain deposition disease of the liver may also be associated with AL type amyloidosis and produce severe cholestasis [4].

There may be a nephrotic syndrome, albuminuria or progressive renal failure.

AA amyloidosis has been associated with hepato-cellular adenoma resulting in nephrotic syndrome which improved after resection of the tumour [5]. Massive spontaneous hepatic haemorrhage has been reported in a patient with the very rare hereditary lysozyme-associated amyloidosis [6].

DIAGNOSTIC METHODS

In patients with AL, *immuno-electrophoresis* can detect a monoclonal protein in serum or urine in about 90% of patients [10].

Bone marrow aspiration and biopsy is done in patients with suspected myeloma. Appropriate staining of the biopsy shows amyloid in 50% [10].

Subcutaneous abdominal fat pad aspiration biopsy is safe and gives a positive result in 50–80% [10].

Rectal biopsy is also safe but is positive for amyloid in only 50–75% of cases depending in part on expertise in the procedure [10, 16].

Aspiration liver biopsy is the most satisfactory but more

invasive technique for diagnosis. In both AA and AL patients liver histology is positive for amyloid in about 95% [10, 16]. Hepatic amyloidosis is diffuse and the sampling error is negligible. The procedure is said to be dangerous, but this has been over-emphasized.

Histologically, the amyloid is shown as homogeneous, amorphous, eosinophilic material (fig. 23.14). It stains with Congo red or methyl violet (fig. 23.15) and reddish-brown with iodine. All these reactions are transient and remain for only a few weeks. Polarization microscopy of Congo red stained sections shows the amyloid as green birefringent fibrils [8]. Amyloid may also be shown by fluorescent microscopy.

The amyloid is deposited between the columns of liver cells and the sinusoidal wall in the space of Disse. The liver cells themselves are not involved but are compressed to a variable extent. The mid-zonal and portal areas are most heavily infiltrated.

Occasionally, in AL primary amyloidosis or that complicating multiple myeloma, the amyloid is found only in the portal tracts in the walls of hepatic arterioles, around the interlobular arteries and lying free in clumps.

Electron microscopy confirms fibrils 10 nm long that do not branch.

Percutaneous renal biopsy is used for the diagnosis of renal involvement.

Scanning. Multiple filling defects may simulate metastases on hepatic scans.

Recently a method for imaging amyloid tissue has been developed using radiolabelled serum amyloid P component (SAP) [7]. This is a normal circulating plasma

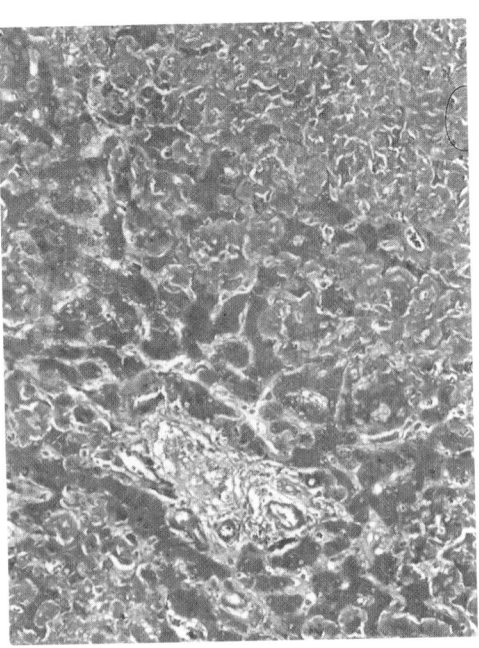

Fig. 23.15. Amyloid is shown as amorphous dark staining material between liver cells and sinusoids. (Stained methyl violet, ×40.)

protein synthesized by hepatocytes, which is also contained in all amyloid. Radiolabelled SAP can be used for imaging or metabolic clearance studies. Imaging gives a whole body picture of the distribution of amyloid and permits quantitation. Patients may be studied serially to show the effect of treatment. This method is, however, at present a specialized tool with restricted availability.

PROGNOSIS

This depends on the causative condition and on the extent of the kidney involvement. Ninety per cent of patients with reactive 'secondary' amyloid disease (AA) are dead within 2 years of diagnosis, usually from the toxaemia of their chronic infection. In the few patients who live long enough, death occurs from secondarily contracted amyloid kidneys. These patients never die of liver failure.

The median survival of a series of 474 patients with AL amyloidosis was 13 months. Seven per cent survived for 5 years or more; only 1% were alive at 10 years [10]. Survival was worse for those presenting with congestive cardiac failure.

TREATMENT

AA amyloid is treated by controlling the underlying disease. If tuberculosis is cured then amyloid may disappear. Similarly, clinical improvement in rheumatoid

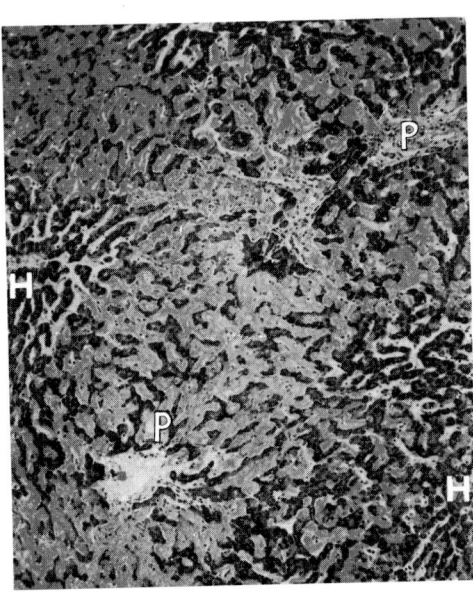

Fig. 23.14. Amyloid material is deposited in the sinusoidal wall, especially in the peri-portal zones. The liver cell trabeculae are narrowed. H = central hepatic veins; P = portal tracts. (Best's carmine, ×70.)

arthritis may be paralleled by disappearance of clinical signs of amyloidosis. There is no specific treatment.

Prophylactic colchicine prevents the development of amyloidosis in all cases of FMF [16].

AL amyloid may be treated by melphalan and prednisone which reduce the synthesis of precursor proteins [11].

Liver transplantation is the definitive treatment for familial amyloidotic polyneuropathy. This condition is characterized by progressive peripheral and autonomic neuropathy and varying degrees of cardiac, renal and other visceral involvement. It is due in most cases to point mutations in the gene for plasma transthyretin, which is synthesized in the liver. Liver transplantation results in disappearance of the variant TTR from plasma, and regression of some disease. Recovery from autonomic neuropathy is greater than peripheral neuropathy [14, 15].

References

1 Bion E, Brenard R, Pariente EA *et al.* Sinusoidal portal hypertension in hepatic amyloidosis. *Gut* 1991; **32**: 227.

2 Cohen AS, Connors LH. The pathogenesis and biochemistry of amyloidosis. *J. Pathol.* 1987; **151**: 1.

3 Dinarello CA. Interleukin-I and the pathogenesis of the acute phase response. *N. Engl. J. Med.* 1984; **311**: 1413.

4 Faa G, Van Eyken P, De Vos R *et al.* Light chain deposition disease of the liver associated with AL-type amyloidosis and severe cholestasis. *J. Hepatol.* 1991; **12**: 75.

5 Fievet P, Sevestre H, Boudjelal M *et al.* Systemic AA amyloidosis induced by liver cell adenoma. *Gut* 1990; **31**: 361.

6 Harrison RF, Hawkins PN, Roche WR *et al.* 'Fragile' liver and massive hepatic haemorrhage due to hereditary amyloidosis. *Gut* 1996; **38**: 151.

7 Hawkins PN, Pepys MB. Imaging amyloidosis with radio-labelled SAP. *Eur. J. Nucl. Med.* 1995; **22**: 595.

8 Heller H, Missmahl H-P, Sohar E *et al.* Amyloidosis: its differentiation into perireticulin and pericollagen types. *J. Path. Bact.* 1964; **88**: 15.

9 Kanel GC, Uchida T, Peters RL. Globular hepatic amyloid— an unusual morphologic presentation. *Hepatology* 1981; **1**: 647.

10 Kyle RA, Gertz MA. Primary systemic amyloidosis: clinical and laboratory features in 474 cases. *Semin. Haematol.* 1995; **32**: 45.

11 Kyle RA, Greipp PR, Garton JP *et al.* Primary systemic amyloidosis. Comparison of melphalan/prednisone versus colchicine. *Am. J. Med.* 1985; **79**: 708

12 Peters RA, Koukoulis G, Gimson A *et al.* Primary amyloidosis and severe intrahepatic cholestatic jaundice. *Gut* 1994; **35**: 1322.

13 Pras E, Aksentijevich I, Gruberg L *et al.* Mapping of a gene causing familial Mediterranean fever to the short arm of chromosome 16. *N. Engl. J. Med.* 1992; **326**: 1509.

14 Skinner M, Lewis WD, Jones LA *et al.* Liver transplantation as a treatment for familial amyloidotic polyneuropathy. *Ann. Intern. Med.* 1994; **120**: 133.

15 Steen L, Holmgren G, Suhr O *et al.* World-wide survey of liver transplantation in patients with familial amyloidotic polyneuropathy. *Amyloid* 1994; **1**: 138.

16 Tan SY, Pepys MB, Hawkins PN. Treatment of amyloidosis. *Am. J. Kidney Dis.* 1995; **26**: 267.

17 Virchow R. Über den Gang der Amyloiden Degeneration. *Virchows Archiv.* 1855; **8**: 364.

α_1-Antitrypsin deficiency [18]

α_1-Antitrypsin is synthesized in the rough endoplasmic reticulum of the liver. It comprises 80–90% of the serum α_1-globulin and is an inhibitor of trypsin and other proteases. Deficiency results in the unopposed action of these enzymes, in particular neutrophil elastase. The lungs are the major target, with damage to alveoli and resulting emphysema.

The gene for α_1-antitrypsin is on chromosome 14. There are about 75 different alleles at this locus which can be distinguished by isoelectric focusing or agarose electrophoresis at acid pH, or by PCR analysis. M is the common normal allele. Z and S are the most frequent abnormal alleles which put the individual at risk of disease. One gene is derived from each parent. The combination results in normal, intermediate, low or zero serum α_1-antitrypsin levels. Pi (protease inhibitor) MM gives a serum α_1-antitrypsin value of 20–53 μmol/l—the normal state. PiZZ results in a low concentration of 2.5–7 μmol/l and PiNull-Null gives zero levels. Both give a high risk of emphysema. PiSS and PiMZ give levels 50–60% of normal with no increased risk of lung disease. PiSZ gives α_1-antitrypsin levels of 8–19 μmol/l with a mildly increased risk.

Mutation of the gene can give deficiency of circulating α_1-antitrypsin by a number of mechanisms. Liver disease, however, only occurs with mutations where α_1-antitrypsin accumulates in hepatocytes. The classical type is PiZZ but the M_{malton} and M_{duarte} variants may do the same [5].

PATHOGENESIS OF LIVER DISEASE [18]

Only the PiZZ phenotype has been clearly associated with liver disease. This is not due to the low circulating levels of α_1-antitrypsin arriving at the liver since other phenotypes with a low circulating level do not develop hepatic damage. Intrahepatic accumulation of α_1-antitrypsin seems to be responsible. Studies of the molecular structure have shown that with the ZZ mutation there is polymerization of protein units. Normally the reactive loop (fig. 23.16) swings in between the β helices of the so-called A sheet of the protein, where it interacts with elastase and other enzymes. In the ZZ mutant protein the reactive loop cannot do this. It remains on the outside and is then available to insert into the A sheet of an adjacent ZZ unit [14]. The polymers formed prevent export of most of the protein.

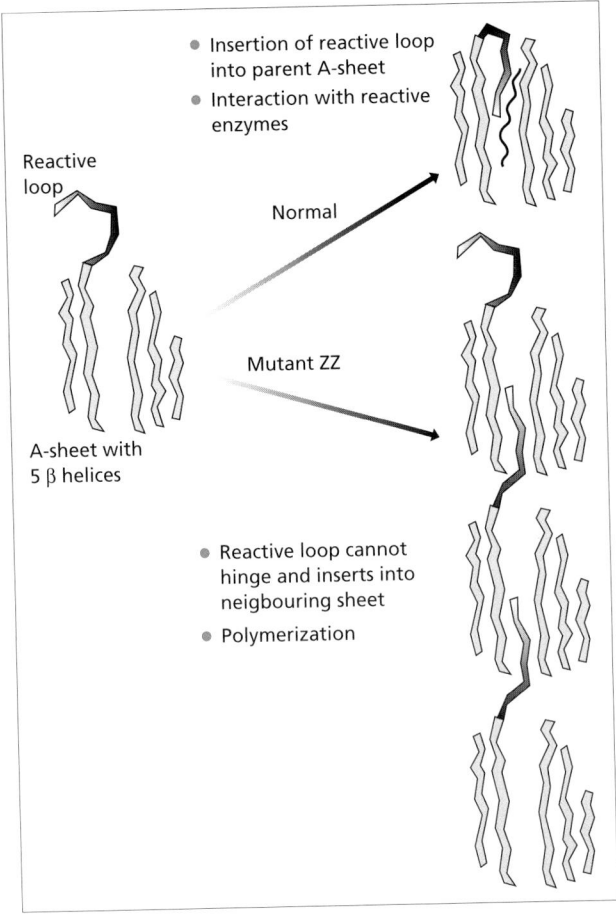

- Insertion of reactive loop into parent A-sheet
- Interaction with reactive enzymes

Reactive loop

Normal

Mutant ZZ

A-sheet with 5 β helices

- Reactive loop cannot hinge and inserts into neigbouring sheet
- Polymerization

Fig. 23.16. Proposed mechanism of polymerization of ZZ α_1-antitrypsin.

Accumulation is thought to be responsible for liver damage but the mechanism is still unclear. Polymerization of ZZ protein occurs spontaneously or following minor perturbations such as a rise in temperature. However, the mutation of the α_1-antitrypsin protein is not the only reason for its retention. Cells from individuals with α_1-antitrypsin liver disease also have a reduction in the degradatory pathways in the endoplasmic reticulum [18]. The variation in clinical disease therefore appears to depend not only on the abnormal protein produced in PiZZ but also other cellular mechanisms as yet poorly understood. Transgenic mice carrying the human ZZ type may provide a useful experimental setting in which to dissect the mechanisms involved [2].

CLINICAL PICTURE

α_1-Antitrypsin deficiency has a wide spectrum of disease. The number of patients with recognized liver or lung disease is much less than expected from calculations made from the gene frequency. The spectrum for liver disease stretches from liver failure and the need for transplantation in childhood, to individuals at 18 years old having no evidence of liver disease—the outcome in the majority of patients [17]. The explanation may be environmental and other as yet unknown genetic influences.

Emphysema is the most common manifestation of α_1-antitrypsin deficiency but takes decades to become apparent [6, 17]. There is a threshold of serum α_1-antitrypsin level below which the risk is increased. Cigarette smoking accelerates the development of emphysema and shortens survival. Symptoms of α_1-antitrypsin-related emphysema do not usually begin until the third decade of life. However, there is a wide variability in the incidence and severity of disease, with some smokers remaining asymptomatic or only developing disease in the seventh or eighth decade of life. Overall patients with α_1-antitrypsin deficiency have a shortened life span of 10–15 years compared to the normal population [6].

Most patients with PiZZ develop liver disease at some stage. In the first year of life 75% of infants have an elevated serum alanine transaminase level [17]. Some develop severe hepatitic-cholestatic jaundice in the first few months of life which may be fatal or lead to transplantation. However, the majority recover. In a series of 127 PiZZ Swedish children detected in a screening programme, 22 had clinical liver disease in infancy (neonatal cholestasis or hepatosplenomegaly). Two of these died early in life of cirrhosis. Two died of other causes and liver histology showed cirrhosis/fibrosis. This agrees with a calculation of 3% of α_1-antitrypsin children coming to liver transplantation [16]. Follow-up of the Swedish group at the age of 18 years showed that the remainder were clinically well. Abnormal liver function tests were found in only two patients [17].

Cirrhosis may remain compensated for many years but can pursue a relentless course with 25% dying during childhood [1]. The incidence of liver disease at age 50 years is about 15%, more frequent in men [4]. The patient may present as a problem of portal hypertension or ascites.

In an adult liver clinic, only five homozygotes (ZZ phenotype) α_1-antitrypsin-deficient patients were found in 469 patients with chronic liver disease and all five gave a history of neonatal jaundice [9].

Rarely, both pulmonary and hepatic disease affect the same patient with α_1-antitrypsin deficiency [10].

Hepato-cellular carcinoma may be a complication particularly in males [8].

There is an increased gene frequency of α_1-antitrypsin in patients with genetic haemochromatosis but the reason for the association is unexplained [7].

An increased prevalence of heterozygotes (MZ) has been found in patients with cryptogenic cirrhosis or chronic hepatitis [3]. The significance is unknown.

Hepato-cellular carcinoma can develop in cirrhotic patients heterozygous for α_1-antitrypsin deficiency but this may be more related to other factors, such as hepatitis C or alcohol, than the metabolic disease itself [15].

Partial deficiency of α_1-antichymotrypsin, another proteinase inhibitor, may also be associated with liver disease [13].

LIVER HISTOLOGY

The acute picture is of neonatal hepatitis except that giant cells are not prominent. After 12 weeks, intracellular globules which are diastase resistant and stain brilliantly with PAS are seen in *peri-portal* liver cells (fig. 23.17). The globules stain positively with the specific α_1-antitrypsin immunoperoxidase method. The liver contains increased amounts of copper.

Electron microscopy shows clumps of protein in dilated rough endoplasmic reticulum. These fluoresce when exposed to an antibody against α_1-antitrypsin.

DIAGNOSIS

The condition should be suspected with neonatal jaundice. It should also be considered in any patient with cirrhosis, whatever the age, particularly with a past history of infantile liver disease or with associated chest infections. α_1-Antitrypsin deficiency can present as cryptogenic cirrhosis in persons over the age of 50 [19].

Confirmation comes by measuring serum α_1-antitrypsin. The exact phenotype should be determined.

There is a 75% chance that a subsequent affected child will run the same clinical course.

The deficiency may be diagnosed prenatally by amniotic fluid or cultured amniotic cells using synthetic oligomer probes for DNA analysis [12].

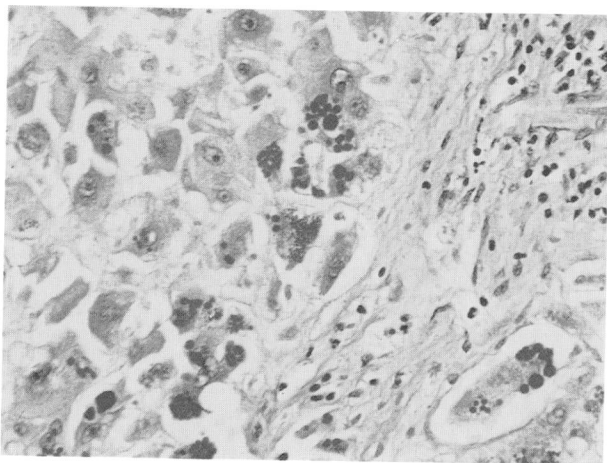

Fig. 23.17. α_1-Antitrypsin deficiency. Liver biopsy shows bright red deposits in peri-portal liver cells when stained by periodic acid–Schiff after diastase digestion. (PAS, ×100.)

First trimester prenatal diagnosis is also possible by analysis of fetal DNA [11]. This is justified in families where there is a history of severe disease.

TREATMENT

Replacement therapy with plasma-derived or synthetic α_1-antitrypsin has been used to treat the pulmonary disease [6].

α_1-Antitrypsin deficiency is the second most common chronic childhood liver disease for which liver transplantation is performed [16]. Survival and complications are similar to that for other indications. The recipient's phenotype rapidly changes to that of the donor [20].

Increasing understanding of the molecular mechanism of hepatocyte injury may lead to new approaches to treatment, such as peptides to prevent ZZ polymerization by filling the cleft in the A sheet, but these remain speculative [18].

References

1 Alagille D. Alpha-1-antitrypsin deficiency. *Hepatology* 1984; **4**: 115.

2 Ali R, Perfumo S, della Rocca C *et al.* Evaluation of a transgenic mouse model for α_1-antitrypsin related liver disease. *Ann. Hum. Genet.* 1994; **58**: 305.

3 Brind AM, Bassendine MF, Bennett MK *et al.* Alpha-1-antitrypsin granules in the liver—always important? *Q. J. Med.* 1990; **279**: 699.

4 Cox DW, Smyth S. Risk of liver disease in adults with α_1-antitrypsin deficiency. *Am. J. Med.* 1983; **74**: 221.

5 Crowley JJ, Sharp HL, Freier E *et al.* Fatal liver disease associated with alpha 1-antitrypsin deficiency PiM$_1$ PiM$_{duarte}$. *Gastroenterology* 1987; **93**: 242.

6 Crystal RG. α_1-Antitrypsin deficiency, emphysema and liver disease: genetic basis and strategies for therapy. *J. Clin. Invest.* 1990; **85**: 1343.

7 Elzouki A-NY, Hultcrantz R, Stal P *et al.* Increased PiZ gene frequency for α_1-antitrypsin in patients with genetic haemochromatosis. *Gut* 1995; **36**: 922.

8 Eriksson S, Carlson J, Velez R. Risk of cirrhosis and primary liver cancer in alpha 1-antitrypsin deficiency. *N. Engl. J. Med.* 1986; **314**: 736.

9 Fisher RL, Taylor L, Sherlock S. α_1-Antitrypsin deficiency in liver disease: the extent of the problem. *Gastroenterology* 1976; **71**: 646.

10 Glasgow JFT, Lynch MJ, Hercz A *et al.* Alpha$_1$ antitrypsin deficiency in association with both cirrhosis and chronic obstructive lung disease in two sibs. *Am. J. Med.* 1973; **54**: 181.

11 Hejtmancik JF, Ward PA, Sifers RN *et al.* Prenatal diagnosis of alpha 1-antitrypsin deficiency by restriction fragment length polymorphisms, and comparison with oligonucleotide probe analysis. *Lancet* 1984; **ii**: 767.

12 Kidd VJ, Golhus MS, Wallace RB *et al.* Prenatal diagnosis of alpha-1-antitrypsin deficiency by direct analysis of the mutation site in the gene. *N. Engl. J. Med.* 1984; **310**: 639.

13 Lindmark B, Eriksson S. Partial deficiency of α-1-antichymotrypsin is associated with chronic cryptogenic

liver disease. *Scand. J. Gastroenterol.* 1991; **26**: 508.

14 Lomas DA. Loop-sheet polymerization: the structural basis of Z α_1-antitrypsin accumulation in the liver. *Clin. Sci.* 1994; **86**: 489.

15 Propst T, Propst A, Dietze O *et al.* Prevalence of hepatocellular carcinoma in α_1-antitrypsin deficiency. *J. Hepatol.* 1994; **21**: 1006.

16 Sharp HL. Wherefore art thou liver disease associated with α_1-antitrypsin deficiency? *Hepatology* 1995; **22**: 666.

17 Sveger T, Eriksson S. The liver in adolescents with α_1-antitrypsin deficiency. *Hepatology* 1995; **22**: 514.

18 Teckman J, Perlmutter DH. Conceptual advances in the pathogenesis and treatment of childhood metabolic liver disease. *Gastroenterology* 1995; **108**: 1263.

19 Thatcher BS, Winkelman EI, Tuthill RJ. Alpha-1-antitrypsin deficiency presenting as cryptogenic cirrhosis in adults over 50. *J. Clin. Gastroenterol.* 1985; **7**: 405.

20 Van Furth R, Kramps JA, Van Der Putten ABMM *et al.* Change in alpha-1-antitrypsin phenotype after orthotopic liver transplant. *Clin. Exp. Immunol.* 1986; **66**: 669.

Hereditary tyrosinaemia [5]

This autosomal recessive disorder is due to lack of the enzyme fumaryl acetoacetate hydrolase, an enzyme that catalyses the last step of tyrosine degradation. Abnormal metabolites of tyrosine accumulate, which are toxic to both liver and kidney. The main clinical features are progressive liver disease and renal tubular abnormalities.

The acute type, usually seen in early infancy, results in death from hepatic failure within the first year of life. The chronic form leads to growth retardation, cirrhosis, severe hypophosphataemic rickets, renal tubular defects and a derangement of tyrosine metabolism with hyper-aminoacidaemia. Hepato-cellular carcinoma is a complication occurring in over 40% of patients. Episodes of severe acute peripheral neuropathy are reported [4].

Diagnosis is confirmed by the presence of elevated plasma and urinary tyrosine, phenylalanine and methionine levels and increased levels of succinyl acetone in the urine. The prognosis is related to the time of presentation [5]. Survival when symptoms develop before 2 months of age, between 2 and 6 months, and after 6 months is 38, 74 and 96%, respectively.

The chronic type will respond to dietary avoidance of aromatic amino acids and methionine but this does not prevent the liver disease or the appearance of hepato-cellular carcinoma. Without liver transplantation death occurs within the first decade of life. Treatment with an inhibitor of an enzyme preceding the metabolic defect has produced benefit [2] but awaits further study.

CT scanning shows the progression of liver disease from cirrhosis, to macronodular disease and finally hepato-cellular carcinoma.

Liver transplantation for both acute and chronic disease.can be successful and virtually corrects the metabolic disease [3]. A mild metabolic abnormality persists probably due to continued abnormal renal metabolism but this is not a clinical problem. Because of the difficulty in predicting or preventing complications, including hepato-cellular carcinoma, early liver transplantation has been advocated [1].

References

1 Freese DK, Tuchman M, Schwarzenberg SJ *et al.* Early liver transplantation is indicated for tyrosinemia type I. *J. Pediatr. Gastroenterol. Nutr.* 1991; **13**: 10.

2 Lindstedt S, Holme E, Lock EA *et al.* Treatment of hereditary tyrosinemia type I by inhibition of 4-hydroxyphenylpyruvate dioxygenase. *Lancet* 1992; **340**: 813.

3 Mieles LA, Esquivel CO, Van Thiel DH *et al.* Liver transplantation for tyrosinemia: a review of 10 cases from the University of Pittsburgh. *Dig. Dis. Sci.,* 1990; **35**: 153.

4 Mitchell G, Larochelle J, Lambert M *et al.* Neurologic crises in hereditary tyrosinemia. *N. Engl. J. Med.* 1990; **322**: 432.

5 van Spronsen FJ, Thomasse Y, Smit GPA *et al.* Hereditary tyrosinemia type I: a new clinical classification with difference in prognosis on dietary treatment. *Hepatology* 1994; **20**: 1187.

Cystic fibrosis [3, 10]

This condition is inherited with an autosomal recessive pattern. The prevalence is approximately 1 in 2000. The carrier rate is about 5%. The gene responsible, on chromosome 7, has been cloned and the product is a transmembrane protein regulating ion conductance. The mutation in the majority of patients with cystic fibrosis is of three bases, removing phenylalanine 508 from the protein. The result is a secretion containing an abnormal sodium, chloride and calcium content with increased viscosity. Lungs and pancreas are the major targets of pathology.

Postnatal jaundice is associated with meconium ileus.

Approximately 20% of patients develop liver disease including fatty change, focal biliary fibrosis [1] and portal fibrosis followed by multi-lobular biliary cirrhosis. The pathogenesis of the liver disease is thought to be the plugging of intra-hepatic bile ducts with inspissated bile. The loss of cystic fibrosis transmembrane regulator (CFTR) gene expression, normally present in bile duct epithelial cells [2], is thought to lead to abnormally concentrated bile and loss of mucous protection. An increase in hepato-toxic bile acids may play a role. It is not certain why some patients develop liver disease and others do not. Histocompatibility antigens have been implicated, HLA-DQ6 being more frequent in those with liver disease [5]. The liver damage may lead to portal hypertension. Cholangiography shows features consistent with intra-hepatic sclerosing cholangitis [7]. The sclerotic bile duct changes are usual in patients with hepatomegaly and biochemical abnormalities. With improved management of the respiratory disease, patients are living longer and this may be responsible for the increased recognition of liver disease.

Gallbladder disease, including gallstones, is seen in 3.6% [9]. Chclecystectomy is safe.

Clinical features of cirrhosis rarely become apparent until pulmonary and pancreatic diseases have been overt for many years. The cirrhosis is usually clinically silent but may cause portal hypertension.

Scintigraphy with DISIDA may show focal retention of isotope despite normal liver function tests and ultrasound [8].

The prognosis seems to be determined by the respiratory state rather than the liver. Ursodeoxycholic acid therapy is associated with biochemical improvement, but further studies are needed to assess long-term benefit [3]. Liver transplantation is successful in 70% of patients, either alone for those with end-stage hepatic disease but preserved respiratory function [3, 6] or combined with lung transplantation for those with late-stage pulmonary disease [4].

References

1 Bodian M. *Fibrocytic Disease of the Pancreas*, p. 104. Heinemann, London, 1952.

2 Cohn JA, Strong TV, Picciotto MR *et al.* Localization of the cystic fibrosis transmembrane conductance regulator in human bile duct epithelial cells. *Gastroenterology* 1993; **105**: 1857.

3 Colombo C, Battezzati PM, Podda M. Hepatobiliary disease in cystic fibrosis. *Semin. Liver Dis.* 1994; **14**: 259.

4 Couctil JPA, Houssin DP, Soubrane O *et al.* Combined lung and liver transplantation in patients with cystic fibrosis. *J. Thorac. Cardiovasc. Surg.* 1995; **110**: 1415.

5 Duthie A, Doherty DG, Donaldson PT *et al.* The major histocompatibility complex influences the development of chronic liver disease in male children and young adults with cystic fibrosis. *J. Hepatol.* 1995; **23**: 532.

6 Noble-Jamieson G, Valente J, Barnes ND *et al.* Liver transplantation for hepatic cirrhosis in cystic fibrosis. *Arch. Dis. Child.* 1994; **71**: 349.

7 O'Brien S, Keogan M, Casey M *et al.* Biliary complications of cystic fibrosis. *Gut* 1992; **33**: 387.

8 O'Connor PJ, Southern KW, Bowler IM *et al.* The role of hepatobiliary scintigraphy in cystic fibrosis. *Hepatology* 1996; **23**: 281.

9 Stern RC, Rothstein FC, Doershuk CF. Treatment and prognosis of symptomatic gallbladder disease in patients with cystic fibrosis. *J. Pediatr. Gastroenterol. Nutr.* 1986; **5**: 35.

10 Tanner MS, Taylor CJ. Liver disease in cystic fibrosis. *Arch. Dis. Child.* 1995; **72**: 281.

Liver and thyroid

The liver metabolizes thyroxine by oxidative deamination, deiodination, conjugation and finally biliary excretion. There is an entero-hepatic circulation, but only about 3% of thyroxine is reabsorbed.

The liver contains 35% of the body's exchangeable thyroxine (T4), and 5% of the tri-iodothyronine (T3)—there is a ready exchange with the bound hormone in plasma. The liver converts T4 to T3 [6]. Reversed T3 (rT3) is probably produced in extra-hepatic tissues [8]. The liver also produces thyroxine-binding globulin.

Thyrotoxicosis

Minor abnormalities of liver function are seen in hyperthyroidism [2]. There is little evidence of significant hepatic functional and structural changes in an otherwise normal liver. Jaundice in thyrotoxic patients may be due to heart failure [4]. In addition, thyrotoxicosis may cause severe cholestasis in patients without heart failure [11], and result in reversible exacerbation of cholestasis in primary biliary cirrhosis [9].

Thyrotoxicosis may also aggravate an underlying defect in serum bilirubin metabolism, such as Gilbert's syndrome, by decreasing bilirubin UDP–glucuronosyl-transferase activity [10].

Liver biopsy is normal in those not in congestive failure. Electron microscopy shows enlarged mitochondria, hypertrophied smooth endoplasmic reticulum and decreased glycogen.

Myxoedema

Ascites without congestive heart failure in patients with myxoedema has been attributed to centrizonal congestion and fibrosis. The pathogenesis is unknown. It disappears on giving thyroxine. There is a high ascitic protein content of greater than 25 g/l [3].

Jaundice may be related to neonatal thyroid deficiency.

Changes in hepato-cellular disease

Most patients with liver disease are clinically euthyroid although standard function tests may give misleading results [5]. The radio-iodine uptake may be abnormally low. Serum total T4 may be raised or decreased in association with varying levels of thyroid hormone binding proteins. The free thyroxine index is usually normal.

In *alcoholic liver disease* raised serum levels of thyrotrophin (TSH) and free T4 are associated with normal or low T3 values [7]. The conversion of T4 to T3 is reduced. This suggests a compensatory increase in TSH in response to relative T3 deficiency. The total and free T3 levels are reduced in proportion to the degree of liver damage. Plasma rT3 levels are high.

In *primary biliary cirrhosis* and *chronic hepatitis* thyroxine-binding globulins are increased and these may be markers of inflammatory activity [8]. Although average total T4 and T3 should be increased, the corresponding free hormone concentrations are reduced, probably because of decreased thyroid function associated with the high incidence of thyroiditis in these patients [1].

References

1 Babb RR. Associations between diseases of the thyroid and the liver. *Am. J. Gastroenterol.* 1984; **79**: 421.

2 Beckett GJ, Kellett HA, Gow SM *et al.* Subclinical liver damage in hyperthyroidism and in thyroxine replacement therapy. *Br. Med. J.* 1985; **291**: 427.

3 De Castro F, Bonacini M, Walden JM *et al.* Myxedema ascites: report of two cases and review of the literature. *J. Clin. Gastroenterol.* 1991; **13**: 411.

4 Fong TL, McHutchison JG, Reynolds TB. Hyperthyroidism and hepatic dysfunction. A case series analysis. *J. Clin. Gastroenterol.* 1992; **14**: 240.

5 Huang MJ, Liaw YF. Clinical associations between thyroid and liver diseases. *J. Gastroenterol. Hepatol.* 1995; **10**: 344.

6 Klachko DM, Johnson ER. The liver and circulating thyroid hormones. *J. Clin. Gastroenterol.* 1983; **5**: 465.

7 Nomura S, Pittman CS, Chambers JB Jr *et al.* Reduced peripheral conversion of thyroxine to triiodothyronine in patients with hepatic cirrhosis. *J. Clin. Invest.* 1975; **56**: 643.

8 Schussler GC, Schaffner F, Korn F. Increased serum thyroid hormone binding and decreased free hormone in chronic active liver disease. *N. Engl. J. Med.* 1978; **299**: 510.

9 Thompson NP, Leader S, Jamieson CP *et al.* Reversible jaundice in primary biliary cirrhosis due to hyperthyroidism. *Gastroenterology* 1994; **106**: 1342.

10 Van Steenbergen W, Fevery J, De Vos R *et al.* Thyroid hormones and the hepatic handling of bilirubin. I. Effects of hypothyroidism and hyperthyroidism on the hepatic transport of bilirubin mono- and diconjugates in the Wistar rat. *Hepatology* 1989; **9**: 314.

11 Yao JDC, Gross JB, Ludwig J *et al.* Cholestatic jaundice in hyperthyroidism. *Am. J. Med.* 1989; **86**: 619.

Liver and adrenal

Undiagnosed Addison's disease can be associated with mild elevation of transaminase levels [1]. These return to normal after treatment with corticosteroids. The mechanism is not known.

Reference

1 Boulton R, Hamilton MI, Dhillon AP *et al.* Subclinical Addison's disease: a cause of persistent abnormalities in transaminase values. *Gastroenterology* 1995; **109**: 1324.

Liver and growth hormone

The liver and kidney degrade growth hormone. Basal and stimulated growth hormone concentrations are elevated in cirrhotic patients and correlate with the degree of liver dysfunction [2]. These increased levels may contribute to insulin resistance and glucose intolerance in cirrhosis [5]. Acromegaly does not develop despite the chronic elevation of growth hormone.

Insulin-like growth factor I (IGF-I), which mediates the effects of growth hormone and whose production by the liver is stimulated by growth hormone, is reduced in the serum of cirrhotics [1]. The serum levels of the major binding proteins are also altered, which may affect the bioavailability of IGF-I. Administration of recombinant growth hormone to patients with alcoholic cirrhosis results in a rise in IGF-I, but there appears to be no clinical or biochemical benefit [3].

In *acromegaly* the liver enlarges in line with other viscera. The splanchnic blood flow is normal so that tissue perfusion must be reduced relative to the increment in hepatic mass [4].

References

1 Donaghy A, Ross R, Gimson A *et al.* Growth hormone, insulin-like growth factor, and insulin-like growth factor binding proteins 1 and 3 in chronic liver disease. *Hepatology* 1995; **21**: 680.

2 Moller S, Becker U. Insulin-like growth factor I and growth hormone in chronic liver disease. *Dig. Dis.* 1992; **10**: 239.

3 Moller S, Becker U, Gronbaek M *et al.* Short-term effect of recombinant human growth hormone in patients with alcoholic cirrhosis. *J. Hepatol.* 1994; **21**: 710.

4 Preisig R, Morris TQ, Shaver JC *et al.* Volumetric, hemodynamic and excretory characteristics of the liver in acromegaly. *J. Clin. Invest.* 1966; **65**: 1379.

5 Shankar TP, Fredi JL, Himmelstein S *et al.* Elevated growth hormone levels and insulin resistance in patients with cirrhosis of the liver. *Am. J. Med. Sci.* 1986; **291**: 248.

Hepatic porphyrias [20, 28]

Porphyrias are caused by defects in the biosynthesis of haem (fig. 23.18). The clinical features are the result of accumulation of porphyrins due to the enzyme defect. In addition the lack of haem increases ALA and PBG production because of loss of negative feedback on ALA-synthetase activity. Accumulation of early precursors (ALA/PBG) results in neurological features, with the acute pattern of attack (table 23.6) including abdominal pain, peripheral neuropathy, autonomic dysfunction and psychosis. Accumulation of substrates later in the pathway gives the cutaneous pattern, in particular photosensitivity. Some types of porphyria give both neurological and cutaneous features.

Most porphyrias are inherited as autosomal dominant [7], but there is low penetrance. The majority of carriers have latent porphyria and are clinically asymptomatic. Attacks are precipitated by drugs, hormonal factors and endogenous metabolic changes.

The product of this metabolic pathway, haem, is an important component of haemoglobin, myoglobin and haem-requiring enzymes, for example the cytochrome

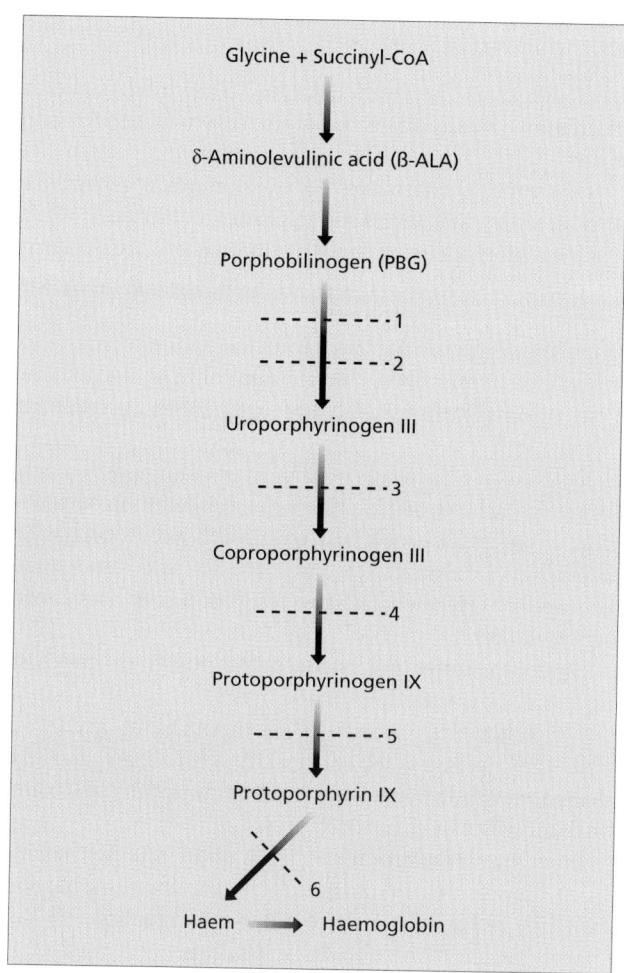

Fig. 23.18. Porphyria and the biosynthesis of porphyrins. Numbers indicate site of enzyme defect leading to: 1, acute intermittent porphyria; 2, congenital erythropoietic porphyria; 3, porphyria cutanea tarda and hepatoerythropoietic porphyria; 4, hereditary coproporphyria; 5, variegate porphyria; 6, erythropoietic protoporphyria.

Table 23.6. Classifications of porphyria

Acute	
neuroporphyria	*Acute intermittent porphyria*
neurocutaneous	*Hereditary coproporphyria*
	Variegate porphyria
Non-acute (cutaneous)	*Porphyria cutanea tarda*
	Erythropoietic protoporphyria
	Congenital erythropoietic porphyria

Hepatic in italics; erythropoietic in roman.

P450 oxidase system. Protoporphyrin synthesis is therefore most pronounced in hepatic cells and erythrocytes, which gives a further classification of hepatic and erythropoietic porphyrias (table 23.6).

The acute hepatic porphyrias include *acute intermittent porphyria*, *hereditary coproporphyria* and *variegate porphyria*. All are marked by neuropsychiatric attacks with vomiting, abdominal colic, constipation and peripheral neuropathy. All are exacerbated by countless enzyme-inducing drugs including barbiturates, sulphonamides, oestrogens, oral contraceptives, griseofulvin, chloroquine and possibly alcohol.

Hormones are important inducers and women develop attacks in pregnancy and pre-menstrually.

During the attacks, large amounts of the colourless porphyrin precursors, porphobilinogen and delta aminolaevulinic acid (ALA) are excreted in the urine. In all three, an acute attack is treated by glucose loading. Infusions of haematin which repress or inhibit hepatic ALA synthetase may also be valuable [2].

Haem arginate which suppresses overproduction of haem precursors and improves hepatic oxidative metabolism may be useful [11]. Cimetidine has been effective in treating acute porphyria [13].

The fourth type of hepatic porphyria, *porphyria cutanea tarda*, is probably hereditary and may be associated with hepato-cellular disease. It is not exacerbated by barbiturates and acute neurological attacks are not seen.

The erythropoietic porphyrias are congenital erythropoietic porphyria (autosomal recessive) and erythropoietic protoporphyria (dominant).

ACUTE INTERMITTENT PORPHYRIA [28]

The basic deficiency is in hepatic porphobilinogen deaminase. A diagnostic deficiency may be shown in red cells. The enzyme delta aminolaevulinic acid-synthetase (ALA-S) is secondarily induced in the liver because of loss of the normal negative feedback mechanism due to haem. Over-production of ALA and PBG follows. The clinical features are of acute porphyria.

Photosensitivity is absent. The urine darkens on standing and gives a positive urobilinogen test. It contains slight increases in ALA and porphobilinogen. Latent cases develop acute attacks on various drugs and in the later stages of pregnancy.

General anaesthesia for major surgery can be done safely in known patients with the appropriate choice of drugs; the danger of anaesthesia is in those in whom the diagnosis has not been made [6].

Hepato-cellular carcinoma occurs in 8% during long-term follow-up [14].

HEREDITARY COPROPORPHYRIA

The deficiency is in coproporphyrinogen oxidase. Attacks may be neurological or cutaneous with lesions like porphyria cutanea tarda. ALA-S activity is increased in the liver. Faecal and urinary coproporphyrin are increased with a corresponding increase in protoporphyrin.

PORPHYRIA VARIEGATA

The defect is in protoporphyrinogen oxidase. ALA-S is increased in the liver. This variant is frequently encountered in South Africa and New England [21]. The features are intermediate between acute intermittent porphyria and hereditary coproporphyria. Protoporphyrin and porphyrins may be increased in the stool between attacks. Biliary porphyrin estimation may be diagnostic in the asymptomatic patient [17].

PORPHYRIA CUTANEA TARDA

This is the most common porphyria and is usually latent and the patient symptom-free.

Uroporphyrinogen decarboxylase (URO-D) activity is reduced. Two forms are described: familial with point mutations in the URO-D gene, and sporadic where there is a URO-D defect restricted to the liver perhaps due to an inhibitor rather than mutation [9]. Sensitivity to drugs such as barbiturates is absent. Exposure to alcohol and oestrogens may precipitate attacks. A background of hepatic siderosis appears necessary for clinical expression of disease [26].

Porphyria cutanea tarda is characterized clinically by photosensitive skin, blistering and scarring, pigmentation and hypertrichosis. Acute neurological attacks with abdominal pain are absent. There is usually evidence of liver dysfunction. Uroporphyrin is increased in the urine.

Liver biopsy [16] shows subacute hepatitis or cirrhosis. Iron overload has never been adequately explained and may or may not be related to coexistent HLA-linked haemochromatosis [1]. Uroporphyrin can be shown by red fluorescence in ultraviolet light.

A high prevalence of hepatitis C has been found in patients with porphyria cutanea tarda, although varying greatly (8–80%) between different countries [8, 27]. This virus may contribute to the liver disease, but does not necessarily play a role in the pathogenesis of porphyria cutanea tarda.

The incidence of hepato-cellular carcinoma is increased [25].

Exacerbation of symptoms accompanies deterioration of liver function. At this time, porphyrins that would normally be excreted into the bile may be directed via the kidneys to the urine. When the liver is healthy, the porphyrin is excreted harmlessly into the bile; when it is diseased, it is retained in the blood. The porphyrin itself may be hepato-toxic.

Venesection has a good effect, probably related to removal of excess iron.

ERYTHROPOIETIC PROTOPORPHYRIA [22]

The defect is in ferrochelatase. The inheritance is dominant. Protoporphyrin is increased in tissues and urine.

This type is characterized by skin photosensitivity. Protoporphyrin is increased in tissues and urine.

Liver biopsies examined by fluorescent microscopy or phase microscopy show focal deposits of pigment containing protoporphyrin crystals. Electron microscopy shows abnormalities of nuclei, endoplasmic reticulum and membranes, despite normal light microscopy [23]. Complications include gallstones containing protoporphyrin.

Deaths have been reported in liver failure particularly after alcohol excess [5]. These are related to accumulation of the protoporphyrin within the hepatocyte with subsequent damage [15]. In patients with end-stage protoporphyric liver disease neurotoxicity has been reported [24].

Haematin infusions, by reducing porphyrin production, may be useful therapeutically [3].

Cholestyramine increases protoporphyrin excretion and may reduce hepato-toxicity [18]. Iron therapy decreases erythrocyte and stool protoporphyrin levels and improves liver function [10].

Liver transplantation has been successful for severe liver disease [4, 19] although precautions should be taken to reduce the risk of cutaneous reactions at the time of surgery. The metabolic defect is not corrected in bone marrow so that long-term follow-up will be necessary to assess whether hepatic injury recurs.

CONGENITAL ERYTHROPOIETIC PORPHYRIA

The major clinical problem in this rare type is photosensitivity. Neurological symptoms do not occur. The liver may be enlarged and contain excess iron. Uroporphyrinogen III cosynthase is deficient.

HEPATOERYTHROPOIETIC PORPHYRIA

This very rare type presenting within the first year of life with skin disease is due to homozygous deficiency of uroporphyrinogen decarboxylase [30]. It is marked by hepato-splenomegaly and cirrhosis. Liver biopsies fluoresce but there is no iron excess. The acute presentation may be preceded by acute viral hepatitis [12].

SECONDARY COPROPORPHYRIAS

Heavy metal intoxication, especially with lead, causes porphyria with ALA and coproporphyrin in the urine. Erythrocyte protoporphyrins are increased. Coproporphyrinuria may also be seen with sideroblastic anaemia, various liver diseases, the Dubin–Johnson syndrome and as a complication of drug therapy.

A patient has been described with a *hepatic adenoma* who developed photosensitivity with skin blisters and showed uroporphyrin and coproporphyrin in the urine [29]. Family history was negative. The tumour was removed and contained considerable quantities of proto-, copro- and uroporphyrin. Post-operatively the skin lesions disappeared and the urinary excretion of porphyrins returned to normal.

References

1 Beaumont C, Fauchet R, Phung LN *et al.* Porphyria tarda and HLA-linked hemochromatosis: evidence against a systematic association. *Gastroenterology* 1987; **92**: 1833.

2 Bissell DM. Treatment of acute hepatic porphyria with hematin. *J. Hepatol.* 1988; **6**: 1.

3 Bloomer JR, Pierach CA. Effect of hematin administration to patients with protoporphyria and liver disease. *Hepatology* 1982; **2**: 817.

4 Bloomer JR, Weimer MK, Bossenmaier IC *et al.* Liver transplantation in a patient with protoporphyria. *Gastroenterology* 1989; **97**: 188.

5 Bonkovsky HL, Schned AR. Fatal liver failure in protoporphyria: synergism between ethanol excess and the genetic defect. *Gastroenterology* 1986; **90**: 91.

6 Dover SB, Plenderleith L, Moore MR *et al.* Safety of general anaesthesia and surgery in acute hepatic porphyria. *Gut* 1994; **35**: 1112.

7 Elder GH. Molecular genetics of disorders of haem biosynthesis. *J. Clin. Pathol.* 1993; **46**: 977.

8 Fargion S, Piperno A, Cappellini MD *et al.* Hepatitis C virus and porphyria cutanea tarda: evidence of a strong association. *Hepatology* 1992; **16**: 1322.

9 Garey JR, Franklin KF, Brown DA *et al.* Analysis of uroporphyrinogen decarboxylase complementary DNAs in sporadic porphyria cutanea tarda. *Gastroenterology* 1993; **105**: 165.

10 Gordeuk VR, Brittenham GM, Hawkins CW *et al.* Iron therapy for hepatic dysfunction in erythropoietic protoporphyria. *Ann. Intern. Med.* 1986; **105**: 27.

11 Herrick A, McColl KEL, McLellan A *et al.* Effect of haem arginate therapy on porphyrin metabolism and mixed function oxygenase activity in acute hepatic porphyria. *Lancet* 1987; **ii**: 1178.

12 Hift RJ, Meissner PN, Todd G. Hepatoerythropoietic porphyria precipitated by viral hepatitis. *Gut* 1993; **34**: 1632.

13 Horie Y, Norimoto M, Tajima F *et al.* Clinical usefulness of cimetidine treatment for acute relapse in intermittent porphyria. *Clin. Chim. Acta* 1995; **234**: 171.

14 Kauppinen R, Mustajoki P. Prognosis of acute porphyria: occurrence of acute attacks, precipitating factors, and associated diseases. *Medicine* 1992; **71**: 1.

15 Koningsberger JC, Rademakers LHPM, van Hattum J *et al.* Exogenous protoporphyrin inhibits Hep G2 cell proliferation, increases the intracellular hydrogen peroxide concentration and causes ultrastructural alterations. *J. Hepatol.* 1995; **22**: 57.

16 Lefkowitch JH, Grossman ME. Hepatic pathology in por-

phyrea cutanea tarda. *Liver* 1983; **3**: 19.

17 Logan GM, Weimer MK, Ellefson M *et al.* Bile porphyrin analysis in the evaluation of variegate porphyria. *N. Engl. J. Med.* 1991; **324**: 1408.

18 McCullough AJ, Barron D, Mullen KD *et al.* Fecal protoporphyrin excretion in erythropoietic protoporphyria: effect of cholestyramine and bile acid feeding. *Gastroenterology* 1988; **94**: 177.

19 Mion FBC, Faure J-L, Berger F *et al.* Liver transplantation for erythropoietic protoporphyria. Report of a new case with subsequent medium-term follow-up. *J. Hepatol.* 1992; **16**: 203.

20 Moore MR. Biochemistry of porphyria. *Int. J. Biochem* 1993; **25**: 1353.

21 Muhlbauer JE, Pathak MA, Tishler PV *et al.* Variegate porphyria in New England. *JAMA* 1982; **247**: 3095.

22 Nordmann Y. Erythropoietic protoporphyria and hepatic complications. *J. Hepatol.* 1992; **16**: 4.

23 Rademakers LHPM, Cleton MI, Kooijman C *et al.* Early involvement of hepatic parenchymal cells in erythrohepatic protoporphyria? An ultrastructural study of patients with and without overt liver disease and the effect of chenodeoxycholic acid treatment. *Hepatology* 1990; **11**: 449.

24 Rank JM, Carithers R, Bloomer J *et al.* Evidence of neurological dysfunction in end-stage protoporphyric liver disease. *Hepatology* 1993; **18**: 1404.

25 Salata H, Cortes JM, Enriquez de Salamanca R *et al.* Porphyria cutanea tarda and hepatocellular carcinoma — frequency of occurrence and related factors. *J. Hepatol.* 1985; **1**: 477.

26 Siersema PD, Rademakers LHPM, Cleton MI *et al.* The difference in liver pathology between sporadic and familial forms of porphyria cutanea tarda: the role of iron. *J. Hepatol.* 1995; **23**: 259.

27 Stölzel U, Köstler E, Koszka C *et al.* Low prevalence of hepatitis C virus infection in porphyria cutanea tarda in Germany. *Hepatology* 1995; **21**: 1500.

28 Tefferi A, Colgan JP, Solberg LA. Acute porphyrias: diagnosis and management. *Mayo Clin. Proc.* 1994; **69**: 991.

29 Tio Tiong Hoo, Leijnse B, Jarrett A *et al.* Acquired porphyria from a liver tumour. *Clin. Sci.* 1957; **16**: 517.

30 Toback AC, Sassa S, Poh-Fitzpatrick MB *et al.* Hepatoerythropoietic porphyria: clinical, biochemical, and enzymatic studies in a three-generation family lineage. *N. Engl. J. Med.* 1987; **316**: 645.

Hereditary haemorrhagic telangiectasia [3]

Hepatomegaly is a common feature of this rare autosomal dominant disease. There are mutations in endothelium-related proteins which may cause vascular dysplasia but the pathogenetic mechanism is uncertain [3, 4]. The liver may show telangiectasia and cirrhosis. Bands of fibrous tissue surrounding the regenerative nodules contain numerous thin-walled telangiectases (fig. 23.19) [5]. It has been suggested that the telangiectases interfere with the nutrition of liver cells.

Diagnosis of liver involvement can be made by dynamic CT scan or coeliac angiography [2].

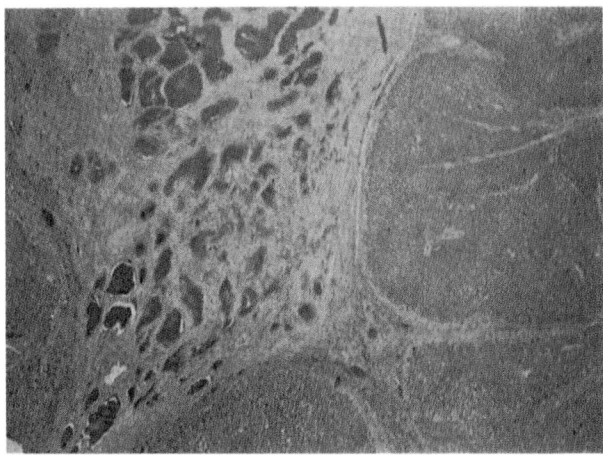

Fig. 23.19. The cirrhosis accompanying hereditary haemorrhagic telangiectasia. Note spaces filled with blood at the periphery of the lobules.

There may be high output cardiac failure due to the intra-hepatic arterio-portal fistulae. Portal hypertension and bleeding varices (due to the hepatic artery/portal venous fistulae rather than cirrhosis) can be treated by hepatic arterial ligation [6]. Intra-hepatic bile duct calculi may form due to stenosis of the ducts secondary to bands of fibrous tissue [1].

References

1 Ball NJ, Duggan MA. Hepatolithiasis in hereditary hemorrhagic telangiectasia. *Arch. Pathol. Lab. Med.* 1990; **114**: 423.
2 Bernard G, Mion F, Henry L. Hepatic involvement in hereditary hemorrhagic telangiectasia: clinical, radiological, and hemodynamic studies of 11 cases. *Gastroenterology* 1993; **105**: 482.
3 Guttmacher AE, Marchuk DA, White RI. Hereditary hemorrhagic telangiectasia. *N. Engl. J. Med.* 1995; **333**: 918.
4 Johnson DW, Berg JN, Baldwin MA *et al.* Mutations in the activin receptor-like kinase 1 gene in hereditary haemorrhagic telangiectasia type 2. *Nature Genet.* 1996; **13**: 189.
5 Martini GA. The liver in hereditary haemorrhagic telangiectasia: an inborn error of vascular structure with multiple manifestations: a reappraisal. *Gut* 1978; **19**: 531.
6 Zentler-Munro PL, Howard ER, Karani J *et al.* Variceal haemorrhage in hereditary haemorrhagic telangiectasia. *Gut* 1989; **30**: 1293.

Chapter 24
The Liver in Infancy and Childhood

Biochemical tests in infancy

Fractionation into unconjugated and conjugated *serum bilirubin* is important in neonates. Because of overlap, the proportion of serum bilirubin conjugates does not distinguish between extra-hepatic biliary obstruction and hepato-cellular disease [105].

Serum bilirubin levels are a guide to the development of kernicterus. Serial levels are useful in the assessment of prolonged jaundice.

Serum cholesterol. Extremely high levels may be recorded in prolonged cholestasis, particularly intra-hepatic cholestasis.

Serum alkaline phosphatase levels are influenced by bone metabolism as well as by cholestasis. Levels are increased in the first month of life as well as around puberty.

Serum gamma glutamyl transpeptidase levels are useful indicators of bile duct damage and in the diagnosis of cholestatic syndromes [78].

Serum transaminase values are about twice the normal adult level during the first month of life.

Bile acid metabolism [125]. Bile acid secretion evolves during the final trimester of pregnancy and in the early neonatal period. In the infant, conjugation and pool size are reduced, as are secretion, intraluminal concentration and ileal active transport. Serum bile acids are increased.

The main bile acid in neonates is glycocholic. After 1–3 months, glycochenodeoxycholic predominates. Secretion of bile acids by the hepatocyte may be reduced and atypical bile acids produced which may not be functionally adequate. A primitive pathway for the synthesis of fetal bile acids may be responsible for excretion of cholestatic bile acids during the immaturity of hepatic excretory function which lasts in infants from birth until 3 months [62]. This picture of *'physiological cholestasis'* is enhanced in the low birth-weight neonate. It may contribute to cholestasis produced by other factors, for instance, infection or prolonged parenteral nutrition.

Liver size

Liver span in normal infants and children is measured by percussion of the upper border and percussion/palpation of the lower border (table 24.1) [90].

Circulatory factors and hepatic necrosis

In the fetus the right lobe of the liver is supplied largely by the portal vein whereas the left receives highly oxygenated, placental blood. In the fetal mouse, higher levels of cytochrome P450 gene expression are found in the left lobe [22]. This lobar heterogeneity disappears as the adult pattern of liver circulation develops.

At the time of birth, loss of placental blood can be followed by atrophy of the left lobe of the liver.

Right-sided hepatic necrosis may be seen in postmature infants dying about the time of birth. This is related to poor placental blood supply and anoxia at the time of delivery.

Disseminated mid-zonal necrosis is found with congenital cardiac defects [115]. This may be due to a decrease in total hepatic blood flow. In others the zone 3 changes of congestive heart failure may be seen. Cholestasis in the first week can be related to congenital cardiac defects and 'shock'.

Localized necrosis of the liver may be due to trapping in defects of the anterior abdominal wall.

Copper is increased in the fetal liver, more so in the left lobe than the right [34].

Table 24.1. Approximate mean liver span of infants and children based on four studies on 470 subjects [90]

Age	Span (cm)
Birth	5.6–5.9
2 months	5
1 year	6
2 years	6.5
3 years	7
4 years	7.5
5 years	8
12 years	9

Neonatal hyperbilirubinaemia

Unconjugated hyperbilirubinaemia (tables 24.2, 24.3)

Jaundice, reaching its peak within 2–5 days of birth and disappearing in 2 weeks, is common in normal infants (*physiological jaundice*). It is a benign self-limited process (table 24.3). It is more serious in low birth-weight infants where it may persist for as long as 2 weeks. The urine contains both urobilin and bilirubin and the stools are paler than normal.

Hepatic conjugating and transport systems for bilirubin are delayed in the neonate. Absorption of bilirubin from the intestine is increased. Bilirubin binding to albumin is reduced particularly in premature infants [105]. The jaundice is enhanced by factors which depress liver function such as hypoxia and hypoglycaemia. Drugs such as water-soluble vitamin K analogues add to the jaundice.

Serum bilirubin levels may be *lower* in infants with circulatory failure, asphyxia and sepsis. Bilirubin may be a physiological antioxidant providing protection against perinatal ischaemia-reperfusion tissue injury [10, 38].

The bilirubinaemia is *not* physiological if the level exceeds 5 mg (86 μmol/litre) on the first day, 10 mg (171 μmol/litre) on the second day, or 12–13 mg (206–223 μmol/litre) at any time.

Table 24.2. Unconjugated hyperbilirubinaemia in neonates related to time of onset

Birth to 2 days
Haemolytic disease

3–7 days
Physiological ± prematurity
　　　　　　hypoxia
　　　　　　acidosis

1–8 weeks
Congenital haemolytic disorders
Breast milk jaundice
Lucey–Driscoll
Crigler–Najjar
Hypothyroidism
Perinatal complications: haemorrhage, sepsis
Upper gastrointestinal obstruction

Table 24.3. Investigations of the jaundiced newborn

Total and direct serum bilirubin
Blood group
Rhesus status
Coombs' test
Haematocrit
Blood smear for morphology
Blood culture
Urine culture

Unconjugated hyperbilirubinaemia in the neonatal period is complicated by bilirubin encephalopathy (*kernicterus*).

Management

Phototherapy. Hyperbilirubinaemia may be prevented or controlled by exposure of the infant to light of wavelength near 450 nm. The light converts bilirubin IXα photochemically to a relatively stable geometric isomer. Structural isomerization also takes place with the production of a non-reversible product called *lumirubin* [32]. Side-effects include increased insensible water loss, haemolysis and bronzing of the skin. The eyes must be protected.

Phototherapy should not be routine but is of value in selected cases. It is also useful in the Crigler–Najjar syndrome.

Phototherapy is being grossly overused in full-term infants, mainly for medicolegal reasons. This particularly applies to home phototherapy.

Exchange transfusion is rarely necessary with the advent of phototherapy which is as effective [110].

Enzyme induction, using phenobarbitone, is effective when given to the mother. Antipyrine, similarly, reduces serum bilirubin levels but without causing drowsiness.

Tin-protoporphyrin is a potent, competitive inhibitor of haem oxygenase, the rate-limiting enzyme for haem catabolism to bilirubin. It has been used to treat neonates with jaundice and ABO incompatibility with a reduction in peak bilirubin levels and total bilirubin production [57]. It may be too toxic to be the final drug of choice.

Haemolytic disease of the newborn

The fetal–maternal incompatibility usually concerns the rhesus blood factors and rarely the ABO or other blood groups.

Characteristically, the first-born escapes the disease unless the mother's blood has been sensitized by a previous transfusion of Rh-positive blood. A normal first pregnancy sensitizes the mother's blood sufficiently to provoke haemolytic disease in subsequent infants. The clinical forms of the disease vary in severity, but the underlying pathological lesions are essentially similar.

The infant is jaundiced during the first 2 days of life. Serum unconjugated bilirubin is increased. The critical period is in the first few days when the more deeply jaundiced infants may develop *kernicterus*.

Diagnosis may be suspected by antenatal examination of the mother's blood for specific antibodies and confirmed by a positive Coombs' test in the infant and by blood-typing on mother and child.

The risk of mental or physical impairment is low until the serum bilirubin increases well above 20 mg/342 μmol/l.

KERNICTERUS (BILIRUBIN ENCEPHALOPATHY)

This grave condition is a complication of prematurity jaundice, haemolytic disease and neonatal hepatitis. Management with phototherapy, exchange transfusion and phenobarbitone has significantly reduced its occurrence.

Within the first 5 days of life, the jaundiced infant becomes restless or lethargic and febrile, developing a stiff neck and head retraction which proceeds to opisthotonus. There is stiffness of the limbs with pronated arms, eye squinting, lid retraction, twitching or convulsions and a high-pitched cry.

Death may supervene rapidly in 12 hours and 70% of affected infants die within 7 days of onset. The remaining 30% may survive, but are maimed by mental defect, cerebral palsy or athetosis, until they eventually die from intercurrent infections.

Bilirubin neurotoxicity may occur at relatively low bilirubin levels and be recognized only by new neurophysiological techniques [97].

Autopsy reveals yellow staining of the basal ganglia and other areas of the brain and spinal cord with unconjugated bilirubin which, being lipid-soluble, has an affinity for nervous tissue.

Kernicterus is related to circulating free bilirubin crossing the blood–brain barrier. Reduction of serum bilirubin–albumin binding may play a part and indeed albumin infusions have been used therapeutically.

The classical definition of kernicterus requires both bilirubin staining in the brain and neuronal damage. Limited animal studies suggest that functional brain toxicity and even death from hyperbilirubinaemia may occur in the absence of both visible yellow staining and cellular damage [38]. Mechanisms of the bilirubin toxicity and the neurone damage are unknown. Bilirubin however, does inhibit neuronal function [45]. Each molecule of haem releases one molecule of carbon monoxide. This can be measured in less than 1 minute on expired air using a nasal catheter. This may be helpful in identifying the baby at risk of kernicterus.

Kernicterus is potentiated by hypoxia, metabolic acidosis and septicaemia [45]. Organic anions which compete for bilirubin binding sites on albumin increase kernicterus although the serum bilirubin level falls. Such anions include salicylates, sulphonamides, free fatty acids and haematin.

CONGENITAL HAEMOLYTIC DISORDERS

These can all lead to unconjugated hyperbilirubinaemia in the first 2 days of life. They include the red cell enzyme deficiencies (glucose-6PD and pyruvate kinase) congenital spherocytosis and pyknocytosis.

Glucose-6-phosphate dehydrogenase deficiency. Infants develop jaundice, usually on the second or third day of life. The precipitating haemolytic agent may be a drug such as salicylate, phenacetin, or sulphonamides transmitted in the maternal breast milk. This condition is frequent in the Mediterranean area, in the Far East and in Nigeria.

BREAST MILK JAUNDICE

Hyperbilirubinaemia (serum bilirubin more than 12 mg/dl) affects 34% of newborn breast-fed babies compared with only 15% of those who are formula-fed [96]. It may be due to increased β-glucuronidase in breast milk which leads to increased unconjugated bilirubin in the intestine and to its subsequent absorption [40]. Increased free fatty acids in breast milk might inhibit conjugation.

The condition lasts from 2 weeks to more than 2 months. Discontinuation of breast-feeding results in a fall of the bilirubin level.

TRANSIENT FAMILIAL HYPERBILIRUBINAEMIA (LUCEY–DRISCOLL TYPE) [77]

This appears in the first few days and persists into the second or third week. It affects every sibling. It is believed to be due to an inhibitor of bilirubin conjugation present in maternal and infantile serum.

CRIGLER–NAJJAR HYPERBILIRUBINAEMIA (Chapter 12)

This may present in the first few days of life.

HYPOTHYROIDISM

This is three times more common in girls than boys. Mild anaemia is common and the infant is sluggish. The diagnosis is confirmed by finding low serum thyroxine and tri-iodothyronine levels with high thyroid-stimulating hormone and by observing the effects of therapy. The mechanism of the jaundice is unknown.

PERINATAL COMPLICATIONS

Haemorrhage with release of blood into the tissues provides a bilirubin load which may exacerbate jaundice, particularly in the premature. Anaemia depresses hepato-cellular function. Cephalohaematoma is a common association. The prothrombin time should be measured and vitamin K given.

Sepsis, whether umbilical or elsewhere, leads to unconjugated hyperbilirubinaemia in the first few days of life. Blood, urine and, if necessary, cerebrospinal fluid are cultured and appropriate antibodies given.

458   *Chapter 24*

UPPER GASTROINTESTINAL OBSTRUCTION [35]

About 10% of infants with congenital pyloric stenosis are jaundiced due to unconjugated bilirubin. The mechanism may be similar to that postulated for the increase in jaundice when patients with Gilbert's syndrome are fasted.

Hepatitis and cholestatic syndromes (conjugated hyperbilirubinaemia)

The reaction of the neonatal liver to different insults is similar. Proliferation of giant cells is always a part and this reflects increased regenerative ability. In some instances the condition may be the so-called 'idiopathic' hepatitis formerly called giant cell hepatitis. In others a specific virus such as type B or another infection can be identified. Metabolic disturbances, such as galactosaemia, can cause a giant cell reaction. Cholestatic syndromes are also seen which may be associated with hepatitis and, in these, hepatic histology may include a giant cell reaction. In all these conditions the conjugated 'direct reacting' bilirubin is more than 30% of the total (table 24.4).

Some are immediately treatable, such as congenital syphilis or bacterial infections—which will respond to antibiotics—and galactosaemia or tyrosinosis—which will require exclusion diets. The main bile duct atresias,

Table 24.4. Conjugated hyperbilirubinaemia in neonates

Infection
Viruses (CMV rubella, Coxsackie, herpes, hepatitis A, B and C)
 (Chapter 16)
Syphilis
Bacteria (*Escherichia coli*)

Metabolic (Chapter 23)
Galactosaemia
α_1-Antitrypsin deficiency
Tyrosinosis
Cystic fibrosis
Hereditary fructose intolerance
Total parenteral nutrition
Niemann–Pick disease

Idiopathic
'Neonatal' hepatitis
Congenital hepatic fibrosis
Byler's disease

Biliary atresia
Intra-hepatic
Extra-hepatic

Erythroblastosis with cholestasis

which may benefit from surgical treatment, must be diagnosed early.

Diagnosis of the hepatitic–cholestatic syndromes
(tables 24.4, 24.5)

Family history is important in diagnosing galactosaemia, α_1-antitrypsin deficiency, tyrosinosis, cystic fibrosis and hereditary fructose intolerance.

Virus infections in the mother during pregnancy, such as rubella, hepatitis, or genital herpes, must be recorded.

At the onset it is valuable to test the blood of mother, father and other siblings by appropriate methods and to store the sera for later use. The *routine biochemical tests* of the adult are of little value in the diagnosis of jaundice in infancy and childhood. A serum alkaline phosphatase level three times normal and a serum cholesterol value exceeding 250 mg/100 ml suggest intra-hepatic biliary atresia. A serum γ-glutamyl transpeptidase value exceeding 300 iu/litre, particularly if rising, is also suggestive, but not diagnostic, of atresia [37]. A direct reacting bilirubin value exceeding 4 mg (68 μmol) suggests extra-hepatic biliary obstruction.

Serum tyrosine is measured if tyrosinosis is suspected and serum α_1-antitrypsin values noted for the diagnosis of α_1-antitrypsin deficiency.

Biliary isotopic scanning (HIDA) is useful in establishing patency of the biliary passages [25].

Serological methods. The serum is tested for HBsAg, IgM anti-HBc, IgM anti-HAV, anti-HCV, HCV RNA and for syphilis. Antibodies to herpes simplex, rubella, toxoplasma, cytomegala, adenovirus and Coxsackie viruses are estimated in both baby and mother. Blood cultures are performed if *Escherichia coli* infection is suspected.

Urine tests. Cultures are taken for Gram-negative organisms and for cytomegala infection. Aminoaciduria

Table 24.5. Aetiology of cholestasis in neonates

Week 1
Inspissated bile syndrome (erythroblastosis with cholestasis)
Bacterial infections
Vascular causes
 'shock'
 congenital heart disease

After week 1
Bile duct anomalies
Genetic
 galactosaemia
 α_1-antitrypsin deficiency
 others
Infections (same as immune deficiency in adults)
 TORCH screen (toxoplasmosis, rubella, cytomegala, herpes)
Parenteral hyperalimentation

is noted. Reducing substances are sought if galactosaemia is suspected.

Liver biopsy. Needle biopsy of the liver is easy and well tolerated in neonates, infants and children. Interpretation is always difficult due to the overlap between hepatitis and cholestatic syndromes, both of intra-hepatic and extra-hepatic origin. Neonatal changes in the liver include giant cells and extra-medullary erythropoiesis. These subside by about 3 months.

Portal zone duct proliferation and a biliary type of fibrosis are helpful in diagnosing extra-hepatic atresia. A relative paucity of portal zone bile ducts supports the diagnosis of intra-hepatic cholestasis but is not constant.

The PAS-positive bodies of α_1-antitrypsin deficiency may be seen after 2 months.

Electron microscopy is essential if metabolic disease is suspected.

Ultrasonography shows absence of the gallbladder in biliary atresia [25]. It can also diagnose choledochal cyst.

CT scan is also of value.

Percutaneous and endoscopic cholangiography. The percutaneous technique is of great value when liver biopsy findings are equivocal and the HIDA test suggests biliary atresia. Endoscopic cholangiography is employed using suitably sized instruments [15].

Viral hepatitis

Immunity is reduced in the neonate and virus infections similar to those seen in the immunodeficient adult are frequent. The infection is very liable to persist and chronic hepatitis and cirrhosis ensue. Similarly, older children with immunological deficits such as agammaglobulinaemia or who are receiving treatment with immunosuppressive drugs are at risk.

HEPATITIS B

This disease develops in babies of mothers who suffer the acute disease during the later part of pregnancy, within 2 months of delivery, or who are chronic carriers. The mother is usually, but not always, hepatitis B 'e' antigen positive. Antigenaemia is usually found between 6 weeks and 6 months of birth, suggesting transmission from the mother's blood during delivery or later during her care of the infant. The condition is probably not spread by breast milk.

Umbilical cord sera may rarely be positive for HBsAg. Placental transmission is rare.

The natural history of hepatitis B contracted at birth and in early life is very variable. Fulminant hepatitis is rare and the precore mutant was found in only two of seven patients and one of three with acute hepatitis B [51].

Hepatitis B is a frequent cause of chronic hepatitis par-

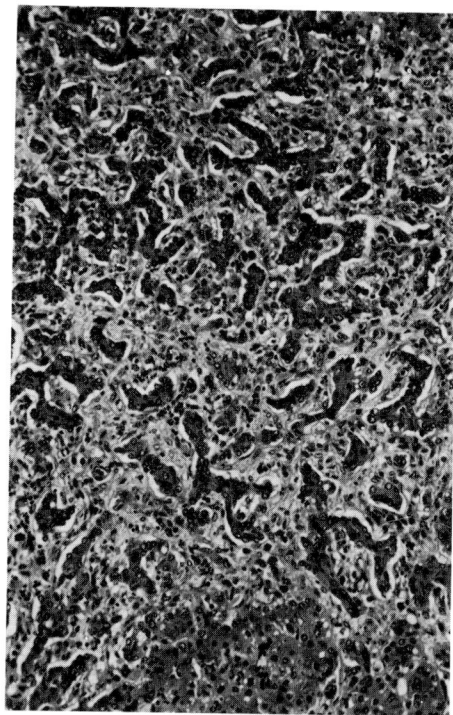

Fig. 24.1. Viral hepatitis in an infant of 3 months. Necrosis of liver cells and multinucleated giant liver cells are seen. Bile thrombi stained very darkly. (Stained H & E, ×115.)

ticularly in Italy and in the Far East [12]. Spread is perinatal and in the family. The liver disease is usually mild and stable reflecting immunological tolerance to the virus [75]. High levels of virus replication are found. Histological regression is associated with conversion from HBeAg-positive to anti-HBe [21]. Others, particularly males, develop cirrhosis and hepato-cellular cancer. Core antigen is detected in the cytoplasm of the hepatocyte in those with aggressive disease compared with presence in the nuclei or absence in the inactive. In Italy, superinfection with hepatitis delta virus may influence the progression towards cirrhosis.

Liver biopsy in the acute stage shows a giant cell hepatitis (fig. 24.1). Later, the picture is of chronic persistent hepatitis and only occasionally of chronic active hepatitis and cirrhosis.

Prophylaxis

See Chapter 16.

Treatment

Interferon is well tolerated and the efficacy in Caucasian infants is similar to that of adults [7, 8, 107, 109]. This is in contrast to Chinese children where the results are poor [75]. Interferon is more effective in horizontally transmitted disease than in those infected at birth [16, 17]. Predictive factors of good response are similar to those found in adults, particularly transaminases more than twice the upper limit of normal and histological activity on liver biopsy [107].

HEPATITIS A

Asymptomatic hepatitis A can spread in nurseries for neonates. The source may be infected blood [91] or a nurse carrier [64]. The babies spread the hepatitis A to adults in the nursery and to the community.

HEPATITIS C

Babies born to anti-HCV-positive mothers show passively transmitted antibody for the first 6 months.

Mothers who are HCV-RNA-positive can transmit HCV-RNA-positive disease to their infants [103], but this is infrequent [79]. There is probably no difference between transmission from HIV-positive or HIV-negative mothers. Those with a high serum HCV-RNA are more likely to transmit the disease [93] (fig. 24.2). Breast-feeding seems safe [74].

Hepatitis C virus disease is predominantly seen in those who have received multiple transfusions, are thalassaemic, or on renal dialysis [55].

Approximately one-third will have a response to interferon therapy [108].

CYTOMEGALOVIRUS

This is a very common virus infection (Chapter 27). The incidence in small children is 5–10% in those living in good hygienic conditions, rising to 80% in the underprivileged.

It is usually acquired placentally from an asymptomatic mother. It can also be transmitted in breast milk and from blood products. Many congenital infections are asymptomatic.

The disease may, however, be fulminant with intense jaundice, purpura, hepatosplenomegaly and neurological and pulmonary defects. Survivors may run a long course with persistent jaundice, hepatomegaly and disappearing bile ducts [36].

Intranuclear viral inclusions are seen in bile duct epithelium and rarely in hepatocytes. Diagnosis is made on urine or tissue *in situ* using PCR [20].

HERPES SIMPLEX

The liver may be involved in the course of a fulminating viraemia, contracted at birth from maternal genital herpes. Jaundice is due to viral involvement of the liver, which shows white nodules. Histologically, these represent necrosis with little or no inflammatory reaction. Giant cells are absent, but inclusion bodies may be found.

Human herpes virus VI has caused fulminant hepatitis in a baby [5].

Gancyclovir is often given too late, when massive hepatic necrosis and chronic cholestasis have developed and the mortality is 70% [80].

CONGENITAL RUBELLA SYNDROME

This disease, if contracted in the first trimester of pregnancy, may cause fetal malformations. It may also persist through the neonatal period and into later life. The liver with the brain, lung, heart and other organs are involved in the generalized virus infection.

Jaundice commences within the first 1 or 2 days with hepatosplenomegaly. The picture is sometimes cholestatic. Serum transaminase levels are slightly elevated.

Hepatic histology shows bile in swollen Kupffer cells and ductules with a focal hepato-cellular necrosis and portal fibrosis. Erythroid haemopoietic tissue is relatively increased. A typical giant cell hepatitis can be seen [123]. The virus can be identified from the liver at necropsy or biopsy.

Usually the hepatitis resolves completely.

Intra-uterine *parvovirus* B19 can cause severe giant cell hepatic disease in the neonate [81], also fulminant liver failure and aplastic anaemia [69].

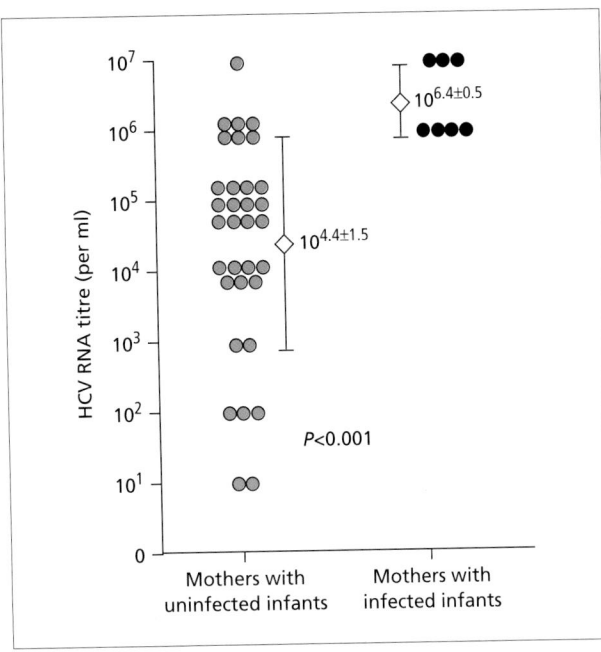

Fig. 24.2. Mean (± SD) serum HCV-RNA titres in seven mothers with HCV-infected infants and the 33 mothers with uninfected infants (from [93] with permission).

ADENOVIRUSES

These may disseminate in babies with decreased resistance due to thymic alymphoplasia and agammaglobulinaemia. A marked coagulative necrosis with inclusion-bearing cells may be seen. Under similar circumstances this lesion can also complicate *varicella*.

Acquired immuno-deficiency syndrome (AIDS)

Babies and children with AIDS have a very similar picture to that seen in the adult with the same spectrum of infections, primary lymphoma and Kaposi's sarcoma. Hepatic histology shows more giant-cell transformation and fewer granulomas [54]. Diffuse, lymphoplasmocytic infiltration is associated with lymphoid interstitial pneumonia.

Non-viral causes of hepatitis

CONGENITAL SYPHILIS

This condition is very rare. Visceral involvement is late in acquired syphilis but common in fetal infection [76]. Tremendous numbers of treponemas can be found in the liver. Such involvement leads to a fine peri-cellular cirrhosis with a marked connective tissue reaction. Jaundice is usual. The diagnosis is made serologically.

CONGENITAL TOXOPLASMOSIS

Infection is intra-uterine. Jaundice develops within a few hours of birth with hepatomegaly, encephalomyelitis, choroidoretinitis and intra-cerebral calcification. Toxoplasmosis may develop later in the neonatal period [26]. It is diagnosed by finding toxoplasma IgM antibodies.

The liver shows infiltration of portal zones with mononuclear cells. Extramedullary haemopoiesis with increased stainable iron is conspicuous. Histiocytes containing toxoplasma may be present. The jaundice is difficult to relate to the extent of liver damage and haemolysis may be contributory. The liver disease is generally mild.

BACTERIAL INFECTION

In the neonate, an immature reticulo-endothelial system with decreased complement and opsonins impairs the ability of the liver and spleen to phagocytose bacteria.

The upsurgence of Gram-negative infections, particularly *E. coli*, in nurseries, has led to an increase in cholestatic jaundice due to this cause.

The origins include umbilical sepsis, pneumonia, otitis media or even gastroenteritis. Diagnosis may be difficult as focal signs are minimal or absent. Jaundice appears suddenly in a baby who does not look ill. Hepatomegaly need not be present and splenomegaly is never great. The leucocyte count exceeds 12 000. A blood culture is usually positive. The umbilical stump should be cultured. Liver function tests are of little value.

Hepatic histology is non-contributory. It shows non-specific changes with Kupffer cell hypertrophy and portal zone infiltrates. Culture of liver biopsies is usually negative. The jaundice seems to be due to a combination of haemolysis, hepato-cellular dysfunction and even cholestasis, presumably due to endotoxaemia.

Prognosis depends on early treatment and age of onset, the mortality being 80% below the age of 1 week and 25% later. Antibiotics are appropriate.

Portal vein occlusion may be diagnosed years later.

Liver abscesses in older children are associated with blood-spread organisms. A third have acute blastic leukaemia.

URINARY TRACT INFECTIONS

Jaundice may be associated with urinary tract infections both in infants and children. Infants are usually affected in the first week of life. They are often male, but have no underlying abnormality of the renal tract. Endotoxin is believed to contribute to the hepatic dysfunction.

The infants fail to thrive, show fever, jaundice and moderate hepatomegaly. Bilirubinuria is found. Liver biopsy shows a non-specific hepatitis. Urine culture is an essential investigation in any jaundiced child or infant.

'Idiopathic' neonatal hepatitis

Aetiology

After specific infections and metabolic causes have been identified, the number of cases being diagnosed has diminished. The condition is often familial, the inheritance being autosomal recessive. The familial incidence may reflect defects in bile acid metabolism, hitherto unrecognized. The familial type has a worse prognosis than the sporadic.

Clinical features

The infant may be stillborn or die soon after or before jaundice has had time to develop. More usually a fluctuant jaundice appears during the first 2 weeks or even up to 4 months. The liver and sometimes the spleen are enlarged and the stools pale. The child may appear well and continue to gain weight, or may fail to thrive. Serum transaminase is usually above 800 iu/litre. Hypoprothrombinaemia may be profound. Stools are pale and urine contains bilirubin. Serum α-fetoprotein levels correlate with severity [70].

Histology

This is non-specific with giant cell transformation, extra-medullary haematopoiesis and portal inflammatory exudate. Bile duct proliferation is minimal and there may be canalicular cholestasis.

Prognosis and treatment

The hepatitis resolves slowly over a matter of months or may blend imperceptibly with the intra-hepatic cholestases (bile duct paucity or hypoplasia). In a 10-year follow-up of 29 patients, two had died and only two had signs of persisting liver disease [31].

Treatment is symptomatic. Medium-chain triglycerides may be useful to promote nutrition. The haemorrhagic diathesis must be controlled. Corticosteroid therapy is useless.

Infantile cholangiopathies

Cholestasis in infancy can have numerous causes (fig. 24.3) [7]. A broad classification is made into extra-hepatic, including such lesions as choledochal cyst or biliary atresia, and intra-hepatic, subdivided into neonatal hepatitis and the bile duct diseases such as syndromatic or non-syndromic biliary atresia. Idiopathic hepatitis and non-syndromic biliary atresia may overlap.

Biliary atresia

Biliary atresia commences in intra-uterine life (fig. 24.4). It is often classified as congenital, although, in most instances, the abnormality is due to an extraneous, often infectious, cause acting during the normal process of intra-uterine development or shortly after birth. This is supported by the histology of ductular tissue showing acute and chronic inflammation with bile duct oblit-

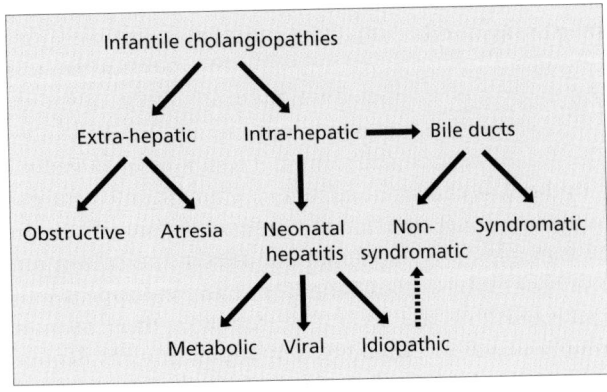

Fig. 24.3. An algorithm for managing infantile cholangiopathies (after [7] with permission).

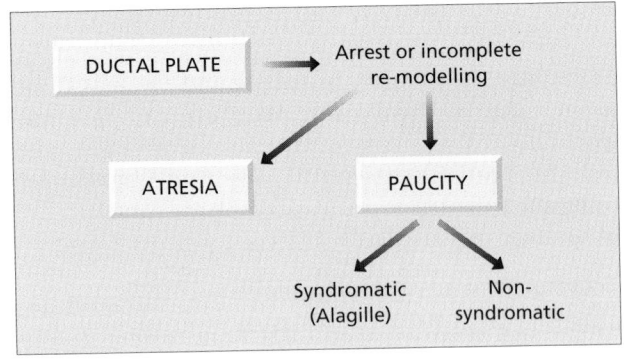

Fig. 24.4. Infantile cholangiopathy. Intra-uterine mechanisms of biliary atresia.

eration. Reovirus 3 causes liver parenchymal damage and biliary tract necrosis in young mice and has been invoked [86], but this could not be confirmed by PCR analysis of preserved tissue from infants with cholestatic liver disease [121]. Other possible infective causes include cytomegalovirus [36, 46] and rubella [123].

Vascular malformations of the hepatic artery might cause ischaemic fibrosis of the extra-hepatic biliary tree [50].

The biliary atresias are rarely familial [66].

A chromosomal abnormality, namely trisomy 17–18, and Down's syndrome have been associated with neonatal hepatitis and atresia [4], but these are rare.

The atresias result not from the failure of bile ducts to form, but from their destruction at some moment during embryonic development [131]. Hepatic histology indicates the stage at which the damage started. At the early stage of the ductal plate, abnormal cylindrical ducts show atrophy or necrosis of lining cells; later the changes are of regression and involution in normally shaped ducts.

There are grades of destruction from complete absence of bile ducts, termed *atresia*, to drastic reduction of numbers, termed *paucity of bile ducts*. The extent of the process and its continuation into extra-uterine life is reflected in the prognosis. The baby with complete atresia is usually dead by 5 years old. The baby with paucity of bile ducts may survive into adult life.

Finally, there is the Alagille syndromatic form of paucity of bile ducts [3]. Here the characteristic facies, skeletal defects, cardiovascular and eye changes make the diagnosis.

Extra-hepatic biliary atresia

The abnormality may be in any part of the biliary system. 25% show errors in other organs [68, 83]. In some, bile ducts are absent at birth, but in others the ducts may have been formed but sclerosis starts in the perinatal period and there is a dynamic evolution to bile duct destruction. There is acquired progressive disease of the biliary system.

Developmental aspects

The biliary passages may fail to develop from the primitive foregut bud. The gallbladder may be absent or the biliary tract represented only by a gallbladder connecting directly with the duodenum. The more usual defect is failure of vacuolation of the solid biliary bud. This is usually partial and rarely extends throughout the biliary tree.

Pathology

The ducts may be absent or replaced by fibrous strands. The site and extent of the atresia are variable. Bile is absent from the extra-hepatic biliary system including the gallbladder.

The cystic duct only may be involved, the gallbladder becoming a mucous cyst; this has no clinical significance. Involvement of the common bile duct or hepatic duct gives rise to the characteristic syndrome of biliary atresia with deep cholestatic jaundice.

Liver biopsy shows cholestasis with a variable number of giant cells; proliferated bile ductules are conspicuous with biliary-type fibrosis. There is paucity of interlobular ducts. The picture is virtually diagnostic.

Clinical features

Extra-hepatic biliary atresia complicates one in 10 000 live births. There are more females than males, and all races are affected. The condition is not inherited.

The baby becomes icteric by the first week and this continues unremittingly. Pruritus is severe and increasing. The urine is dark. The stools are pale, although some pigment may reach the intestine, presumably through the intestinal secretions. Serum transaminase values rarely exceed 300 iu/dl. Nutrition is well maintained for the first 2 months and then falls off, the child usually dying before 3 years. The serum cholesterol level may be very high and skin xanthomas appear (fig. 24.5). The prolonged steatorrhoea can result in osteomalacia (*biliary rickets*).

Death is usually due to intercurrent infection, to liver cell failure, or to bleeding related to vitamin K deficiency or to oesophageal varices. Ascites is a late and terminal event.

Prognosis

Prognosis is poor unless the cystic duct only is involved or the bile ducts are hypoplastic and not entirely obliter-

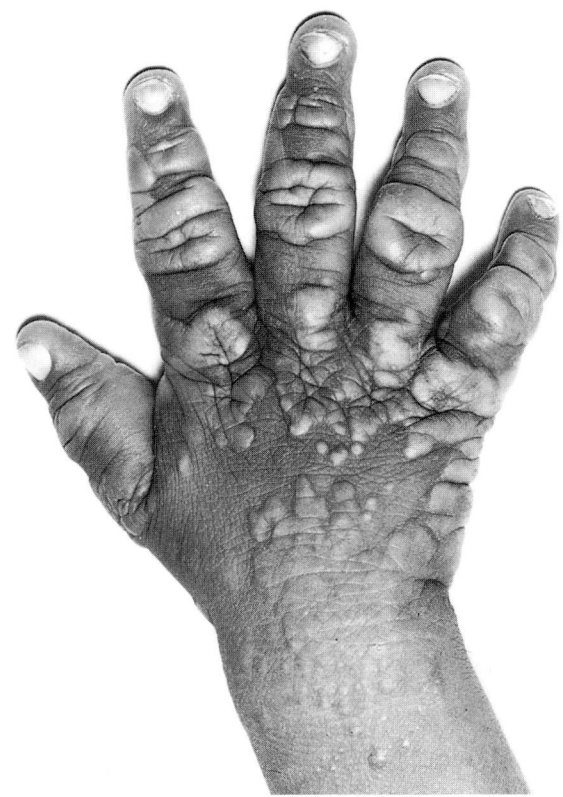

Fig. 24.5. Intra-hepatic biliary atresia (Alagille's syndrome) in a child of 4 years of age. Cholesterol deposits are noted on the hands, particularly on the extensor surfaces. Note also skin pigmentation and white nailbeds. This child spontaneously lost the xanthomas and is alive and reasonably well at 19 years.

ated. Very few patients are amenable to curative surgical treatment.

Surgery

If the proximal bile ducts are patent but end blindly before the duodenum the condition is *correctable* by Roux-en-Y jejunal anastomosis to the common hepatic duct. This is an exceedingly rare circumstance (<5%).

In the vast majority of infants the atresia is *non-correctable* because extra-hepatic ducts are not patent. The *Kasai operation (hepatic porto-enterostomy)* must be considered. The entire ductal system is resected in the porta hepatis and proximal transected common hepatic duct anastomosed to the intestine. The basis for subsequent biliary drainage is the presence of minuscule biliary ductules in the scarred 'non-patent' extra-hepatic bile ducts. These communicate with the intra-hepatic biliary system and when surgically transected may drain bile from the liver into the interposed intestine.

Biliary atresia is strongly suggested if a newborn baby remains jaundiced for 6 weeks with pale stools and dark urine. A full work-up is done to ensure that the baby is not suffering from the biliary hypoplasia syndrome, where the prognosis is relatively good and jaundice will lessen without porto-enterostomy. The Kasai procedure is performed at 2 months. After 5 months it is useless as the small hilar bile ducts will have disappeared. If performed early, 86% will develop bile flow [83]. A successful early Kasai operation allows growth before hepatic transplant becomes necessary. Post-operative complications include cholangitis, progressive portal hypertension and liver failure. Success depends on early age, the size of residual ducts, the absence of ascending cholangitis and the rate of progression of the hepatic and ductular disease.

In a post-Kasai 10-year follow-up of 122 patients, one-third were alive but only 11 had normal biochemical tests and no portal hypertension. At the age of 10–23 years, only 10 of 71 survivors of 241 porto-enterostomies had no clinical features of liver disease [130]. 80% of survivors will eventually undergo liver transplantation [69] which is not compromised by a previous Kasai procedure provided that complex loops and enterostomies are avoided.

Liver transplant is indicated if the serum bilirubin exceeds 10 mg/dl (170 μmol/litre) or 5 mg/dl accompanied by severe oesophageal varices [58]. Prolongation of prothrombin time and episodes of bleeding are other indications [92]. Hepatic transplantation is discussed further in Chapter 35.

Intra-hepatic atresia (paucity of bile ducts) syndrome

Intra-hepatic cholestasis in early life may be related to a known cause such as α_1-antitrypsin deficiency. The characteristic PAS-positive cells can be seen in a liver biopsy from the age of 2 months. Congenital abnormalities of bile salt metabolism can present in the first 6 months of life.

In the majority, however, no clear aetiology is evident. The early histological appearances may resemble 'idiopathic neonatal hepatitis'. This progresses histologically to bile duct disappearance and biliary cirrhosis. This suggests that hepatitis, often viral, in the neonatal period or even *in utero* may be the first change, ultimately leading to biliary hypoplasia [47]. In most instances the causative virus cannot be identified, although occasionally an association with congenital cardiac defects, nerve deafness or rising titres of rubella antibody suggests that this virus is at fault. Reovirus 3 [86], Epstein–Barr and cytomegalovirus [36] have also been incriminated.

Clinical presentation

Jaundice usually appears within 3 days of birth, but may be delayed to 3–4 weeks.

Idiopathic adulthood ductopenia, presenting at age 16–22 years, may be a late onset form of the non-syndromic paucity of interlobular bile ducts seen in children [17].

Biochemical changes

The findings are those of chronic cholestasis with very high serum gamma-glutamyl transpeptidase levels. Serum cholesterol levels are very high and xanthomas appear after about the first year of life (fig. 24.5). Serum bile acids are increased.

Hepatic histology [56]

The early changes, at less than 90 days, are those of cholestasis, bile duct paucity, inflammation and fibrosis. Giant cells may be conspicuous. Electron microscopy shows abnormal bile ducts.

Later the picture is of hypoplasia of intra-hepatic bile ducts, increasing portal fibrosis and eventually cirrhosis.

ARTERIO-HEPATIC DYSPLASIA (ALAGILLE'S SYNDROME) [3]

This is sometimes called syndromatic or syndromic paucity of intra-hepatic bile ducts. It is seen worldwide.

Chronic intra-hepatic cholestasis presents in infancy or early childhood [116]. Inheritance is autosomal dominant with variable expression and penetrance. A deletion of the short arm of chromosome 20 has been demonstrated [44].

The face is triangular with a prominent broad forehead, deep set eyes, a flattened nose and a pointed mandible (fig. 24.6). Hepato-splenomegaly is usual. Skeletal changes include short distal phalanges and butterfly vertical bodies. The eyes show various abnormalities including retinal pigmentation and posterior embryotoxon [13]. Renal abnormalities have been noted [127]. Peripheral pulmonary stenosis is usual [83].

Liver biopsy shows few, if any, interlobular bile ducts with a reduced number of portal zones [43]. There is little fibrosis so that neither cirrhosis nor secondary portal hypertension develop. However, the liver biopsy appearances are not diagnostic of the Alagille syndrome.

Patients survive into adult life with varying degrees of growth and mental retardation, xanthomatosis and pruritus (fig. 24.7) [47]. Hepato-cellular carcinoma may be a complication [60, 61]. This can be familial [101]. On the whole, the condition improves with time. Long-term

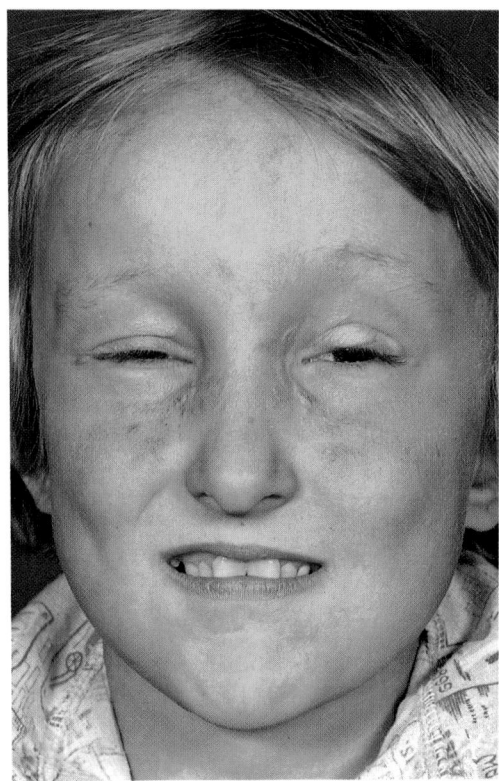

Fig. 24.6. Alagille's syndrome of biliary atresia. A 5-year-old boy showing triangular facies, deep set eyes and a flattened nose. This patient had poor vision. At 19 years he is well with normal intelligence but dwarfed.

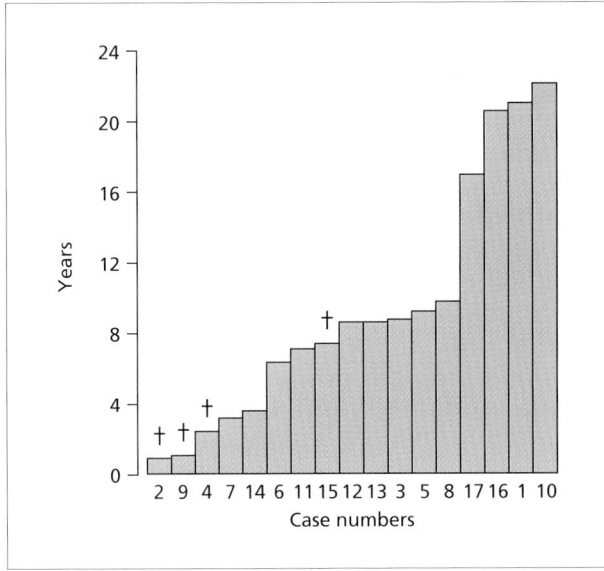

Fig. 24.7. Histogram showing the ages to date of 17 children with chronic intra-hepatic cholestasis. † = patient died [47].

follow-up of 80 patients, showed 21 had died, liver failure being responsible in only four [2]. The patient can have normal children.

Associated cardiovascular abnormalities make hepatic transplantation hazardous [129].

SYMPTOMATIC TREATMENT OF CHOLESTATIC SYNDROMES [1]

Calcium and vitamin D are not absorbed and biliary rickets results. Vitamin A deficiency is frequent. Hepatic storage is normal and faulty absorption is the cause [94]. Vitamin A (50 000 units), vitamin D (50 000 units) and vitamin K_1 (5 mg) must be given by intramuscular injection every 4 weeks. The child is encouraged to drink skimmed milk.

Vitamin E deficiency is particularly important in cholestatic infants (Chapter 13). It results in a degenerative neuromuscular syndrome with areflexia. Vitamin E 10 mg/kg should be given intramuscularly every 2 weeks. Oral D-α-tocopheryl polyethylene glycol-1000 succinate 15–25 iu/kg/day may also be useful [119]. Once a neurological condition has developed, it is arrested, but not reversed, by intramuscular vitamin E [118].

Medium chain triglyceride (coconut oil) is added to puréed fruit and vegetables and used in cooking.

The tendency to bone thinning absolutely contraindicates the use of corticosteroids, which also stunt growth. In any case they are not of permanent value.

In partial cholestasis, cholestyramine is given flavoured with apple purée, tomato juice or chocolate syrup. It is valuable in controlling pruritus and in reducing skin xanthomas. Serum lipids, bile salts and bilirubin are reduced.

Ursodeoxycholic acid (10 mg/kg body weight) is given in two doses after the mid-day and evening meals. It reduces serum enzyme levels and may relieve pruritus.

PROLONGED PARENTERAL NUTRITION

The cholestasis affects premature low birth-weight or severely compromised babies. Diagnosis is made by exclusion as the infants usually have other causes of cholestasis. Diseases with impaired intestinal passage and the presence of infections predispose to hyperbilirubinaemia [65].

After 1–2 weeks, serum conjugated bilirubin rises steadily, increasing with duration of therapy.

Liver biopsy shows non-specific changes with features of extra-hepatic biliary obstruction. Biliary sludge and gallstones develop.

Cholestasis continues for as long as the parenteral nutrition. It usually resolves within weeks or months of stopping. In some patients, enteral feeding will not halt the liver disease once jaundice develops [88]. If therapy cannot be stopped, biliary cirrhosis develops and this may be fatal. The use of amino-acid free parenteral nutrition with enteral whey amino acids may prevent the cholestasis [14].

The cholestasis is related to loss of the entero-hepatic circulation of bile acids and consequent reduced bile formation, biliary stasis and sludging.

ABNORMAL BILE ACID BILE SYNTHESIS

Primary bile acids are the driving force for bile acid-dependent secretion of bile. Defects can cause diminished bile flow and abnormal transport processes and so cholestasis [114]. Errors of bile acid metabolism may account for as many as 2–5% of the idiopathic cholestatic liver diseases in children [124].

3β-hydroxy-C27-steroid dehydrogenase-isomerase deficiency results in cholestasis without pruritus and with normal serum gamma GT and bile acids [53]. Cholestasis has also resulted from *δ4-3-oxosteroid-5β-reductase deficiency* [28].

Abnormal synthesis of labile *sulphated cholenoic acids* has been associated with cholestasis and giant cell hepatitis in a 3-month-old boy [24]. Inheritance was autosomal recessive.

Coprostanicacidaemia results from a defect in the conversion of coprostanic to varinic acid. It is associated with progressive cholestasis and death by 2 years.

Zellweger's cerebro-hepato-renal syndrome is a fatal autosomal recessive condition with severe cholestasis. It is probably related to defective peroxisomal β-oxidation.

Treatment

Replacement of exogenous bile acids results in the generation of bile acid-dependent flow and a decrease in the synthesis of toxic bile salts. Remarkable benefit has followed the administration of chenodeoxycholic acid, ursodeoxycholic acid and cholic acid [24, 52, 124]. Pruritus is reduced and transaminases and serum bilirubin levels fall.

BYLER'S DISEASE (PROGRESSIVE FAMILIAL INTRA-HEPATIC CHOLESTASIS)

See Chapter 13 [133].

IDIOPATHIC HYPOPITUITARISM

This is associated with severe hypoglycaemia, hepatomegaly and persistent direct hyperbilirubinaemia during the neonatal period [59].

NEONATAL LUPUS ERYTHEMATOSUS SYNDROME

This presents as neonatal cholestasis and hepatitis [106]. Cutaneous lupus erythematosus and congenital heart block are associated.

SPONTANEOUS PERFORATION OF THE BILE DUCTS

This occurs between birth and 3 months, usually in the anterior wall of the common bile duct close to the junction with the cystic duct. The child develops non-bile-stained vomiting and acholic stools. Jaundice is mild, intermittent and variable. Abdominal hernias develop and the scrotum becomes green. Cholangiography shows the blocked cystic duct with the hepatic duct leak. The results of surgery are good.

GALLBLADDER DISEASE AND GALLSTONES [102]

Total parenteral nutrition is frequently accompanied by biliary sludge in the gallbladder and cholestasis. Phytosterolaemia may predispose to biliary sludge and liver damage if bile salts are deficient [23]. Bile duct perforation is associated with gallstones secondary to bile stasis.

Pigment gallstones may be found in the lower common bile duct without obvious cause. Acute gastroenteritis with bacterial overgrowth, dehydration or a minor atypical termination of the common bile duct may contribute.

A similar picture may complicate neonatal jaundice due to such conditions as hepatic prematurity or haemolytic disease. This has been termed the *inspissated bile syndrome*.

Surgical or endoscopic washing of the bile ducts is curative without the need for cholecystectomy.

In older children, cholecystitis and gallstones may be associated with blood dyscrasias or congenital anomalies of the biliary tract, such as choledochal cysts or biliary atresia. Immunoglobulin A deficiency has been linked with biliary sludge and gallstones in children [27].

Older children with gallstones often have a strong family history.

Sclerosing cholangitis may present in early infancy as intra-hepatic cholestasis progressing to end-stage biliary cirrhosis in childhood [29]. There may be an autosomal recessive inheritance. Associations include ulcerative colitis, autoimmune hepatitis, histiocytosis X and immune deficiencies [117]. The prognosis is poor (see Chapter 15).

Reye's syndrome

In 1963 Reye and associates described this syndrome of acute encephalopathy and fatty change in the viscera [104].

Aetiology and epidemiology

The syndrome has followed almost any known viral disease and can be encountered in epidemic form, often in winter or spring. There are two phases, an infective followed by an encephalopathic. Influenza B or A or varicella are the commonest antecedent infections.

The role of salicylates is controversial. A large survey related the risk of Reye's syndrome to the dose consumed [99] and numbers have certainly fallen since salicylates have been avoided for respiratory infections in children. However, in Australia, the incidence has fallen unrelated to salicylate ingestion [95].

Other possible exogenous factors include aflatoxin, multiple hornet stings [132] and insecticides.

There are geographic differences in Reye's syndrome. In the USA, the incidence is in late childhood and early adolescence, whereas in Australia and the UK two-thirds are less than 3 years old [95]. The disease is milder in the USA than in the UK and Australia.

Clinical features

Sexes are equally affected, usually below 14 years old; young adults have been described [82]. Three to 7 days after a viral-type illness the child develops intractable vomiting and progressive neurological deterioration. The encephalopathy is marked by erratic behaviour, irritability and listlessness progressing through lethargy to stupor and coma. Jaundice is rare.

Milder (grade 1) Reye's syndrome presents simply as vomiting with abnormal liver function tests after an upper respiratory infection or varicella [73].

In severe cases, medullary coning and brain death result 4–60 hours after the onset.

Liver biopsy

This shows microvesicular fat. Electron microscopy shows swelling and distortion of the mitochondria to be followed by showers of peroxisomes.

Succinate dehydrogenase activity is low or absent.

Other organs

The kidneys show proximal tubular fat. The myocardium is fatty and there is marked cerebral oedema. Electron microscopy of the neurones shows similar mitochondrial changes to those seen in the liver.

Laboratory findings

There is an acute mitochondrial insult with decreased activity of mitochondrial enzymes in the liver. A rise in blood ammonia with low citrulline values can be related to reduction in Krebs' cycle enzymes. The serum amino-acid profile shows a high glutamine, alanine and leucine. Hypoglycaemia is found in about 50%—usually in those seriously ill and less than 2 years old; it may reflect inhibition of the citric acid cycle. Mitochondrial injury also depresses fatty acid oxidation and plasma free fatty acids are increased. Serum transaminases are raised. A prothrombin time more than 3 seconds prolonged, together with a serum ammonium value greater than $100\,\mu g/dl$, predict a serious course [49]. Coagulopathy is constant.

Reye's syndrome is one of the mitochondrial cytopathies (see Chapter 25). Some paediatricians doubt the existence of Reye's syndrome and consider that all cases could be due to some underlying metabolic defect.

Treatment

The patient presents as a problem in liver disease, but the cerebral oedema is lethal. Treatment is directed towards this, combined with intense supportive care. There is no specific treatment.

Reye-like syndromes

A number of metabolic defects produce a picture clinically, biochemically and histologically resembling Reye's syndrome [39].

In younger children it is particularly important to exclude urea cycle defects, disturbances in the mitochondrial β-oxidation pathway of fatty acids and particularly deficiencies of medium- and long-chain acyl-co-A-dehydrogenase [41, 128]. Exclusion of these metabolic defects demands special diagnostic facilities. Specimens of urine and serum should be obtained and frozen so that they may be subsequently analysed in specialist centres. Electron microscopy of a liver biopsy may also be useful, as, in contrast to Reye's syndrome, mitochondrial morphology in the metabolic cases is normal.

Cirrhosis in infancy and childhood

The cirrhosis of infants and children has many aetiologies. Many are cryptogenic.

A number, presenting in later childhood and at puberty, show the picture of *chronic autoimmune hepatitis*. These patients usually respond to prednisolone treatment (Chapter 17).

Neonatal 'giant cell' hepatitis may be followed by cirrhosis and this may also apply to some of the neonatal virus infections such as hepatitis B or C.

Neonatal haemochromatosis is probably of autosomal recessive inheritance. It may be associated with abnormal bile acids and with mitochondrial oxidative phosphorylation deficiency [112]. It may present as fulminant liver failure in the newborn [84].

Iron overload is usually related to transfusion in anaemic children, often thalassaemic. However, hereditary haemochromatosis can affect children as early as 2 years [33]. Females and males are equally affected. Cardiac involvement is often fatal. Hypogonadism is frequent.

Wilson's disease, galactosaemia, Fanconi's disease, type IV glycogen disease and *fibro-cystic disease* may be followed by cirrhosis.

In the tropics the kwashiorkor syndrome is not followed by cirrhosis whereas *veno-occlusive disease* is followed by zone 3 fibrosis and finally a cirrhosis.

Congenital hepatic fibrosis may cause portal hypertension but the hepatic lesion is not a cirrhosis.

Cholestatic syndromes are followed by biliary cirrhosis and this is also true of *α-antitrypsin deficiency.*

Cardiac cirrhosis is unusual in childhood except complicating constrictive pericarditis.

Clinical features

Portal hypertension is usually prominent. The spleen tends to be larger than in the adult. Presentation with splenomegaly and hepatomegaly at a school medical examination or while in hospital for another condition is not unusual. Vascular spiders are conspicuous. Growth is uninterrupted; indeed the adolescent growth spurt may be particularly great so that the child is above normal height (fig. 24.8).

At puberty, both sexes may show acne and facial mooning with cutaneous striae; girls have amenorrhoea and boys gynaecomastia.

This relatively inactive stage can continue for years. Decompensation is followed by deepening jaundice and very high serum globulin and transaminase values. When pre-coma appears it is accompanied by mania, screaming, fits and psychic outbursts. Ascites is usual at this late stage. Sclerotherapy of oesophageal varices is well tolerated.

The prognosis is very variable depending on the aetiology. The outlook is bettter than for an adult with an equivalent degree of clinical decompensation.

Indian childhood cirrhosis

This condition is seen in rural, middle-class Hindu families throughout India. Both sexes are affected between the ages of 1 and 3 years. The familial incidence suggests genetic factors are involved although it may indicate a common environmental origin. Death is usually due to liver failure and occurs within 1 year of diagnosis.

Hepatic histology shows profound injury to liver cells which may contain Mallory's hyaline and are sur-

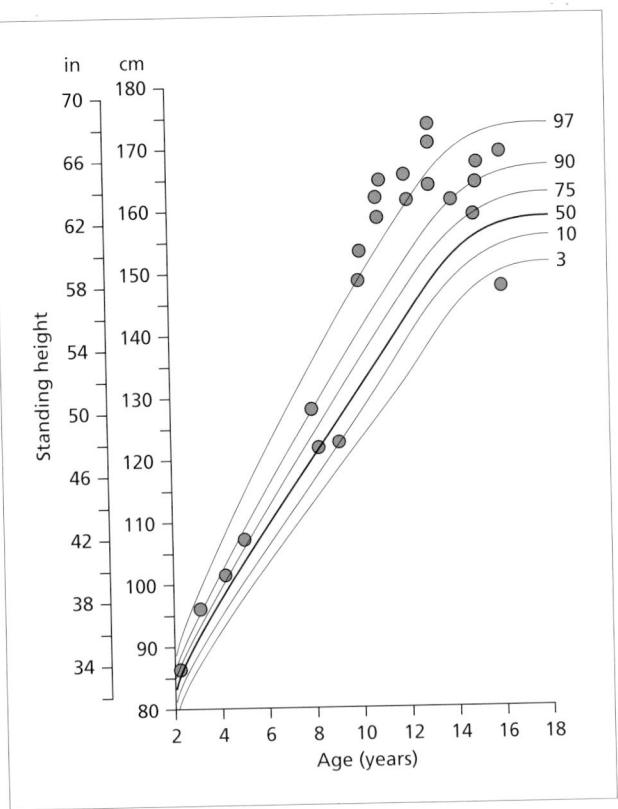

Fig. 24.8. Cirrhosis in female children. Note that children between 10 and 13 years are taller than 90% of the population.

rounded by polymorphs. A micronodular cirrhosis results. The picture resembles acute alcoholic hepatitis but without the fatty change.

Hepatic copper is markedly increased, and this is largely located in the cytoplasm. The livers of unaffected siblings do not show excess copper.

Ingestion of animal milk contaminated by brass and copper household utensils provides the excess copper [11]. Prevention is by changing the feeding of the child.

Alkaloids may play a part [87].

Wilson's disease is excluded by absence of Kayser–Fleischer rings and normal serum caeruloplasmin values.

D-penicillamine prolongs life and results in marked reduction in histological liver activity [100, 126].

Non-Indian childhood cirrhosis (copper-associated liver disease) [5]

A childhood disorder indistinguishable from Indian childhood cirrhosis has been reported from other countries [71, 89, 111] and termed copper-associated liver disease [5]. It seems not to be related to increased copper ingestion in drinking water. A genetic defect seems likely [111]. Excess copper and zinc have been reported in Canadian native children with cirrhosis [98].

Fetal alcohol syndrome

Hepatomegaly and raised transaminase values may be found. The liver may show fatty changes with portal and perisinusoidal fibrosis resembling those seen in the adult with alcoholic liver disease [72].

Idiopathic steato-hepatitis

This affects obese, peripubertal children and is diagnosed by liver biopsy [6].

Hamartomas

These benign, congenital lesions present as an abdominal mass in the first 2 years of life. They may be an incidental finding at autopsy and must be distinguished from malignant tumours. They consist of abnormal arrangements of all the cells of the normal liver, particularly bile ducts and fibroblasts. They contain central veins and are nearly always cystic. They require no treatment.

Nodular regenerative hyperplasia

The children present with hepatomegaly or splenomegaly with or without portal hypertension. Associations include neoplasms or consumption of drugs such as anti-convulsants [85].

Tumours of the liver

See also Chapter 28. Primary tumours in infants and children are rare; two-thirds are diagnosed before the second year of life. They may arise from liver cells and/or from supporting structures. Secondary tumours are extremely rare and are usually associated with a neuroblastoma of the adrenals.

Diagnosis

Biochemical tests may be normal. The most usual abnormality is an increase in serum gammaglutamyl transpeptidase and α_2-globulin levels. Serum α-fetoprotein may be increased. The site and extent of the tumour must be defined by ultrasound, CT and, if necessary, angiography.

Guided liver biopsy is usually a safe method of confirming the diagnosis.

Mesenchymal hamartoma

This is a rare developmental anomaly, largely of bile ducts, seen in children less than 2 years old. It is treated conservatively, or if necessary by surgical excision [30].

Malignant mesenchymoma (undifferentiated sarcoma)

This is seen in older children (6–12 years). Histology is that of sarcoma with PAS-positive intra-cytoplasmic pink globules. The tumour should be resected surgically with subsequent chemotherapy [18]. Long-term survivors are reported [122].

Adenomas

These rare tumours do not become malignant, and over the years may even regress. They consist of sheets of liver cells and have a fibrous capsule. They should be treated conservatively.

Hepato-cellular carcinoma

These usually present after 5 years old. Males are more frequently affected than females. The tumours are often single, large and metastasize late. Cirrhosis may be absent.

Hepatitis B and C are the usual causes especially in the Far East [19, 134]. Hepato cellular carcinoma may also complicate giant cell hepatitis, biliary atresia and the polycystic diseases (including congenital hepatic fibrosis), tyrosinosis and glycogen storage diseases.

The patients present with weight loss, abdominal swelling usually in the right upper quadrant, pain, ascites and jaundice. Calcification in the tumour may be noted.

Treatment

The only hope is surgical resection and this is rarely possible. However, following lobectomy, growth and development are normal. Chemotherapy may be useful in reducing tumour size before resection.

The fibrolamellar form has a much better prognosis and resection is more often possible.

Hepatoblastoma [67]

This rare tumour with epithelial and mesenchymal elements usually presents before 3 years of age and is usually fatal within 5 years.

It has been reported in association with hemihypertrophy, Wilms' tumour, fetal alcohol syndrome and with polyposis coli in the mother [63]. It may produce human chorionic gonadotrophins resulting in precocious puberty.

Hypercholesterolaemia can be associated.

Chemotherapy may prolong life so that resection may be possible. Hepatic transplantation has led to falls of human chorionic gonadotrophins [48].

The prognosis depends on the degree of differentiation [42].

Infantile haemangio-endothelioma

This, usually benign, vascular tumour of infancy consists of endothelium-lined channels of capillary size [117]. It may be associated with skin haemangiomas. It presents before 6 months of age as an abdominal mass. Cardiac failure may be related to arteriovenous shunts within the tumour. A systolic bruit may be heard in the epigastrium. Rupture can cause haemoperitoneum. Associated congenital defects are frequent.

Severe anaemia and thrombocytopenia have been attributed to microangiopathic haemolysis related to the abnormal, tortuous, narrow vessels within the tumour.

CT shows typical features of haemangioma. Ultrasound is used to monitor progress [120].

Treatment is symptomatic with hepatic arterial embolization for refractory heart failure or rupture [9]. The prognosis is good.

Treatment

The only procedure offering hope of cure in the primary carcinoma group is resection. This will cure the benign lesions. Cure may even follow in the malignant group for the tumour is usually single, often large and metastasizes late. In any case palliation is usual. Subsequent growth and development are normal after hepatic lobectomy.

The prognosis is very poor if resection is impossible.

Hepatic transplantation

This is particularly important in children with liver disease and is considered in Chapter 35.

References

1 Alagille D. Management of paucity of interlobular bile ducts. *J. Hepatol.* 1985; **1**: 561.
2 Alagille D, Estrada A, Hadchouel M *et al.* Syndromic paucity of interlobular bile ducts (Alagille syndrome or arteriohepatic dysplasia): review of 80 cases. *J. Pediatr.* 1987; **110**: 195.
3 Alagille D, Odièvre M, Gautier M *et al.* Hepatic ductular hypoplasia associated with characteristic facies, vertebral malformations, retarded physical, mental and sexual development and cardiac murmur. *J. Pediatr.* 1975; **86**: 63.
4 Alpert LI, Strauss L, Hirschhorn K. Neonatal hepatitis and biliary atresia associated with trisomy 17–18 syndrome. *N. Engl. J. Med.* 1969; **270**: 16.
5 Baker A, Gormally S, Saxena R *et al.* Copper-associated liver disease in childhood. *J. Hepatol.* 1995; **23**: 538.
6 Baldridge AD, Perez-Atayde AR, Graeme-Cook F *et al.* Idiopathic steatohepatitis in childhood: a multicenter retrospective study. *J. Pediat.* 1995; **127**: 700.
7 Balistreri WF. Neonatal cholestasis — medical progress. *J. Pediatr.* 1985; **106**: 171.
8 Barbera C, Bortolotti F, Crivellaro C *et al.* Recombinant interferon-α$_{2a}$ hastens the rate of HBeAg clearance in children with chronic hepatitis B. *Hepatology* 1994; **20**: 287.
9 Becker JM, Heitler MS. Hepatic hemangioendotheliomas in infancy. *Surg. Gynecol. Obstet.* 1989; **168**: 189.
10 Benaron DA, Bowen FW. Variation of initial serum bilirubin rise in new born infants with type of illness. *Lancet* 1991; **338**: 78.
11 Bhave SA, Pandit AN, Tanner MS. Comparison of feeding history of children with Indian childhood cirrhosis and paired controls. *J. Pediatr. Gastroenterol. Nutr.* 1987; **6**: 562.
12 Bortolotti F. Chronic hepatitis B acquired in childhood: unanswered questions and evolving issues. *J. Hepatol.* 1994; **21**: 904.
13 Brodsky MC, Cunniff C. Ocular anomalies in the Alagille syndrome (arteriohepatic dysplasia). *Ophthalmology* 1993; **100**: 1767.
14 Brown MR, Thunberg BJ, Golub L *et al.* Decreased cholestasis with enteral instead of intravenous protein in very low-birth-weight infant. *J. Pediatr. Gastroenterol. Nutr.* 1989; **9**: 21.
15 Brown CW, Werlin SL, Geenen JE *et al.* The diagnostic and therapeutic role of endoscopic retrograde cholangiopancreatography in children. *J. Pediatr. Gastroenterol. Nutr.* 1993; **17**: 19.
16 Bruguera M, Amat L, Garcia O *et al.* Treatment of chronic hepatitis B in children with recombinant alfa interferon. Different response according to age at infection. *J. Clin. Gastroenterol.* 1993; **17**: 296.
17 Bruguera M, Llach J, Rodés J. Nonsyndromic paucity of intrahepatic bile ducts in infancy and idiopathic ductopenia in adulthood: the same syndrome? *Hepatology* 1992; **15**: 830.
18 Case Records of the Massachussetts General Hospital. *N. Engl. J. Med.* 1990; **322**: 1378.
19 Chang M-H, Chen D-S, Hsu H-C *et al.* Maternal transmission of hepatitis B virus in childhood hepatocellular carcinoma. *Cancer* 1989; **64**: 2377.
20 Chang M-H, Huang HH, Huang ES *et al.* Polymerase chain reaction to detect human cytomegalovirus in livers of infants with neonatal hepatitis. *Gastroenterology* 1992; **103**: 1022.
21 Chang M-H, Hwang L-Y, Hsu H-C *et al.* Prospective study of asymptomatic HBsAg carrier children infected in the perinatal period: clinical and liver histologic studies. *Hepatology* 1988; **8**: 374.
22 Chianale J, Dvorak C, Farmer DL *et al.* Cytochrome P-450 gene expression in the functional units of the fetal liver. *Hepatology* 1988; **8**: 318.
23 Clayton PT, Bowron A, Mills KA *et al.* Phytosterolemia in children with parenteral nutrition-associated cholestatic liver disease. *Gastroenterology* 1993; **105**: 1806.
24 Clayton PT, Mills KA, Johnson AW *et al.* 4-3-oxosteroid 5β-reductase deficiency: failure of ursodeoxycholic acid treatment and response to chenodeoxycholic acid plus cholic acid. *Gut* 1996; **38**: 623.
25 Cox KL, Stadalnik RC, McGahan JP *et al.* Hepatobiliary scintigraphy with technetium-99m disoferin in the evaluation of neonatal cholestasis. *J. Pediatr. Gastroenterol. Nutr.* 1987; **6**: 885.

26 Daffos F, Forestier F, Capella-Pavlovsky M *et al.* Prenatal management of 746 pregnancies at risk for congenital toxoplasmosis. *N. Engl. J. Med.* 1988; **318**: 271.

27 Danon YL, Dinari G, Garty B-Z *et al.* Cholelithiasis in children with immunoglobulin A deficiency: a new gastroenterologic syndrome. *J. Pediatr. Gastroenterol. Nutr.* 1983; **2**: 663.

28 Daugherty CC, Setchell KDR, Heubi JE *et al.* Resolution of liver biopsy alterations in three siblings with bile acid treatment of an inborn error of bile acid metabolism (Δ4-3-oxosteroid 5β-reductase deficiency). *Hepatology* 1993; **18**: 1096.

29 Debray D, Pariente D, Gauthier F *et al.* Cholelithiasis in infancy: a study of 40 cases. *J. Pediatr.* 1993; **122**: 385.

30 DeMaioribus CA, Lally KP, Sim K *et al.* Mesenchymal hamartoma of the liver. A 35-year review. *Arch. Surg.* 1990; **125**: 598.

31 Dick MC, Mowat AP. Hepatitis syndrome in infancy — an epidemiological survey with 10 year follow up. *Arch. Dis. Child.* 1985; **60**: 512.

32 Ennever J, Costarino AT, Polin RA *et al.* Rapid clearance of a structural isomer of bilirubin during phototherapy. *J. Clin. Invest.* 1987; **79**: 1674.

33 Escobar GJ, Heyman MB, Smith WB *et al.* Primary hemochromatosis in childhood. *Pediatrics* 1987; **80**: 549.

34 Faa G, Liguori C, Columbano A *et al.* Uneven copper distribution in the human newborn liver. *Hepatology* 1987; **7**: 838.

35 Felsher BF, Carpio NM, Woolley MM *et al.* Hepatic bilirubin glucuronidation in neonates with unconjugated hyperbilirubinaemia and congenital gastrointestinal obstruction. *J. Lab. Clin. Med.* 1974; **83**: 90.

36 Finegold MJ, Carpenter RJ. Obliterative cholangitis due to cytomegalovirus: a possible precursor of paucity of intrahepatic bile ducts. *Hum. Pathol.* 1982; **13**: 662.

37 Fung KP, Lau SP. Gamma-glutamyl transpeptidase activity and its serial measurement in differentiation between extra-hepatic biliary atresia and neonatal hepatitis. *J. Pediatr. Gastroenterol. Nutr.* 1985; **4**: 208.

38 Gartner LM, Catz CS, Yaffe SJ. Neonatal bilirubin workshop. *Pediatrics* 1994; **94**: 537.

39 Glasgow JFT, Moore R. Reye's syndrome 30 years on. Possible marker of inherited metabolic disorders. *Br. Med. J.* 1993; **367**: 950.

40 Gourley GR, Arend RA. β glucuronidase and hyperbilirubinaemia in breast-fed and formula-fed babies. *Lancet* 1986; **i**: 644.

41 Greene CL, Blitzer MG, Shapira E. Inborn errors of metabolism and Reye's syndrome: differential diagnosis. *J. Pediatr.* 1988; **113**: 156.

42 Haas JE, Muczynski KR, Krailo M *et al.* Histopathology and prognosis in childhood hepatoblastoma and hepatocarcinoma. *Cancer* 1989; **64**: 1082.

43 Hadchouel M, Hugon RN, Gautier M. Reduced ratio of portal tracts to paucity of intrahepatic bile ducts. *Arch. Pathol. Lab. Med.* 1978; **102**: 402.

44 Hadchouel M, Zhang FR, Aurias A *et al.* Deletion of the short arm of chromosome 20 in arterio-hepatic dysplasia (Alagille syndrome). *Hepatology* 1989; **10**: 603 (abstract).

45 Hansen TWR. Bilirubin in the brain. Distribution and effects on neurophysiological and neurochemical processes. *Clin. Pediatr.* 1994; **33**: 452.

46 Hart MH, Kaufman SS, Vanderhoof JA *et al.* Neonatal hepatitis and extra-hepatic biliary atresia associated with cytomegalovirus infection in twins. *Am. J. Dis. Child.* 1991; **145**: 302.

47 Heathcote J, Deodhar KP, Scheuer PJ *et al.* Intrahepatic cholestasis in childhood. *N. Engl. J. Med.* 1976; **295**: 801.

48 Heimann A, White PF, Riely CA *et al.* Hepatoblastoma presenting as sexual precocity. *J. Clin. Gastroenterol.* 1987; **9**: 105.

49 Heubi JE, Daughterty CC, Partin JS *et al.* Grade 1 Reye's syndrome — outcome and predictors of progression to deeper coma grades. *N. Engl. J. Med.* 1984; **311**: 1539.

50 Ho C-W, Shioda K, Shirosaki K *et al.* The pathogenesis of biliary atresia: a morphological study of the hepatobiliary system and the hepatic artery. *J. Pediatr. Gastroenterol. Nutr.* 1993; **16**: 53.

51 Hsu H-Y, Chang M-H, Lee C-Y *et al.* Precore mutant of hepatitis B virus in childhood fulminant hepatitis B: an infrequent association. *J. Infect. Dis.* 1995; **171**: 776.

52 Ichimiya H, Nazer H, Gunasekaran T *et al.* Treatment of chronic liver disease caused by 3 beta-hydroxy-5-C27-steroid dehydrogenase deficiency with chenodeoxycholic acid. *Arch. Dis. Child.* 1990; **65**: 1121.

53 Jacquemin E, Setchell KDR, O'Connell NC *et al.* A new cause of progressive intrahepatic cholestasis: 3β-hydroxy-C_{27}-steroid dehydrogenase/isomerase deficiency. *J. Pediatr.* 1994; **125**: 379.

54 Jonas MM, Roldan EO, Lyons HJ *et al.* Histopathologic features of the liver in pediatric acquired immune deficiency syndrome. *J. Pediatr. Gastroenterol. Nutr.* 1989; **9**: 73.

55 Jonas MM, Zilleruelo GE, LaRue SJ *et al.* Hepatitis C infection in a pediatric dialysis population. *Pediatrics* 1992; **89**: 707.

56 Kahn E, Daum F, Markowitz J *et al.* Nonsyndromatic paucity of interlobular bile ducts: light and electron microscopic evaluation of sequential liver biopsies in early childhood. *Hepatology* 1986; **6**: 890.

57 Kappas A, Drummond GS, Mannola T *et al.* Sn-protoporphyrin use in the management of hyperbilirubinemia in term newborns with direct Coombs-positive ABO incompatibility. *Pediatrics* 1988; **81**: 485.

58 Kasai M, Mochizuki I, Ohkohchi N *et al.* Surgical limitation for biliary atresia: indication for liver transplantation. *J. Pediatr. Surg.* 1989; **24**: 851.

59 Kaufman FR, Costin G, Thomas DW *et al.* Neonatal cholestasis and hypopituitarism. *Arch. Dis. Child.* 1984; **59**: 787.

60 Kaufman SS, Wood RP, Shaw B Jr *et al.* Hepato-carcinoma in a child with the Alagille syndrome. *Am. J. Dis. Child.* 1987; **141**: 698.

61 Keeffe EB, Pinson CW, Ragsdale J *et al.* Hepatocellular carcinoma in arteriohepatic dysplasia. *Am. J. Gastroenterol.* 1993; **88**: 1446.

62 Kimura A, Yamakawa R, Ushijima K *et al.* Fetal bile acid metabolism during infancy: analysis of 1β-hydroxylated bile acids in urine, meconium and feces. *Hepatology* 1994; **20**: 819.

63 Kingston JE, Herbert A, Draper GJ *et al.* Association between hepatoblastoma and polyposis coli. *Arch. Dis. Child.* 1983; **38**: 959.

64 Klein BS, Michaels JA, Rytel MW *et al.* Nosocomial hepatitis A: a multinursery outbreak in Winsconsin. *JAMA* 1984; **252**: 2716.

65 Kubota A, Okada A, Nezu R *et al.* Hyperbilirubinemia in neonates associated with total parenteral nutrition. *J. Par-*

enter. Enteral. Nutr. 1988; **12**: 602.

66 Lachaux A, Descos B, Plchau H *et al.* Familial extrahepatic biliary atresia. *J. Pediatr. Gastroenterol. Nutr.* 1988; **7**: 280.

67 Lack EE, Neave C, Vawter GF. Hepatoblastoma: a clinical and pathologic study of 54 cases. *Am. J. Surg. Pathol.* 1982; **6**: 693.

68 Landing BH. Considerations of the pathogenesis of neonatal hepatitis, biliary atresia and choledochal cyst — the concept of infantile obstructive cholangiopathy. *Prog. Paediatr. Surg.* 1974; **6**: 113.

69 Langnas AN, Markin RS, Cattral MS *et al.* Parvovirus B19 as a possible causative agent of fulminant liver failure and associated aplastic anemia. *Hepatology* 1995; **22**: 1661.

70 Lee P-I, Chang M-H, Chen D-S *et al.* Prognostic implications of serum alpha-fetoprotein levels in neonatal hepatitis. *J. Pediatr. Gastroenterol. Nutr.* 1990; **11**: 27.

71 Lefkowitch JH, Honig CL, King ME *et al.* Hepatic copper overload and features of Indian childhood cirrhosis in an American sibship. *N. Engl. J. Med.* 1982; **307**: 271.

72 Lefkowitch JH, Rushton AR, Feng-Chen K-C. Hepatic fibrosis in fetal alcohol syndrome. Pathologic similarities to adult alcoholic liver disease. *Gastroenterology* 1983; **85**: 951.

73 Lichtenstein PK, Heubi JE, Daughterty CC *et al.* Grade I Reye's syndrome: a frequent cause of vomiting and liver dysfunction after varicella and upper-respiratory-tract infection. *N. Engl. J. Med.* 1983; **309**: 133.

74 Lin H-H, Kao J-H, Hsu H-Y *et al.* Absence of infection in breast-fed infants born to hepatitis C virus-infected mothers. *J. Pediatr.* 1995; **126**: 589.

75 Lok ASF, Lai C-L. A longitudinal follow-up of asymptomatic hepatitis B surface antigen-positive Chinese children. *Hepatology* 1988; **8**: 1130.

76 Long WA, Ulshen MH, Lawson EE. Clinical manifestations of congenital syphilitic hepatitis: implications for pathogenesis. *J. Pediatr. Gastroenterol. Nutr.* 1984; **3**: 551.

77 Lucey JF, Arias IM, McKay RJ Jr. Transient familial neonatal hyperbilirubinemia. *Am. J. Dis. Child.* 1960; **100**: 787.

78 Maggiore G, Bernard O, Hadchouel M *et al.* Diagnostic value of serum γ-glutamyl transpeptidase activity in liver disases in children. *J. Pediatr. Gastroenterol. Nutr.* 1991; **12**: 21.

79 Manzini P, Saracco G, Cerchier A *et al.* Human immunodeficiency virus infection as risk factor for mother-to-child hepatitis C virus transmission; persistance of anti-hepatitis virus in children is associated with the mother's anti-hepatitis C virus immunoblotting pattern. *Hepatology* 1995; **21**: 328.

80 Marret S, Buffet-Janvresse C, Metayer J *et al.* Herpes simplex hepatitis with chronic cholestasis in a newborn. *Acta Paediatr.* 1993; **82**: 321.

81 Metzman R, Anand A, DeGiulio PA *et al.* Hepatic disease associated with intrauterine parvovirus B19 infection in a newborn premature infant. *J. Pediatr. Gastroenterol. Nutr.* 1989; **9**: 112.

82 Meythaler JM, Varma RR. Reye's syndrome in adults. Diagnostic considerations. *Arch. Intern. Med.* 1987; **147**: 61.

83 Mieli-Vergani G, Howard ER, Portman B *et al.* Late referral for biliary atresia — missed opportunities for effective surgery. *Lancet* 1989; **i**: 421.

84 Moerman P, Pauwels P, Vandenberghe K *et al.* Neonatal haemochromatosis. *Histopathology* 1990; **17**: 345.

85 Moran CA, Mullick FG, Ishak KG. Nodular regenerative hyperplasia of the liver in children. *Am. J. Surg. Pathol.* 1991; **15**: 449.

86 Morecki R, Glaser JH, Cho S *et al.* Biliary atresia and reovirus type 3 infection. *N. Engl. J. Med.* 1982; **307**: 481.

87 Morris P, O'Neill D, Tanner S. Synergistic liver toxicity of copper and retrorsine in the rat. *J. Hepatol.* 1994; **21**: 735.

88 Moss RL, Das JB, Raffensperger JG. Total parenteral nutrition-associated cholestasis: clinical and histopathologic correlation. *J. Pediatr. Surg.* 1993; **28**: 1270.

89 Muller T, Feichtinger H, Berger H *et al.* Endemic Tyrolean infantile cirrhosis: an ecogenetic disorder. *Lancet* 1996; **347**: 877.

90 Naveh Y, Berant M. Assessment of liver size in normal infants and children. *J. Pediatr. Gastroenterol. Nutr.* 1984; **3**: 346.

91 Noble RC, Kane MA, Reeves SA *et al.* Post transfusion hepatitis A in a neonatal intensive care unit. *JAMA* 1984; **252**: 2711.

92 Ohkohchi N, Chiba T, Ohi R *et al.* Long-term follow-up study of patients with cholangitis after successful Kasai operation in biliary atresia: selection of recipients for liver transplantation. *J. Pediatr. Gastroenterol. Nutr.* 1989; **9**: 416.

93 Ohto H, Terazawa S, Sasaki N *et al.* Transmission of hepatitis C virus from mothers to infants. *N. Engl. J. Med.* 1994; **330**: 744.

94 Ong DE, Amédée-Manesme O. Liver levels of vitamin A and cellular retinol-binding protein for patients with biliary atresia. *Hepatology* 1987; **7**: 253.

95 Orlowski JP, Gillis J, Kilham HA. A catch in the Reye. *Pediatrics* 1987; **80**: 638.

96 Osborn LM, Reiff MI, Bolus R. Jaundice in the full-term neonate. *Pediatrics* 1984; **73**: 520.

97 Perlman M, Frank JW. Bilirubin beyond the blood–brain barrier. *Pediatrics* 1988; **81**: 304.

98 Phillips MJ, Ackerley CA, Superina RA *et al.* Excess zinc associated with severe progressive cholestasis in Cree and Ojibwa-Cree children. *Lancet* 1996; **347**: 866.

99 Pinsky F, Hurwitz ES, Schonberger LB *et al.* Reye's syndrome and aspirin. *JAMA* 1988; **260**: 657.

100 Pradhan AM, Bhave SA, Joshi VV *et al.* Reversal of Indian childhood cirrhosis by D-penicillamine therapy. *J. Pediatr. Gastroenterol. Nutr.* 1995; **20**: 28.

101 Rabinovitz M, Imperial JC, Schade RR *et al.* Hepatocellular carcinoma in Alagille's syndrome: a family study. *J. Pediatr. Gastroenterol. Nutr.* 1989; **8**: 26.

102 Reif S, Sloven DG, Lebenthal E *et al.* Gallstones in children. Characterization by age, etiology, and outcome. *Am. J. Dis. Child.* 1991; **145**: 105.

103 Resti M, Azzari C, Lega L *et al.* Mother-to-infant transmission of hepatitis C virus. *Acta. Paediatr.* 1995; **84**: 251.

104 Reye RDK, Morgan G, Baral J. Encephalopathy and fatty degeneration of the viscera. A disease entity in childhood. *Lancet* 1963; **ii**: 749.

105 Rosenthal P, Henton D, Felber S *et al.* Distribution of serum bilirubin conjugates in pediatric hepatobiliary diseases. *J. Pediatr.* 1987; **110**: 201.

106 Rosh JR, Silverman ED, Groisman F *et al.* Intrahepatic cholestasis in neonatal lupus erythematosus. *J. Pediatr. Gastroenterol. Nutr.* 1993; **17**: 310.

107 Ruiz-Moreno M, Camps T, Jimenez J *et al.* Factors predictive of response to interferon therapy in children with chronic hepatitis B. *J. Hepatol.* 1995; **22**: 540.

108 Ruiz-Moreno M, Rua MJ, Castillo I *et al.* Treatment of chil-

dren with chronic hepatitis C with recombinant interferon-α: a pilot study. *Hepatology* 1992; **16**: 882.

109 Ruiz-Moreno M, Rua MJ, Molina J *et al.* Prospective, randomized controlled trial of interferon-alpha in children with chronic hepatitis B. *Hepatology* 1991; **13**: 1035.

110 Scheidt PC, Bryla DA, Nelson KB *et al.* Phototherapy for neonatal hyperbilirubinemia: six-year follow-up of the National Institute of Child Health and Human Development clinical trial. *Pediatrics* 1990; **85**: 455.

111 Scheinberg IH, Sternlieb I. Is non-Indian childhood cirrhosis caused by excess dietary copper? *Lancet* 1994; **344**: 1002.

112 Schneider BL, Setchell KDR, Whittington PF *et al.* Delta 4-3 oxosteroid 5-beta-reductase deficiency causing neonatal liver failure and hemochromatosis. *J. Pediatr.* 1994; **124**: 234.

113 Selby DM, Stocker JT, Waclawiw MA *et al.* Infantile hemangioendothelioma of the liver. *Hepatology* 1994; **20**: 39.

114 Setchell KDR, Suchy FJ, Welsh MB *et al.* Delta-4-3 oxosteroid 5 beta-reductase deficiency described in identical twins with neonatal hepatitis. *J. Clin. Invest.* 1988; **82**: 2148.

115 Shiraki K. Hepatic cell necrosis in the newborn: a pathogenic study of 147 cases with particular reference to congenital heart disease. *Am. J. Dis. Child.* 1970; **119**: 395.

116 Shulman SA, Hyams JS, Gunta R *et al.* Arterio-hepatic dysplasia (Alagille syndrome): extreme variability among affected family members. *Am. J. Med. Genet.* 1984; **19**: 325.

117 Sisto A, Feldman P, Garel L *et al.* Primary sclerosing cholangitis in children: study of five cases and review of the literature. *Pediatrics* 1987; **80**: 918.

118 Sokol RJ, Guggenheim MA, Iannaccone ST *et al.* Improved neurologic function after long-term correction of vitamin E deficiency in children with chronic cholestasis. *N. Engl. J. Med.* 1985; **313**: 1580.

119 Sokol RJ, Heubi JE, Butler-Simon N *et al.* Treatment of vitamin E deficiency during chronic childhood cholestasis with oral alpha-tocopheryl polyethylene glycol-1000 succinate. *Gastroenterology* 1987; **93**: 975.

120 Stanley P, Geer GD, Miller JH *et al.* Infantile hepatic hemangiomas. Clinical features, radiologic investigations, and treatment of 20 patients. *Cancer* 1989; **64**: 936.

121 Steele MI, Marshall CM, Lloyd RE *et al.* Reovirus 3 not detected by reverse transcriptase-mediated polymerase chain reaction analysis of preserved tissue from infants with cholestatic liver disease. *Hepatology* 1995; **21**: 697.

122 Steiner M, Bostrum B, Leonard AS *et al.* Undifferentiated (embryonal) sarcoma of the liver. A clinicopathologic study of a survivor treated with combined technique therapy. *Cancer* 1989; **64**: 1318.

123 Stern H, Williams BM. Isolation of rubella virus in a case of neonatal giant-cell hepatitis. *Lancet* 1966; **i**: 293.

124 Suchy FJ. Bile acids for babies? Diagnosis and treatment of a new category of metabolic liver disease. *Hepatology* 1993; **18**: 1274.

125 Suchy FJ, Bucuvalas JC, Novak DA. Determinants of bile formation during development: ontogeny of hepatic bile acid metabolism and transport. *Semin. Liver Dis.* 1987; **7**: 77.

126 Tanner MS, Bhave SA, Pradhan AM *et al.* Clinical trials of penicillamine in Indian childhood cirrhosis. *Arch. Dis. Child.* 1987; **62**: 1118.

127 Tolia V, Dubois RS, Watts FB Jr *et al.* Renal abnormalities in paucity of interlobular bile ducts. *J. Pediatr. Gastroenterol. Nutr.* 1987; **6**: 971.

128 Treem WR, Witzleben CA, Piccoli DA *et al.* Medium-chain and long-chain acyl CoA dehydrogenase deficiency: clinical, pathologic and ultrastructural differentiation from Reye's syndrome. *Hepatology* 1986; **6**: 1270.

129 Tzakis AG, Reyes J, Tepetes K *et al.* Liver transplantation for Alagille's syndrome. *Arch. Surg.* 1993; **128**: 337.

130 Valayer J, Gauthier F, Yandza T *et al.* Biliary atresia: results of long-term conservative treatment and of liver transplantation. *Transplant Proc.* 1993; **25**: 3290.

131 Van Eyken P, Sciot R, Callea F *et al.* The development of the intra-hepatic bile ducts in man: a keratin-immunohistochemical study. *Hepatology* 1988; **8**: 1586.

132 Weizman Z, Mussafi H, Ishay JS *et al.* Multiple hornet stings with features of Reye's syndrome. *Gastroenterology* 1985; **89**: 1407.

133 Whitington PF, Freese DK, Alonso EM *et al.* Clinical and biochemical findings in progressive familial intrahepatic cholestasis. *J. Pediatr. Gastroenterol. Nutr.* 1994; **18**: 134.

134 Wu TC, Tong MJ, Hwang B *et al.* Primary hepato-cellular carcinoma and hepatitis B infection during childhood. *Hepatology* 1987; **7**: 46.

Chapter 25
The Liver in Pregnancy

Normal pregnancy

Physical examination may show palmar erythema and vascular spiders. The liver is impalpable. Serum biochemical tests in the last trimester show modest increases in alkaline phosphatase, cholesterol and α_1- and α_2-globulins. Most of the alkaline phosphatase is of placental origin and the serum γ-GT value is normal. Serum bile acids are slightly increased [18]. The transport maximum for bromsulphalein (BSP) is reduced [7]. These results, taken together, suggest that a normal pregnancy is mildly cholestatic. Bilirubin and transaminase levels are within normal limits. Serum albumin, urea and uric acid concentrations are reduced.

Needle liver biopsy in normal pregnancy gives virtually normal histological appearances. Electron microscopy shows some increase in endoplasmic reticulum.

Liver blood flow is within the normal range [22]. In pregnancy, blood volume and cardiac output increase. The liver blood flow comprises 35% of the cardiac output in non-pregnant females and only 28% of the cardiac output in pregnancy. The excess blood volume is shunted through the placenta.

Liver disease in pregnancy

Jaundice may be peculiar to pregnancy, such as acute fatty liver, cholestatic jaundice, or jaundice complicating the toxaemias. The jaundice may be an intercurrent one affecting the pregnant woman such as virus hepatitis or gallstones. Finally, the effect of pregnancy on underlying chronic liver disease must be considered (table 25.1).

Hyperemesis gravidarum

This is an extension of the morning sickness of the first trimester. Increases in serum bilirubin and decreases in albumin are recorded in about one-third of sufferers. Liver dysfunction is found in up to two-thirds of severe cases [35]. Half the patients show increases in serum transaminases to between 600 and 1000. Liver biopsies are virtually normal.

Table 25.1. Jaundice in pregnancy

	Notes
Peculiar to pregnancy	
Acute fatty liver	Presents vomiting, variable prognosis
Recurrent cholestasis	Good prognosis, familial, recurs, fetal wastage
Toxaemias	Rare cause of jaundice
	Hepatic haemorrhage may be a complication
Hyperemesis	Rare cause of jaundice
Intercurrent	
Viral hepatitis	Prognosis as in non-pregnant
	A—no effect on fetus
	B—rarely transmitted to fetus
	E—often fatal in Africa and Asia
Gallstones	Rare cause of jaundice, ultrasound diagnosis
Underlying chronic liver disease	Rare to become pregnant, prognosis variable, stillbirths increased

Acute fatty liver of pregnancy

The first full description is usually attributed to Sheehan [41] who, in 1940, described obstetric acute liver atrophy as a specific cause of jaundice in pregnancy.

It is still rare, but recognition of milder cases and knowledge of the wide spectrum of illness has resulted in more patients being diagnosed. The incidence in an American study published in 1984 was 1 per 13 328 deliveries [26].

Clinical features

The onset is between the 30th and 38th week of pregnancy and is marked by nausea, repeated vomiting and abdominal pain followed by jaundice (table 25.2). It is commoner with twins and male births and in primiparae. In those severely affected, the course is marked by coma, renal failure and haemorrhages.

Table 25.2. Acute fatty liver of pregnancy. Symptoms and signs recorded before hospital admission in 12 patients [5]

Patient	1	2	3	4	5	6	7	8	9	10	11	12
Malaise	+	+	+	+	+	+	+	+	+	+	+	+
Anorexia		+		+		+		+	+			
Nausea/vomiting	+	+	+	+	+	+	+	+	+	+	+	+
Coffee-ground vomiting	+					+				+		
Heartburn						+	+	+	+			
Abdominal pain/tenderness			+	+	+	+	+	+	+	+		
Hypertension	+		+	+	+			+	+		+	
Peripheral oedema	+		+	+	+		+		+	+	+	+
Proteinuria	+		+		+	+			+	+		+
Jaundice (days from onset of symptoms)	10	7	16	8	2	14	7	15	8	18	11	postdelivery

Ascites is found in 50%, perhaps related to portal hypertension.

Polydipsia and polyuria with transient diabetes insipidus have been reported [30].

Serum biochemical changes

Serum ammonia and amino-acid levels are increased reflecting mitochondrial failure. This is also suggested by lactic acidosis. High serum uric acid levels are usual and may be related to the tissue destruction and lactic acidosis [5].

Hypoglycaemia can be profound.

Hyperbilirubinaemia is found without haemolysis in contradistinction to pregnancy toxaemia where jaundice is rare except for haemolysis. Serum transaminase values are variable, usually less than 1000 and may be normal.

Haematological findings

Leucocytosis and thrombocytopenia are common but the blood film may be leucoerythroblastic [5].

Prothrombin time and partial prothrombin time are increased. Fibrinogen levels are decreased. Severe bleeding is frequent, but disseminated intravascular coagulation is found in only 10%.

Liver histology

Liver biopsy is not usually necessary for diagnosis but can be performed by the transjugular route. The histological picture is of microvesicular and macrovesicular fat droplets with ballooned hepatocytes containing dense, central nuclei (fig. 25.1). Zone 1 (peri-portal) is relatively spared. The microvacuoles may be clearly recognized only on fresh sections stained for fat with such methods as oil red O (fig. 25.2) [4, 38].

Foci of inflammation and necrosis may be seen; also

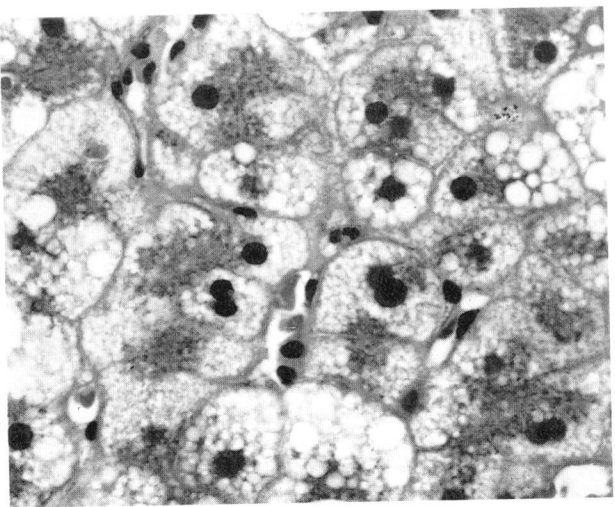

Fig. 25.1. Acute fatty liver of pregnancy. Hepatocytes have a foamy appearance with a central dense nucleus. (Stained H & E, ×120.)

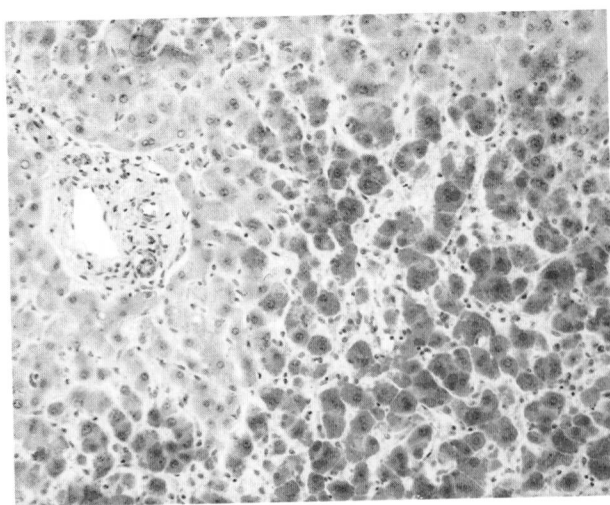

Fig. 25.2. Acute fatty liver of pregnancy: zone 3 hepatocytes are full of microvesicular fat droplets. Portal zones are normal and inflammation is minimal. (Stained oil red, ×40.)

cholestasis with bile canalicular plugs and bile-stained Kupffer cells. Liver architecture is normal.

Electron microscopy confirms vacuoles and may show a honeycomb appearance in the smooth endoplasmic reticulum. Mitochondria are large, pleomorphic with paracrystalline inclusions [30].

Multi-organ involvement is shown by fatty infiltration of the renal tubules and renal lesions typical of pre-eclampsia [34]. Fatty infiltration of the pancreas and the heart have been reported [38].

Ultrasonography of the liver may show a diffuse increased echogenicity which is very suggestive of acute fatty liver of pregnancy [6]. A normal sonogram does not exclude the diagnosis. *CT* is hypodense in 30% [19].

Course and prognosis

Acute fatty liver of pregnancy used to be considered a catastrophic illness of the third trimester with a maternal and fetal mortality of 80–90%. Early recognition with prompt treatment has allowed diagnosis of milder cases and the current fetal and maternal mortality is 0–20% [34]. Fetal mortality remains high.

Death is usually due to extra-hepatic causes such as disseminated intravascular coagulation with massive haemorrhage and to renal failure. These features are not seen in the less severe cases.

Subsequent pregnancies are usually normal but there have been three recurrences reported. In one, a black woman presented with the disease in her fourth and fifth pregnancies [2, 3]. From Australia, a woman had acute fatty liver of pregnancy in her first and second pregnancies [40]. A Chilean report describes acute fatty liver of pregnancy in two consecutive pregnancies [30, 31].

Management

The management of the average mild case is careful observation of mother and fetus in hospital. If the mother's status deteriorates (intractable vomiting, increased jaundice and features of a coagulopathy) the pregnancy should be terminated by either caesarean section or vaginal delivery. The appropriate cover is given for any coagulopathy or hypoglycaemia. One particularly severe case required liver transplantation [23].

Post-partum care should include monitoring for coagulopathy, hypoglycaemia, renal failure or progression of liver dysfunction.

Oesophagitis with bleeding is a frequent complication and omeprazole or a similar drug should be given.

Aetiology

Acute fatty liver of pregnancy can be regarded as a member of the *mitochondrial cytopathy family* (table 25.3).

Table 25.3. The mitochondrial cytopathies

Causes
Acute fatty liver of pregnancy
Reye's syndrome
Genetic defects in mitochondrial function
Drug-related

Features
Vomiting and apathy
Lactic acidosis
Hypoglycaemia
Hyperammonaemia
Microvesicular fat in organs

Members include Reye's syndrome, genetic defects in mitochondrial enzymes and drug reactions, especially to sodium valproate and nucleoside analogues (e.g. FIAU) [20].

Apart from the breakdown of carbohydrate, nearly all the reactions involved in energy production take place in mitochondria. Some of oxidative phosphorylation includes the oxidation of fuel molecules by oxygen and simultaneous energy transduction into ATP. Fatty acids are broken down in the mitochondria into shorter derivative fatty acids and acyl-co-A. This cycle of repeated fatty acid cleavage requires a series of specific enzymes.

The mitochondrial cytopathies are marked by vomiting and weakness. Lactic acidosis and metabolic acidosis are related to defective mitochondrial energy supply and defects in oxidative phosphorylation. Hypoglycaemia may be related to failure of mitochondrial citric acid cycle function. Raised blood ammonia relates to defects in mitochondrial Krebs' cycle enzymes. Microvesicular fat is seen in the organs.

Young people are predominantly affected in Reye's disease and in genetic defects of mitochondrial enzymes. Patients with acute fatty liver of pregnancy are usually reasonably young. Adverse hepatic effects of sodium valproate are roughly twice as frequent in children than in adults. This has led to the hypothesis that all these diseases primarily affect patients having an underlying defect in mitochondrial function. A woman with acute fatty liver of pregnancy gave birth to a seemingly normal full-term infant who later developed hypoglycaemia, coma and profound hepatic steatosis. The infant had a defect in fatty acid oxidation (long chain 3-hydroxyacyl coenzyme A deficiency) and the mother proved to be heterozygous for this metabolic condition. The interaction of an affected fetus with a female who is heterozygous for the defect in fatty acid oxidation in the last trimester may account for some cases of acute fatty liver of pregnancy [47]. In another report, 11 pregnancies complicated by features of fatty liver and the HELLP syndrome were followed by six babies with long chain

3-hydroxyacyl coenzyme A dehydrogenase deficiency. The mothers might be heterozygotes for this deficiency because they can have uneventful pregnancies when the fetus is unaffected [51].

Pregnancy *per se* may affect mitochondrial function. In mice, late pregnancy is associated with failure of mitochondrial oxidation of fatty acids as a consequence of both decreased mitochondrial β-oxidation of medium chain fatty acids and decreased activity of the tricarboxylic acid cycle [10].

The mode of initiation of the mitochondrial cytopathies, apart from the genetic enzyme defects, is uncertain. It might be viral, as speculated in Reye's syndrome. It might be toxic and acute fatty liver of pregnancy has followed exposure to toluene [25]. Nutritional factors have also been suggested.

Acute fatty liver of pregnancy should be regarded as part of systemic mitochondrial dysfunction affecting particularly liver, muscle, nervous system, pancreas and kidneys.

Pregnancy toxaemias

These conditions are of unknown aetiology and classically are characterized by hypertension, proteinuria and fluid retention. The term 'pregnancy toxaemia' includes a spectrum of conditions (table 25.4). The target organs are the uterus, kidney and brain. Hepatic damage is only seen in patients with severe pre-eclampsia and eclampsia.

The aetiology of pre-eclampsia is unknown. The patients have an increased vascular sensitivity to endogenous pressor agents and to catecholamine. Plasma levels of E_1 prostaglandins are decreased, and this may be a trigger for vasospasm and systemic hypertension. Arteriolar constriction accounts for the renal glomerular lesions. Vascular endothelial damage leads to platelet deposition, thrombocytopenia and fibrin deposition in sinusoids. The resultant ischaemia accounts for the focal and diffuse hepato-cellular necrosis and haemorrhages in zone 1 (fig. 25.3).

In mild cases increases in serum alkaline phosphatase and transaminase values are frequent. Minor signs of disseminated intravascular coagulation, such as a reduction in platelets, are also common.

Jaundice is infrequent and often terminal. It is usually haemolytic with disseminated intravascular coagu-

Table 25.4. Spectrum of toxaemias

Pre-eclampsia
HELLP syndrome
Infarction
Bleeding and rupture

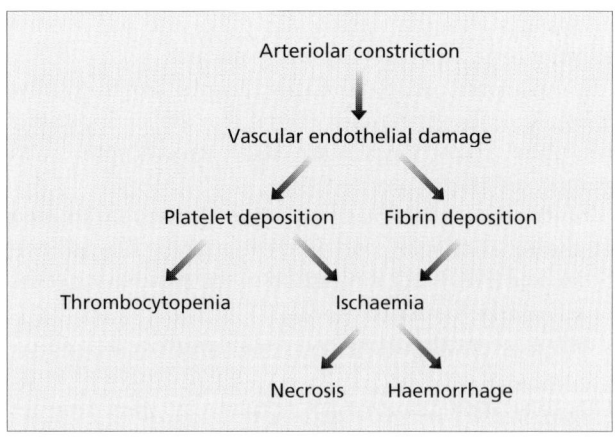

Fig. 25.3. The liver in eclampsia. Hepato-cellular necrosis and haemorrhage follow ischaemia related to vascular endothelial damage.

lation. Failure of renal bilirubin excretion may contribute. Serum bilirubin is less than 6 mg/dl.

Severe toxaemia may present with epigastric pain, nausea, vomiting, right upper quadrant tenderness and hypertension.

Hepatic histology. Peri-portal (zone 1) fibrin deposits [36] and haemorrhage progress to small necrotic foci, infarcts and haematomas. Zone 3 necrosis and haemorrhage represent shock. An inflammatory reaction is characteristically absent (fig. 25.4). Capillary and hepatic arterial thrombi and, rarely, intra-hepatic portal venous thrombi may be noted. *Serum transaminases* are usually more than 10 times elevated.

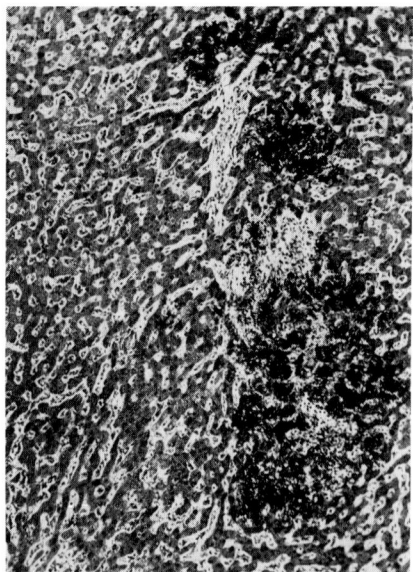

Fig. 25.4. The liver in eclampsia. Focal peri-portal necrosis of liver cells; the lesion contains fibrin. (Stained Mallory's phosphotungstic acid, ×80.)

Rupture of the liver is associated with shock.

Ultrasound and CT show focal filling defects.

The *treatment* of severe toxaemia is by termination of the pregnancy and by supportive care.

The HELLP syndrome

This is a rare variant of toxaemia. It consists of haemolysis, elevated liver enzymes and low platelet count [49]. It often affects multipara. The blood pressure may be normal and proteinuria may be absent.

Liver histology shows fibrin deposition [2]. This suggests severe pre-eclamptic liver disease and calls for immediate delivery. The laboratory results do not reflect hepatic histology [2]. Perinatal mortality is 10–60% and the maternal mortality 1.5–5% [43].

Toxaemia and HELLP syndrome

There is considerable overlap between acute fatty liver of pregnancy and the pregnancy toxaemias and also the HELLP syndrome (table 25.5). Some features of toxaemia are present in 50–100% of patients with acute fatty liver of pregnancy [5, 13]. The features include proteinuria and even some peri-sinusoidal fibrin deposition but hypertension is unusual. The patient with clear pregnancy toxaemia may lack proteinuria and hypertension and yet the liver biopsy, in addition to fibrin deposition, shows some microvesicular fat. Multiparous patients with acute fatty liver of pregnancy often have a history of pre-eclampsia [34].

Hepatic haemorrhage

This usually complicates pre-eclampsia or eclampsia and the HELLP syndrome with accompanying disseminated intravascular coagulation and intra-hepatic vascular lesions [9]. The picture includes infarction [16], subcapsular haemorrhage and ruptured liver. Clinically this catastrophe is suspected by sudden constant right upper quadrant or epigastric pain with vomiting and circulatory collapse. The diagnosis is confirmed by ultra-

sound, CT and angiography. Treatment varies with the severity. Subcapsular haemorrhage is usually treated conservatively. Surgery may be required. Hepatic arterial embolization with gelfoam has been used to control haemorrhage [46].

Hepatic adenomas, often with peliosis hepatitis, and often associated with oral contraceptives, may rupture during pregnancy.

Cholestasis of pregnancy

This intra-hepatic cholestasis appears in the last trimester of pregnancy [27].

In its mildest form, pruritus is the only abnormality. It accounts for generalized itching in the last weeks of pregnancy. Pruritus usually commences in the last trimester, but can start as early as the second or third month. Jaundice is rarely deep. The urine is dark and the stools pale. General health is preserved and there is no pain. Weight loss may be great. The liver and spleen are impalpable. After delivery, jaundice disappears and within 1–2 weeks the pruritus has ceased. The condition usually recurs with subsequent pregnancies. Consecutive pregnancies in multiparous patients are associated with variability in the severity and in the time of onset.

Laboratory changes

Serum shows an increase in conjugated bilirubin and alkaline phosphatase values. Serum transaminases are normal or slightly increased, although occasionally very high values are found. These changes return to normal after delivery. Increased serum bile acid levels are common in pregnant women, particularly in those of Mediterranean or Asian origin [18]. They predict pruritus in pregnancy.

Steatorrhoea is usual. It correlates with the severity of the cholestasis.

The prothrombin time is prolonged due to vitamin K deficiency. Cholestyramine enhances the hypoprothrombinaemia.

Hepatic histology shows mild focal and irregular cholestasis. Electron microscopy shows the changes in the microvilli of the bile canaliculi common to all forms of cholestasis.

Aetiology

Multiple factors probably interact with a genetic predisposition to alter the canalicular and hepatic membranes, increasing their sensitivity to sex steroids. Overproduction of oestrogens may reduce bile flow in normal pregnancy. However, there is no evidence that any specific oestrogenic steroid or oestrogen metabolite is responsible for the cholestasis. Hormonal factors are

Table 25.5. Acute fatty liver of pregnancy and toxaemias contrasted: overlaps exist

	Acute fatty liver	Toxaemia
Abdominal pain	50%	100%
Jaundice	100%	40%
Serum transaminases (× normal)	< 10	> 10
Scans	Diffuse change	Focal abnormalities
Liver biopsy	Microvesicular fat	Fibrin (peri-sinusoidal)
Liver failure	Present	Absent

suggested by worsening with multiple pregnancies and recurrences with menstruation or oestrogen therapy.

Seasonal variation suggests that environmental factors could be important.

The aetiology of cholestasis of pregnancy remains unknown.

Epidemiology

Cholestasis of pregnancy is often familial, and has been reported in mothers, sisters and daughters, some of whom develop pruritus when given oral contraceptives [11, 28]. Male family members may show the cholestatic tendency when given oestrogens [29]. Findings support a Mendelian dominant inheritance.

This condition is particularly common in Scandinavia, Northern Europe, Chile, Bolivia and China. It is very rare in Asiatic or Black women [27]. Prevalence varies widely and figures from 1 in 750 to 1 in 7000 pregnancies have been quoted. The prevalence is decreasing markedly in Chile and Sweden.

In Chile, cholestasis seems to be associated with Araucanial Indian descent, rather than with Chilean Caucasians.

Family history is associated with increased frequency of HLA-B8 and HLA-Bw 16 histocompatibility antigens [32].

Diagnosis

In the first pregnancy, the diagnosis from viral hepatitis and other conditions causing jaundice may be difficult. Absence of constitutional symptoms, prominent pruritus and biochemical tests suggesting cholestasis are helpful. Ultrasound helps to exclude obstruction to main bile ducts. Liver biopsy is rarely necessary, but the appearances are diagnostic. Failure of the pruritus to stop after delivery, with continuing high serum alkaline phosphatase values, suggests underlying primary biliary cirrhosis, and liver biopsy and serum mitochondrial antibody tests should be performed. After delivery, the woman may show a cholestatic response to small dose of oestrogens [11].

Prognosis and management

Prognosis for the mother is excellent. The fetus however, is at increased risk of distress, prematurity and death [37]. The fetus must be carefully monitored and termination is indicated for fetal distress [7]. The mother should be delivered at 38 weeks but at 36 weeks if cholestasis is severe.

Nutritional support is essential. Vitamin K supplements are necessary as post-partum haemorrhage is increased. Management of pruritus includes cholestyramine and ursodeoxycholic acid [7, 24]. S-adenosyl-L-methionine (SAMe) is said to be beneficial but this could not be confirmed in a double-blind, placebo-controlled trial [33].

The mother is warned that the condition will usually return in a subsequent pregnancy and that she may develop pruritus if she takes oral contraceptive drugs.

Viral hepatitis

Viral hepatitis causes about 50% of jaundice in pregnancy [44]. It is particularly serious in developing countries with a mortality ranging from 10 to 45%. In Ethiopia it ranks among the leading causes of maternal mortality, coming third to septic abortion and puerperal sepsis [17]. In developed countries, the course and mortality of acute hepatitis in pregnancy are about the same as in the non-pregnant. Fetal abnormalities are not recorded, but stillbirths may be increased.

Hepatitis A

The disease is usually passed to the mother by contact with the excreta of older children attending nursery schools.

Pregnant women exposed should receive immunoglobulin and vaccine immediately. The course is similar to that in the non-pregnant even in the last trimester. It is rarely transmitted to the fetus.

Hepatitis B

Pregnant women in close contact with persons carrying hepatitis B must receive hepatitis B vaccine, which is safe in pregnancy, and also hepatitis B immunoglobulin. An acute attack of hepatitis B usually runs the same course in the pregnant as in the non-pregnant woman. The chances of the disease progressing to chronic hepatitis are less than 10%. In underdeveloped countries the mortality is high and fetal wastage and stillbirths are increased. The effect on the baby of a mother carrying hepatitis B is very serious (see Chapter 24).

Screening of mothers for hepatitis B viral markers should be universal and not simply directed to those at increased risk of hepatitis B carriage, such as drug abusers, those of Chinese and African origin and those working in the health-care professions [12].

The *hepatitis δ virus* can be transmitted to the fetus from a mother who is carrying both hepatitis B and delta. This results in more serious hepatitis. A baby vaccinated against hepatitis B will be protected from δ virus infection.

Hepatitis C

Pregnant women having difficult deliveries and receiving blood transfusions (often unnecessarily) are at particular risk of developing hepatitis virus C related chronic liver disease. Anti-HCV passes the placenta, and babies born to anti-HCV mothers remain positive for anti-HCV for 6 months, the life of circulating maternal antibody. Babies born to hepatitis C positive mothers rarely develop the disease unless they are HIV positive.

Hepatitis E

Hepatitis E has a striking 20% mortality in the last trimester of pregnancy [14]. This might be related to malnutrition. In underdeveloped countries, almost all maternal deaths from hepatitis are probably due to this virus. Hopefully, in the future, a vaccine will be available which can be offered to pregnant women in areas of poor water supply.

Herpes simplex (HSV type II)

This infection is usually reported in the immunocompromised, but has been reported in pregnant women [15]. This might be related to a defect in cell-mediated immunity thought to exist in pregnant women. The hepatitis can mimic acute fatty liver of pregnancy. It is marked by very high serum transaminase levels but without jaundice. Herpetic lesions can usually be detected on the vulva or cervix. Liver biopsy shows extensive hepatocellular necrosis and intranuclear herpetic inclusions. The treatment is with acyclovir.

Biliary tract disease

During pregnancy the bile becomes more lithogenic and gallbladder emptying is impaired. Gallstones form [8]. Immediately, post-partum, gallbladder ultrasound examinations have shown sludge in 26.2% and gallstones in 5.2%. One year later, only two of 45 patients with sludge and 13 of 15 with gallstones still had abnormal ultrasound findings. In spite of these observations, symptoms of gallbladder disease during pregnancy are rare.

Patients with choledocholithiasis can be successfully relieved by ERCP and sphincterotomy. This may be performed as early as the second trimester and with minimal exposure to radiation [1]. Cholecystectomy, whether by open operation [45] or the laparoscopic technique [21] is safe during pregnancy.

Hepato-toxic drugs and the pregnant woman

The pregnant woman can react to drugs causing jaundice in a similar fashion to the non-pregnant. Drugs may potentiate jaundice or kernicterus in the newborn. In particular, drugs such as sulphonamides which displace bilirubin from its binding site to serum albumin should be avoided. Drugs such as phenacetin given to the mother may precipitate jaundice in an infant with glucose-6-phosphate dehydrogenase deficiency.

Effect of pregnancy on pre-existing chronic liver disease

The full-time parturition of a woman suffering from hepatic cirrhosis is unusual. It is rare for such a patient to conceive. The liver disease *per se* is not an indication for termination. Patients with chronic hepatitis (autoimmune hepatitis) are younger, often physically attractive women. Amenorrhoea is usual at the onset but, as the disease becomes less active with corticosteroid therapy, menses return and they may become pregnant [50]. Liver function may deteriorate during pregnancy, but after delivery soon returns to its previous level. The fetal loss rate is about 33% and babies may be born prematurely, but will be normal. The coincidence of liver disease with pregnancy should not *per se* indicate termination. Corticosteroids must be continued. Management in a specialist obstetric unit with hepatological back-up is essential.

Bleeding from oesophageal varices is a risk in those with portal hypertension, whether due to cirrhosis or a portal vein obstruction. Patients who have previously bled are at particular risk. It is treated along similar lines to those adopted in the non-pregnant.

Pregnancy is not contraindicated in those with well-treated Wilson's disease, and penicillamine does not pose an undue risk to the fetus [48].

Primary biliary cirrhosis may present as cholestatic jaundice in, or shortly after, pregnancy.

Successful pregnancy has been reported in a patient with Alagille's syndrome [39].

Pregnancy in liver transplant recipients

Pregnancy can be allowed after 1 year post-transplant, and if the condition of the graft is stable. Successful outcomes are recorded, but the pregnancy must be regarded as high risk. Immunosuppression must be continued. There is a high risk of premature delivery and of low birth-weight infants. Rarely, the mother loses the graft and re-transplantation is necessary.

References

1 Baillie J, Cairns SR, Putnam WS *et al.* Endoscopic management of choledocholithiasis during pregnancy. *Surg. Gynecol. Obstet.* 1990; **171**: 1.
2 Barton JR, Riely CA, Adamec TA *et al.* Hepatic histopathologic condition does not correlate with laboratory abnormalities in HELLP syndrome (hemolysis, elevated liver enzymes, and low platelet count). *Am. J. Obstet. Gynecol.* 1992; **167**: 1538.

3 Barton JR, Sibai BM, Mabie WC *et al.* Recurrent acute fatty liver of pregnancy. *Am. J. Obstet. Gynecol.* 1990; **163**: 534.

4 Bernuau J, Degott C, Nouel O *et al.* Non-fatal acute fatty liver of pregnancy. *Gut* 1983; **24**: 340.

5 Burroughs AK, Seong NH, Dojcinov DM *et al.* Idiopathic acute fatty liver of pregnancy in 12 patients. *Q. J. Med.* 1982; **51**: 481.

6 Campillo B, Bernuau J, Witz M-O *et al.* Ultrasonography in acute fatty liver of pregnancy. *Ann. Intern. Med.* 1986; **105**: 383.

7 Davis MH, da Silva RCMA, Jones SR *et al.* Fetal mortality associated with cholestasis and the potential benefit of therapy with ursodeoxycholic acid. *Gut* 1995; **37**: 580.

8 Everson GT. Pregnancy and gallstones. *Hepatology* 1993; **17**: 159.

9 Greenstein D, Henderson JM, Boyer TD. Liver hemorrhage: recurrent episodes during pregnancy complicated by preeclampsia. *Gastroenterology* 1994; **106**: 1668.

10 Grimbert S, Fromenty B, Fisch C *et al.* Decreased mitochondrial oxidation of fatty acids in pregnant mice: possible relevance to development of acute fatty liver of pregnancy. *Hepatology* 1993; **17**: 628.

11 Holzbach RT, Sivak DA, Braun WE. Familial recurrent intrahepatic cholestasis of pregnancy: a genetic study providing evidence for transmission of a sex-limited, dominant trait. *Gastroenterology* 1983; **85**: 175.

12 Jonas MM, Schiff ER, O'Sullivan MJ *et al.* Failure of centers for disease control criteria to identify hepatitis B infection in a large municipal obstetrical population. *Ann. Intern. Med.* 1987; **107**: 335.

13 Kaplan MM. Current concepts. Acute fatty liver of pregnancy. *N. Engl. J. Med.* 1985; **313**: 367.

14 Khuroo MS, Teli MR, Skidmore S *et al.* Incidence and severity of viral hepatitis in pregnancy. *Am. J. Med.* 1981; **70**: 252.

15 Klein NA, Mabie WC, Shaver DC *et al.* Herpes simplex virus hepatitis in pregnancy: two patients successfully treated with acyclovir. *Gastroenterology* 1991; **100**: 239.

16 Krueger KJ, Hoffman BJ, Lee WM. Hepatic infarction associated with eclampsia. *Am. J. Gastroenterol.* 1990; **85**: 588.

17 Kwast BE, Stevens JA. Viral hepatitis as a major cause of maternal mortality in Addis Ababa, Ethiopia. *Int. J. Gynaecol. Obstet.* 1987; **25**: 99.

18 Lunzer M, Barnes P, Byth K *et al.* Serum bile acid concentrations during pregnancy and their relationship to obstetric cholestasis. *Gastroenterology* 1986; **91**: 825.

19 Mabie WC, Dacus JV, Sibai BM *et al.* Computed tomography in acute fatty liver of pregnancy. *Am. J. Obstet. Gynecol.* 1988; **158**: 142.

20 McKenzie R, Fried MW, Sallie R *et al.* Hepatic failure and lactic acidosis due to fialuridine (FIAU) an investigational nucleoside analogue for chronic hepatitis B. *N. Engl. J. Med.* 1995; **333**: 1099.

21 Morrell DG, Mullins JR, Harrison PB. Laparoscopic cholecystectomy during pregnancy in symptomatic patients. *Surgery* 1992; **112**: 856.

22 Munnell EW, Taylor HC Jr. Liver blood flow in pregnancy—hepatic vein catheterization. *J. Clin. Invest.* 1947; **26**: 952.

23 Ockner SA, Brunt EM, Cohn SM *et al.* Fulminant hepatic failure caused by acute fatty liver of pregnancy treated by orthotopic liver transplantation. *Hepatology* 1990; **11**: 59.

24 Palma J, Reyes H, Ribalta J *et al.* Effects of ursodeoxycholic acid in patient with intrahepatic cholestasis of pregnancy. *Hepatology* 1992; **15**: 1043.

25 Paraf F, Lewis J, Jothy S. Acute fatty liver of pregnancy after exposure to toluene. A case report. *J. Clin. Gastroenterol.* 1993; **17**: 163.

26 Pockros PJ, Peters RL, Reynolds TB. Idiopathic fatty liver of pregnancy: findings in ten cases. *Medicine (Baltimore)* 1984; **63**: 1.

27 Reyes H. The enigma of intrahepatic cholestasis of pregnancy: lessons from Chile. *Hepatology* 1982; **2**: 87.

28 Reyes H, Ribalta J, Gonzáles-Cerón M. Idiopathic cholestasis of pregnancy in a large kindred. *Gut* 1976; **17**: 709.

29 Reyes H, Ribalta J, Gonzáles MC *et al.* Sulfobromophthalein clearance tests before and after ethinyl estradiol administration, in women and men with familial history of intrahepatic cholestasis of pregnancy. *Gastroenterology* 1981; **81**: 226.

30 Reyes H, Sandoval L, Wainstein A *et al.* Acute fatty liver of pregnancy: a clinical study of 12 episodes in 11 patients. *Gut* 1994; **35**: 101.

31 Reyes H, Simon FR. Intraepatic cholestasis of pregnancy: an estrogen-related disease. *Semin. Liver Dis.* 1993; **13**: 289.

32 Reyes H, Wegmann ME, Segovia N *et al.* HLA in Chileans with intrahepatic cholestasis of pregnancy. *Hepatology* 1982; **2**: 463.

33 Ribalta J, Reyes H, Gonzalez MC *et al.* S-adenosyl-L-methionine in the treatment of patients with intrahepatic cholestasis of pregnancy: a randomized, double-blind, placebo-controlled study with negative results. *Hepatology* 1991; **13**: 1084.

34 Riely CA. Acute fatty liver of pregnancy. *Semin. Liver Dis.* 1987; **7**: 47.

35 Riely CA. Hepatic disease in pregnancy. *Am. J. Med.* 1994; **96**: 117–185.

36 Riely CA, Romero R, Duffy TP. Hepatic dysfunction with disseminated intravascular coagulation in toxaemia of pregnancy: a distinct clinical syndrome. *Gastroenterology* 1981; **80**: 1346.

37 Rioseco AJ, Ivankovic MB, Manzur A *et al.* Intrahepatic cholestasis of pregnancy: a retrospective case-control study of perinatal outcome. *Am. J. Obstet. Gynecol.* 1994; **170**: 890.

38 Rolfes DB, Ishak KG. Acute fatty liver of pregnancy: a clinicopathologic study of 35 cases. *Hepatology* 1985; **5**: 1149.

39 Romero R, Reece EA, Riely C *et al.* Arteriohepatic dysplasia in pregnancy. *Am. J. Obstet. Gynecol.* 1983; **147**: 108.

40 Schoeman MN, Batey RG, Wilcken B. Recurrent acute fatty liver of pregnancy associated with a fatty-acid oxidation defect in the offspring. *Gastroenterology* 1991; **100**: 544.

41 Sheehan HL. The pathology of acute yellow atrophy and delayed chloroform poisoning. *J. Obstet. Gynaecol. Br. Emp.* 1940; **47**: 49.

42 Sherlock S. Acute fatty liver of pregnancy and the microvesicular fat diseases. *Gut* 1983; **24**: 265.

43 Sibai BM, Taslimi MM, El-Nazer A *et al.* Maternal–perinatal outcome associated with the syndrome of hemolysis, elevated liver enzymes, and low platelets in severe preeclampsia-eclampsia. *Am. J. Obstet. Gynecol.* 1986; **155**: 501.

44 Simms J, Duff P. Viral hepatitis in pregnancy. *Semin. Perinatol.* 1993; **17**: 384.

45 Swisher SG, Schmit PJ, Hunt KK *et al.* Biliary disease during pregnancy. *Am. J. Surg.* 1994; **168**: 576.

46 Terasaki KK, Quinn MF, Lundell CJ *et al.* Spontaneous hepatic hemorrhage in preeclampsia: treatment with hepatic arterial embolization. *Radiology* 1990; **174**: 1039.

47 Treem WR, Rinaldo P, Hale DE *et al*. Acute fatty liver of pregnancy and long-chain 3-hydroxyacyl-coenzyme A dehydrogenase deficiency. *Hepatology* 1994; **19**: 339.

48 Walshe JM. Pregnancy in Wilson's disease. *Q. J. Med.* 1977; **46**: 73.

49 Weinstein L. Syndrome of hemolysis, elevated liver enzymes, and low platelet count: a severe consequence of hypertension in pregnancy. *Am. J. Obstet. Gynecol.* 1982; **142**: 159.

50 Whelton MJ, Sherlock S. Pregnancy in patients with hepatic cirrhosis. Management and outcome. *Lancet* 1968; **ii**: 995.

51 Wilcken B, Leung K-C, Hammond J *et al*. Pregnancy and fetal long-chain 3-hydroxyacylcoenzyme A dehydrogenase deficiency. *Lancet* 1993; **341**: 407.

Chapter 26
The Liver in Systemic Disease; Hepatic Trauma

The liver in the collagen diseases

If hepatomegaly is present, it is probably due to amyloidosis in chronic rheumatoid arthritis, or to cardiac failure with rheumatic fever or systemic lupus erythematosus. Splenomegaly reflects reticulo-endothelial hyperplasia rather than portal hypertension.

Primary biliary cirrhosis is associated with collagen diseases.

Biochemistry

Serum α- and β-globulins may be elevated and serum albumin values slightly depressed. Serum bilirubin, transaminase and alkaline phosphatase levels are normal or mildly disturbed.

Diseases

Polyarteritis nodosa. The hepatic arterioles may show characteristic lesions with, occasionally, small hepatic infarcts [14]. Hepatic arteriography may be useful in diagnosis. Hepatic arterial aneurysms are sometimes found. Nodular regenerative hyperplasia may be a complication [9].

Hepatitis B carriage may be associated with polyarteritis nodosa with migrating arthralgias or with polymyositis [7]. Immune complexes containing HBsAg can be shown in the tissues.

Giant cell arteritis can be found with granulomatous liver disease and with hepatic arteritis [10].

Polymyalgia rheumatica. Changes include granulomatous hepatitis and lymphocytic infiltration. These usually remit with corticosteroid treatment.

Rheumatoid arthritis. The liver shows non-specific changes such as mild fatty infiltration, focal necroses, sinusoidal dilatation [3] or complicating amyloidosis. Kupffer cells are hyperplastic. Serum alkaline phosphatase increases. Serum bilirubin and transaminases are normal [12].

Felty's syndrome. Lymphocytic infiltration of the sinusoids with nodular regenerative hyperplasia may lead to portal hypertension and variceal bleeding [13].

Cryoglobulinaemia and vasculitis. Hepatomegaly and increased hepatic enzymes are found in patients with mixed cryoglobulinaemia. Histology varies from mild non-specific changes to chronic active hepatitis and cirrhosis. Some patients have serological evidence of hepatitis B or C [1, 4] infection. Mixed cryoglobulinaemia is also a feature of primary liver disease such as acute and chronic hepatitis and primary biliary cirrhosis.

Weber–Christian disease. Severe fatty change may be seen with Mallory's hyaline. These changes are related to reduced lipoprotein synthesis in the deformed rough endoplasmic reticulum [2].

Systemic lupus erythematosus (SLE)

Subclinical liver disease, as measured by liver enzyme increases, is seen in about a quarter, but in only 8% are these unexplained, and possibly related to SLE itself [8]. Liver biopsy shows no serious lesions, and only rarely has chronic hepatitis been described [6, 11].

Autoimmune 'lupoid' chronic hepatitis is not SLE but belongs in the spectrum of chronic active hepatitis [14].

Rarely a severe hepatic arteritis is present. Rupture of the liver has been reported [5].

Jaundice with SLE is usually haemolytic.

References

1 Cacoub P, Fabiani FL, Musset L *et al.* Mixed cryoglobulinemia and hepatitis C virus. *Am. J. Med.* 1994; **96**: 124.
2 Kimura H, Kako M, Yo K *et al.* Alcoholic hyalins (Mallory bodies) in a case of Weber–Christian disease: electron microscopic observations of liver involvement. *Gastroenterology* 1980; **78**: 807.
3 Laffón A, Moreno A, Gutierrez-Bucero A *et al.* Hepatic sinusoidal dilatation in rheumatoid arthritis. *J. Clin. Gastroenterol.* 1989; **11**: 653.
4 Levey JM, Bjornsson B, Banner B *et al.* Mixed cryoglobulinemia in chronic hepatitis C infection. A clinicopathologic analysis of 10 cases and review of recent literature. *Medicine (Baltimore)* 1994; **73**: 1.
5 Levitin PM, Sweet D, Brunner CM *et al.* Spontaneous rupture of the liver; an unusual complication of SLE. *Arthritis Rheum.* 1977; **20**: 748.
6 Matsumoto T, Yoshimine T, Shimouchi K *et al.* The liver in systemic lupus erythematosus: pathologic analysis of 52 cases and review of the Japanese Autopsy Registry Data.

Hum. Pathol. 1992; **23**: 1151.

7 Mihas AA, Kirby D, Kents P. Hepatitis B antigen and polymyositis. *JAMA* 1978; **239**: 221.

8 Miller MH, Urowitz MB, Gladman DD *et al.* The liver in systemic lupus erythematosus. *Q. J. Med.* 1984; **53**: 401.

9 Nakanuma Y, Ohta G, Sasaki K. Nodular regenerative hyperplasia of the liver associated with polyarteritis nodosa. *Arch. Path. Lab. Med.* 1984; **108**: 133.

10 Ogilvie AL, James PD, Toghill PJ. Hepatic artery involvement in polymyalgia arteritica. *J. Clin. Pathol.* 1981; **34**: 769.

11 Runyon BA, La Brecque DR, Anuras S. The spectrum of liver disease in systemic lupus erythematosus. *Am. J. Med.* 1980; **69**: 187.

12 Thompson PW, Houghton BJ, Clifford C *et al.* The source and significance of raised serum enzymes in rheumatoid arthritis. *Q. J. Med.* 1990; **76**: 869.

13 Thorne C, Urowitz MB, Wanless I *et al.* Liver disease in Felty's syndrome. *Am. J. Med.* 1982; **73**: 35.

14 Weinblatt ME, Teser JRP, Gilliam JH, III. The liver in rheumatic diseases. *Semin. Arthritis Rheum.* 1982; **11**: 399.

Hepatic granulomas

Hepatic granulomatous lesions, having a common histological pattern but sometimes differing in detail, are found in a number of diseases (table 26.1). Although seen anywhere in the liver they are most frequent near the portal tracts. They are sharply defined and do not disturb the normal pattern of the liver. They consist

Table 26.1. Differential diagnosis of some diseases with hepatic granulomas

Disease	Diagnostic aids
Sarcoidosis	Chest X-ray. Kveim. SACE. Broncho-alveolar lavage
Tuberculosis	Tuberculin skin test. Broncho-alveolar lavage. Isolation of organism. Acid-fast staining
Brucellosis	Blood culture. Agglutinin titre
Berylliosis	Industrial exposure. Chest X-ray
Syphilis	*Treponema* test
Leprosy	Race. Lepromin skin test
Histoplasmosis	Complement fixation test. Chest X-ray
Infectious mononucleosis	Blood film. Monospot. IgM EB antibodies
AIDS	Poorly formed granulomas. Acid-fast and fungal stains
Primary biliary cirrhosis	Mitochondrial antibody
Lymphomas	Chest X-ray. Lymph node biopsy. CT scan
Drug reaction	History

basically of pale-staining, epithelioid cells with surrounding lymphocytes (fig. 26.1). Giant cells, central caseation and necrosis may be present. Older lesions may be surrounded by a fibrous capsule, and healing is accompanied by hyaline change (figs 26.2, 26.3). They cause little hepatic functional disturbance.

Granulomas express a cell-mediated immune response comprising Th-1-type CD4 lymphocytes, macrophages and cytokines including interleukin 1 and 2, interferon-γ and tumour necrosis factor. Fibronectin and pro-collagen encourage fibroblast proliferation to end-stage fibrosis.

The importance of granulomas is as a means of diagnosing the causative condition. Hepatic biopsy can be

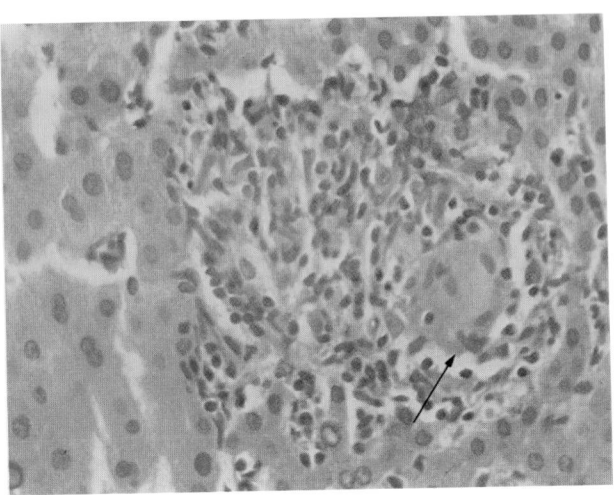

Fig. 26.1. A well-demarcated hepatic granuloma in zone 1 shows a giant cell (arrow) pale-staining epithelioid cells and a rim of lymphocytes. (Stained H & E, ×160.)

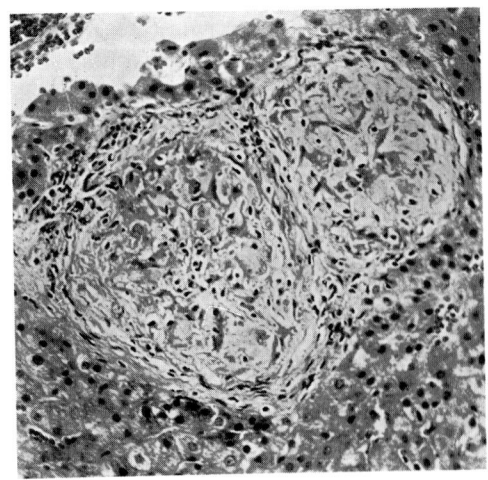

Fig. 26.2. Healing hepatic sarcoid. Two adjacent lesions are acquiring a structureless hyaline appearance and are surrounded by a connective tissue capsule. (Stained H & E, ×90.)

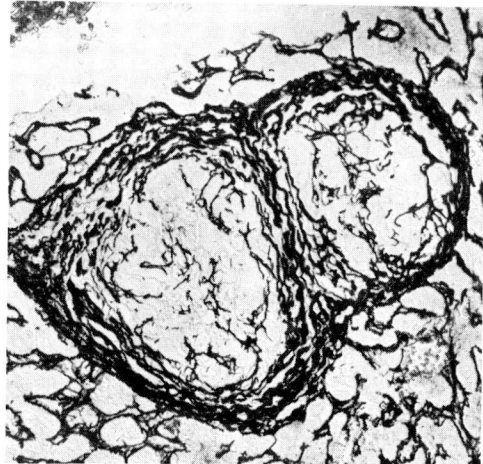

Fig. 26.3. Same section as in fig. 26.2 stained to show reticulin formation around the granulomas. (Stained modified silver, ×90.)

Table 26.2. Hepatic granulomas in patients with AIDS

Infections
Mycobacterium avium-intracellulare
Mycobacterium tuberculosis
Cytomegalovirus
Histoplasmosis
Toxoplasmosis
Cryptococcosis

Neoplasms
Hodgkin's and non-Hodgkin's lymphoma

Drugs
Sulphonamides
Antibiotics
Antifungals
Isoniazid
Tranquillizers

used to obtain confirmation of the diagnosis. The percentage of granulomas obtained is surprisingly high considering the random scattering of lesions and the small size of the biopsy sample.

Aetiology

Hepatic granulomas are found in 4–10% of needle liver biopsies. In 10% of these no cause is found even after noting specific histological characteristics, staining for possible causative organisms, and culture of the specimen [5]. The granulomas vary in size, between 50 and 300 μm. This must be related to the diameter of an aspiration liver biopsy specimen of about 100 μm. Serial sections must therefore be cut and stained if granulomas are to be identified.

Hepatic granulomas are always part of a generalized disease process. They are associated with a multitude of diseases (table 26.1). Sarcoidosis and tuberculosis account for 50–65%.

Drug reactions may be granulomatous and causes include sulphonamides, allopurinol [28], carbamazepine [13] and quinine [10].

They are frequent with AIDS (table 26.2).

The granulomas may be found by chance in a needle biopsy specimen. The interpretation is difficult. Many of these patients may be suffering from sarcoidosis or tuberculosis with minimal clinical evidence. In symptomless patients the granuloma must be ignored but the patient should be observed over the next year or so.

Necrotizing or caseating granulomas are small to large, well formed with a necrotic centre. The histiocytic rim often has a palisade pattern and fibrosis is variable. They are associated with fungal infections and rarely with tuberculosis or Hodgkin's lymphoma [8].

A hepatitis-like background should be sought and in particular note made of infections including AIDS and hepatitis A, B and C [5].

Clinical syndrome of hepatic granulomas

Granulomas are often asymptomatic [14]. Overt hepatic insufficiency is rare. The liver is palpable in only 20% of patients. Very rarely the picture is of active liver disease with marked hepatic functional abnormalities and liver cell destruction and fibrosis on liver biopsy [14]. In general, however, the evidence of hepatic involvement arises from the results of the liver biopsy.

Serum IgG and alkaline phosphatase may be raised. Serum bilirubin level is normal. Serum angiotensin-converting enzyme (SACE) is increased.

'GRANULOMATOUS HEPATITIS'

Hepatic granulomas may be associated with a prolonged, febrile syndrome [24]. Some patients are eventually diagnosed as having an infection, such as tuberculosis, histoplasmosis or Q fever or a lymphoma. Those that defy diagnosis are labelled 'granulomatous hepatitis'. They accounted for 50% of hepatic granulomas in one series [22]. The sufferer is often a middle-aged or elderly male. The granulomas are not widespread and pulmonary involvement is unusual. Biochemical tests of liver function are moderately impaired with increases in serum alkaline phosphatase, and slight increases in serum transaminases and globulins. Serum bilirubin is normal. The condition may subside spontaneously or necessitate short- or long-term prednisolone treatment. The ultimate prognosis is excellent [32]. Those not responding to, or unwilling to take, corticosteroids may benefit from low-dose, oral pulse methotrexate [11].

SARCOIDOSIS

Sarcoidosis is a disease of unknown aetiology, characterized by widespread granulomatous lesions involving most organs [7]. Involvement of lungs, lymph nodes, eyes, skin and the neurological system may be associated with well-recognized clinical features, although this is not always so.

The liver is frequently affected although granulomas are often asymptomatic [23]. Overt hepatic insufficiency is rare. The liver is palpable in only 20% of patients. Occasionally the picture is of active liver disease with marked hepatic functional abnormalities and liver cell destruction, and fibrosis on liver biopsy [14]. The evidence of hepatic involvement arises not by the clinical picture but from the result of liver biopsy. This technique confirms sarcoidosis in about 60%. This agrees with autopsy figures showing hepatic involvement in about two-thirds.

Liver biopsy is indicated when another more accessible tissue, such as lymph gland or skin, is not available.

Hepatic histology

Rounded, well-demarcated lesions can occur anywhere, but most often in the portal zones. The pallor makes them distinctive even in H&E-stained sections.

The granulomas are repetitively monotonous, all being at the same stage of development. Classically the granuloma is small and well formed with clusters of histiocytes with ill-defined cell cytoplasm. Multinucleated giant cells may be present (fig. 26.1). In the liver, these rarely contain asteroid bodies, Schaumann bodies or crystalline inclusions. Occasionally, there is a central area of eosinophilic necrosis. Lymphocytes often surround or mix with the histiocytes. Caseation is absent. Granulomas can coalesce to form large aggregates. As the granuloma heals, reticulin fibres are deposited and it is replaced or surrounded by a fibrous reaction (fig. 26.2). The granuloma may only be seen as a nodule of collagen (fig. 26.3).

Proliferation of Kupffer cells demonstrates the widespread reticulo-endothelial activity.

The granuloma is converted into an acellular mass of hyaline material with a fibrous capsule (figs 26.2, 26.3); many disappear.

Since the hepatic lesions are focal, and fibrosis is restricted to healing lesions, sarcoidosis does not produce the diffuse fibrosis and nodular regeneration of cirrhosis. It is, therefore, difficult to accept the occasional reports of cirrhosis following sarcoidosis, and a fortuitous combination seems more likely. The association with jaundice and hepatic failure is very rare and unexpected.

Corticosteroid therapy seems to have little effect on the liver biopsy appearances.

Biochemical changes. Serum IgG is raised and alkaline phosphatase may be slightly raised. Serum bilirubin level is normal. SACE is increased.

CT scanning shows discrete upper abdominal glandular enlargement in about 60% of patients with sarcoidosis [2] (fig. 26.4). Hepatic CT changes are found only in 38% of those with known hepatic involvement. This is shown by multiple, small low-attenuation areas on a bolus contrast-enhanced CT scan [16]. CT may be useful in confirming hepatosplenomegaly.

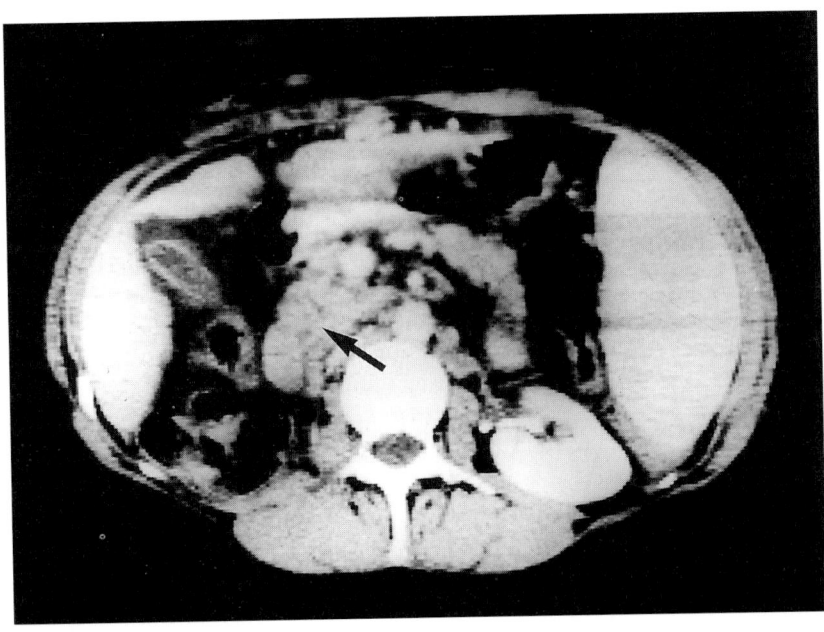

Fig. 26.4. Contrast-enhanced CT scan from a patient with chronic sarcoidosis shows retroperitoneal lymphadenopathy (arrow).

MRI shows multiple diffuse densely packed islands of iso-intense or slightly hyper-intense parenchyma on proton density images and corresponding foci of hypo-intensity on T$_2$-weighted images. This finding effectively excludes metastatic or inflammatory disease which would exhibit hyper-intense signals on T$_2$-weighted images.

Broncho-alveolar lavage shows lymphocyte excess with activated macrophages [25].

Portal hypertension

The patients are usually young, Black people of both sexes, or females greater than 40 years. The portal hypertension is pre-sinusoidal due to portal (zone 1) granulomas (figs 26.5, 26.6). Sinusoidal block may be superimposed due to fibrosis [26, 27]. Corticosteroids do not prevent the portal hypertension.

In some, thrombotic occlusion of a portal or splenic vein may be found. Rarely, oesophageal bleeding is a real problem. These patients tolerate surgical shunts well.

Budd–Chiari syndrome

Sarcoidosis has been reported in association with hepatic vein occlusion. The hepatic veins are narrowed by sarcoid granulomas leading to venous stasis and extensive thrombotic occlusions [21]. Similar Budd–Chiari syndrome has been caused by idiopathic granulomatous venulitis involving hepatic vein radicles [31].

Cholestasis

Rarely patients with sarcoidosis, usually male and Black,

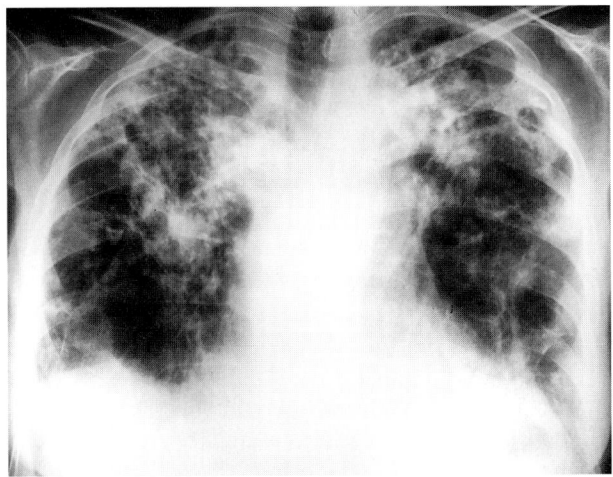

Fig. 26.5. Chronic sarcoidosis with portal hypertension. Chest X-ray of a woman aged 45 shows bilateral, severe, end-stage pulmonary fibrosis.

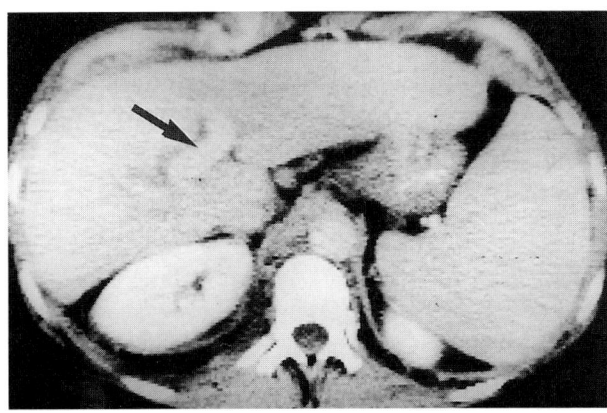

Fig. 26.6. Contrast-enhanced abdominal CT scan from same patient as in fig. 26.5 shows a patent portal vein (arrow) and a large spleen.

show features of chronic intra-hepatic cholestasis [1, 15]. They present with fever, malaise, weight loss, jaundice and usually pruritus. Serum alkaline phosphatase levels are very high and transaminases increased about 2–5 times. Hepatosplenomegaly is usual. Liver biopsy usually shows granulomas. Portal areas contain hepatic arteries but show damaged or even absence of bile ducts (fig. 26.7). The ductopenia can be related to the extent of the fibrosis which may be massive. Sequential liver biopsies show relentless progression of the fibrosis and bile duct loss [15].

ERCP shows tortuous stretched ducts due to the disturbed liver architecture [15]. Rarely the common hepatic duct is involved [12].

The prognosis is poor. The patients usually die within 2–18 years from the onset.

Corticosteroids are not helpful. The usual regime for chronic cholestasis, including ursodeoxycholic acid is used. Eventually hepatic transplantation may be necessary and is well tolerated [3].

The condition may resemble, and even be indistinguishable from, primary biliary cirrhosis (table 14.2).

TUBERCULOSIS

Miliary dissemination accompanies the primary complex, and is also common with chronic adult tuberculosis. Aspiration liver biopsies in patients with tuberculosis have shown positive results in about 25%.

Aspiration biopsy has been used in the diagnosis of tuberculous meningitis when other methods have failed, and also in miliary tuberculosis at the stage of an indeterminate pyrexia. In such cases, Ziehl–Neelsen stains should be performed, and an unfixed portion of the biopsy cultured for tubercle bacilli.

The distinction between these granulomas and those of sarcoidosis may be impossible. Distinctive features of

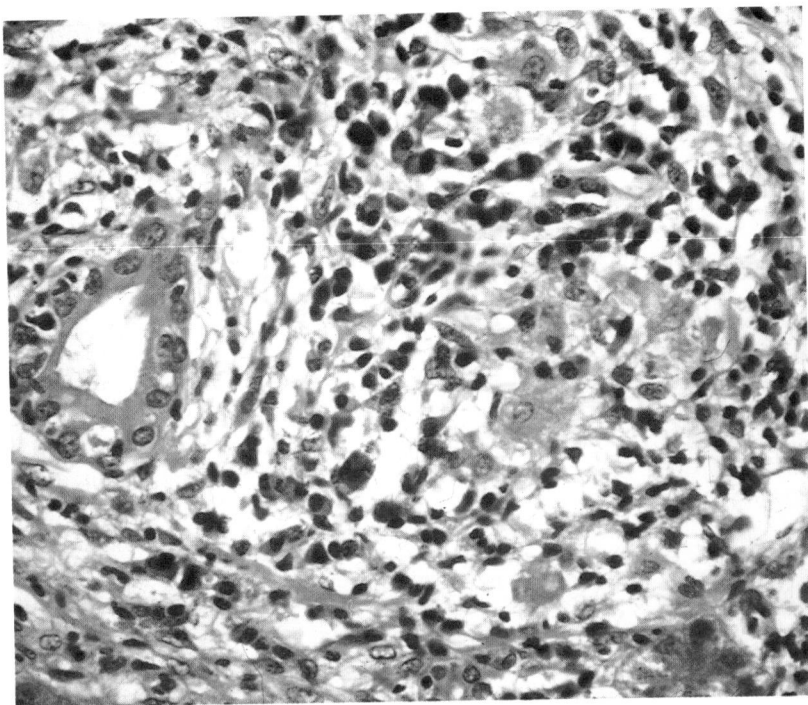

Fig. 26.7. Chronic cholestasis in sarcoidosis. A damaged bile duct is surrounded by an inflammatory infiltrate including lymphocytes. (Stained H & E, ×160.)

tuberculosis are the presence of acid-fast bacilli and caseation with destruction of the reticulin framework. There is irregularity of the contour with a particularly dense cuff of lymphocytes. Less numerous lesions with a tendency to coalesce also suggest tuberculosis.

Miliary granulomas are found after BCG vaccination, especially in the immunosuppressed [6].

Granulomas containing *atypical mycobacteria*, usually *M. avium-intracellulare*, may complicate AIDS (Chapter 27).

BRUCELLOSIS

Hepatic granulomas complicate *Br. abortus* infection. *Br. suis* is more invasive with hepatic suppuration sometimes followed by calcification in the liver and spleen.

Hepatic tenderness and mild elevations of transaminases and alkaline phosphatase may be found in the acute stage [4].

Hepatic histology usually shows a non-specific reactive hepatitis. Granulomas may be associated. These cannot be distinguished from those of sarcoidosis, although they tend to be smaller and less clearly demarcated (fig. 26.8). Healing results in scarring. Brucellosis leads to miliary granulomas and the subsequent healing is never diffuse enough to justify the term cirrhosis.

In *Br. melitensis* the picture may be of scattered inflammatory cells and necrotic hepatocytes without granulomas. *Br. suis* can lead to hepatic abscesses after years of dormancy [30].

A small portion of the unfixed biopsy specimen

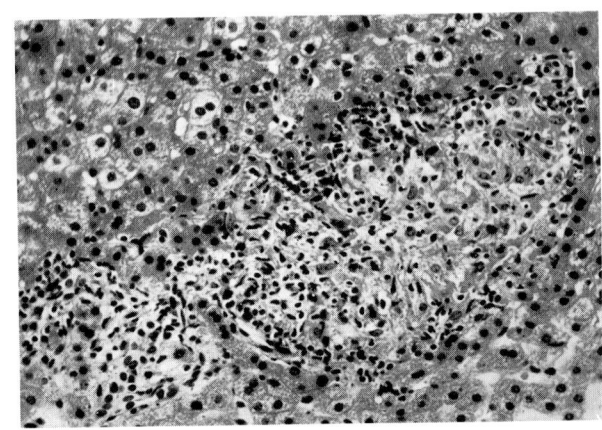

Fig. 26.8. Brucellosis. Granulomas in the liver. The smaller is little more than a collection of round cells. (Stained H & E, ×170.)

should be cultured and is occasionally positive for *Br. abortus* or *Br. melitensis*.

INDUSTRIAL CAUSES

Beryllium poisoning leads to pulmonary granulomas. Hepatic involvement consists of miliary granulomas, as in sarcoidosis.

Pulmonary and hepatic granulomas may be due to inhalation of *cement* and *mica dust* [19] and in vineyard sprayers to *copper* [18].

OTHER CONDITIONS WITH HEPATIC
GRANULOMAS

Similar granulomas are found in the livers of patients suffering from acquired secondary *syphilis*.

In lepromatous *leprosy*, hepatic granulomas indistinguishable from sarcoidosis may be found in 62% of patients compared with the tuberculoid form when only 21% are positive [9]. Lepra bacilli are sometimes present [9].

Histoplasmosis. The liver is second only to the spleen in frequency of involvement. In the granulomatous form, the lesions are histologically identical with those of sarcoidosis, except for the presence of the intra-cellular fungus in the Kupffer cells. Liver biopsy can be used in the diagnosis of histoplasmosis. Sections should be stained for *Histoplasma capsulatum* and an unfixed portion of the biopsy should be cultured. Histoplasmosis leads to discrete hepatic calcification.

Toxoplasmosis may be associated with granulomas, usually without giant cells [17].

Coccidioidomycosis and *blastomycosis* also produce sarcoid-like hepatic granulomas and the organism may be demonstrated.

Q fever. Characteristic 'doughnut' granulomas are seen (see Chapter 27).

Hepatic granulomas can be due to migrating larvae of *Ascaris lumbricoides*. Hepatic granulomas may also be found in children suffering from *Toxocara canis*.

Acute *cytomegalovirus* infection produces a mononucleosis syndrome. Transient well-formed hepatic granulomas may be associated.

Hepatic granulomas may also be seen in *schistosomiasis*, but the presence of ova usually makes the diagnosis easy.

In the early stages of *primary biliary cirrhosis* the liver may show widespread hepatic granulomas. This histological picture may be indistinguishable from sarcoidosis.

Whipple's disease may be accompanied by hepatic granulomas, with bacillary inclusions negative for PAS stain after protein digestion.

NON-SPECIFIC RETICULO-ENDOTHELIAL
PROLIFERATIONS: 'REACTIVE HEPATITIS' [5]

Focal accumulations of mononuclear and epithelioid cells are found in a great variety of diseases. They are perhaps most frequent in virus infections, including infectious mononucleosis, during the recovery phase of virus hepatitis when they contain iron, and in influenza. Occasionally, they are noted in pyogenic infections and septicaemias where polymorphonuclear leucocytes are also present.

Their distinction from small sarcoid granulomas may

be difficult, especially since they may also be seen in sarcoidosis. If such an accumulation of cells is found in a liver biopsy section, the whole block should be sectioned serially to identify typical granulomas.

Generalized proliferation of Kupffer cells is another frequent finding occurring in infections and in malignant disease arising in any part of the body. Generalized Kupffer cell proliferation is also seen in a liver containing local lesions—such as malignant deposits or an amoebic abscess.

The lipogranuloma consists of poorly formed perivenular aggregates of histiocytes and macrophages, some containing fat [29] which can be identified in the granuloma. It is often associated with fatty liver. They are due to deposition of mineral oils used in the food industry.

Microgranulomas consist only of a cluster of six or less histiocytes. They have many associations and probably represent a non-specific reaction to cell necrosis.

Fibrin-ring granulomas are typical of Q fever, but are also seen as a drug reaction to such agents as carbamazepine [13], allopurinol [28], and are also described with acute hepatitis A [20].

Necrotizing or caseating granulomas are small to large, well formed with a necrotic centre. The histiocytic rim often has a palisade pattern and fibrosis is variable. They are associated with fungal infections and rarely with tuberculosis.

References

1 Bass NM, Burroughs AK, Scheuer PJ *et al*. Chronic intrahepatic cholestasis due to sarcoidosis. *Gut* 1982; **23**: 417.

2 Britt AR, Francis IR, Glazer GM *et al*. Sarcoidosis: abdominal manifestations at CT. *Radiology* 1991; **178**: 91.

3 Casavilla FA, Gordon R, Wright HI *et al*. Clinical course after liver transplantation in patients with sarcoidosis. *Ann. Intern. Med.* 1993; **118**: 865.

4 Cervantes F, Bruguera A, Carbonell J *et al*. Liver disease in brucellosis. A clinical and pathological study of 40 cases. *Postgrad. Med. J.* 1982; **58**: 346.

5 Ferrell LD. Hepatic granulomas: a morphologic approach to diagnosis. *Surg. Path.* 1990; **3**: 87.

6 Flipping T, Mukherji B, Dayal Y. Granulomatous hepatitis as a late complication of BCG immunotherapy. *Cancer* 1980; **46**: 1759.

7 James DG. Definition and classification. In: James DG, ed. *Sarcoidosis and Other Granulomatous Disorders*. Marcel Dekker, New York, 1994; 19.

8 Johnson LN, Iseri O, Knodell RG. Caseating hepatic granulomas in Hodgkin's lymphoma. *Gastroenterology* 1990; **99**: 1837.

9 Karat ABA, Job CK, Rao PSS. Liver in leprosy: histological and biochemical findings. *Br. Med. J.* 1971; **i**: 307.

10 Katz B, Weetch M, Chopra S. Quinine-induced granulomatous hepatitis. *Br. Med. J.* 1983; **286**: 264.

11 Knox TA, Kaplan MM, Gelfand JA *et al*. Methotrexate treatment of idiopathic granulomatous hepatitis. *Ann. Intern.*

Med. 1995; **122**: 592.

12 Kusielewicz D, Duchatelle V, Valeyre D *et al.* Obstructive jaundice by granulomatous stenosis of the extrahepatic biliary tract due to sarcoidosis. *Gastroenterol. Clin. Biol.* 1988; **12**: 664.

13 Levy M, Goodman MW, van Dyne BJ *et al.* Granulomatous hepatitis secondary to carbamazepine. *Ann. Intern. Med.* 1981; **95**: 64.

14 Maddrey WC, Johns CJ, Boitnott JK *et al.* Sarcoidosis and chronic hepatic disease: a clinical and pathological study of 20 patients. *Medicine (Baltimore)* 1970; **49**: 375.

15 Murphy JR, Sjogren MH, Kikendall JW *et al.* Small bile duct abnormalities in sarcoidosis. *J. Clin. Gastroenterol.* 1990; **12**: 555.

16 Nakata K, Iwata K, Kujima K *et al.* Computed tomography of liver sarcoidosis. *J. Comput. Assist. Tomogr.* 1989; **13**: 707.

17 Ortego TJ, Robey B, Morrison D *et al.* Toxoplasma chorioretinitis and hepatic granulomas. *Am. J. Gastroenterol.* 1990; **85**: 1418.

18 Pimentel JC, Menezes AP. Liver granulomas containing copper in vineyard sprayer's lung. *Ann. Rev. Respir. Dis.* 1975; **111**: 189.

19 Pimentel JC, Menezes AP. Pulmonary and hepatic granulomatous disorders due to the inhalation of cement and mica dusts. *Thorax* 1978; **33**: 219.

20 Ponz E, García-Pagán JC, Bruguera M *et al.* Hepatic fibrin-ring granulomas in a patient with hepatitis A. *Gastroenterology* 1991; **100**: 268.

21 Russe EW, Bansky G, Pfaltz M *et al.* Budd–Chiari syndrome in sarcoidosis. *Am. J. Gastroenterol.* 1986; **81**: 71.

22 Sartin JS, Walker RC. Granulomatous hepatitis: a retrospective review of 88 cases. *Mayo Clin. Proc.* 1991; **66**: 914.

23 Sherlock S. The liver in sarcoidosis. In: James DG, ed. *Sarcoidosis and Other Granulomatous Disorders.* Marcel Dekker, New York, 1994; 375.

24 Simon HB, Wolff SM. Granulomatous hepatitis and prolonged fever of unknown origin: a study of 13 patients. *Medicine (Baltimore)* 1973; **52**: 1.

25 Spiteri MA, Johnson M, Epstein O *et al.* Immunological features of lung lavage cells from patients with primary biliary cirrhosis may reflect those seen in pulmonary sarcoidosis. *Gut* 1990; **31**: 208.

26 Tekeste H, Latour F, Levitt RE. Portal hypertension complicating sarcoid liver disease: case report and review of the literature. *Am. J. Gastroenterol.* 1984; **79**: 389.

27 Valla D, Pessegueiro-Miranda H, Degott C *et al.* Hepatic sarcoidosis with portal hypertension. A report of seven cases with a review of the literature. *Q. J. Med.* 1987; **63**: 531.

28 Vanderstigel M, Zafrani ES, Lejonc JL *et al.* Allopurinol hypersensitivity syndrome as a cause of hepatic fibrin-ring granulomas. *Gastroenterology* 1986; **9**: 188.

29 Wanless IR, Geddie WR. Mineral oil lipogranulomata in liver and spleen. *Path. Lab. Med.* 1985; **109**: 283.

30 Williams PK, Crossley K. Acute and chronic hepatic involvement of brucellosis. *Gastroenterology* 1982; **83**: 455.

31 Young ID, Clark RN, Manley PN *et al.* Response to steroids in Budd–Chiari syndrome caused by idiopathic granulomatous venulitis. *Gastroenterology* 1988; **94**: 503.

32 Zoutman DE, Ralph ED, Frei JV. Granulomatous hepatitis and fever of unknown origin. An 11-year experience of 23 cases with three years' follow-up. *J. Clin. Gastroenterol.* 1991; **13**: 69.

Hepato-biliary associations of inflammatory bowel disease

In one large clinic over half the patients with ulcerative colitis showed liver functional abnormalities.

The surgeon sees acute fatty liver when operating on patients with fulminant colitis, biliary strictures in those with sclerosing cholangitis, or gallstones in patients with ileal resection. In treating ulcerative colitis the physician sees chronic active (autoimmune) hepatitis or chronic cholestasis in those with peri-cholangitis and sclerosing cholangitis. The pathologist may encounter hepatic granulomas or amyloidosis in a liver biopsy from a patient with inflammatory bowel disease. Involvement of the liver in patients with malabsorption has been discussed in Chapter 23.

Sclerosing cholangitis (Chapter 15) presents in many forms. *Gallstones* are present in up to a third of patients with Crohn's disease of the terminal ileum.

Ulcerative colitis, rarely, has been complicated by the *Budd–Chiari syndrome* [1].

Fatty change. This is very frequent. As with other types of fatty infiltration, the incidence is higher when autopsy rather than biopsy material is used for diagnosis. It may be focal but usually starts in zone 1 and spreads to zone 3. Cirrhosis is not a sequel.

This change is related to the anorexia, anaemia, faecal protein loss and malnutrition of severe colitis.

Carcinoma of the bile ducts (Chapter 34). This has been reported in ulcerative colitis, usually with sclerosing cholangitis. The ulcerative colitis is usually of long standing. The bile duct carcinoma develops independently of the extent and severity of the colitis. It may develop many years after proctocolectomy. It must be considered in any patient with ulcerative colitis developing deep, persistent cholestatic jaundice.

Chronic active hepatitis and cirrhosis. Five per cent of cirrhotic patients have ulcerative colitis, a greater incidence than in the general population. In some the cirrhosis is of chronic autoimmune type. The colitis is then part of the general spectrum of this *multi-system disease.* In these patients, and in contrast to sclerosing cholangitis, the colitis tends to present with the cirrhosis and to be severe but often not subsequently relapsing. The recognition of the cirrhosis may precede the diarrhoea.

In others the cirrhosis is inactive and is diagnosed after many years of chronic relapsing colitis. Initially the colitis is predominant and the cirrhosis mild, but as the years pass the positions reverse.

The cirrhosis might be related to the long course of the illness, many hospital attendances, injections, infusions and blood transfusions, all carrying the hazard of viral hepatitis. This cannot be the whole answer because the cirrhosis may precede the colitis.

The later stages of pericholangitis and sclerosing cholangitis may be associated with piecemeal necrosis of liver cells and scar formation. This can proceed to a biliary cirrhosis.

Primary sclerosing cholangitis is a much more common association than is autoimmune chronic active hepatitis.

Liver abscess. Patients with Crohn's disease may develop liver abscesses, usually multiple and with a predisposing abdominal focus of infection rather than a biliary one [3]. Streptococci, especially *S. milleri*, are often responsible.

Coeliac disease. Non-specific liver lesions are frequent and improve with a gluten-free diet [2]. Chronic hepatitis is also found and shows no dietary response. Steatosis may be massive [4].

References

1 Chesner IM, Muller S, Newman J. Ulcerative colitis complicated by Budd–Chiari syndrome. *Gut* 1986; **27**: 1096.
2 Jacobsen MB, Fausa O, Elgjo K *et al.* Hepatic lesions in adult coeliac disease. *Scand. J. Gastroenterol.* 1990; **25**: 656.
3 Mir-Madjlessi SH, McHenry MC, Farmer RG. Liver abscess in Crohn's disease. Report of four cases and review of the literature. *Gastroenterology* 1986; **91**: 987.
4 Naschitz JE, Yeshurun D, Zuckerman E *et al.* Massive hepatic steatosis complicating adult celiac disease: report of a case and review of the literature. *Am. J. Gastroenterol.* 1987; **82**: 1186.

Hepatic trauma

This is usually due to road traffic accidents, to penetrating wounds from stabbing or to gun shots. It may follow birth injury. Spontaneous rupture can complicate the last trimester of pregnancy usually with toxaemia.

Blunt injury may be due to deceleration (leading to splits and tears from shearing) or to direct violence causing contusion or disruption of the liver substance. It may complicate cardiopulmonary resuscitation [1].

Injury to the hepatic parenchyma is the main problem, and injuries to portal vein, hepatic artery, hepatic vein or retro-hepatic vena cava are rare [6].

Extra-hepatic bile duct injuries are rare, but all types can follow both blunt and penetrating abdominal trauma and of course laparoscopic or conventional cholecystectomy [4].

Diagnosis

This may be difficult as physical signs may be minimal.

Pattern bruising of the abdominal wall indicates severe abdominal compression.

Diagnostic peritoneal aspiration [5], ultrasonography and CT scanning are invaluable. CT may show laceration, sub-capsular fluid (blood or bile) and fragmentation (fig. 26.9). Hepatic parenchymal gas may indicate infection but may also be seen simply after blunt trauma [13].

The possibility of other organs being damaged, such as spleen, intestines, lungs, kidneys, or the coincidence of head injuries and fractures, must be remembered.

Blunt abdominal trauma may lead to haemobilia, usually secondary to hepatic arterial aneurysm (see Chapter 11) [14]. Angiography is a necessary investigation.

HIDA biliary scans show bile leaks (Chapter 29).

In children, blunt abdominal trauma results in injury to the liver, usually the right lobe and frequently posteriorly [19]. Associated thoracic injuries are common.

Management

This depends on the type of injury, the extent and the haemodynamic stability of the patient (table 26.3) [2, 12]. Gun shot wounds require abdominal exploration. Stable patients with anterior stab wounds require local exploration followed by laparotomy if the anterior fascia is violated. Indications for surgery following blunt trauma include positive peritoneal lavage, abnormal CT scan and abdominal tenderness. Surgery can be avoided in some patients if observation is close and the patient haemodynamically stable [3].

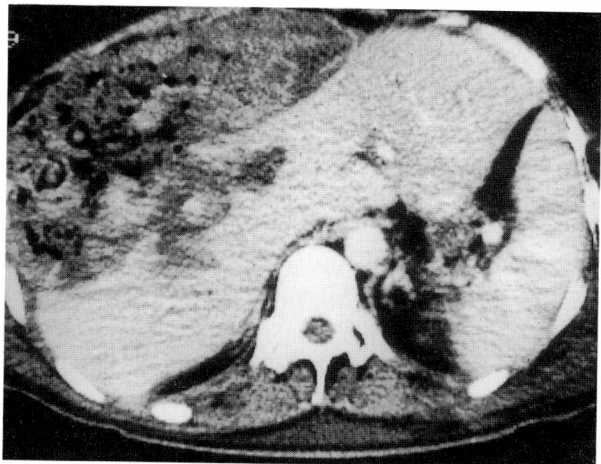

Fig. 26.9. CT (intravenous contrast enhanced) of a patient with a gun shot injury to the anterior part of the liver. A low attenuation haematoma with disorganized liver tissue and gas indicates infection. Successful treatment was by drainage of pus, debridement, and gel foam angiographic embolization of a feeding hepatic artery branch.

Table 26.3. Severity of liver injury graded according to the American Association for the Surgery of Trauma hepatic injury scale [2]

Grade*		Injury description†
I	Haematoma	Subcapsular, non-expanding, <10% surface area
	Laceration	Capsular tear, non-bleeding, <1 cm parenchymal depth
II	Haematoma	Subcapsular, non-expanding, 10–50% surface area
	Laceration	Capsular tear, active bleeding; 1–3 cm parenchymal depth, <10 cm in length
III	Haematoma	Subcapsular, >50% surface area or expanding; ruptured subcapsular haematoma with active bleeding; intraparenchymal haematoma >2 cm or expanding
	Laceration	>3 cm parenchymal depth
IV	Haematoma	Ruptured intraparenchymal haematoma with active bleeding
	Laceration	Parenchymal disruption involving 25–50% of hepatic lobe
V	Laceration	Parenchymal disruption involving >50% of hepatic lobe
	Vascular	Juxtahepatic venous, injuries, i.e. retrohepatic vena cava/major hepatic veins
VI	Vascular	Hepatic avulsion

* Advance one grade for multiple injuries to the same organ.
† Based on most accurate assessment at autopsy, laparotomy or radiological study.

Most liver injuries require only minor therapy. Mild splits, lacerations and penetrating wounds can usually be managed by simple haemostasis and drainage. If CT shows minimal or absent haemoperitoneum and an intact or nearly intact hepatic capsule surgical intervention will not be necessary. Deeper lacerations with tearing of intra-hepatic vessels and bile ducts are treated by ligating the bleeding vessels and repairing the liver with deep sutures. Omental packing may be helpful, and gauze used when omentum is unavailable.

If surgical treatment is impossible at a local centre, the patient should be transferred immediately to a specialized unit where definitive operative treatment can be carried out. In general, packing should be avoided as this increases the mortality, particularly from abscess.

Porta-hepatis injuries are rare and control of bleeding is of prime importance [17]. Bleeding is controlled by digital compression of the hepatic artery and portal vein in the lesser omentum. Selective hepatic arteriography is useful in defining treatment. Hepatic arterial embolization with gel foam must be considered (fig. 26.9).

Repair of major venous injuries requires adequate exposure. The mid-line abdominal incision is extended, cephalad, and a median sternal split made. This allows control of the hepatic vein and any tear of the subdiaphragmatic inferior vena cava. Repairs of the inferior vena cava or hepatic vein are sutured or side-clamped. Portal vein injuries are rare and are nearly always associated with pancreatic rupture [7]. They have the worst prognosis. They are treated by suture or end-to-side portal-caval anastomosis or, if necessary, acute portal vein ligation [9].

In the majority of cases hepatic trauma can be managed by local pressure and aggressive debridement with hepatic segmentectomy. With damaged liver exposed, ragged areas of questionable viability can be excised, local haemostasis obtained and efficient drainage established. Excellent results have been noted after resection of as much as 400 g of liver tissue. Hepatic resection and lobectomy are required in only a small number of cases.

Repeated ultrasound examinations are important in following the patient.

Post-operative complications include coagulopathy, sepsis, biliary fistula and stricture and late haemorrhage [10]. Abscess is a late and often fatal complication [15]. Diagnosis of bile duct injuries is difficult and may be delayed [4]. Endoscopic therapy with sphincterotomy and biliary stenting is usually effective, but more serious injuries require surgical relief [11].

Prognosis

The overall mortality is 10.5% with 78.1% of all deaths occurring in the post-operative period from shock or coagulopathies [6]. Penetrating wounds have a lower mortality than blunt ones. This is largely due to the greater magnitude of associated injury [2]. The mortality following major penetrating liver injury in an urban setting is 17% [10].

The prognosis depends on the extent of the injury and the number of organs involved. Injuries to the hepatic veins, portal vein or retro-hepatic inferior vena cava are highly lethal. Hepatic venous injuries, usually due to blunt trauma, have a 61% mortality usually due to blood loss [8].

Abscess is related to increase in severity of trauma and to transfusion requirements [2].

RUPTURE OF THE GALLBLADDER

Rupture or contusion of the gallbladder can follow blunt trauma [18]. It is rare because the gallbladder is cushioned by surrounding bony and visceral structures. The gallbladder is usually distended at the time of rupture. Early diagnosis is difficult. The condition is recognized by fever, jaundice, increasing distension and ascites.

Paracentesis shows bile-stained fluid. Later, encysted bile accumulations are recognized by ultrasound and CT scanning. The perforation is confirmed by percutaneous or endoscopic cholangiography. HIDA scanning is useful.

Treatment is by cholecystectomy.

References

1 Adler SN, Klein RA, Pellechia C *et al.* Massive hepatic hemorrhage associated with cardiopulmonary resuscitation. *Arch. Intern. Med.* 1983; **143**: 813.

2 Fabian TC, Croce MA, Stanford GG *et al.* Factors affecting morbidity following hepatic trauma. A prospective analysis of 482 injuries. *Ann. Surg.* 1991; **213**: 540.

3 Federico JA, Horner WR, Clark DE *et al.* Blunt hepatic trauma: Nonoperative management in adults. *Arch. Surg.* 1990; **125**: 905.

4 Feliciano DV. Biliary injuries as a result of blunt and penetrating trauma. *Surg. Clin. North Am.* 1994; **74**: 897.

5 Feliciano DV, Bitondo CG, Steed G *et al.* Five hundred open taps or lavages in patients with abdominal stab wounds. *Am. J. Surg.* 1984; **148**: 772.

6 Feliciano DV, Jordan GL Jr, Bitondo CG *et al.* Management of 1000 consecutive cases of hepatic trauma (1979–1984). *Ann. Surg.* 1986; **204**: 438.

7 Henne-Bruns D, Kremer B, Lloyd DM *et al.* Injuries of the portal vein in patients with blunt abdominal trauma. *HPB Surg.* 1993; **6**: 163.

8 Hollands MJ, Little JM. Hepatic venous injury after blunt abdominal trauma. *Surgery* 1990; **107**: 149.

9 Ivatury RR, Nallathambi M, Gunduz Y *et al.* Liver packing for uncontrolled haemorrhage: a reappraisal. *J. Trauma* 1986; **26**: 744.

10 Knudson MM, Lim RC, Olcott EW. Morbidity and mortality following major penetrating liver injuries. *Arch. Surg.* 1994; **129**: 256.

11 Kozarek RA. Endoscopic techniques in management of biliary tract injuries. *Surg. Clin. North Am.* 1994; **74**: 883.

12 Moore EE, Shackford SR, Pachter HL *et al.* Organ injury scaling: spleen, liver, and kidney. *J. Trauma* 1989; **29**: 1664.

13 Panicek DM, Paquet DJ, Clark KG *et al.* Hepatic parenchymal gas after blunt trauma. *Radiology* 1986; **159**: 343.

14 Sax SL, Athey PA, Lamki N *et al.* Sonographic findings in traumatic hemobilia: report of two cases and review of the literature. *J. Clin. Ultrasound* 1988; **16**: 29.

15 Scott CM, Grasberger RC, Heeran TF. Intra-abdominal sepsis after hepatic trauma. *Am. J. Surg.* 1988; **155**: 284.

16 Shanmuganathan K, Mirvis SE. CT evaluation of the liver with acute blunt trauma. *Crit. Rev. Diagn. Imaging* 1995; **36**: 73.

17 Sheldon GF, Lim RC, Yee ES *et al.* Management of injuries to the porta hepatis. *Ann. Surg.* 1985; **202**: 539.

18 Soderstrom CA, Maekawa K, Du Priest RW Jr *et al.* Gallbladder injuries resulting from blunt abdominal trauma. *Ann. Surg.* 1981; **193**: 60.

19 Stalker HP, Kaufman RA, Towbin R. Patterns of liver injury in childhood: CT analysis. *Am. J. Roentgenol.* 1986; **147**: 1199.

Chapter 27
The Liver in Infections

Pyogenic liver abscess

Pyogenic liver abscess used to be due to portal infection, often in young people secondary to acute appendicitis. This is less frequent, because of earlier diagnosis and treatment. Abscesses secondary to obstruction and infection of the biliary tree, and affecting an older age group, have, however, continued to increase. Immunosuppression as in AIDS, intensive chemotherapy or transplant recipients is increasing the number due to opportunist organisms.

Earlier diagnosis has followed increased use of scanning and cholangiographic techniques. Failures are usually due to the clinician not considering the diagnosis.

Classification

Portal pyaemia

Pelvic or gastrointestinal infection may result in portal pylephlebitis or in septic emboli. This may follow appendicitis [4], empyema of the gallbladder, diverticulitis, regional enteritis [19], *Yersinia* ileitis [9], perforated gastric or colonic ulcers, leaking anastomoses, pancreatitis [1] or infected haemorrhoids.

Neonatal umbilical vein sepsis may spread to the portal vein with subsequent hepatic abscesses.

Biliary

The biliary tree is the commonest source of infection. Septic cholangitis can complicate any form of biliary obstruction, especially if partial. The abscesses are commonly multiple. Causes include gallstones, cancer, sclerosing cholangitis and congenital biliary anomalies especially Caroli's disease. Abscess may follow biliary procedures such as stent insertion, stricture repair [17] or reflux of intestinal contents following biliary/enteric anastomoses [13, 18] when it may be surprisingly indolent.

Direct infection

Solitary liver abscess may follow a penetrating wound or direct spread from an adjacent septic focus such as a perinephric abscess. It may follow secondary infection of an amoebic abscess, metastasis, cyst or intrahepatic haematoma. Automobile accidents or other blunt trauma may lead to hepatic abscess formation.

Miscellaneous

Iatrogenic causes include liver biopsy, percutaneous biliary drainage or hepatic artery injury or perfusion. It may affect patients with haematological diseases such as leukaemia who are receiving chemotherapy [3]. Underlying malignancy is important and may be associated with fungal infection; amphotericin may be useful [11].

Where there is no obvious cause diabetes, often with gas-forming organisms (*Klebsiella*), must be considered [20].

Severe dental disease can be associated [6].

About one half have no obvious predisposing cause. This is especially so in the elderly.

Bacteriology

The commonest infecting organisms are Gram-negative. *Escherichia coli* is found in two-thirds. *Streptococcus faecalis*, *Klebsiella* and *Proteus vulgaris* are also frequent. Recurrent pyogenic cholangitis may be due to *Salmonella typhi*.

Anaerobic organisms have become increasingly important.

Streptococcus milleri Lancefield group F, which is neither a true anaerobe nor a microaerobe, is a very common cause [16].

Staphylococci are found in nearly half, especially in those who have received chemotherapy, when they are usually resistant. Friedländer's bacillus, *Pseudomonas* and *Clostridium welchii* may also be found.

Rare causes include *Yersinia enterocolitica* [9] septicaemic melioidosis and *Pasteurella multocida* [5].

Infection is often multiple.

The abscess may be sterile, but this is usually due to

lack of adequate, particularly anaerobic, culture techniques or to previous antibiotics.

Pathology

The enlarged liver may contain multiple yellow abscesses, 1 cm in diameter, or a single abscess encased in fibrous tissue.

When there is an associated pylephlebitis, the portal vein and its branches may contain pus and blood clots (fig. 27.1). The abscesses are particularly in the right lobe. There may be peri-hepatitis or adhesion formation.

In bacteroides infections, the pus has a foul odour and the abscess wall is ill defined.

When infection is spread by the bile ducts, multiple foci correspond to the bile duct system.

A chronic solitary liver abscess may persist for as long as 2 years before death or diagnosis.

There may be small pyaemic abscesses elsewhere, such as lungs, kidneys, brain and spleen. Direction extension from the liver may lead to subphrenic or pleuro-pulmonary suppuration. Extension to the peritoneum or rupture of a sinus pointing under the skin are rare. A small amount of ascites is present in about a third of patients.

Histologically, areas remote from the abscess show infection in the portal tracts surrounding disintegrating liver cells being infiltrated by polymorphs.

Clinical features

In the pre-antibiotic era, the picture was of spiking fever and right upper quadrant pain, often with prostration and shock. Nowadays the presentation is less acute, with malaise, low-grade fever and dull abdominal pain increased by movement. It is particularly likely to be occult in the elderly.

The onset may be insidious and the duration at least one month before diagnosis. Multiple abscesses are associated with more acute systemic features and the cause is more often identified. The single abscess is more insidious and often 'cryptogenic'. If there is subdiaphragmatic irritation or pleuro-pulmonary spread of infection, the patient may complain of right shoulder pain and an irritating cough. The liver is enlarged and tender, and pain may be accentuated by percussion over the lower rib cage.

The spleen is palpable in chronic cases. Detectable ascites is rare. Jaundice is late unless there is suppurative cholangitis.

Recovery may be followed by portal hypertension due to thrombosis of the portal vein.

Investigations

Jaundice is usually mild except in the cholangitic types. It is more common than with amoebic abscess.

Serum alkaline phosphatase is usually raised. The ESR is very high. Polymorph leucocytosis is usual.

Blood cultures show the causative organism or organisms in 50% [2].

Fluoroscopic examination

This may show a high, immobile, right diaphragm, with alterations in contour and a pleural effusion. A penetrated film may show a fluid level, indicating gas-producing organisms.

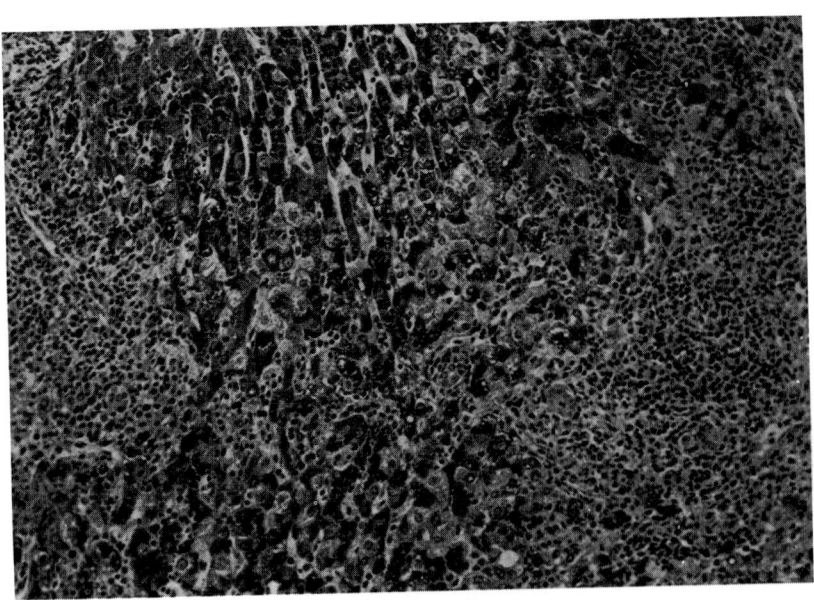

Fig. 27.1. Pylephlebitis complicating acute appendicitis. The portal tracts show an acute inflammatory exudate in which polymorphonuclear leucocytes are conspicuous. The walls of the portal vein radicles are thickened and the lining epithelium is desquamating. The inflammatory cells are invading the adjoining liver parenchyma and the periportal liver cells are necrosing. Culture of this biopsy grew *E. coli*. (Stained Best's carmine, ×145.)

Localization of the abscess

Ultrasound distinguishes a solid from a fluid-filled lesion (fig. 27.2). *CT scanning* is particularly valuable although false-negatives can be due to lesions near the dome of the liver and to micro-abscesses (figs 27.3, 27.4, 27.5). Multiple small abscesses aggregate suggesting the beginning of coalescence into single larger abscesses (*cluster sign*) [8].

Endoscopic or percutaneous cholangiography may be used to diagnose cholangitic abscesses.

MRI shows a raised lesion with sharp borders, hypo-intense on T_1-weighting, hyper-intense on a T_2-weighted

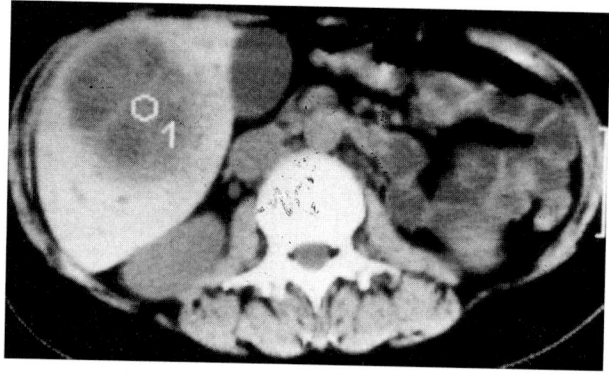

Fig. 27.3. Thalassaemic Greek patient post-splenectomy. CT scan shows a filling defect in the right lobe of the liver with marker over it (1).

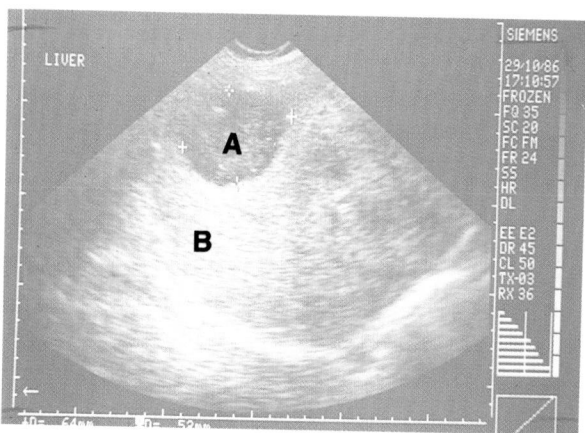

Fig. 27.2. Ultrasound of a pyogenic liver abscess shows a low-density lesion (A) containing echogenic material which is pus and necrotic tissue. Acoustic enhancement (B) beyond the lesion is characteristic.

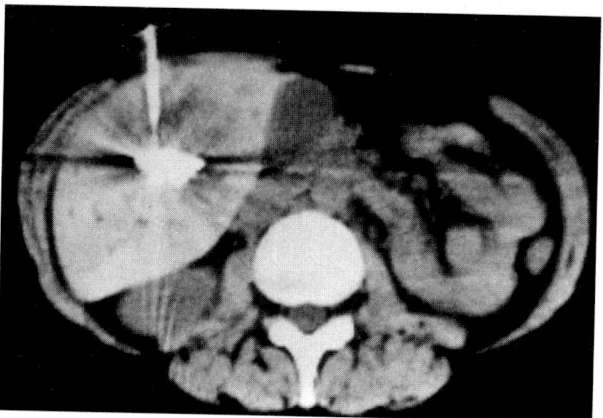

Fig. 27.4. Same patient as in fig. 27.3 with directed puncture of the abscess which resolved without surgery.

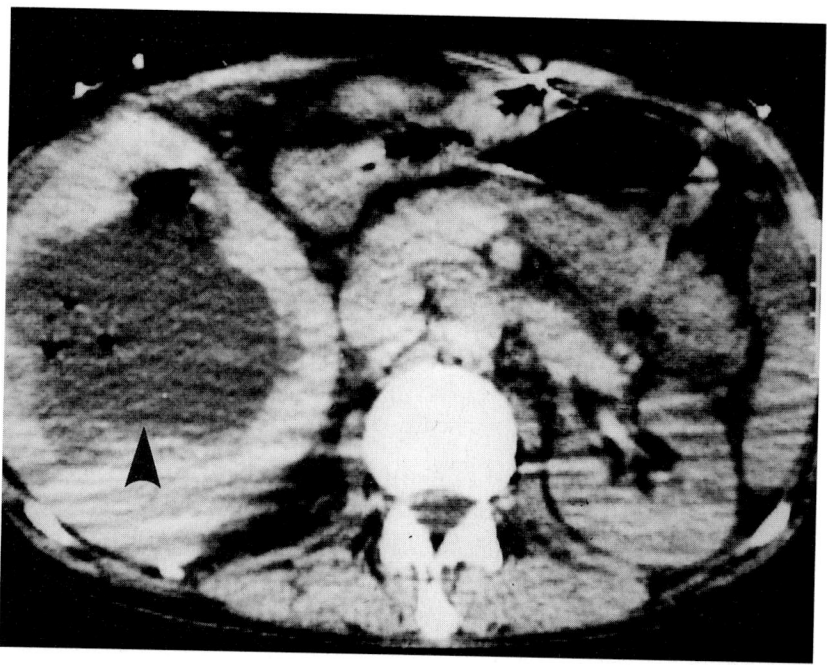

Fig. 27.5. CT shows a large pyogenic abscess with thick shaggy walls in the inferior part of the right lobe of the liver (arrow). The abscess contains gas.

image. Appearances are not specific or diagnostic of biliary or haematogenous origin [14].

Aspirated material is positive in 90% [2]. It should be cultured aerobically, anaerobically and in carbon dioxide enriched media for *Strep. milleri*. Ultrasound or CT guided percutaneous needle (22–16 gauge) aspiration is usually effective. It is repeated if necessary every 3–7 days [7].

Treatment

Prevention is by early treatment of acute biliary and abdominal infections and the adequate drainage, usually percutaneous, of intra-abdominal purulent collections under antibiotic cover.

Intravenous antibiotics are rarely effective alone, and should not postpone mandatory drainage. The choice is dependent on the causative organism.

Once a single abscess is localized, it must be drained. If amoebiasis is suspected, metronidazole should be given before aspiration [7].

Sometimes a percutaneously inserted pigtail catheter is necessary for drainage.

With multiple abscesses, the largest is aspirated and the smaller lesions usually resolve with chemotherapy. Occasionally, percutaneous drainage of each is necessary.

High-dose antibiotics alone, given for at least 6 months, may be successful particularly if the infection is streptococcal [12].

Open surgical drainage is rarely indicated. However, solitary left-sided abscess requires surgical drainage especially in children [15].

Biliary obstruction must be relieved. This is usually done by ERCP, papillotomy and stone removal. If necessary a biliary endoprosthesis is inserted (Chapter 29).

Even with eventual cure, fever may continue for 1–2 weeks [2].

Prognosis

The advent of needle aspiration and antibiotic therapy has lowered the mortality to 16% [3]. The prognosis is better for a unilocular abscess in the right lobe where survival is 90%. The outcome for multiple abscesses throughout the liver, especially if biliary, is very poor: only 20% survive.

The prognosis is made worse by delay in diagnosis, continued fever, multiple infections shown by blood culture, hyperbilirubinaemia, associated diseases, hypoalbuminaemia, pleural effusion and old age [10].

References

1 Ammann R, Münch R, Largiadèr F *et al.* Pancreatic and hepatic abscesses: a late complication in 10 patients with chronic pancreatitis. *Gastroenterology* 1992; **103**: 560.

2 Barnes PF, DeCock KM, Reynolds TN *et al.* A comparison of amebic and pyogenic abscesses of the liver. *Medicine (Baltimore)* 1987; **66**: 472.

3 Branum GD, Tyson GS, Branum MA *et al.* Hepatic abscess. Changes in etiology, diagnosis, and management. *Ann. Surg.* 1990; **212**: 655.

4 Case Records of the Massachusetts General Hospital. *N. Engl. J. Med.* 1991; **324**: 1575.

5 Cortez JC, Shapiro M, Awe RJ. *Pasteurella multocida* liver abscess. *Am. J. Med. Sci.* 1986; **292**: 107.

6 Crippin JS, Wang KK. An unrecognised etiology for pyogenic hepatic abscesses in normal hosts: dental disease. *Am. J. Gastroenterol.* 1992; **7**: 1740.

7 Giorgio A, Tarantino L, Mariniello N *et al.* Pyogenic liver abscesses: 13 years of experience in percutaneous needle aspiration with US guidance. *Radiology* 1995; **195**: 122.

8 Jeffrey RB Jr, Tolentino CS, Chang FC *et al.* CT of small pyogenic hepatic abscesses: the cluster sign. *Am. J. Roentgenol.* 1988; **151**: 487.

9 Khanna R, Levendoglu H. Liver abscess due to *Yersinia enterocolitica*: case report and review of the literature. *Dig. Dis. Sci.* 1989; **34**: 636.

10 Lee K-T, Sheen P-C, Chen J-S *et al.* Pyogenic liver abscess: multivariate analysis of risk factors. *World J. Surg.* 1991; **15**: 372.

11 Marcus SG, Walsh TJ, Pizzo PA *et al.* Hepatic abscess in cancer patients. Characterization and management. *Arch. Surg.* 1993; **128**: 1358.

12 Matlow A, Vellend H. Medical treatment of multiple streptococcal liver abscesses. *J. Clin. Gastroenterol.* 1983; **5**: 143.

13 Matthews JB, Gertsch P, Baer HU *et al.* Hepatic abscess after biliary tract procedures. *Surg. Gynecol. Obstet.* 1990; **170**: 469.

14 Méndez RJ, Schiebler ML, Outwater EK *et al.* Hepatic abscesses: MR imaging findings. *Radiology* 1994; **190**: 431.

15 Moore SW, Millar AJ, Cywes S. Conservative initial treatment for liver abscesses in children. *Br. J. Surg.* 1994; **81**: 872.

16 Moore-Gillon JC, Eykyn SJ, Phillips I. Microbiology of pyogenic liver abscess. *Br. Med. J.* 1981; **283**: 819.

17 Reddy KR, Jeffers L, Livingstone AS *et al.* Pyogenic liver abscess complicating common bile duct stenosis secondary to chronic calcific pancreatitis. *Gastroenterology* 1984; **86**: 953.

18 Rumans MC, Katon RM, Lowe DK. Hepatic abscesses as a complication of the sump syndrome: combined surgical and endoscopic therapy. Case report and review of the literature. *Gastroenterology* 1987; **92**: 791.

19 Vakil N, Hayne G, Sharma A *et al.* Liver abscess in Crohn's disease. *Am. J. Gastroenterol.* 1994; **89**: 1090.

20 Yang CC, Chen CY, Lin XZ *et al.* Pyogenic liver abscess in Taiwan: emphasis on gasforming liver abscess in diabetics. *Am. J. Gastroenterol.* 1993; **88**: 1911.

Other infections

Giardiasis is rarely associated with hepatic granulomas and cholangitis [4].

Campylobacter colitis can be related to a non-specific acute hepatitis [3].

Cat scratch disease is believed to be due to a pleomorphic bacillus. It causes hepatic nodules, biopsy of which reveals necrotizing granulomas containing the organism [2]. CT shows focal hepatic defects and mediastinal and peri-portal lymphadenopathy [5].

Listeria monocytogenes can cause liver abscesses [1].

References

1 Jenkins D, Richards JE, Rees Y *et al.* Multiple listerial liver abscesses. *Gut* 1987; **28**: 1661.
2 Lenoir AA, Storch GA, De Schryver-Kecskemeti K *et al.* Granulomatous hepatitis associated with cat scratch disease. *Lancet* 1988; **i**: 1132.
3 Reddy KR, Farnum JB, Thomas E. Acute hepatitis associated with campylobacter colitis. *J. Clin. Gastroenterol.* 1983; **5**: 259.
4 Roberts-Thomas JC, Anders RF, Bhathal PS. Granulomatous hepatitis and cholangitis associated with giardiasis. *Gastroenterology* 1982; **83**: 480.
5 Rocco VK, Roman RJ, Eigenbrodt EH. Cat scratch disease. Report of a case with hepatic lesions and a brief review of the literature. *Gastroenterology* 1985; **89**: 1400.

Hepatic amoebiasis

Entamoeba histolytica exists in a vegetative form and as cysts, which survive outside the body and are highly infectious. The cystic form passes unharmed through the stomach and small intestine and changes into the vegetative, trophozoite form in the colon. Here, it invades the mucosa, forming typical flask-shaped ulcers. Amoebae are carried to the liver in the portal venous system. Occasionally, they pass through the hepatic sinusoids into the systemic circulation with the production of abscesses in lungs and brain.

Amoebae multiply and block small intra-hepatic portal radicles with consequent focal infarction of liver cells. They contain a proteolytic enzyme which destroys the liver parenchyma. The lesions produced are single or multiple and of variable size.

The amoebic abscess is usually about the size of an orange. The most frequent site is in the right lobe, often supero-anteriorly, just below the diaphragm. The centre consists of a large necrotic area which has liquefied into thick, reddish-brown pus. This has been likened to anchovy or chocolate sauce. It is not strictly pus because it is produced by lysis of liver cells. Fragments of liver tissue may be recognized in it. Initially, the abscess has no well-defined wall, but merely shreds of shaggy, necrotic liver tissue. Histologically, the necrotic areas consist of degenerate liver cells, leucocytes, red blood cells, connective tissue strands and debris. Amoebae may be identified in scrapings from the wall.

Small lesions heal with scars, but larger abscesses show a chronic wall of connective tissue of varying age.

The lesion is focal and liver away from the abscess or micro-abscesses is normal.

Many factors determine the balance between healing and progression. The virulence and resistance of the host must play a part. In isolates, pathogenic amoebae may be distinguished from non-pathogenic by DNA markers to antigens on the surface [6].

Only 10% of asymptomatic subjects harbouring pathogenic *E. histolytica* will develop invasive amoebiasis.

Secondary bacterial infection occurs in about 20%. The pus then becomes green or yellow and foul smelling.

Epidemiology

Colonic amoebae have a world-wide distribution, but hepatic amoebiasis is a disease of the tropics and sub-tropics. Endemic areas are Africa, South-East Asia, Mexico, Venezuela and Colombia.

In temperate climates, symptomless carriers of toxic strains are found but colonic ulcers are not seen. It is a frequent commensal in homosexual men [3].

In the tropics a new arrival is heavily exposed. Spread of infection by faeces is easier when sanitation is poor. Locals are less prone to hepatic amoebiasis than Europeans, presumably because of partial immunity induced by repeated contact.

The latent period between the intestinal infection and hepatic involvement has not been explained.

Clinical features

Note must be made of any residence or illness suffered in tropical or subtropical areas. Amoebic dysentery is present in only 10% and cysts in the stool of only 15% of patients with hepatic amoebiasis. A past history of dysentery is rare. Hepatic amoebiasis has been recorded as long as 30 years after the primary bowel infection. It is most frequent in young males aged 28–50. Multiple abscesses are frequent in such areas as Mexico and Taiwan.

The onset is usually *sub-acute* with symptoms lasting up to 6 months. Rarely it may be *acute* with rigors and sweating and a duration of less than 10 days. Fever is variously intermittent, remittent or even absent unless an abscess becomes secondarily infected; it rarely exceeds 40°C. Deep abscesses may present simply as fever without signs referable to the liver.

Jaundice is unusual and, if present, mild. Bile duct compression with large and multiple abscesses may lead to jaundice as a presentation.

The patient looks ill, with a peculiar sallowness of the skin, like faded suntan.

Pain in the liver area may commence as a dull ache, later becoming sharp and stabbing. If the abscess is near the diaphragm, there may be referred shoulder pain accentuated by deep breathing or coughing. Alcohol makes the pain worse, as do postural changes. The patient tends to lean to the left side; this opens up the right intercostal spaces and diminishes the tension on the liver capsule. The pain increases at night.

A swelling may be visible in the epigastrium or bulging the intercostal spaces. Hepatic tenderness is virtually constant. It may be elicited over a palpable liver edge or by percussion over the lower right chest wall. The spleen is not enlarged.

The lungs may show consolidation of the right lower zone, pleurisy or an effusion. Pleural fluid may be blood stained.

Examination of faeces. Cysts and vegetative forms are rare.

Serological tests

These remain positive for some time after a clinical cure. However, an amoebic abscess is unlikely to be present if serological tests are negative [5]. The indirect haemagglutination test is sensitive and valuable in community surveys.

Biochemical tests

In chronic cases, serum alkaline phosphatase values are usually about twice normal. Increases in transaminases are found only in those who are acutely ill or with severe complications. A rise in serum bilirubin is unusual except in those with superinfection or rupture into the peritoneum.

Radiological features

Chest radiographs may show a high right diaphragm, obliteration of the costo-phrenic and cardio-phrenic angles by adhesions, pleural effusions or right basal pneumonia. Perpendicular string-like adhesions may pass from the diaphragm to the lung base. A right lateral abscess may cause widening of the intercostal spaces. A central or inferior abscess may show few signs. The liver shadow may be enlarged with a raised immobile right diaphragm (fig. 27.6). The abscess commonly causes a bulge in the antero-medial part of the right diaphragm.

An abscess in the left lobe of the liver may show a crescentic deformity of the lesser curve of the stomach.

Ultrasound (fig. 27.7) is most useful in diagnosis and in following progress [9]. *CT* shows the abscess with a somewhat irregular edge and lower attenuation than the surrounding liver. It is more sensitive than ultrasound for small abscesses. It is particularly useful for showing extra-hepatic involvement, for instance in the lung [7]. *MR* imaging can be used for diagnosis and to follow treatment [2]. Liquefaction of the cavity may be shown as early as 4 days after starting treatment [2].

Arteriography shows an avascular mass, with distortion of the normal vascular architecture.

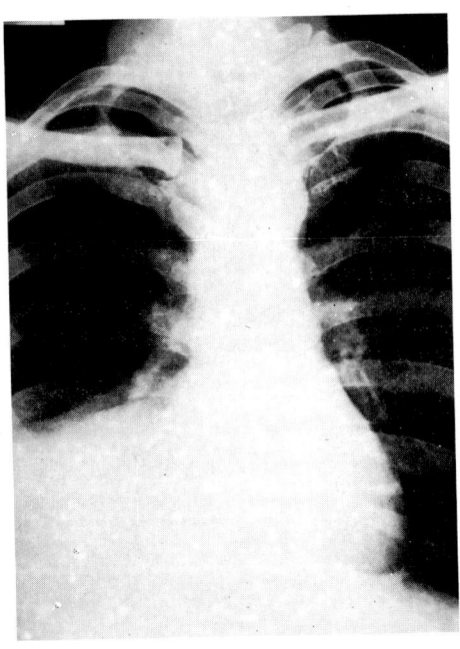

Fig. 27.6. Amoebic abscess of liver. Note the elevated right diaphragm with overlying reaction in the lung field.

Diagnostic criteria

1 History of residence in an endemic area.
2 An enlarged tender liver in a young male.
3 Response to metronidazole.
4 Leucocytosis without anaemia in those with a short history, and less marked leucocytosis and anaemia with a long history.
5 Suggestive postero-anterior and lateral chest X-ray.
6 Scanning showing a filling defect.
7 A positive amoebic indirect haemagglutination test.

Complications

Two-thirds of ruptures are intra-peritoneal and one-third intra-thoracic [4].

Rupture into the lungs or pleura causes empyema, hepato-bronchial fistula or pulmonary abscess. The patient coughs up pus, develops pneumonitis or lung abscess or a pleural effusion.

Rupture into the pericardium is a complication of amoebic abscess in the left lobe.

Intra-peritoneal rupture results in acute peritonitis. If the patient survives the initial effect, long-term results are good. Abscesses of the left lobe may perforate into the lesser sac.

Rupture into the portal vein, bile ducts or gastrointestinal tract is rare.

Secondary infection is suspected if prostration is particularly great, and fever and leucocytosis high. Aspira-

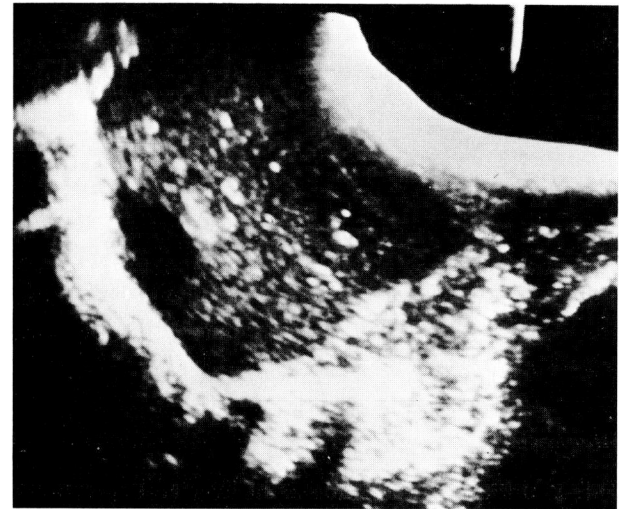

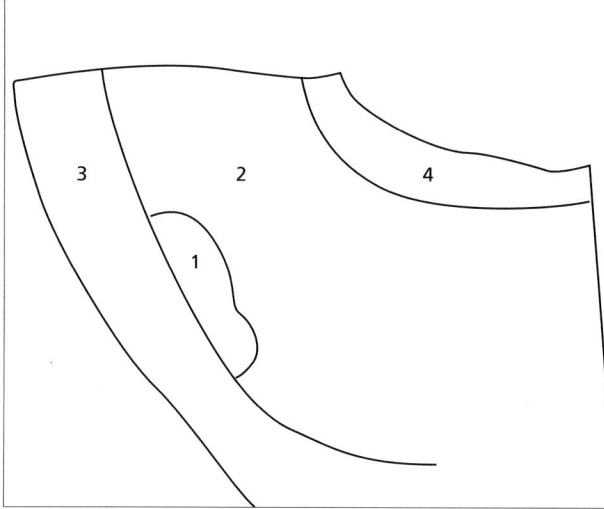

Fig. 27.7. Amoebic liver abscess. Ultrasound demonstrates an amoebic abscess (1) in the liver (2) lying posteriorly against the diaphragm (3). The anterior abdominal wall (4) is also shown.

tion reveals yellowish, often fetid, pus and culture reveals the causative organism.

Treatment

Metronidazole, 750 mg three times a day for 5–10 days, is the treatment of choice having a 95% success rate. An intravenous preparation is available. The time to defervescence is 3–5 days [1]. Failures may be related to persistence of intestinal amoebiasis, drug resistance or inadequate absorption.

The time taken for the abscess to disappear depends on its size and varies from 10 to 300 days [9].

A controlled trial showed no advantage of metronidazole with needle aspiration over metronidazole alone [8].

Aspiration may be necessary with very large abscesses or where there is lack of response to 5 days of metronidazole treatment; it should be done under ultrasound or CT guidance. The needle should be at least 10 cm long of 1–2 mm diameter and with a fitted stilette. A tense abscess in the left lobe that is likely to rupture into the peritoneum demands aspiration. The mortality for amoebic liver abscess should be zero [1].

A course of a luminal amoebocide such as diloxanide furoate (500 mg three times a day for 10 days) or iodoquinol (650 mg three times a day for 20 days) should be given to cover amoebae persisting in the gut.

References

1 Barnes PF, De Cock KM, Reynolds TB *et al.* A comparison of amebic and pyogenic abscess of the liver. *Medicine* 1987; **66**: 472.

2 Elizondo G, Weissleder R, Stark DD *et al.* Amebic liver abscess: diagnosis and treatment evaluation with MR imaging. *Radiology* 1987; **165**: 795.

3 Goldmeier D, Sargeaunt PG, Price AB *et al.* Is *Entamoeba histolytica* in homosexual men a pathogen? *Lancet* 1986; **i**: 641.

4 Greaney GC, Reynolds TB, Donovan AJ. Ruptured amebic liver abscess. *Arch. Surg.* 1985; **120**: 555.

5 Greenstein AJ, Sachar DB. Pyogenic and amebic abscesses of the liver. *Semin. Liver Dis.* 1988; **8**: 210.

6 Katwinkel-Wladarsch S, Lascher T, Rinder H. Direct amplification and differentiation of pathogenic and non-pathogenic *Entamoeba histolytica* DNA from stool specimens. *Am. J. Trop. Med. Hyg.* 1994; **51**: 115.

7 Radin DR, Ralls PW, Colletti PM *et al.* CT of amebic liver abscess. *Am. J. Roentgenol.* 1988; **150**: 1297.

8 Sharma MP, Rai RR, Acharya SK *et al.* Needle aspiration of amoebic liver abscess. *Br. Med. J.* 1989; **299**: 1308.

9 Simjee AE, Patel A, Gathiram V *et al.* Serial ultrasound in amoebic liver abscess. *Clin. Radiol.* 1985; **36**: 61.

Tuberculosis of the liver

Abdominal tuberculosis is suspected in immigrants from Third World countries and also increasingly in patients with AIDS [6].

The liver may be involved as part of miliary tuberculosis or as local tuberculosis where evidence of extra-hepatic disease is not obvious [5]. Rarely hepatic tuberculosis can cause fulminant liver failure [7].

The basic lesion is the *granuloma* which is very frequent in the liver in both pulmonary and extra-pulmonary tuberculosis (fig. 27.8) (Chapter 26). The lesions usually heal without scarring but sometimes with focal fibrosis and calcification.

Pseudo-tumoral hepatic *tuberculomas* are rare [1]. There may be no evidence of extra-hepatic tuberculosis [3]. They may be multiple, consisting of a white, irregular, caseous abscess surrounded by a fibrous capsule (fig. 27.9). Their naked eye distinction from Hodgkin's

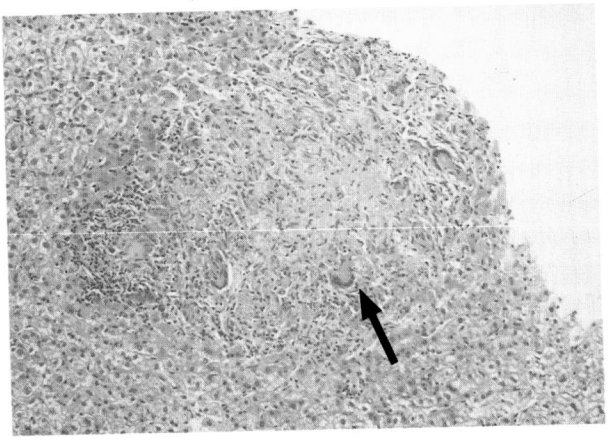

Fig. 27.8. Miliary tuberculosis: a caseating granuloma contains lymphocytes, epithelial cells and numerous giant cells (arrow). There is central caseation.

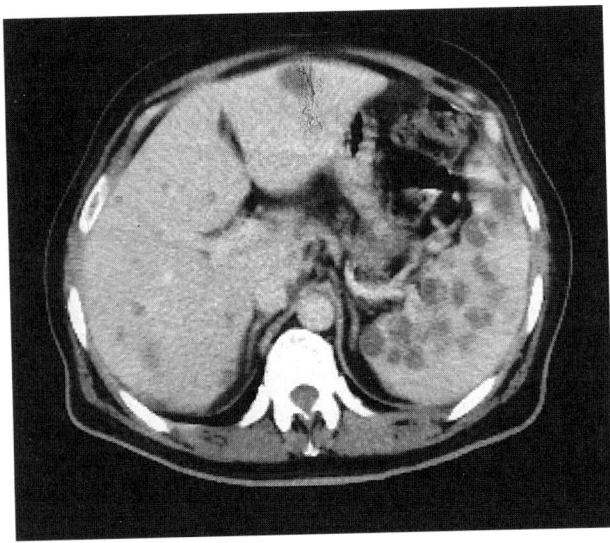

Fig. 27.9. Hepato-splenic tuberculosis. CT shows scattered filling defects in liver and spleen. Aspirate showed acid-fast bacilli and the culture was positive.

disease, secondary carcinoma or actinomycosis may be difficult. Occasionally, the necrotic area calcifies.

Tuberculous cholangitis is extremely rare, resulting from spread of caseous material from the portal tracts into the bile ducts.

Biliary stricture is a rare complication [4].

Tuberculous pylephlebitis results from rupture of caseous material. It is usually rapidly fatal although chronic portal hypertension can result [10].

Tuberculous glands at the hilum may lead rarely to biliary stricture.

Clinical features

These may be few or absent. The condition may present

as a pyrexia of unknown origin. Jaundice may appear in overwhelming miliary tuberculosis, particularly in the racially susceptible. Rarely multiple caseating granulomas lead to massive hepatosplenomegaly and death in liver failure [7].

Biochemical tests

The serum albumin : globulin ratio may be reduced with a disproportionate rise in serum alkaline phosphatase. Hyperglobulinaemia reflects chronic infection and hepatic granulomas.

Diagnosis

This is difficult. Tuberculomas in liver and spleen are difficult to differentiate from lymphoma. Liver biopsy is essential. The indications are unexplained fever and weight loss with hepatomegaly or hepatosplenomegaly. A portion of the biopsy should be stained for acid-fast bacilli and cultured. Positives are obtained in about 50%.

A *plain X-ray* of the abdomen may reveal hepatic calcification. This may be multiple and confluent in tuberculoma, discrete and scattered and of uniform size, or large and chalky adjoining a stricture in the common bile duct [8].

CT may show a lobulated mass or multiple filling defects in liver and spleen (fig. 27.9).

Extra-hepatic features of tuberculosis may not be obvious.

Treatment is that for haematogenous tuberculosis and is very effective.

The effect on the liver of tuberculosis elsewhere

Amyloidosis may complicate chronic tuberculosis. Fatty change is due to wasting and toxaemia. Drug jaundice may follow therapy, especially with isoniazid, rifampicin and pyrazinamide.

Other mycobacteria

Atypical mycobacteria can produce a granulomatous hepatitis, particularly as part of the AIDS syndrome (Chapter 26). *Mycobacterium scrofulaceum* can cause a granulomatous hepatitis, characterized by a rise in alkaline phosphatase, tiredness and low-grade fever. Liver biopsy culture produces the organism [9].

References

1 Achem SR, Kolts BE, Grisnik J *et al*. Pseudotumoral hepatic tuberculosis. Atypical presentation and comprehensive review of the literature. *J. Clin. Gastroenterol.* 1992; **14**: 72.

2 Asada Y, Hayashi T, Sumiyoshi A *et al*. Miliary tuberculosis

presenting as fever and jaundice with hepatic failure. *Hum. Pathol.* 1991; **22**: 92.

3 Chien R-N, Lin P-Y, Liaw Y-F. Hepatic tuberculosis: comparison of miliary and local form. *Infection* 1995; **23**: 5.

4 Fan ST, Ng IOL, Choi TK *et al.* Tuberculosis of the bile duct: a rare cause of biliary stricture. *Am. J. Gastroenterol.* 1989; **84**: 413.

5 Gallinger S, Strasberg SM, Marcus HI *et al.* Local hepatic tuberculosis, the cause of a painful hepatic mass: case report and review of the literature. *Can. J. Surg.* 1986; **29**: 451.

6 Guth AA, Kim U. The reappearance of abdominal tuberculosis. *Surg. Gynecol. Obstet.* 1991; **172**; 432.

7 Hussain W, Mutimer D, Harrison R *et al.* Fulminant hepatic failure caused by tuberculosis. *Gut* 1995; **36**: 792.

8 Maglinte DDT, Alvarez SZ, Ng AC *et al.* Patterns of calcifications and cholangiographic findings in hepatobiliary tuberculosis. *Gastrointest. Radiol.* 1988; **13**: 331.

9 Patel KM. Granulomatous hepatitis due to *Mycobacterium scrofulaceum*: report of a case. *Gastroenterology* 1981; **81**: 156.

10 Ruttenberg D, Graham S, Burns D *et al.* Abdominal tuberculosis—a cause of portal vein thrombosis and portal hypertension. *Dig. Dis. Sci.* 1991; **36**: 112.

Hepatic actinomycosis

Hepatic involvement due to *Actinomyces israeli* is a sequel to intestinal actinomycosis, especially of the caecum and appendix. It spreads by direct extension or, more often, by the portal vein, but can be primary. Large greyish-white masses, superficially resembling malignant metastases, soften and form collections of pus, separated by fibrous tissue bands, simulating a honeycomb. The liver becomes adherent to adjacent viscera and to the abdominal wall, with the formation of sinuses. These lesions contain the characteristic 'sulphur granules', which consist of branching filaments with eosinophilic, clubbed ends.

Clinical features

The patient is toxic, febrile, sweating, wasted and anaemic. There is local, sometimes irregular, enlargement of the liver with tenderness of one or both lobes. The overlying skin may have the livid, dusky hue seen over a taut abscess that is about to rupture. Multiple irregular sinus tracks develop. Similar sinuses may develop from the ileo-caecal site or from the chest wall if there is pleuro-pulmonary extension.

Diagnosis

The diagnosis is obvious at the stage of sinus tracts, because the organism can be isolated from the pus. If actinomycosis is suspected before this stage, percutaneous liver biopsy may reveal sulphur granules with organisms [1].

In the early stages the condition presents as pyrexia with hepatosplenomegaly, anaemia, and non-specific hepato-cellular infiltrates [2]. It may be months before multiple abscesses are detected, often by ultrasound or CT [3]. Anaerobic blood cultures may be positive.

Treatment

Intravenous penicillin should be given in massive doses. Because of the thick fibrous capsule, parenterally administered penicillin may reach the abscess with difficulty.

References

1 Bhatt BD, Zuckerman MJ, Ho H *et al.* Multiple actinomycotic abscesses of the liver. *Am. J. Gastroenterol.* 1990; **85**: 309.

2 Meade RH III. Primary hepatic actinomycosis. *Gastroenterology* 1980; **78**: 355.

3 Mongiardo N, De Rienzo B, Zanchetta G *et al.* Primary hepatic actinomycosis. *J. Infect.* 1986; **12**: 65.

Other fungal infections

These usually affect the immunocompromised, including sufferers from AIDS, acute leukaemia [6], cancer [10] and following liver transplant.

The liver is involved, together with other organs, particularly kidney, spleen, heart, lungs and brain. Fever with a raised serum transaminase or alkaline phosphatase indicates needle liver biopsy.

Ultrasound shows multiple hypoechoic areas throughout the liver and spleen, often with a target (bulls-eye) configuration [8]. *CT* shows multiple, non-enhancing, low-attenuation lesions [6]. The scanning appearances are not diagnostic.

The histological picture is usually granulomatous and the causative organism can be identified by appropriate stains and cultures, so allowing selection of appropriate anti-fungal treatment [4, 5].

Candidiasis. The liver is affected in up to three-quarters of those with disseminated *Candida albicans* infection who come to autopsy [5]. Hepatic granulomas and micro-abscesses are the commonest histological lesions. *Candida* can be demonstrated in the liver [2]. The treatment is with fluconazole.

Disseminated aspergillosis may attack the immunocompromised patients with respiratory, renal or hepatic failure [7].

Hepatic cryptococcosis usually affects the immunocompromised but sometimes it may be seen in the otherwise normal. Liver biopsy shows granulomas with yeast-like organisms.

The picture may resemble sclerosing cholangitis when bile is positive for the fungus (Chapter 15).

Disseminated coccidioidomycosis may involve the liver and be diagnosed by liver biopsy [3].

Torulopsis glabrata hepatic abscesses and fungaemia have developed in a severely diabetic patient with biliary stricture due to chronic pancreatitis [1].

Blastomyces dermatitidis can cause cholangitis in the elderly or immunocompromised [9].

References

1 Friedman E, Blahut RJ, Bender MD. Hepatic abscesses and fungemia from *Torulopsis glabrata*. Successful treatment with percutaneous drainage and amphotericin B. *J. Clin. Gastroenterol.* 1987; **9**: 711.

2 Gordon SC, Watts JC, Veneri RJ *et al.* Focal hepatic candidiasis with perihepatic adhesions: laparoscopic and immunohistologic diagnosis. *Gastroenterology* 1990; **98**: 214.

3 Howard PF, Smith JW. Diagnosis of disseminated coccidioidomycosis. *Arch. Intern. Med.* 1983; **143**: 1335.

4 Korinek JK, Guarda LA, Bolivar R *et al.* Trichosporon hepatitis. *Gastroenterology* 1983; **85**: 732.

5 Lewis JH, Patel HR, Zimmerman HJ. The spectrum of hepatic candidiasis. *Hepatology* 1982; **2**: 479.

6 Maxwell AJ, Mamtora H. Fungal liver abscesses in acute leukaemia—a report of two cases. *Clin. Radiol.* 1988; **39**: 197.

7 Park GR, Drummond GB, Lamb D *et al.* Disseminated aspergillosis occurring in patients with respiratory, renal and hepatic failure. *Lancet* 1982; **i**: 179.

8 Pastakia B, Shawker TH, Thaler M *et al.* Hepatosplenic candidiasis: wheels within wheels. *Radiology* 1988; **166**: 417.

9 Ryan ME, Kirchner JP, Sell T *et al.* Cholangitis due to *blastomyces* dermatitidis. *Gastroenterology* 1989; **96**: 1346.

10 Thaler M, Pastakia FB, Shawker TH *et al.* Hepatic candidiasis in cancer patients: the evolving picture of the syndrome. *Ann. Intern. Med.* 1988; **108**: 88.

Syphilis of the liver

Congenital

The liver is heavily infected by any trans-placental infection. It is firm, enlarged and swarming with spirochaetes. Initially, there is a diffuse hepatitis, but gradually fibrous tissue is laid down between the liver cells and in the portal tracts, and this leads to a true pericellular cirrhosis.

Since hepatic involvement is but an incident in a widespread spirochaetal septicaemia, the clinical features are seldom those of the liver disease. The fetus may be stillborn or die soon after birth. If the infant survives, other manifestations of congenital syphilis are obvious, apart from the hepatosplenomegaly and mild jaundice. Syphilis nowadays is a very rare cause of neonatal jaundice.

In older children who have survived without this florid neonatal picture, the hepatic lesion may be a gumma.

Diagnosis can be confirmed by blood serology which is always positive. Needle liver biopsy has been used for diagnosis and to assess the effects of treatment.

Secondary

In the secondary septicaemic stage, spirochaetes invade the liver with the production of miliary granulomas [1].

Fifty per cent of sufferers have raised serum enzyme levels [3]. Clinical hepatitis is rare. However, sometimes the picture is of severe cholestatic jaundice [2].

Serology is positive. Serum alkaline phosphatase levels are high. The M1 cardiolipin fluorescent antimitochondrial antibody is positive and becomes normal with recovery [2].

Liver biopsy shows non-specific changes with moderate infiltration with polymorphs and lymphocytes, some hepato-cellular disarray but cholestasis is absent or mild except in the severely cholestatic patients [2]. Portal-to-central zone necrosis can be seen (fig. 27.10). Spirochaetes are sometimes detected in the liver biopsy by appropriate stains.

Tertiary

Gummas may be single or multiple. They are usually situated in the right lobe. They consist of a caseous mass, circumscribed by a fibrous capsule, from which fibrous tissue spreads out interstitially. Healing is followed by deep scars and coarse lobulation (*hepar lobatum*). Despite this distortion, the liver architecture is not disturbed and the lesion is not a true cirrhosis.

Hepatic gummas are usually discovered incidentally at laparotomy or autopsy. Occasionally, the enlarged nodular liver may be confused with cirrhosis or hepatic metastases. Liver function tests are unhelpful and the presence of positive serology is insufficient evidence of hepatic syphilis. Aspiration liver biopsy of an accessible nodule provides histological confirmation. Adequate penicillin results in diminution in size over a prolonged period of time.

Jaundice complicating penicillin treatment

Rarely, the patient shows an idiosyncrasy to penicillin. Jaundice, chills and fever, often with a rash (*erythema of Milan*), occur about 9 days after starting therapy. This is part of the Herxheimer reaction. The mechanism of the jaundice is unclear.

References

1 Case Records of the Massachusetts General Hospital Case 27, 1983. *N. Engl. J. Med.* 1983; **309**: 35.

2 Comer GM, Mukherjee S, Sachdev RK *et al.* Cardiolipin-fluorescent (M1) antimitochondrial antibody and cholestatic hepatitis in secondary syphilis. *Dig. Dis. Sci.* 1989; **34**: 1298.

3 Schlossberg D. Syphilitic hepatitis: a case report and review of the literature. *Am. J. Gastroenterol.* 1987; **82**: 552.

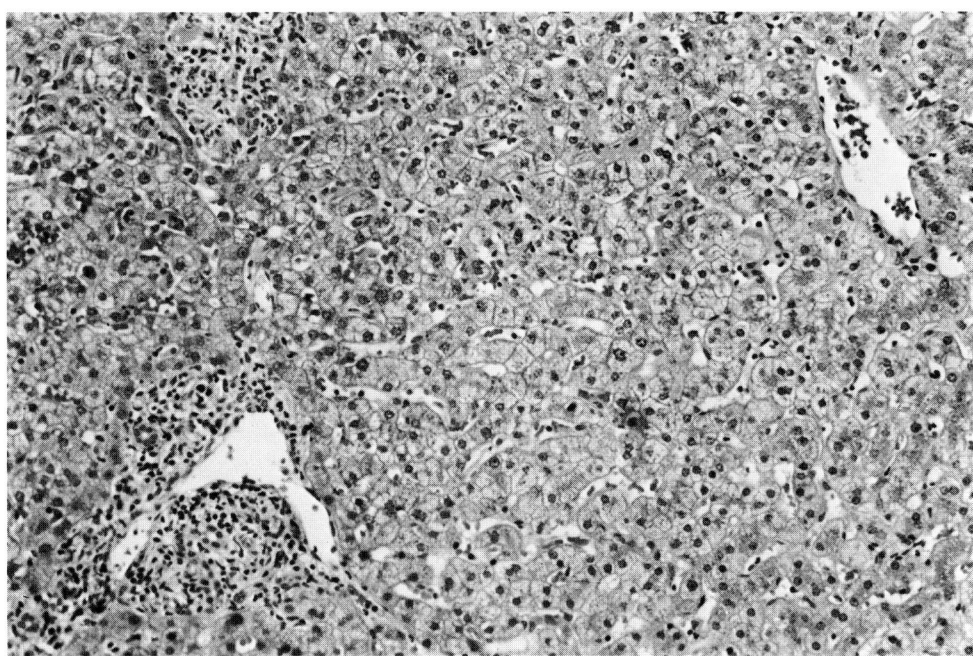

Fig. 27.10. Liver in secondary syphilis. Mononuclear cell infiltration can be seen in portal zones and in the sinusoids. (Stained H & E, ×160.)

Leptospirosis

In 1886, Weil [4] described a disease characterized by intense prostration, fever, jaundice, renal injury and a haemorrhagic tendency. This was later shown to be due to a leptospira, *L. icterohaemorrhagiae*, and to be transmitted by rats. Later various other leptospira were related to human disease. These do not cause a distinct clinical pattern and the whole group should be designated leptospirosis.

A genetic classification, mainly by DNA–DNA homology, has yielded eight genomic species of pathogenic leptospiras.

Weil's disease

Mode of infection

Living leptospira are continually excreted in the urine of infected rats and are capable of surviving for months in pools, canals or damp soil. The patient is infected by immersion in contaminated water or by direct occupational contact with rat carriers. The highest incidence is therefore in adult males, particularly agricultural workers, sewer workers, coal miners, soldiers and fish cutters.

Pathology

The primary lesion is a cell membrane defect of small blood vessels.

Liver [1] necrosis is minimal and focal. Dissociation of the cells one from another is probably a post-mortem phenomenon. Zone 3 necrosis is absent. Active hepato-cellular regeneration, shown by mitoses and nuclear polyploidy, is out of proportion to cell damage. Swollen Kupffer cells contain leptospiral debris.

Peri-portal leucocyte infiltration and bile thrombi are prominent in zone 3 in the deeply jaundiced. The histological changes do not parallel the severity of icterus. Cirrhosis is not a sequel.

Kidney shows tubular necrosis. *Skeletal muscles* show punctate haemorrhages and focal necrosis of muscle fibres. *Heart* may show haemorrhages in all layers.

Haemorrhage into tissues, especially skin and lungs, is due to capillary injury and thrombocytopenia.

The *jaundice* is complex. It is related to hepato-cellular dysfunction magnified by renal failure impairing urinary bilirubin excretion. Tissue haemorrhages and intravascular haemolysis increase the bilirubin load on the liver. Hypotension with diminished hepatic blood flow contributes.

The *uraemia* is related to pigment in the tubules, to a direct effect of the spirochaetes on the kidney and to lowered renal blood flow.

Clinical features (fig. 27.11)

The clinical picture is not pathognomonic and the disease is heavily underdiagnosed. The disease is most

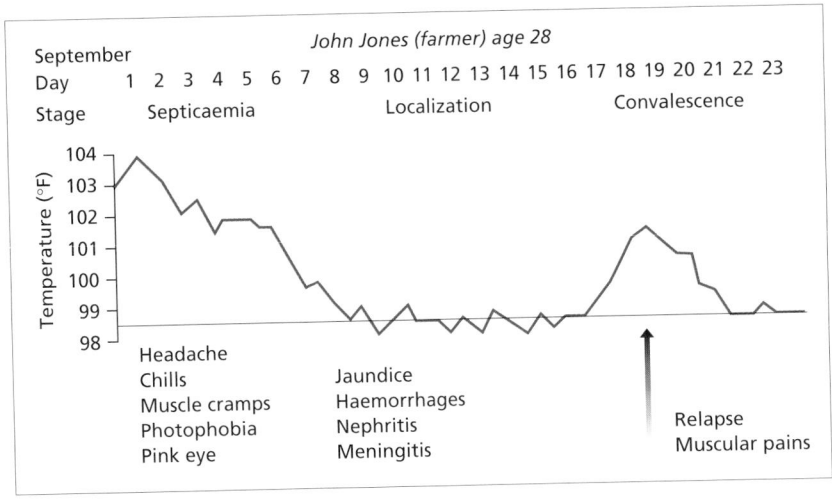

John Jones (farmer) age 28

| September Day | 1 2 3 4 5 6 7 8 9 10 11 12 13 14 15 16 17 18 19 20 21 22 23 |
| Stage | Septicaemia   Localization   Convalescence |

Temperature chart (°F, 98–104)

Headache
Chills
Muscle cramps
Photophobia
Pink eye

Jaundice
Haemorrhages
Nephritis
Meningitis

Relapse
Muscular pains

Blood								
organisms	+ + + + + + ± 0							
antibodies			1:75	1:300		1:2400		
WBC	18 000 (80% polys)							8000
Bilirubin (mg)	2	5	10	14	3	2		0.5
Urea (mg)	30	70	130	210	50	40		30
BP	130/60	130/70	100/60	90/50	110/60	120/70		
Urine volume (ml)	700	800	500	100	1100	900	1500
albumin	+	++	+++	+++	++	+	++
organisms			0	+	++	+	0

Fig. 27.11. The clinical course of a patient with Weil's disease.

prevalent in late summer and autumn. The incubation period is 6–15 days. The course may be divided into three stages: the first or septicaemic phase lasts for about 7 days, the second or toxic stage for a similar period, and the third or convalescent period begins in the third week.

The first or septicaemic stage is marked by the presence of the spirochaete in the circulating blood.

The onset is abrupt, with prostration, high fever, and even rigors. The temperature rises rapidly to 39.5–40.5°C and falls by lysis within 3–10 days.

Abdominal pain, nausea and vomiting may simulate an acute abdominal emergency, and severe muscular pains, especially in the back or calves, are common.

Central nervous system involvement is shown by severe headache, mental confusion and sometimes meningism. The cerebrospinal fluid confirms the meningeal infection, there being an increase in protein, with a leucocytosis. If jaundice is present, there is xanthochromia, the infection increasing the permeability of the meninges to bile pigments.

The eyes show a characteristic suffusion.

There is a haemorrhagic tendency, usually in those with a severe attack. Bleeding may occur from nose, gut or lung, with skin petechiae or ecchymoses.

Pneumonitis with cough, sore throat and rhonchi occurs in 40% of sufferers.

Jaundice appears between the fourth and seventh day in 80% of patients. It is a grave sign, for the disease is never fatal in the absence of icterus. The liver is enlarged, but not the spleen.

The urine shows albumin and bile pigment. The stools are well coloured.

There is a leucocytosis of 10 000–30 000/mm³ with a relative increase in polymorphs. Thrombocytopenia may be profound.

The second or immune stage in the second week is characterized by a normal temperature but without clinical improvement. This is the stage of deepening jaundice, with increasing renal and myocardial damage. Albuminuria persists, there is a rising blood urea, and oliguria may proceed to anuria. Death may be due to renal failure. A markedly elevated creatinine phosphokinase level reflects myositis.

Severe prostration is accompanied by a low blood pressure and a dilated heart. There may be transient cardiac arrhythmias and electrocardiograms may show a prolonged P–R or Q–T interval, with T-wave changes. Death may be due to circulatory failure.

During this stage, the leptospira can be found in the urine, and rising antibody titres demonstrated in the serum.

The third or convalescent stage starts at the beginning of the third week. Clinical improvement is shown by a brightening of the mental state, fading of the jaundice, a rise in blood pressure and an increased urinary volume, with a drop in the blood urea concentration. Albuminuria is slow to disappear. Permanent renal and hepatic damage have not been reported.

Temperature may rise during the third week (fig. 27.11), associated with muscle pains. Such relapses occur in 20% of cases.

There is great variation in the clinical course ranging from a mild illness, clinically indistinguishable from influenza, to a prostrating, fatal disease with anuria.

Investigations

In the first week, the spirochaetes are found in the blood, becoming less evident with the development of antibodies at the end of the first week. Thereafter, they may be isolated from the urine.

Diagnosis in the first week

1 Thick, dry, blood films are used for staining for spirochaetes and for dark field examination.
2 Blood culture is performed but results take several days.
3 Acute-phase serological antibodies are measured as a base line for subsequent rising titres.
4 The leucocyte count is raised — a point of distinction from viral hepatitis.
5 Blood is injected intra-peritoneally into guinea-pigs, who develop jaundice and fever within a few days. Spirochaetes are demonstrated in liver and other tissues.

Diagnosis after the first week

From the 10th to the 20th day, leptospira may be shown in the urine. Injection into a guinea-pig may be positive, but the organisms are not often viable from urine.

Serological antibodies appear after the first week and usually reach a peak in the fourth week. They may persist for years.

The IgM specific dot-ELISA technique is useful for rapid serodiagnosis [2].

The leptospiral agglutination test is usually positive in a titre of at least 1 in 300 and a rising titre can be demonstrated. The microscopic agglutination test (MAT) utilizes a battery of test-antigen suspensions that represent all the common serotypes.

Aspiration liver biopsy. In spite of the bleeding tendency, biopsies have been performed. The histological picture is not specific for leptospirosis. However, it is quite distinct from acute virus hepatitis. A portion of the liver biopsy may be used for culture.

Liver function tests are non-contributory. The serum bilirubin level is raised and the alkaline phosphatase and transaminases slightly increased.

Table 27.1. The diagnosis of Weil's disease from viral hepatitis during the first week of illness

	Weil's disease	Viral hepatitis
Onset	Sudden	Gradual
Headache	Constant	Occasional
Muscle pains	Severe	Mild
Conjunctival injection	Present	Absent
Prostration	Great	Mild
Disorientation	Common	Rare
Haemorrhagic diathesis	Common	Rare
Nausea and vomiting	Present	Present
Abdominal discomfort	Common	Common
Bronchitis	Common	Rare
Albuminuria	Present	Absent
Leucocyte count	Polymorph leucocytosis	Leucopenia with lymphocytosis
Inoculation of blood into guinea-pig	Spirochaetes present	Spirochaetes absent

Differential diagnosis

In the early stages, Weil's disease is confused with septicaemic bacterial infections or typhus fever. When jaundice is evident acute viral hepatitis must be excluded (table 27.1). Important distinguishing points are the sudden onset and albuminuria of Weil's disease.

Spirochaetal jaundice would be diagnosed more often if blood samples for agglutinins were taken from patients with obscure icterus and fever.

Prognosis

Mortality is about 5%. This depends on the depth of jaundice, renal and myocardial involvement, and the extent of haemorrhages. Death is usually due to renal failure. The mortality is negligible in non-icteric patients, and is lower in those under 30 years old. Since many mild infections are probably unrecognized, the overall mortality may be considerably less.

Although transient relapses in the third and fourth weeks are common, final recovery is complete.

Prevention

Specific immune serum has proved preventative in exposed laboratory workers.

Protective clothing, such as rubber boots and gloves, should be provided for workers in industries with a high incidence of Weil's disease, and adequate measures taken to control rodents. Bathing in stagnant water should be avoided.

Treatment

Penicillin, 6 million units intravenously for 7 days, in severe and even late leptospirosis shortens hospital stay, and reduces duration of fever and rises in creatinine [3]. It will be less effective after the first 4 days of illness, i.e. at the time when the diagnosis is usually made and treatment instituted.

Prognosis is improving with earlier diagnosis, attention to fluid and electrolyte balance, renal dialysis, antibiotics and circulatory support.

Other types of leptospirosis

There are many species of leptospira pathogenic to man, varying in antigenic constitution and geographic distribution. In general these infections are less severe than those due to *L. icterohaemorrhagiae*. *L. canicola* infection, for instance, is characterized by headache, meningitis and conjunctival infection. Albuminuria is only found in 40%, and jaundice in only 18% of patients. The frequent presentation is that of 'benign aseptic meningitis'. The disease affects young adults who have usually been in close contact with an infected dog. Fatalities in man are virtually unknown.

Diagnosis is confirmed in a similar way to Weil's disease. A convenient method is rising antibody titres. The spinal fluid shows a lymphocytic picture in most cases.

References

1 Arean VM. The pathologic anatomy and pathogenesis of fatal human leptospirosis (Weil's disease). *Am. J. Pathol.* 1962; **40**: 393.
2 Pappas MG, Ballou WR, Gray MR *et al*. Rapid serodiagnosis of leptospirosis using the IgM-specific Dot-ELISA. Comparison with the microscopic agglutination test. *Am. J. Trop. Med. Hyg.* 1985; **34**: 346.
3 Watt G, Padre LP, Tuazon ML *et al*. Placebo-controlled trial of intravenous penicillin for severe and late leptospirosis. *Lancet* 1988; **i**: 433.
4 Weil A. Über eine eigenthumliche mit Milztumor, Icterus and Nephritis einhergehene, acute Infektionskrankheit. *Dtsch. Arch. Klin. Med.* 1886; **39**: 209.

Relapsing fever

This arthropod-borne infection is caused by spirochaetes of the species *Borrelia recurrentis*. It is encountered throughout the world except in New Zealand, Australia and some parts of the west Pacific.

The *Borrelia* multiply in the liver, invading liver cells and causing focal necrosis. Just before the crisis the *Borrelia* roll up and are ingested by reticulo-endothelial cells. This effect is related to immunologically competent lymphocytes. Surviving *Borrelia* remain in the liver, spleen, brain and bone marrow until the next relapse [2].

Clinical features [1]

The incubation period is 3–15 days. The onset is acute with chills, a continuous high temperature, headache, muscle pains and profound prostration. The patient is flushed, sometimes with injected conjunctivae, and epistaxes. In severe attacks, tender hepatosplenomegaly and jaundice develop. The jaundice is similar to that of Weil's disease. Sometimes a rash develops on the trunk. There may be bronchitis.

These symptoms continue for 4–9 days and then the temperature falls, often with collapse of the patient. This peripheral collapse may be fatal, but more usually the symptoms and signs then rapidly abate, the patient remains afebrile for about 1 week, when there is a relapse. There may be a second or even a third milder relapse before the disease ends.

Diagnosis

Spirochaetes can rarely be found in thick blood films. Agglutination and complement fixation tests are available [2]. Organisms may be identified by lymph node aspiration, or from the insect bite site.

Treatment

Tetracyclines and streptomycin are more effective than penicillin. Mortality is 5%.

References

1 Bryceson ADM, Parry EHO, Perine PL *et al*. Louse-born relapsing fever: a clinical and laboratory study of 62 cases in Ethiopia and a reconsideration of the literature. *Q. J. Med.* 1970; **39**: 129.
2 Felsenfeld O, Wolf RH. Immunoglobulins and antibodies in borrelia turicetae infections. *Acta Trop.* 1969; **26**: 156.

Lyme disease

This is due to a tick-borne spirochaete, *Borrelia burgdorferi* [2]. It has caused hepatitis with numerous liver cell mitoses [1]. It responds to oral doxycycline therapy.

References

1 Goellner MH, Agger WA, Burgess JH *et al*. Hepatitis due to recurrent Lyme disease. *Ann. Intern. Med.* 1988; **108**: 707.
2 Rahn DW, Malawista SE. Lyme diseases: recommendations for diagnosis and treatment. *Ann. Intern. Med.* 1991; **114**: 472.

Q fever

This rickettsial disease has predominantly pulmonary manifestations. Occasionally hepatitis may be prominent and clinical features may mimic anicteric virus hepatitis [2, 3].

The liver shows a granulomatous hepatitis. Portal areas contain abundant lymphocytes and the limiting plate is destroyed. Kupffer cells are hypertrophied. The granulomas have a characteristic ring of fibrinoid necrosis surrounded by lymphocytes and histiocytes. In the centre of the granuloma is a clear space giving a 'doughnut' appearance (fig. 27.12). The diagnosis is made by showing a rising titre of complement-fixing antibodies to *Coxiella burnetii* 2–3 weeks after the infection.

Rocky mountain spotted fever

Jaundice and rises in serum enzymes sometimes occur. Liver histology shows portal zone inflammation with large mononuclear cells. Hepato-cellular necrosis is inconspicuous but erythrophagocytosis is marked. Rickettsiae may be demonstrated in the portal zones by immunofluorescence microscopy [1].

References

1 Adams JS, Walker DH. The liver in rocky mountain spotted fever. *Am. J. Clin. Pathol.* 1981; **75**: 156.
2 Dupont HL, Hornick RB, Levin HS *et al*. Q fever hepatitis. *Ann. Intern. Med.* 1971; **74**: 198.
3 Tissot-Dupont H, Raoult D, Brouquil P *et al*. Epidemiologic features and clinical presentation of acute Q fever in hospitalized patients: 323 French cases. *Am. J. Med.* 1992; **93**: 427.

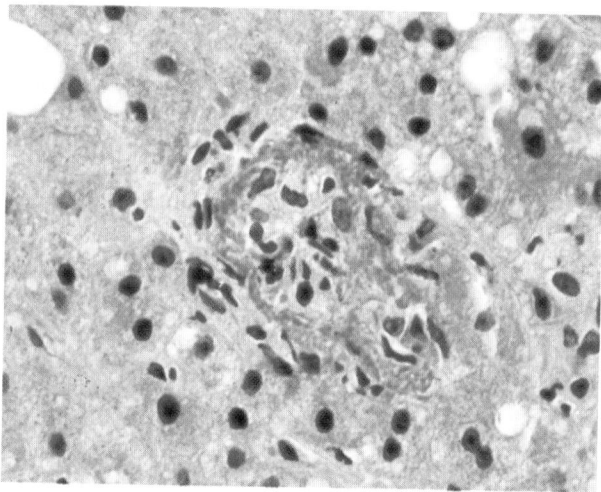

Fig. 27.12. Liver biopsy in Q fever showing a granuloma with fibrin rings having a clear centre. (Stained martius scarlet blue, ×350.)

Schistosomiasis (bilharziasis)

Hepatic schistosomiasis is usually a complication of the intestinal disease, since emboli of schistosoma ova reach the liver from the intestines via the mesenteric veins. *Schistosoma mansoni* and *S. japonicum* affect the liver. *S. haematobium* can sometimes involve the liver.

Schistosomiasis affects more than two hundred million people in 74 countries. *S. japonicum* is prevalent in Japan, China, Indonesia and the Philippines. *S. mansoni* is found in Africa, the Middle East, the Caribbean and Brazil.

Pathogenesis

Eggs, excreted in the faeces, hatch out in water to release free-swimming embryos which enter appropriate snails and develop into fork-tailed cercariae. These re-enter human skin in contact with infected water. They burrow down to the capillary bed, whence there is widespread haematogenous dissemination. Those reaching the mesenteric capillaries enter the intra-hepatic portal system, where they grow rapidly.

The extent and severity of chronic liver disease correlates with the intensity and duration of egg production and hence with the number of eggs excreted. Adult male and female worms can exist for about 5 years producing 300 to 3000 eggs daily in portal venules. If liver disease is advanced, faecal egg counts may fall because of senescence of adult worms or previous therapy.

S. japonicum is more pathogenic than *S. mansoni* and produces hepatosplenic schistosomiasis more often and faster.

In the liver, the ova penetrate and obstruct the portal branches and are deposited either in the large radicles, producing the coarser type of bilharzial hepatic fibrosis, or in the small portal tracts, producing the fine diffuse form.

The granulomatous reaction to the *Schistosoma* ovum is of delayed hypersensitivity type, related to antigen released by the egg. TH0- and TH2-type helper lymphocytes play an important role in granuloma formation [15].

Portal fibrosis is related to the adult worm load. The classic, clay-pipestem cirrhosis is due to fibrotic bands originating from the granulomas. The collagen deposited is type 1, 3 and B [3].

Early on, cytokines, formed from granulomas around ova, may play a central role in fibrogenesis [10]. Fibrosis may be slowly reversible with treatment [6].

Wide, irregular, thin-walled arteriolar spaces are found in 85% of cases in the thickened portal tracts. These angiomatoids are useful in distinguishing the bilharzial liver from other forms of hepatic fibrosis. Remnants of ova are also diagnostic. There is little or no bile duct proliferation. The extent of nodular regeneration and disturbance of the hepatic architecture is not sufficient to justify the term 'cirrhosis'.

In areas where schistosomiasis, virus B and virus C coexist, a mixed picture of schistosomal fibrosis with cirrhosis may be seen.

Splenic enlargement is mainly due to portal venous hypertension and reticulo-endothelial hyperplasia. Very few ova are found in the spleen. Porto-systemic collateral channels are numerous.

There are associated bilharzial lesions in the intestines and elsewhere. Fifty per cent of patients with rectal schistosomiasis have granulomas in the liver.

Clinical features

Schistosomiasis shows three stages of infection. Itching follows the entry of the cercariae through the skin. This is followed by a stage of fever, urticaria and eosinophilia. Finally, the third stage of deposition of ova results in intestinal, urinary and hepatic involvement.

Initially liver and spleen are firm, smooth and easily palpable. This is followed by hepatic fibrosis and eventually portal hypertension which may appear years after the original infection.

Oesophageal varices develop. Bleeding episodes are recurrent but rarely fatal.

The liver shrinks in size and the spleen becomes much larger. Dilated abdominal wall veins and a venous hum over the liver are indications of the portal venous obstruction. Ascites and oedema may develop. The blood shows leucopenia and anaemia. The faeces at this stage contain few, if any, parasites.

Patients tolerate blood loss well and hepatic encephalopathy is unusual. This is because hepato-cellular function remains good although there is a large porto-systemic collateral circulation.

Aspiration liver biopsy (fig. 27.13) [5]. Eggs or their remnants are seen in 94% of livers from those with faecal eggs.

Remnants of ova may be seen but appearances are not usually diagnostic and the liver biopsy mainly excludes other types of liver disease.

Diagnostic tests

Active infection is detected by stool examination. In long-standing or treated infections, very few eggs may be found. The rectal mucosal biopsy, crushed in saline (rectal snip), is helpful in detecting very light or recently treated infections (fig. 27.14). Bleeding may be a complication in those with portal hypertension.

Serological tests indicate past exposure without specifying the time. A negative ELISA excludes schistosomal infection. An ELISA for detecting circulating soluble egg

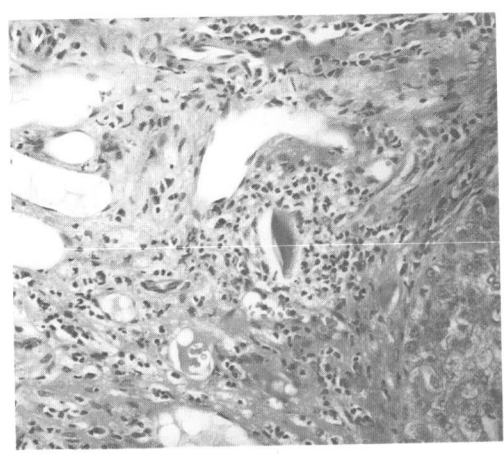

Fig. 27.13. Bilharzial liver. An ovum of *S. mansoni* has lodged in a portal tract which shows a granulomatous reaction. (Stained H & E, ×64.)

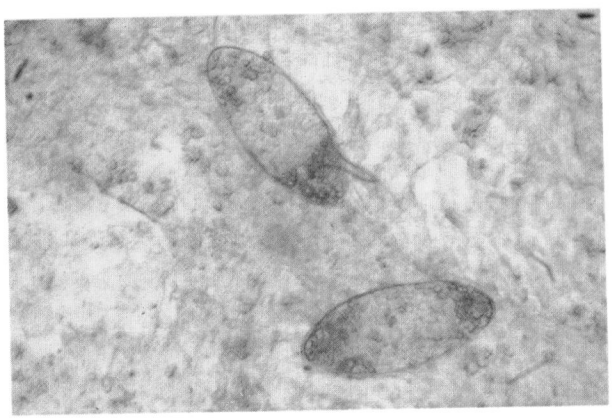

Fig. 27.14. Rectal ('snip') biopsy in schistosomiasis mansoni. A 'squash' preparation in glycerol reveals the ova of *S. mansoni.*

antigens in serum correlates with egg output [90]. A reagent strip assay is based on glycoconjugates for adult schistosomes [14].

CT shows dense bands following the portal vein from the porta to the liver edge; these enhance with contrast [6].

Ultrasound shows greatly thickened portal veins (fig. 27.15). It may be used to grade fibrosis [1]. Liver, spleen, peri-portal and pancreatic lymph nodes are diffusely enlarged without evidence of portal hypertension.

Portal hypertension

This is pre-sinusoidal and presumably related to the portal zone reaction. As the portal venous blood flow falls, hepatic arterial blood flow increases so that total hepatic blood flow is not significantly reduced. Retrograde flow develops in the portal vein [2].

At the stage of haemorrhage from varices the granulo-

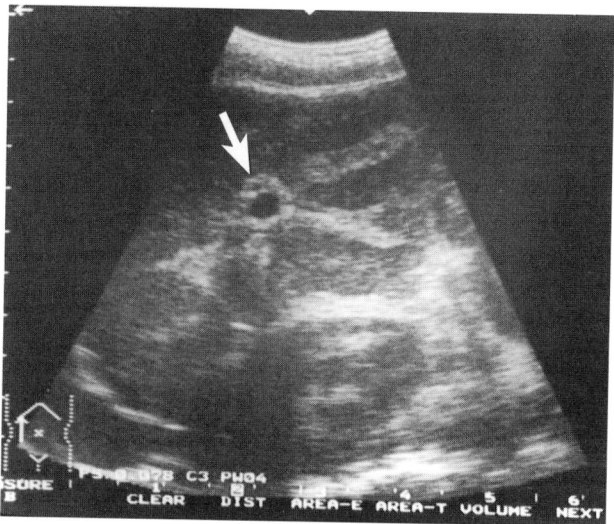

Fig. 27.15. Schistosomiasis: ultrasound shows bright portal tracts and a portal vein with greatly thickened walls (arrowed).

matous reaction may have subsided and the picture is predominantly that of fibrosis.

Biochemical changes

Serum alkaline phosphatase may be raised. Hypoalbuminaemia can be related to poor nutrition and to the effects of repeated gastrointestinal haemorrhages. Serum transaminases are virtually normal.

Serum procollagen 3 peptide levels can be used to assess activity and a degree of fibrosis [13].

Treatment

Chemotherapy

Praziquantel, 40–75 mg/kg once only, is the drug of choice for all forms of schistosomiasis. Side-effects are few. In murine schistosoma-induced fibrosis, praziquantel decreased messenger RNA levels of the major proteins associated with fibrosis [8].

Oxamniquine 20 mg/kg per day for 3 days is effective only against *S. mansoni*. Drowsiness, giddiness and headaches are side-effects.

Control is by mass education on hygiene and on the avoidance of infected water. Killing the snails is very difficult. Community-based chemotherapy, with praziquantel, of all infected children or adults will eventually reduce the numbers of persons responsible for transmitting the disease. This is under trial [4].

In former days, the use of unsterile syringes and needles to administer tartar emetic set the stage for subsequent HCV and HBV infections which are still being diagnosed.

Bleeding oesophageal varies

This is rarely fatal and can usually be controlled by endoscopic sclerotherapy.

In the later stages, a haemorrhage from oesophageal varices may be treated by a distal spleno-renal shunt. Survival is longer and rebleeding and encephalopathy (4.4%) less than when performed in other forms of chronic liver disease. Hepatic encephalopathy is more frequent after proximal or distal spleno-renal shunt than with oesophago-gastric devascularization [11]. Rebleeding is rare, but is more frequent with devascularization plus splenectomy but this is the best operation because of the low mortality and encephalopathy rates. Transjugular intra-hepatic portal-systemic stent shunt (TIPS) also reduces portal pressure. However, hyperbilirubinaemia is frequent after shunts for schistosomiasis and this is exaggerated by TIPS.

References

1 Abdel-Wahab MF, Esmat G, Farrag A *et al*. Grading of hepatic schistosomiasis by the use of ultrasonography. *Am. J. Trop. Med. Hyg.* 1992; **46**: 403.
2 Alves CAP, Alves AR, Abreu ION *et al*. Hepatic artery hypertrophy and sinusoidal hypertension in advanced schistosomiasis. *Gastroenterology* 1977; **72**: 126.
3 Biempica L, Dunn MA, Kamel IA *et al*. Liver collagen-type characterization in human schistosomiasis. *Am. J. Trop. Med. Hyg.* 1983; **32**: 316.
4 Capron A, Riveau G, Gryzch JM *et al*. Development of a vaccine strategy against human and bovine schistosomiasis: background and update. *Trop. Geogr. Med.* 1994; **46**: 242.
5 Case records of the Massachusetts General Hospital. *N. Engl. J. Med.* 1989; **319**; 37.
6 Fataar S, Bassiony H, Satyanath S. CT of hepatic schistosomiasis mansoni. *Am. J. Roentgenol.* 1985; **145**: 63.
7 Kremsner PG, Enyong P, Krijger FW. Circulating anodic and cathodic antigen in serum and urine from *Schistosoma haematobium*-infected Cameroonian children receiving praziquantel: a longitudinal study. *Clin. Infect. Dis.* 1994; **18**: 408.
8 Kresina TF, Qing HE, Esposti SD *et al*. Gene expression of transferring growth factor β 1 and extra-cellular matrix proteins in muring *Schistosoma mansoni* infection. *Gastroenterology* 1994; **107**: 773.
9 Nourel Din MS, Nibbeling R, Rotmans JP *et al*. Quantitative determination of circulating soluble egg antigen in urine and serum of *Schistosoma mansoni*-infected individuals using a combined two-site enzyme-linked immunosorbent assay. *Am. J. Trop. Med. Hyg.* 1994; **50**: 585.
10 Prakash S, Postlethwaite AE, Wyler DJ. Alterations in influence of granuloma-derived cytokines on fibrogenesis in the course of murine *Schistosomal mansoni* infection. *Hepatology* 1991; **13**: 970.
11 Raia S, Dasilua LC, Gayotto LCC *et al*. Portal hypertension in schistosomiasis: a long-term follow-up of a randomized trial comparing three types of surgery. *Hepatology* 1994; **20**: 398.
12 Rabello ALT, Pinto da Silva RA, Rocha RS *et al*. Abdominal

ultrasonography in acute clinical schistosomiasis mansoni. *Am. J. Trop. Med. Hyg.* 1994; **50**: 748.

13 Shahin M, Schuppan D, Waldherr R *et al.* Serum procollagen peptides and collagen type VI for the assessment of activity and degree of hepatic fibrosis in schistosomiasis and alcoholic liver disease. *Hepatology* 1992; **15**: 637.

14 Van Etten L, Folman CC, Eggeltte TA *et al.* Rapid diagnosis of schistosomiasis by antigen detection in urine with a reagent strip. *J. Clin. Microbiol.* 1994; **32**: 2404.

15 Zhu Y, Lukacs NW, Botos DL. Cloning of TH0- and TH2-type helper lymphocytes from liver granulomas of *Schistosoma mansoni*-infected mice. *Infect. Immun* 1994; **62**: 994.

Malaria [1]

In the *erythrocytic stage*, the parasite is engulfed by reticulo-endothelial cells. The liver suffers from the general effects of the toxaemia and pyrexia [2].

In the *pre-erythrocytic* (exo-erythrocytic) stage, schizogony takes place in the liver without obvious effect on its function. The hepatocyte is invaded by the sporozoite. The nucleus of the parasite divides many times and, at last (in 6–12 days according to the species), a spherical or irregular body containing thousands of ripe merozoites is formed. This pre-erythrocytic schizont bursts and the merozoites are discharged into the sinusoids and invade red blood corpuscles. In quartan or benign tertian malaria, a few merozoites return to the liver cells to initiate the exo-erythrocytic or relapse cycle. In malignant tertian this does not happen and there are no true relapses. So far only *Plasmodium falciparum* and *P. vivax* have been found in the liver of man. The tissue stage of human malaria is confined to the liver cells.

Pathological changes

The liver shows reticulo-endothelial proliferation, both of Kupffer cells and in zone 1. Focal accumulations of histiocytes, forming non-specific granulomatous lesions, may be seen in the sinusoids. Brown 'malarial' pigmentation (iron and haemofuscin) is seen in Kupffer cells. Malarial parasites are not demonstrable. Hepato-cellular change is slight. The cells may be swollen, with nuclei of variable size and shape and increased mitoses.

Zone 3 necrosis described in malignant (*P. falciparum*) malaria is probably a post-mortem phenomenon. Sinusoids may contain parasitized clumped erythrocytes.

The reaction of the liver to the malarial parasite is reticulo-endothelial, with minor effects on the liver cells. Fibrosis does not follow. The high incidence of cirrhosis in malarial areas may be attributed to other factors operating in the region.

Clinical features

There are usually no specific hepatic features. Occasionally, in acute malignant malaria, there may be mild jaundice, hepatomegaly and tenderness over the liver.

Hepatic function changes

Increases in serum bilirubin concentration are rarely above 3 mg/dl. Serum transaminases increase slightly.

Reticulo-endothelial proliferation is associated with a rise in the serum globulin concentration.

References

1 Cook GC. Malaria in the liver. *Postgrad. Med. J.* 1994; **70**: 780.
2 Hollingdale MR. Malaria and the liver. *Hepatology* 1985; **5**: 327.

Kala-azar (leishmaniasis)

Leishmaniasis is a reticulo-endothelial disease. Periportal cellular infiltrations and macrophage accumulations are scattered throughout the liver and within them the Leishman–Donovan bodies may be identified (fig. 27.16). There is some portal zone fibrosis [1]. The picture is similar in the American, Mediterranean and Oriental types [1].

Kala-azar presents with fever, splenomegaly, a firm, tender liver, pancytopenia, anaemia and very high serum globulins. Aspiration of the bone marrow is usually positive.

Reference

1 Da Silva JR, De Paola D. Hepatic lesions in American kala-azar: a needle-biopsy study. *Ann. Trop. Med. Parasitol.* 1961; **55**: 249.

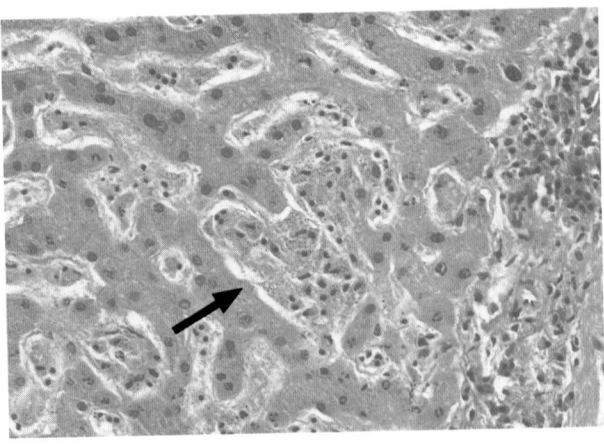

Fig. 27.16. Kala-azar. Liver biopsy shows enlarged Kupffer cells (arrowed) distending the sinusoids. These contain Leishman–Donovan bodies. (H & E, ×100.)

Hydatid disease

Hydatid disease is due to the larval or cyst stage of infection by the tapeworm, *Echinococcus granulosus*, which lives in dogs. Man, sheep and cattle are intermediate hosts.

Biology (fig. 27.17)

Man is infected by the excreta of dogs, often during childhood. The dog is infected by eating the viscera of sheep, which contain hydatid cysts. Scolices, contained in the cysts, adhere to the small intestine of the dog and become adult taenia which attach to the intestinal wall. Each worm sheds 500 ova into the bowel. The infected faeces of the dog contaminate grass and farmland, and the contained ova are ingested by sheep, pigs, camels or man. The ova adhere to the coats of dogs, so man is infected by handling dogs, as well as by eating contaminated vegetables.

The ova have chitinous envelopes which are dissolved by gastric juice. The liberated ovum burrows through the intestinal mucosa and is carried by the portal vein to the liver, where it develops into an adult cyst. Most cysts are caught in the hepatic sinusoids and 70% of hydatid cysts form in the liver. A few ova pass through the liver and heart and are held up in the pulmonary capillary bed causing pulmonary cysts. A few ova reach the general circulation causing spleen, brain and bone cysts.

Development of the hepatic cyst (fig. 27.18)

The adult cyst develops slowly from the ovum and provokes a cellular response in which three zones can be distinguished: a peripheral zone of fibroblasts, an intermediate layer of endothelial cells and an inner zone of

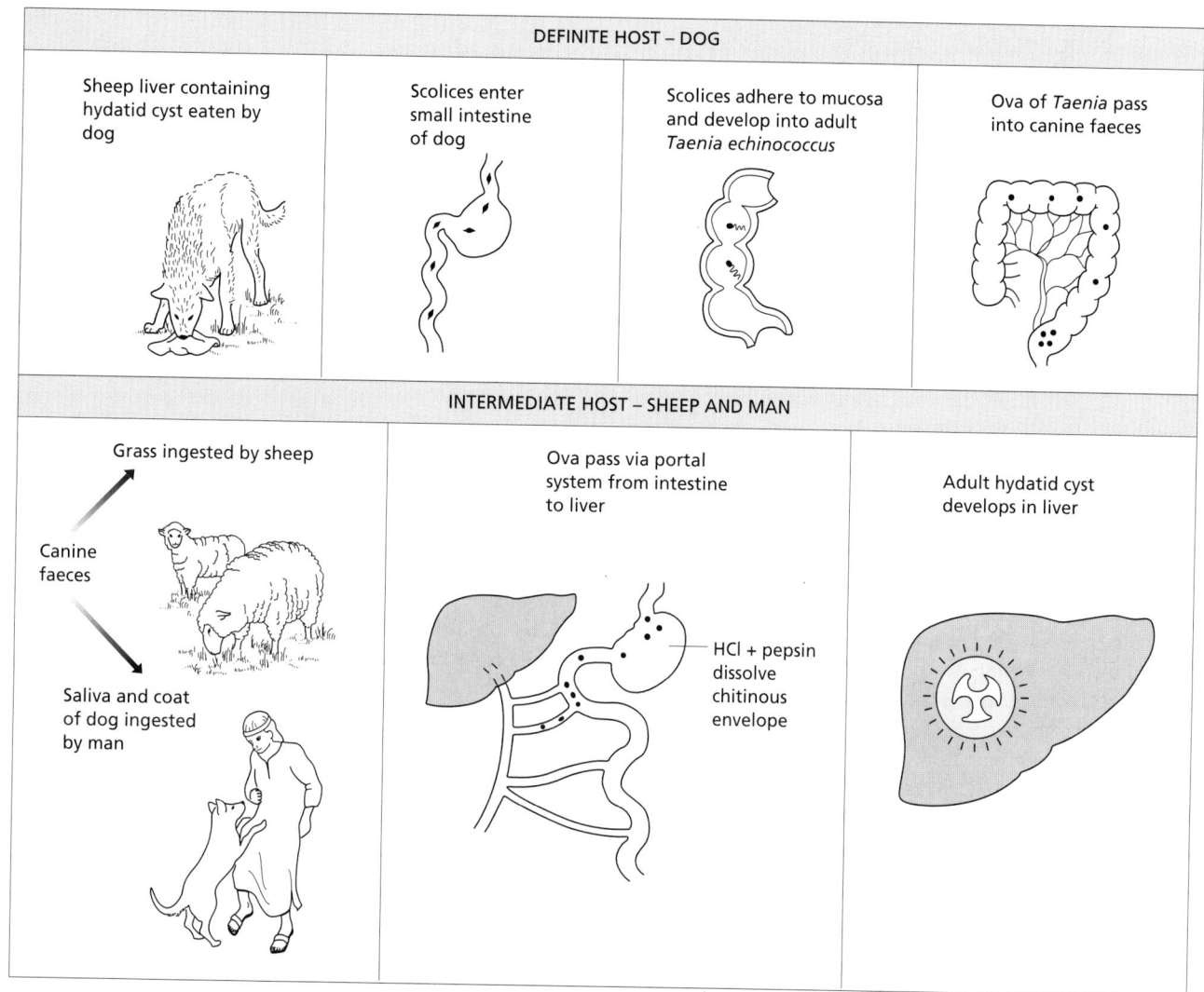

Fig. 27.17. The life cycle of the hydatid parasite.

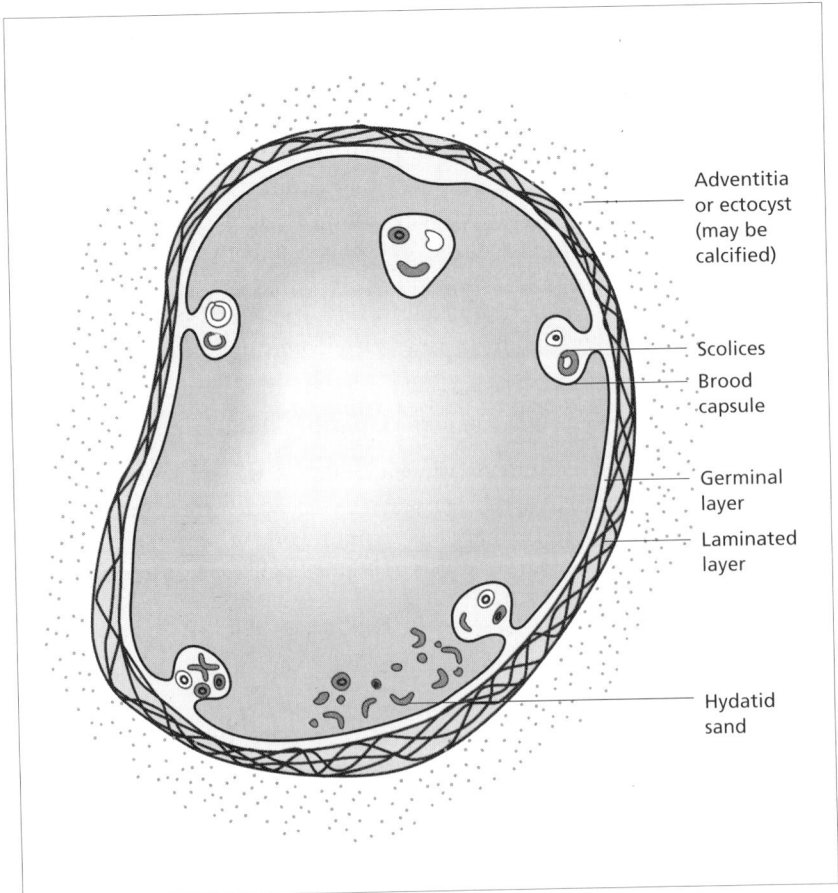

Adventitia
or ectocyst
(may be
calcified)

Scolices

Brood
capsule

Germinal
layer

Laminated
layer

Hydatid
sand

Fig. 27.18. The basic constitution of a
hydatid cyst.

round cells and eosinophils. The peripheral zone, derived from the host tissues, becomes the *adventitia* or ectocyst, a thick layer which may calcify. The intermediate and inner zones become hyalinized (the *laminated layer*). Finally, the cyst becomes lined with the *germinal layer*, which gives rise to pedunculated nodes of multiplying cells which project into the lumen of the cyst as *brood capsules*. Scolices develop from the brood capsules and eventually indent it. The attachment of the brood capsules to the germinal layer becomes progressively thinner until the capsule bursts, releasing the scolices into the cyst fluid. These fall to the bottom by gravity and are termed *hydatid sand*. When ingested by the dog, the cycle begins again.

The cyst fluid is a transudate of serum. It contains protein and is antigenic. If released into the circulation eosinophilia or anaphylaxis may result.

Daughter and even grand-daughter cysts develop by fragmentation of the germinal layer. The majority of cysts in adult patients are thus multilocular.

Endemic regions

The disease is common in sheep-raising countries, where dogs have access to infected offal. These include South Australia, New Zealand, Africa, South America, southern Europe, especially Cyprus, Greece and Spain, and the Middle and Far East. The disease is rare in Britain, apart from some areas in Wales.

Distribution of cysts in the liver

Hydatid cysts usually involve the right lobe on its antero-inferior or postero-inferior surface. If the right lobe is involved anteriorly, the costal margin is pushed forward; if posteriorly, the diaphragm is pushed upwards. When the left lobe is involved, the swelling presents in the epigastrium.

Clinical features

These depend on the site, the stage of development and whether the cyst is alive or dead.

The rest of the liver hypertrophies and hepatomegaly results.

The *uncomplicated hydatid cyst* may be silent and found incidentally at autopsy. It should be suspected if a rounded, smooth swelling, continuous with the liver, is found in a patient who is not obviously ill. The only complaints may be a dull ache in the right upper quadrant and sometimes a feeling of abdominal distension. The tension in the cyst is high and fluctuation is never marked.

Complications

Rupture. Intra-peritoneal rupture is frequent and leads to multiple cysts throughout the peritoneal cavity with intestinal obstruction and gross abdominal distension.

The pressure in the cyst greatly exceeds that in bile and rupture into bile ducts is frequent. This may lead to cure or to cholestatic jaundice with recurrent cholangitis.

Colonic rupture leads to elimination per rectum and to secondary infection.

The cysts may adhere to the diaphragm, rupture into the lungs and result in expectoration of daughter cysts. Pressure on and rupture into the hepatic veins leads to the Budd–Chiari syndrome. Secondary involvement of the lungs may follow.

Infection. Secondary invasion by pyogenic organisms follows rupture into biliary passages, giving the picture of a pyogenic abscess; the parasite dies. Occasionally, the entire cyst content undergoes aseptic necrosis and again the parasite dies. This amorphous yellow debris must be distinguished from the pus of secondary infection.

Other organs. Cysts can occur in lung, kidney, spleen, brain or bone, but mass infestation is rare in man; the liver is usually the only organ involved. If a hydatid cyst is found elsewhere, there is always concomitant infestation of the liver.

Hydatid allergy. Cyst fluid contains a foreign protein which sensitizes the host. This may lead to severe anaphylactic shock but more commonly leads to recurrent urticaria or 'hives'.

Membranous glomerulitis may be related to glomerular deposits of hydatid antigen [10].

Diagnosis

Serological tests

Hydatid fluid contains specific antigens, leakage of which sensitizes the patient with the production of antibodies.

ELISA with whole hydatid fluid gives positive results in about 85% [3].

All serological tests can give false negative and false positive results.

Results may be negative for all tests if the cyst has never leaked, if it contains no scolices or if the parasite is dead.

Eosinophilia of greater than 7% is found in about 30% of patients.

Radiological changes

These include a raised, poorly moving right diaphragm, hepatomegaly and calcification. Calcium is laid down in the ectocyst as a distinct round or oval opacity (fig. 27.19) or merely as shreds. Calcification in adjacent structures such as adrenal, kidney, gallbladder, peritoneum, diaphragm, costal cartilages and in an old subphrenic abscess must be excluded.

Floating bodies within hydatid cysts indicate the presence of free-moving daughter cysts. Infected gas-containing cysts may show a fluid level.

Hepatic cysts may cause displacement of the stomach or hepatic flexure of the colon.

Characteristic radiological changes may be seen in the lungs, spleen, kidney or bone.

Selective coeliac angiography shows stretching and elongation of the hepatic arteries and avascular areas in the hepatogram.

Ultrasound or *CT scanning* demonstrates single or multiple cysts which may be uni- or multi-loculated, thin or thick walled (figs 27.20, 27.21, 27.22). Appearances may be classified (table 27.2) [7]. Infected cysts are poorly defined.

MRI may show a characteristic intense rim, daughter cysts and detachment of the membranes [14]. Intra-hepatic and extra-hepatic rupture can be defined.

ERCP may show cysts in the bile ducts (figs 27.23, 27.24).

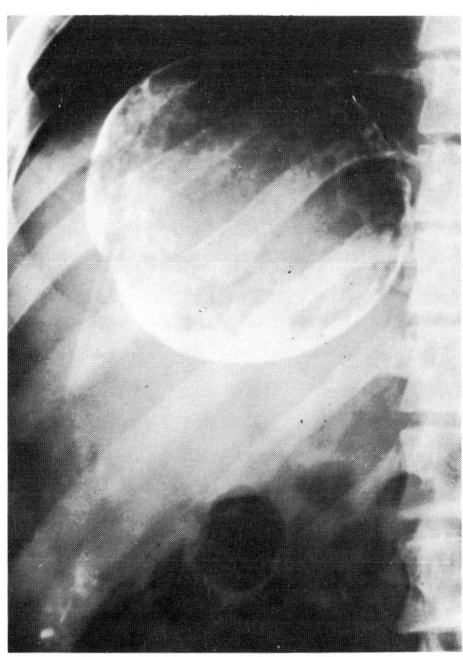

Fig. 27.19. X-ray of the abdomen shows a calcified hydatid cyst in the liver.

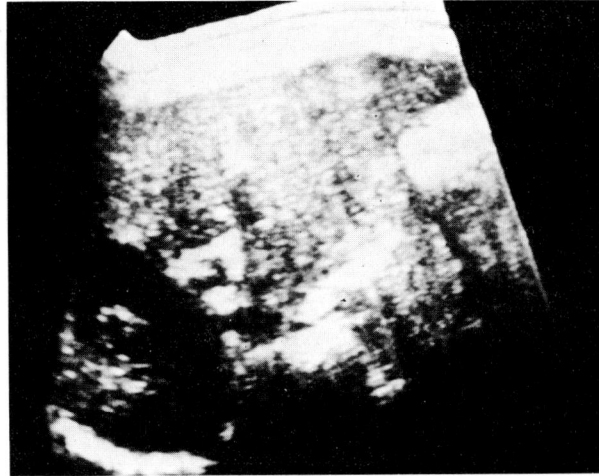

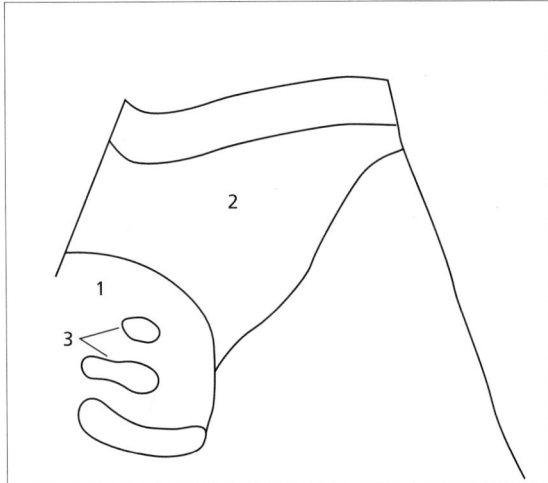

Fig. 27.20. Ultrasound shows a hydatid cyst (1) in the right lobe of the liver (2). Daughter cysts (3) can be seen inside the larger cyst.

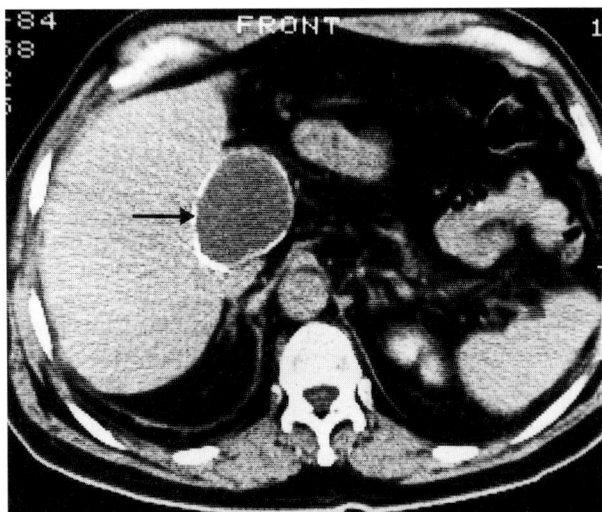

Fig. 27.21. CT scan shows calcified hydatid cyst (arrowed) in quadrate lobe of the liver (contrast-enhanced scan).

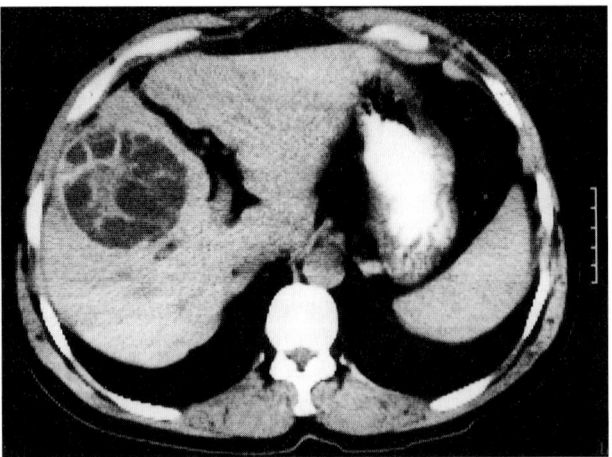

Fig. 27.22. CT scan. Hydatid cyst in right lobe of liver showing patchy calcification of the wall and containing multiple septae produced by daughter cysts (contrast-enhanced scan).

Table 27.2. Classification of ultrasound appearances in hydatid disease [7]

Type	Description
I	Purely cystic
II	Detached membrane
III	Undulating in cyst cavity Multiseptate cyst
IV	Heterogenous complex mass (dead parasite) Calcified mass (eggshell) (dead parasite)

Prognosis

The uncomplicated hepatic hydatid cyst carries a reasonably good prognosis. The risk of complications is, however, always present. Intra-peritoneal or intra-pleural rupture is grave, but rupture into the biliary tree is not so serious because spontaneous cure may follow the biliary colic. Infection used to be fatal, but the outlook is now improved by antibiotics. Calcification is unwelcome if surgery is attempted because of the difficulty in collapsing the cyst cavity.

Treatment

Dogs are denied access to infected offal and hands are washed after handling dogs [6]. Dogs in affected areas must be regularly de-wormed.

Surgery

The risks of rupture and secondary infection are so great that, unless they are small and multiple, hepatic

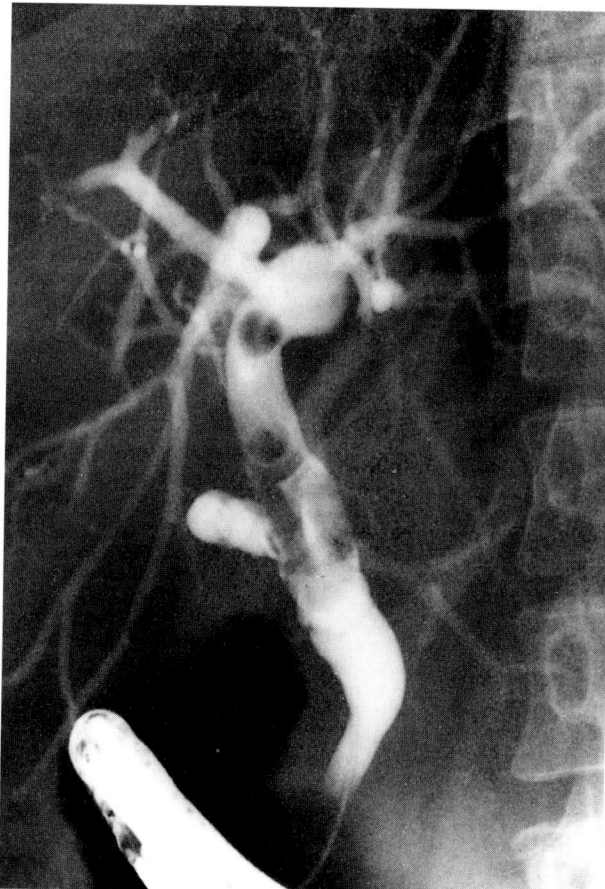

Fig. 27.23. Endoscopic cholangiography shows hydatid cysts in the common bile duct.

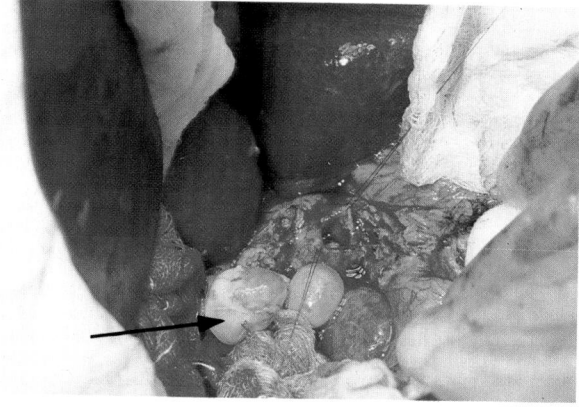

Fig. 27.24. Four glistening hydatid cysts were removed surgically from the common bile duct of the patient shown in fig. 27.23 (arrow).

hydatids should be treated surgically if the patient's condition permits.

There is no completely satisfactory surgical approach but the operation is best performed by an expert. The object is to remove the cyst completely, without soiling and infecting the peritoneum, and with complete obliteration of the resulting dead space. Complete removal of the cyst, with its adventitia, is ideal to avoid spilling the contents.

The cyst is first aspirated through its most superficial part (detected by scanning) and 90% alcohol, 20% saline or silver nitrate injected into it as a scolicidal agent. Sclerosing cholangitis can complicate injection of these agents particularly if formalin is used [17].

The usual operation is cystectomy with removal of the germinal and laminated layers and preservation of the host-derived ectocyst [13]. The ectocyst cavity, left after removal of the parasitic endocyst, is difficult to obliterate. The choice lies between leaving it open (with or without a drain), tightly closing it after filling it with saline, or performing omentoplasty.

Radical pericystectomy includes removal of the pericyst and has a high mortality.

The operative mortality for these operations is 2.2% and the morbidity rate 23.7% [13].

Occasionally, the cyst is removed by hemihepatectomy or segmentectomy.

Recurrence is the major complication and is usually due to spillage at operation. Serial scans are used in follow-up.

Cholangitis is treated by biliary drainage, usually by endoscopy with papillotomy and cyst removal. Otherwise, surgical biliary drainage may be necessary. The technical problem is great (figs 27.23, 27.24).

Rupture into the peritoneal cavity

The cyst contents are removed from the peritoneal cavity as far as possible by sucking and swabbing. The scolices, however, usually settle down in the peritoneal cavity and form daughter cysts so that recurrence is almost inevitable.

Urgent surgery has a substantial morbidity and mortality [16]. Chemotherapy is essential.

Medical treatment

Mebendazole diffuses through the cyst membrane and interferes with glucose metabolism and microtubular function in the parasite. Viable cysts can persist even after 12 months of therapy. Recurrence is not unusual and the concentration of drug achieved in large cysts is very uncertain.

Albendazole freely diffuses across parasitic membranes [15]. It is more satisfactory than mebendazole. 10% per kg body weight for 3 months results in non-viable cysts [8]. This should be the initial therapy for uncomplicated cysts. Asymptomatic, small ones may respond to this therapy, but larger ones require surgery.

Aspiration

Formerly, this was contraindicated because of the risk of dissemination and of anaphylaxis. Aspiration under ultrasound guidance using a 22 gauge 0.7 mm needle now appears safe and has been used both diagnostically and therapeutically. The aspirated fluid can be stained to show fragments of laminated membrane, hooklets and scolices [9]. Therapeutic transhepatic aspiration and 95% alcohol or hypertonic saline injection under albendazole cover seems safe and effective [1]. The cyst should be univesicular (Gharbi type I or II) [7]. The fluid must not be bile stained as a fall in cyst pressure might prevent closure of a biliary fistula. This technique is largely confined to those who refuse surgery or are unsuitable for it.

Percutaneous drainage with albendazole is more effective on cyst-size reduction than albendazole alone or aspiration alone [12].

Echinococcus multilocularis (alveolar echinococcosis)

This is found in the northern hemisphere. Rodents are intermediate and foxes definitive hosts. The larvae grow indefinitely and produce liver necrosis and a major granulomatous reaction. It may be diagnosed by PCR [11]. The disease behaves like a locally malignant tumour. The echinococcus invades liver and biliary tissue, hepatic veins, inferior vena cava and diaphragm. Chemotherapy is effective but not curative [2]. It is fatal unless completely removed by surgery [18]. Hepatic transplant may be necessary [4].

References

1 Acunas B, Rozanes I, Çalik L *et al.* Purely cystic hydatid disease of the liver: treatment with percutaneous aspiration and injection of hypertonic saline. *Radiology* 1992; **182**: 541.

2 Ammann RW, Ilitsch N, Marincek B *et al.* Effect of chemotherapy on the larval mass and the long-term course of alveolar echinococcosis. *Hepatology* 1994; **19**: 735.

3 Babba H, Messedi A, Masmoudi S *et al.* Diagnosis of human hydatidosis: comparison between imaging and six serologic techniques. *Am. J. Trop. Med. Hyg.* 1994; **50**: 64.

4 Bresson-Hadni S, Franza A, Miguet JP *et al.* Orthotopic liver transplantation for incurable alveolar echinococcosis of the liver: report of 17 cases. *Hepatology* 1991; **13**: 1061.

5 Filice C, Pirola F, Brunetti E *et al.* A new therapeutic approach for hydatid liver cysts. Aspiration and alcohol injection under sonographic guidance. *Gastroenterology* 1990; **98**: 1366.

6 Gemmell MA, Lawson JR, Roberts MG. Control of echinococcosis/hydatidosis: present status of worldwide progress. *Bull. World Health Organ.* 1986; **64** (3): 333.

7 Gharbi HA, Hassine W, Brauner MW *et al.* Ultrasound examination of the hydatic liver. *Radiology* 1981; **139**: 459.

8 Gil-Grande LA, Rodriguez-Caabeiro F, Prieto JG *et al.* Randomized controlled trial of efficacy of albendazole in intra-abdominal hydatid disease. *Lancet* 1993; **342**: 1269.

9 Hira PR, Shweiki H, Lindberg LG *et al.* Diagnosis of cystic hydatid disease: role of aspiration cytology. *Lancet* 1988; **2**: 655.

10 Ibarrola AS, Sobrini B, Guisantes J *et al.* Membranous glomerulonephritis secondary to hydatid disease. *Am. J. Med.* 1981; **70**: 311.

11 Kern P, Frosch P, Helbig M *et al.* Diagnosis of *Echinococcus multilocularis* infection by reverse-transcription polymerase chain reaction. *Gastroenterology* 1995; **109**: 596.

12 Khuroo MS, Dar MY, Yattoo GN *et al.* Percutaneous drainage versus albendazole therapy in hepatic hydatidosis: a prospective randomized study. *Gastroenterology* 1993; **104**: 1452.

13 Magistrelli P, Masetti R, Coppola R *et al.* Surgical treatment of hydatid disease of the liver. A 20 year experience. *Arch. Surg.* 1991; **126**: 518.

14 Marani SA, Canossi GC, Nicoli FA *et al.* Hydatid disease: MR imaging study. *Radiology* 1990; **175**: 701.

15 Morris DL, Chinnery JB, Georgiou G *et al.* Penetration of albendazole sulphoxide into hydatid cysts. *Gut* 1987; **28**: 75.

16 Schaefer JW, Khan MY. Echinococcosis (hydatid disease): lessons from experience with 59 patients. *Rev. Infect. Dis.* 1991; **13**: 243.

17 Teres J, Gomez-Moli J, Bruguera M *et al.* Sclerosing cholangitis after surgical treatment of hepatic echinococcal cysts: report of three cases. *Am. J. Surg.* 1984; **148**: 694.

18 Wilson JF, Rausch RL, Wilson FR *et al.* Alveolar hydatid disease. Review of the surgical experience in 42 cases of active disease among Alaskan Eskimos. *Ann. Surg.* 1995; **221**: 315.

Ascariasis

Ascaris infection is particularly common in the Far East, India and South Africa. Ova of the round worm *Ascaris lumbricoides* arrive in the liver by retrograde flow in the bile ducts. They exert an immunological reaction and eggs, giant cells and granulomas are surrounded by a dense eosinophil infiltrate (fig. 27.25). The adult worm is 10–20 cm long but occasionally may lodge in the common bile duct producing partial bile duct obstruction, and secondary cholangitic abscesses [2]. The ascaris may be a nucleus for intra-hepatic gallstones [4]. Biliary colic is a complication.

A plain abdominal X-ray may show calcified worms.

Clinical presentation is as acute cholecystitis, acute cholangitis, biliary colic, acute pancreatitis and, rarely, hepatic abscess [2].

Ultrasound shows long linear echogenic structures or strips which characteristically move. It can be used to monitor migration of the worms. It cannot diagnose duodenal ascariasis.

ERCP shows the ascaris as a linear filling defect (fig. 27.26). Worms can be seen moving into and out of the biliary tree from the duodenum [1].

Treatment is by ERCP with endoscopic worm extraction with or without sphincterotomy [3]. Failures need surgical treatment.

Treatment with piperazine citrate, mebendazole or

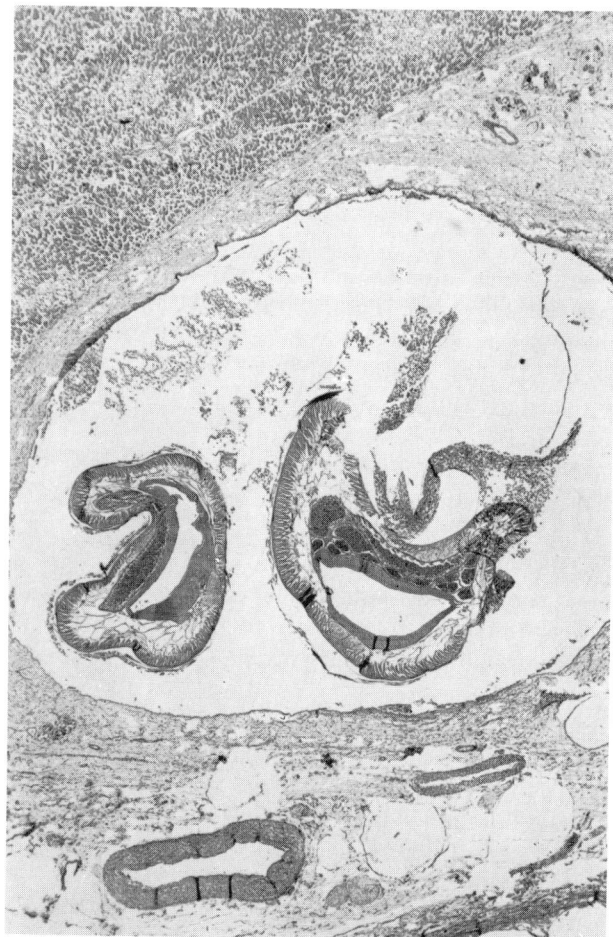

Fig. 27.25. Section shows a dead ascaris in an intra-hepatic blood vessel in a portal zone. There is surrounding fibrous tissue reaction. (Stained H & E, ×40.)

albendazole will usually kill the ascaris but it remains in the bile ducts. Re-invasion is common.

References

1 Kamath PS, Joseph DC, Chandran R *et al.* Biliary ascariasis: ultrasonography, endoscopic retrograde cholangiopancreatography, and biliary drainage. *Gastroenterology* 1986; **91**: 730.
2 Khuroo MS, Zargar SA, Mahajan R. Hepatobiliary and pancreatic ascariasis in India. *Lancet* 1990; **335**: 1503.
3 Manialawi MS, Khattar NY, Helmy MM *et al.* Endoscopic diagnosis and extraction of biliary ascaris. *Endoscopy* 1986; **18**: 204.
4 Shulman A. Non-Western patterns of biliary stones and the role of ascariasis. *Radiology* 1987; **162**: 425.

Strongyloides stercoralis

This soil-transmitted intestinal nematode is common in tropical countries. It is usually asymptomatic but can cause biliary obstruction due to biliary stenosis [1]. Thiabendazole is effective treatment.

Reference

1 Delarocque Astagneau E, Hadengue A, Degott C *et al.* Biliary obstruction resulting from *Strongyloides stercoralis* infection: report of a case. *Gut* 1994; **35**: 705.

Trichiniasis

This disease is caused by eating raw, infected pork with subsequent dissemination of *Trichinella* larvae throughout the body.

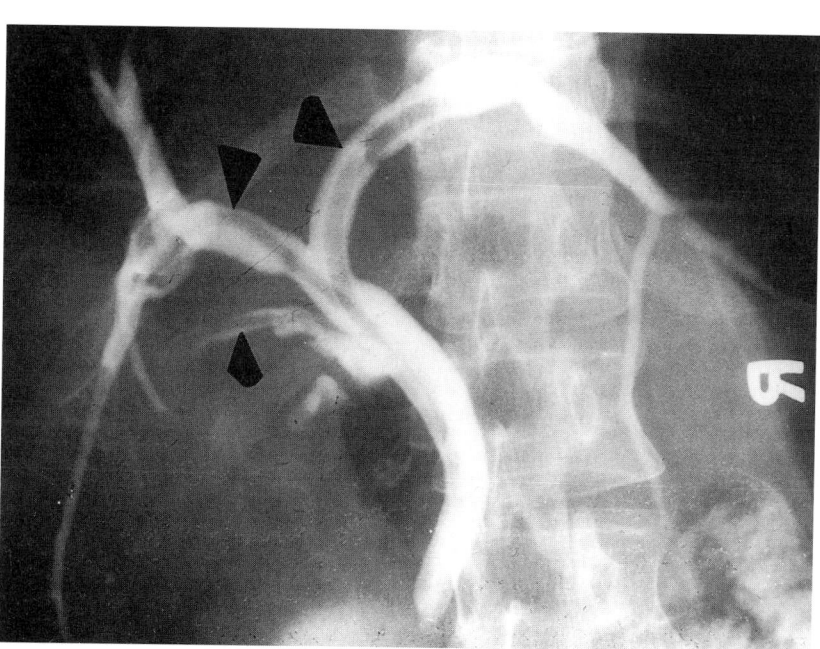

Fig. 27.26. Ascariasis: endoscopic cholangiography shows linear filling defects in the bile ducts due to ascaris worms (arrows).

Hepatic histology may show invasion of hepatic sinusoids by *Trichinella* larvae and fatty change [1].

Diagnosis is difficult unless in an epidemic. Eosinophilia is suggestive. Muscle pain and tenderness may warrant muscle biopsy.

Treatment. ERCP is indicated if the biliary tract is obstructed. Treatment is unsatisfactory. Mebendazole may be effective in the migratory stage but is of doubtful value later.

Reference

1 Guattery JM, Milne J, House RK. Observations on hepatic and renal dysfunction in trichinosis. Anatomic changes in these organs occurring in cases of trichinosis. *Am. J. Med.* 1956; **21**: 567.

Toxocara canis (visceral larva migrans)

This parasite is spread by cats and dogs. The second stage can infect the liver of man, forming granulomas [1]. Hepatomegaly, recurrent pneumonia, eosinophilia and hypergammaglobulinaemia are associated findings. The serum fluorescent antibody test is positive.

Treatment may be tried with diethyl carbamazine or thiabendazole.

Reference

1 Zinkham WH. Visceral larva migrans. *Am. J. Dis. Child.* 1978; **132**: 627.

Liver flukes

Cysts are consumed and larvae develop in the duodenum and eventually reach the bile ducts. The flukes probably invade the liver through its peritoneal coat and are carried via the parenchyma to the bile ducts. During the migratory phase they cause fever and eosinophilia. When they reach the biliary passages they may cause obstruction with complicating suppurative cholangitis.

Clonorchis sinensis

The Chinese liver fluke is found mainly in eastern Asia. It can present years after the patient has left his country of origin as the biliary flukes persist for decades. Cysts are ingested with improperly cooked or raw, fresh-water fish. The cyst wall is destroyed by trypsin in the duodenum and the larvae migrate from the duodenum into the peripheral intra-hepatic bile ducts where they mature to adult worms. In uncomplicated cases, the changes are confined to the bile duct walls with abundant adenomatous formation; fibrosis increases with time [4]. Cholangio-carcinoma is a serious complication [7].

Clinical manifestations depend on the number of flukes, the period of infestation and the complications. With heavy infestation, the patient suffers weakness, epigastric discomfort, weight loss and diarrhoea. Jaundice is due to obstruction to the intra-hepatic biliary tree by worms or inflammation. Infection leads to fever, chills and abdominal pain. Cholangio-carcinoma is marked by progressive jaundice and pruritus.

Diagnosis is based on finding ova in the stool or aspirated bile. Laboratory findings include eosinophilia and an increased serum alkaline phosphatase.

ERCP shows filamentous filling defects in the bile ducts which have blunted tips [5]. The defects are of uniform size and change in position.

Ultrasound and *CT* changes are based on flukes within dilated ducts and periductal changes without evidence of extra-hepatic biliary obstruction [1, 5].

The *therapeutic response* to praziquantel is poor and relapses may follow bithionol. Triclabendazole, used in veterinary fascioliasis, has been tried in human chronic fascioliasis with encouraging results.

Fasciola hepatica

The common sheep fluke is found mostly in mid- and western Europe and in the Caribbean. The animal infestation rate in Britain is high: 30–90% of all sheep and cattle excrete the ova. This increases in wet summers when the intermediate host, the snail *Lymnaea trunculata*, is also more numerous. The encysted cercariae from these snails survive on herbage and patients are affected usually by eating contaminated watercress.

The clinical picture in the acute stage is of cholangitis with fever, right upper quadrant pain and hepatomegaly. Eosinophilia and a raised serum alkaline phosphatase are noted. The picture may simulate choledocholithiasis.

ERCP shows several irregular linear or rounded filling defects in the bile ducts or segmental stenosis, with an inflammatory pattern. Worms can be aspirated [6].

Liver biopsy shows infiltration of the portal zones with histiocytes, eosinophils and polymorphs. Hepatic granulomas and ova in the liver may occasionally be seen.

Diagnosis is suspected by finding the clinical picture of biliary tract disease with eosinophilia. It is confirmed by finding ova in the faeces. These, however, may not be detected until 12 weeks after the infection when parasites have attained sexual maturity. They disappear later.

The diagnosis may be confirmed by ELISA testing of circulating antibodies to *Fasciola hepatica* excretory-secretory antigens [2].

CT shows peripheral filling defects, sometimes crescentic, in the liver due to the migrating fluke (fig. 27.27) [8].

Treatment of all liver flukes is by praziquantel, bithionol or albendazole.

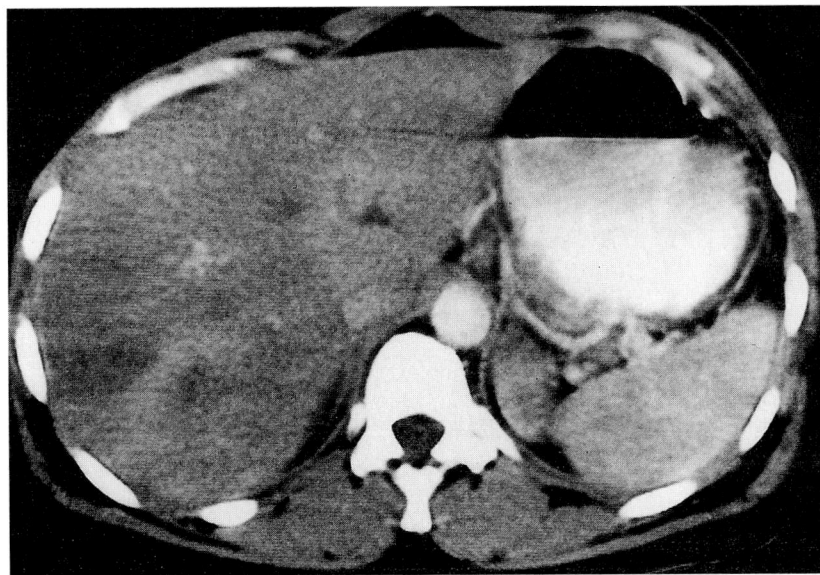

Fig. 27.27. *Fasciolia hepatica*: CT in the migratory stage shows multiple, sometimes linear, filling defects at the periphery of the liver (courtesy P.A. McCormick).

Treatment of intra-hepatic stones is difficult. They are unaffected by biliary solvents. Endoscopic papillotomy may be useful in high-risk patients. Endoprostheses inserted trans-hepatically or endoscopically may be useful to treat biliary obstruction [9]. Surgery may be necessary.

Recurrent pyogenic cholangitis

This is a common disease in South-East Asia. The initial cause is uncertain, but may be *clonorchis* or enteric micro-organisms. Biliary stone and stricture formation follow recurrent bacterial infections. Treatment is by antibiotics following biliary drainage either endoscopic or surgical [2, 3, 6].

References

1 Choi BI, Kim HJ, Han MC *et al*. CT findings of clonorchiasis. *Am. J. Roentgenol*. 1989; **152**: 281.
2 Espino AM, Marcet R, Finlay CM. Detection of circulating excretory secretory antigens in human fascioliasis by sandwich enzyme-linked immunosorbent assay. *J. Clin. Microbiol*. 1990; **28**: 2637.
3 Fan ST, Choi TK, Wong J. Recurrent pyogenic cholangitis: current management. *World J. Surg*. 1991; **15**: 248.
4 Hou PC, Pang LSC. *Clonorchis sinensis* infestation in man in Hong Kong. *J. Pathol. Bact*. 1964; **87**: 245.
5 Lim JH. Radiologic findings of clonorchiasis. *Am. J. Roentgenol*. 1990; **155**: 1001.
6 Lopez Roses L, Alonso D, Iniguez F *et al*. Hepatic fasciliasis of long-term evolution: diagnosis by ERCP. *Am. J. Gastroenterol*. 1993; **88**: 2118.
7 Ona FV, Dytoc JNT. Clonorchis-associated cholangiocarcinoma: a report of two cases with unusual manifestations. *Gastroenterology* 1991; **101**: 831.
8 Pagola Serrano MA, Vega A, Ortega E *et al*. Computed tomography of hepatic fascioliasis. *J. Comp. Assist. Tomogr*. 1987; **11**: 269.
9 Van Sonnenberg E, Casola G, Cubberley DA *et al*. Oriental cholangio-hepatitis: diagnostic imaging and interventional management. *Am. J. Roentgenol*. 1986; **146**: 327.

Peri-hepatitis

This upper abdominal peritonitis is associated with genital infections, particularly *Chlamydia trachomatis* and less often with *Neisseria gonorrhoeae* [2]. It affects young, sexually active women and simulates biliary tract disease. Diagnosis is by laparoscopy. The liver surface shows white plaques, tiny haemorrhagic spots and 'violin string' adhesions.

CT may also show the 'violin string' adhesions [1] (fig. 27.28). Treatment is with tetracycline.

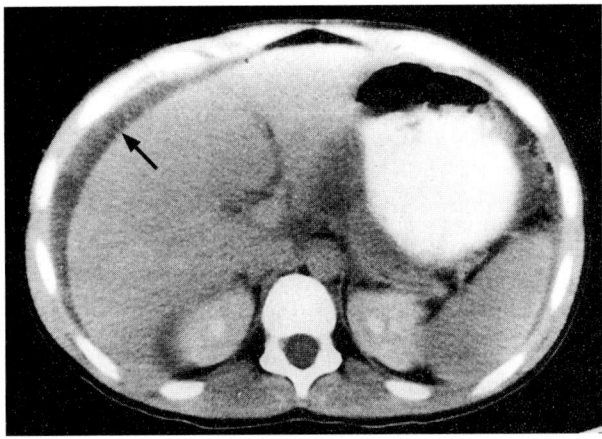

Fig. 27.28. CT in chlamydial peri-hepatitis shows 'violin string' adhesions between liver and anterior abdominal wall (arrowed) and ascites.

References

1 Haight JB, Ockner SA. *Chlamydia trachomatis* perihepatitis with ascites. *Am. J. Gastroenterol.* 1988; **83**: 323.

2 Simson JNL. Chlamydial perihepatitis (Curtis–Fitz Hugh syndrome) after hydrotubation. *Br. Med. J.* 1984; **289**: 1146.

Hepato-biliary changes in AIDS

There are probably no direct effects of HIV on the liver. Many diseases, however, affect the immunodeficient and provide a confusing picture. All parts of the hepato-biliary system can show changes and may be involved by more than one process (table 27.3). In general, there is little difference in the hepato-biliary disease seen in homosexual, drug abuser, or blood-product-related AIDS except for the prevalence of virus B and C markers.

The liver is involved as part of a disseminated disease and isolated hepatic disease is rare. Hepatomegaly is seen in two-thirds or more of patients and 80% show abnormal liver function tests. In most instances, a blood culture is more helpful than a liver biopsy.

Hepatic histology is seldom normal, showing macrovesicular fat and mild portal and peri-portal lymphocytes [18]. Occasionally Kupffer cells contain iron and focal necrosis may be seen. On the whole, lymphocytes are deficient. Liver biopsy is particularly helpful in showing granulomas of mycobacterial infection, whether *Mycobacterium tuberculosis* or *M. avium intracellulare*. The findings of hepatitis B or C may be shown [6]. Despite the frequency of hepatic changes, there is virtually no morbidity or mortality attributed to the liver disease [24]. The liver is usually involved as part of a disseminated infection or neoplastic process. Treatment is usually ineffective. An exception can be made for AIDS-related biliary tract disease, where relief of biliary obstruction may be possible, and for *M. tuberculosis*.

A high serum alkaline phosphatase level is an indication for US or CT (fig. 27.29). Those with dilated bile ducts should proceed to ERCP to confirm biliary obstruction. Those with a focal lesion should have a guided liver biopsy. In the absence of a focal or bile duct lesion a liver biopsy should be performed to exclude mycobacteria [4].

In those with a predominant increase in serum transaminases, drug toxicity should be considered and therapy withdrawn. Liver biopsy may be necessary.

Table 27.3. Hepato-biliary changes in AIDS

Non-specific
Hepatomegaly
Abnormal biochemistry
Histology
    fatty change
    portal inflammation
    Kupffer cell iron
    diminished lymphocytes

Infections
Mycobacterium avium intracellulare
Mycobacterium tuberculosis
Cytomegalovirus*
Herpes simplex
Epstein–Barr
*Cryptococcus neoformans**
Histoplasmosis
*Candida albicans**
Coccidiomycosis
*Microsporidia**
Toxoplasmosis
Bacillary peliosis

Hepatitis B
Impaired response to vaccine and antiviral therapy
Fulminant (rare)

Hepatitis C

Tumours
Hodgkin's and non-Hodgkin's lymphoma
Kaposi's sarcoma (rare)

Hepato-toxic drugs
Sulphonamides
Antibiotics
Isoniazid
Antifungals
Tranquillizers
Nucleoside analogues

*Associated biliary tract disease.

Infections

These are largely opportunistic and part of generalized infection. Liver biopsy in patients with hepatomegaly, fever and abnormal biochemical tests gives the cause in about 25%.

Mycobacterium avium intracellulare is the most commonly diagnosed hepatic infection. It is shown by poorly formed granulomas without lymphocyte cupping, giant cells or central caseation. Acid-fast bacilli are present in large numbers in clusters of foamy histiocytes or within Kupffer cells (figs 27.30, 27.31). If *Mycobacterium avium* is seen in liver biopsies, the mean survival is only 69 days. *Mycobacterium tuberculosis* leads to granulomas and is part of miliary tuberculosis [6].

Cytomegalovirus and *herpes simplex virus* infections are usually part of disseminated disease. Granulomas can be seen. Diagnosis is made by demonstrating the large intranuclear and small cytoplasmic inclusions in Kupffer cells, bile duct epithelium and, occasionally, hepatocytes.

Epstein–Barr virus can cause hepatitis, particularly in

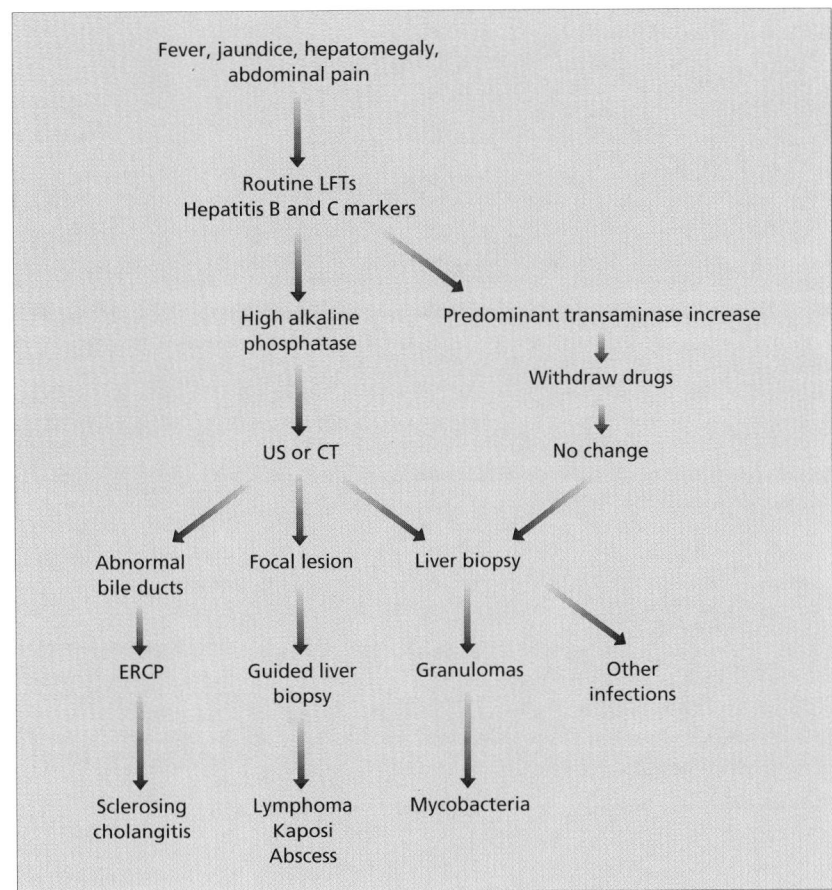

Fig. 27.29. The management of the patient with hepato-biliary AIDS.

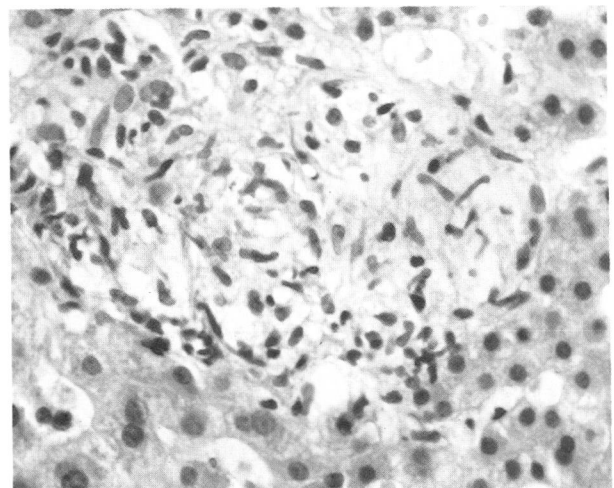

Fig. 27.30. An ill-defined poorly cellular granuloma in the liver of a patient with AIDS. (Stained H & E, ×220.)

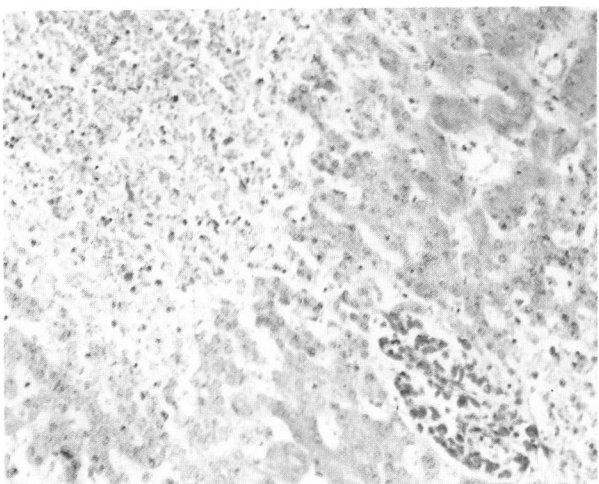

Fig. 27.31. Same patient as in fig. 27.30. Liver stained for acid-fast bacilli shows two granulomas containing many red-staining bacilli (*Mycobacterium avium intracellulare*).

children [8]. Occasionally the picture may be markedly cholestatic.

Pneumocystis carinii can rarely cause hepatitis [22].

Fungal infections are usually part of disseminated disease. They include *Cryptococcus neoformans* where yeast can be shown in the liver [2] (fig. 27.32). Similarly *histoplasmosis* (fig. 27.33), *coccidiomycosis* [27] and *Candida albicans* may involve the liver. Those with low CD4 counts exposed to cryptosporidium are at risk of biliary disease and death within 1 year [28].

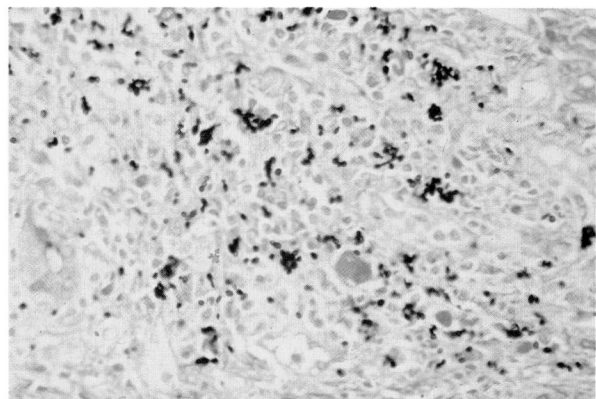

Fig. 27.32. Cryptococcal hepatitis in a patient with AIDS. Many yeast forms of *Cryptococcus neoformans* are stained black. (Methenamine silver, ×350.)

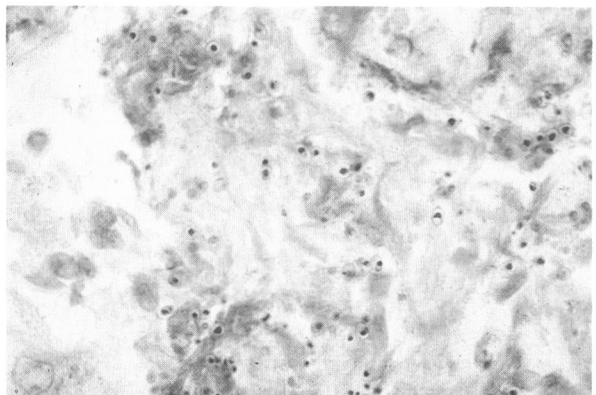

Fig. 27.33. Histoplasmosis hepatitis in a patient with AIDS. Many intracellular forms of *Histoplasma capsulatum* are stained red. (PAS diastase, ×500.)

The protozoan, *Microsporidia*, can cause hepatitis and is diagnosed only by electron microscopy.

Abnormalities of the biliary tract

These include intra- and extra-hepatic sclerosing cholangitis [5], papillary stenosis and acalculous cholecystitis.

Infecting organisms are usually cryptosporidia (fig. 27.34), cytomegalovirus (fig. 27.35) or microsporidial infections [3, 23]. The infective agent probably involves vascular endothelium causing ischaemic vasculitis and bile duct damage. The mechanism is similar to that seen in hepatic transplant recipients. The agent can be found in gallbladder wall and bile.

The patient presents with intermittent upper abdominal pain and tenderness and diarrhoea, cholestatic liver function tests, but normal serum bilirubin. Presentation may also be as painless cholestasis or as acute bacterial cholangitis.

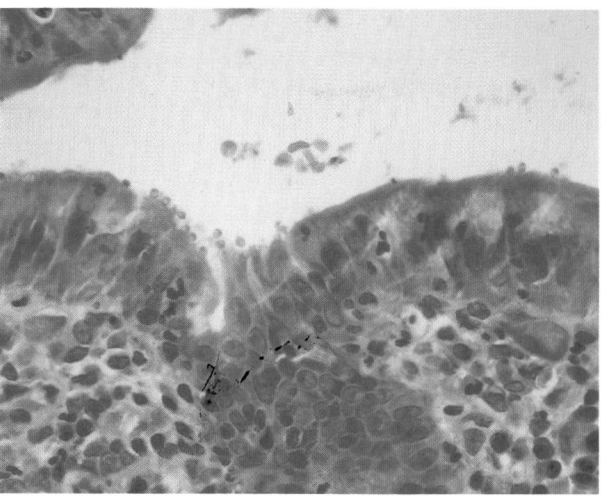

Fig. 27.34. Cryptosporidiosis of the gallbladder in a patient with AIDS. (Stained H & E, ×160.)

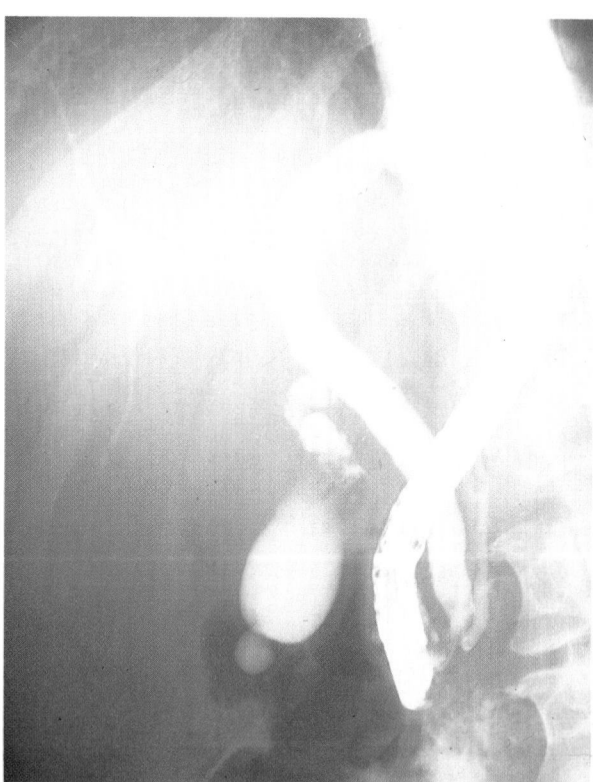

Fig. 27.35. Ampullary stenosis and sclerosing cholangitis due to cytomegalovirus infection in a patient with AIDS.

CT and *US* show biliary dilatation, thickening of the bile duct and/or the gallbladder. Filling defects adjacent to bile ducts simulate metastases [14].

Ultrasound may show an echogenic nodule at the lower end of the common bile duct, probably oedematous papilla [7].

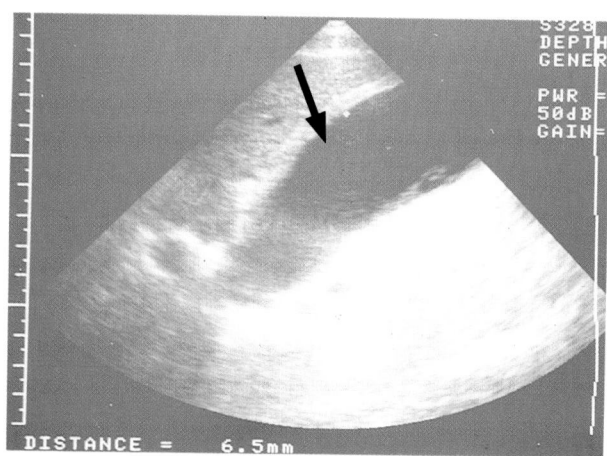

Fig. 27.36. Cryptosporidial biliary infection in a patient with AIDS. Ultrasound shows greatly thickened gallbladder wall (arrowed) and bile ducts.

ERCP shows an irregularly dilated common bile duct with papillary stenosis. Better yield of the causative agent is obtained if multiple (duodenal and papillary) biopsies are taken and the bile sampled [3].

Prognosis and treatment. The patient with hepato-biliary AIDS has the same overall outcome (mean survival 7.5 months) as in matched AIDS controls [11]. Only 14% survive 1 year [3].

The papillary stenosis is treated by endoscopic sphincterotomy which relieves the pain. Balloon dilatation and stents may be needed.

Acalculous cholecystitis can be due to cytomegalovirus or cryptosporidia. It can be gangrenous. Ultrasound shows a thickened gallbladder wall, air in the gallbladder and pericholecystic fluid [1] (fig. 27.36).

Bacillary angiomatosis and peliosis

Sinusoidal abnormalities, dilatation and peliosis hepatis are probably due to injury to endothelial cells.

Peliosis can accompany cutaneous bacillary angiomatosis when Gram-negative *Rochalimaea* can be isolated from the cutaneous lesions and from liver [16, 25]. The patient presents with massive hepatomegaly. Anaemia can be due to sequestration of blood in the lesion [12].

Erythromycin is effective treatment.

Relation to hepatitis B and C co-infection

In homosexual men or drug abuser patients with AIDS, markers of past or present HBV infection are found in approximately 90%. Those positive for HBsAg tend to be HBe-antigen positive despite having minimal biochemical and histological evidence of inflammation. Seroconversion from HBV e-antigen positive to HBe-antibody

positive can occur despite severe immunodeficiency [15]. Delta is present depending on the location [26]. These patients respond poorly to hepatitis B vaccination [13] and to antiviral treatment [21].

HIV infected patients who also carry the hepatitis C virus tend to have chronic hepatitis or even fulminant disease. Liver failure was reported in 9% of HCV-HIV infected haemophiliacs compared with 0% of HIV patients who were not co-infected [9]. Mothers who are HIV-HCV positive are likely to transmit both infections to their babies.

Drug-related liver injury

AIDS patients are exposed to many potential hepatotoxins including sulphonamides, antibiotics, antifungals and tranquillizers. Trimethoprim-sulfamethoxazole is a common offender causing granulomatous hepatitis and jaundice [17]. Hepatomegaly and steatosis may be related to nucleoside-analogue retroviral therapy [11]. The multiplicity of drug exposure in patients with AIDS presenting with fever and abnormal biochemical tests of liver function offers a diagnostic challenge.

Tumours

Kaposi's sarcoma frequently involves the liver, but is usually detected at autopsy rather than by biopsy. It is shown macroscopically as purple-brown, soft nodules. Histology shows multifocal areas of vascular endothelial proliferation with pleomorphic spindle cells and extravasated erythrocytes (fig. 27.37). The patient is usually asymptomatic.

Ultrasound shows small hyper-echoic nodules and dense peripheral bands. *CT* shows hypo-attenuated lesions enhanced after contrast [20].

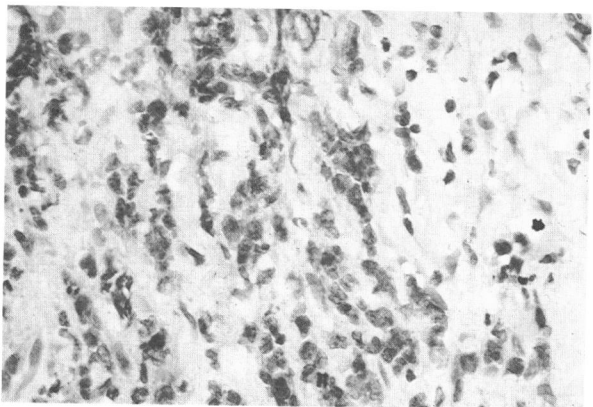

Fig. 27.37. Kaposi's sarcoma in a patient with AIDS. Portal zones show expansion with spindle cell tumour cells which are forming vascular clefts. (Stained H & E, ×150.)

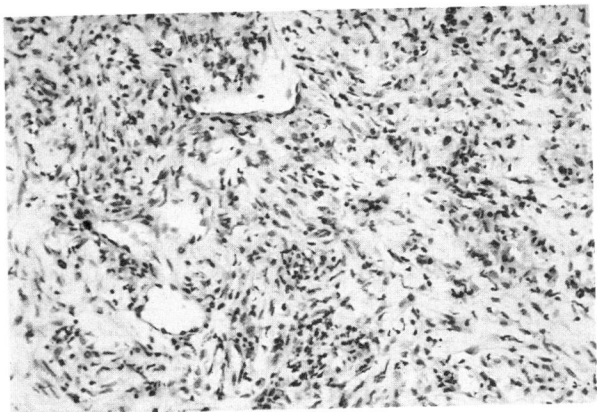

Fig. 27.38. B-cell lymphoma in a patient with AIDS. Sinusoids are infiltrated with large pleomorphic lymphoid cells. (Stained H & E, ×350.)

Non-Hodgkin's lymphoma

B-cell lymphoma is usually metastatic but can be primary [19] (fig. 27.38). It may develop in asymptomatic patients as a first manifestation of HIV, in patients with AIDS-related complex or in those with established AIDS. Lymphoma presents as fever, weight loss, night sweats, abdominal pain with a rise in serum transaminases and especially serum alkaline phosphatase. Large hepatic lesions present with jaundice and pruritus.

US and *CT* show large, usually multifocal, solid space-occupying lesions. Guided liver biopsy is diagnostic.

The survival is short and response to chemotherapy poor.

References

1 Aaron JS, Wynter CD, Kirton OC *et al.* Cytomegalovirus associated with acalculous cholecystitis in a patient with acquired immune deficiency syndrome. *Am. J. Gastroenterol.* 1988; **83**: 879.

2 Bonacini M, Nussbaum J, Ahluwalia C. Gastrointestinal, hepatic, and pancreatic involvement with *Cryptococcus neoformans* in AIDS. *J. Clin. Gastroenterol.* 1990; **12**: 295.

3 Bouche H, Housset C, Dumont J-L *et al.* AIDS-related cholangitis: diagnostic features and course in 15 patients. *J. Hepatol.* 1993; **17**: 34.

4 Cappell MS. Hepatobiliary manifestations of the acquired immune deficiency syndrome. *Am. J. Gastroenterol.* 1991; **86**: 1.

5 Cello JP. Acquired immunodeficiency syndrome cholangiopathy: spectrum of disease. *Am. J. Med.* 1989; **86**: 539.

6 Comer GM, Mukherjee S, Scholes JV *et al.* Liver biopsies in the acquired immune deficiency syndrome: influence of endemic disease and drug abuse. *Am. J. Gastroenterol.* 1989; **84**: 1525.

7 Da Silva F, Boudghene F, Lecomte I *et al.* Sonography in AIDS-related cholangitis: prevalence and cause of an echogenic nodule in the distal end of the common bile duct. *Am. J. Roentgenol.* 1993; **160**: 1205.

8 Duffy LF, Daum F, Kahn E *et al.* Hepatitis in children with acquired immune deficiency syndrome. *Gastroenterology* 1986; **90**: 173.

9 Eyster ME, Diamondstone LS. Natural history of hepatitis C virus infection in multi-transfused hemophiliacs: effect of coinfection with human immunodeficiency virus. *J. AIDS* 1993; **6**: 602.

10 Forbes A, Blanshard C, Gazzard B. Natural history of AIDS-related sclerosing cholangitis: a study of 20 cases. *Gut* 1993; **34**: 116.

11 Fortgang IS, Belitsos PC, Chaisson RE *et al.* Hepatomegaly and steatosis in HIV-infected patients receiving analog anti-retroviral therapy. *Am. J. Gastroenterol.* 1995; **90**: 1433.

12 Garcia-Tsao G, Panzini L, Yoselevitz M *et al.* Bacillary peliosis hepatitis as a cause of acute anemia in a patient with the acquired immunodeficiency syndrome. *Gastroenterology* 1992; **102**: 1065.

13 Hadler SC, Judson FN, O'Malley PM *et al.* Outcome of hepatitis B virus infection in homosexual men and its relation to prior human immunodeficiency virus infection. *J. Infect. Dis.* 1991; **163**: 454.

14 Hasan FA, Jeffers LJ, Dickinson G *et al.* Hepatobiliary cryptosporidiosis and cytomegalovirus infection mimicking metastatic cancer to the liver. *Gastroenterology* 1991; **100**: 1743.

15 Housset C, Pol S, Carnot F *et al.* Interactions between human immunodeficiency virus-1, hepatitis delta virus and hepatitis B virus infections in 260 chronic carriers of hepatitis B virus. *Hepatology* 1992; **15**: 578.

16 Koehler JE, Quinn FD, Berger TG *et al.* Isolation of *Rochalimaca* species from cutaneous and osseous lesions of bacillary angiomatosis. *N. Engl. J. Med.* 1992; **327**: 1625.

17 Kreisberg R. Clinical problem-solving. We blew it. *N. Engl. J. Med.* 1995; **332**: 945.

18 Lefkowitch JH. Pathology of AIDS-related liver disease. *Dig. Dis. Sci.* 1994; **12**: 321.

19 Lisker-Melman M, Pittaluga S, Pluda JM *et al.* Primary lymphoma of the liver in a patient with acquired immune deficiency syndrome and chronic hepatitis B. *Am. J. Gastroenterol.* 1989; **84**: 1445.

20 Luburich P, Bru C, Ayuso MC *et al.* Hepatic Kaposi sarcoma in AIDS: US and CT findings. *Radiology* 1990; **175**: 172.

21 McDonald JA, Caruso L, Karayiannis P *et al.* Diminished responsiveness of male homosexual chronic hepatitis B carriers with HTLV-111 antibodies to recombinant alpha interferon. *Hepatology* 1987; **7**: 719.

22 Poblete RB, Rodriguez K, Foust RT *et al. Pneumocystis carinii* hepatitis in the acquired immunodeficiency syndrome (AIDS). *Ann. Intern. Med.* 1989; **110**: 737.

23 Pol S, Romana CA, Richard S *et al.* Microsporidia infection in patients with the human immunodeficiency virus and unexplained cholangitis. *N. Engl. J. Med.* 1993; **328**: 95.

24 Schneiderman DJ, Arenson DM, Cello JP *et al.* Hepatic disease in patients with the acquired immune deficiency syndrome (AIDS). *Hepatology* 1987; **7**: 925.

25 Slater LN, Welch DT, Min KW. *Rochalimaea henselae* causes bacillary angiomatosis and peliosis hepatitis. *Arch. Intern. Med.* 1992; **152**: 602.

26 Soloman RE, Kaslow RA, Phair JP *et al.* Human immunodeficiency virus and hepatitis delta virus in homosexual men. A study of four cohorts. *Ann. Intern. Med.* 1988; **108**: 51.

27 Stevens DA. Current concepts. Coccidiomycosis. *N. Engl. J. Med.* 1995; **332**: 1077.

28 Vakil NB, Schwartz SM, Buggy BP *et al.* Biliary cryptosporidiosis in HIV-infected people after the waterborne outbreak of cryptosporidiosis. *N. Engl. J. Med.* 1996; **334**: 19.

Jaundice of infections

Bacterial pneumonia

Jaundice is an unusual complication of pneumonia. It is, however, still frequent in Africans, where it may be related partly to haemolysis in those deficient in glucose 6-phosphate dehydrogenase [6]. The jaundice is also both hepato-cellular and cholestatic.

Liver biopsy shows non-specific changes; electron microscopy shows cholestasis. There is also evidence of toxic liver injury. Increased numbers of fat-storing lipocytes are seen during the acute stage.

Septicaemia and septic shock

Liver function abnormalities, including modest increases in serum alkaline phosphatase, transaminases and bile salts, are not uncommon in patients with severe infections, septicaemia, toxic shock and endotoxaemia [1, 5]. In two-thirds, jaundice is a feature and, if it persists, carries a bad prognosis.

Hepatic histology shows non-specific hepatitis including mid-zonal and peripheral necrosis. Cholestasis may be marked and in severe cases is shown as inspissated bile within dilated and proliferated portal and periportal bile ductules [2]. Cultures of the liver are sterile.

The causes are multifactorial. Hepatic hypoperfusion plays a part. The cholangiolar lesions might be related to interference with canalicular exchange of water and electrolytes, to endotoxaemia, to staphylococcal exotoxin [4] or to interference with the peribiliary vascular plexus as a result of shock [1]. Tumour necrosis factor-α may mediate endotoxin-induced cholestasis [7]. Endotoxin interferes with bile acid transport [3].

The syndrome of jaundice associated with extrahepatic infection is functional and reversible upon control of the infection.

References

1 Gourley GR, Chesney PJ, Davis JP *et al.* Acute cholestasis in patients with toxic-shock syndrome. *Gastroenterology* 1981; **81**: 928.
2 Lefkowitch JH. Bile ductular cholestasis: an ominous histopathologic sign related to sepsis and 'cholangitis tenta'. *Hum. Pathol.* 1982; **13**: 19.
3 Moseley RH, Wang W, Takeda H *et al.* Effect of endotoxin on bile acid transport in rat liver: a potential model for sepsis-associated cholestasis. *Am. J. Physiol*; **271**: G137.
4 Quale JM, Mandel LJ, Bergasa NV *et al.* Clinical significance and pathogenesis of hyperbilirubinemia associated with staphylococcus aureus septicemia. *Am. J. Med.* 1988; **85**: 615.
5 Sikuler E, Guetta V, Keynan A *et al.* Abnormalities in bilirubin and liver enzyme levels in adult patients with bacteremia. *Arch. Intern. Med.* 1989; **149**: 2246.
6 Tugwell P, Williams AO. Jaundice associated with lobar pneumonia. *Q. J. Med.* 1977; **46**: 97.
7 Whiting JF, Green RM, Rosenbluth AB *et al.* Tumor necrosis factor-alpha decreases hepatocyte bile salt uptake and mediates endotoxin-induced cholestasis. *Hepatology* 1995; **22**: 1273.

Chapter 28
Hepatic Tumours

The liver is affected by both benign and malignant tumours (table 28.1). The simple ones are usually anatomical curiosities of no clinical importance. Malignant disease of the liver, however, is common, secondary deposits in the liver being at least 30 times commoner than primary cancers.

Hepato-cellular carcinoma

This causes an estimated 1 250 000 deaths every year worldwide. It is the seventh commonest cause of cancer in men. The frequency depends on the geographical area (table 28.2). The highest frequency is in the African and Oriental races in whom there is nearly always an associated cirrhosis. It is the second commonest cancer encountered in South-East Asia. The condition is increasing in the West, perhaps related to the prevalence of hepatitis B and C virus infections, the commonest associations of hepato-cellular cancer.

Experimental liver cancer

A bewildering number of carcinogens can initiate

Table 28.1. Primary tumours of the liver

	Benign	Malignant
Hepato-cellular	Adenoma	HCC Fibro-lamellar Hepatoblastoma
Biliary	Adenoma Cystadenoma Papillomatosis	Cholangiocarcinoma Combined hepato-cellular– cholangiocarcinoma Cystadenocarcinoma

Mesodermal	Haemangioma	Angiosarcoma
		  (haemangio-endothelioma)
		Epithelioid
		  haemangio-endothelioma
		Sarcoma

Other	Mesenchymal hamartoma Lipoma Fibroma	

Table 28.2. Worldwide incidence of primary liver cancer reported by cancer registries

Area	Rate per 100 000 males per year
Group 1	
Mozambique	98.2
China	17.0
South Africa	14.2
Hawaii	7.2
Nigeria	5.9
Singapore	5.5
Uganda	5.5
Group 2	
Japan	4.6
Denmark	3.4
Group 3	
England and Wales	3.0
USA	2.7
Chile	2.6
Sweden	2.6
Iceland	2.5
Jamaica	2.3
Puerto Rico	2.1
Columbia	2.0
Yugoslavia	1.9

tumours in animals, but their relevance to man is uncertain. They include *p*-dimethyl-amino-azobenzene (butter yellow), nitrosamines, aflatoxin and senecio alkaloids.

There are multiple steps from initiation to progression and finally to expression of the cancer. The carcinogen binds covalently to DNA. The development of cancer depends on the ability of the host to repair the DNA or on its tolerance to the carcinogen.

Relation to cirrhosis

Cirrhosis may be a premalignant condition irrespective of the aetiology. The nodular hyperplasia progresses to carcinoma. Liver cell *dysplasia*, marked by cellular enlargement, nuclear pleomorphism and multi-nucleate cells affecting groups or whole nodules, may be an intermediate step [4]. This is found in 60% of cirrhotic livers containing hepato-cellular carcinoma (HCC) and in only 10% of non-cirrhotic livers. Patients with cirrhosis and high cell proliferation rates are at increased risk of developing cancer [8]. Alternatively, caranogenesis may be monoclonal with genetic alteration [1].

In one series of 1073 HCCs, 658 (61.3%) also showed cirrhosis. However, in 30% of African patients with hepatitis B-related hepato-cellular cancer, cirrhosis was not present. In the UK, about 30% of patients with HCC have no cirrhosis and survival is significantly better.

There are pronounced geographical differences in the frequency of cancer in cirrhotic livers. There is a particularly high association in South Africa and Indonesia, where cancer is reported in more than 30% of cirrhotic livers, whereas frequencies of 10–20% are reported from India, Britain and North America.

Relation to viruses

The relation of the virus to the development of HCC is through chronic hepatitis and cirrhosis (fig. 28.1). Almost all patients with virus-related HCC have an underlying cirrhosis. The hepatocyte necrosis and mitosis of chronic hepatitis favour nodular regeneration which, in appropriate circumstances, is followed by hepatocyte dysplasia and carcinoma [159]. Although nodular regeneration and cirrhosis remain the most important antecedents, the tumour can develop in the absence of cirrhosis. In this case, and by analogy with the hepatitis B-like woodchuck chronic hepatitis, necro-inflammatory activity may be an important requisite [126].

Relation to hepatitis B virus

Worldwide, the problem of hepatitis B virus (HBV) carriage correlates with the frequency of HCC [9, 10, 142]. The geographical distribution of those affected is related to the prevalence of the HBV carrier state in that area [40]. Chronic carriers of HBV are at greater risk of HCC than the general population [10]. Hepadna viruses, such as the woodchuck hepatitis virus, are also associated with HCC [130]. HBV DNA has been found in HCC tissue.

Carcinogenesis is a multi-stage process in which both virus and host play a part [46, 141]. The end result is the disorganization and rearrangement of hepatocyte DNA (fig. 28.2). The molecular mechanism for the postulated hepato-carcinogenic role of HBV is not known. During the course of HBV, the virus becomes integrated with host chromosomal DNA but the method by which this leads to cancer is uncertain. Integration is accompanied by chromosomal deletions and translocations, which affect cell growth and differentiation (*insertional mutagenesis*). The deletions are not related to the sites of integration, however, and in 15% of cancers integrated sequences are not found in the tumour [46]. The semi-random integration of HBV DNA into the host genome has not been associated with the over-expression of a particular proto-oncogene or with deletion of a specific region of the genome harbouring a potential anti-oncogene [46]. Inconsistent patterns of integration have emerged and the viral genome may integrate in different sites in tumours from different subjects.

The hepatitis B X-antigen (HBX) has been suggested as a transactivator increasing the rate of transcription of oncogenes [36].

The pre-S HBV envelope protein may accumulate in toxic amounts sufficient for carcinogenesis. Thus, in transgenic mice, over-production of HBV pre-S results in severe hepatic inflammation and regeneration which is followed by neoplasia [25]. Dysregulation of HBV envelope expression might be a consequence of integration.

Translocation of tumour suppressor genes located on chromosome 17 have been associated with HBV DNA integration. Thus tumour suppressor genes, such as the P53 oncogene on chromosome 17, may be crucial in HBV-related hepato-carcinogenesis [65, 101]. TGF-α is expressed at a high value in 80% of human HCC [64] and may be a co-factor. Histochemistry shows that it is localized with HBsAg to the same hepatocyte but not in the cancer cell.

Chronic hepatitis, progressing to cirrhosis, remains the most important pre-cancerous factor. HBV induces the cancer through integration, transactivation, muta-

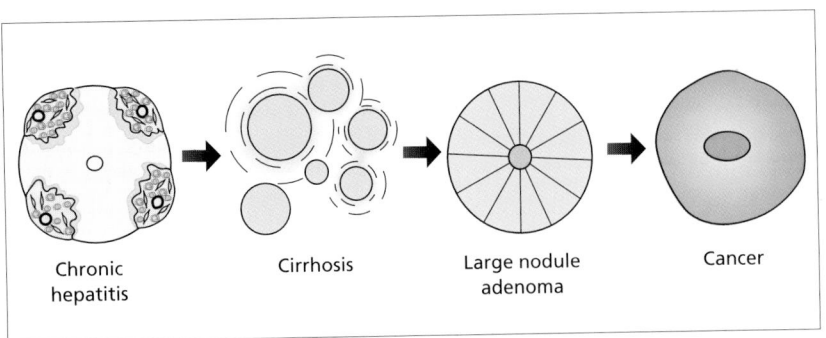

Chronic hepatitis   Cirrhosis   Large nodule adenoma   Cancer

Fig. 28.1. Stages in the evolution of HCC from chronic hepatitis through cirrhosis and large nodules [141].

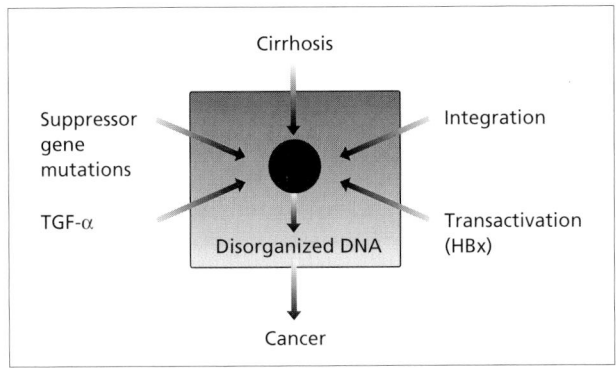

Fig. 28.2. Factors in the production of hepato-cellular cancer [141].

tions in tumour suppressor genes and increases in TGF-α.

HBsAg-positive patients infected with the δ agent have a reduced incidence of hepato-cellular cancer perhaps because the δ virus suppresses HBV.

Relation to hepatitis C virus (HCV)

Worldwide there is a strong association between chronic HCV infection and HCC. In Japan, the majority of patients with HCC are serum anti-HCV positive and about half of these give a history of blood transfusion [113]. Strong association is also found in Italy [33], Spain [16], South Africa [83] and the USA. HCV is of comparatively minor epidemiological importance in areas such as Hong Kong where HBV infection is overwhelming [93]. Sophisticated techniques for serum HCV DNA, as opposed to first-generation antibody tests, have altered the statistics. Thus, the relationship of HCV to HCC in South Africa changed from 46.1 to 19.5% [20]. In the USA, 43% hepatitis B surface antigen negative patients with HCC had second-generation positivity for HCV antibody or HCV RNA in the serum, liver or both [95]. Hepatitis C may be more important than hepatitis B in the aetiology of HCC. There is a four times higher incidence of liver cancer among anti-HCV positive patients than among HBsAg carriers. HCV genotypes are similar to those found in chronic HCV [158].

The low prevalence of HCV-related HCC in the USA compared with Japan might be related to the age of the patient. HCC only develops some 10–29 years after infection [84]. The Japanese probably acquired HCV infection in early childhood through unsterile syringes and injections. The Americans largely contracted it in adult life from drug abuse or infected blood transfusions and so they must wait for the full impact of HCV-related HCC to strike them.

In contrast to HBV, HCV is an RNA virus that lacks a reverse transcriptase enzyme and does not integrate into the host genome. The mode of carcinogenesis is uncertain, but is presumably through cirrhosis [44, 143]. HCV genomes, however, can be detected in the tumour and surrounding liver tissue [50].

There may be an interaction between hepatitis B and C infections as patients who are anti-HCV positive have HCC more often if they are HBsAg positive [33].

Carriers of hepatitis C should be regularly screened for HCC by ultrasound and serum α-fetoprotein in the same way as carriers of hepatitis B.

Relation to alcohol

In Northern Europe and North America there is a four-fold risk of primary hepato-cellular cancer in alcoholics particularly in older patients [59]. Cirrhosis is always present and alcohol is probably not a hepatic carcinogen *per se*.

Alcohol may be a co-carcinogen with HBV. Hepatitis B markers are highly prevalent in alcoholic cirrhotic patients complicated by hepato-cellular cancer. Alcohol-mediated enzyme induction may increase the conversion of co-carcinogens to carcinogens. Alcohol may also promote carcinogenesis through depression of immune responses. Carcinogen-mediated DNA alkylation is impaired by alcohol.

Hepato-cellular cancer in alcoholic cirrhotics is sometimes accompanied by the finding of integrated HBV DNA in malignantly transformed hepatocytes. However, hepato-cellular cancer can develop in alcoholics without past or present hepatitis B infection.

Mycotoxins

The most important mycotoxin is *aflatoxin* produced by a contaminating mould, *Aspergillus flavus* [41]. It is highly carcinogenic to the rainbow trout, mouse, guinea-pig and monkey. There is species variation in susceptibility. Aflatoxin and similar toxic moulds can readily contaminate food such as ground nuts or grain especially when stored in tropical conditions.

Estimated aflatoxin intake from foods in various areas of Africa correlates with the frequency of HCC (table 28.3) [98]. Aflatoxin may act as a co-carcinogen with hepatitis B.

Mutations in P53, a tumour suppressor gene, have been found in human cancers from Mozambique, South Africa and China, and have been linked to increased intake of aflatoxin [30]. Such mutations were a rare event in hepato-carcinogenesis in the UK, an area of low aflatoxin exposure.

Race and sex

There is no clear evidence of genetic predisposition.

Table 28.3. Aflatoxin ingestion and hepatoma incidence

Country	Locale	Aflatoxin intake (ng/kg/day)	Hepatoma rate (per 10^5/year)
Kenya	High altitude	3.5	1.2
Thailand	Songkhla	5.0	2.0
Swaziland	High veld	5.1	2.2
Kenya	Mid-altitude	5.9	2.5
Swaziland	Mid-veld	8.9	3.8
Kenya	Low altitude	10.0	4.0
Swaziland	Lebombo	15.4	4.3
Thailand	Ratburi	45.6	6.0
Swaziland	Low veld	43.1	9.2
Mozambique	Inhambane	222.4	13.0

Worldwide, hepato-cellular cancer is three times more frequent in males than females. This may partly be due to the higher carriage rate of hepatitis B in males. Expression of androgen receptors on cancerous hepatocytes may be augmented and oestrogen receptors suppressed [115]. The significance of this remains uncertain.

Sex hormone therapy

See Chapter 18.

Miscellaneous factors

Hepato-cellular cancer is a rare complication of auto-immune chronic hepatitis and cirrhosis [19].

It is also rare in patients with Wilson's disease or primary biliary cirrhosis [169].

Hepato-cellular cancer is a frequent cause of death in haemochromatosis [112]. It is increased in α_1-antitrypsin deficiency [42], type 1 glycogen storage disease and porphyria cutanea tarda.

Hepato-cellular cancer can complicate massive immunosuppressive therapy in patients having renal transplants.

Clonorchiasis may be followed by hepato-cellular and cholangio-carcinoma.

The relationship between schistosomiasis and liver cancer has not been established.

In Africa and Japan, hepato-cellular cancer is associated with membranous obstruction to the inferior vena cava [144].

Conclusions

Worldwide, hepatitis B and C are the most important factors for the development of hepato-cellular cancer. Co-factors contribute. However, in low prevalence areas, other factors are concerned [175]. The mechanisms in such cases and in particular the role of cirrhosis *per se* remain obscure.

Pathology

The tumour is usually white, sometimes necrotic, bile stained or haemorrhagic. Large hepatic or portal veins within the liver are often thrombosed and contain tumour. The morphological division is into three types: *expanding* with discrete margins, *spreading* (infiltrative) and *multifocal* [118]. The expanding type tends to affect the non-cirrhotic liver and in Japan may be encapsulated. In the West and Africa, most tumours are either spreading or multifocal [121].

Hepato-cellular carcinoma (figs 28.3, 28.4)

The cells resemble normal liver, with compact finger-like processes or solid trabeculae. The tumour simulates normal liver with varying degrees of success. The cells sometimes secrete bile and contain glycogen. There is no intercellular stroma and the tumour cells line the blood spaces.

The tumour cell is usually smaller than the normal liver cell; it is polygonal, with granular cytoplasm. Occasionally, atypical giant cells are found. The cytoplasm is eosinophilic, becoming basophilic with increasing malignancy. The nuclei are hyperchromatic and vary in size. Predominantly eosinophilic tumours may sometimes be seen. The centres of the tumours are often necrotic. Peri-portal lymphatic involvement with malignant cells is an early feature. PAS positive, diastase-resistant globular inclusions are found in about 15%, usually in those with high α-fetoprotein (AFP) levels. They may represent hepatocyte-produced glycoproteins. α_1-Antitrypsin and AFP have also been shown.

All gradations exist from benign regenerative nodules to malignant tumours. Dysplasia is an intermediate appearance [4]. The small dysplastic cell may be particularly pre-cancerous. Nuclear density more than 1.3 times that of controls suggests well-differentiated HCC [110].

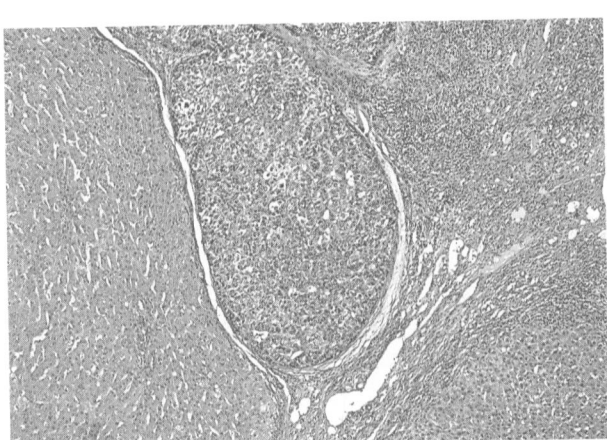

Fig. 28.3. Cirrhosis and very small HCC. This tumour was resected. (Stained H & E, ×60.)

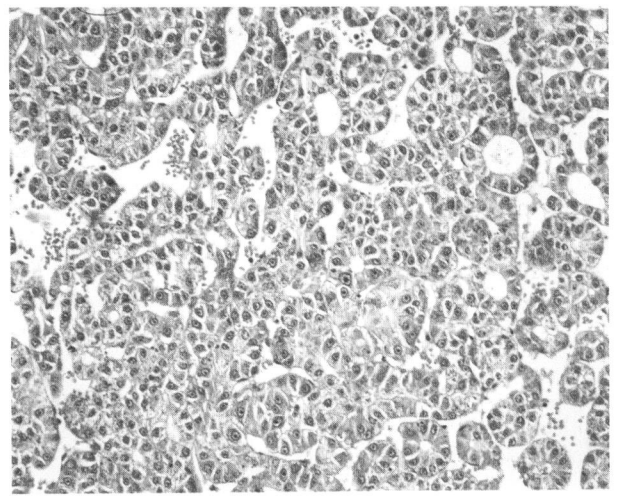

Fig. 28.4. HCC. The tumour cells are smaller than normal with granular cytoplasm and large hyperchromatic nuclei. Mitoses are conspicuous. Atypical giant cell may be seen. Stroma is scanty and the tumour cells have blood spaces between them. (Stained H & E, ×90.)

Electron microscopy. 'Cytoplasmic' hyaline is described in human HCC cells [79]. The cytoplasmic inclusions are filamentous bodies and also autophagic vacuoles.

Clear cell HCC

Tumour cells have clear non-staining cytoplasm, often foamy. Lipids and sometimes glycogen are present in excess abundant cytoplasm. The condition is often associated with hypoglycaemia and hypercholesterolaemia and has a variable prognosis [133].

HCC with giant cells

This rare entity shows osteoclast-like giant cells in sheets with a background of mononuclear cells [63]. Other areas show typical features of HCC.

Spread

Intra-hepatic. Metastases in the liver may be multiple or in one lobe. Spread is by the blood vessels, for the tumour cells abut on vascular spaces. Lymphatic permeation and direct infiltration also occur.

Extra-hepatic. Involvement of small or large hepatic or portal veins or the vena cava may be seen. Metastases have also been found in oesophageal varices even if sclerosed. Lung metastases, usually small, may develop by this route [5]. Tumour emboli result in pulmonary thrombosis. Systemic spread results in deposits anywhere, but especially in bone. Regional lymph nodes at the porta hepatis are frequently involved

and the mediastinal and cervical chains can also be infiltrated.

The tumour may involve the peritoneum with resulting haemorrhagic ascites; this may be terminal.

The histology of metastases. The secondary tumour may faithfully reproduce the structure of the primary, even forming bile. Sometimes, however, the cell type diverges widely. Bile or glycogen in cells of a metastasis suggests a hepatic primary.

Clinical features

The clinical picture is very variable. The patient may be completely asymptomatic with no physical signs other than those of cirrhosis. The tumour may have been diagnosed incidentally (see screening). Alternatively the presentation may be so florid and liver failure so great that the picture resembles a liver abscess. There are all intervening stages.

Age. All ages are affected. In races such as the Chinese and the Bantu the sufferers are often below 40 years. In temperate climates the patients are usually over 40.

Sex. Males exceed females in a ratio of 4–6:1.

Associated cirrhosis must be established. Primary carcinoma of the liver should be suspected if a patient with cirrhosis deteriorates or develops right upper-quadrant pain, or if a local lump can be palpated in the liver. It should be considered if there is no improvement when ascites, bleeding varices or pre-coma is adequately treated.

Rapid decline in a patient with haemochromatosis or with chronic liver disease and a positive HBsAg or anti-HCV suggests a complicating carcinoma.

The patient complains of malaise and abdominal fullness. He loses weight. The temperature is rarely higher than 38°C.

Pain is frequent but rarely severe and is felt as a non-specific, continuous dull ache in the epigastrium, right upper quadrant or back. Severe pain is due to perihepatitis or involvement of the diaphragm.

Gastrointestinal symptoms such as anorexia, flatulence and constipation are common. Diarrhoea may be a presenting symptom. This might be due to cholestasis or production of active substances, such as prostaglandins, by the tumour.

Dyspnoea is late and due to the large size of the tumour compressing or directly involving the diaphragm, or to pulmonary metastases.

Jaundice is rarely deep and has little relation to the extent of hepatic involvement. Rarely, the tumour presents as an intra-biliary, pedunculated polyp causing obstructive jaundice [161]. The tumour may rupture into the common bile duct [24]. Intra-bile duct tumour casts may be seen and haemobilia may be the immediate cause of death.

Occasionally the tumour presents with pyrexia and leucocytosis and with a necrotic centre. The picture resembles pyogenic liver abscess [119].

The liver is enlarged, not only downwards into the abdomen but also into the thorax. A hard irregular lump may be felt in the right upper quadrant, continuous with the liver. If the left lobe is involved, the mass is epigastric. Sometimes multiple masses are palpable. Tenderness may be so severe that the patient cannot tolerate palpation.

A friction rub, due to peri-hepatitis, is occasionally heard over the tumour. An arterial murmur (fig. 28.5) [29] is due to increased arterial vascularity. In the absence of acute alcoholic hepatitis this is diagnostic of HCC.

Ascites is found in about half the patients. The protein content is high. Malignant cells may be found but interpretation of these in peritoneal fluid is difficult. LDH and carcino-embryonic antigen may be increased. The fluid may be blood stained. Rupture causes *haemo-peritoneum*. This may present insidiously or as an acute abdomen with severe pain [105]. Prognosis is very poor.

Portal vein thrombosis adds to ascites. *Hepatic vein block* may occcur. Tumour may grow into the right atrium or oesophageal varices. [5].

Haemorrhage from oesophageal varices is frequent and usually terminal. Failure to control variceal bleeding in a cirrhotic patient is often due to a complicating HCC with portal vein invasion.

Clinical features of metastases

Lymph glands may be felt, especially in the right supra-clavicular region [82]. *Pulmonary metastases* may result in a pleural effusion. Massive pulmonary emboli may lead to dyspnoea and to pulmonary hypertension [170]. Massive arterio–portal fistulae can develop [137]. *Osseous metastases* may appear in ribs and vertebrae. *Brain secondaries* give the features of a brain tumour (see fig. 28.16).

Systemic effects

Florid endocrine changes are associated more often with the hepatoblastoma of childhood than with adult primary liver cell carcinoma.

Painful *gynaecomastia* [156] with increased secretion of oestrogen may be seen.

Hypercalcaemia is sometimes due to pseudo-hyperparathyroidism. The tumour may contain a parathormone-like material and serum parathormone levels are raised. Hepatic arterial embolization may be useful therapeutically [6].

Hypoglycaemia can be found in up to 30% of patients. This may be due to demand for glucose by an enormous

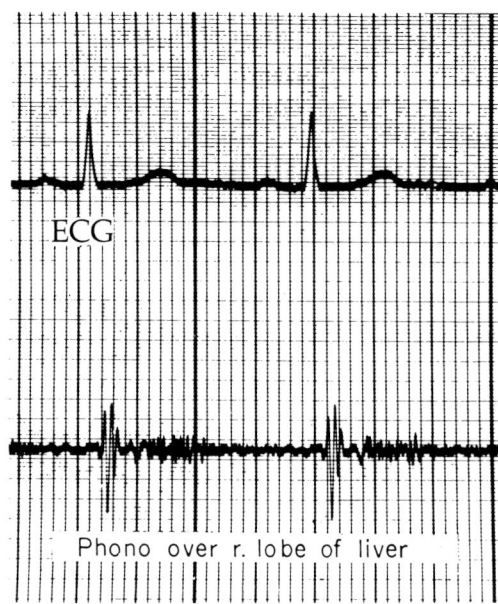

Fig. 28.5. HCC in the right lobe. Phonogram of the right lobe of the liver showing a systolic murmur [29].

tumour mass and so is often associated with an undifferentiated, rapidly progressing tumour. Rarely the hypoglycaemia is seen with a slowly progressive cancer. In this type glucose-6-phosphatase and phosphorylase are reduced or absent in the tumour while the glycogen content in tumour and adjacent tissues is increased. This suggests an acquired glycogen storage disease as the mechanism of the hypoglycaemia. In this group, control is difficult even with an enormous carbohydrate intake.

In patients with severe recurrent hypoglycaemia, the tumour tissue contains 10–20-fold more high molecular weight insulin-like growth factor II (IGF-II) than normal liver [139]. This might mediate the hypoglycaemia.

Hyperlipidaemia is rare, but about a third have increased serum cholesterol levels when maintained on a low cholesterol diet. In one patient, the hyperlipidaemia and the hypercholesterolaemia were caused by production of an abnormal lipoprotein with β mobility.

Hyperthyroidism may be due to inappropriate thyroid-stimulating hormone production [61].

Pseudo-porphyria with markedly elevated levels of porphobilinogen in urine and serum may be related to porphyrin production by the carcinoma [125].

Biochemical changes

Biochemical changes may be only those of cirrhosis. The serum alkaline phosphatase is markedly elevated and serum transaminase levels increase.

Electrophoresis of serum proteins may show a γ and an α_2 component. A serum macroglobulin of myeloma type is a rare finding.

Serological markers

Serum α₁-fetoprotein

AFP is a normal fetal serum protein. The adult value of up to 20 ng/ml is reached 10 weeks after birth. Progressive increases are found in some patients with HCC although values can be normal [160]. Raised levels at presentation in a cirrhotic patient predict development of HCC at follow-up [32]. Patients with levels greater than 20 ng/ml or who have transient increases over 100 ng/ml particularly with hepatitis B- or C-related cirrhosis, are in a super high risk group for HCC [116]. Those with repeated values greater than 100 ng/ml show a 36% incidence of HCC during a 5-year follow-up [116].

Slight increases are usual in acute hepatitis, chronic hepatitis and cirrhosis and overlaps can cause diagnostic difficulties.

The level usually correlates with tumour size but there are exceptions. However, AFP doubling time is closely related to tumour doubling time. Resection of the primary tumour, or hepatic transplantation, results in a fall in serum AFP. Persisting low levels indicate residual tumour and increases indicate rapid tumour growth. Serial values are useful in assessing therapy.

The structure of circulating AFP differs in patients with HCC from those with cirrhosis. Measurement of the AFP fractions may be useful in diagnosing HCC from cirrhosis and be predictive of HCC developing during follow-up [138].

Fibrolamellar tumours and cholangio-carcinomas usually give normal AFP results. Values can be very high with hepatoblastoma.

Carcino-embryonic antigen values are particularly high with hepatic metastases. Because of lack of specificity it is of little value in the diagnosis of hepato-cellular cancer. Lack of specificity also applies to increases of serum α₁-antitrypsin and *α-acid glycoprotein*.

Serum ferritin increase is due to production of ferritin by the tumour rather than to liver necrosis. Ferritin is increased in active hepato-cellular disease; increases do not necessarily mean hepato-cellular cancer.

Des-γ-carboxyprothrombin is a vitamin K dependent prothrombin precursor synthesized in the normal hepatocyte and also by HCC [166].

Values greater than 100 ng/ml are highly suggestive of HCC. Values are normal in chronic hepatitis, cirrhosis and metastases. Specificity is superior to AFP but the test is not sensitive enough to detect small tumours.

Serum α-L-fucosidase is increased in HCC but the mechanism is not known [157]. It may be useful in early detection of HCC in patients with cirrhosis.

Haematological changes

The leucocyte count is usually raised to about 10 000 per mm³ with 80% polymorphonuclears. Eosinophilia is an occasional finding. The platelet count may be high—an unusual feature of uncomplicated cirrhosis.

The erythrocyte count is usually normal and anaemia is mild. Erythrocytosis is seen in 1%. It is probably due to increased erythropoietin production by the tumour. Increased serum erythropoietin levels may even be found with a normal haemoglobin and packed cell volume.

Blood coagulation may be disturbed. Fibrinolytic activity tends to be decreased. This may be due to liberation by the tumour of an inhibitory substance. Increase in plasma fibrinogen levels may be secondary to this effect.

Dysfibrinogenaemia may represent reversion to a fetal form of fibrinogen [53]. Ground-glass cells in HCC may contain fibrinogen and be producing it [154].

Hepatitis markers

Tests for HBV and HCV should be done (fig. 28.6).

Tumour localization

Plain X-ray may show calcification (sunburst lesion) (fig. 28.7).

Hepatic scanning

Isotope scan shows tumours larger than 3 cm in diameter as filling defects.

The *ultrasound pattern* may show increased or decreased reflectivity or a mixed echo picture. The tumour is hypo-echoic with ill-defined margins and non-uniform echoes. The diagnosis may be confirmed by guided biopsy. Sensitivity and specificity are high. False positives in cirrhosis are due to increased echogenicity in large nodules. The method is particularly suitable for screening. Lesions less than 2 cm in diameter can be detected (fig. 28.8).

CT scan shows a hypodense lesion (fig. 28.9) [152]. It frequently fails to depict the size and number of the tumours, especially when cirrhosis is present [103]. Contrast enhancement is essential [124]. The picture is of a mosaic pattern with multiple nodules of differing attenuation with enhancing septa within the masses. The tumour may or may not be encapsulated. Fatty change is frequent. There may be invasion of the portal vein and arterio-portal shunting.

Lipiodol introduced into the hepatic artery is cleared from non-cancerous tissue but remains in the tumour almost permanently so that lesions as small as 3 mm may be detected by CT some 2 weeks later (figs 28.10, 28.11, 28.12). Tumours as small as 0.2–0.3 cm can be identified.

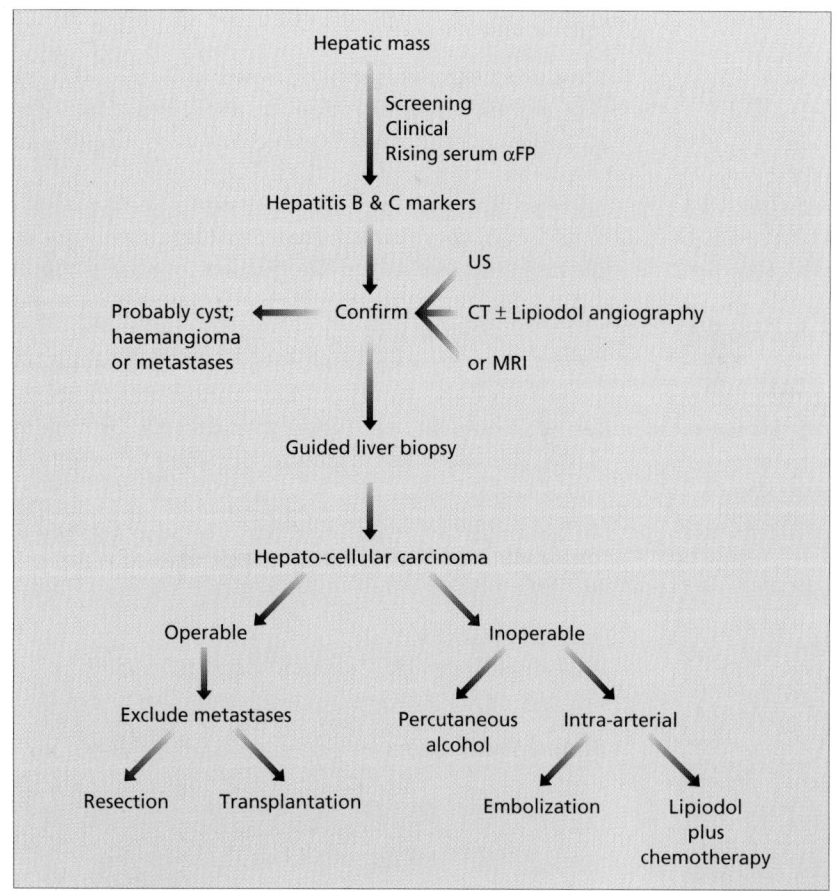

Fig. 28.6. Management of a patient with cirrhosis with positive screening for HCC.

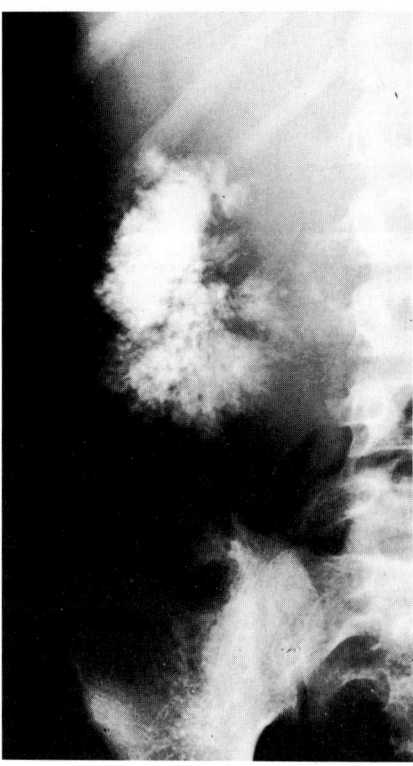

Fig. 28.7. Primary liver cancer. A plain X-ray of the abdomen shows calcification (sunburst lesion).

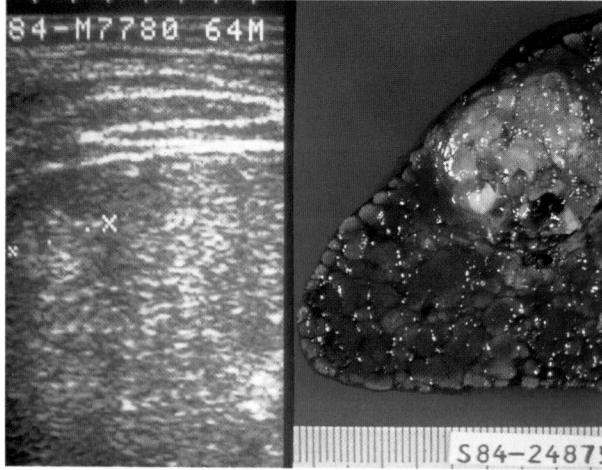

Fig. 28.8. Ultrasound shows a small hepato-cellular carcinoma (marked ××). This was surgically resected and the specimen is shown (courtesy J. F. Liaw).

Lipiodol is taken up by focal nodular hyperplasia, but in contrast to HCC, is washed away within 3 weeks [85].

MRI [135] is slightly better than CT for showing focal lesions. It is particularly useful if fatty liver coexists. T_1-weighted images of the tumour have a hypo-intense peripheral ring and are isodense. T_2-weighted images

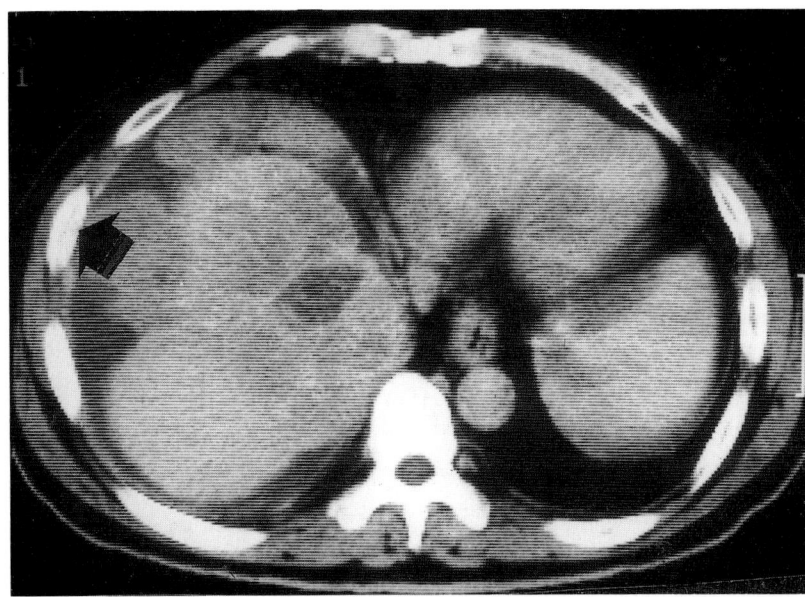

Fig. 28.9. CT scan in hepato-cellular cancer shows tumour bursting through capsule (arrow). Ascites is also present.

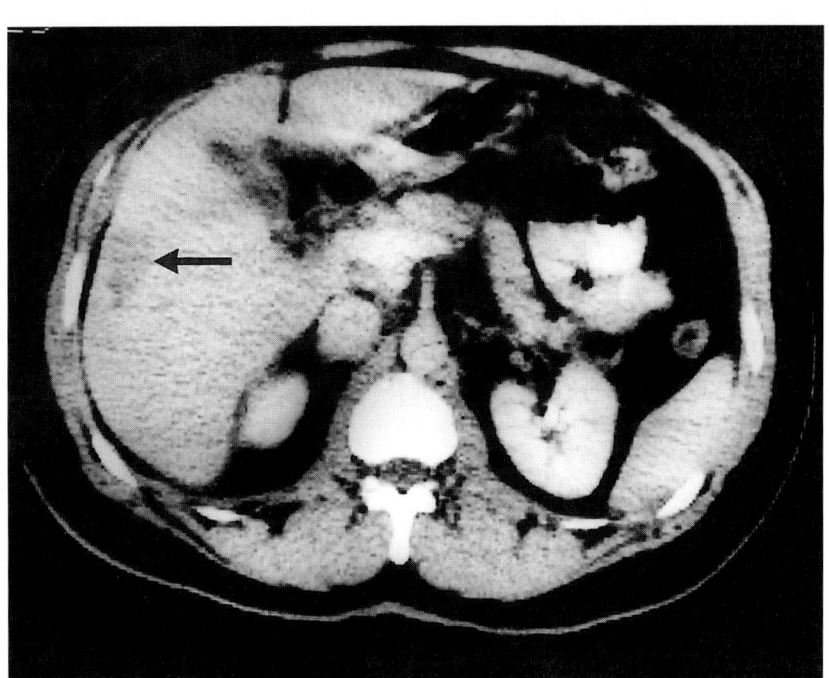

Fig. 28.10. Contrast-enhanced CT scan shows hypodense lesion in the right lobe of the liver (arrow).

show good tumour–liver contrast and can detect vascular invasion and satellite nodules.

Intravenous iodine-containing contrast (gadolinium) or magnesium contrast agents (MndPDP) enhance in HCC [104]. Supermagnetic iron oxide (ferumoxides) are safe and useful in T_2-weighted images [131].

Hepatic angiography

This is valuable for localization, for diagnosis, to determine operability and to follow the effects of therapy. The tumour is suplied by the hepatic artery and selective coeliac and superior mesenteric arteriography may demonstrate the lesion (figs 28.12, 28.13). Super selective contrast infusion angiography is of particular value in identifying small tumours. Selective intraarterial digital substraction angiography (DSA) shows tumours of 2 cm or less which change from isovascular to hypervascular with time [69].

CT arterioportography shows paucity of portal blood flow within the nodule [68].

Difficulty may arise in distinction from regenerative nodules in the cirrhotic liver. The appearances can be related to the gross anatomy of the tumour. The arterial pattern is bizarre with pooling, stretching and displacement of vessels. The vessels may be sclerosed, have an

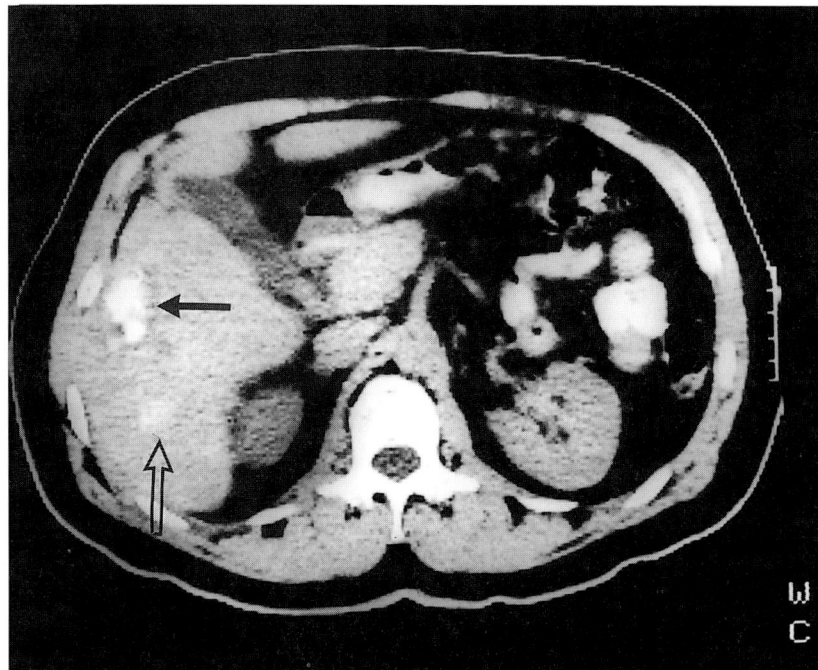

Fig. 28.11. Same patient as in fig. 28.10 with oral contrast CT scan 9 days after intra-hepatic arterial lipiodol shows uptake into the right lobe tumour (arrow) with another possible lesion more posteriorly (open arrow).

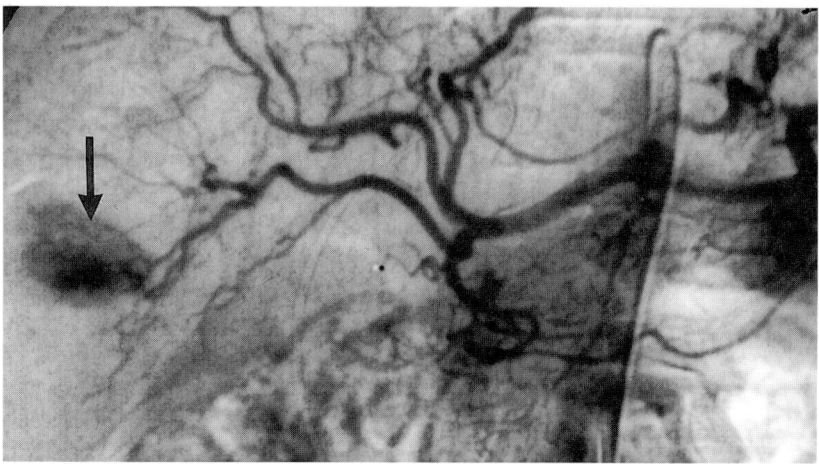

Fig. 28.12. Same patient as in figs 28.10 and 28.11. Selective hepatic arterial angiography confirms tumour in right lobe (arrow).

irregular lumen and be fragmented (fig. 28.14). Arterio-venous shunts can be shown often with retrograde filling of the portal trunk. There may be delayed emptying of the lesion. The portal vein may be distorted if there is tumour invasion.

Doppler ultrasound shows intravascular tumour spread. Portal vein invasion is shown by an intraportal arterial wave form in a hepato-fugal direction [120, 127]. Peak systolic flow velocity is increased, very high values being associated with arteriovenous shunting or portal venous involvement [114]. A distinction can be made from haemangioma.

Needle liver biopsy

Histological confirmation is important if small space-

occupying lesions have been detected by ultrasound or CT. If possible, the biopsy should be done under imaging control (Chapter 3). The possibility that biopsy will facilitate spread along the needle tract exists but is rare.

Fine-needle aspiration, using a 22-gauge needle, yields cytological specimens which will diagnose moderately and poorly differentiated tumours (fig. 28.15), but the cytological diagnosis of well-differentiated tumours is difficult.

Screening

Small, asymptomatic HCC in a cirrhotic liver may be diagnosed during screening of high-risk patients, by chance during imaging or found in a liver removed at

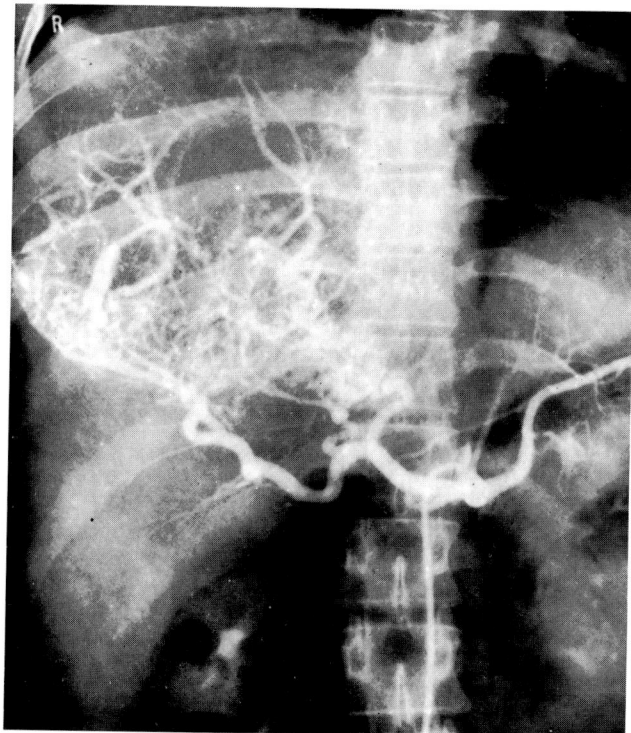

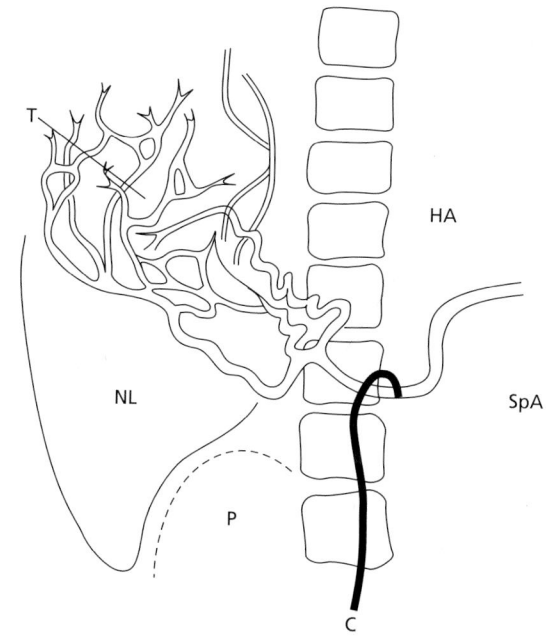

Fig. 28.13. Selective coeliac arteriogram showing catheter in the coeliac axis (C), the splenic artery (SpA) and the hepatic artery (HA). An abnormal arterial pattern (T) is shown in the tumour. The normal liver (NL) is not outlined by contrast media. P = pyelogram.

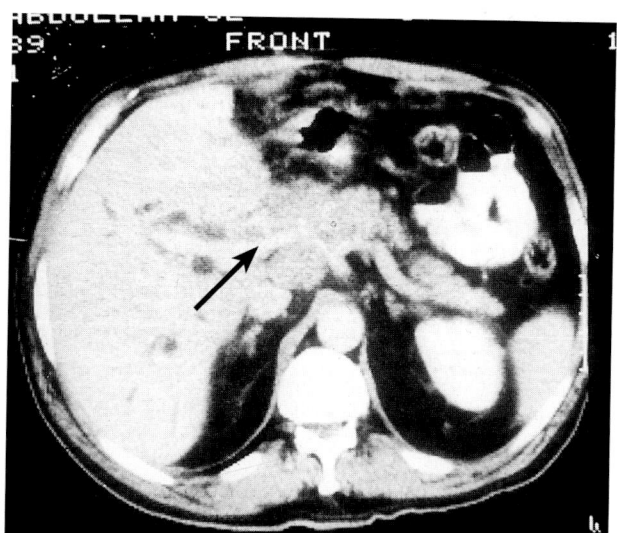

Fig. 28.14. Contrast-enhanced CT shows encasement of the contrast-filled hepatic artery by the tumour (arrow). This is a contraindication to resection or transplantation.

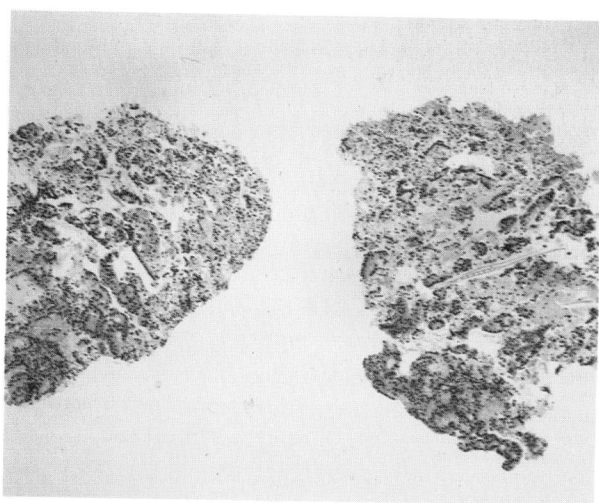

Fig. 28.15. Fine-needle aspiration under ultrasound guidance yielded a clump of HCC cells.

the time of transplantation (fig. 28.6). Early recognition is important as the chances of successful resection or liver transplant are greater. The 1-year survival of untreated patients with well-compensated liver disease (Child's grade A) and having asymptomatic HCC is 90% at 1 year, whereas the 1-year survival of symptomatic patients is only 40% [34]. Success is related to the growth rate of the tumour. It will clearly be more effective with the Japanese slow-growing tumour than with the South African rapidly progressive one.

Screening is indicated for patients at high risk of developing HCC. These are men, HBsAg or anti-HCV positive, more than 40 years old, and with chronic liver disease especially with cirrhosis and large macro-regenerative nodules. Ultrasound is more sensitive than CT. This is usually followed by directed fine-needle biopsy. Specimens must also be taken from non-tumorous tissue to determine the presence or absence of a concomitant cirrhosis and its activity.

Serum AFP estimation should be performed at 4–6 monthly intervals, particularly in those who have an initially increased concentration or where macro-regenerative nodules have been detected. Normal serum AFP does not exclude a tumour [34].

There are geographical differences in the reported value of screening. It is high in areas such as Japan where tumours are small and often encapsulated. In South Africa, tumours are rapidly growing and aggressive and screening is of little value. Europe seems to be in an intermediate position [33]. Economics play a part in the planning of screening programmes. In Japan, such procedures as ultrasound and AFP estimations are routinely available at no cost to the patient. This is clearly not so in most other parts of the world. The prognosis of HCC is so poor that where cost is an important consideration there is probably a reluctance to screen especially as there is no firm consensus that the death rate will be reduced.

Prognosis and risk factors

The outlook is usually hopeless. The time lag between exposure to hepatitis B or C and tumour development can vary from a few years to many decades [32].

The growth rate of the tumour varies greatly and correlates with survival. Asymptomatic Italian patients had a tumour volume doubling time varying from 1 to 19 months with a mean of 6 months [32, 34]. HCC in Africans is much more rapidly growing. Reasons are speculative, perhaps genetic, perhaps related to malnutrition, to co-factors such as aflatoxin or perhaps to late diagnosis in an itinerant African mine worker.

Small tumours (less than 3 cm in diameter) are associated with a 1-year survival of 90.7%, a 2-year survival of 55% and a 3-year survival of 12.8%. Infiltrating tumours have a worse prognosis than expanding ones. The presence of an intact capsule is a good sign. Although cirrhosis is the main risk factor, macro-regenerative nodules (at least 1 cm in diameter) and hypoechoic ones are particularly pre-cancerous [47, 162].

Severity of liver disease correlates with the chances of developing HCC [22, 69]. Patients less than 45 years old survive longer than older ones. A tumour size exceeding 50% of the liver, a serum albumin less than 3 g/dl and a raised serum bilirubin level are ominous features [118].

The risk increases if the patient is HBsAg or anti-HCV positive.

Co-factors are of importance in increasing the development of cirrhosis. In high endemic areas, progression from chronic hepatitis to cirrhosis and to HCC was thought to be increased by double infection with hepatitis B and C. This was based largely on first-generation testing methods. When specific viral markers (HCV RNA and HBV DNA) were measured in Spain, only nine of 63 patients with HCC were co-infected by HBV [134]. Co-infection with HBV and HCV was noted in 15% of USA patients with HCC [95]. In patients with HCV-related cirrhosis, alcohol abuse has been variably reported to have little effect or to increase the risk of carcinoma.

Pulmonary metastases adversely affect survival.

Treatment

Accurate localization is essential, particularly if surgery is planned. This is best done by CT with or without angiography. It may be combined with lipiodol angiography which detects 96% of tumours, but this does add to the complexity of diagnosis and is not always necessary.

The only procedures that offer the possibility of cure are resection or transplantation.

Resection

After partial resection, DNA synthesis increases and the remaining liver cells become larger (*hypertrophy*) and undergo increased mitosis (*hyperplasia*). Up to 90% of a non-cirrhotic liver may be removed with eventual survival.

The resectability rate for HCC is low, only about 3–30%. Successful local resection depends on size (less than 5 cm in diameter), position, particularly in relation to large vessels, presence of vascular invasion, presence of a capsule, absence of satellite lesions and the number of lesions (tables 28.4, 28.5). Multiple lesions have a high recurrence rate and a low survival time [67, 69].

Cirrhosis is not a definite contraindication but is associated with a higher intra-operative and peri-operative morbidity and mortality [45]. The operative mortality in the non-cirrhotic is less than 3% but 23% in the cirrhotic. The cirrhosis should be Child's grade A or B and jaundice is a contraindication. The patients age and general condition must be taken into account.

Metastases must be sought by chest X-ray, CT scan or MRI of the head (fig. 28.16) and isotope bone scan.

Improved results for resection have followed better knowledge of the segmental anatomy of the liver. Also,

Table 28.4. Surgical resection for HCC

Country	Author	No. treated	Op. or hosp. mortality %	% 1-year survival	% resectable
Africa	Kew	—	—	—	5
UK	Dunk	46	—	—	6.5
France	Bismuth	270	15	66	12.9
USA*	Lim	86	36	22.7	22
Hong Kong	Lee	935	20	45	17.6
Japan	Okuda	2411	27.5	33.5	11.9
China	Li	?	11.4	58.6	?
Taiwan	Lees	?	6	84	?

*Chinese-Americans.

Table 28.5. Factors in resection for HCC

- Size <5 cm
- One lobe
- Capsule
- Vascular invasion
- Cirrhosis grade
- Age and general condition

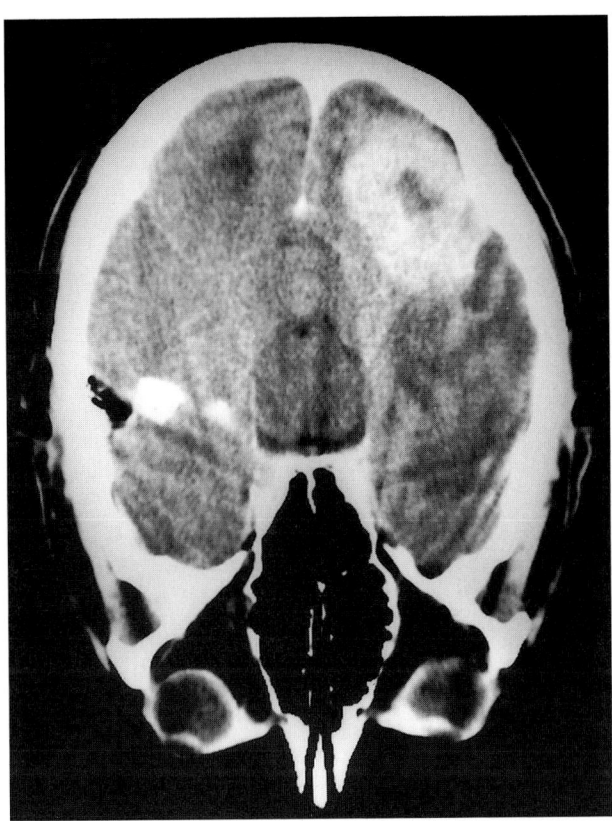

Fig. 28.16. Brain MRI shows large occipital metastasis in a patient with HCC.

this has followed the use of intra-operative diagnostic ultrasound [74]. The left lobe is resected with relative ease. The right lobe is more difficult. Small tumours may be removed by segmentectomy; in others, lobectomy or trisegmentectomy may be necessary and this demands adequate liver function. The post-resection prognosis is related to the resection of a wide margin around the tumour, the absence of tumour thrombosis in hepatic vein or portal vein and no obvious intra-hepatic metastases [155].

About 57% of recurrences within the first 2 years can be expected in the residual liver. In Spain, survival increased from 12.4 months in untreated controls to 27.1 months in those with resected tumours and results were even better for tumours less than 5 cm [18]. Results from recent series show a 1-year survival after resection of 55–80% and a 5-year survival of 25–39%.

Hepatic transplantation

The results are generally unsatisfactory (Chapter 35). If the patient survives the surgery, recurrence and metastasis are usual and this may be enhanced by the immunosuppression necessary to prevent rejection. Transplantation tends to be used for those patients unsuitable for resection, having severe hepato-cellular disease, multifocal and bilateral large lesions and with centrally located tumours. It is not surprising that these patients do worse than those resected; rejected patients should not be transplanted. Liver transplant is effective for single small (5 cm or less) unresectable tumours and no more than three tumour nodules (3 cm or less) [13, 100]. After 4 years the actuarial survival is 75% and recurrence-free survival 83%. Those who are HBsAg positive do considerably worse [28]. Those with cirrhosis have a poor outlook [48].

Results are best for those with tumours discovered at the time of screening or when a transplant is performed for another indication. Since 1963 more than 300 patients have been reported having liver transplantation for the treatment of HCC [45]. The ranges of the 1 and 5 years actuarial survival rates are 42–71% and 20–45%, respectively. However, recurrence rates are as high as 65%. This depends on the size of the tumour. If less than 5 cm in diameter, the survival time is 55 ± 8 months, whereas those with tumours 5 cm or larger have a mean survival time of 24 ± 6 months [174].

Systemic chemotherapy

Mitozantrone given intravenously in courses every 21 days is probably the drug of choice. Results are disappointing with a response rate of only 27.3% [39].

Trans-arterial embolization

Catheterization of the hepatic artery via the femoral artery and coeliac axis allows embolization of the blood supply to the tumour. Chemotherapeutic agents may be delivered in high concentration. The procedures have limited success due to the development of arterial collaterals which ultimately supply the tumour.

Embolization is used for unresectable tumours and occasionally as a preliminary to resection or for recurrence [111]. It may be used as an emergency to control intra-peritoneal haemorrhage from a ruptured HCC [117].

The procedure is performed under local or general anaesthesia and with antibiotic cover. The portal vein must be patent. The hepatic artery branch feeding the tumour is then embolized using gel foam, sometimes with an added agent such as doxorubicin, mitomycin or cysplatin (figs 28.17, 28.18) [68]. The tumour undergoes complete or incomplete necrosis. Gelatine cubes with steel coil embolization exerts an anti-tumoural effect with a moderate increase in survival but prospective controlled trials are needed to confirm this [17].

Side-effects include pain, which can be severe, fever, nausea, encephalopathy, ascites and massive rises in transaminases. The AFP falls. Abscess formation and misplaced embolization are other complications.

Mitomycin C microcapsules can be used with an objective response rate of 43% [7].

Yttrium-90 glass microspheres can be used to deliver large doses of internal radiation to the tumour as long as extra-hepatic venous shunting can be excluded [173].

HCCs are not sensitive to radiotherapy.

The results of embolization are variable from failure to prolongation of survival. Prognosis depends on the tumour type and extension, size, portal vein involvement, presence of ascites and jaundice [172]. All lesions without a capsule are resistant to embolization [164]. The technique is more useful in the treatment of *hepatic carcinoid tumours* where there is marked reduction in symptoms and tumour size (figs 28.19, 28.20) [106].

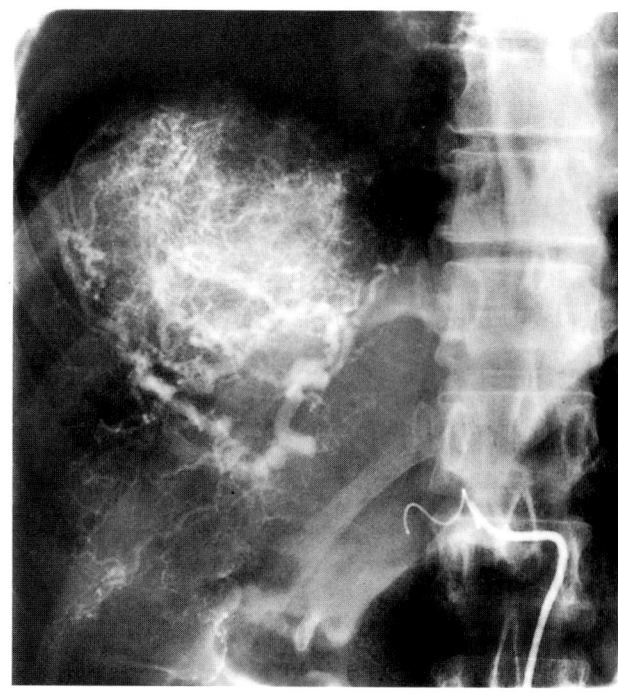

Fig. 28.17. Selective hepatic angiography shows a large HCC in the right lobe of the liver.

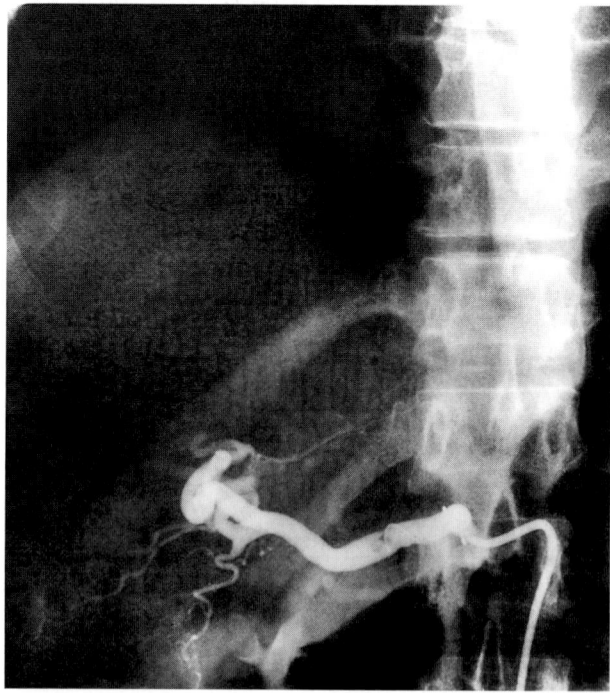

Fig. 28.18. Same patient as fig. 28.17. Hepatic arterial embolization with gel foam occlusion of blood supply to the tumour.

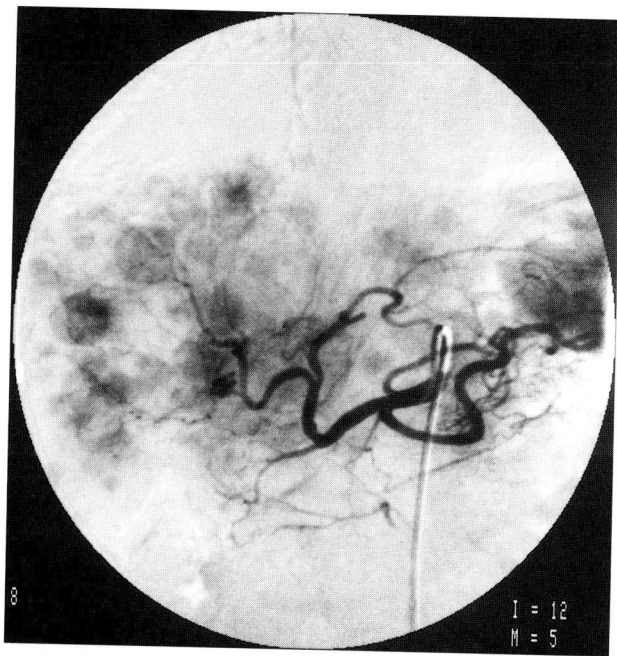

Fig. 28.19. Coeliac angiography in a patient with primary carcinoid tumour of the ileum and multiple, symptomatic liver metastases [139].

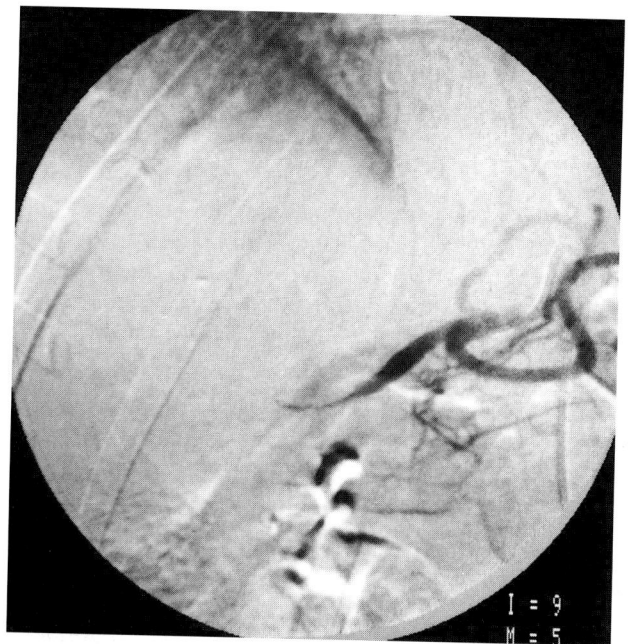

Fig. 28.20. Same patient as fig. 28.19 after selective hepatic arterial embolization to ablate tumour effects [139].

Lipiodized oil

Lipiodol, an iodized poppy seed oil, is retained in the tumour for 7 or more days after hepatic arterial infusion but disappears from non-tumorous liver (fig. 28.11). This is valuable in showing very small tumours. The degree of lipiodol labelling is an important prognostic factor [107]. It is used to target lipophilic anti-cancer drugs such as epirubicin [76], cisplatin [77], or lipiodol I-131 to the tumour [57]. These drugs all seem to prolong survival but there is little difference in the agent used. The treatment can be repeated at 3–6 month intervals. Results are encouraging for small tumours [137].

Trans-arterial oily chemoembolization may be used as adjuvant therapy after hepatic resection [72]. Disease-free survival is increased but the treatment fails to reduce recurrence or prolong life [55].

Unfortunately, viable tumour cells often remain in and around the tumour [86] and a complete cure cannot be expected.

Percutaneous ethanol injection

Small (less than 5 cm) tumours usually not more than three in number may be treated by ultrasound or CT-guided percutaneous injection of absolute alcohol (table 28.6). The patient can be treated as an outpatient twice a week with 2–12 ml absolute alcohol for 3–15 sessions. Alternatively, a single session under general anaesthesia using 57 ml may be used for larger lesions, but it is not advised in the presence of advanced cirrhosis [96]. The treatment results in intra-tumoural arterial thrombosis and coagulative necrosis followed by ischaemia of the tumour. It is only used for encapsulated tumours. Necrosis of the tumour is rarely complete. MRI may be useful for showing the effectiveness of therapy [146].

The injection may be a preliminary to resection and can be repeated if the tumour recurs. Multiple tumours can be treated. Injection is used to control bleeding following rupture of the tumour [27]. The side-effects are similar to those of embolization. Three-year survival for Child's A is 71%, Child's B is 41% [96].

Immuno-targeting

A radio-isotope bound to a monoclonal antibody against antigens on the cell surface of the tumour is given intravenously or into the hepatic artery. This targets anti-tumour drugs such as I^{131} ferritin. At present results are inconclusive [78].

Table 28.6. Percutaneous alcohol injection for HCC

Less than 5 cm
Not more than three lesions
Local anaesthesia
Ultrasound or CT control
2–12 ml absolute alcohol
Side-effects

Immunotherapy

The growth of the cancer may be related to inability of the host to mount an immune response adequate for lysis of sufficient numbers of tumour cells. The immunological response may be stimulated by autologous lymphokine activated killer (LAK) cells plus IL2 [122]. The tumour is then lysed. Treatment is well tolerated but the results are uncertain.

Hormone manipulation

Experimentally, male and female sex steroids influence chemically induced carcinomas. Patients with a hepato-cellular cancer have oestrogen and androgen receptors on the tumour [115]. Tamoxifen (10mg twice daily) significantly improved survival over non-treated patients [23], but this was not confirmed [22].

Conclusions

Hepato-cellular cancer remains a fatal disease. In a large trial of 123 patients with stage 1 HCC, usually with cirrhosis, all treatments increased the probability of survival [15] (fig. 28.21). Results, however, did not differ between resection, liver transplantation and trans-arterial oily embolization. The various procedures have rarely been subjected to prospective clinical trials. Results are compared with historical controls or no treatment and trials are urgently needed.

Fibro-lamellar carcinoma of the liver

This tumour is found in young people (aged 5–35) of both sexes [35]. It presents as an abdominal mass, some-times with pain. It is unrelated to sex hormones. The liver is non-cirrhotic.

Histologically, clumps of large, polygonal deeply eosinophilic tumour cells are interspersed with bands of mature fibrous tissue (fig. 28.22). The cells have cytoplasmic pale bodies representing intra-cellular fibrinogen storage. Occasionally the fibrous stroma is lacking.

Electron microscopy shows the cytoplasm packed with mitochondria and thick compact bands of collagen in parallel arrays. The tumour cells are believed to be oncocytes. The hepatocytes contain excess of copper-associated protein, presumably produced by the cancer cell [91].

Serum AFP is normal. Serum calcium levels may be raised with pseudo-hyperparathyroidism. Serum vitamin B_{12} binding protein [123] and neurotensin [31] may also be increased.

Ultrasound shows hyper-echoic homogeneous lesions. CT shows a hypodense mass which enhances markedly with contrast. Calcification may be noted.

MRI shows that the tumour is iso-intense in T_1- and T_2-weighted images and hypo-intense in T_2-weighted images.

Prognosis is better than for other forms of liver cancer (survival 32–62 months), although the tumour may metastasize to regional lymph nodes.

Treatment is by surgical resection or transplantation [129, 148].

Hepatoblastoma

This rare tumour affects children of both sexes less than 4 years old and very rarely older children and adults [54]. It presents as progressive enlargement of the abdomen with anorexia, failure to thrive, fever and, rarely, jaun-

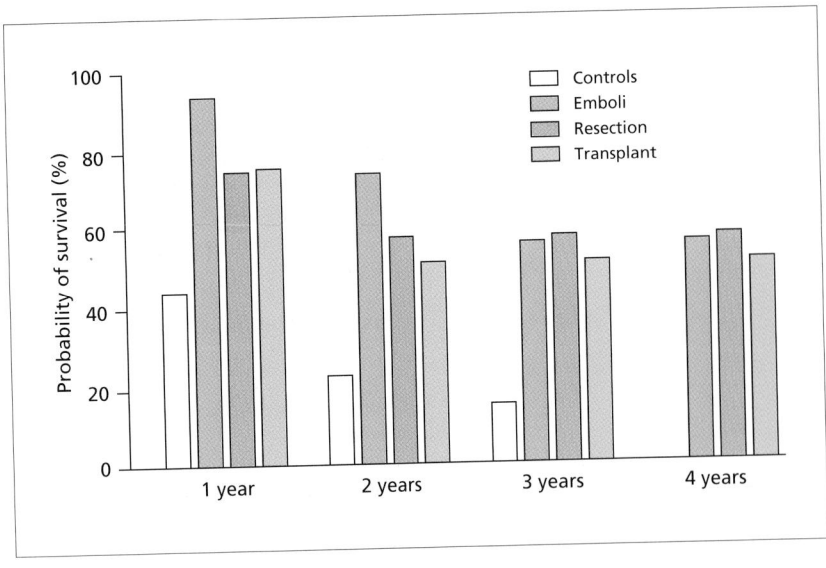

Fig. 28.21. Results of treating early (stage 1) hepato-cellular carcinoma on survival [15].

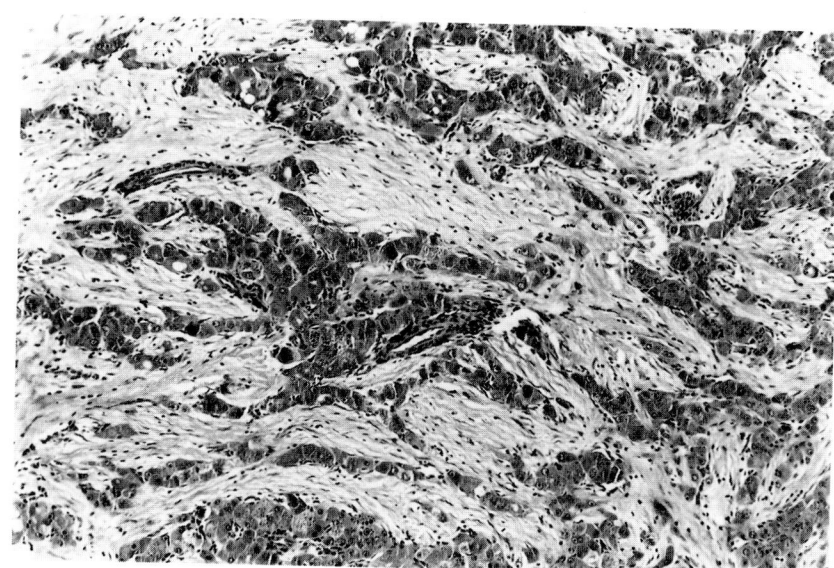

Fig. 28.22. Fibro-lamellar carcinoma: clumps of eosinophilic cells are interspersed with bands of mature connective tissue. (Stained H & E, ×275.)

dice. Associated features include sexual precocity due to secretion of an ectopic gonadotrophin by the tumour, cystathioninuria, hemihypertrophy and renal adenomas. Serum AFP levels are markedly increased. Imaging shows a space-occupying lesion in the liver with displacement of adjacent organs. There may be focal calcification. Angiography shows the features of primary liver cancer with a diffuse parenchymal blush persisting into the venous phase, encasement of vessels, pooling of contrast and an ill-defined margin.

Histological features recapitulate the developmental stages of the liver. Teratoid features may therefore be seen. The usual picture is of fetal type with embryonal cells in acini, pseudo-rosettes or papillary formations [57]. Sinusoids contain haematopoietic cells. The mixed epithelial–mesenchymal type shows primitive mesenchyma, osteoid tissue and, rarely, cartilage, rhabdomyoblasts or squamous foci [56].

A link has been found between familial adenomatous polyposis coli and hepatoblastoma [37]. There are other associations, a gene on chromosome 11 has been associated with hepatoblastoma and other embryonal tumours. Chromosomal abnormalities have been shown by cytogenetic studies [37].

If a resection is possible, the prognosis is better than for primary HCC, 36% of patients surviving 5 years.

Hepatic transplantation has been performed.

Intra-hepatic cholangiocarcinoma

Aetiological factors include clonorchiasis, primary sclerosing cholangitis, the fibrocystic diseases, anabolic steroids and thorotrast.

The tumour is firm to hard and of whitish colour. This is a glandular tumour arising from intra-hepatic bile ducts. The tumour cells resemble bile duct epithelium;

sometimes they have a papillary arrangement. There is no bile secretion. The stroma differs from that of HCC as it consists of fibrous tissue with little or no capillary formation (fig. 28.23). Histological appearances do not allow distinction of intra-hepatic cholangiocarcinoma from metastatic adenocarcinoma.

Keratin is a good marker of biliary epithelium and is found in 90% of cholangiocarcinomas [52].

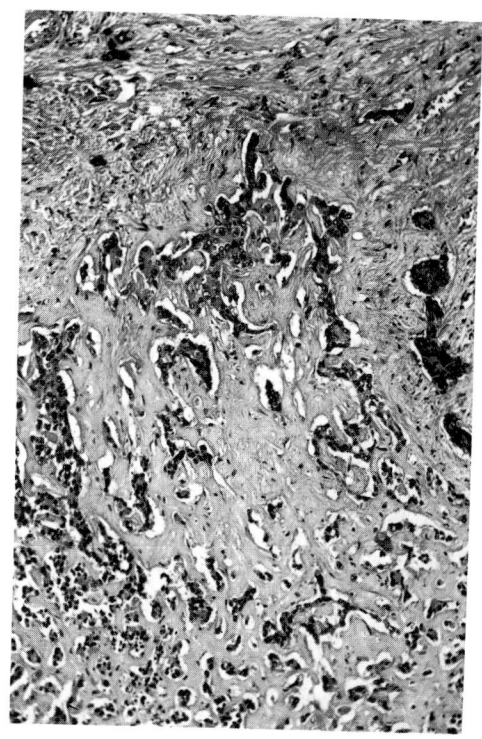

Fig. 28.23. Bile duct carcinoma. The tumour cells are arranged in tubular fashion simulating bile ducts. The cell type is columnar. Stroma is dense, fibrous and avascular. (Stained H & E, ×90.)

The tumour affects older persons. The clinical features are those of hepatic malignancy with jaundice prominent. Serum AFP is not increased.

CT scan shows a space-occupying lesion of low attenuation, sometimes with calcification. It is usually hypovascular [132]. Angiography and MRI may show vascular encasement.

Treatment is unsatisfactory, and there is no response to chemotherapy.

Combined hepato-cellular–cholangiocarcinoma

This primary liver cancer shows the features of both hepato-cellular and biliary epithelial differentiation [52]. Some represent coincidental occurrence of both hepato-cellular and cholangiocarcinoma in the same patient. Some contain transition elements between hepato-cellular and cholangiocarcinoma, and some are examples of fibro-lamellar tumours.

Within the tumour, intra-cellular AFP is found in 29% and keratin markers of bile duct epithelium in 52%.

The *clinical features* are those of HCC. Cirrhosis may or may not be present.

Cystadenocarcinoma

This rare tumour occurs in adults, more often female. It presents as abdominal fullness with pain and weight loss.

The large tumour, usually in the right lobe, is multicystic and contains bile-stained, mucinous material. Histologically, the cysts are lined by malignant epithelial cells with papillary enfoldings and dense fibrous stroma [168]. The origin may be from a benign cystadenoma or even a congenital cyst.

Imaging shows a space-occupying lesion, usually large, with cystic features.

The prognosis is better than for cholangiocarcinoma with survival of up to 5 years after resection. Hepatic transplantation may also be possible.

Angiosarcoma (haemangio-endothelioma)

This very rare and highly malignant tumour is difficult to distinguish from primary hepato-cellular cancer [97]. The liver is enlarged and full of knobbly cavernous growths. Angiosarcoma is part of a spectrum of diseases of the sinusoidal barrier including peliosis and sinusoidal dilatation. All three conditions can be related to vinyl chloride, arsenic, thorotrast and anabolic steroids [43]. It may complicate neurofibromatosis [88].

Histologically, blood-filled cavernous sinuses are lined with layers of highly malignant, anaplastic, endothelial cells which in parts may resemble the earliest stages of embryonic vascular development. Well-differentiated tumours resemble peliosis hepatis.

Giant cell formations, solid sarcomatous foci, and intrasinusoidal spread with invasion of portal venous and hepatic venous radicles are prominent. Adjacent liver shows cholangio-proliferation and hypertrophy of sinusoidal lining cells.

Factor VIII-related antigen, an endothelial cell marker, may be identified in tumour cells.

The disease affects older people. It presents as hepato-cellular liver disease, weight loss and fever. The course is rapidly downhill with cachexia, blood-stained ascites and death within 2 years.

A bruit may be heard over the liver. Platelets may be consumed in the tumour and disseminated intravascular coagulation has been reported. Occasionally the course is chronic with ascites and hepatomegaly over many years [26].

Scanning shows multiple defects in the liver (fig. 28.24). The right diaphragm is high.

The *prognosis* is very poor, and the tumour is only rarely radiosensitive.

Thorotrast

This consists of a colloidal solution of thorium dioxide with the isotope radiothorium which is mainly an α-ray emitter and has a half-life of 1.3×10^6 years. It was formerly used as a contrast medium in radiology. Primary hepatic tumours have developed years after intravascular administration. Hepato-cellular or bile duct carcinoma [136] has a latent period of about 20 years and haemangio-endothelioma about 15 years. Plain X-ray of the abdomen shows continued presence of the isotope in liver and spleen and this is confirmed by autoradiographs of liver tissue. Total body counting may be used to quantitate radioactivity in the patient's body. Cirrhosis can develop even without liver tumours.

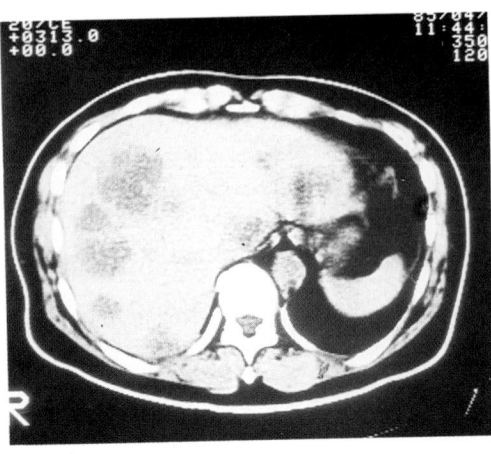

Fig. 28.24. Haemangio-endothelioma. CT shows multifocal nodules.

Epithelioid haemangio-endothelioma [70]

This rare tumour of adults, predominantly female, is usually slow growing with low-grade malignancy but can be rapidly progressive. It presents incidentally with abdominal fullness and pain, with jaundice or with haemoperitoneum.

Microscopically, tumour cells are dendritic and epithelioid and infiltrate sinusoids and intra-hepatic veins of all sizes. The matrix may show inflammation, sclerosis and calcification.

The histochemical demonstration of endothelial markers (factor VIII antigen and lectins: UEA-I) in the tumour cells is diagnostic.

Ultrasound, CT and MRI imaging show coalescent peripheral hepatic masses with capsular retraction due to fibrosis [102]. CT shows the tumours of low attenuation on enhancement, peripheral or alternating attenuations correlate with the hyperaemic rim. MRI shows low signal halos around many lesions which have a high T_2 signal.

The prognosis is more favourable than for angiosarcoma but the tumour can metastasize. Surgical excision and liver transplantation must be considered [80, 100].

Undifferentiated sarcoma of the liver

This is an extremely rare tumour differentiated from anaplastic HCC, angiosarcoma or epithelioid haemangio-endothelioma by hepatic histology. Spread of a sarcoma from a nearby structure such as the thoracic cage, diaphragm or retroperitoneum must be excluded.

The tumour usually affects children (Chapter 24) [94] but can affect the adult [49].

The histology is typical of sarcoma. Reticulin stains show the characteristic uniform distribution of fibres.

The prominent clinical features are pyrexia and an abdominal mass. Hypoglycaemia may develop. The course is rapidly downhill with a survival of about 2 months.

Imaging shows a solid and cystic lesion with multiple loculi. Calcification and invasion of the right atrium and inferior vena cava may be noted. Angiography shows variable vascularity depending on the degree of cystic transformation.

Chemotherapy is useless and hepatic transplantation is rarely possible.

Benign tumours of the liver

Adenoma

These are very rare [9]. They present as right upper-quadrant masses or as acute intra-peritoneal haemorrhage. They have an association with sex hormone therapy (Chapter 18) and with pregnancy.

Cholangioma (bile duct adenoma)

This is a very rare, simple tumour of bile duct origin. It has the structure of a cystadenoma and it must be distinguished from a simple cyst or polycystic disease of the liver. A mixed type of tumour is also recorded with both proliferating bile ducts and hepatic cells.

Biliary cystadenoma

The tumour is usually large and affects the right lobe. It may be pedunculated. The cysts contain clear yellow or mucinous brown material.

This tumour affects largely middle-aged women. Symptoms include abdominal mass and pain. Rarely, the biliary tree is obstructed.

The tumour must be distinguished from fibropolycystic disease and simple cyst.

Resection may be possible.

Biliary papillomatosis

See Chapter 34.

Haemangioma

This is the commonest benign tumour of the liver, being found in about 5% of autopsies. It is increasingly being diagnosed with the greater use of scanning procedures. It is usually single and small, but occasionally may be multiple or very large.

The tumour is commonly subcapsular, on the convexity of the right lobe of the liver, and is occasionally pedunculated. On section it appears round or wedge-shaped, dark red in colour and has a honeycomb pattern, with a fibrous capsule which may be calcified. Histologically, a communicating network of spaces contains red corpuscles. Factor VIII may be expressed.

The tumour is lined by flat endothelial cells and contains scanty fibrous tissue. Occasionally, there is a marked fibrous component.

Clinical features. The majority are asymptomatic and discovered incidentally. Symptoms from giant tumours (>4 cm diameter) include abdominal mass and pain due to thrombosis. Symptoms may be due to pressure on adjacent organs. Rarely, a vascular hum is heard over the lesion.

Radiology [14]

A *plain X-ray* may show a calcified capsule.

Ultrasound shows a solitary echogenic spot with smooth well-defined borders (fig. 5.3). Posterior acoustic enhancement, due to increased sound transmission through the blood of the cavernous sinuses, is characteristic [14].

CT scan, enhanced by contrast, shows distinctive puddling of contrast in venous channels (fig. 28.25). The contrast diffuses from the periphery to the centre, until opacification is homogeneous after 30–60 minutes. Foci of globular enhancement are seen after dynamic bolus CT [128]. Calcification may be seen due to previous bleeding or thrombus formation.

MRI shows the tumour as a markedly high intensity area. T_2 is prolonged over 8 ms (fig. 28.26). MRI is of special value in diagnosing small haemangiomas [71].

Single photon emission CT (*SPECT*) with ^{99m}Tc- labelled red blood cells shows persistent blood pool activity within the lesion [12].

Angiography is only necessary in cases not showing typical CT appearances. Lesions displace large hepatic arterial branches to one side. The hepatic arteries are not enlarged, taper normally and divide to normal small vessels before filling the vascular spaces. The spaces tend to adopt a circular or 'C' shape due to the central fibrosis. Haemangiomas may show prolonged opacification even up to 18 seconds.

Needle liver biopsy (directed). Using a fine-needle biopsy

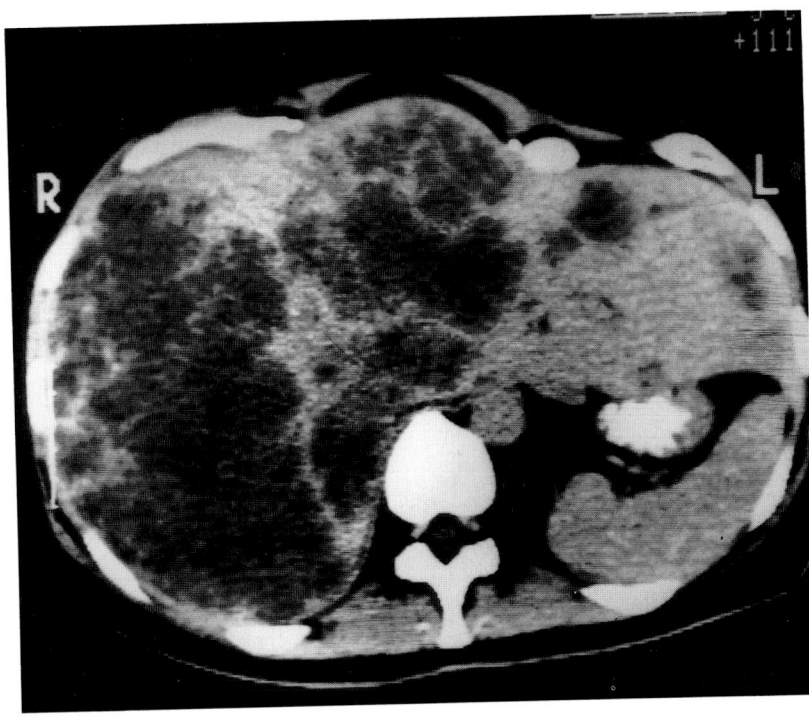

Fig. 28.25. Haemangioma: CT shows a giant benign haemangioma in the right lobe of the liver. A few small lesions are seen in the left lobe. The lesions filled in completely 1 hour after intravenous contrast.

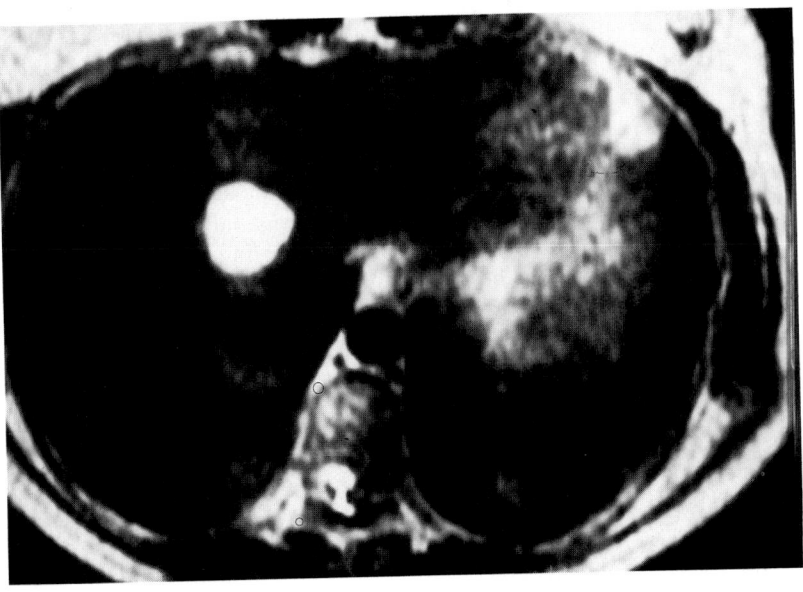

Fig. 28.26. Haemangioma. MRI using long T_2 weighting (echo time) shows a very bright lesion. This finding reflects a profuse and very sluggish blood circulation usually due to a haemangioma.

technique this is usually safe [163] but unnecessary in view of the diagnostic imaging appearances.

Treatment is usually unnecessary as the lesions do not increase in size or in clinical manifestations [109]. The possibility of rupture is not an indication for surgery. If there is severe pain or rapid expansion, resection (usually lobectomy or segmentectomy) is safe [11, 145].

Mesenchymal hamartoma [38]

This usually presents in the first 2 years of life as a massive cystic lesion of the right lobe of liver [87]. It can affect adults. It arises from tissues in the portal zones and histology shows an admixture of hepatocytes, biliary epithelium, mesenchymal elements and cysts. Extra-medullary haematopoiesis may be seen. The lesion probably has an anomalous solitary vascular supply evolving into stromal cysts due to early ischaemic change [92].

Treatment is by surgical resection, but aspiration and careful follow-up may be considered in some cases.

Paraneoplastic hepatopathy

Hepato-splenomegaly with cholestasis, fever, weight loss, increased serum globulins and alkaline phosphatase can complicate hypernephroma without hepatic metastases [153]. Liver biopsy shows non-specific cellular infiltration. It has also been reported with soft tissue sarcomas not involving the liver [140]. The changes may regress if the tumour is resected. The mechanism of the hepatic changes is unknown.

Hepatic metastases

The liver is the most frequent site of blood-borne metastases, irrespective of whether the primary is drained by systemic or portal veins. It is involved in about a third of all cancers, including half of those of stomach, breast, lung and those arising from the colon. Other frequent primary sites include oesophagus, pancreas and those of malignant melanoma. Prostatic and ovarian metastases are exceedingly rare.

Pathogenesis

Invasion from tumours in adjacent organs, retrograde lymphatic permeation and extension along the lumen of blood vessels are all unusual.

Portal emboli come from malignant neoplasms arising in the organs of the portal vascular territory. Primary tumours in the uterus and ovaries, kidneys, prostate or bladder, may involve contiguous tissue drained by the portal vein and hence give embolic metastases to the liver; these are extremely rare.

Microscopically, *hepatic arterial seeding* is difficult to identify, because the picture is confused by the succeeding intra-hepatic metastases. It must be frequent.

Pathology

There may be only one or two microscopic nodules or the whole liver may be enormous and full of metastases. Liver weights of 5000 g are not unusual and one liver is said to have weighed 21 500 g. The deposits are usually white and well demarcated. The consistency depends on the ratio of cancer cells to fibrous stroma. Occasionally the centre may be soft, necrotic and haemorrhagic. On the surface of the liver they show characteristic umbilication; this results from necrosis of the centre, which has outgrown its blood supply. Perihepatitis may be seen over peripheral lesions. A zone of venous hyperaemia may surround the deposits. Portal vein invasion is usual, and arteries are rarely involved by tumour thrombus although they may be encased.

The tumour cells metastasize rapidly and widely through the liver, both by peri-vascular lymphatics and by direct invasion of the portal venous radicles.

Injection studies show that, in contrast to HCC, metastases may have a decreased rather than increased blood supply from the hepatic artery. This is particularly so in those of gastrointestinal origin.

Histology

The secondary deposits in the liver may reproduce the histology of the primary lesions. However, this is not necessarily so, and in many instances the primary tumour may be well differentiated, while the secondary deposits in the liver may be extremely anaplastic and give no hint of their origin (fig. 28.27).

Clinical features

These may be due to the hepatic metastases, to the distant primary growth or more usually to a combination of both.

The patients complain of malaise, lassitude and loss of weight. Abdominal distension and a dragging sensation are due to the enlarged liver. Occasionally the pain is sharp and intermittent, simulating biliary colic. Fever and sweats may occur.

Depending upon the weight loss, the patient may be emaciated, with an enlarged abdomen. The liver may be normal sized or so large that it protrudes visibly in the right upper abdomen. The tumour deposits are hard and may be umbilicated. Friction may be heard over them. The deposits are not vascular, so an arterial bruit is not heard. Splenomegaly is frequent, even in those with a patent portal vein. Jaundice is mild and may be absent. Deep jaundice implies invasion of major bile ducts.

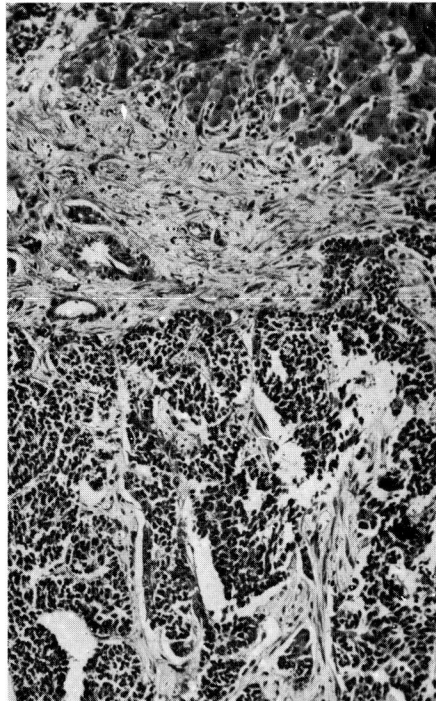

Fig. 28.27. Anaplastic secondary carcinoma of the liver. The tumour is composed of sheets of undifferentiated malignant cells. Normal liver cells are seen at the top. There was a small bronchial primary growth which was not revealed by chest X-ray. (Stained H & E, ×110.)

Oedema of the legs with dilated veins coursing upwards over the abdominal wall suggests that the inferior vena cava is obstructed on the posterior aspect of the liver.

Glands in the right supra-clavicular region may be involved.

A pleural effusion may indicate pulmonary metastases and similar localizing signs may provide clinical evidence of the primary growth.

Ascites reflects peritoneal involvement and occasionally a thrombosed portal vein. Bleeding may be secondary to portal hypertension. Rarely obstructive jaundice may be seen due to metastases from breast, colon, or small cell lung cancer [73].

Secondary malignant deposits are by far the commonest causes of a really large liver.

Hypoglycaemia is a rare complication. The primary is usually a sarcoma. Rarely, extensive tumour infiltration and parenchymal infarction may lead to the picture of fulminant hepatic failure [60].

When *malignant carcinoid* of the small intestine or bronchus is associated with vaso-motor abnormalities and pulmonary stenosis, there are always many hepatic metastases.

Unless the bile ducts are completely obstructed, the faeces are well coloured, and if the primary lesion is in the alimentary tract they may give a positive reaction for blood.

Laboratory investigations

Biochemical tests

Even with an enormous liver, sufficient functioning tissue remains. The smaller intra-hepatic bile ducts may be compressed yet no jaundice develops. The area with uninvolved ducts may excrete the bilirubin from the occluded areas. Serum total bilirubin values greater than $2\,mg/100\,ml$ ($34\,\mu mol/l$) suggest involvement of major bile ducts at the hilum.

Biochemical tests suggesting hepatic metastases include a raised serum alkaline phosphatase or lactic dehydrogenase level. Transaminase levels may be increased. If serum bilirubin, alkaline phosphatase, lactic dehydrogenase and transaminase levels are all normal, there is a 98% probability that metastases are absent [75].

Serum albumin concentration is normal or slightly decreased. The *serum globulin* level may be normal, slightly raised or even, occasionally, very high. Electrophoresis may show a raised α_2- or γ-globulin.

Serum carcino-embryonic antigen may be present.

The *ascitic fluid* shows increased protein, occasionally the presence of carcino-embryonic antigen and increases in lactic dehydrogenase three times over the serum value.

Haematology

A polymorph leucocytosis is fairly common: even values up to $40\,000$–$50\,000$ per mm^3 are sometimes recorded. There may be a mild anaemia.

Needle liver biopsy

The chances of a positive result are increased if the biopsy needle is directed into the lesion under ultrasound, CT or peritoneoscopic guidance. Tumour tissue is characteristically white and friable. If a cylinder of tissue is not obtained it is worth examining any blood clot or debris for malignant cells. Even if tumour cells are not aspirated, the presence of proliferated and abnormal bile ducts and polymorphs in oedematous portal tracts and focal sinusoidal dilatation suggest an adjacent metastasis [51].

Histology will not always allow the site of the primary to be identified especially if the tumour is undifferentiated (fig. 28.27). Cytological examination of aspirated fluid and touch preparations of the biopsy may slightly increase the yield of cancer cells.

Histochemical studies are particularly valuable for

cytology and if the sample is small. Monoclonal antibodies, particularly HEPPARI which reacts with hepatocytes but not bile ducts and non-parenchymal liver cells can be used to distinguish primary from metastatic carcinoma of the liver [167].

The chances of obtaining a positive needle liver biopsy increases with the extent of tumour, size of liver and the presence of a palpable nodule.

Radiology

A *plain film* of the abdomen demonstrates the large liver. The diaphragm may be elevated and its contour irregular. *Calcification* in hepatic tumours is rare but is noted with primary cancer or haemangiomas and in secondaries, for instance from the colon, breast, thyroid or bronchus.

Chest radiograph may show associated pulmonary metastases.

Barium swallow may show oesophageal varices and the *meal* displacement of the stomach to the left and rigidity of the lesser curve. *Barium enema* may reveal depression of the hepatic flexure and transverse colon.

Scanning

Scanning usually detects lesions greater than 2 cm in diameter. Imaging for number, size and location is important for diagnosis, for assessing the possibilities of resection and for follow-up [8].

Ultrasound usually shows echogenic lesions. It is useful, simple and inexpensive. Intra-operative ultrasound is of great value in detecting metastases.

CT shows metastases as low attenuation lesions (fig. 28.28). Those from the colon generally have a large avascular centre with a dense peripheral ring-like accumulation of contrast. About 29% of patients undergoing apparently curative resection for colorectal cancer will have occult hepatic metastases demonstrated by CT scanning. Delayed contrast enhancement adds to the positivity rate. Lipiodol CT scans are also useful.

T_1-*MRI* is the best method of detecting colo-rectal liver metastases [165]. T_2-weighted images show oedema adjacent to the liver metastases [90] (fig. 28.29).

Iron oxide or gadolinium enhanced MRI imaging is better than unenhanced [58]. Duplex colour Doppler sonography shows a lower portal vein congestive index compared with cirrhosis and portal hypertension [89].

Special diagnostic problems

The patient with a known primary growth may be suspected of having liver secondaries but they cannot be confirmed clinically. Suggestive evidence includes slightly increased serum bilirubin, transaminase and

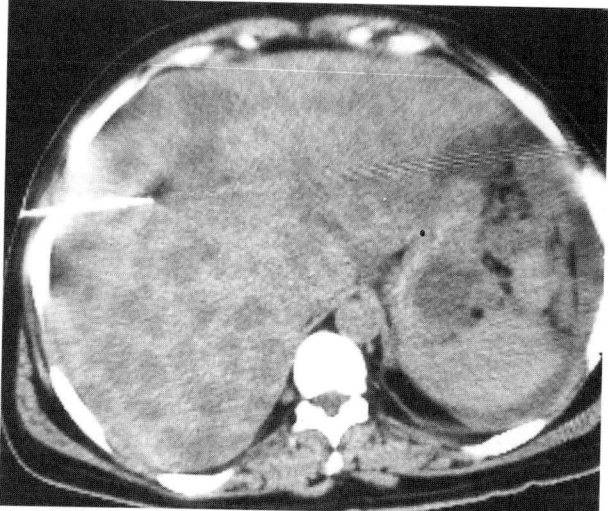

Fig. 28.28. CT scan of widespread hepatic metastases from a primary in the colon. A biopsy needle is directed into one of them.

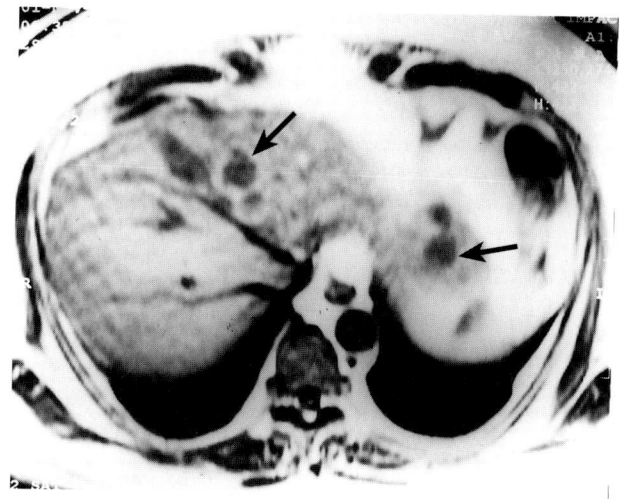

Fig. 28.29. MRI shows multiple hepatic metastases in both lobes but especially along the hepatic vein (arrows).

alkaline phosphatase levels. Aspiration needle biopsy, scanning and peritoneoscopy are useful.

The other problem, of more academic interest, is obvious involvement of the liver when the primary is unknown. Breasts, thyroid and lungs must be considered as possible primaries. Positive stool blood suggests gastrointestinal cancer. Removal of skin tumours and the presence of melanomas suggest malignant melanoma. Suspected carcinoma of the body of the pancreas merits ERCP. Needle liver biopsy is usually positive and may indicate the site of the primary. However, even this may show only the presence of a squamous, scirrhous, columnar or anaplastic growth, the site of the primary remaining unknown.

Prognosis

This depends on the site of the primary and the malignancy. In general, patients die within 1 year of diagnosis of hepatic metastases. Secondaries from tumours of colon and rectum have the best outlook. Patients with hepatic metastases at the time of colonic resection have a mean survival of 12 months with an 8 month median.

Treatment

This remains very unsatisfactory. Those that have the best prognosis without therapy, for instance secondaries from the rectum, do best with therapy. Most of the published results are uncontrolled. Nevertheless, therapy has to be offered if only to give the patient and relatives some hope. Chosen treatment should be the one having the greatest prospect of slowing tumour growth and with the least undesirable side-effects.

Combined therapy uses 5-FU or mitozantrone plus methotrexate and methyl CCNU. Side-effects are great and the results uncontrolled. Best results are associated with breast metastases.

Metastases are resistant to radiation. In the carcinoid syndrome, heroic surgery should be considered. The tumours shell out rather easily. Embolization via the hepatic artery is probably preferable. Embolization with gel foam into a peripheral artery has also been used for other types of hepatic metastases.

Hepatic arterial infusion chemotherapy

Primary and secondary hepatic tumours are supplied mainly by the hepatic artery, although the portal vein may play a small part. Cytotoxic drugs may be delivered directly to the tumour by hepatic artery catheterization. The catheter is usually introduced surgically into the hepatic artery via the gastroduodenal artery. The gallbladder is removed. The agent is usually 5-fluorodeoxy uridine (FUDR), which has an 80–95% extraction rate during the first pass through the liver. It is delivered continuously via an implantable pump for periods of 2 weeks in each month.

This treatment leads to regression of the cancer in 20% and symptomatic improvement in 50%. For colorectal cancer, the survival is 26 months against 8 months in historical controls. A randomized trial showed a higher response rate compared with systemic treatment [81]. Another trial of 69 patients treated with chemoperfusion of the hepatic artery showed 35 with a partial response, nine stable and 25 progressive [151].

Side-effects include sepsis and catheter failure, peptic ulcer, chemical cholecystitis and hepatitis, and sclerosing cholangitis.

Hepatic arterial perfusion may be used as an adjuvant to surgical resection [62].

Hepatic cryotherapy has been combined with regional cytotoxic hepatic arterial perfusion [108].

Interstitial laser photocoagulation has been done with ultrasound monitoring. CT confirms a reduction of the tumour volume by 50% [3].

Surgical resection of colorectal cancer metastases

The secondaries grow slowly, can be single, and are mostly found in the subcapsular regions. Resection may be feasible in about 5–10% of patients. Pre-operative imaging is essential. CT during arterial portography (CTAP) is very sensitive and intra-operative ultrasound is essential [147]. Resection is used when the number of metastases is less than four with no extra-hepatic recurrence or co-morbid disease. The surgeon must be prepared at the time of operation to increase the resection by at least a quarter and to abandon cure in an eighth. A lobectomy or segmentectomy is usually performed.

In a multi-institutional study of 607 patients having metastases resected, 43% showed a recurrence in the liver and 31% in the lungs [66]. 36% recurred in the first year and 25% were alive and disease free at 5 years. In another series, 21% of patients survived 10 years—a most impressive figure. Patients with a carcinogenic embryonic antigen less than 200 ng/ml with 1 cm surgical margins and less than 1000 g liver removed have a greater than 50% estimated 5-year disease-free survival rate [21]. There is an increased risk of recurrence if a resection margin free of tumour is not obtained and if the metastases are bilobar. In another series of 150 patients, curative resection (46%) gave a median survival of 37 months, non-curative resections (12%) survived 21.2 months and the unresectable (42%) survived 16.5 months [149, 150].

The whole picture is confused and controlled trials are required to establish the contribution of surgery to survival of patients with hepatic metastases.

Transplantation

The overall 2-year survival after liver transplantation for metastatic carcinoma averages only 6%.

Metastatic endocrine tumours have been successfully transplanted with additional resection of the pancreatic primary [2].

References

1 Aihara T, Noguchi S, Sasaki Y *et al*. Clonal analysis of precancerous lesion of hepatocellular carcinoma. *Gastroenterology* 1996; **111**: 455.

2 Alsina AE, Bartus S, Hull D *et al*. Liver transplant for

metastatic neuroendocrine tumour. *J. Clin. Gastroenterol.* 1990; **12**: 533.

3 Amin Z, Donald JJ, Masters A *et al.* Hepatic metastases: interstitial laser photo-coagulation with real-time US monitoring and dynamic CT evaluation of treatment. *Radiology* 1993; **187**: 339.

4 Anthony PB. Liver cell dysplasia: what is its significance? *Hepatology* 1987; **7**: 394.

5 Arakawa M, Kage M, Matsumoto S *et al.* Frequency and significance of tumour thrombi in oesophageal varices in hepatocellular carcinoma associated with cirrhosis. *Hepatology* 1986; **6**: 419.

6 Attali P, Houssin D, Roche A *et al.* Hepatic arterial embolization for malignant hypercalcemia in hepatocellular carcinoma. *Dig. Dis. Sci.* 1984; **29**: 466.

7 Audisio RA, Doci R, Mazzaferro V *et al.* Hepatic arterial embolization with microencapsulated mitomycin C for unresectable hepatocellular carcinoma in cirrhosis. *Cancer* 1990; **66**: 228.

8 Baker ME, Pelley R. Hepatic metastases: basic principles and implications for radiologists. *Radiology* 1995; **197**: 329.

9 Ballardini G, Groff P, Zoli M *et al.* Increased risk of hepatocellular carcinoma development in patients with cirrhosis and with high hepatocellular proliferation. *J. Hepatol.* 1994; **20**: 218.

10 Beasley RP. Hepatitis B virus as the etiologic agent in hepatocellular carcinoma — epidemiologic considerations. *Hepatology* 1982; **2**: 215.

11 Belli L, De Carlis L, Beati C *et al.* Surgical treatment of symptomatic giant hemangiomas of the liver. *Surg. Gyn. Obstet.* 1992; **174**: 474.

12 Birnbaum BA, Weinreb JC, Megibow AJ *et al.* Definitive diagnosis of hepatic hemangiomas: MR imaging versus Tc-99m—labeled red blood cell SPECT. *Radiology* 1990; **176**: 95.

13 Bismuth H, Chiche L, Adam R *et al.* Liver resection versus transplantation for hepatocellular carcinoma in cirrhotic patients. *Ann. Surg.* 1993; **218**: 145.

14 Brant WE, Floyd JL, Jackson DE *et al.* The radiological evaluation of hepatic cavernous hemangioma. *JAMA* 1987; **257**: 2471.

15 Bronowicki J-P, Nisand G, Altieri M *et al.* Compared results of resection (RX), orthotopic liver transplantation (OLT) and transcatheter oily chemoembolization (TOCE) in the treatment of Okuda's stage 1 hepatocellular carcinoma (HCC). *Gastroenterology* 1993; **104**: A881.

16 Bruix J, Barrera JM, Calvet X *et al.* Prevalence of antibodies to hepatitis C virus in Spanish patients with hepatocellular carcinoma and hepatic cirrhosis. *Lancet* 1989; **2**: 1004.

17 Bruix J, Castells A, Montanyà X *et al.* Phase II study of transarterial embolization in European patients with hepatocellular carcinoma: need for controlled trials. *Hepatology* 1994; **20**: 643.

18 Bruix J, Ciera I, Calvet X *et al.* Surgical resection and survival in Western patients with hepatocellular carcinoma. *J. Hepatol.* 1992; **15**: 350.

19 Burroughs AK, Bassendine MF, Thomas HC *et al.* Primary liver cell cancer in autoimmune chronic liver disease. *Br. Med. J.* 1981; **282**: 273.

20 Bukh J, Miller RH, Kew MC *et al.* Hepatitis C virus RNA in southern African Blacks with hepatocellular carcinoma. *Proc. Natl. Acad. Sci. USA* 1993; **90**: 1848.

21 Cady B, Stone MD, McDermott WV Jr *et al.* Technical and biological factors in disease-free survival after hepatic resection for colorectal cancer metastases. *Arch. Surg.* 1992; **127**: 561.

22 Castells A, Bruix J, Bru C *et al.* Treatment of hepatocellular carcinoma with tamoxifen: a double-blind placebo-controlled trial in 120 patients. *Gastroenterology* 1995; **109**: 917.

23 Cerezo FJM, Tomas A, Donoso L *et al.* Controlled trial of tamoxifen in patients with advanced hepatocellular carcinoma. *J. Hepatol.* 1994; **20**: 702.

24 Chen M-F, Jan Y-Y, Jeng L-B *et al.* Obstructive jaundice secondary to ruptured hepatocellular carcinoma into the common bile duct. *Cancer* 1994; **73**: 1335.

25 Chisari FV, Klopchin K, Moriyama T *et al.* Molecular pathogenesis of hepatocellular carcinoma in hepatitis B virus transgenic mice. *Cell* 1989; **59**: 1145.

26 Chowdhury AR, Black M, Lorber SH *et al.* Hemangioendotheliomatosis of the liver: a twelve year follow-up. *Gastroenterology* 1977; **72**: 157.

27 Chung SCS, Lee TW, Kwok SPY *et al.* Injection of alcohol to control bleeding from ruptured hepatomas. *Br. Med. J.* 1990; **301**: 421.

28 Chung SW, Toth JL, Rezieg M *et al.* Liver transplantation for hepatocellular carcinoma. *Am. J. Surg.* 1994; **167**: 317.

29 Clain D, Wartnaby K, Sherlock S. Abdominal arterial murmurs in liver disease. *Lancet* 1966; **ii**: 516.

30 Collier JD, Carpenter M, Burt AD *et al.* Expression of mutant p53 protein in hepatocellular carcinoma. *Gut* 1994; **35**: 98.

31 Collier NA, Weinbren K, Bloom SR. Neurotensin secretion by fibrolamellar carcinoma of the liver. *Lancet* 1984; **i**: 538.

32 Colombo M. Hepatocellular carcinoma. *J. Hepatol.* 1992; **15**: 225.

33 Colombo M, De Franchis R, Del Ninno E *et al.* Hepatocellular carcinoma in Italian patients with cirrhosis. *N. Engl. J. Med.* 1991; **325**: 675.

34 Cottone M, Virdone R, Fusco G *et al.* Asymptomatic hepatocellular carcinoma in Child's A cirrhosis. A comparison of natural history and surgical treatment. *Gastroenterology* 1989; **96**: 1566.

35 Craig JR, Peters RL, Edmondson HA *et al.* Fibrolamellar carcinoma of the liver: a tumor of adolescents and young adults with distinctive clinico-pathologic features. *Cancer* 1980; **46**: 372.

36 Diamantis ID, McGandy CE, Chen T-J *et al.* Hepatitis B X-gene expression in hepatocellular carcinoma. *J. Hepatol.* 1992; **15**: 400.

37 Ding S-F, Michail NE, Habib NA. Genetic changes in hepatoblastoma. *J Hepatol.* 1994; **20**: 672.

38 Dooley JS, Li AKC, Scheuer PJ *et al.* A giant cystic mesenchymal hamartoma of the liver: diagnosis management, and study of cyst fluid. *Gastroenterology* 1983; **85**: 958.

39 Dunk AA, Scott SC, Johnson PJ *et al.* Mitoxantrone as a single agent therapy in hepatocellular carcinoma. A phase II study. *J. Hepatol.* 1985; **1**: 395.

40 Dunk AA, Spiliadis, Sherlock S *et al.* Hepatocellular carcinoma and the hepatitis B virus: a study of British patients. *Q. J. Med.* 1987; **62**: 109.

41 Enwonwu CO. The role of dietary aflatoxin in the genesis of hepatocellular cancer in the developing countries. *Lancet* 1984; **ii**: 956.

42 Eriksson S, Carlson J, Velez R. Risk of cirrhosis and primary liver cancer in ATT deficiency. *N. Engl. J. Med.* 1986; 314: 736.

43 Falk H, Thomas LB, Popper H *et al*. Hepatic angiosarcoma associated with androgenic-anabolic steroids. *Lancet* 1979; **ii**: 1120.

44 Farinati F, Fagiuoli S, De Maria N *et al*. Anti-HCV positive hepatocellular carcinoma in cirrhosis. Prevalence, risk-factors and clinical features. *J. Hepatol.* 1992; **14**: 183.

45 Farmer DG, Rosove MH, Shaked A *et al*. Current treatment modalities for hepatocellular carcinoma. *Ann. Surg.* 1994; **219**: 236.

46 Feitelson M. Hepatitis B virus infection and primary hepatocellular carcinoma. *Clin. Microbiol. Rev.* 1992; **5**: 275.

47 Ferrell L, Wright T, Lake J *et al*. Incidence and diagnostic features of macroregenerative nodules vs. small hepatocellular carcinoma in cirrhotic livers. *Hepatology* 1992; **16**: 1372.

48 Fisher A, Miller CM. Ischemic-type biliary strictures in liver allografts: the Achilles heel revisited? *Hepatology* 1995; **21**: 589.

49 Forbes A, Portmann B, Johnson P *et al*. Hepatic sarcomas in adults: a review of 25 cases. *Gut* 1987; **28**: 668.

50 Gerber MA, Shieh YSC, Shim K-S *et al*. Detection of replicative hepatitis C virus sequences in hepatocellular carcinoma. *Am. J. Pathol.* 1992; **141**: 1271.

51 Gerber MA, Thung SN, Bodenheimer HC Jr *et al*. Characteristic histologic triad in liver adjacent to metastatic neoplasm. *Liver* 1986; **6**: 85.

52 Goodman ZD, Ishak KG, Langloss JM *et al*. Combined hepatocellular-cholangiocarcinoma: a histologic and immunohistochemical study. *Cancer* 1985; **55**: 124.

53 Gralnik HR, Givelber H, Abrams E. Dysfibrinogenemia associated with hepatoma. *N. Engl. J. Med.* 1978; **299**: 221.

54 Green LK, Silva EG. Hepatoblastoma in an adult with metastasis to the ovaries. *Am. J. Clin. Pathol.* 1989; **92**: 110.

55 Groupe d'étude et de traitement de carcinome hépatocellulaire. A comparison of chemoembolization and conservative treatment for unresectable hepatocellular carcinoma. *N. Engl. J. Med.* 1995; **332**: 1256.

56 Gururangan S, O'Meara A, MacMahon C *et al*. Primary hepatic tumours in children: a 26-year review. *J. Surg. Oncol.* 1992; **50**: 30.

57 Haas JE, Muczynski KA, Krailo M *et al*. Histopathology and prognosis in childhood hepatoblastoma and hepatocarcinoma. *Cancer* 1989; **64**: 1082.

58 Hamm B, Thoeni RF, Gould RG *et al*. Focal liver lesions: characterization with non-enhanced and dynamic contrast material-enhanced MR imaging. *Radiology* 1994; **190**: 417.

59 Hardell L, Bengtsson NO, Jonsson U *et al*. Aetiological aspects of primary liver cancer with special regard to alcohol, organic solvents and acute intermittent porphyria — an epidemiological investigation. *Br. J. Cancer* 1984; **50**: 389.

60 Harrison HB, Middleton HM III, Crosby JH *et al*. Fulminant hepatic failure: an unusual presentation of metastatic liver disease. *Gastroenterology* 1981; **80**: 820.

61 Helzberg JH, McPhee MS, Zarling EJ *et al*. Hepatocellular carcinoma: an unusual course with hyperthyroidism and inappropriate thyroid-stimulating hormone production. *Gastroenterology* 1985; **88**: 181.

62 Hodgson WJB, Mittelman A, Katz S *et al*. Treatment of colorectal hepatic metastases by intrahepatic chemotherapy alone or as an adjuvant to complete or partial removal of metastatic disease. *Ann. Surg.* 1986; **203**: 420.

63 Hood DL, Bauer TW, Leibel SA *et al*. Hepatic giant cell carcinoma: an ultrastructural and immunohistochemical study. *Am. J. Clin. Pathol.* 1990; **93**: 111.

64 Hsia CC, Axiotis CA, Di Bisceglie AM *et al*. Transforming growth factor-alpha in human hepatocellular carcinoma and coexpression with hepatitis B surface antigen in adjacent liver. *Cancer* 1992; **70**: 1049.

65 Hsu H-C, Huang A-M, Lai P-L *et al*. Genetic alterations at the splice junction of p53 gene in human hepatocellular carcinoma. *Hepatology* 1994; **19**: 122.

66 Hughes KS, Simon R, Songhorabodi S *et al*. Resection of the liver for colorectal carcinoma metastases: a multi-institutional study of patterns of recurrence. *Surgery* 1986; **100**: 278.

67 Ikeda K, Saitoh S, Koida I *et al*. Diagnosis and follow-up of small hepatocellular carcinoma with selective intraarterial digital subtraction angiography. *Hepatology* 1993; **17**: 1003.

68 Ikeda K, Saitoh S, Koida I *et al*. Imaging diagnosis of small hepatocellular carcinoma. *Hepatology* 1994; **20**: 82.

69 Ikeda K, Saitoh S, Koida I *et al*. A multivariate analysis of risk factors for hepatocellular carcinogenesis: a prospective observation of 795 patients with viral and alcoholic cirrhosis. *Hepatology* 1993; **18**: 47.

70 Ishak KG, Sesterhenn IA, Goodman MZD *et al*. Epithelioid hemangioendothelioma of the liver: a clinicopathologic and follow-up study of 32 cases. *Hum. Pathol.* 1984; **15**: 839.

71 Itai Y, Ohtomo K, Furui S *et al*. Non-invasive diagnosis of small cavernous hemangioma of the liver. Advantage of MRI. *Am. J. Roentgenol.* 1985; **145**: 1195.

72 Izumi R, Shimizu K, Iyobe T *et al*. Postoperative adjuvant hepatic arterial infusion of lipiodol containing anticancer drugs in patients with hepatocellular carcinoma. *Hepatology* 1994; **20**: 295.

73 Johnson DH, Hainsworth JD, Greco FA. Extrahepatic biliary obstruction caused by small-cell lung cancer. *Ann. Intern. Med.* 1985; **102**: 487.

74 Jwo S-C, Chiu J-H, Chau G-Y *et al*. Risk factors linked to tumor recurrence of human hepatocellular carcinoma after hepatic resection. *Hepatology* 1992; **16**: 1367.

75 Kamby C, Dirksen H, Vejborg I *et al*. Incidence and methodologic aspects of the occurrence of liver metastases in recurrent breast cancer. *Cancer* 1987; **59**: 1524.

76 Kanematsu T, Furuta T, Takenaka K *et al*. A 5-year experience of lipiodolization: selective regional chemotherapy for 200 patients with hepatocellular carcinoma. *Hepatology* 1989; **10**: 98.

77 Kasugai H, Kojima J, Tatsuta M *et al*. Treatment of hepatocellular carcinoma by transcatheter arterial embolization combined with intraarterial infusion of a mixture of cisplatin and ethiodized oil. *Gastroenterology* 1989; **97**: 965.

78 Keegan-Rogers V, Wu GY. Immunotargeting in the diagnosis and treatment of liver cancer. *Hepatology* 1989; **9**: 646.

79 Keeley AF, Iseri OA, Gottlieb LS. Ultrastructure of hyaline cytoplasmic inclusions in a human hepatoma: relationship to Mallory's alcoholic hyalin. *Gastroenterology* 1972; **62**: 280.

80 Kelleher MB, Iwatsuki S, Sheahan DG. Epithelioid hemangioendothelioma of the liver. Clinicopathological correlation of 10 cases treated by orthotopic liver transplantation. *Am. J. Surg. Pathol.* 1989; **13**: 999.

81 Kemeny N, Daly J, Reichman B *et al*. Intrahepatic or systemic infusion of fluorodeoxyuridine in patients with liver metastases from colorectal carcinoma. *Ann. Intern. Med.* 1987; **107**: 459.

82 Kew MC. Virchow–Troisier's lymph node in hepatocellular carcinoma. *J. Clin. Gastroenterol.* 1991; **13**: 217.

83 Kew MC, Houghton M, Choo Q-L *et al.* Hepatitis C virus antibodies in southern African blacks with hepatocellular carcinoma. *Lancet* 1990; **335**: 873.

84 Kiyosawa K, Sodeyama T, Tanaka E *et al.* Interrelationship of blood transfusion, non-A, non-B hepatitis and hepatocellular carcinoma analysis: by detection of antibody to hepatitis C virus. *Hepatology* 1990; **12**: 671.

85 Kondo S, Nishikawa M, Takami S *et al.* Diagnostic value of lipiodol injection in focal nodular hyperplasia of the liver. *Am. J. Gastroenterol.* 1991; **86**: 779.

86 Kuroda C, Sakurai M, Monden M *et al.* Limitation of transcatheter arterial chemoembolization using iodized oil for small hepatocellular carcinoma. *Cancer* 1991; **67**: 81.

87 Lack EE. Mesenchymal hamartoma of the liver. A clinical and pathological study of nine cases. *Am. J. Pediatr. Hematol/Onocology* 1986; **8**: 91.

88 Lederman SM, Martin EC, Laffey KT *et al.* Hepatic neurofibromatosis, malignant shwannoma and angiosarcoma in von Recklinghausen's disease. *Gastroenterology* 1987; **92**: 234.

89 Leen E, Goldberg JA, Anderson JR *et al.* Hepatic perfusion changes in patients with liver metastases: comparison with those patients with cirrhosis. *Gut* 1993; **34**: 554.

90 Lee MJ, Saini S, Compton CC *et al.* MR demonstration of edema adjacent to a liver metastasis: pathologic correlation. *Am. J. Roentgenol.* 1991; **157**: 499.

91 Lefkowitch JH, Muschel R, Price JB *et al.* Copper and copper-binding protein in fibrolamellar liver cell carcinoma. *Cancer* 1983; **51**: 97.

92 Lennington WJ, Gray GF Jr, Page DL. Mesenchymal hemartoma of liver. A regional ischemic lesion of a sequestered lobe. *Am. J. Dis. Child.* 1993; **147**: 193.

93 Leung NWY, Tam JS, Lai JY *et al.* Does hepatitis C virus infection contribute to hepatocellular carcinoma in Hong Kong? *Cancer* 1992; **70**: 40.

94 Leuschner I, Schmidt D, Harms D. Undifferentiated sarcoma of the liver in childhood. Morphology, flow cytometry and literature review. *Hum. Pathol.* 1990; **21**: 68.

95 Liang TJ, Jeffers LJ, Reddy KR *et al.* Viral pathogenesis of hepatocellular carcinoma in the United States. *Hepatology* 1993; **18**: 1326.

96 Livraghi T, Bolondi L, Buscarini L *et al.* No treatment, resection and ethanol injection in hepatocellular carcinoma: a retrospective analysis of survival in 391 patients with cirrhosis. *J. Hepatol.* 1995; **22**: 522.

97 Locker GY, Doroshaw JH, Zwelling LA *et al.* The clinical features of hepatic angiosarcoma: a report of four cases and a review of the English literature. *Medicine* (*Baltimore*) 1979; **58**: 48.

98 Lutwick LI. Relation between aflatoxins and hepatitis-B virus and hepatocellular carcinoma. *Lancet* 1979; **i**: 755.

99 Marino IR, Todo S, Tzakis AG *et al.* Treatment of hepatic epithelioid hemangioendothelioma with liver transplantation. *Cancer* 1988; **62**: 2079.

100 Mazzaferro V, Regalia E, Doci R *et al.* Liver transplantation for the treatment of small hepatocellular carcinomas in patients with cirrhosis. *N. Engl. J. Med.* 1996; **223**: 693.

101 Meyer M, Wiedorn KH, Hofschneider PH *et al.* A chromosome 17:7 translocation is associated with a hepatitis B virus DNA integration in human hepatocellular carcinoma DNA. *Hepatology* 1992; **15**: 665.

102 Miller WJ, Dodd GD III, Federle MP *et al.* Epithelioid hemangioendothelioma of the liver: imaging findings with pathologic correlation. *Am. J. Roentgenol.* 1992; **159**: 53.

103 Miller WJ, Federle MP, Campbell WL. Diagnosis and staging of hepatocellular carcinoma: comparison of CT and sonography in 36 liver transplantation patients. *Am. J. Roentgenol.* 1991; **157**: 303.

104 Mirowitz SA, Gutierrez E, Lee JKT *et al.* Normal abdominal enhancement patterns with dynamic gadolinium-enhanced MR imaging. *Radiology* 1991; **180**: 637.

105 Miyamoto M, Sudo T, Kuyama T. Spontaneous rupture of hepatocellular carcinoma: a review of 172 Japanese cases. *Am. J. Gastroenterol.* 1991; **86**: 67.

106 Moertel CG, Johnson M, McKusick MA *et al.* The management of patients with advanced carcinoid tumors and islet cell carcinomas. *Ann. Intern. Med.* 1994; **120**: 302.

107 Mondazzi L, Bottelli R, Brambilla G *et al.* Transarterial oily chemoembolization for the treatment of hepatocellular carcinoma: a multivariate analysis of prognostic factors. *Hepatology* 1994; **19**: 1115.

108 Morris DL, Horton MDA, Dilley AV *et al.* Treatment of hepatic metastases by cryotherapy and regional cytotoxic perfusion. *Gut* 1993; **34**: 1156.

109 Mungovan JA, Cronan JJ, Vacarro J. Hepatic cavernous hemangiomas: lack of enlargement over time. *Radiology* 1994; **191**: 111.

110 Nagato Y, Kondo F, Kondo Y *et al.* Histological and morphometrical indicators for a biopsy diagnosis of well-differentiated hepatocellular carcinoma. *Hepatology* 1991; **14**: 473.

111 Nakao N, Kamino K, Miura K *et al.* Recurrent hepatocellular carcinoma after partial hepatectomy: value of treatment with transcatheter arterial chemoembolization. *Am. J. Roentgenol.* 1991; **156**: 1177.

112 Niederau C, Fischer R, Sonnenberg A *et al.* Survival and causes of death in cirrhotic and in noncirrhotic patients with primary hemochromatosis. *N. Engl. J. Med.* 1985; **313**: 1256.

113 Nishioka K, Watanabe J, Furuta S *et al.* A high prevalence of antibody to the hepatitis C virus in patients with hepatocellular carcinoma in Japan. *Cancer* 1991; **67**: 429.

114 Numata K, Tanaka K, Mitsui K *et al.* Flow characteristics of hepatic tumors at color Doppler sonography: correlation with arteriographic findings. *Am. J. Roentgenol.* 1993; **160**: 515.

115 Ohnishi S, Murakami T, Moriyama T *et al.* Androgen and estrogen receptors in hepatocellular carcinoma and in the surrounding non-cancerous liver tissue. *Hepatology* 1986; **6**: 440.

116 Oka H, Tamori A, Kuroki T *et al.* Prospective study of alpha-fetoprotein in cirrhotic patients monitored for development of hepatocellular carcinoma. *Hepatology* 1994; **19**: 61.

117 Okazaki M, Higashihara H, Koganemaru F *et al.* Intraperitoneal hemorrhage from hepatocellular carcinoma: emergency chemoembolization or embolization. *Radiology* 1991; **180**: 647.

118 Okuda K, and Liver Cancer Study Group of Japan. Primary liver cancers in Japan. *Cancer* 1980; **45**: 2663.

119 Okuda K, Kondo Y, Nakano M *et al.* Hepatocellular car-

cinoma presenting with pyrexia and leukocytosis: report of five cases. *Hepatology* 1991; **13**: 695.

120 Okuda K, Obata H, Nakajima Y *et al*. Prognosis of primary hepatocellular carcinoma. *Hepatology* 1984; **4**: 3S.

121 Okuda K, Peters RL, Simson IW. Gross anatomic features of hepatocellular carcinoma from three disparate geographic areas. *Cancer* 1984; **54**: 2165.

122 Onishi S, Saibara T, Fujikawa M *et al*. Adoptive immunotherapy with lymphokine-activated killer cells plus recombinant interleukin 2 in patients with unresectable hepatocellular carcinoma. *Hepatology* 1989; **10**: 349.

123 Paradinas RJ, Melia WM, Wilkinson ML *et al*. High serum vitamin B12 binding capacity as a marker of the fibrolamellar variant of hepatocellular carcinoma. *Br. Med. J.* 1982; **285**: 840.

124 Patten RM, Byun J-Y, Freeny PC. CT of hypervascular hepatic tumors: are unenhanced scans necessary for diagnosis? *Am. J. Roentgenol.* 1993; **161**: 979.

125 Pierach CA, Bossenmaier IC, Cardinal RA *et al*. Pseudoporphyria in a patient with hepatocellular carcinoma. *Am. J. Med.* 1984; **76**: 545.

126 Popper H. Viral versus chemical hepatocarcinogenesis. *J. Hepatol.* 1988; **6**: 229.

127 Pozniak MA, Baus KM. Hepatofugal arterial signal in the main portal vein: an indicator of intravascular tumor spread. *Radiology* 1991; **180**: 663.

128 Quinn SF, Benjamin GG. Hepatic cavernous hemangiomas: simple diagnostic sign with dynamic bolus CT. *Radiology* 1992; **182**: 545.

129 Ringe B, Wittekind C, Weimann A *et al*. Results of hepatic resection and transplantation for fibrolamellar carcinoma. *Surg. Gyn. Obstet.* 1992; **175**: 299.

130 Robinson WS, Klote L, Aoki N. Hepadnaviruses in cirrhotic liver and hepatocellular carcinoma. *J. Med. Virol.* 1990; **31**: 18.

131 Ros PR, Freeny PC, Harms SE *et al*. Hepatic MR imaging with ferumoxides: a multicenter clinical trial of the safety and efficacy in the detection of focal hepatic lesions. *Radiology* 1995; **196**: 481.

132 Ros PR, Buck JL, Goodman ZD *et al*. Intrahepatic cholangiocarcinoma; radiologic-pathologic correlation. *Radiology* 1988; **167**: 689.

133 Ross JS, Kurian S. Clear cell hepatocarcinoma: sudden death from hypoglycemia. *Am. J. Gastroenterol.* 1985; **80**: 188.

134 Ruiz J, Sangro B, Cuende JI *et al*. Hepatitis B and C viral infections in patients with hepatocellular carcinoma. *Hepatology* 1992; **16**: 637.

135 Rummeny E, Weissleder R, Stark DD *et al*. Primary liver tumors: diagnosis by MR imaging. *Am. J. Roentgenol.* 1989; **63**: 72.

136 Rubel LR, Ishak KG. Thorotrast-associated cholangiocarcinoma: an epidemiologic and clinicopathologic study. *Cancer* 1982; **50**: 1408.

137 Ryder SD, Rizzi PM, Metivier E *et al*. Chemoembolization with lipiodol and doxorubicin: applicability in British patients with hepatocellular carcinoma. *Gut* 1996; **38**: 125.

138 Sato Y, Nakata K, Kato Y *et al*. Early recognition of hepatocellular carcinoma based on altered profiles of alphafetoprotein. *N. Engl. J. Med.* 1993; **328**: 1802.

139 Shapiro ET, Bell GI, Polonsky KS *et al*. Tumor hypo-

140 Sharara AI, Panella TJ, Fitz JG. Paraneoplastic hepatopathy associated with soft tissue sarcoma. *Gastroenterology* 1992; **103**: 330.

141 Sherlock S. Viruses and hepatocellular carcinoma. *Gut* 1994; **35**: 828.

142 Sherlock S, Fox FA, Niazi SP *et al*. Chronic liver disease and primary liver-cell cancer with hepatitis-associated (Australia) antigen in serum. *Lancet* 1970; **i**: 1243.

143 Simonetti RG, Camma C, Fiorello F *et al*. Hepatitis C virus infection as a risk factor for hepatocellular carcinoma in patients with cirrhosis. A case-control study. *Ann. Intern. Med.* 1992; **116**: 97.

144 Simpson IW. Membranous obstruction of the inferior vena cava and hepatocellular carcinoma of South Africa. *Gastroenterology* 1982; **82**: 171.

145 Sinanan MN, Marchioro T. Management of cavernous hemangioma of the liver. *Am. J. Surg.* 1989; **157**: 519.

146 Sironi S, Livraghi T, Angeli E *et al*. Small hepatocellular carcinoma: MR follow-up of treatment with percutaneous ethanol injection. *Radiology* 1993; **187**: 119.

147 Soyer P, Levesque M, Elias D *et al*. Detection of liver metastases from colorectal cancer: comparison of intraoperative US and CT during arterial portography. *Radiology* 1992; **183**: 541.

148 Starzl TE, Iwatsuki S, Shaw BW Jr *et al*. Treatment of fibrolamellar hepatoma with partial or total hepatectomy and transplantation of the liver. *Surg. Gyn. Obstet.* 1986; **162**: 145.

149 Steele G Jr, Bleday R, Mayer RJ *et al*. A prospective evaluation of hepatic resection for colorectal carcinoma metastases to the liver: gastrointestinal tumor study group protocol 6584. *J. Clin. Oncol.* 1991; **9**: 1105.

150 Steele G Jr, Ravikumar TS. Resection of hepatic metastases from colorectal cancer. Biologic perspectives. *Ann. Surg.* 1989; **210**: 127.

151 Sterchi JM, Richards F, White DR *et al*. Chemoinfusion of the hepatic artery for metastases to the liver. *Surg. Gyn. Obstet.* 1989; **168**: 291.

152 Stevens WR, Johnson CD, Stephens DH *et al*. CT findings in hepatocellular carcinoma: correlation of tumor characteristics with causative factors, tumor size, and histologic tumor grade. *Radiology* 1994; **191**: 531.

153 Strickland RC, Shenker S. The nephrogenic hepatic dysfunction syndrome: a review. *Am. J. Dig. Dis.* 1977; **22**: 49.

154 Strohmeyer FW, Ishak KG, Gerber MA *et al*. Ground-glass cells in hepatocellular carcinoma may contain fibrinogen. *Am. J. Clin. Pathol.* 1980; **74**: 254.

155 Sugioka A, Tsuzuki T, Kanai T. Postresection prognosis of patients with hepatocellular carcinoma. *Surgery* 1993; **113**: 612.

156 Summerskill WHJ, Adson MA. Gynecomastia as a sign of hepatoma. *Am. J. Dig. Dis.* 1962; **74**: 250.

157 Takahashi H, Saibara T, Iwamura S *et al*. Serum alpha-L-fucosidase activity and tumor size in hepatocellular carcinoma. *Hepatology* 1994; **19**: 1414.

158 Takano S, Yokosuka O, Imazeki F *et al*. Incidence of hepatocellular carcinoma in chronic hepatitis B and C: a prospective study of 251 patients. *Hepatology* 1995; **21**: 650.

159 Takayama T, Makuuchi S, Hirohashi M *et al*. Malignant transformation of adenomatous hyperplasia to hepatocellular carcinoma. *Lancet* 1990; **336**: 1150.

glycemia: relationship to high molecular weight insulin-like growth factor II. *J. Clin. Invest.* 1990; **85**: 1672.

160 Taketa K. Alpha-fetoprotein: reevaluation in hepatology. *Hepatology* 1990; **12**: 1420.

161 Terada T, Nakanuma Y, Kawai K. Small hepatocellular carcinoma presenting as intrabiliary pedunculated polyp and obstructive jaundice. *J. Clin. Gastroenterol.* 1989; **11**: 578.

162 Theise ND, Schwartz M, Miller C *et al.* Macroregenerative nodules and hepatocellular carcinoma in forty-four sequential adult liver explants with cirrhosis. *Hepatology* 1992; **16**: 949.

163 Tung GA, Cronan JJ. Percutaneous needle biopsy of hepatic cavernous hemangioma. *J. Clin. Gastroenterol.* 1993; **16**: 117.

164 Wakasa K, Sakurai M, Kuroda C *et al.* Effect of transcatheter arterial embolization on the boundary architecture of hepatocellular carcinoma. *Cancer* 1990; **65**; 913.

165 Ward BA, Miller DL, Frank JA *et al.* Prospective evaluation of hepatic imaging studies in the detection of colorectal metastases: correlation with surgical findings. *Surgery* 1989; **105**: 180.

166 Weitz IC, Liebman HA. Des-gamma-carboxy (abnormal) prothrombin and hepatocellular carcinoma: a critical review. *Hepatology* 1993; **18**: 990.

167 Wennerberg AE, Nalasnik MA, Coleman WB. Hepatocyte paraffin I: a monoclonal antibody that reacts with hepatocytes and can be used for differential diagnosis of hepatic tumors. *Am. J. Pathol.* 1993; **143**: 1050.

168 Wheeler DA, Edmondson HA. Cystadenoma with mes-enchymal stroma (CMS) in the liver and bile ducts: a clinicopathologic study of 17 cases, 4 with malignant change. *Cancer* 1985; **56**: 1434.

169 Wilkinson ML, Portmann B, Williams R. Wilson's disease and hepatocellular carcinoma: possible protective role of copper. *Gut* 1983; **24**: 767.

170 Willett IR, Sutherland RC, O'Rourke MF *et al.* Pulmonary hypertension complicating hepatocellular carcinoma. *Gastroenterology* 1984; **87**: 1180.

171 Winter TC III, Freeny PC, Nghiem HV *et al.* MR imaging with IV superparamagnetic iron oxide: efficacy in the detection of focal hepatic lesions. *Am. J. Roentgenol.* 1993; **161**: 1191.

172 Yamashita Y, Takahashi M, Koga Y *et al.* Prognostic factors in the treatment of hepatocellular carcinoma with transcatheter arterial embolization and arterial infusion. *Cancer* 1991; **67**: 385.

173 Yan Z-P, Lin G, Zhao H-Y *et al.* An experimental study and clinical pilot trials on yttrium-90 glass microspheres through the hepatic artery for treatment of primary liver cancer. *Cancer* 1993; **72**: 3210.

174 Yokoyama I, Todo S, Iwatsuki S *et al.* Liver transplantation in the treatment of primary liver cancer. *Hepato-Gastroenterol.* 1990; **37**: 188.

175 Zaman SN, Melia WM, Johnson RD *et al.* Risk factors in development of hepatocellular carcinoma in cirrhosis: prospective study of 613 patients. *Lancet* 1985; **i**: 1357.

Chapter 29
Imaging of the Biliary Tract: Interventional Radiology and Endoscopy

Imaging is central to the investigation and diagnosis of biliary tract disease. Upper abdominal pain is a common symptom and imaging of the gallbladder may be necessary to identify or rule out disease. The symptoms of cholestasis—jaundice and itching—are not specific, nor are the physical findings. Biochemical tests only confirm cholestasis. Common bile duct obstruction, for example from stones and tumour, must be distinguished from intra-hepatic cholestasis such as that caused by drugs. An algorithm helps (fig. 13.20). Non-invasive tests (ultrasound, CT, IDA scans) provide important data on which to choose more invasive and definitive techniques (ERCP, PTC, liver biopsy). Angiography is used to assess resectability of tumours. Interventional endoscopy and radiology provide an alternative therapeutic approach to surgery. Aspiration cytology or biopsy are done to give a tissue diagnosis.

Plain film of the abdomen

Diagnostic yield is low and this test is tending to be omitted. However, it may reveal gallstones, a calcified gallbladder, pancreatic calcification or, rarely, the outline of a distended gallbladder.

With obstruction to the cystic duct, calcium carbonate may be excreted with the bile (milk of calcium bile or 'limey bile'). The wall of the gallbladder may also calcify (porcelain gallbladder).

Gas in the biliary tree ('aerobilia') may be seen after endoscopic sphincterotomy or surgical bile duct/bowel anastomosis. In such a patient with cholestasis or fever, however, this finding should not be used as evidence of unobstructed bile drainage, since it may occur above a significant stricture, or stone (fig. 29.1) [26]. Rarely, biliary infection with gas-forming organisms produces aerobilia.

Ultrasound

Bile ducts

Ultrasonography (US) is the most important screening investigation in patients with cholestasis. The major intra-hepatic bile ducts are normally 2 mm in diameter,

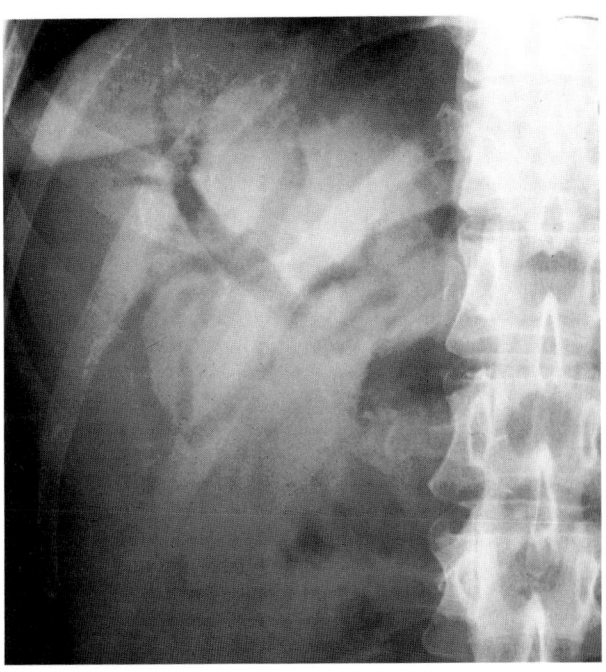

Fig. 29.1. Plain abdominal X-ray showing gas in the intra-hepatic biliary tree.

the common hepatic duct <4 mm and the common bile duct <5–7 mm in diameter. The presence of dilated ducts characterizes large bile duct obstruction (fig. 29.2). The technique is 95% accurate if the serum bilirubin level exceeds 170 μmol/litre (10 mg/dl). False negatives are seen if the obstruction is of short duration or intermittent. US diagnoses the correct level and cause of the obstruction in about 60% and <50% of cases respectively, largely due to failure to visualize the complete biliary tract. The lower end particularly may not be seen because of overlying gas in the duodenum and bowel. Endoscopic US shows this area much better and very small lesions can be detected. For common duct stones, endoscopic US is more accurate than percutaneous US or CT [2]. It is only available, however, in a few centres.

Gallbladder

The gallbladder is ideal for sonography which has a high

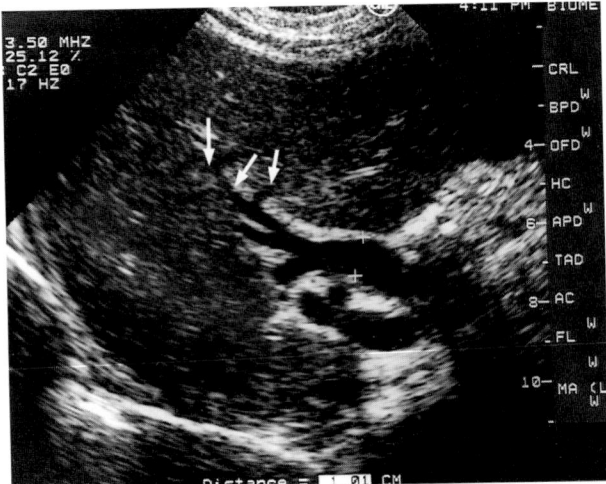

Fig. 29.2. Ultrasound scan showing dilated intra-hepatic ducts (arrowed) and common bile duct (marked ++).

accuracy in detecting disease. The examination should be performed after fasting which should result in a distended gallbladder full of bile. Failure to identify the gallbladder (no fluid-filled lumen and shadowing in the gallbladder bed) may be as important as finding an abnormality. Gallstones cast intense echoes with obvious posterior acoustic shadows (fig. 29.3). They change in position with that of the patient. Stones 3 mm in size and upwards may be visualized. Diagnostic accuracy is said to be 96% but less experienced operators will not achieve this success and there are many diagnostic pitfalls [69].

Acute calculous cholecystitis is suggested by the finding of stones in the gallbladder together with other signs indicative of inflammation [10, 29]. These include a thickened wall of the gallbladder (>5 mm) (fig. 29.4) and a positive sonographic Murphy sign — the presence of

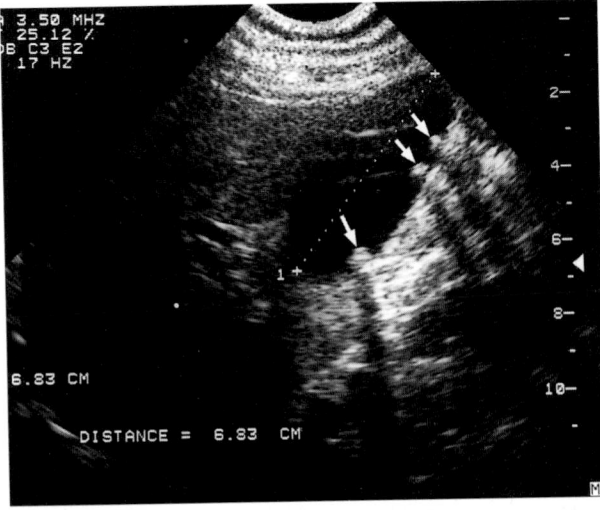

Fig. 29.3. Ultrasound scan of gallbladder showing three stones (arrowed) which cast acoustic shadows.

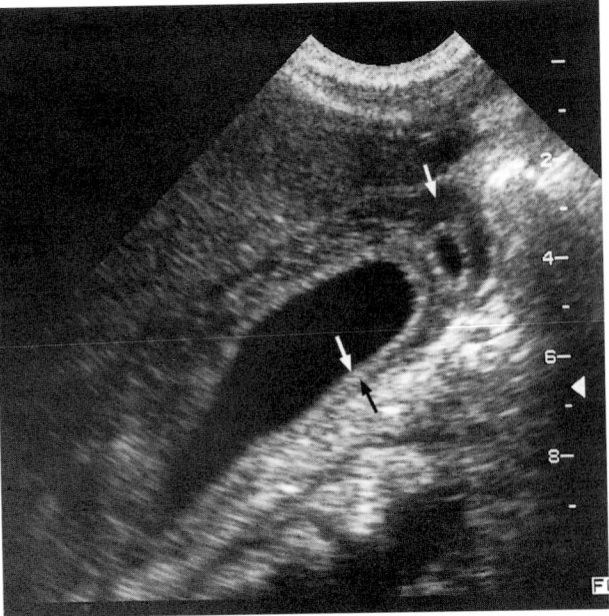

Fig. 29.4. Ultrasound scan in acute cholecystitis. Note the thickened wall of the gallbladder (between black and white arrows) with some peri-cholecystic fluid (single arrow).

maximum tenderness, elicited by direct pressure of the transducer, over a sonographically localized gallbladder. Distention, peri-cholecystic fluid, subserosal oedema (without ascites), intramural gas or a sloughed mucosal membrane are also important signs. The same features of gallbladder inflammation hold for the diagnosis of acute acalculous cholecystitis [13].

Ultrasonographic examination of the gallbladder and liver may detect gallbladder polyps or carcinoma, or congenital biliary anomalies such as Caroli's disease or choledochal cysts.

Ultrasound allows guided percutaneous access to the gallbladder for drainage, antegrade cholangiography, and even gallstone dissolution or removal.

Computed tomography

CT also shows dilated bile ducts distinguishing obstructive from non-obstructive jaundice in 90% of cases. But as a screening procedure it has no advantage over ultrasound. It is, however, more likely than ultrasound to show the level and cause of obstruction. The lower end of a dilated bile duct is usually seen; pancreatic lesions if large enough will be shown (fig. 29.5). Hilar cholangiocarcinoma is rarely demonstrated. Routine CT is not accurate in detecting duct and gallbladder stones. CT may be used, however, to distinguish cholesterol-rich gallbladder stones from calcium-containing stones (based on the attenuation value) — useful information if extracorporeal shock wave lithotripsy is being considered.

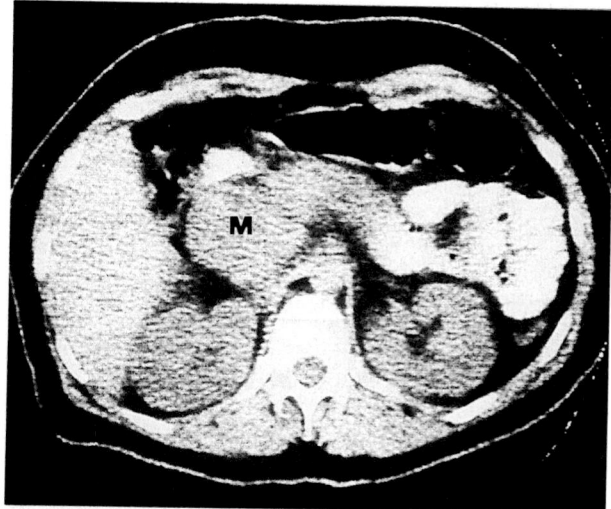

Fig. 29.5. CT scan showing mass (M) in head of pancreas due to carcinoma.

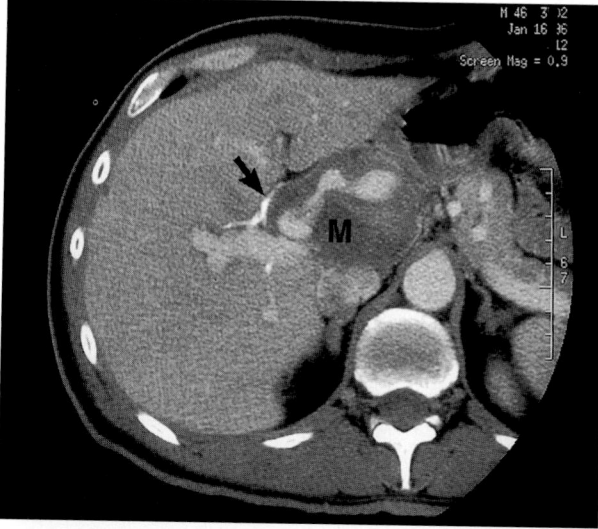

(a)

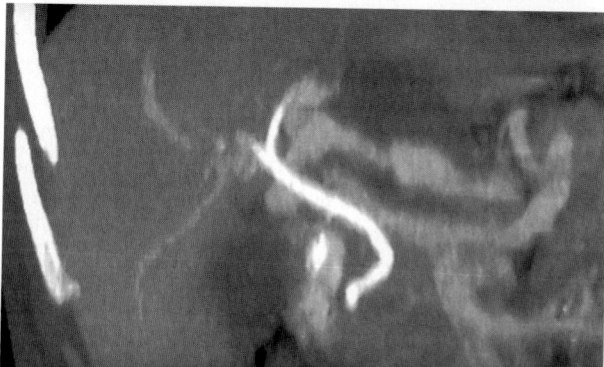

(b)

Fig. 29.6. (a) Spiral CT with intravenous cholangiographic contrast medium showing common hepatic duct (arrowed) between liver and vascular mass (M), known to be a hepatic artery aneurysm. (b) Three-dimensional reconstruction (maximum intensity projection, MIP) of normal bile duct using spiral CT cholangiography.

Spiral CT allows scanning to be completed quickly (15–30 seconds) during a single breath hold [75]. The major advantage is that the scan can be completed while there is a high concentration of contrast in the blood vessels of interest, and before significant contrast equilibration has occurred. Detail of small vessels is remarkable — particularly useful in the assessment of tumour resectability [7].

CT cholangiography (fig. 29.6) with or without contrast is possible. The disadvantages of cholangiography with contrast are the well-recognized risk of fatal anaphylaxis, and restriction of this technique to patients with normal or near normal liver function. However, three-dimensional reconstruction is possible [71]. Normal and abnormal intra- and extra-hepatic ducts are seen as well as the site of obstruction. In patients with bile duct obstruction three-dimensional spiral CT without contrast can be used [76]. These techniques, however, await comparison with MR cholangiography, which at present is more widely used than the CT method.

Magnetic resonance imaging

Cross-sectional (two-dimensional) MRI has a place where US and CT have been inconclusive, and can show dilated bile ducts, masses and stones. As with spiral CT, three-dimensional reconstruction of MRI of the biliary tree has been developed (MR cholangiography) (fig. 29.7) [3, 42]. No contrast agent is required. The pancreatic duct is seen. This technique is highly accurate in the diagnosis of bile duct obstruction and its cause [27, 64]. Its performance versus ERCP needs further study to establish its role in the work-up of patients with biliary tract disease. However, it is likely to be restricted to selected patients where non-invasive cholangiography is preferred or there is complex anatomy.

Biliary scintigraphy

The technetium-labelled compound is cleared from the plasma by hepato-cellular organic anion transport and excreted in the bile (fig. 29.8a). Biliary radiopharmaceuticals have so improved that one of the newest, iododiethyl IDA (Iodida), is easily prepared and is taken up by the liver and excreted into bile efficiently with only 5% of the injected dose excreted in the urine. Effective concentration in the bile duct is achieved in patients with total serum bilirubin levels exceeding 340 μmol/l (20 mg/dl). Resolution is much less than with other forms of bile duct visualization and the role of cholescintigraphy is therefore limited.

The method may be used to determine patency of the cystic duct in suspected *acute cholecystitis* (fig. 29.8b). The radioactivity is followed until it reaches the duodenum.

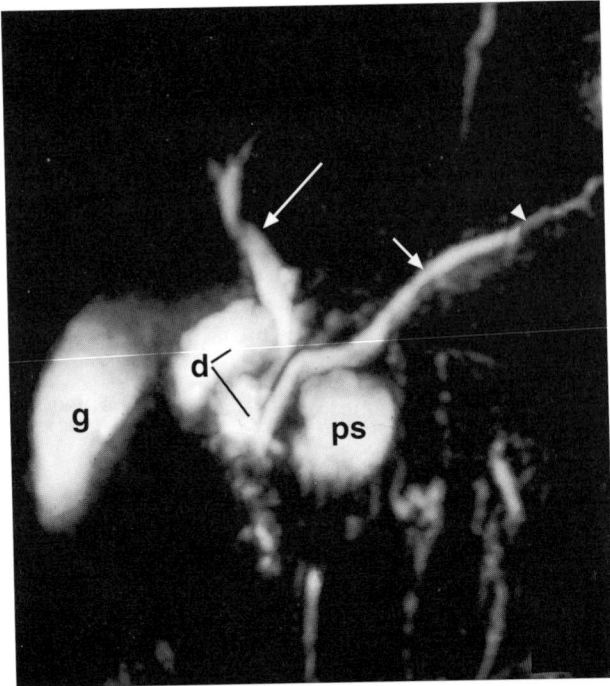

Fig. 29.7. MR cholangiopancreatography. The common bile duct appears normal (large arrow). The pancreatic duct (small arrow) is wider than expected and irregular in the tail (arrowhead). There is a pseudocyst (ps) in the head of the pancreas. ERCP confirmed the normal biliary tree, and features of chronic pancreatitis in both body and tail (g = gallbladder; d = duodenum).

If the gallbladder fails to visualize, despite common bile duct patency and intestinal visualization, the probability of acute cholecystitis is 99%. Cholescintigraphy combined with morphine (to promote gallbladder filling) is useful in the evaluation of suspected acalculous cholecystitis [20].

The gallbladder ejection fraction can be calculated from the loss of isotope from the gallbladder after a standard infusion of sincalide (the C-terminal octapeptide of CCK) [77]. This technique identifies gallbladder disease in some patients who have gallbladder-like pain but a normal ultrasound [74].

Cholescintigraphy can show whether the bile duct is obstructed, but in most units US serves this role.

In the more complicated patient, analysis of the pattern of radioactivity, or the combination of scintigraphy with US can differentiate intra-hepatic cholestasis from bile duct obstruction [41]—useful, for example, in the patient with a biliary stricture, who remains cholestatic despite insertion of a biliary endoprosthesis. Scintigraphy is also useful in assessing the patency of biliary-enteric anastomoses, and may show biliary leaks after cholecystectomy (fig. 29.8c) and liver transplantation.

Choledochal cysts can be diagnosed although ultrasound or CT scanning are just as satisfactory.

In the *neonate*, IDA scanning is used to differentiate between biliary atresia and neonatal hepatitis (fig. 29.8d). It may be combined with ultrasound.

Functional obstruction of the sphincter of Oddi after cholecystectomy may be suggested by delayed and reduced excretion of activity with slower emptying of the biliary tree.

Oral cholecystography

The contrast materials are iodine-containing, conjugated with glucuronic acid by the liver, and excreted in the bile. With renal disease hepato-biliary excretion increases. Reabsorption of water by the gallbladder mucosa leads to a rise in concentration of the contrast and gallbladder opacification. Complications such as hypersensitivity and renal changes are extremely rare particularly with the newer contrast agents.

Three X-ray films are necessary: control, fasting after oral contrast, and after gallbladder contraction by a fatty meal or CCK. The gallbladder will be shown in 85% of patients. Films are taken in erect and prone (fig. 29.9) positions. The erect film is useful in demonstrating translucent stones.

Normal visualization, without stones, gives a 95% probability that the gallbladder is normal.

Cholecystography should not be done if the serum conjugated bilirubin level is above 34 μmol/litre (2 mg/dl). Failure of gallbladder filling within 14 hours may be due to defective intestinal absorption of contrast, poor liver function, a diseased gallbladder, an obstructed cystic duct or previous cholecystectomy.

Uses of cholecystography [45]

Gallstones will be detected with an accuracy of 85–90%. US, however, is 15–20% more sensitive with a lower false negative rate and is the first-line test to detect stones.

Oral cholecystography remains of value to establish the number and size of stones, the patency of the cystic duct and the ability of the gallbladder wall to concentrate bile and contract. These features are important when non-surgical management is being considered. The technique is also of particular value in showing lesions of the gallbladder wall, seen after gallbladder contraction stimulated by fat. Examples are the radiolucent zones unaffected by posture caused by cholesterol deposits. *Adenomyomatosis* is seen as small fundal outpouchings. *Rokitansky–Aschoff sinuses* are shown as a dotted second contour around the gallbladder. Finally, anomalies of the gallbladder may be visualized.

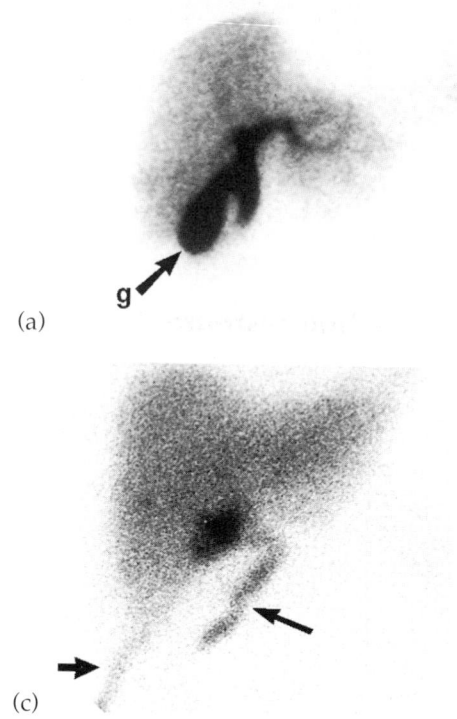

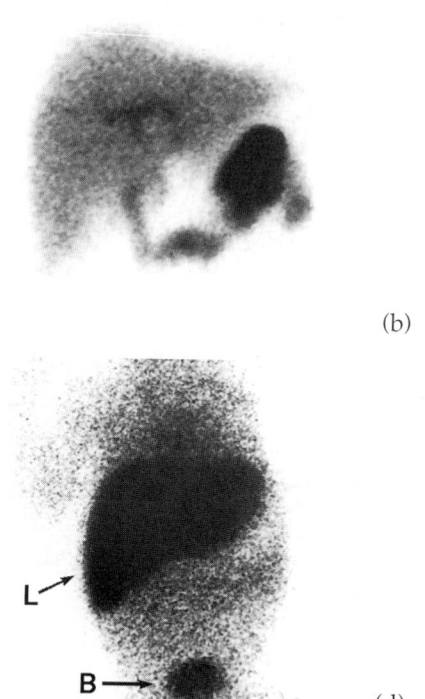

(a)

(b)

(c)

(d)

Fig. 29.8. Cholescintigraphy: (^{99m}Tc Iodida). (a) Normal scan. At 30 minutes the gallbladder (g) has filled. Isotope has already entered the bowel (not shown). (b) Acute cholecystitis. Gallbladder has not filled by 60 minutes. (c) Post-cholecystectomy bile leak. Isotope tracks laterally from gallbladder bed (short arrow) and T-tube track (long arrow). (d) Two-week-old infant with severe jaundice. Radioactivity concentrated in liver (L) and did not enter bowel. Biliary atresia was confirmed. B = bladder.

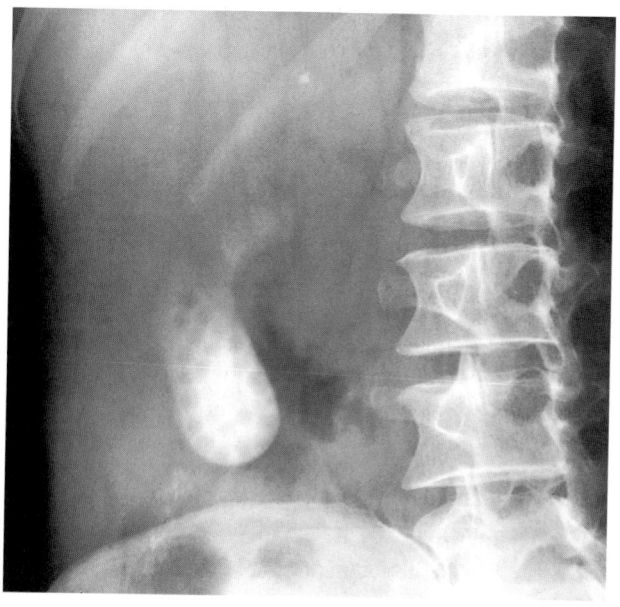

Fig. 29.9. Oral cholecystogram showing gallbladder packed with stones.

Intravenous cholangiography

The contrast (meglumine iotroxate; biliscopin) is concentrated by the liver so that hepatic and common bile ducts are regularly demonstrated. Tomography is used.

Intravenous cholangiography had become obsolete because of its poor diagnostic accuracy, its morbidity and the advent of percutaneous and endoscopic retrograde cholangiography. Some units, however, are now using it to screen for common duct stones before laparoscopic cholecystectomy. In one series of patients without risk factors for duct stones, intravenous cholangiography detected stones in only 1.8% [53]. Such a low yield argues against its routine use in this group of patients.

Endoscopic retrograde cholangiopancreatography (ERCP) [14, 62]

The ampulla of Vater is visualized endoscopically, the common bile duct or pancreatic duct is cannulated and contrast material injected (fig. 29.10).

Patients with suspected biliary obstruction, a history of cholangitis or a pancreatic pseudocyst are at risk of procedure-related sepsis, and require antibiotic premedication [9]. The elderly are also at greater risk. Microorganisms responsible include colonic flora (*Escherichia coli*, *Klebsiella*, *Proteus*, *Pseudomonas*, *Streptococcus faecalis*) and the antibiotic choice should reflect this and the hospital policy. Oral ciprofloxacin is as effective as intravenous cefuroxime, and more cost-effective [49].

The patient is starved for 6 hours. The procedure is done under sedation with a benzodiazepine (diazepam, midazolam) with an opiate as necessary.

At ERCP, diseases of oesophagus, stomach, duodenum, pancreas and biliary tract including duodenal diverticula and fistulae may be diagnosed. Manometry of the sphincter area is possible. Immediate treatment may be instituted, for example sphincterotomy for common duct stones. However, endoscopes are costly and the technique demands an experienced team. Usually the patient must be under observation for 24 hours after the procedure. Outpatient ERCP may, however, be done for selected patients [35]. Two of 115 patients required readmission.

The side-viewing duodenoscope is passed. The stomach and duodenum are inspected and biopsy and cytology specimens taken if indicated. The papilla is identified. Duodenal ileus is maintained by intermittent intravenous hyoscine *N*-butylbromide (Buscopan) or glucagon. Any lesion in the area is biopsied. The cannula is then introduced under direct vision into the papilla and contrast (e.g. iopromide) injected under fluoroscopic control. Preferential catheterization of bile duct and pancreatic duct is helped by directing the catheter towards 11 and 12 o'clock respectively, with the ampullary area *en face* seen as a clock face.

The intra-hepatic biliary tree, cystic and common bile ducts and gallbladder are filled (fig. 29.10). Changes in the position of the patient and tilting of the screening table after injection encourage distribution of contrast material throughout the duct system. In difficult cases, such as after sphincterotomy, a balloon catheter in the duct may be used to prevent reflux of contrast into the duodenum and so obtain better filling. The pancreatic duct is similarly cannulated and X-ray films taken.

An aseptic technique is maintained throughout. Cannulas are sterilized with ethylene oxide gas and the endoscopes thoroughly cleansed with soap and water and disinfected with *activated* glutaraldehyde. The danger of introducing infection is shown by a single endoscope which, although cleaned in an automatic machine, remained contaminated with *Pseudomonas aeruginosa* so resulting in biliary infection in ten patients, with one fatality [1]. This could have been prevented by manually suctioning alcohol through the working channel of the endoscope.

A history of minor reactions to intravenous contrast is not important but those who have had a major allergic reaction to iodinated contrast should be premedicated with corticosteroids and antihistamines [50].

The success rate for ERCP is 80–90% but depends on experience. Other causes of failure include a periampullary diverticulum or an ampullary tumour or stricture. A Billroth II gastrectomy poses difficulties

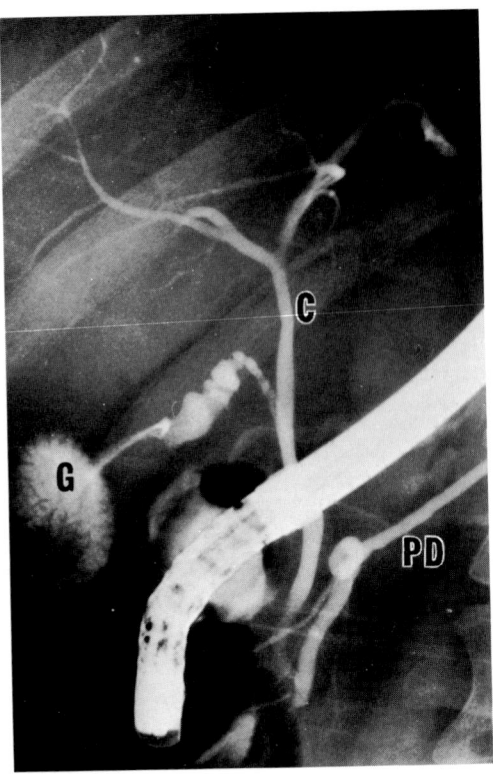

Fig. 29.10 ERCP, normal appearances. PD = pancreatic duct; G = gallbladder; C = common bile duct.

which may be overcome by an experienced endoscopist often using a forward viewing endoscope.

Interpretation of the cholangiogram is not always easy. Contrast may obscure small stones. Air bubbles may cause confusion. Failure to fill the biliary tree, particularly in non-dependent parts, may add to the difficulty.

Complications [68]

The complication rate is 2–3% and mortality 0.1–0.2%. Complications are directly related to the skill and experience of the operator and to the presence of underlying pancreatic or biliary disease.

Serum amylase levels rise considerably after ERCP and acute pancreatitis is the commonest complication. It almost always follows successful pancreatic cannulation and injection, usually in those with pancreatic disease. The volume of contrast injected should be kept to a minimum. Non-ionic lower osmolarity contrast media have not been proven to carry a lower risk of acute pancreatitis [40]. Pancreatic pseudo-cyst is a relative contraindication to ERCP.

Cholangitis is the second most common complication but the commonest cause of death. Bacteraemia is reported in 0–14% [61]. Pre-existing biliary infection and obstruction are important risk factors. Prophylactic antibiotics are important in prevention together with early decompression of any biliary obstruction.

In patients with primary sclerosing cholangitis and advanced disease, there may be deterioration after ERCP [6].

Clinical indications

ERCP adds to the speed of diagnosis of the jaundiced patient as it can be performed irrespective of depth of icterus or state of liver function. It outlines the site of any biliary obstruction and in many instances indicates the cause.

It can be used to diagnose gallbladder and common bile duct stones, and duct strictures (figs 29.11, 29.12). It is of particular value in those with biliary disease and undilated intra-hepatic ducts. Diagnoses include primary sclerosing cholangitis, Caroli's disease and other congenital anomalies.

ERCP may be performed after biliary surgery in the investigation of benign post-cholecystectomy symptoms or to define and treat more serious sequelae such as residual calculi, leaks and biliary strictures [5].

ERCP may be used to diagnose pancreatic disease, particularly in those with coincident hepato-biliary problems such as carcinoma of the pancreas and alcoholic pancreatitis with biliary obstruction.

ERCP is used in the investigation of the patient with obscure epigastric pain. It allows visualization of stomach and duodenum as well as pancreatic and biliary ducts, all at one sitting.

Pure bile or pancreatic juice may be obtained for culture, aspiration cytology or chemical analysis.

Strictures may be brushed for cytology or biopsied [37].

Endoscopic sphincterotomy [14]

Normal coagulation is a prerequisite for endoscopic sphincterotomy and the result of platelet count and pro-thrombin time as well as haemoglobin should be known. Serum is taken for blood group analysis and saved in case transfusion is necessary. Premedication with anti-biotic is routine in most units. A skilled team is required with adequate equipment, in a hospital with facilities to treat any complication.

After the diagnostic ERCP has shown a stone, the ampulla is catheterized with a sphincterotome appropriate in length and design to the anatomy found. Fluo-

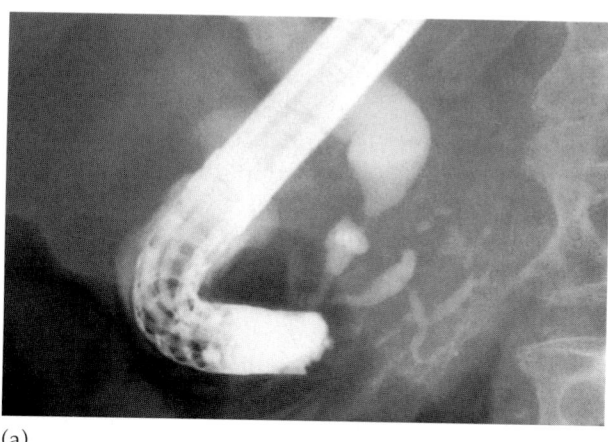

(a)

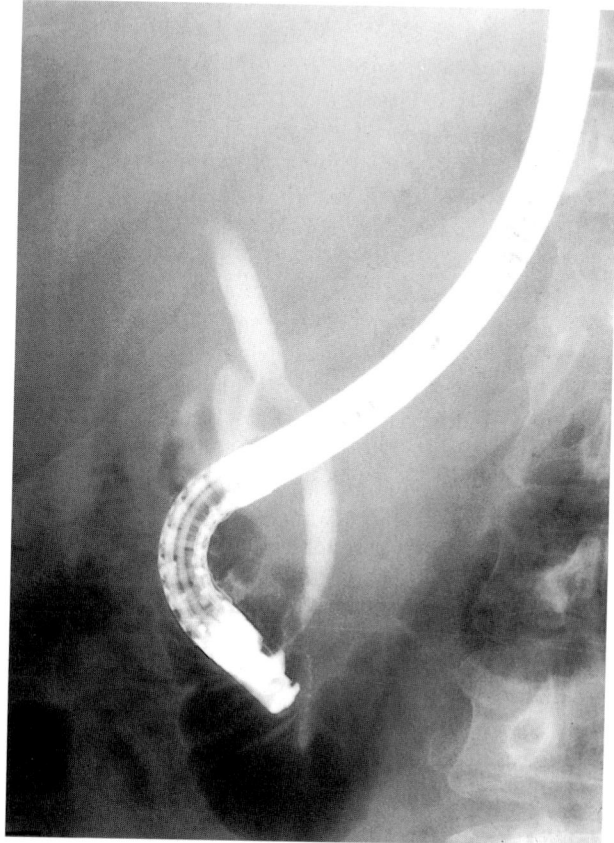

(b)

Fig. 29.11. ERCP showing: (a) dilated bile duct above a stricture. The pancreatic duct comes to an abrupt halt in the head of the pancreas. Appearances are of carcinoma of the pancreas; (b) common bile duct filling as far as a hilar stricture due to a cholangiocarcinoma.

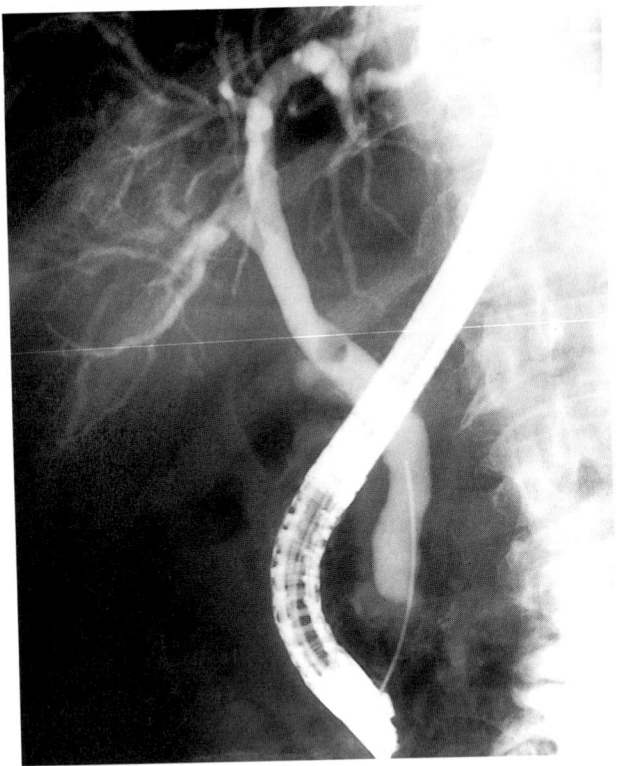

Fig. 29.12. ERCP showing common bile duct stone. A sphincterotome has been passed into the lower end of the bile duct.

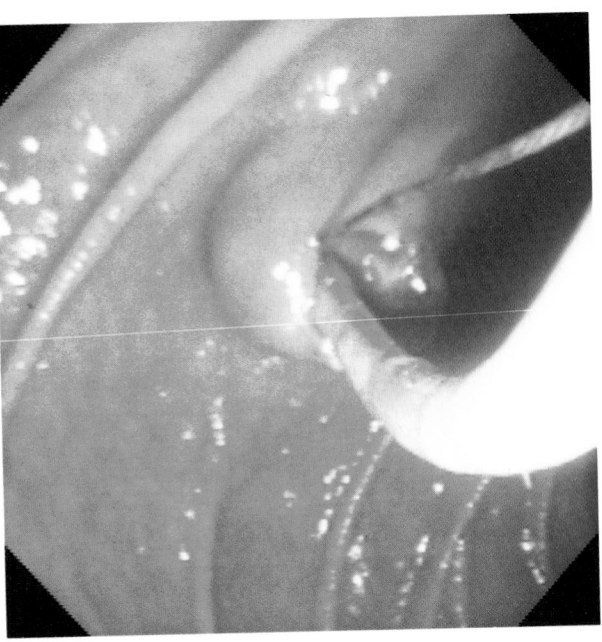

Fig. 29.13. Sphincterotome inserted into ampulla of Vater. The wire has been bowed and the sphincterotomy cut has begun.

roscopy is used to establish that this has entered the bile duct. The sphincterotome is then withdrawn leaving approximately 1 cm of the wire within the ampulla, the wire is bowed and, under direct vision, a cut is made using a blend or cutting current from the cautery unit (fig. 29.13). The length of cut depends upon the anatomy of the ampulla and the supra-ampullary area, and the size of the stone. If sphincterotomy is being done as a preliminary to endoprosthesis insertion only a small cut is needed. For stone removal, the aim is to cut through the biliary sphincter, shown by the release of bile. Air refluxes up the bile duct.

The success rate is above 90% [30] reaching 97% in an expert unit [70]. Causes of failure include a large peri-ampullary diverticulum, a Billroth II partial gastrectomy and an impacted stone at the ampulla.

Related techniques which may be helpful include needle knife papillotomy [21] but this should only be used by experienced endoscopists.

Complications [22, 68]

These occur in about 10% and include haemorrhage, cholangitis, pancreatitis, duodenal perforation, Dormia basket impaction and Gram-negative shock. They are life threatening in 2–3%. Mortality is 0.4–0.6%.

Bleeding, usually from the retro-duodenal artery, is the most serious potential problem. It usually settles but, if not, surgery can be difficult. Successful treatment by arterial embolization has been reported [58].

Cholangitis occurs if biliary decompression (stone removal) is unsuccessful. Prevention is by insertion of a nasobiliary tube or endoprosthesis.

Late results show that two-thirds of patients have air in the biliary tract and free reflux of duodenal juice. Bacterial colonization of the bile is present whether or not there are symptoms; the significance of this is unknown. Late complications (5–10% over 5 years) include sphincter stenosis and recurrent stones. The long-term effects of loss of sphincter function are unresolved.

Indications

Choledocholithiasis is the commonest indication. Emergency ERCP with endoscopic sphincterotomy is the treatment of choice for patients with *acute suppurative obstructive cholangitis* [38] which is almost always caused by a stone. Where there is *acute cholangitis* of lesser severity elective ERCP is done after a period of antibiotic treatment. Whether or not the gallbladder is in place, sphincterotomy is the treatment of choice.

In patients with *common duct stones without cholangitis* the choice depends on the clinical situation. For *post-cholecystectomy retained bile duct stones* sphincterotomy is clearly the best treatment in elderly frail patients and those with other medical problems. In this group of patients it is also the accepted treatment even when the gallbladder is still *in situ*. After removal of the common duct stone(s), the gallbladder need not be removed, long-term studies showing subsequent cholecystectomy to be required in less than 20% followed for up to 10 years [19].

In younger, fit patients with retained stones after cholecystectomy, sphincterotomy is preferred to surgical bile duct exploration. With the gallbladder in place, however, it is not clear whether cholecystectomy should be preceded by endoscopic sphincterotomy or accompanied by duct exploration and stone removal at the time of surgery.

The evolution of laparoscopic cholecystectomy and duct exploration adds to the therapeutic choice.

Acute gallstone pancreatitis, particularly if severe and non-resolving, is an indication for emergency ERCP and sphincterotomy if a stone is found (Chapter 31).

Stone extraction is done with wire baskets or balloon catheters (fig. 29.14a,b). In 90% the common bile duct is successfully cleared of stones. If all the stones cannot be extracted from a patient with cholangitis a naso-biliary catheter or endoprosthesis must be left to drain the duct (fig. 29.14c). Stones larger than 15 mm may be difficult to extract. Mechanical lithotripsy may be used to crush stones with success in 92% of patients [60]. Alternatively an endoprosthesis may be inserted [47]. This prevents the stone obstructing the bile duct, and is a quicker procedure than lithotripsy. Endoprosthesis insertion may be temporary until another attempt at stone removal, or used for long-term drainage. Administration of oral ursodeoxycholic acid while the endoprosthesis is in place appears to make later clearance of stones from the duct more successful [33]. With the availability of these techniques, there is little place for intra-biliary infusion of solvents such as methyl-tert-butyl ether [34].

Extracorporeal shock wave lithotripsy of common bile duct stones fragments them and allows them to pass through the sphincterotomy [59]. Laser lithotripsy is also being developed.

Sphincterotomy is often done before *endoscopic endoprosthesis* insertion. This was originally recommended to reduce the risk of pancreatic duct obstruction and pancreatitis, but carries the risk of bleeding and is not essential.

Sphincterotomy at the main papilla may be used to treat the rare *sump syndrome* following choledochoduodenostomy. *Papillary stenosis* (see Chapter 31) can also be treated by sphincterotomy.

Stone removal without sphincterotomy

Small stones (<8 mm) may be removed through an intact ampulla, with or without balloon dilatation [48]. Larger stones have been removed using the combination of mechanical lithotripsy and balloon dilatation of the sphincter of Oddi [43]. Pancreatitis is a complication in about 4%. Trials of these techniques versus sphincterotomy are awaited.

Naso-biliary drainage

A sphincterotomy is not usually necessary. After ERCP, the common bile duct is cannulated and a guide wire passed deep into an intra-hepatic duct. The cannula is

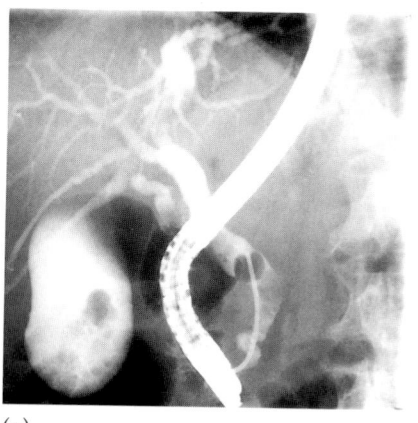

(a)

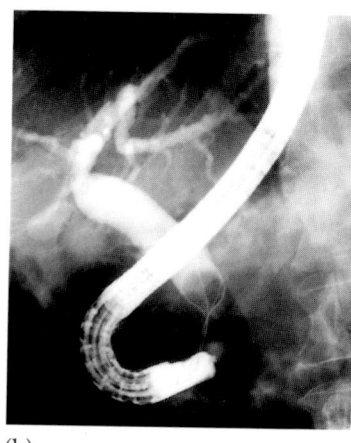

(b)

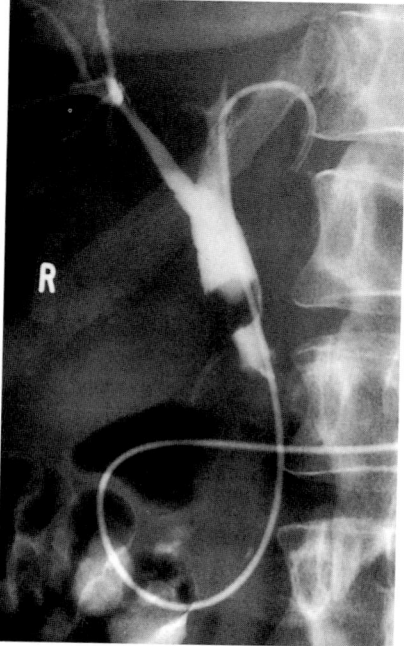

(c)

Fig. 29.14. (a) ERCP showing trawling of bile duct with balloon catheter to remove stones. (b) Removal of duct stone with basket. (c) Naso-biliary tube with stones in the common bile duct.

removed and a 300 cm 5 French (F) pigtail catheter with multiple side holes is threaded over the wire which is then removed (fig. 29.14c). The catheter is rerouted through the nose. This technique allows decompression of the biliary tree.

There are fewer complications than with percutaneous biliary drainage in terms of infection, bile leak and bleeding.

Naso-biliary drainage can be used as a preliminary to later sphincterotomy in poor risk patients with choledocholithiasis and acute suppurative cholangitis especially if coagulation is abnormal.

A naso-biliary drain may be left in position when, after sphincterotomy, it has been impossible to clear all the stones from the common bile duct. Later cholangiography through the tube shows whether the stones have passed. The naso-biliary drain also allows perfusion of the common bile duct with gallstone solvents such as mono-octanoin and methyl-tert-butyl ether.

Endoscopic biliary endoprostheses

After catheterization of the ampulla and demonstration of the stricture by contrast, a guide wire is passed through the catheter and an attempt made to pass through the stricture. At the first session this is possible in 60–70% of patients. Using a combination of an inner tube and pushing tube, an endoprosthesis is railroaded into position across the stricture. A 3.3 mm diameter (10 F) tube requires an endoscope with a 4.2 mm channel and provides effective decompression (fig. 29.15). Barbs on the endoprosthesis prevent it passing all the way up into bile duct or down into duodenum. Two endoprostheses may be used if necessary, for example to left and right hepatic ducts when there is a hilar stricture. Overall success rate of endoprosthesis insertion is 85–90% in skilled hands [31].

Early complications include cholangitis and pancreatitis, and haemorrhage if sphincterotomy is done.

Late complications include cholangitis and recurrent jaundice due to blockage of the tube, which can easily be removed and replaced endoscopically. To reduce this complication, a mesh metal endoprosthesis has been developed which, after insertion in compressed form, expands when released to a diameter of up to 1 cm (fig. 29.16) [25].

Results and indications

Endoscopic plastic endoprostheses successfully decompress the bile duct and relieve symptoms in about 70–80% of patients. The method carries fewer complications than the percutaneous route [65], and has a lower morbidity and mortality than surgical palliative bypass in patients with peri-ampullary carcinoma [63]. Block-

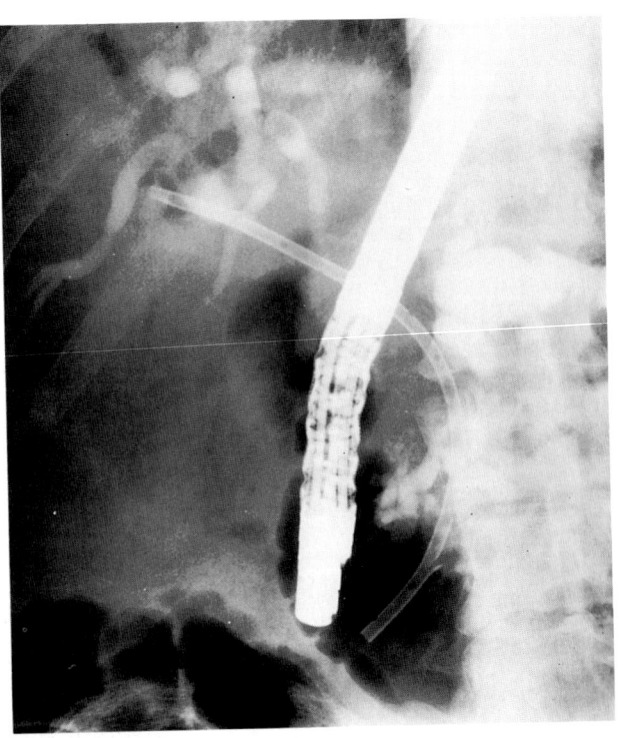

Fig. 29.15. ERCP: polyethylene stent inserted to relieve obstruction due to peri-ampullary tumour.

age of polyethylene endoprostheses occurs in 25–30% at 3–6 months. Antibiotic and ursodeoxycholic acid administration do not prevent this [24]. However, the patency of expandable metal mesh endoprostheses is significantly longer than plastic types (fig. 29.17) [15, 36], but the metal type is more expensive. Present experience suggests that a plastic type be placed first, and when it blocks, a metal endoprosthesis is inserted in those patients who are progressing more slowly and are expected to survive longer [52].

Inoperable malignant biliary obstruction from carcinoma of pancreas, ampulla and hilum can be relieved. For a malignant hilar obstruction, drainage of only one lobe provides good palliation. A second endoprosthesis is only needed if cholestasis is not relieved sufficiently or there is sepsis in the undrained side [55].

Benign strictures, whether due to primary sclerosing cholangitis or post-cholecystectomy, can be treated in this way, although balloon dilatation is an alternative. Surgery remains the first choice for the post-cholecystectomy stricture.

Failed endoscopic removal of common duct stones. A stent may be introduced into the common bile duct where it has been impossible to remove all stones and when the patient is unfit for surgery.

External biliary fistulas. Post-operative leaks from the cystic duct or injuries to the common bile duct may be treated by introduction of a biliary stent. The leak

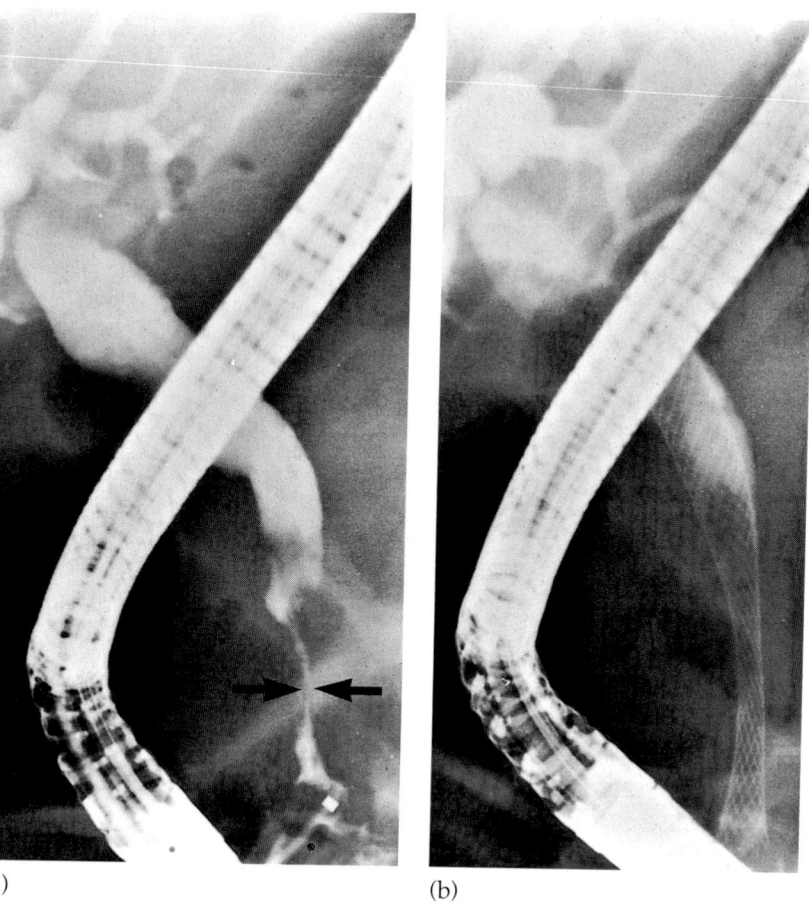

(a)

(b)

Fig. 29.16. (a) ERCP showing malignant stricture (arrows) at lower end of bile duct. (b) Mesh metal stent (Wallstent) placed across the stricture (courtesy of Dr Kees Huibregtse).

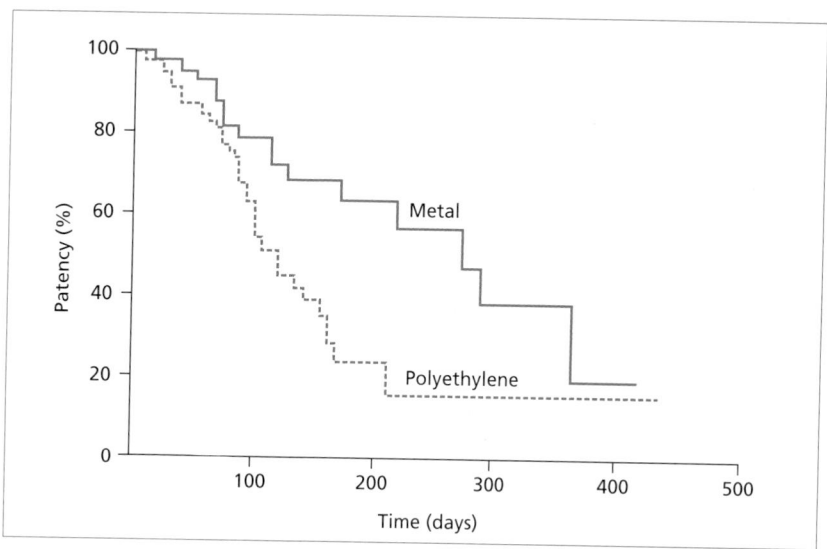

Fig. 29.17. Kaplan–Meier life table analysis of stent polyethylene: randomized trial of metal versus polythylene stent (reproduced with permission from [15]).

usually seals making re-operation unnecessary. The stent is removed after a few weeks [5].

Balloon dilatation

Following endoscopic cholangiography, a balloon catheter may be introduced into the common bile duct and inflated. This may be used for a benign stricture (fig.

29.18), whether traumatic or secondary to primary sclerosing cholangitis. It may be a useful preliminary step before insertion of an endoprosthesis [23].

Peroral cholangioscopy

The bile duct interior can be inspected using a 'baby' endoscope introduced via a large channel ('mother')

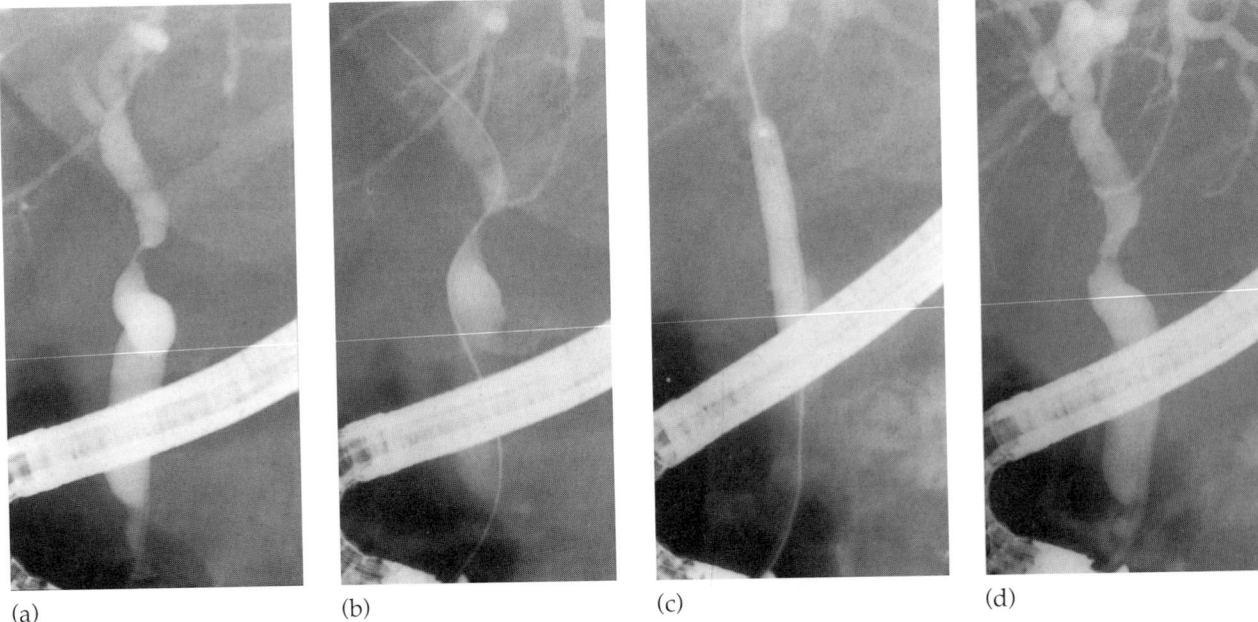

(a)   (b)   (c)   (d)

Fig. 29.18. Endoscopic balloon dilatation of bile duct stricture following liver transplantation. (a) Cholangiogram showing stricture. (b) Wire passed into intra-hepatic ducts. (c) Balloon dilatation to 8 mm diameter. (d) Final cholangiogram with good result.

duodenoscope. This may provide additional information [56], but the thin scopes are fragile, the system expensive, and the technique requires two endoscopists.

Percutaneous trans-hepatic cholangiography [73]

Contrast is injected percutaneously into a bile duct within the liver (fig. 29.19). The procedure is done in the radiology department with intravenous diazepam premedication and under local anaesthesia. Antibiotics are given 0.5–1 hour before the procedure. The 'skinny' Chiba needle is 0.7 mm (22 gauge) outside diameter. It is very flexible so that the patient is able to breathe normally with it *in situ*.

The needle is introduced in the seventh, eighth or ninth right intercostal space at the point of maximal dullness to percussion in the midaxillary line. Ultrasound guidance adds to the success [39]. It is advanced parallel to the table top to about 1 inch from the spine, bisecting a sagittal line between the dome of the diaphragm and the duodenal cap identified by its gas shadow. Contrast is injected continuously as the needle is withdrawn. Bile ducts are identified by the persistence of contrast in tube-like branching structures. Portal and hepatic veins are recognized by the peripheral direction of flow and rapid disappearance of contrast medium. Lymphatics can be filled and the contrast takes 5–10 minutes to be cleared.

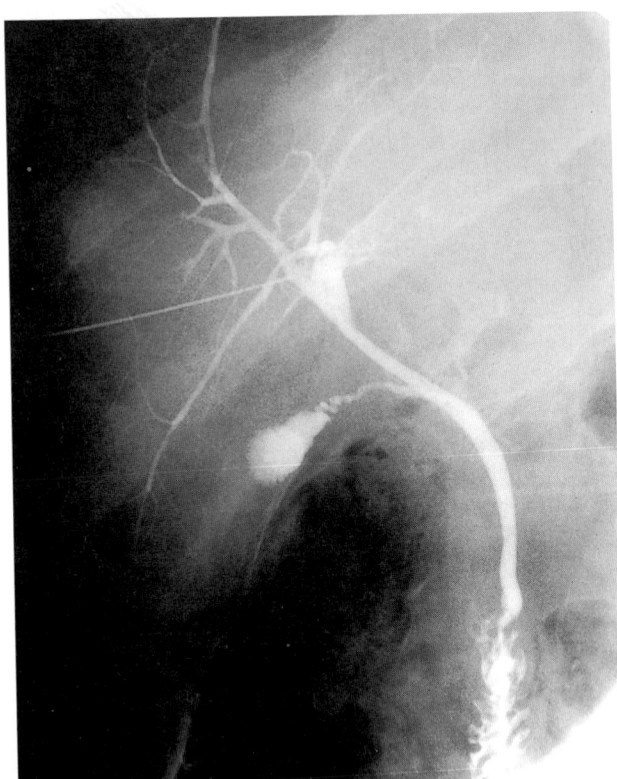

Fig. 29.19. Diagnostic percutaneous trans-hepatic cholangiogram showing normal right and left intra-hepatic ducts and common bile duct, and free flow of contrast into duodenum. The gallbladder is beginning to fill.

Up to six needle 'passes' are allowed before the procedure is abandoned.

After successful injection into obstructed and dilated ducts the patient may need to be tilted so that the common bile duct has an opportunity to fill. If hilar obstruction prevents communication between the right and left hepatic duct, a percutaneous cholangiogram from both sides should be done. The technique is relatively safe so that surgery need not inevitably follow immediately. If dilated ducts are encountered, they should be catheterized and external or internal biliary drainage established. Trans-hepatically aspirated bile should be cultured. The patient must be observed carefully in hospital.

The technique is easy and the success rate is 100% if intra-hepatic bile ducts are dilated. With undilated ducts, such as in primary sclerosing cholangitis or with some cases of choledocholithiasis, the success rate drops to 90% but can rise to 95% in specially skilled hands.

Complications

The complication rate is less than 5% and includes bleeding, bile peritonitis and septicaemia (usually Gram negative) in those with cholangitis or unsuspected bacteria in the bile [51].

Clinical indications

For the majority of patients percutaneous cholangiography is the *second choice* to show the biliary system, used only after ERCP has failed. This practice is based less on the relative complication rates of the two diagnostic procedures, and more on the greater therapeutic potential of ERCP, with a lower risk. Thus the endoscopic approach allows sphincterotomy for stones, and safer stent insertion. Percutaneous cholangiography comes into its own, however, when endoscopic access is difficult or impossible (*hepatico-enterostomy, Billroth II*). It is also important in the work-up of hilar cholangiocarcinoma, where detail of both right- and left-sided duct systems is needed. Brush cytology and biliary biopsy may be performed by the percutaneous as well as endoscopic route [66].

Percutaneous bile drainage

Bile duct catheterization

A sheathed needle is directed under antero-posterior and lateral fluoroscopy into a selected intra-hepatic duct already opacified by the 'skinny' needle cholangiogram. The needle is withdrawn and a guide wire passed through the sheath into common bile duct or peripheral intra-hepatic duct.

External biliary drainage

A drainage catheter is exchanged for the sheath over the guide wire, secured to skin and connected to a drainage bag. Theoretically, external bile drainage would be expected to bring the patient with biliary obstruction, particularly malignant, to surgery in better condition and so lessen the incidence of post-operative renal failure. There are, however, many complications including fluid and electrolyte loss, sepsis and dislodgement of the drainage tube [44]. Several randomized control trials have now shown that short-term (1–2 weeks) preoperative external bile drainage does not reduce the post-operative mortality and morbidity in patients having surgery for malignant bile duct obstruction [28, 44, 54]. Long-term external drainage should be avoided, having both physical and psychological side-effects. It is now rarely necessary, since either endoscopic or percutaneous stenting, or surgical bypass is possible.

Internal/external biliary drainage

After bile duct catheterization, a guide wire can usually be manipulated through the stricture and into low bile duct or bowel. A catheter (8–9 F) can then be placed across the stricture with side holes above and below. Bile can then drain into bowel, or, if the external limb is not spigotted, into an external bag. This technique is usually used as the first stage before endoprosthesis insertion a few days later. It is occasionally used in its own right for long-term relief of obstruction but commits the patient to a permanent external tube even if closed off.

Percutaneous biliary endoprosthesis

Following percutaneous cholangiography, bile duct catheterization and manipulation of a guide wire through the stricture, an endoprosthesis (10–14 F) is inserted over the guide wire across the stricture allowing free drainage of bile into bowel (fig. 29.20). Sometimes an external drain is left temporarily above the endoprosthesis for 24–48 hours to guarantee biliary decompression and to allow check cholangiography. The external tube is then removed. Endoprostheses made of polyethylene and other plastics have been used for many years [16, 17]. As with endoscopic stents, these also block with time. Metal stents have been developed including the metal wire zigzag (Gianturco) and metal mesh type (Wallstent) [25, 32]. The longer patency of mesh metal stents is based on endoscopic trials (see above).

Results and complications

Success rate for endoprosthesis insertion is 85%. Failures are due to inability to find the lumen of the stricture with the guide wire. Hilar strictures are more difficult than low common duct obstruction [17]. There is complete relief of bile duct obstruction in 65–70% of patients, a

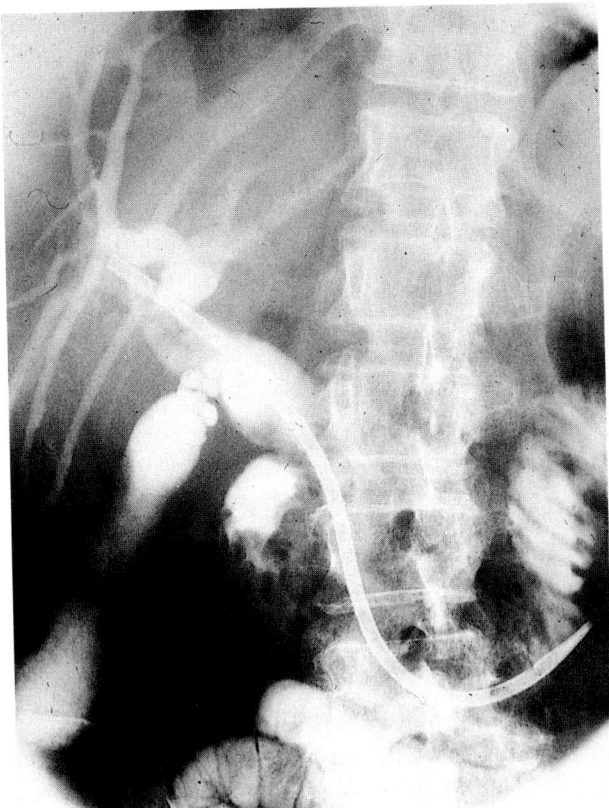

Fig. 29.20. Percutaneous trans-hepatic insertion of Carey–Coons stent.

further 15% having partial decompression. Major complications (haemorrhage and bile leakage with peritonitis) occur in 3% of patients. Deaths due to the procedure are reported rarely. Other early complications include septicaemia and pleural effusion. Late complications are stent blockage with cholangitis and recurrent jaundice, and passage of the stent out of the bile duct.

Indications

When endoscopic access to the biliary tree is possible, ERCP and endoscopic stent insertion is the first choice to relieve irresectable malignant biliary obstruction. When this fails or endoscopic access is impossible, percutaneous insertion is indicated. An alternative is a *combined approach* with percutaneous catheterization of the stricture, placement of the guide wire tip in the duodenum, and endoscopic retrograde insertion of the stent over the wire. This approach still carries an appreciable mortality and morbidity [18]. Since percutaneous metal mesh stents can be inserted on a 7F catheter, this technique may replace the more complicated combined approach [46].

Re-stenosis of hepatico-enteric anastomoses may be treated by percutaneous stenting or balloon dilatation if surgical revision is not appropriate.

Percutaneous balloon dilatation

Benign strictures of the bile duct have been successfully treated by percutaneous trans-hepatic balloon dilatation [12] (see Chapter 32).

Resectability of tumours

Pancreatic carcinomas and hilar cholangiocarcinomas are rarely resectable, but this possibility should be assessed particularly in the middle-aged and younger patient.

For pancreatic carcinoma, US and CT are capable of predicting irresectability with a high degree of accuracy [7] based on hepatic metastases, local extension, vascular encasement or invasion, and lymphadenopathy (Chapter 33), but both depend on good technique and experience. Laparoscopy may show hepatic metastases or peritoneal seedlings. Each unit will have its preferred approach. Angiography is worth while but may not provide extra information on resectability. It gives a road map which some surgeons value greatly.

For cholangiocarcinoma, many imaging techniques have a place in the assessment of resectability, including cholangiography, US, CT, hepatic arteriography and portography (see Chapter 34).

With ampullary carcinomas, the treatment is surgical resection if there is no medical contraindication.

Choice between surgical and non-surgical palliation of malignant obstruction

Randomized control trials have shown that percutaneous stenting has a similar outcome to bypass surgery [8]. Endoscopic insertion has a lower morbidity and mortality than either the percutaneous route [65] or palliative bypass surgery [63]. The disadvantage of plastic stents is that they block, but many patients die from their malignant disease before this problem occurs.

Less well-defined clinical features influence choice of therapy and in general it is the older, poorer risk patient who receives the non-surgical endoprosthesis and the younger, fitter patient who may still have surgery, especially if a tissue diagnosis has not been made. Exfoliative bile cytology, brush cytology and percutaneous aspiration cytology should be done in an attempt to establish a tissue diagnosis.

Choice between endoscopic and percutaneous approach (table 29.1)

Using ERCP or PTC the biliary tree can be visualized in virtually every patient in whom mechanical cholestasis has to be excluded. Any large hospital should have both

Table 29.1. Comparison of percutaneous trans-hepatic cholangiography (PTC) and endoscopic retrograde cholangiopancreatography (ERCP)

	PTC	ERCP
Technique	Easy	Difficult
Time taken (minutes)	15–30	15–60
Anatomical difficulties	Few	Many
Cost	Low	High
Complications (%)	5	5
	Biliary leak	Pancreatitis
	Cholangitis	Cholangitis
	Haemorrhage	
Success (%)		
Overall	95	80–90
Dilated ducts	100	85
Undilated ducts	90	85
Pancreatic duct	–	85
Endoprosthesis insertion (%)		
Overall	85	80
High stricture	70	80
Low stricture	90	80

techniques available and a surgeon should always have a cholangiogram in front of him when exploring the biliary tract. ERCP is the first choice. PTC is used after failed ERCP or when the ampulla is inaccessible. Both techniques may be necessary, for example when ERCP has shown a hilar stricture but the intra-hepatic ducts have not filled. PTC is indicated, left and right sided if necessary, to show the anatomy. The techniques are complementary rather than competitive. Intervention by both routes is now used widely. ERCP offers sphincterotomy and is the safer method for duct drainage.

Percutaneous cholecystostomy

The gallbladder is punctured percutaneously under real-time ultrasound or fluoroscopic control, and drained. This technique has been used successfully as an emergency for high-risk patients with acute calculous and acalculous cholecystitis [72]. Access is either direct across the peritoneal cavity or trans-hepatic. The latter is generally safer since the point of gallbladder puncture is sealed by adjacent liver. The transperitoneal route is preferred if gallstones are to be removed [11]. The trans-hepatic approach is best for drainage of empyema and instillation of solvents for stone dissolution (Chapter 31).

Operative and post-operative cholangiography

Routine operative cholangiography is not necessary at cholecystectomy unless there are indications suggesting

that stones are present in the common bile duct [4]. These include a history of jaundice, dilated bile ducts, palpable gallstones or a raised serum bilirubin, alkaline phosphatase or gamma GT level. After exploration of the common bile duct, cholangiography should always be performed using high kVp technique and full strength contrast [67].

Debris may cause filling defects less sharply defined than those caused by gallstones. Air bubbles may simulate stones. Small stones may be obliterated by the contrast medium.

During laparoscopic cholecystectomy, laparoscopic ultrasound successfully detects duct stones [57] and may obviate the need for intra-operative cholangiography.

Post-operative cholangiography, using contrast injected gently, should be undertaken routinely before final removal of a T-tube draining the biliary tree. During the injection, bile duct contents, including bacteria, probably regurgitate into the blood. This is particularly marked in the presence of biliary obstruction.

A surprising number of operative and post-operative cholangiograms are technically unsatisfactory, through failure to visualize intra-hepatic bile ducts or the trans-duodenal or sphincteric segment of the ducts. It is essential not to use too dense contrast to fill the biliary tree and to ensure correct positioning and exposure.

T-tube extraction of gallstones

See Chapter 31.

References

1 Allen JI, Allen MO, Olson MM *et al.* Pseudomonas infection of the biliary system resulting from the use of a contaminated endoscope. *Gastroenterology* 1987; **92**: 759.

2 Amouyal P, Amouyal G, Lévy P *et al.* Diagnosis of choledocholithiasis by endoscopic ultrasonography. *Gastroenterology* 1994; **106**: 1062.

3 Barish MA, Yucel EK, Soto JA *et al.* MR cholangiopancreatography: efficacy of three-dimensional turbo spin–echo technique. *Am. J. Roentgenol.* 1995; **165**: 295.

4 Barkun AN, Barkun JS, Fried GM *et al.* Useful predictors of bile duct stones in patients undergoing laparoscopic cholecystectomy. *Ann. Surg.* 1994; **220**: 32.

5 Bergman JJGHM, van den Brink GR, Rauws EAJ *et al.* Treatment of bile duct lesions after laparoscopic cholecystectomy. *Gut* 1996; **38**: 141.

6 Beuers U, Spengler U, Sackmann M *et al.* Deterioration of cholestasis after endoscopic retrograde cholangiography in advanced primary sclerosing cholangitis. *J. Hepatol.* 1992; **15**: 140.

7 Bluemke DA, Cameron JL, Hruban RH *et al.* Potentially resectable pancreatic adenocarcinoma: spiral CT assessment with surgical and pathologic correlation. *Radiology* 1995; **197**: 381.

8 Bornman PC, Tobias R, Harries-Jones EP *et al.* Prospective controlled trial of transhepatic biliary endoprosthesis

versus bypass surgery for incurable carcinoma of head of pancreas. *Lancet* 1986; **i**: 69.

9 Byl B, Devière J, Struelens MJ *et al.* Antibiotic prophylaxis for infectious complications after therapeutic endoscopic retrograde cholangiopancreatography: a randomized, double-blind, placebo-controlled study. *Clin. Infect. Dis.* 1995; **20**: 1236.

10 Carroll BA. Preferred imaging techniques for the diagnosis of cholecystitis and cholelithiasis. *Ann. Surg.* 1989; **210**: 1.

11 Chiverton SG, Inglis JA, Hudd C *et al.* Percutaneous cholecystolithotomy: the first 60 patients. *Br. Med. J.* 1990; **300**: 1310.

12 Citron SJ, Martin LG. Benign biliary strictures: treatment with percutaneous cholangioplasty. *Radiology* 1991; **178**: 339.

13 Cornwell EE, Rodriguez A, Mirvis SE *et al.* Acute acalculous cholecystitis in critically injured patients. *Ann. Surg.* 1989; **210**: 52.

14 Cotton PB, Williams CB. *Practical Gastrointestinal Endoscopy*, 4th edn. Blackwell Science, Oxford, 1996.

15 Davids PHP, Groen AK, Rauws EAJ *et al.* Randomised trial of self-expanding metal stents versus polyethylene stents for distal malignant biliary obstruction. *Lancet* 1992; **340**: 1488.

16 Dick R, Platts A, Gilford J. The Carey-Coons percutaneous biliary endoprosthesis: a three centre experience in 87 patients. *Clin. Radiol.* 1987; **38**: 175.

17 Dooley JS, Dick R, George P *et al.* Percutaneous transhepatic endoprosthesis for bile duct obstruction: complications and results. *Gastroenterology* 1984; **86**: 905.

18 Dowsett JF, Vaira D, Hatfield ARW *et al.* Endoscopic biliary therapy using the combined percutaneous and endoscopic technique. *Gastroenterology* 1989; **96**: 1180.

19 Dowsett JF, Vaira D, Polydorou A *et al.* Intervention endoscopy in the pancreatobiliary tree. *Am. J. Gastroenterol.* 1988; **83**: 1328.

20 Flancbaum L, Alden SM, Trooskin SZ. Use of cholescintigraphy with morphine in critically ill patients with suspected cholecystitis. *Surgery* 1989; **106**: 668.

21 Foutch PG. A prospective assessment of results for needle-knife papillotomy and standard endoscopic sphincterotomy. *Gastrointest. Endosc.* 1995; **41**: 25.

22 Freeman ML, Nelson DB, Sherman S *et al.* Complications of endoscopic biliary sphincterotomy. *N. Engl. J. Med.* 1996; **335**: 909.

23 Geenen DJ, Geenen JE, Hoagen WJ *et al.* Endoscopic therapy for benign bile duct strictures. *Gastrointest. Endosc.* 1989; **35**: 367.

24 Ghosh S, Palmer KR. Prevention of biliary stent occlusion using cyclical antibiotics and ursodeoxycholic acid. *Gut* 1994; **35**: 1757.

25 Gillams A, Dick R, Dooley JS *et al.* Self-expandable stainless steel braided endoprosthesis for biliary strictures. *Radiology* 1990; **174**: 137.

26 Gillams A, Dick R, Rubin G *et al.* The false security of aerobilia. *Gut* 1989; **30**: A1460.

27 Guibaud L, Bret PM, Reinhold C *et al.* Bile duct obstruction and cholelithiasis: diagnosis with MR cholangiography. *Radiology* 1995; **197**: 109.

28 Hatfield ARW, Terblanche J, Fataar S *et al.* Pre-operative external biliary drainage in obstructive jaundice: a prospective controlled clinical trial. *Lancet* 1982; **ii**: 896.

29 Health and Policy Committee, American College of Physicians. How to study the gallbladder. *Ann. Intern. Med.* 1988; **109**: 752.

30 Horton RC, Lauri A, Dooley JS. Endoscopic removal of common duct stones: current indications and controversies. *Postgrad. Med. J.* 1991; **67**: 107.

31 Huibregtse K. *Endoscopic Biliary and Pancreatic Drainage*. George Thieme Verlag, Stuttgart, New York, 1988.

32 Irving JD, Adam A, Dick R *et al.* Gianturco expandable metallic biliary stents: results of a European clinical trial. *Radiology* 1989; **172**: 321.

33 Johnson GK, Geenen JE, Venu RP *et al.* Treatment of non-extractable common bile duct stones with combination ursodeoxycholic acid plus endoprostheses. *Gastrointest. Endosc.* 1993; **39**: 528.

34 Kaye GL, Summerfield JA, McIntyre N *et al.* Methyl tert butyl ether dissolution therapy for common duct stones. *J. Hepatol.* 1990; **10**: 337.

35 Kelly SM, Page J, Kennedy HJ. ERCP as a daycase procedure —safe, and well tolerated. *Gut* 1995; **37** (Suppl. 2): A11.

36 Knyrim K, Wagner HJ, Pausch J *et al.* A prospective, randomized, controlled trial of metal stents for malignant obstruction of the common bile duct. *Endoscopy* 1993; **25**: 207.

37 Kurzawinski TR, Deery A, Dooley JS *et al.* A prospective study of biliary cytology in 100 patients with bile duct strictures. *Hepatology* 1993; **18**: 1399.

38 Lai ECS, Mok FPT, Tan ESY *et al.* Endoscopic biliary drainage for severe acute cholangitis. *N. Engl. J. Med.* 1992; **326**: 1582.

39 Lameris JS, Obertop H, Jeekel J. Biliary drainage by ultrasound-guided puncture of the left hepatic duct. *Clin. Radiol.* 1985; **36**: 269.

40 Lehman GA. Contrast media in ERCP. *Gastrointest. Endosc.* 1988; **34**: 295.

41 Lieberman DA, Krishnamurthy GT. Intrahepatic versus extrahepatic cholestasis. Discrimination with biliary scintigraphy combined with ultrasound. *Gastroenterology* 1986; **90**: 734.

42 Macaulay SE, Schulte SJ, Sekijima JH. Evaluation of a non-breath-hold MR cholangiography technique. *Radiology* 1995; **196**: 227.

43 Macmathuna P, White P, Lennon J *et al.* Endoscopic sphincteroplasty: a novel and safe alternative to papillotomy in the management of bile duct stones. *Gut* 1994; **35**: 127.

44 McPherson GAD, Benjamin IS, Hodgson HJF *et al.* Pre-operative percutaneous transhepatic biliary drainage: the results of a controlled trial. *Br. J. Surg.* 1984; **71**: 371.

45 Maglinte DDT, Torres WE, Laufer I. Oral cholecystography in contemporary gallstone imaging: a review. *Radiology* 1991; **178**: 49.

46 Martin DF. Combined percutaneous and endoscopic procedures for bile duct obstruction. *Gut* 1994; **35**: 1011.

47 Maxton DG, Tweedle DEF, Martin DF. Retained common bile duct stones after endoscopic sphincterotomy: temporary and long-term treatment with biliary stenting. *Gut* 1995; **36**: 446.

48 May GR, Cotton PB, Edmunds SEJ *et al.* Removal of stones from the bile duct at ERCP without sphincterotomy. *Gastrointest. Endosc.* 1993; **39**: 749.

49 Mehal WZ, Culshaw KD, Tillotson GS *et al.* Antibiotic prophylaxis for ERCP: a randomised clinical trial comparing ciprofloxacin and cefuroxime in 200 patients at high risk of cholangitis. *Eur. J. Gastroenterol. Hepatol.* 1995; **7**: 841.

50 Moreira VF, Meroño E, Larraona JL *et al.* ERCP and allergic reactions to iodized contrast media. *Gastrointest. Endosc.* 1985; **31**: 293.

51 Mueller PR, Van Sonnenberg E, Simeone JF. Fine needle transhepatic cholangiography. Indications and usefulness. *Ann. Intern. Med.* 1982; **97**; 567.

52 O'Brien S, Hatfield ARW, Craig PI *et al.* A three-year follow-up of self-expanding metal stents in the endoscopic palliation of long-term survivors with malignant biliary obstruction. *Gut* 1995; **36**: 618.

53 Patel JC, McInnes GC, Bagley JS *et al.* The role of intravenous cholangiography in pre-operative assessment for laparoscopic cholecystectomy. *Br. J. Radiol.* 1993; **66**: 1125.

54 Pitt HA, Gomes AS, Lois JF *et al.* Does preoperative percutaneous biliary drainage reduce operative risk or increase hospital cost? *Ann. Surg.* 1985; **201**: 545.

55 Polydorou AA, Cairns SR, Dowsett JF *et al.* Palliation of proximal malignant biliary obstruction by endoscopic endoprosthesis insertion. *Gut* 1991; **32**: 685.

56 Riemann JF, Kohler B, Harloff M *et al.* Peroral cholangioscopy—an improved method in the diagnosis of common bile duct disease. *Gastrointest. Endosc.* 1989; **35**: 435.

57 Röthlin MA, Schlumpf R, Largiadèr F. Laparoscopic sonography. An alternative to routine intraoperative cholangiography? *Arch. Surg.* 1994; **129**: 694.

58 Saeed M, Kadir S, Kaufman SL *et al.* Bleeding following endoscopic sphincterotomy: angiographic management by transcatheterisation embolization. *Gastrointest. Endosc.* 1989; **35**: 300.

59 Sauerbruch T, Holl J, Sackmann M *et al.* Fragmentation of bile duct stones by extracorporeal shock-wave lithotripsy: a five-year experience. *Hepatology* 1992; **15**: 208.

60 Shaw MJ, Mackie RD, Moore JP *et al.* Results of a multicentre trial using a mechanical lithotripter for the treatment of large bile duct stones. *Am. J. Gastroenterol.* 1993; **88**: 730.

61 Shorvon PJ, Eykyn SJ, Cotton PB. Progress report: gastrointestinal instrumentation, bacteraemia, and endocarditis. *Gut* 1983; **24**: 1078.

62 Siegel JH. *Endoscopic Retrograde Cholangio-pancreatography. Technique, Diagnosis and Therapy.* Raven Press, New York 1992.

63 Smith AC, Dowsett JF, Russell RCG *et al.* Randomised trial of endoscopic stenting versus surgical bypass in malignant low bileduct obstruction. *Lancet* 1994; **344**: 1655.

64 Soto JA, Barish MA, Yucel EK *et al.* Magnetic resonance cholangiography: comparison with endoscopic retrograde cholangiopancreatography. *Gastroenterology* 1996; **110**: 589.

65 Speer AG, Cotton PB, Russell RCG *et al.* Randomised trial of endoscopic versus percutaneous stent insertion in malignant obstructive jaundice. *Lancet* 1987; **ii**: 57.

66 Terasaki K, Wittich GR, Lycke G *et al.* Percutaneous transluminal biopsy of biliary strictures with a bioptome. *Am. J. Roentgenol.* 1991; **156**: 77.

67 Thompson WM, Halvorsen RA, Foster WL *et al.* Optimal cholangiographic technique for detecting bile duct stones. *Am. J. Roentgenol.* 1986; **146**: 537.

68 Thornton J, Axon A. Towards safer endoscopic retrograde cholangiopancreatography. *Gut* 1993; **34**: 721.

69 Turner MA. Diagnostic methods and pitfalls in the gallbladder. *Semin. Roentgenol.* 1991; **26**: 197.

70 Vaira D, Ainley C, Williams S *et al.* Endoscopic sphincterotomy in 1000 consecutive patients. *Lancet* 1989; **ii**: 431.

71 Van Beers BE, Lacrosse M, Trigaux M *et al.* Non-invasive imaging of the biliary tree before or after laparoscopic cholecystectomy: use of three-dimensional spiral CT cholangiography. *Am. J. Roentgenol.* 1994; **162**: 1331.

72 Verbanck JJ, Demol JW, Ghillebert GL *et al.* Ultrasound-guided puncture of the gallbladder for acute cholecystitis. *Lancet* 1993; **341**: 1132.

73 Wilkinson M, Adam A. Hepatobiliary intervention. In: Watkinson A, Adam A (eds). *Interventional Radiology: A Practical Guide.* Radcliffe Medical Press, Oxford. 1996; 59.

74 Yap L, Wycherley AG, Morphett AD *et al.* Acalculous biliary pain: cholecystectomy allieviates symptoms in patients with abnormal cholescintigraphy. *Gastroenterology* 1991; **101**: 786.

75 Zeman RK, Silverman PM, Cooper C *et al.* Helical (spiral) computed tomography: implications for imaging of the abdomen. *Gastroenterol. Clin. North Am.* 1995; **24**: 183.

76 Zeman RK, Berman PM, Silverman PM *et al.* Biliary tract: three-dimensional helical CT without cholangiographic contrast material. *Radiology* 1995; **196**: 865.

77 Ziessman HA, Fahey FH, Hixson DJ. Calculation of a gallbladder ejection fraction: advantage of continuous sincalide infusion over the three-minute infusion method. *J. Nucl. Med.* 1992; **33**: 537.

Chapter 30
Cysts and Congenital Biliary Abnormalities

Fibropolycystic disease

Cystic lesions of the liver and bile ducts are increasingly being diagnosed. This can be related to the improved methods of imaging the liver and bile ducts and of liver biopsy. Application of such methods makes it clear that the fibropolycystic diseases do not exist as single entities, but as members of a family [43]. The members are found in various combinations (fig. 30.1). They consist of polycystic liver disease, microhamartoma, congenital hepatic fibrosis, congenital intra-hepatic biliary dilatation (Caroli's disease) and choledochal cysts (fig. 30.2). Clinically, fibropolycystic diseases have three effects, again present in different proportions: those of a space-occupying lesion, of portal hypertension and of cholangitis. They are usually inherited. Fibrocystic disease of the kidneys is associated to a variable extent. Embryologically the hepato-biliary abnormalities are thought

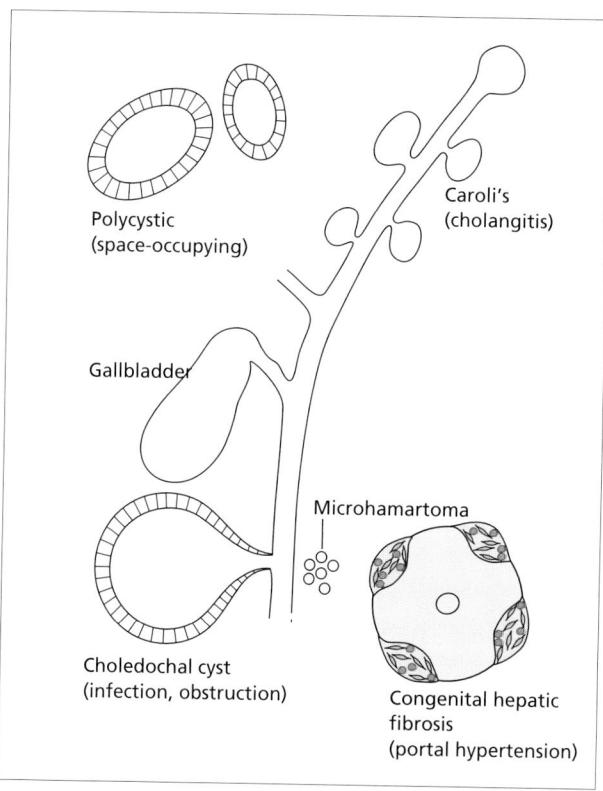

Fig. 30.2. Fibropolycystic disease: spectrum of pathology.

to stem from ductal plate maldevelopment in different parts of the biliary tree [11].

Malignant change may complicate congenital hepatic fibrosis, bile duct cysts and Caroli's syndrome [4, 39].

Childhood fibropolycystic diseases

These are recessively inherited and may be perinatal, neonatal or infantile (table 30.1). Prognosis depends on the extent of renal involvement. Morphometry shows that the neonatal and infantile forms represent one disorder [25]. In individual patients the relative renal and hepatic manifestations may change with time. Choledochal cysts may coexist.

The importance of the renal relative to the hepatic problem varies from patient to patient.

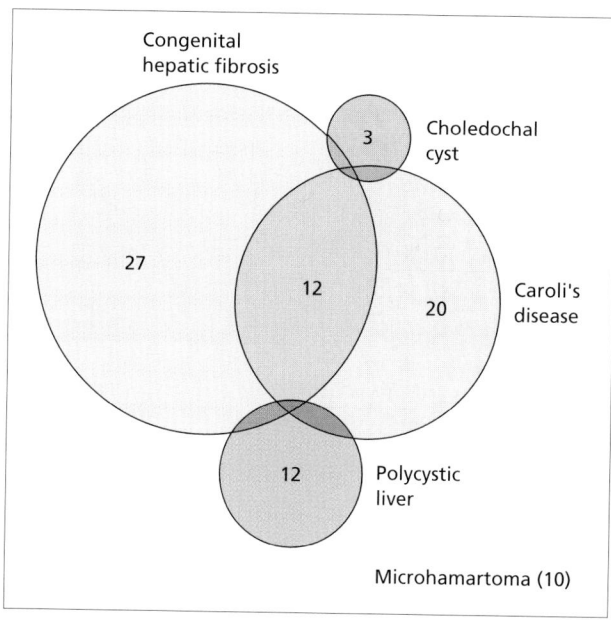

Fig. 30.1. Venn diagram showing one series of 51 patients in which many had more than one fibropolycystic disease. The combination of congenital hepatic fibrosis and Caroli's disease was most striking. Microhamartomas, although reported in only 10 patients in this series, are common [43].

Table 30.1. Hepatic fibropolycystic disease

Subtype	Inheritance	Presentation	Hepatic	Portal hypertension	Renal*
Childhood fibropolycystic					
Perinatal	Recessive	Birth	Fibrosis ± Ducts dilated +	—	90%
Neonatal	Recessive	1 month	Fibrosis ++ Ducts dilated +	—	60%
Infantile	Recessive	3–6 months	Fibrosis ++ Ducts dilated +	Common	25%
Congenital hepatic fibrosis	Recessive	Child or adult	Fibrosis +++ Ducts dilated +	Usual	0–10%
Adult polycystic	Dominant	Adult	Cysts	Rare	Cysts
Intra-hepatic biliary dilatation (Caroli's)	See text	Cholangitis any age	Dilated ducts only	—	—

* Percentage of tubules with cystic change.

Adult polycystic disease

The liver cysts are probably developmental and similar to and frequently associated with autosomal dominant polycystic kidneys. Isolated polycystic liver disease also inherited as autosomal dominant but without renal cysts is reported [34].

The cysts may arise from defective development of the intra-hepatic bile ducts in the portal tracts. This may occur at about the 23 mm stage of fetal life, when the original segment of blind bile ducts is being replaced by a second generation of highly active, proliferating bile ducts. The original group may become distorted and degenerate into cysts. These, frequently localized, cystic areas are accompanied by normal second-generation bile ducts elsewhere, so there is no biliary dysfunction.

Pathology

Depending on the number and size of the cysts, the liver may be normal or greatly enlarged. Cysts may be scattered diffusely or restricted to one lobe, usually the left. The outer surface may be considerably deformed. A cyst may vary in size from a pin's head to a child's head, the largest having a capacity of over a litre. They are rarely greater than 10 cm in diameter. The larger ones are probably formed by rupture of septa between adjacent cysts, and the cut liver may display a honeycomb appearance. The cavities are thin walled and contain clear or brown fluid due to altered blood. They never contain bile because they are not in continuity with the biliary tract. They may be complicated by haemorrhage or infection.

Histologically (fig. 30.3) the lobular architecture is unchanged and the liver cells are normal. The cystic areas are related to the bile ducts and to biliary micro-hamartomas in the portal areas [36]. They are sur-

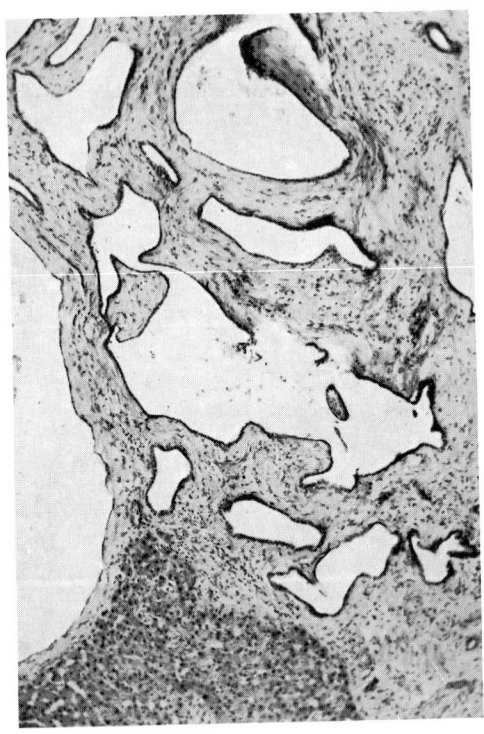

Fig. 30.3. Polycystic disease of the liver. The cysts vary in size and are lined by flattened epithelium. (H & E, ×63.)

rounded by a fibrous tissue capsule and lined by columnar or cuboidal epithelium.

Frequently, there is cystic disease of other organs, including kidneys, spleen, pancreas, ovary and lungs. About half the patients with polycystic disease of the liver have polycystic kidneys. The majority (50–88%) of patients with polycystic kidneys have a polycystic liver [18, 21]. The prevalence increases with age [18].

Cyst fluid

Fluid has been obtained using needle aspiration under ultrasound guidance [16]. The constituents and response to secretin support the concept that the cyst fluid is formed by functioning bile duct epithelium lining the cysts.

Clinical features

In many patients the liver lesion is diagnosed incidentally during scanning or at autopsy. Sometimes the patient presents with some other disease or with polycystic kidneys.

Patients with symptoms and signs are usually in the fourth or fifth decade. Cysts tend to be larger in women who have been pregnant [19]. The patient complains of abdominal distension and dull abdominal pain. Pressure on the stomach and duodenum causes epigastric discomfort, nausea, flatulence and occasional vomiting. Acute pain may be due to rupture of or haemorrhage into a cyst.

Ascites, obstructive jaundice [51] and hepatic venous outflow obstruction [48] are rare.

Symptoms are more often due to associated polycystic kidney disease.

On examination the liver may be impalpable or so large that it seems to fill the whole abdomen. The edge is firm and nodules can be palpated. There may be difficulty in distinguishing cysts from other types of liver nodule.

Bilaterally enlarged irregular *kidneys* may suggest associated renal cysts.

Hepatic function is excellent because the liver cells are preserved. Serum alkaline phosphatase and γ-GT may be increased but bilirubin is normal.

Portal venous obstruction is usually absent, but occasionally can result in oesophageal varices with bleeding. The spleen is not enlarged.

Imaging

Ultrasound is the most satisfactory method of diagnosis (fig. 30.4). CT scanning is also useful (fig. 30.5). The space-occupying lesion does not enhance with intravenous contrast.

Differential diagnosis

Polycystic liver should be suspected in an apparently well person, often over 30 years of age, with nodular hepatomegaly, but no evidence of hepatic dysfunction, associated with polycystic kidney or a family history of this condition.

The condition may be confused with *hydatid disease* (Chapter 27).

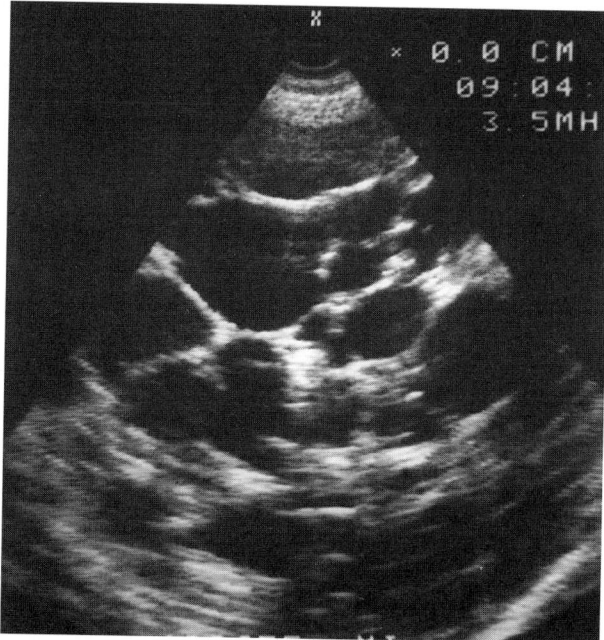

Fig. 30.4. Adult polycystic liver: ultrasound shows numerous echo-free space-occupying lesions.

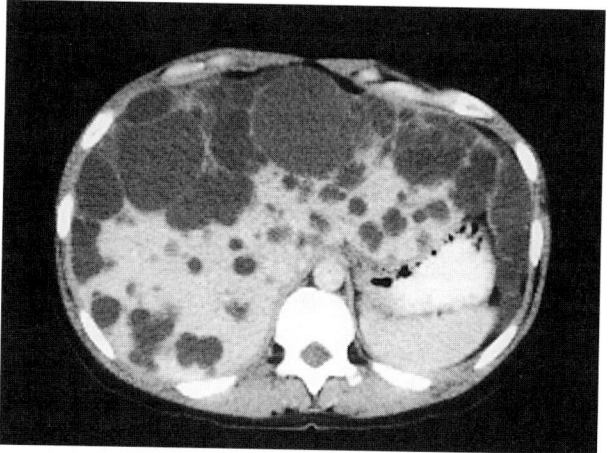

Fig. 30.5. CT scan (contrast enhanced) showing polycystic liver.

Metastases are accompanied by malaise, weight loss, rapid increase in size of the liver, and, possibly, evidence of a primary neoplasm.

Cirrhosis may be accompanied by signs of hepatocellular disease and the spleen is usually enlarged.

Prognosis and treatment

Polycystic disease of the liver is compatible with long life.

The prognosis is determined by the extent of associated renal cystic disease. Carcinoma is very rare. Surgery is rarely necessary and aspiration under ultrasound control is easy and effective in controlling acute symptoms. However, the fluid usually returns.

Large cysts, greater than 10 cm, may be excised if symptomatic and accessible. In patients incapacitated by massive liver enlargement, operative fenestration of cysts with or without hepatic resection produces symptomatic improvement in the majority [17, 35, 49]. Liver transplantation may be successful [42]. Both approaches carry a mortality.

Congenital hepatic fibrosis [23]

This condition consists, histologically, of broad, densely collagenous fibrous bands surrounding otherwise normal hepatic lobules (fig. 30.6) [23]. The bands contain large numbers of microscopic, well-formed bile ducts (fig. 30.7), some containing bile. Arterial branches are normal or hypoplastic, while the veins appear reduced in size. Inflammatory infiltration is not seen. Caroli's syndrome may be associated, also choledochal cyst.

The disease appears both sporadically and in a familial form. It is inherited as autosomal recessive. A ductal plate malformation of interlobular bile ducts has been suggested as the pathogenetic mechanism [15].

Portal hypertension is common. Occasionally this may be due to defects in the main portal veins. More often it is

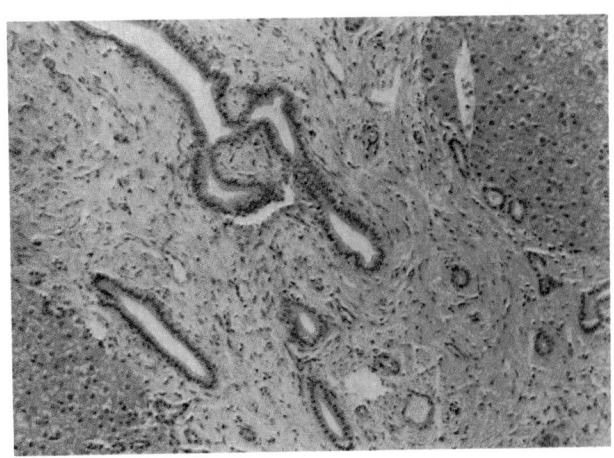

Fig. 30.7. Congenital hepatic fibrosis. Portal area shows dense mature fibrous tissue with a number of abnormal bile ducts. (Stained H & E, ×40.)

caused by hypoplasia or fibrous compression of portal vein radicles in the fibrous bands surrounding the nodules.

Associated renal conditions include renal dysplasia, adult type polycystic kidneys [9] and nephronophthisis (medullary cystic disease) [5].

Clinical features

The condition is often misdiagnosed as cirrhosis. The patient is usually diagnosed between the ages of three and 10 years but recognition may be delayed until adult life. Sexes are equal. The patient presents with haemorrhage from oesophageal varices, a symptomless, large, very hard liver or splenomegaly (fig. 30.8; table 30.2).

There may be other congenital anomalies, especially of the biliary system with cholangitis [14].

Carcinoma, both hepato-cellular and cholangiolar, may be a complication [2, 39] as may adenomatous hyperplasia [3].

Investigations

Serum protein, bilirubin and transaminase levels are usually normal, but serum alkaline phosphatase values are sometimes increased.

Liver biopsy is essential for diagnosis. Because of the tough consistency of the liver this may be difficult.

Ultrasound shows very bright areas of echogenicity due to the dense bands of fibrous tissue. Percutaneous or endoscopic *cholangiography* shows tapered intra-hepatic radicles, suggesting fibrosis.

Portal venography reveals the collateral circulation and a normal or distorted intra-hepatic portal tree [23].

Ultrasound, CT and *intravenous pyelography* may show cystic renal changes or medullary sponge kidney.

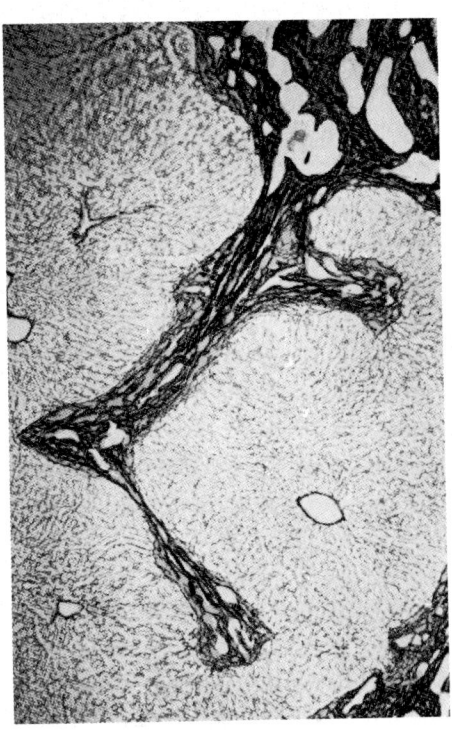

Fig. 30.6. Congenital hepatic fibrosis. Broad bands of fibrous tissue containing bile ducts separate and surround liver lobules. (Silver impregnation, ×36) [23].

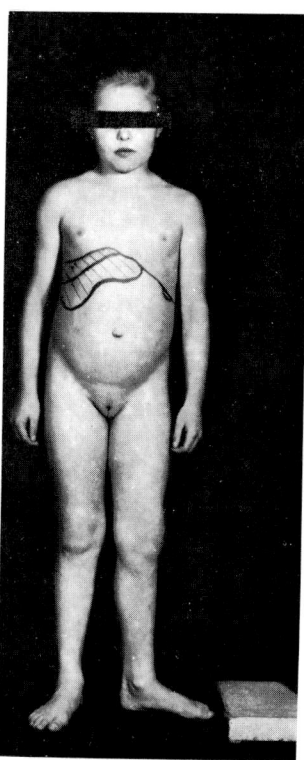

Fig. 30.8. Girl of 8 years. Hepatosplenomegaly discovered at routine examination. Liver biopsy showed congenital hepatic fibrosis. Note normal development.

Table 30.2. The presentation of 16 patients with congenital hepatic fibrosis

Presentation	No.	Age (years)
Large abdomen	9	2.5–9
Haematemesis or melaena	5	3–6
Jaundice	1	10
Anaemia	1	16

Prognosis and treatment

Congenital hepatic fibrosis must be distinguished from cirrhosis since hepato-cellular function is preserved and the prognosis is considerably better.

Following haemorrhage these patients are excellent candidates for porta-caval anastomosis.

Death can be due to renal failure, but renal transplantation has been successful.

Congenital intra-hepatic biliary dilatation (Caroli's disease) [7]

This rare disease is characterized by congenital, segmental, saccular dilatations of the intra-hepatic bile ducts without other hepatic histological abnormalities. The dilated ducts connect with the main duct system and are liable to become infected and contain stones (fig. 30.9).

The inheritance of Caroli's disease is uncertain [46]. Kidney lesions are usually absent, but renal tubular ectasia and larger cysts have been associated.

Clinical features

The condition presents at any age, but usually in childhood or early adult life, as abdominal pain, hepatomegaly, and fever with Gram-negative septi-caemia [28]. About 75% are male.

Jaundice is mild or absent but may increase during the episodes of cholangitis. Portal hypertension is absent.

Biliary drainage may be excessive, and flow increased by an infusion of secretin which stimulates ductular secretion. It is likely that the high resting flow arises from the cysts [47].

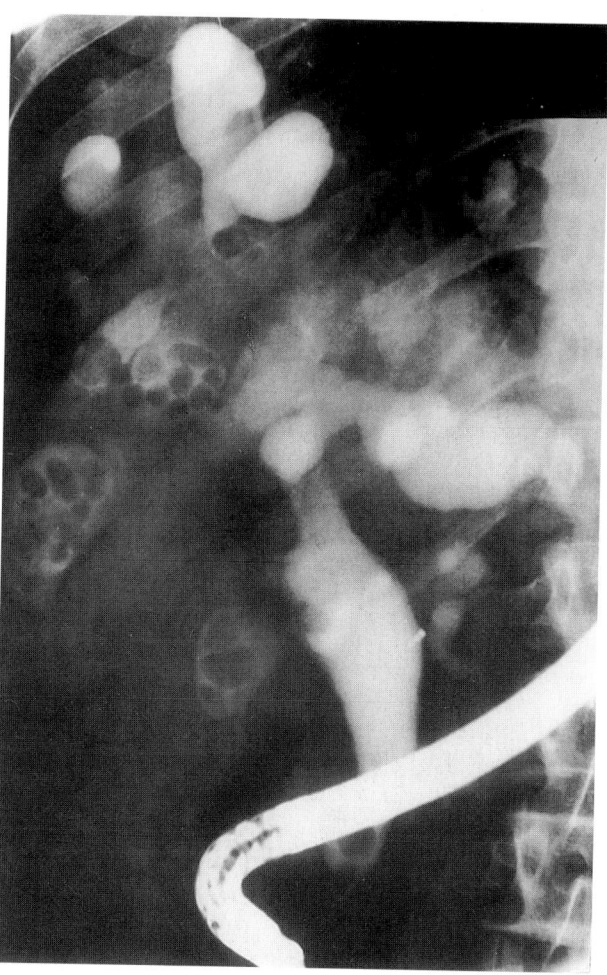

Fig. 30.9. Caroli's disease. Endoscopic cholangiography shows bulbous dilatations of the intra-hepatic bile ducts, some of which contain multiple gallstones.

Imaging

Ultrasound may be helpful as may CT scanning (fig. 30.10) where portal vein radicles can be seen after enhancement within dilated intra-hepatic bile ducts (the 'central dot' sign) [8]. Endoscopic or percutaneous cholangiography is diagnostic (fig. 30.9). The common bile duct is normal, but the intra-hepatic ducts are marked by bulbous dilatations with normal ducts between. The abnormality may be unilateral [29]. The appearances contrast with those of primary sclerosing cholangitis where the common bile duct is irregular with strictures and the intra-hepatic ducts show irregularities with dilatations. The changes in cirrhosis are smooth distortion of main bile ducts around regeneration nodules.

Cholangiocarcinoma may be a complication, reported in about 7% of patients [13].

Treatment

Antibiotics are given to treat the cholangitis as it appears, and drainage of the common bile duct, whether endoscopic or surgical, may be required to remove calculi. Intra-hepatic stones have been successfully treated with ursodeoxycholic acid [38].

Unilateral involvement may be treated by hepatic resection [29]. Hepatic transplantation must be considered, but the infection is usually a contraindication.

The prognosis is poor but episodes of cholangitis can extend over many years.

Death from renal failure is very unusual.

Congenital hepatic fibrosis and Caroli's disease

Caroli's disease often coexists with congenital hepatic fibrosis [43] and is then designated Caroli's syndrome. Both result from similar malformations of the embryonic ductal plate at different levels of the biliary tree. Inher-

itance is autosomal recessive. Presentation may be as abdominal pain and cholangitis or as haemorrhage from oesophageal varices (fig. 30.11).

A neonate, at autopsy, showed the features of congenital hepatic fibrosis, Caroli's disease and the infantile type of polycystic disease of the kidneys [12].

Choledochal cyst

This is a dilatation of the common bile duct. The gall-bladder, cystic duct and hepatic ducts above the dilatation are not distended, as distinct from the pattern of dilatation of the whole biliary tree above a stricture. Caroli's disease may coexist. Histologically the cyst wall consists of fibrous tissue lacking epithelium or smooth muscle. An anomalous pancreatico-biliary ductal anatomy (with a long common segment) is reported in patients with choledochal cyst. Biliary reflux of pancreatic enzymes is suggested as an aetiology [24].

Choledochal cysts are *classified* (fig. 30.12) [26] into:

Type I: segmental or diffuse fusiform dilatation of the extrahepatic bile duct.

Type II: the cyst forms a diverticulum from the extrahepatic bile duct.

Type III: this is a choledochocele of the distal common bile duct lying mostly within the duodenal wall.

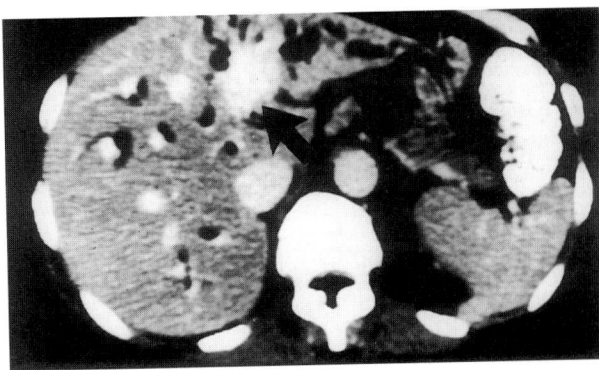

Fig. 30.10. Caroli's disease. CT scan after intravenous contrast shows dilated intra-hepatic bile ducts with adjacent enhanced radicles of the portal vein.

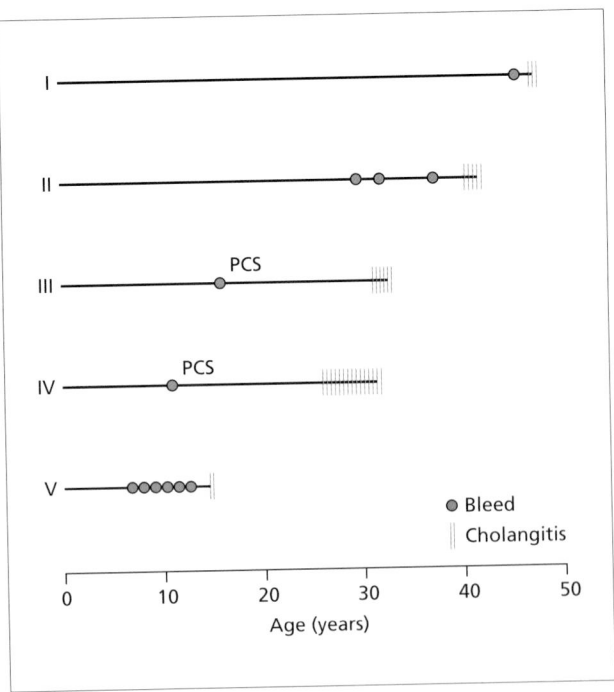

Fig. 30.11. The evolution of symptoms in five patients with coexistent congenital hepatic fibrosis and Caroli's disease who had both variceal haemorrhages and cholangitis. Haemorrhage always occurred first, followed, a mean of 10 years later, by cholangitis. PCS = porta-caval shunt [43].

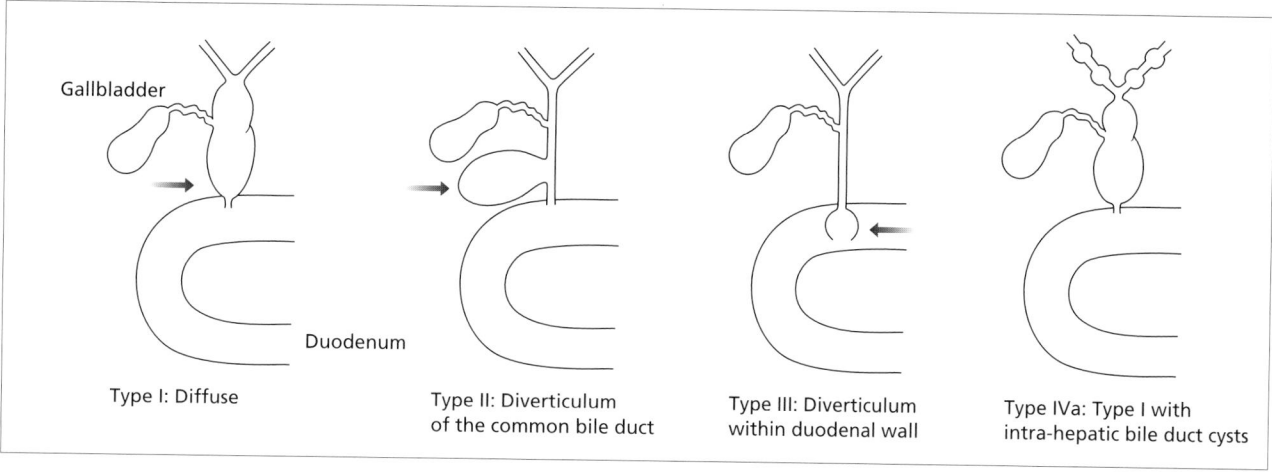

Gallbladder

Duodenum

Type I: Diffuse

Type II: Diverticulum of the common bile duct

Type III: Diverticulum within duodenal wall

Type IVa: Type I with intra-hepatic bile duct cysts

Fig. 30.12. Classification of congenital biliary dilatation (choledochal cyst) (IVb is type I plus III).

Type IV: this comprises type I anatomy with an intra-hepatic bile duct cyst (IVa) (Caroli's) or a choledochocele (IVb). When used, type V denotes Caroli's disease.

The fusiform extra-hepatic form (I) is the most common, with the combined intra- and extra-hepatic form (IVa) next most frequent [20, 26]. Whether choledochocele (III) should be classified as a choledochal cyst has been questioned [41].

Rarely a solitary cystic dilatation of an intra-hepatic bile duct is seen [44].

The type I lesion presents as a partially retroperitoneal, cystic tumour varying from 2 to 3 cm in size, to a capacity of 8 litres. The cyst contains thin, dark brown fluid. It is sterile but may become secondarily infected. The cyst can burst.

Biliary cirrhosis is a late complication. Choledochal cysts may obstruct the portal vein leading to portal hypertension. Malignant tumours in the cyst or bile ducts may develop [26]. Biliary papillomatosis with a K-*ras* gene mutation is reported [32].

Clinical features

The infantile form presents as prolonged cholestasis. In infancy the cyst may perforate causing bile peritonitis. Later the classical symptoms are intermittent jaundice, pain and an abdominal tumour. Children are more likely to have two or more of this 'classical' triad than adults (82 versus 25%) [26]. Although formerly regarded as a childhood disease, the diagnosis is now more often made in adult life. One-quarter of individuals affected present with symptoms and signs of pancreatitis [26]. Choledochal cysts appear more frequently in the Japanese and other Oriental races.

The jaundice is intermittent, of cholestatic type, and associated with fever. The pain is colicky and mainly experienced in the right upper abdomen. The tumour is cystic and in the right upper quadrant of the abdomen. It characteristically varies in size and in tenseness.

Choledochal cysts may be associated with congenital hepatic fibrosis or Caroli's disease. Anomalous pancreatico-biliary drainage is important particularly if the duct junction is right angular or acute [33].

Imaging

Plain X-ray of the abdomen may show a soft tissue mass. In infants the cyst may sometimes be revealed by HIDA scanning or ultrasound which allows diagnosis *in utero* and after delivery. In older children and adults, ultrasound and CT can show the cystic lesion. False negatives are found with all techniques [40]. The diagnosis is confirmed by percutaneous or endoscopic cholangiography (fig. 30.13).

Treatment

Because of the risk of subsequent adenocarcinoma or squamous cell carcinoma, excision is the method of choice [26]. Biliary tract continuity is maintained by choledochojejunostomy with Roux-en-Y anastomosis.

Anastomosis of the cyst to the intestinal tract without excision is simpler but post-operative cholangitis and subsequent biliary stricturing and stone formation are frequent. The risk of carcinoma remains, perhaps related to dysplasia and metaplasia of the epithelium [45].

Microhamartoma (von Meyenberg complexes)

These are usually asymptomatic, diagnosed incidentally or found at autopsy. Rarely, they may be associated with portal hypertension. Kidneys may show medullary

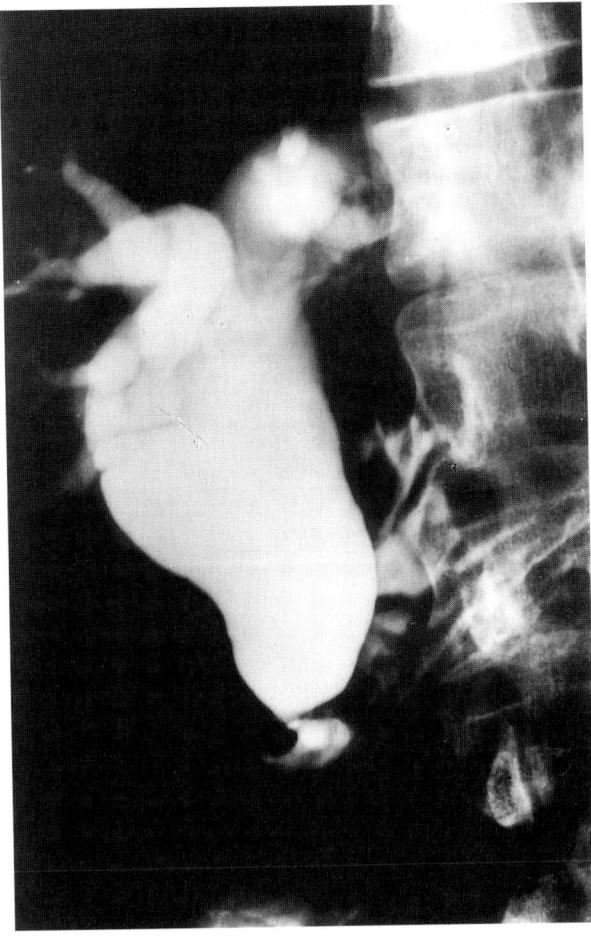

Fig. 30.13. Endoscopic cholangiogram in a 21-year-old woman with type I choledochal cyst showing a grossly dilated common bile duct from which contrast medium drained freely. This patient presented with acute pancreatitis.

sponge change. Microhamartomas can be associated with polycystic disease.

Histologically, microhamartomas consist of groups of rounded biliary channels, lined by cuboidal epithelium and often containing inspissated bile (fig. 30.14). These biliary structures are embedded in mature collagenous stroma. They are usually located in, or near, portal tracts. The appearances suggest congenital hepatic fibrosis, but in a localized form.

Imaging

In a hepatic arteriogram, multiple microhamartomas lead to stretching of the arteries and blushing in the venous phase.

Carcinoma secondary to fibropolycystic disease

Tumours may arise in association with microhamartomas, congenital hepatic fibrosis, Caroli's disease [13], and choledochal cyst [26]. Carcinoma is rare in association with non-parasitic cysts [31] or polycystic liver disease. Malignant change is more likely where epithelium is exposed to bile.

Solitary non-parasitic liver cyst

This is being increasingly diagnosed due to the increase in various scanning techniques. It is probably a variant of polycystic disease.

The lining wall has partitions, which suggest an origin from conglomerate polycystic disease. The fibrous capsule contains aberrant bile ducts and blood vessels. The contents vary from colourless to brown altered

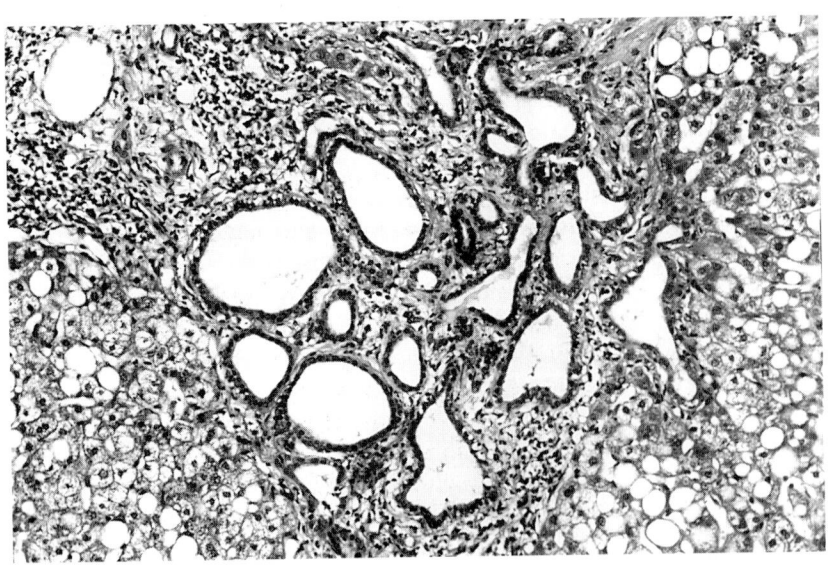

Fig. 30.14. Microhamartoma of the liver. Groups of biliary channels are lined by cuboidal epithelium and are embedded in mature fibrous tissue [43]. (Stained H & E, ×180.)

blood. The cyst appears as a smooth, glistening, greyish-blue tumour usually on the antero-inferior aspect of the right lobe. The tension is low in contrast to the high pressure of hydatid cysts.

Symptoms are rare and related to abdominal distension, or pressure effects on adjacent organs including the bile ducts causing intermittent jaundice. The patient should be reassured.

Symptoms follow rupture [1] or haemorrhage into the cyst. These events are extremely rare. Surgical excision is indicated only for complications.

Other cysts

These are all very rare, small and superficial. Their contents vary with the cause. Bile cysts may follow prolonged extra-hepatic biliary obstruction of all types.

Hepatic cysts can arise from glands adjacent to bile ducts especially in patients with portal hypertension [50]. These can cause obstructive jaundice.

Blood cysts follow haemorrhage into a simple cyst. They can also follow trauma to the liver. Small cystic spaces containing blood may follow needle biopsy.

Lymphatic cysts are due to obstruction or congenital dilatation of liver lymphatics. They are usually on the surface of the liver.

Biliary cystadenoma and cystadenocarcinoma are rare (Chapter 28). Malignant pseudocysts from degeneration and softening of secondary malignant growths also occur.

Congenital anomalies of the biliary tract

The liver and biliary tract develop from a bud-like outpouching of the ventral wall of the primitive foregut just cranial to the yolk sac. Two solid buds of cells form the right and left lobes of the liver while the original elongated diverticulum forms the hepatic and common bile duct. The gallbladder arises as a smaller bud of cells from this same diverticulum. The biliary tract is patent in early intra-uterine life but becomes solid later by epithelial proliferation within the lumen. Eventually revacuolization takes place, starting simultaneously in different parts of the solid gallbladder bud and spreading until the whole system is recanalized. At 5 weeks the ductal communications of gallbladder, cystic duct and hepatic ducts are completed and at 3 months the fetal liver begins to secrete bile.

The majority of the congenital anomalies can be related to alterations in the original budding from the foregut or to failure of vacuolization of the solid gallbladder and bile diverticulum (table 30.3).

These congenital defects are usually of no importance and cannot be related to symptoms. Occasionally bile duct anomalies lead to bile stasis, inflammation and gall-

Table 30.3. Classification of congenital anomalies of the biliary tract

---

Anomalies of the primitive foregut bud
Failure of bud
   Absent bile ducts
   Absent gallbladder
Accessory buds or splitting of bud
   Accessory gallbladder
   Bilobed gallbladder
   Accessory bile ducts
Bud migrates to left instead of right
   Left-sided gallbladder

Anomalies of vacuolization of the solid biliary bud
Defective bile duct vacuolization
Congenital obliteration of bile ducts
Congenital obliteration of cystic duct
Choledochal cyst
Defective gallbladder vacuolization
   Rudimentary gallbladder
Fundal diverticulum
Serosal type of Phrygian cap
Hour-glass gallbladder

Persistent cysto-hepatic duct
Diverticulum of body or neck of gallbladder

Persistence of intra-hepatic gallbladder

Aberrant folding of gallbladder anlage
Retroserosal type of Phrygian cap

Accessory peritoneal folds
Congenital adhesions
Floating gallbladder

Anomalies of hepatic and cystic arteries
Accessory arteries
Abnormal relation of hepatic artery to cystic duct

---

stones [10]. They are of importance to the radiologist and to the biliary and hepatic transplant surgeon.

Anomalies of the biliary tree and liver may be associated with congenital lesions elsewhere, including cardiac defects, polydactyly and polycystic kidneys. They can also be related to maternal virus infections, such as rubella.

Absence of the gallbladder [37]

This is a rare congenital anomaly. Two types can be recognized.

Type I is the failure of the gallbladder and cystic duct to develop as an outgrowth from the hepatic diverticulum of the foregut. This type is often found with other anomalies of the biliary passages.

Type II is the failure of the gallbladder to vacuolize from its solid state. This is usually associated with atresia of the extra-hepatic ducts. The gallbladder is not absent but *rudimentary*. This type is therefore found in infants who present the picture of congenital biliary atresia.

Most cases occur in infants with other major congenital anomalies. Adults are usually healthy and without other anomalies. Some have right upper quadrant pain or jaundice. The inability to show the gallbladder on ultrasound may be interpreted as gallbladder disease and lead to surgery. The possibility of agenesis or an ectopic location must be considered. Cholangiography should be diagnostic. Failure to identify the gallbladder at operation is not proof of its absence. The gallbladder may be intra-hepatic, buried in extensive adhesions, or atrophied following previous cholecystitis.

An intra-operative cholangiogram should be done.

Double gallbladder

Double gallbladder is very rare. In embryonic life, little pockets often arise from the hepatic or common bile ducts. Occasionally these persist and form a second gall-bladder having its own cystic duct (fig. 30.15). This may enter the hepatic substance directly. If the pouch forms from the cystic duct the two gallbladders share a Y-shaped cystic duct.

Double gallbladder can be recognized by imaging. The accessory organ is frequently diseased.

Bilobed gallbladder [27] is an extremely rare congenital

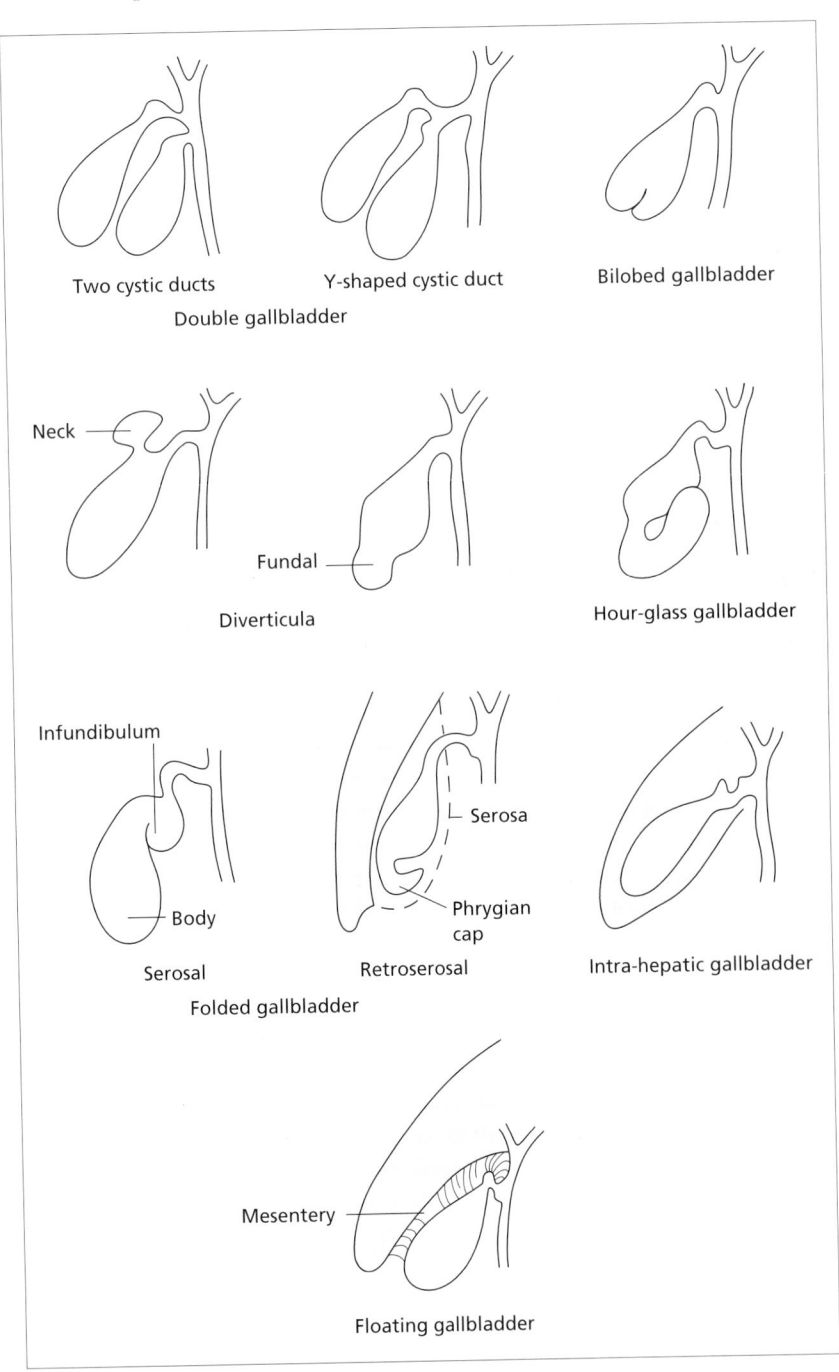

Fig. 30.15. Congenital anomalies of the gallbladder.

anomaly. Embryologically, the single bud forming the gallbladder becomes paired but primary connection is maintained, thus forming two separate and distinct fundi with a single cystic duct.

The anomaly is of no clinical significance.

Accessory bile ducts

These are rare. The extra duct is usually a subdivision of the right hepatic system and joins the common hepatic duct somewhere between the junction of the main right and left hepatic ducts and the entry of the cystic duct (see fig. 32.1c). It may, however, join the cystic duct, the gallbladder or the common bile duct.

Cholecysto-hepatic ducts are due to persistence of fetal connections between the gallbladder and the liver parenchyma with failure of re-canalization of the right and left hepatic ducts [22]. Continuity is maintained by the cystic duct entering a remaining hepatic duct or common hepatic duct or the duodenum directly.

Accessory ducts are of importance to the biliary and transplant surgeon as they may be inadvertently ligated or cut with resultant biliary stricture or fistula.

Left-sided gallbladder

In this rare anomaly the gallbladder lies under the left lobe of the liver to the left of the falciform ligament [30]. The embryonic bud from the hepatic diverticulum migrates to the left instead of to the right. Alternatively, it may be due to independent development of a second gallbladder from the left hepatic duct with failure of development or regression of the normal structure on the right side.

In transposition of the viscera, the gallbladder bears its normal relationship to the liver but lies on the left side of the abdomen.

A left-sided gallbladder is of little clinical significance.

Rokitansky–Aschoff sinuses of the gallbladder

These consist of hernia-like protrusions of the gallbladder mucosa through the muscular layer (intra-mural diverticulosis). Although potentially congenital they are particularly prominent with chronic cholecystitis when intraluminal pressure rises. They may be seen in an oral cholecystogram as a halo-like stippling surrounding the gallbladder.

Folded gallbladder

The gallbladder is deformed so that the fundus appears folded 'bent down to the breaking point after the manner of a *Phrygian cap*' [6]. A Phrygian cap is a conical cap or bonnet, with the peak bent or turned over in front, worn by the ancient Phrygians, and identified with the Cap of Liberty (*Oxford English Dictionary*).

Two varieties are recognized:
1 *Kinking between body and fundus (retroserosal; Phrygian cap)* (fig. 30.15). This is due to aberrant folding of the gallbladder within the embryonic fossa.
2 *Kinking between body and infundibulum (serosal)* (fig. 30.15). This is due to aberrant folding of the fossa itself in the early stages of development. The bend in the gallbladder is fixed by development of fetal ligaments, vestigial septa or constrictions of the lumen following delayed vacuolization of the solid epithelial anlage.

These kinked gallbladders empty at a normal rate and are of no clinical significance [6]. The importance lies in the correct interpretation of cholecystograms.

Hour-glass gallbladder. This probably represents an exaggerated form of Phrygian cap, presumably of the serosal type. The constancy of position of the fundus during contraction and the small size of the opening between the two parts indicate that this is probably a fixed, congenital malformation.

Diverticula of the gallbladder and ducts

Diverticula of body and neck may arise from persistent cysto-hepatic ducts which run in embryonic life between the gallbladder and the liver.

The fundal variety arises from incomplete vacuolization of the solid gallbladder of embryonic life. An incomplete septum pinches off a small cavity at the tip of the gallbladder (fig. 30.15).

These diverticula are rare and of no clinical significance. The congenital variety should be distinguished from *pseudo-diverticula* developing in the diseased gallbladder as a result of partial perforation. The pseudo-diverticulum in these cases usually contains a large gallstone.

Intra-hepatic gallbladder

The gallbladder is included and buried in hepatic tissue up to the second month of intra-uterine life, thereafter assuming an extra-hepatic position. In some instances the intra-hepatic condition may persist. The gallbladder is higher than normal and more or less buried but never entirely covered by liver tissue. It is frequently diseased, for the embedded organ has difficulty in contracting and so becomes infected, with subsequent gallstone formation.

Congenital adhesions to the gallbladder

These are very frequent. Developmentally these peritoneal sheets are due to an extension of the anterior mesentery, which forms the lesser omentum. The sheet may run from the common bile duct laterally over the gallbladder down to the duodenum, to the hepatic flexure of the colon and even to the right lobe of the liver, perhaps closing the foramen of Winslow. In a milder form, a band of tissue runs from the lesser omentum across to the cystic duct and anterior to the gallbladder; or a loose veil forms a mesentery to the gallbladder ('floating gallbladder').

These adhesions are of no clinical importance. Surgically, their presence should be remembered, so that they are not mistaken for inflammatory adhesions.

Floating gallbladder and torsion of the gallbladder

The gallbladder possesses a supporting membrane in 4–5% of specimens. The peritoneal coat surrounding the gallbladder continues as two approximated leaves to form a fold or mesentery to support the gallbladder from under the surface of the liver. This fold may allow the gallbladder to hang for as much as 2–3 cm below the inferior hepatic surface.

The mobile gallbladder is apt to twist, and *torsion* results. The blood supply is impaired in the small pedicle and infarction follows.

The condition usually occurs in thin, elderly women. With ageing, omental fat lessens and there is a great caudal displacement of abdominal viscera due to loss of tone in the abdominal and pelvic muscles. The gallbladder with mesentery becomes more pendulous and can twist. It can affect all ages, including children.

Torsion is followed by sudden, severe, constant epigastric and right costal margin pain passing through to the back with vomiting and collapse. Characteristically a palpable tumour appears, having the features of an enlarged gallbladder. Within a few hours it may disappear. The treatment is cholecystectomy.

Recurrent partial torsion leads to acute episodes. Ultrasound or CT shows a gallbladder situated low in the abdomen and even in the pelvis. It is suspended by a very long, down-curved cystic duct. Early cholecystectomy is indicated.

Anomalies of the cystic duct and cystic artery

In 20% of subjects the *cystic duct* does not join the common hepatic duct directly but first runs parallel to it, lying in the same sheath of connective tissue. Occasionally it makes a spiral turn around the duct.

These variations are extremely important to the surgeon. Unless the cystic duct is carefully dissected and its union with the common hepatic duct identified, the common hepatic duct may be ligated, with disastrous consequences.

The *cystic artery* can arise not, as normally, from the right hepatic artery but from the left hepatic artery or even from the gastroduodenal artery. Accessory cystic arteries usually arise from the right hepatic artery. Again, the surgeon must be careful to identify the cystic artery precisely.

References

1 Akriviadis EA, Steindel H, Ralls P *et al.* Spontaneous rupture of nonparasitic cyst of the liver. *Gastroenterology* 1989; **97**: 213.

2 Bauman ME, Pound DC, Ulbright TM. Hepatocellular carcinoma arising in congenital hepatic fibrosis. *Am. J. Gastroenterol.* 1994; **89**: 450.

3 Bertheau P, Degott C, Belghiti J *et al.* Adenomatous hyperplasia of the liver in a patient with congenital hepatic fibrosis. *J. Hepatol.* 1994; **20**: 213.

4 Bloustein PA. Association of carcinoma with congenital cystic conditions of the liver and bile ducts. *Am. J. Gastroenterol.* 1977; **67**: 40.

5 Boichis H, Passwell J, David R *et al.* Congenital hepatic fibrosis and nephronophthisis. A family study. *Q. J. Med.* 1973; **42**: 221.

6 Boyden EA. 'Phrygian cap' in cholecystography. A congenital anomaly of the gall bladder. *Am. J. Roentgenol.* 1935; **33**: 589.

7 Caroli J, Corcos V. La dilatation congénitale des voies biliaries intrahépatiques. *Rev. Medicochir. Mal. Foie* 1964; **39**: 1.

8 Choi BI, Yeon KM, Kim SH *et al.* Caroli disease: central dot sign in CT. *Radiology* 1990: **174**: 161.

9 Cobben JM, Breuning H, Schoots C *et al.* Congenital hepatic fibrosis in autosomal-dominant polycystic kidney disease. *Kidney Int.* 1990; **38**: 880.

10 Cullingford G, Davidson B, Dooley J *et al.* Case report: hepatolithiasis associated with anomalous biliary anatomy and a vascular compression. *H.P.B. Surg.* 1991; **3**: 129.

11 D'Agata IDA, Jonas MM, Perez-Atayde AR *et al.* Combined cystic disease of the liver and kidney. *Semin. Liver Dis.* 1994; **14**: 215.

12 Davies CH, Stringer DA, Whyte H *et al.* Congenital hepatic fibrosis with saccular dilatation of intrahepatic bile ducts and infantile polycystic kidneys. *Pediatr. Radiol.* 1986; **16**: 302.

13 Dayton MT, Longmire WP Jr, Tompkins PK. Caroli's disease: a premalignant condition? *Am. J. Surg.* 1983; **145**: 41.

14 De Vos M, Barbier F, Cuvelier C. Congenital hepatic fibrosis. *J. Hepatol.* 1988; **6**: 222.

15 Desmet VJ. What is congenital hepatic fibrosis? *Histopathology* 1992; **20**: 465.

16 Everson GT, Emmett M, Brown WR *et al.* Functional similarities of hepatic cystic and biliary epithelium: studies of fluid constituents and in vivo secretion in response to secretin. *Hepatology* 1990; **11**: 557.

17 Farges O, Bismuth H. Fenestration in the management of polycystic liver disease. *World J. Surg.* 1995; **19**: 25.

18 Gabow PA. Autosomal dominant polycystic kidney disease. *N. Engl. J. Med.* 1993; **329**: 332.

19 Gabow PA, Johnson AM, Kaehny WD *et al.* Risk factors for the development of hepatic cysts in autosomal dominant polycystic kidney disease. *Hepatology* 1990; **11**: 1033.

20 Hewitt PM, Krige JEJ, Bornman PC *et al.* Choledochal cysts in adults. *Br. J. Surg.* 1995; **82**: 382.

21 Itai Y, Ebihara R, Eguchi N *et al.* Hepatobiliary cysts

in patients with autosomal dominant polycystic kidney disease: prevalence and CT findings. *Am. J. Roentgenol.* 1995; **164**: 339.

22 Jackson JB, Kelly TR. Cholecystohepatic ducts: case report. *Ann. Surg.* 1964; **159**: 581.

23 Kerr DNS, Harrison CV, Sherlock S *et al.* Congenital hepatic fibrosis. *Q. J. Med.* 1961; **30**: 91.

24 Komi N, Takehara H, Kunitomo K. Choledochal cyst: anomalous arrangement of the pancreatico-biliary ductal system and biliary malignancy. *J. Gastroenterol. Hepatol.* 1989; **4**: 63.

25 Landing BH, Wells TR, Claireaux AE. Morphometric analysis of liver lesions in cystic diseases of childhood. *Hum. Pathol.* 1980; **11**: 549.

26 Lipsett PA, Pitt HA, Colombani PM *et al.* Choledochal cyst disease: a changing pattern of presentation. *Ann. Surg.* 1994; **220**: 644.

27 Martinoli C, Derchi LE, Pastorino C *et al.* Case report: imaging of a bilobed gallbladder. *Br. J. Radiol.* 1993; **66**: 734.

28 Murray-Lyon IM, Shikin KB, Laws JW *et al.* Non-obstructive dilatation of the intrahepatic biliary tree with cholangitis. *Q. J. Med.* 1972; **41**: 477.

29 Nagasue N. Successful treatment of Caroli's disease by hepatic resection: report of six patients. *Ann. Surg.* 1984; **200**: 718.

30 Newcombe JF, Henley FA. Left-sided gallbladder. *Arch. Surg.* 1964; **88**: 494.

31 Nieweg O, Sloof MJH, Grond J. A case of primary squamous cell carcinoma of the liver arising in a solitary cyst. *H.P.B. Surgery* 1992; **5**: 203.

32 Ohta H, Yamaguchi Y, Yamakawa O *et al.* Biliary papillomatosis with the point mutation of K-*ras* gene arising in congenital choledochal cyst. *Gastroenterology* 1993; **105**: 1209.

33 Oguchi Y, Okada A, Nakamura T *et al.* Histopathologic studies of congenital dilatation of the bile duct as related to an anomalous junction of the pancreatico-biliary ductal system: clinical and experimental studies. *Surgery* 1988; **103**: 168.

34 Pirson Y, Lannoy N, Peters D *et al.* Isolated polycystic liver disease as a distinct genetic disease, unlinked to polycystic kidney disease 1 and polycystic kidney disease 2. *Hepatology* 1996; **23**: 249.

35 Que F, Nagorney DM, Gross JB *et al.* Liver resection and cyst fenestration in the treatment of severe polycystic liver disease. *Gastroenterology* 1995; **108**: 487.

36 Ramos A, Torres VE, Holley KE *et al.* The liver in autosomal dominant polycystic kidney disease. *Arch. Pathol. Lab. Med.* 1990; **114**: 180.

37 Richards RJ, Raubin H, Wasson D. Agenesis of the gallbladder in symptomatic adults: a case and review of the literature. *J. Clin. Gastroenterol.* 1993; **16**: 231.

38 Ros E, Navarro S, Bru C *et al.* Ursodeoxycholic acid treatment of primary hepatolithiasis in Caroli's syndrome. *Lancet* 1993; **342**: 404.

39 Scott J, Shousha S, Thomas HC *et al.* Bile duct carcinoma: a late complication of congenital hepatic fibrosis. Case report and review of literature. *Am. J. Gastroenterol.* 1980; **73**: 113.

40 Sherman P, Kolster E, Davies C *et al.* Choledochal cysts: heterogeneity of clinical presentation. *J. Pediatr. Gastroenterol. Nutr.* 1986; **5**: 867.

41 Spier LN, Crystal K, Kase DJ *et al.* Choledochocele: newer concepts of origin and diagnosis. *Surgery* 1995; **117**: 476.

42 Starzl TE, Reyes, J, Tzakis A *et al.* Liver transplantation for polycystic liver disease. *Arch. Surg.* 1990; **125**: 575.

43 Summerfield JA, Nagafuchi Y, Sherlock S *et al.* Hepatobiliary fibropolycystic disease: a clinical and histological review of 51 patients. *J. Hepatol.* 1986; **2**: 141.

44 Terada T, Nakanuma Y. Solitary cystic dilation of the intrahepatic bile duct: morphology of two autopsy cases and a review of the literature. *Am. J. Gastroenterol.* 1987; **82**: 1301.

45 Todani T, Watanabe Y, Toki A *et al.* Carcinoma related to choledochal cysts with internal drainage operations. *Surg. Gynecol. Obstet.* 1987; **164**: 61.

46 Tsuchida Y, Sato T, Sanjo K *et al.* Evaluation of long-term results of Caroli's disease: 21 years' observation of a family with autosomal 'dominant' inheritance, and review of the literature. *Hepato-gastroenterology* 1995; **42**: 175.

47 Turnberg LA, Jones EA, Sherlock S. Biliary secretion in a patient with cystic dilation of the intrahepatic biliary tree. *Gastroenterology* 1968; **54**: 1155.

48 Uddin W, Ramage JK, Portmann B *et al.* Hepatic venous outflow obstruction in patients with polycystic liver disease: pathogenesis and treatment. *Gut* 1995; **36**: 142.

49 Vauthey J-N, Maddern GJ, Blumgart LH. Adult polycystic disease of the liver. *Br. J. Surg.* 1991; **78**: 524.

50 Wanless IR, Zahradnik J, Heathcote EJ. Hepatic cysts of periductal gland origin presenting as obstructive jaundice. *Gastroenterology* 1987; **93**: 894.

51 Williams AJK, Wild SR, Palmer KR. Adult hepatic fibropolycystic disease presenting as obstructive jaundice. *Gut* 1990; **31**: 1082.

Chapter 31
Gallstones and Inflammatory Gallbladder Diseases

Composition of gallstones

There are three major types of gallstone: cholesterol, black pigment and brown pigment (table 31.1, fig. 31.1). In the Western world most are cholesterol stones. Although these consist predominantly of cholesterol (51–99%) they, along with all types, have a complex content and contain a variable proportion of other components including calcium carbonate, phosphate, bilirubinate and palmitate, phospholipids, glycoproteins and mucopolysaccharides [124]. Crystallography confirms that the cholesterol is in monohydrate and anhydrous forms. The nature of the nucleus of the stone is uncertain — pigment, glycoprotein and amorphous material have all been suggested.

The problem is to explain how in normal persons insoluble cholesterol is kept in solution in bile, and what leads in other people to its precipitation to form gallstones.

Composition of bile

Biliary cholesterol is in the free unesterified form. Concentration is unrelated to serum cholesterol level and depends only to a limited extent on the bile acid pool size and bile acid secretory rate.

Biliary phospholipids. These are insoluble in water and include lecithin (90%) with small quantities of lysolecithin (3%) and phosphatidyl ethanolamine (1%). Phospholipids are hydrolysed in the gut and there is no entero-hepatic circulation. Bile acids determine excretion and enhance synthesis.

Bile acids. The primary bile acids are the trihydroxy, cholic acid, and the dihydroxy, chenodeoxycholic acid. These are conjugated with glycine and taurine. They are converted by bacterial action, usually in the colon, to the secondary bile acids, deoxycholic acid and lithocholic acid. Cholic, cheno- and deoxycholic acids are absorbed and undergo an entero-hepatic circulation which takes place 6–10 times daily [38]. Lithocholic acid is poorly absorbed and there is little to be found in the bile. The total bile acid pool is normally 2.5 g and the average daily production of cholic acid is about 330 mg and chenodeoxycholic acid 280 mg.

The control of bile acid synthesis is complex; it is probably a negative feedback mechanism through the amount of bile salts and cholesterol reaching the liver from the gut. Bile acid synthesis is decreased by administration of bile salts and increased by interruption of the entero-hepatic circulation.

Factors in cholesterol gallstone formation

Three major factors determine the formation of cholesterol gallstones (fig. 31.2). These are: altered hepatic bile which becomes supersaturated with cholesterol, nucleation of cholesterol monohydrate crystals and impaired function of the gallbladder.

Altered hepatic bile composition

Bile is 85–95% water. Cholesterol, which is insoluble in water and must be maintained in solution, is secreted

Table 31.1. Classification of gallstones

	Cholesterol	Black pigment	Brown pigment
Location	Gallbladder, ducts	Gallbladder, ducts	Ducts
Major constituents	Cholesterol	Bilirubin pigment polymer	Calcium bilirubinate
Consistency	Crystalline with nucleus	Hard	Soft, friable
% Radio-opaque	15%	60%	0%
Associations			
Infection	Rare	Rare	Usual
Other diseases	See fig. 31.2	Haemolysis, cirrhosis	Chronic partial biliary obstruction

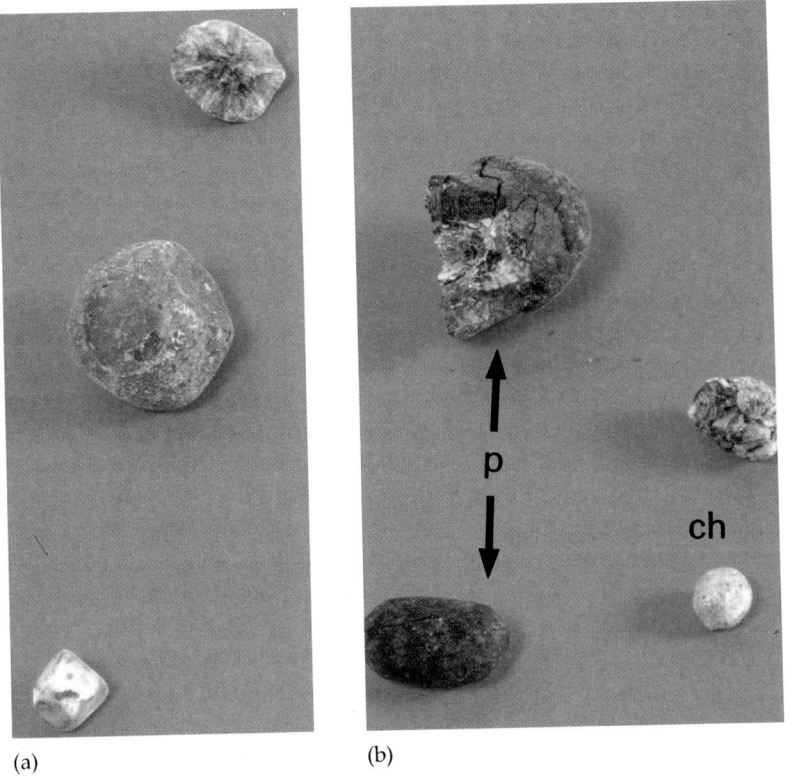
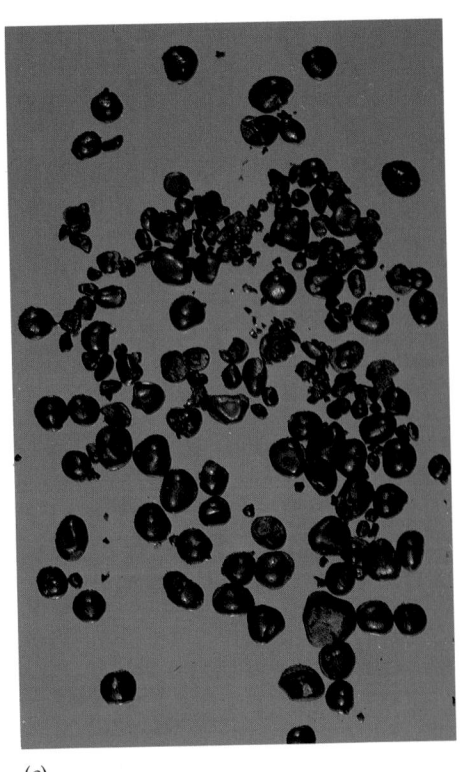

(a)   (b)   (c)

Fig. 31.1. (a) Two faceted cholesterol gallstones. The fragment above shows the concentric structure formed as layer upon layer of cholesterol crystal aggregates. (b) Stones removed from common bile duct (p = brown pigment stone; ch = cholesterol gallstone). (c) Black pigment gallstones.

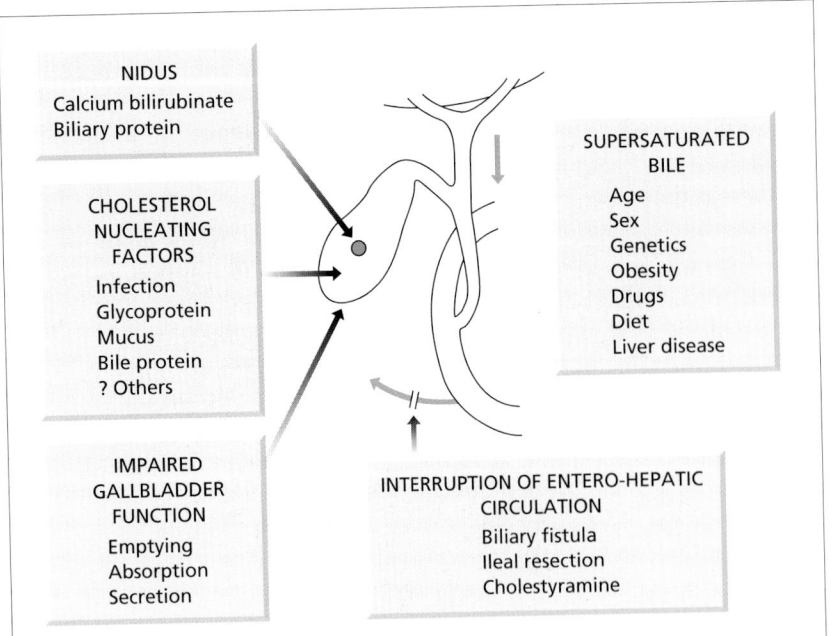

Fig. 31.2. Factors in cholesterol gallstone formation are supersaturation of the bile, the nidus, cholesterol crystal nucleation, impaired gallbladder function, and interruption of the entero-hepatic circulation of bile salts.

from the canalicular membrane in unilamellar phospholipid *vesicles* [81, 182] (fig. 31.3). In hepatic bile unsaturated with cholesterol and containing sufficient bile acid, the vesicles are solubilized into mixed lipid *micelles*. These have a hydrophilic external surface and a hydrophobic interior. Cholesterol is incorporated into the hydrophobic interior. Phospholipids are inserted into the walls of the micelles so that they grow. These 'mixed micelles' are thus able to hold cholesterol in a stable thermodynamic state [21]. This is the situation with a low cholesterol saturation index (derived from the molar ratio of cholesterol, bile acid and phospholipids).

When bile is supersaturated with cholesterol, or bile acid concentrations are low (a high cholesterol saturation index), the excess cholesterol cannot be transported in mixed micelles and unilamellar phospholipid vesicles remain (fig. 31.4) [132]. These are not stable and can aggregate [58]. They fuse to form large multilamellar vesicles from which cholesterol monohydrate crystals may *nucleate* [161].

The process of aggregation and fusion of vesicles and its control remains unclear, as do the factors controlling nucleation [130]. The importance of these processes is demonstrated by the finding that although cholesterol supersaturation is a prerequisite for gallstone formation it does not alone explain the pathogenesis. Other factors must be important since bile supersaturated with cholesterol is frequently found in individuals *without* cholesterol gallstones [70].

Nevertheless, in most gallstone sufferers in the Western world, gallstone formation can be related to supersaturation of bile with cholesterol due to an increased proportion of cholesterol to bile acids. In the majority of patients a diminished hepatic secretion of bile acids is the primary defect, and this is related to a reduced total body pool of bile acids [190]. The bile acids circulate more frequently within the entero-hepatic circulation, thereby suppressing synthesis.

Cholesterol nucleation

Nucleation of cholesterol monohydrate crystals from multilamellar vesicles is a crucial step in the process leading to gallstone formation. The distinguishing feature between those who form gallstones and those who do not, is the ability of the bile to promote or inhibit nucleation rather than the degree of cholesterol supersaturation. The time taken for this process ('nucleation time') is significantly shorter in those with gallstones

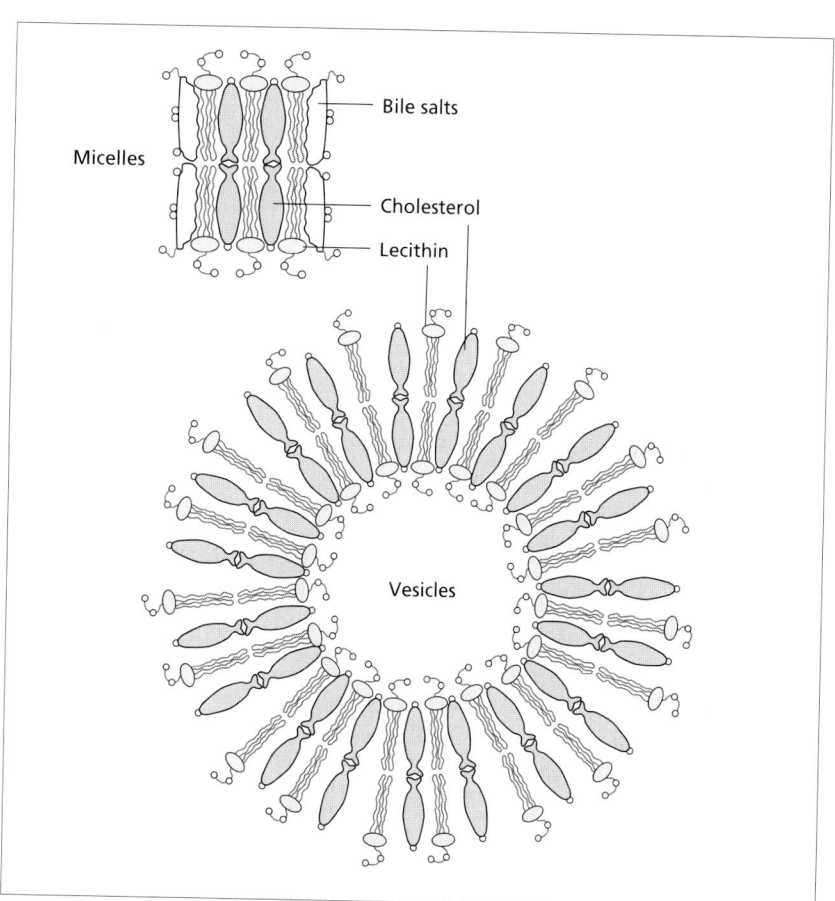

Fig. 31.3. Structure of mixed micelles and cholesterol/phospholipid vesicles.

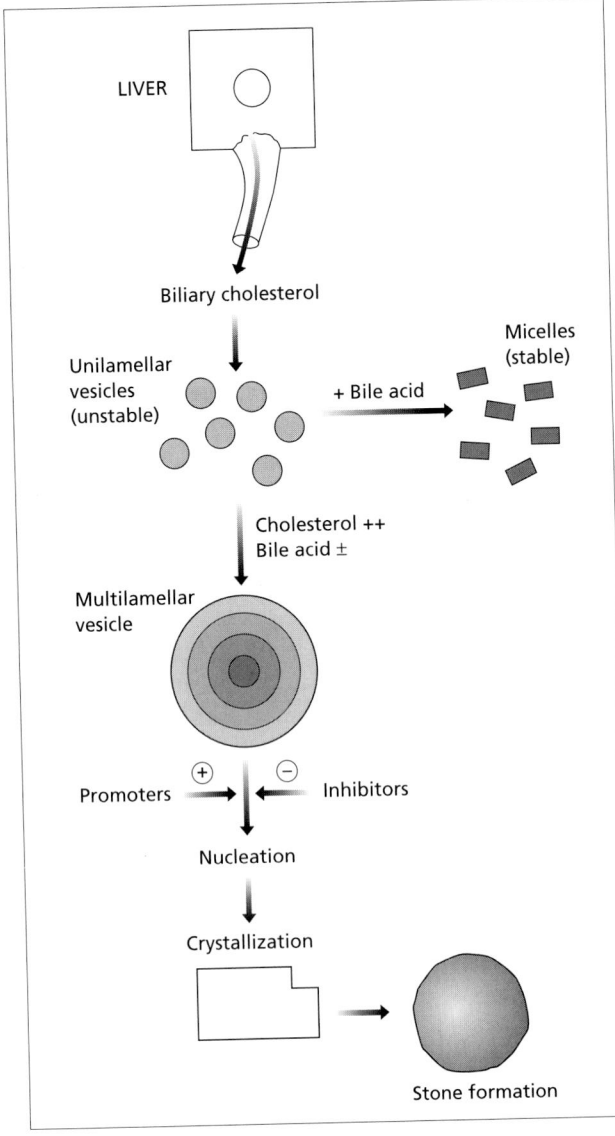

Fig. 31.4. Pathway for cholesterol crystallization in bile.

than in those without [69] and in those with multiple as opposed to solitary stones [83]. The interactions resulting in nucleation are complex. Biliary protein concentration is increased in lithogenic bile [172]. Proteins which accelerate nucleation (pro-nucleators) are gallbladder mucin [4], amino-peptidase-*N* [126, 128], an α_1 acid glycoprotein [2], immunoglobulin and phospholipase C [130]. Aspirin reduces mucus biosynthesis by gallbladder mucosa [146] which explains why this drug and other non-steroidal anti-inflammatory drugs inhibit gallstone formation [71]. Factors that slow nucleation (inhibitors) include apolipoprotein A1 and A2 [87] and a 120 kDa glycoprotein [129]. The interplay of pH and calcium iron concentration in stone formation *in vivo* remains to be established [139].

Ursodeoxycholic acid, as well as decreasing choles-terol saturation, also prolongs the nucleating time, which may have implications in the prevention of gall-stone recurrence [82].

Cholesterol gallstones have bilirubin at their centre, and the protein pigment complex might provide a surface for nucleation of cholesterol crystals from gall-bladder bile.

Gallbladder function

The gallbladder fills with hepatic bile during fasting, concentrates the bile and injects the concentrated bile into the duodenum during a meal. It must be capable of emptying to clear itself of sludge and debris that might initiate stone formation, particularly in the patient with bile supersaturated with cholesterol and a short nucle-ation time. Hepatic bile is stored in the gallbladder and concentrated by the absorption of Na^+, Cl^- and HCO_3^- with a nearly isotonic amount of water. Active transport of sodium and chloride by the mucosa is coupled to osmotic water absorption via intercellular and paracel-lular routes. The biliary concentration of bile salts, biliru-bin and cholesterol, for which the gallbladder wall is essentially impermeable, may rise 10-fold or more. Con-stituents do not, however, rise in parallel and the choles-terol saturation index may decrease with concentration of bile because of the absorption of some cholesterol. The calcium carbonate saturation index also falls because of acidification [167].

Gallbladder contraction is under cholinergic and hor-monal control [100]. *Cholecystokinin* (CCK), derived from the intestine, contracts and empties the gallbladder and increases fluid secretion with dilution of gallbladder contents. *Atropine* reduces the contractile response of the gallbladder to CCK [73]. *Loxiglumide*, a selective CCK antagonist, inhibits both post-prandial gallbladder emp-tying and gallbladder contraction induced by the CCK analogue ceruletide. Other hormones found to have an influence on the gallbladder include *motilin* (stimula-tory) and *somatostatin* (inhibitory).

The relationship between impaired gallbladder emp-tying and the increased incidence of gallstones in patients on long-term parenteral nutrition and in preg-nant women has suggested that gallbladder stasis has a role in the formation of gallstones. Studies of gallbladder motor function in patients with cholesterol stones have been conflicting. This probably relates to the technique used (ultrasound versus scintigraphy) and patient varia-tion. In general, patients with gallbladder stones have increased fasting and post-prandial gallbladder volumes [141]. Detailed analysis using simultaneous ultrasound and scintigraphy has challenged the conventional view of gallbladder function and shown a difference between normal and gallstone patients [80]. The concept of the gallbladder emptying after eating and then subsequently refilling to await the next meal appears oversimplified. Calculations from ultrasound and scintigraphic studies suggest continuous turnover of bile due to concurrent filling and emptying of the gallbladder. This turnover of gallbladder bile is reduced in patients with gallbladder disease [80] encouraging bile stasis and an environment in which nucleation and crystallization of cholesterol is likely to occur. Whether these changes are due to an alteration in gallbladder wall contractility and tone, or cystic duct resistance is not clear.

Gallbladder muscle strips exposed to bile containing excess cholesterol have a reduced contractile response to CCK [12]. Reduced contraction relates to the presence of fewer receptors for CCK in the muscle of the gallbladder wall.

Cholesterol crystallization and the formation of biliary sludge pre-date gallstone formation and therefore whatever the mechanism may be, impaired gallbladder emptying will encourage stone formation.

Biliary sludge

Biliary sludge is a viscous suspension of a precipitate which includes cholesterol monohydrate crystals, calcium bilirubinate granules and other calcium salts [91]. After formation, it disappears in 70% of patients [79]. 20% of patients develop complications of gallstones or acute cholecystitis. Whether treatment of sludge would reduce the incidence of complications is not known.

Role of infection

Although infection is thought to be of little importance in cholesterol stone formation, bacterial DNA is found by polymerase chain reaction in stones containing less than 90% cholesterol [174]. Conceivably bacteria might deconjugate bile salts, allowing their absorption and reducing cholesterol solubility.

Biliary infection plays a role in brown-pigment stone formation, the majority containing bacteria on electron microscopy [95].

Age

There is a steady increase in gallstone prevalence with advancing years, probably due to the increased cholesterol content in bile. By age 75, 20% of men and 35% of women have gallstones [143]. The presentation is usually in the 50s and 60s.

Gallstones of both pigment and cholesterol type are reported in childhood [88].

Genetics

Relatives of patients with gallstones have an increased frequency of gallstones, irrespective of their age, weight or diet [50, 157]. The increase is 2–4 times that expected.

Sex and oestrogens

Gallstones are twice as common in women as in men, and this is particularly so before the age of 50.

The incidence is higher in multiparous than in nulliparous women. Incomplete emptying of the gallbladder in late pregnancy leaves a large residual volume and thus retention of cholesterol crystals; this favours gallstone formation. Biliary sludge occurs frequently in pregnancy but is generally asymptomatic and disappears spontaneously after delivery in two-thirds [110]. In the post-partum period gallstones are present in 8–12% of women (nine times that in a matched group) [183]. One-third are symptomatic in those with a functional gallbladder. Small stones disappear spontaneously in 30%.

The bile becomes more lithogenic when women are placed on birth control pills [13]. Women on long-term oral contraceptives have a twofold increased incidence of gallbladder disease over controls [17]. Post-menopausal women taking oestrogen-containing drugs have a highly significant (2.5 times) increase in gallbladder disease [18]. Men given oestrogen for prostatic carcinoma develop gallstones and their bile becomes saturated with cholesterol [64]. Oestrogen and progesterone receptors have been found in the human gallbladder wall.

Obesity

This seems to be more common among gallstone sufferers than in the general population [103] and is a particular risk factor in women less than 50 years old. Obesity is associated with increased cholesterol synthesis and excretion [162] but there are no consistent changes in post-prandial gallbladder volume. 50% of markedly obese patients have gallstones at surgery [5].

Dieting (2100 kJ/day) can result in symptomatic gallbladder stone formation and biliary sludge in obese individuals [97]. There is a coincident increase in gallbladder mucin and calcium concentration during weight loss [166]. Gallstone formation after rapid weight loss following gastric bypass surgery for obesity is prevented by giving ursodeoxycholic acid [173].

Dietary factors

In Western countries, gallstones have been linked to dietary fibre deficiency and a longer intestinal transit time [63]. This would increase the secondary bile acids such as deoxycholic acid in bile, and render it more lithogenic. Carbohydrate in refined form increases biliary cholesterol saturation. A moderate amount of alcohol seems to protect against gallstones [179]. Vegetarians get fewer gallstones irrespective of their tendency to be slim [138].

Increasing dietary cholesterol increases biliary cholesterol but there is no epidemiological or dietary data to link cholesterol intake with gallstones. Indeed, newly synthesized cholesterol is probably a more important source of biliary cholesterol.

Serum factors

The highest risk of gallstones (both cholesterol and pigment) is associated with low HDL levels and high triglyceride levels which may be more important than body mass [176]. High serum cholesterol is not a determinant of gallstone risk.

Epidemiology (table 31.2)

In the Western world the prevalence of gallbladder stones is about 10%. Black Africans and the Eastern world are largely free of stones. The prevalence, however, is rising as life styles change. In Japan, the change from traditional to Western diets has been associated with a change from bilirubin to cholesterol gallstones.

American Indians have the highest known prevalence. This is related to supersaturation of the bile with cholesterol [191].

Cirrhosis of the liver

About 30% of patients with cirrhosis have gallstones [19]. The risk of developing stones is most strongly associated with Child's grade C and alcoholic cirrhosis with a yearly incidence of about 5% [46]. The mechanisms are uncertain. All patients with hepato-cellular disease show a variable degree of haemolysis. Although bile acid secretion is reduced, the stones are usually of the black

pigment type. Phospholipid and cholesterol secretion are also lowered so that the bile is not supersaturated.

Cholecystectomy and bile duct exploration are poorly tolerated, liver failure being frequently precipitated. Such operations should be done only for life-threatening complications of biliary tract disease, such as empyema or perforation. Endoscopic drainage is indicated for ascending cholangitis.

Other factors

Ileal resection breaks the entero-hepatic circulation of bile salts, reduces the total bile salt pool and is followed by gallstone formation. The same is found in subtotal or total colectomy [109].

Gastrectomy increases the incidence of gallstones [76].

Long-term cholestyramine therapy increases bile salt loss with a reduced bile acid pool size and gallstone formation.

Cholesterol-lowering diets high in unsaturated fat and plant sterols but low in saturated fats and cholesterol result in increased gallstone formation.

Clofibrate enhances biliary cholesterol excretion and makes the bile more lithogenic.

Parenteral nutrition leads to a dilated, sluggish gallbladder containing stones [150].

Long-term *octreotide* treatment induces gallbladder stones in 13–60% of acromegalic patients. The bile is supersaturated with cholesterol, the nucleation time abnormally rapid and the stones formed are cholesterol rich [74]. Additionally, gallbladder emptying is impaired [44].

Summary

The formation of cholesterol gallstones depends on the production of bile in which cholesterol cannot be maintained in solution. This might be related to increased secretion of cholesterol or perhaps a reduction in total bile acid pool. There are nucleation promoting and inhibiting factors in bile. Imbalance between these appears to generate an environment favouring cholesterol crystallization and stone formation. The gallbladder acts as a reservoir allowing growth of the stone. Changes in motor and other functions of the gallbladder increase the risk of stone formation.

Pigment gallstones

This term is used for stones containing less than 30% cholesterol. There are two types: black and brown (table 31.1) [96].

Black pigment stones are largely composed of an insoluble black pigment polymer mixed with calcium phosphate and carbonate. There is no cholesterol. The

Table 31.2. Comparison of gallstone prevalence between countries and races [10]

Very high	High	Moderate	Low
North American Indians	USA Whites	USA Blacks	Greece
Chile	Great Britain	Japan	Egypt
Sweden	Norway		Zambia
Czechoslovakia	Australia		
	Italy		

mechanism of formation is not well understood, but supersaturation of bile with unconjugated bilirubin, changes in pH and calcium, and overproduction of an organic matrix (glycoprotein) play a role [96]. Overall 20–30% of gallbladder stones are black. The incidence rises with age. They may pass into the bile duct. Black stones accompany chronic haemolysis, usually hereditary spherocytosis or sickle cell disease, and mechanical prostheses in the circulation. They show an increased prevalence with all forms of cirrhosis particularly alcoholic [19, 46]. Chemical dissolution therapy of pigment stones remains experimental [96].

Brown pigment stones contain calcium bilirubinate, calcium palmitate, and stearate, as well as cholesterol. The bilirubinate is polymerized to a lesser extent than in black stones. Brown stones are rare in the gallbladder. They form in the bile duct and are related to bile stasis and infected bile, and are usually radiolucent. Their formation is related to the deconjugation of bilirubin diglucuronide by bacterial β-glucuronidase [96]. Insoluble unconjugated bilirubinate precipitates. Brown pigment stones form above biliary strictures in sclerosing cholangitis, and in the dilated segments of Caroli's disease. In the absence of bile duct disease there is an association with juxta-papillary duodenal diverticula [156]. Bacteria are present in greater than 90%. In oriental countries, these stones are associated with parasitic infestations of the biliary tract such as *Clonorchis sinensis* and *Ascaris lumbricoides*. These stones are frequently intra-hepatic [120]. Removal from the common bile duct is by endoscopy sphincterotomy and from intra-hepatic ducts by lithotripsy techniques, percutaneous extraction or surgery.

Radiology of gallstones (see Chapter 29)

Only about 10% of gallstones are radio-opaque, compared with 90% of renal calculi (fig. 31.5). Visualization is due to the calcium content of the stone. Mixed stones may or may not have sufficient calcium to be rendered visible.

Gallstones are usually multiple and faceted, although a single, round stone may fill the whole gallbladder.

They usually have a peripheral rim of calcium and a clear centre. Occasionally the structure is laminated due to alternate deposition of cholesterol and calcium bilirubinate. Rarely, gallstones contain gas which shows stellate, translucent areas (*Mercedes–Benz sign*).

Ultrasound is the technique of choice to detect gallbladder stones [62] having a diagnostic accuracy of 90–95%. They are seen as echogenic foci within the gallbladder and cast acoustic shadows (see fig. 29.3). Ultrasound may also show a thickened gallbladder wall (>5 mm) as well as other features of gallbladder disease such as a tender gallbladder (sonographic Murphy sign)

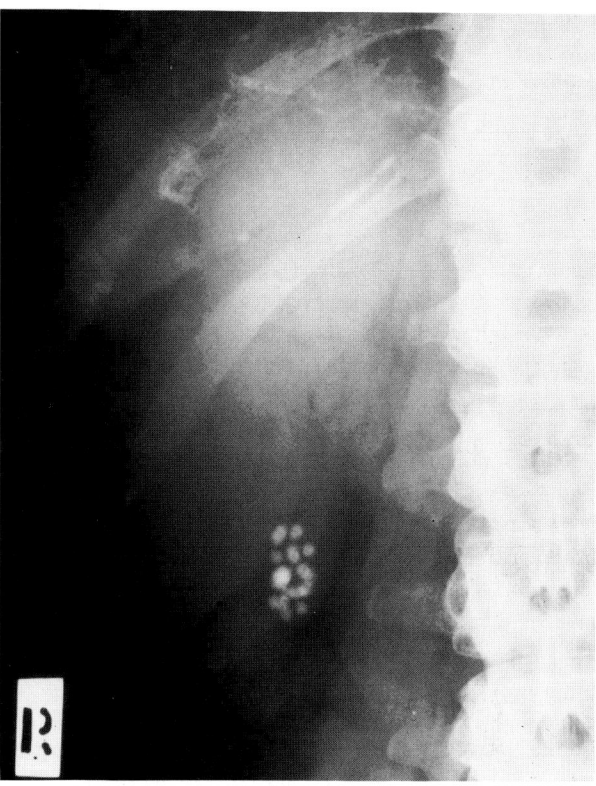

Fig. 31.5. Plain abdominal X-ray showing radio-opaque gallstones. Oral bile acid therapy is contraindicated.

and pericholecystic fluid. Non-visualization of the gallbladder also suggests disease.

With the availability of ultrasound, *oral cholecystography* is now rarely used to look for gallbladder stones. With this technique they appear as negative shadows which usually move with a change in position. In the erect position they may float on the contrast medium as a translucent layer ('floating gallstones'). Although oral cholecystography has only a slightly lower accuracy in showing stones than ultrasound (85–90%), it is more inconvenient for the patient, takes longer, has a higher prevalence of side-effects (nausea, diarrhoea, dysuria) and exposes the patient to radiation. However, because it is more successful than ultrasound in assessing the size and number of stones and the patency of the cystic duct, it does have a role in assessing patients for oral dissolution therapy and lithotripsy.

CT may show gallstones but is not the best test to assess their presence or absence. It has a role, however, in demonstrating the degree of calcification of cholesterol stones in patients who are being considered for nonsurgical therapy with oral bile acid or shock wave lithotripsy.

Imaging is basic to the diagnosis of gallstones and acute cholecystitis since there is not a good relationship between the 'characteristic' upper abdominal pain and the presence of gallbladder stones.

Natural history of gallstones (fig. 31.6)

Disease of the gallbladder is rare unless it complicates gallstones.

Gallstones can be dated from the atmospheric radio-carbon produced by nuclear bomb explosions. This suggests a time lag of about 12 years between initial stone formation and symptoms culminating in cholecystectomy [119].

Stones in the gallbladder are symptomless (*silent gallstones*) unless they migrate into the neck of the gallbladder or into the common bile duct.

Migration of a stone to the neck of the gallbladder causes *obstruction of the cystic duct* resulting in chemical irritation of the gallbladder mucosa by the retained bile, followed by bacterial invasion. According to the severity of the changes, *acute* or *chronic cholecystitis* results. Acute cholecystitis may gradually subside or progress to acute gangrene and perforation of the gallbladder or to empyema. Death is, however, rare at the first presentation of gallstone disease [30].

If the acute attack subsides spontaneously, chronic inflammatory changes persist with subsequent acute exacerbations.

Chronic cholecystitis can be silent. Usually, however, there are dyspeptic symptoms, and the patient may eventually come to cholecystectomy. This is usually curative, but may be followed by further episodes of pain, the *post-cholecystectomy syndrome*, or the unfortunate sequel of *traumatic stricture of the bile duct*.

Internal biliary fistula follows the migration of a gallstone from the acutely, or more usually chronically, inflamed gallbladder into an adjacent viscus. The stone may be passed in the faeces, or impact in the alimentary tract, causing *gallstone ileus*.

Gallstones entering the common bile duct may pass uneventfully into the duodenum, cause acute pancreatitis, or remain clinically silent in the duct, but they usually result in partial *obstruction to the common bile duct* with intermittent obstructive jaundice. Infection behind the obstruction is common with consequent *cholangitis*, and this may ascend to the liver, giving rise to abscesses.

Silent gallstones

Gallbladder stones may be symptomless and diagnosed by chance by imaging or during investigation for some other condition. Physicians usually believe in leaving such stones well alone. The surgeon is more likely to intervene. Follow-up studies, however, show that only a small proportion develop symptoms. In one study only about 10% of patients with asymptomatic gallstones developed symptoms within 5 years and only 5% required surgery [107]. Only about half the patients with symptomatic gallstones come to cholecystectomy within 6 years of diagnosis. Patients with gallstones seem to tolerate their symptoms for long periods of time, preferring this to cholecystectomy. If symptoms develop, they are unlikely to present as an emergency.

Prophylactic cholecystectomy should not be performed [144]. It should not be done to prevent gallbladder cancer, a tumour associated with gallstones, as the risk is small and less than that of cholecystectomy [36].

Treatment of gallstones in the gallbladder [143]

Cholecystectomy

This removes the gallstones and the factory making them. About 500 000 cholecystectomies are performed yearly in the USA and this operation is a billion dollar industry.

Laparoscopic cholecystectomy, introduced in the late 1980s has replaced open cholecystectomy in the majority

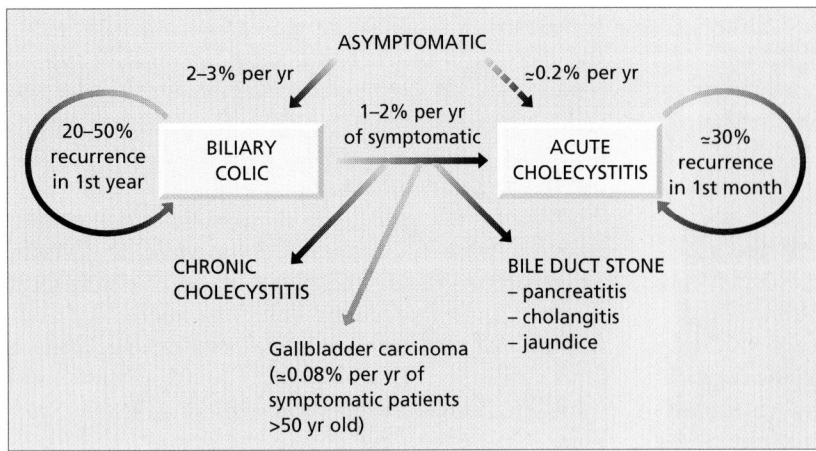

Fig. 31.6. The natural history of gallstones.

of patients [67, 102, 121]. *Open cholecystectomy* is still required where the laparoscopic approach fails, or is not possible. Thus expertise is still needed for the open operation.

The mortality rate of elective open cholecystectomy is 0.03% in patients under 65 years and 0.5% in those over 65 [149]. It is a safe and effective treatment for gallstones. There is a higher risk in those needing common duct exploration and in elderly patients (over 75 years old) having emergency surgery, often with gallbladder perforation and biliary peritonitis. To prevent this, early elective surgery is recommended in patients with *symptomatic* gallstones, especially if elderly.

The operation demands adequate assistance, exposure, illumination and the facilities for operative cholangiography if necessary. This is performed only if clinical, radiological and operative findings predict that stones will be found in the common bile duct [59]. When the common duct is explored, choledochoscopy is useful and reduces the chance of overlooking common duct calculi.

Laparoscopic cholecystectomy

Under general anaesthesia the abdominal cavity is insufflated with CO_2 and the laparoscope and operating channels inserted (fig. 31.7). Cystic duct and vessels to the gallbladder are carefully identified and clipped. Haemostasis is achieved by electrocautery or laser. The gallbladder is dissected from the gallbladder bed on the liver and removed whole. When necessary large stones are fragmented while they are still within the gallbladder to allow its delivery through the anterior abdominal wall.

Success

Laparoscopic cholecystectomy is successful in about 95% of patients. In the remainder, the operation has to be converted to open cholecystectomy. This is more likely if there is acute cholecystitis (34% conversion) particularly with empyema (83%) [27]. In these cases initial laparoscopic assessment is appropriate, and conversion to open operation made if indicated. Expertise is essential for the laparoscopic approach in acute cholecystitis.

Outcome

Most trials between laparoscopic and mini-cholecystectomy show that the laparoscopic approach has a significantly shorter hospital stay, duration of convalescence and delay before the patient returns to normal activities [7, 105] (fig. 31.8). Patients stay in hospital for 2–3 days and need about 2 weeks of convalescence, which compares with 7–14 days and up to 2 months, respectively,

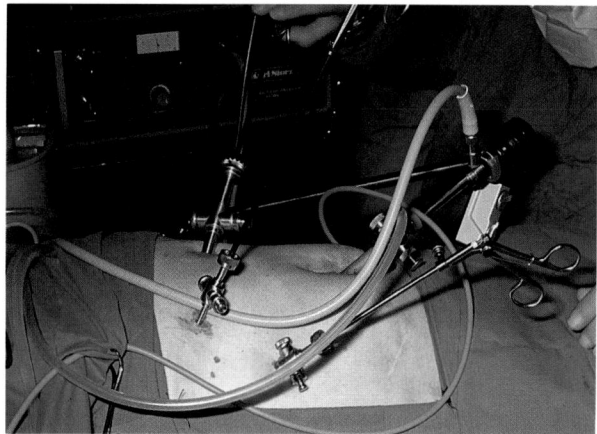

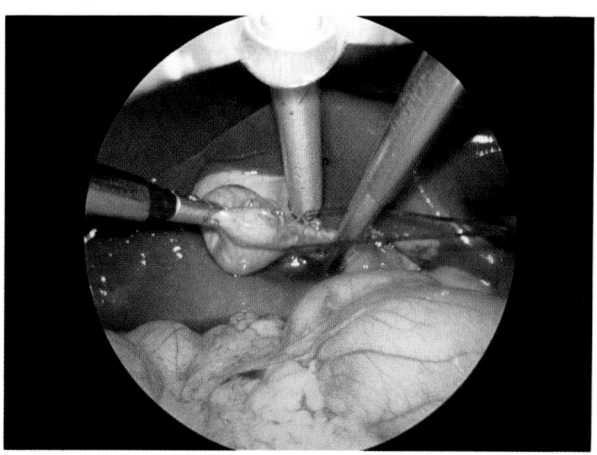

Fig. 31.7. Laparoscopic cholecystectomy. (a) Cannulae and endoscope in position. (b) Ligation of the cystic duct while the gallbladder is held [31].

for conventional open cholecystectomy. However, similar results have been reported for laparoscopic and 'small incision cholecystectomy' [108]. Hospital costs are greater for the laparoscopic approach but despite this the advantages have led to it becoming the method of choice. Symptomatic improvement is similar for the two approaches [187].

Complications

The complication rate is 1.6–8%, including wound infection, bile duct injury (0.1–0.9%; mean 0.5%) [40, 104] and retained duct stones. The rate of bile duct damage falls with increasing operator experience, although duct injury may occur even with an experienced surgeon. The mortality rate is less than 0.1% and this compares favourably with open cholecystectomy.

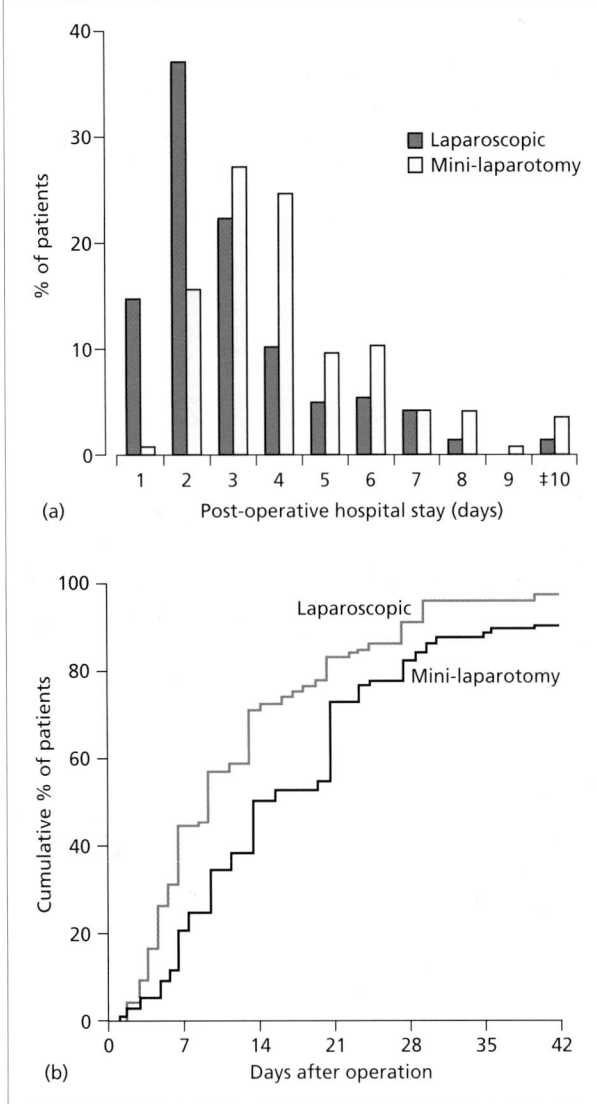

(a)

(b)

Fig. 31.8. Laparoscopic versus mini-cholecystectomy. (a) Post-operative hospital stay. (b) Return to work in the home. (Reproduced with permission from [105].)

Cholangiography

Ten to 15% of patients having cholecystectomy have common duct stones. Pre-operative ERCP is appropriate for patients with criteria suggestive of a duct stone — recent jaundice, cholangitis, pancreatitis, abnormal liver function tests, or duct dilatation on ultrasound. The duct stone is removed after sphincterotomy [193]. The 'duct stone' criteria need further refinement, to reduce the number of normal ERCPs done and the accompanying complications.

The strategy used to define or exclude duct stones depends on local endoscopic expertise, which will change with time. Greater expertise allows reliance on laparoscopic exploration or post-operative ERCP alone

(the present trend); lesser expertise favours pre-operative ERCP and open operation [171].

Intravenous cholangiography using improved contrast agents provides good quality images with a reduced risk of hypersensitivity. Stones can be detected but ERCP is preferred having the potential for sphincterotomy.

Intra-operative cholangiography at laparoscopic cholecystectomy needs experience [184]. Some advocate its routine use to define bile duct anatomy, anomalies and stones [14], but this prevents only the minority of bile duct injuries [8].

Laparoscopic common bile duct exploration

In experienced hands duct stones can be removed in 90% of patients [117]. This technique is not, however, widespread because of lack of expertise and the need for special equipment.

Treatment of bile duct injury

Injuries include bile leak from cystic duct or gallbladder bed, complete transection of the duct, and complete or partial stricture due to clips or damage during dissection. Optimal investigation and treatment depends upon a multidisciplinary approach between endoscopist, interventional radiologist and biliary surgeon. Leaks can be successfully treated by endoscopic stenting [9, 15, 33]. Complete transection and complete stricture are best treated surgically [169]. Results are significantly better if patients are referred to and managed in a specialist biliary unit. Whether incomplete strictures are better managed endoscopically by stenting [33] or by surgical operation [169] awaits study with longer follow up.

Conclusions

The major advantage of laparoscopic cholecystectomy is that there is a reduction in post-operative pain, hospital stay and recovery time, allowing earlier return to work than after open cholecystectomy. The latter, however, is still needed in some patients so that the laparoscopic surgeon must be 'fully trained' in general biliary surgery — a problem if laparoscopic cholecystectomy becomes the standard approach in the future.

Dissolution therapy

Oral bile salts [68]

The total bile salt pool is reduced in gallstone patients. This finding led to successful studies of oral bile acid therapy to treat gallbladder stones. The mechanism, however, is not an increase in biliary bile acid but rather a reduction in biliary cholesterol. After chenodeoxycholic acid, intestinal absorption of cholesterol falls and hepatic cholesterol synthesis is suppressed. Ursodeoxycholic acid also decreases cholesterol absorption but in contrast only inhibits the normal compensatory increase in cholesterol biosynthesis. During treatment with these agents bile acid secretion into bile remains relatively unchanged, but because of the reduced cholesterol secretion bile is desaturated. Also, ursodeoxycholic acid prolongs nucleation time.

Indications

Oral bile acid therapy is usually reserved for patients unfit for or unwilling to undergo surgery. The patient must be compliant and prepared for at least 2 years of treatment. Symptoms must be mild to moderate and silent stones should not be treated. On cholecystography the stones must be radiolucent, preferably floating, and the cystic duct patent. Stones should be less than 15 mm in diameter. Best results are for stones less than 5 mm diameter.

Unfortunately no imaging technique accurately determines the composition of gallstones. Ultrasound is of little value in assessing stone solubility. CT is useful and, because of the expense of bile acid therapy, cost effective in assessing stones. Stones with an attenuation value of less than 100 Hounsfield units (reflecting low calcium content) are more likely to dissolve [192].

Chenodeoxycholic acid

The dose is 12–15 mg/kg per day in the the non-obese. The markedly obese have increased biliary cholesterol and so require 18–20 mg/kg per day. Diarrhoea is a side-effect and the dose should be increased gradually starting with 500 mg daily. A bedtime dose gives the maximum effect. Other side-effects include a dose-dependent rise in serum aspartate transaminase levels which usually subside. Values must be monitored monthly for 3 months, then at 6, 12, 18 and 24 months.

Ursodeoxycholic acid

This is derived from the Japanese white-collared bear. It is the the 7-beta epimer of chenodeoxycholic acid. The dose is 8–10 mg/kg per day with more being needed if the patient is markedly obese. It dissolves about 20–30% of radiolucent gallstones completely [51] and does so more rapidly than chenodeoxycholic acid [43]. Side-effects are absent.

During treatment the stones may undergo surface calcification [11], but this is probably of little significance.

Combination therapy

A combination of chenodeoxycholic acid (6–8 mg/kg per day) and ursodeoxycholic acid (6–8 mg/kg per day) is more effective than ursodeoxycholic acid alone [114, 140] and avoids the side-effects of the higher dose of chenodeoxycholic acid.

Results

The overall success rate for oral bile acid therapy is approximately 40% rising to 60% with careful patient selection. Stones of 5 mm or less in diameter that float, dissolve more quickly (80–90% complete dissolution by 12 months). Larger non-floating stones take longer or never disappear. Careful evaluation with CT to show the degree of calcification of the stone may avoid inappropriate bile acid therapy.

Gallstone dissolution can be shown by ultrasound examination or by oral cholecystography. Ultrasound is more sensitive as residual small fragments may be present after the oral cholecystogram shows no stones. These fragments may provide the nidus for new stone formation.

The effect of bile acid therapy on symptoms is variable and inconsistent. Recurrences develop in 25–50% of patients at a rate of 10% per year. They are most likely in the first 2 years and unlikely after the first 3 years.

Low-dose ursodeoxycholic acid (200–300 mg/day) may be effective in reducing the frequency of gallstone recurrence [72]. Recurrence is higher in those with multiple rather than solitary stones.

Conclusions

The disadvantages of oral bile acid therapy for gallbladder stones include restriction to non-calcified and, if possible, pure cholesterol stones. Dissolution is slow. Combined cheno- and ursodeoxycholic acid therapy appears to be the first choice. Therapy should be reserved for those who are symptomatic and will cooperate. They should have small, lucent gallstones in a functioning gallbladder and poor general health, including obesity, age or associated conditions preventing surgery.

Direct solvent dissolution

A percutaneous trans-hepatic catheter (7 French diameter) is inserted under real-time ultrasound guidance into the gallbladder and solvent pumped in and out (fig. 31.9) [178]. The solvent used is *methyl tert-butyl ether* (MTBE), a gasoline additive of low viscosity and with power to dissolve cholesterol stones rapidly [178]. The solvent (3–7 ml) envelops the stone but should not over-

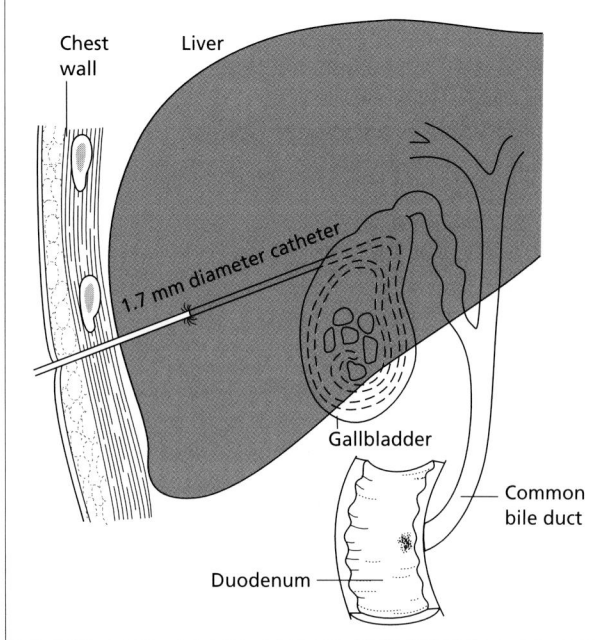

Fig. 31.9. Technique of percutaneous trans-hepatic gallbladder catheter placement for MBTE dissolution of cholesterol gallstones [178].

flow into the cystic duct. Computer-assisted pumps have been devised. These eliminate the tedium of manually filling and emptying the gallbladder.

The gallstones are dissolved in 4–16 hours and the catheter removed the same day or within 2–3 days in most cases. Side-effects include pain and nausea. The risk of bile leakage (which is small) can be reduced by plugging the trans-hepatic tract with gelfoam.

Duodenitis and haemolysis are serious consequences of spill of solvent into the duodenum. Morphological changes in the gallbladder mucosa are mild. An ether smell develops on the breath and the patient may become drowsy. This method may be useful to remove fragments remaining after such procedures as shock-wave therapy.

Shock-wave therapy

Gallstones can be fragmented by shock waves generated extracorporeally by spark gap (electro-hydraulic), electromagnetic or piezo electric lithotripter machines using the same principle as that developed for kidney stones (fig. 31.10). By various methods the shock waves are directed towards a focal point. Ultrasound is usually used to compute the exact position of machine and patient such that the gallbladder stone lies at the point of highest energy (the focus). The waves pass through soft tissue with little absorption of energy but the solid stone absorbs the energy and is fragmented. Although the early prototypes used required the patient to have a general anaesthetic, this is no longer necessary. Fragments, if small enough, may pass down the cystic and common bile duct into bowel and faeces [55]. Oral bile acid therapy is given to dissolve those fragments remaining in the gallbladder. The gallbladder shows bruising and oedema after the shock waves but these are reversible.

Results

There are now numerous reports of the results for shock-wave lithotripsy and these vary from one machine, centre and protocol, to another [175]. Only 20–25% of patients referred satisfy the treatment criteria which included: three or fewer radiolucent gallbladder stones with a total diameter of less than 30 mm, in a functioning gallbladder (on cholecystography), in a symptomatic patient who is otherwise healthy. The stones must be visible on ultrasound and are pin-pointed by this technique for the lithotripter. The shock-wave path should avoid any lung field or bone.

Shock waves successfully fragment stones in the majority of patients although with some machines, particularly the piezo-electric system, several sessions may be necessary. The latter system, however, carries a benefit of less patient discomfort and patients may be treated as outpatients [135]. Adjuvant therapy with *oral*

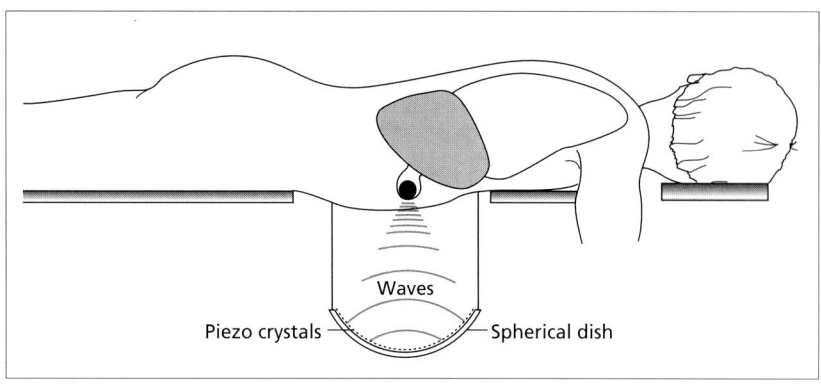

Fig. 31.10. Extracorporeal shock-wave lithotripsy (piezo-electric model). Patient lies face down and the shock waves are transmitted through a water-filled cushion to focus on a stone in the gallbladder.

bile acids (ursodeoxycholic acid 10–12 mg/kg per day) has been found to increase the rate of stone/fragment disappearance from 9% to 21% at 6 months [159]. This therapy or the combination of urso- and cheno-deoxycholic acid has been used routinely in other studies. It is started a few weeks before lithotripsy and is continued for 3 months after complete clearance of the fragments.

Studies have shown overall complete clearance rates at 6 and 12 months of approximately 40–60% and 70–90%, respectively [154]. Fragmentation and clearance is greater with solitary stones less than 20 mm diameter and with high energy lithotripsy. Patients compliant to bile acid therapy have a better outcome. Success also correlates with unimpaired post-prandial gallbladder contraction (ejection fraction >60%) [133]. As after chole-cystectomy, non-specific abdominal symptoms (disten-tion, flatulence, nausea) are not relieved despite successful lithotripsy [170]. Stone recurrence 5 years after stopping bile acids is 30% [152]. Two-thirds are symptomatic. Stone recurrence relates to incomplete gallbladder emptying and excessive deoxycholic acid in the bile acid pool [16].

Some centres accept patients with stones having a rim of calcification, but the success rate is lower [153].

Complications

Side-effects of treatment include biliary colic (30–60%), skin petechiae, haematuria and pancreatitis (2%) due to fragments wedging in the low common bile duct.

Conclusions

Problems include the small percentage of patients who prove suitable, the need for several sessions of lithotripsy and the long commitment to bile acid therapy. The advent of laparoscopic cholecystectomy has reduced the contribution of this method to the treatment of gallbladder stones.

Percutaneous cholecystolithotomy

Developed from percutaneous nephrolithotomy, this technique removes stones from the gallbladder trans-peritoneally. An oral cholecystogram is performed, timed to coincide with surgery. Under general anaesthe-sia the gallbladder is catheterized trans-peritoneally using fluoroscopy and ultrasound screening. The track is dilated to take a sheath wide enough to take the rigid operating cystoscope. The stones are removed after frag-mentation by electro-hydraulic or laser lithotripsy if nec-essary. This technique also allows stones to be removed from a non-functioning gallbladder with catheterization being done under ultrasound. After the stones have been removed a balloon catheter is placed within the gallblad-der and the balloon inflated so that there is drainage with little risk of leakage of bile. The catheter is removed after about 10 days.

Results

In a series of 113 patients, this method was successful in 90% with complications in 13%, but no mortality [22]. Stones recurred in 31% of patients at a mean follow-up of 26 months [37].

Conclusions

The procedure of choice for symptomatic gallstones is cholecystectomy. The laparoscopic method is now con-sidered first and is acceptable to many patients who pre-viously requested non-surgical treatment because of fear of open operation. For the patient who refuses any surgery, or who is judged unfit for general anaesthesia, oral bile acid therapy (with extracorporeal shock-wave lithotripsy if available) is appropriate if the treatment criteria are met. Direct solvent dissolution therapy and percutaneous cholecystolithotomy are rarely used, and are best restricted to the expert enthusiastic operator.

Acute cholecystitis

Aetiology

In 96% of patients the cystic duct is obstructed by a gall-stone. The imprisoned bile salts have a toxic action on the gallbladder wall. Lipids may penetrate the Rokitan-sky–Aschoff sinuses and exert an irritant reaction. The rise in pressure compresses blood vessels in the gallblad-der wall; infarction and gangrene may follow.

Pancreatic enzymes may also cause acute cholecyst-itis, presumably by regurgitation in the presence of obstruction of a common biliary and pancreatic channel. Such pancreatic regurgitation may account for some instances of acute cholecystitis developing in the absence of gallbladder stones.

Bacterial inflammation is an integral part of acute cholecystitis. Bacterial deconjugation of bile salts may produce toxic bile acids which can injure the mucosa.

Pathology

The gallbladder is greyish-red in colour with a lustreless surface. There are vascular adhesions to adjacent struc-tures. The gallbladder is usually distended, but after pre-vious inflammation the wall becomes thickened and contracted. It contains turbid fluid which may be frankly purulent (*empyema of the gallbladder*). A gallstone may be lodged in the neck.

Histology shows haemorrhage and moderate oedema reaching a peak by about the fourth day and diminishing by the seventh day. As the acute reaction subsides it is replaced by fibrosis.

Related lymph glands at the neck of the gallbladder and along the common bile duct are enlarged.

Bacteriology. Cultures of both gallbladder wall and bile usually show organisms of intestinal type, including anaerobes, in about three-quarters of cases.

Clinical features

These vary from those of mild inflammation to fulminating gangrene of the gallbladder wall. The acute attack is often an exacerbation of underlying chronic cholecystitis.

The sufferers are often obese, female and over 40, but no type, age or sex is immune.

Pain often occurs late at night or in the early morning, usually in the right upper abdomen or epigastrium and is referred below the angle of the right scapula, the right shoulder, or rarely to the left side. It may simulate angina pectoris.

The pain usually rises to a plateau and can last 30–60 minutes without relief, unlike the short spasm of biliary colic. Attacks may be precipitated by late-night, heavy meals or fatty food, or even by such simple acts as abdominal palpation or yawning. The wretched, perspiring sufferer lies motionless in a curled-up posture, often with local heat applied to the abdomen.

Distension pain is due to the gallbladder contracting to overcome the blocked cystic duct. This visceral pain is deep seated, central and unaccompanied by muscular rigidity and superficial or deep tenderness.

Peritoneal pain is superficial with skin tenderness, hyperaesthesia and muscular rigidity. The fundus of the gallbladder is in apposition to the diaphragmatic peritoneum, which is supplied by the phrenic and last six intercostal nerves. Stimulation of the anterior branches produces right upper quadrant pain and of the posterior cutaneous branch leads to the characteristic right infrascapular pain.

The spinal nerves extend a short distance into the mesentery and gastro-hepatic ligament around the major bile ducts, and stimulation of these nerves is interpreted as pain and referred to the back and right upper quadrant. This explains the pain of stones in the common bile duct and of cholangitis.

Digestive system. Flatulence and nausea are common, but vomiting is unusual, unless there is a stone in the common bile duct.

Examination

The patient appears ill, with shallow, jerky respirations.

The temperature rises with bacterial invasion. Jaundice usually indicates associated stones in the common bile duct.

The abdomen moves poorly. Spread of infection to peritoneal surfaces leads to gastric and duodenal distension. Hyperaesthesia is maximal in the 8th and 9th right thoracic segments, and the right upper abdominal muscles are rigid. The gallbladder is usually impalpable; occasionally a tender mass of gallbladder and adherent omentum may be felt. *Murphy's sign* is positive. The liver edge is tender.

The *leucocyte count* is raised to about $10 \times 10^9/l$, with moderate increase in polymorphs. In the febrile patient blood cultures may be positive.

For the patient with acute abdominal pain of uncertain cause, a plain X-ray will be taken during the work-up, but if acute cholecystitis is suspected other imaging is of greater value.

Ultrasound (Chapter 29) may show gallstones, a thickened gallbladder wall (fig. 31.11), a sonographic Murphy's sign and peri-cholecystic fluid. *Cholescintigraphy* is also of value. Visualization of a completely normal gallbladder rules out acute cholecystitis whereas radioactivity in the common bile duct and intestine without filling of the gallbladder is reasonable evidence of an obstructed cystic duct (fig. 29.8b). These two tech-

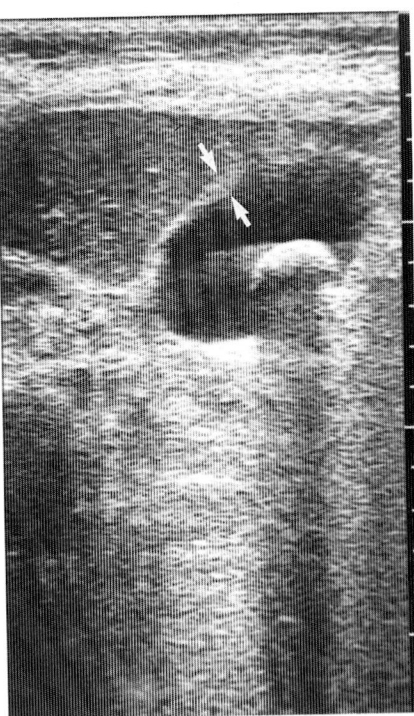

Fig. 31.11. Ultrasound scan of gallbladder in patient with right upper quadrant pain and fever. The gallbladder wall (arrowed) is irregularly thickened and a gallstone is present. There is a fluid–fluid level due to obstruction. Diagnosis: acute cholecystitis.

niques have a similar accuracy in diagnosis of acute cholecystitis and the technique used will depend upon local facilities and expertise.

Differential diagnosis

Acute cholecystitis is liable to be confused with other causes of sudden pain and tenderness in the right hypochondrium. Below the diaphragm, acute retro-caecal appendicitis, intestinal obstruction, a perforated peptic ulcer or acute pancreatitis may produce similar clinical features.

Diaphragmatic pleurisy may be associated with tenderness in the gallbladder area and this is also characteristic of Bornholm disease. Myocardial infarction should always be considered.

Referred pain from muscular and spinal root lesions may cause similar pain.

Prognosis

Spontaneous recovery follows disimpaction of the stone in 85% of patients. However, the gallbladder remains shrunken, fibrotic, full of stones and non-functioning. Recurrent acute cholecystitis may follow, approximately a 30% chance over the next 3 months [143].

Rarely, acute cholecystitis proceeds rapidly to gangrene or empyema of the gallbladder, fistula formation, hepatic abscesses or even generalized peritonitis. The acute fulminating disease is becoming less common because of earlier antibiotic therapy and more frequent cholecystectomies for recurrent gallbladder symptoms.

Acute emergency surgery in the aged (over 74 years old) carries a bad prognosis with many complications [28].

Treatment

General measures include bed rest, intravenous fluids, a light diet and relief of pain with pethidine (demerol) and buscopan.

Antibiotics

Antibiotics are given to treat septicaemia and prevent peritonitis and empyema. During the first 24 hours, 30% of gallbladder cultures are positive. This rises to 80% after 72 hours.

Common infecting organisms are *Escherichia coli*, *Streptococcus faecalis* and *Klebsiella*, often in combination. Anaerobes are present, if sought, and are usually found with aerobes. They include *Bacteroides* and *Clostridia*.

Antibiotic(s) should have a spectrum to cover the colonic type micro-organisms which are usually found with infection of the biliary tree. The choice depends upon the clinical picture. Ampicillin or a cephalosporin is usually adequate for the stable patient with pain and mild fever. The severely septicaemic patient is better treated with a combination of aminoglycoside (gentamicin or netilmicin), ureidopenicillin (azlocillin or piperacillin) and metronidazole. These antibiotics are primarily given to treat septicaemia. They may penetrate and sterilize tissue but eradication of infection from the gallbladder should not be assumed, recurrent sepsis being possible later.

Surgery

There is much to be said for early cholecystectomy, morbidity, mortality and cost being less than with medical management followed by elective cholecystectomy 6–8 weeks later. If performed during the first 3 days, cholecystectomy has a mortality of about 0.5%. In about 50% of patients the acute attack of cholecystitis will resolve without surgery. However, 20% have to be admitted later and may require urgent surgery. Emergency surgery is known to carry a higher risk than elective operation particularly in elderly patients over 75 years old [28] and in the diabetic patient where elective cholecystectomy is preferred once symptoms have developed [66].

About 10% of patients with acute cholecystitis will have associated common duct stones. These are diagnosed by jaundice, dark urine and pale stools, fever, a raised serum bilirubin and alkaline phosphatase with operative findings of a large cystic and common bile duct with possible palpable stones [59]. These indicate exploration of the common duct unless inflammation around the porta hepatis renders dissection and identification of structures difficult.

Percutaneous cholecystostomy

In the very severely ill patient, percutaneous transhepatic cholecystostomy is a safe and effective technique. It has a particular application in the elderly patient with acute complicated cholecystitis [188]. The method can either be done under ultrasound control or fluoroscopy after initial opacification using a skinny needle. A drainage catheter can be left to drain the gallbladder, or aspiration of the fluid and pus can be done without continued drainage [189]. This approach is combined with intensive antibiotic therapy. Bile/pus is sent for culture. There is usually rapid relief of clinical symptoms. The technique may allow the patient to be brought to elective surgery in a better clinical condition. In the inoperable patient, after recovery, the catheter can be removed and the patient treated conservatively often without recurrence [188].

Empyema of the gallbladder

If the cystic duct remains blocked by a stone and infection sets in, empyema may develop. This can occur in cholangitic patients after endoscopic sphincterotomy particularly if duct clearance is not achieved [34].

Symptoms may be of an intra-abdominal abscess (fever, rigors, pain), although the elderly patient may appear relatively well [41].

Treatment is with antibiotics and surgery. There is a high post-operative rate of septic complications [180]. Percutaneous cholecystostomy is a valuable alternative.

Perforation of the gallbladder

Acute calculous cholecystitis may proceed to complete necrosis of the gallbladder wall and perforation. The gallstone may erode the necrotic wall; alternatively, dilated infected Rokitansky–Aschoff sinuses may provide a weak point for rupture.

Rupture usually takes place at the fundus which is the least well vascularized part of the gallbladder. Rupture into the free peritoneal cavity is rare and, more usually, adhesions form between adjacent organs with local abscess formation. Rupture into adjacent viscera leads to internal biliary fistula.

The patient presents with nausea, right upper quadrant pain and vomiting. A right upper quadrant mass is palpable in 50%, and a similar number are febrile. The diagnosis is often overlooked. CT and ultrasound are of value in showing peritoneal fluid, abscess and gallstones.

There are three clinical types [151].

1 *Acute with bile peritonitis*. A history of gallbladder disease is rare. Associated systemic conditions include vascular insufficiency or immunodeficiency such as atherosclerosis, diabetes mellitus, collagen diseases, corticosteroid use or decompensated cirrhosis. The diagnosis should be suspected in any immunocompromised patient such as an AIDS sufferer with an acute abdomen. Prognosis is poor with a mortality of about 30%. Treatment is by massive antibiotics and restoration of the fluid balance. The gangrenous gallbladder wall is removed or drained percutaneously or surgically. Any abscess must also be drained.

2 *Subacute with pericholecystic abscess*. These patients have chronic gallstone disease and the picture is intermediate between the acute and chronic types.

3 *Chronic* with cholecystenteric fistula formation, such as between gallbladder and colon.

Emphysematous cholecystitis

The term is used to denote infection of the gallbladder with gas-producing organisms, *Escherichia coli, Clostrid-*

ium welchii, or anaerobic streptococci. The primary lesion is occlusion of the cystic duct or cystic artery. Infection is secondary [115].

The condition classically affects male diabetics who develop features of severe, toxic, acute cholecystitis. An abdominal mass may be palpable.

Radiology. In the plain film the gallbladder is seen as a sharply outlined pear-shaped gas shadow. Occasionally air may be seen infiltrating the wall and surrounding tissue. Gas is not apparent in the cystic duct which is blocked by a gallstone. In the erect position, a fluid level is seen in the gallbladder; this is never seen with an internal biliary fistula.

CT may also show the gas. Ultrasound has been less useful in diagnosis [60].

Treatment. Antibiotics are given in large doses. Cholecystostomy and drainage are done either surgically or by the percutaneous method.

Chronic calculous cholecystitis

This is the commonest type of clinical gallbladder disease. The association of chronic cholecystitis with stones is almost constant.

Aetiological factors, therefore, include all those related to gallstones. The chronic inflammation may follow acute cholecystitis, but usually develops insidiously.

Pathology

The gallbladder is usually contracted with a thickened, sometimes calcified, wall. The contained bile is turbid with a sediment of debris, called biliary sludge. Stones are seen lying loosely embedded in the wall or in meshes of an organizing fibrotic network. One stone is usually lodged in the neck. The mucosa is ulcerated and scarred. Histologically the wall is thickened and congested with lymphocytic infiltration and occasionally complete destruction of the mucosa.

Clinical features

Chronic cholecystitis is difficult to diagnose because of the ill-defined symptoms. A familial incidence of gallstones, previous attacks of jaundice, multiparity and obesity form a suggestive background. Rarely, episodes of acute cholecystitis punctuate the course. The patient may experience episodes of biliary colic.

Abdominal distension or epigastric discomfort, especially after a fatty meal, may be temporarily relieved by belching. Nausea is common, but vomiting is unusual unless there are stones in the common bile duct. Apart from a constant dull ache in the right hypochondrium and epigastrium, pain may be experienced in the right scapular region, substernally or at the right shoulder. Post-prandial pain may be relieved by alkalis.

Local tenderness over the gallbladder and a positive Murphy sign are very suggestive.

Investigations

The temperature, leucocyte count, haemoglobin and erythrocyte sedimentation rate are within normal limits. A plain abdominal X-ray may show calcified gallstones. However, the imaging technique of first choice is ultrasound, which may show gallstones within a fibrosed gallbladder with a thickened wall. Non-visualization of the gallbladder is also a significant finding. On oral cholecystography the gallbladder is usually non-functioning. CT scan may show gallstones but this technique is not appropriate in the diagnostic work-up of chronic cholecystitis.

Differential diagnosis

Fat intolerance, flatulence and post-prandial discomfort are common symptoms. Even if associated with imaging evidence of gallstones, the calculi are not necessarily responsible, for stones are frequently present in the symptom-free.

Other disorders producing a similar clinical picture must be excluded before cholecystectomy is advised, otherwise symptoms persist post-operatively. These include peptic ulceration, hiatus hernia, irritable bowel syndrome, chronic urinary tract infections and functional dyspepsias. A careful appraisal of the patient's psychological make-up is necessary.

Since approximately 10% of young to middle-aged adults have gallstones which can be shown by imaging, it is possible that symptomatic gallbladder disease may be over-diagnosed. On the other hand ultrasound and oral cholecystography are only about 95% accurate and symptomatic gallbladder disease may therefore sometimes be unrecognized.

Prognosis

This chronic disease is compatible with good life expectancy. However, once symptoms, particularly biliary colic, are experienced, the patients tend to remain symptomatic with about a 40% chance of recurrence within 2 years [177]. Gallbladder cancer is a very rare, later development.

Treatment

Medical measures may be tried if the diagnosis is uncertain and a period of observation is desirable. This is especially so when indefinite symptoms are associated with a well-functioning gallbladder. The general condition of the patient may contraindicate surgery. The place of medical dissolution and shock-wave lithotripsy of radiolucent stones has already been discussed.

Obesity should be corrected. Fat intake will depend upon the functional state of the gallbladder: if it is non-functioning, a low-fat diet is advisable. Cooked fats are badly tolerated and should be avoided.

Cholecystectomy

This is indicated if the patient is symptomatic, particularly with repeated episodes of pain. If laparoscopic cholecystectomy is planned but there is a suspicion of a common duct calculus, preoperative endoscopic cholangiography and sphincterotomy with removal of the stone is indicated. This is because laparoscopic removal of common duct stones is difficult, requires special equipment and is not yet within the capability of most operators. The same management applies if open cholecystectomy is planned and common duct stones are suspected. Operative cholangiography, exploration of the bile duct and stone removal is the alternative, with insertion of a T-tube.

The T-tube is in position in the common bile duct for about 2 weeks. Culture of the bile is done, for post-operative complications are often due to sepsis. Cholangiography precedes removal of the T-tube.

Slight and transient increases in serum bilirubin and transaminase levels can be expected in the normal post-operative cholecystectomy course [57]. Greater increases indicate such complications as a retained duct stone or injury to the bile ducts.

Acalculous cholecystitis [194]

Acute

About 5–10% of acute cholecystitis in adults and about 30% in children occurs in the absence of stones. The most frequent predisposing cause is an associated critical condition such as after major non-biliary surgery, multiple injuries, major burns, recent childbirth, severe sepsis, mechanical ventilation and parenteral nutrition. A severe form was seen in American soldiers seriously wounded in Vietnam, and suffering from bacteraemia [99].

The pathogenesis is unclear and probably multifactorial, but bile stasis (lack of gallbladder contraction), increased bile viscosity and lithogenicity, and gallbladder ischaemia are thought to play a role. Administration of opiates which increase sphincter of Oddi tone may also reduce gallbladder emptying. Shock impairs cystic arterial blood flow.

Clinical features should be those of acute calculous

cholecystitis with fever, leucocytosis and right upper quadrant pain but diagnosis is often difficult because of the overall clinical state of the patient who may be intubated, ventilated and receiving narcotic analgesics.

There may be laboratory evidence of cholestasis with a raised bilirubin and alkaline phosphatase. Cholescintigraphy is less accurate (about 40%) than in calculous cholecystitis having a high false positive rate. Ultrasound and CT are complementary and useful in showing a thickened gallbladder wall (>4 mm), pericholecystic fluid or subserosal oedema without ascites, intramural gas, or a sloughed mucosal membrane [26]. Because of the difficulties of diagnosis a high index of suspicion is needed particularly in patients at risk. Males are more affected than females and the mortality is twice as high as in acute calculous cholecystitis [52]. Gangrene and perforation of the gallbladder are common.

Treatment is emergency cholecystectomy. In the critically ill patient percutaneous cholecystostomy under ultrasound guidance may be life saving.

Chronic

This is a difficult diagnosis as the clinical condition resembles others, particularly the irritable bowel syndrome and the functional dyspepsias. Ultrasound scans and oral cholecystograms are normal. Nevertheless, chronic inflammation can be present in the gallbladder without gallstones and relief will follow cholecystectomy.

Cholescintigraphy with measurement of the gallbladder ejection fraction 15 minutes after CCK infusion is valuable. Normal individuals have an ejection fraction of 70% [25]. In those with an ejection fraction less than 40%, cholecystectomy relieved symptoms in 10 of 11 patients [195]. In 10 patients who did not undergo cholecystectomy, symptoms persisted. Gallbladders removed showed chronic cholecystitis, muscle hypertrophy and/or a narrowed cystic duct. CCK infusion reproduces pain in some patients. This technique may help define which patients with this syndrome will benefit from cholecystectomy.

Typhoid cholecystitis

Circulating typhoid bacilli are filtered by the liver and excreted in the bile. The biliary tract, however, is infected in only about 0.2% of patients with typhoid fever.

Acute typhoid cholecystitis is becoming very rare. Signs of acute cholecystitis appear at the end of the second week or even during convalescence, and are sometimes followed by perforation of the gallbladder.

Chronic typhoid fever cholecystitis and the typhoid carrier state. The typhoid carrier passes organisms in the faeces derived from a focus of infection in the gallbladder or biliary tract. Chronic typhoid cholecystitis is symptomless.

The carrier state is not cured by antibiotic therapy. Cholecystectomy is successful if there is not an associated infection of the biliary ducts. Chronic typhoid cholecystitis is not an important cause of gallstones.

Biliary carriers of other salmonellae have been reported and treated with ampicillin and cholecystectomy.

Acute cholecystitis in AIDS

Four per cent of 904 patients with AIDS needed an abdominal operation over a 4-year period [142]. One-third of these cases had cholecystectomy for acute acalculous cholecystitis. This is thought to occur because of gallbladder stasis and increased bile lithogenicity in the critically ill patient, opportunistic pathogens, such as cytomegalovirus (CMV) and cryptosporidia, or vascular insufficiency due to oedema or infection.

Patients present with fever, right upper quadrant pain and tenderness. The white cell count is often normal but with a left shift of neutrophils. Ultrasound shows features of acute cholecystitis (without stones). The cystic duct is usually patent although cholecystography may fail to show the gallbladder [1].

Treatment is by cholecystectomy with a mortality of around 30% due to sepsis.

Other infections

Actinomycosis can very rarely involve the gallbladder. *Giardiasis* can result in biliary dysfunction [53]. *Staphylococcus* infection [181] and *Vibrio cholerae* [54] can be associated with acalculous cholecystitis.

Other associations

A *chemical cholecystitis* may follow long-term infusion of cytotoxic drugs, such as FUDR, into the hepatic artery [165].

Diseases involving the *cystic artery*, such as polyarteritis nodosa, may lead to cholecystitis [131].

The gallbladder may be involved in *Crohn's disease* [101].

Cholesterolosis of the gallbladder

Cholesterol esters and other lipids are deposited in the submucosal and epithelial cells as small, yellow, lipid specks and, together with the intervening red bile-stained mucosa, give the appearance of a ripe strawberry. The deposits are at first found only on the mucosal ridges but later they extend into the troughs. As more lipid is deposited, it projects into the lumen as polyps which may become pedunculated. The change is confined to the gallbladder and never extends to the ducts.

The lipid is seen in reticulo-endothelial xanthoma cells of the mucosa, which is not inflamed. The cholesterolosis is related to the biliary, not blood, cholesterol concentration.

The aetiology is uncertain [77]. The bile is supersaturated with cholesterol and indeed half the patients do develop gallstones. The gallbladder mucosa may simply be taking up excess cholesterol from bile. Other possibilities are a defect in submucosal macrophages or synthesis of surplus lipid by the mucous membrane.

Cholesterolosis is common, being found in about 10% of autopsies, most frequently in middle-aged women.

There is controversy concerning the relation of cholesterolosis to symptoms. However, cholesterolosis may sometimes cause right upper quadrant pain and features causing confusion with the irritable bowel syndrome. Diagnosis is difficult. Oral cholecystography, preferably with CCK, shows filling defects in the gallbladder in only a third, and ultrasonography is usually negative.

The pain is reproduced by intravenous CCK in those patients who will be relieved by cholecystectomy [93].

Xanthogranulomatous cholecystitis

This is an uncommon inflammatory disease of the gallbladder characterized by a focal or diffuse destructive inflammatory process with lipid-laden macrophages. Macroscopically, areas of xanthogranulomatous cholecystitis appear as yellow masses within the wall of the gallbladder [147]. The gallbladder wall is invariably thickened and cholesterol or mixed gallstones are usually present.

The pathogenesis is uncertain, but an inflammatory response to extravasated bile, possibly from ruptured Rokitansky–Aschoff sinuses, is likely.

Symptoms often begin as an episode of acute cholecystitis and persist for up to 5 years. There is extension of yellow tissue into adjacent organs. Fistulae from gallbladder to skin or duodenum may develop [147]. At operation, carcinoma seems likely and frozen sections are usually required to make the differentiation.

Adenomyomatosis

This may affect the gallbladder wall profusely or locally. There is epithelial proliferation with muscular hypertrophy and mural diverticulae (Rokitansky–Aschoff sinuses), which may be seen as spots of contrast medium outside the lumen of the gallbladder on oral cholecystography after a fatty meal. Adenomyomatosis (*cholecystitis glandularis proliferans*) may cause chronic symptoms which are relieved by cholecystectomy [116].

Porcelain gallbladder

This rare condition (0.4–0.8% at cholecystectomy) is due to extensive calcification of the gallbladder wall. Circumferential calcification is seen on abdominal X-ray or CT. Ultrasound is helpful in showing the extent of involvement of the gallbladder wall. The condition is associated with a high frequency of cancer (12–61%) [168].

Post-cholecystectomy problems

Poor results after cholecystectomy can be expected in about one-third of patients. These may be due to wrong diagnosis. About 95% of those *with gallstones* are freed of symptoms or improved post-operatively. The absence of stones questions the original diagnosis. The patients may have been suffering from a psychosomatic or some other disorder including non-visceral pain [163]. Results of surgery are poor when done for vague symptoms such as flatulence or dyspepsia [148, 187]. A biliary cause is likely if stones are found at cholecystectomy and if a period of relief follows the operation. The colon and pancreas are common alternative culprits.

Symptoms may be related to technical difficulties at the time of surgery. These include traumatic *biliary stricture* (Chapter 32) and *residual calculi*. A *cystic duct remnant*, greater than 1 cm, is very frequent after cholecystectomy. It is an infrequent cause of symptoms in the absence of common duct stones. These patients benefit from removal of the cystic duct or gallbladder remnant.

Amputation neuromas can be demonstrated in some patients but removal offers no relief and this seems unlikely to be the cause of the symptoms.

Chronic pancreatitis, a common association of *choledocholithiasis* may persist post-operatively.

Endoscopic cholangiography is of particular value in the investigation of post-cholecystectomy symptoms. Residual calculi, stricture, ampullary stenosis, a cystic duct stump or normal appearances are significant findings.

Sphincter of Oddi dysfunction [25]

This has been an area of controversy but now appears to be a cause of post-cholecystectomy pain in some patients. Two forms exist.

Papillary stenosis is defined as narrowing of all or part of the sphincter of Oddi. There is fibrosis. It may follow injury due to stones [65], operative instrumentation, biliary infection or pancreatitis. There may be episodes of pain associated with abnormal liver function tests. On ERCP the bile duct is dilated and drains slowly. The basal sphincter tone is raised on manometry and is not reduced by smooth muscle relaxants.

Sphincter of Oddi (biliary) dyskinesia is a more diffi-

Table 31.3 Sphincter of Oddi dysfunction: classification

Group I (definite)	
Biliary-type pain	
Abnormal liver function tests (SGOT; alkaline phosphatase >2× normal) documented on two or more occasions	
Dilated common bile duct >12 mm	
Delayed drainage of ERCP contrast >45 minutes	(Manometry unnecessary)
Group II (presumptive)	
Biliary-type pain and one or two of other group I criteria	(Manometry essential)
Group III (possible)	
Biliary-type pain only. No other abnormalities	(Manometry essential if intervention contemplated)

cult area. Biliary manometry shows a range of abnormalities including sphincter spasm, increased phasic contraction frequency (tachyoddia), paradoxical contraction response to CCK, and abnormal propagation of phasic waves.

There are clinical features (table 31.3) which are valuable in management decisions in patients with sphincter of Oddi dysfunction. Group I benefit from sphincterotomy in 90% of cases. In group II manometry is important. Patients with an elevated basal sphincter pressure have greater benefit from sphincterotomy than those with a normal pressure (91 versus 42%) [48]. Studies continue in group III. Sphincterotomy in those with abnormal manometry may be beneficial in only 50% of patients [25]. Drug treatment with nitrates, nitroglycerin and calcium channel blockers which relax the sphincter are worth a trial, although the vasodilating side-effects limit their therapeutic use.

Gallstones in the common bile duct (choledocholithiasis)

The majority of stones in the common bile duct have migrated from the gallbladder and are associated with calculous cholecystitis. Migration is related to the size of the stone relative to the cystic and common bile duct. The stones grow in the common bile duct so causing biliary obstruction and facilitating the migration of further stones from the gallbladder.

Secondary stones that are not of gallbladder origin usually follow partial biliary obstruction due to such causes as residual calculus, traumatic stricture, sclerosing cholangitis or congenital biliary abnormalities. Infection may be the initial event. Stones are brown, single or multiple, oval and conforming to the long axis of the duct (fig. 31.1b). They tend to impact in the ampulla of Vater.

Effects of common bile duct stones

Bile duct obstruction is usually partial and intermittent since the calculus exerts a ball-valve action at the lower end of the common bile duct. In the anicteric, hepatic histology is virtually normal. In the icteric, it shows cholestasis. In chronic cases, the bile ducts show concentric scarring (fig. 31.12) and eventually secondary sclerosing cholangitis and biliary cirrhosis.

Cholangitis. The stagnant bile is readily infected, probably from the intestines. The bile becomes opaque and dark brown (*biliary sludge*). Rarely the infection is more acute and the bile is purulent. The common bile duct is thickened and dilated, with desquamated or ulcerated mucosa, especially in the ampulla of Vater. The cholangitis may spread to the intra-hepatic bile ducts and, in severe and prolonged infections, cholangitic liver

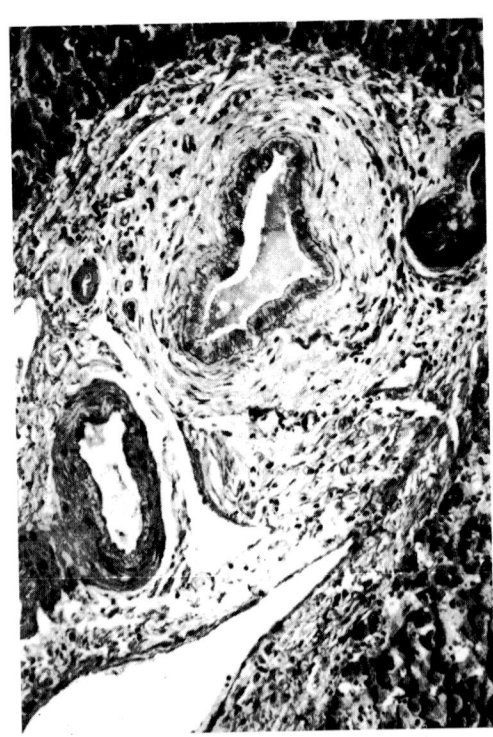

Fig. 31.12. Portal zone from operative liver biopsy of a patient with sclerosing cholangitis secondary to choledocholithiasis. The duct wall shows concentric fibrosis and the whole portal area is fibrosed. (Stained PAS, ×126).

abscesses are seen. The cut section of liver shows cavities containing bile-stained pus, communicating with the bile ducts. *Escherichia coli* is the commonest infecting organism. Others include *Klebsiella, Streptococcus, Bacteroides* and *Clostridia* .

Acute or *chronic pancreatitis* may result from stones wedged in or passing through the ampulla of Vater.

Clinical syndromes

Choledocholithiasis may be silent and symptomless, discovered only by imaging at the time of a routine cholecystectomy for chronic calculous cholecystitis. Alternatively, the stones may cause an acute cholangitis with jaundice, pain and fever. In the elderly, they may present simply as mental and physical debility [24]. Residual stones detected early or late after cholecystectomy can be silent or symptomatic.

Acute jaundice and cholangitis

The classical picture is of an elderly, obese woman, with a previous history of flatulent indigestion, fat intolerance and mid-epigastric pain, presenting with jaundice, abdominal pain, chills and fever.

The cholestatic *jaundice* is usually mild, but may be deep or absent. Bile duct obstruction is rarely complete and the amount of pigment fluctuates in the stools.

Pain occurs in about three-quarters of the patients, is usually severe, colicky, and intermittent and needs analgesics for its relief. Sometimes it is a constant, sharp, severe pain. The site may be right upper quadrant or epigastric. It radiates to the back and to the right scapula. It is associated with vomiting. Palpation of the epigastrium is painful. *Fever* occurs in about a third of the patients, and there may be rigors. *Urine* is dark according to the degree of obstruction.

The *bile* shows a mixed growth of intestinal organisms, predominantly *E. coli.*

The *serum* has the changes of cholestasis with raised alkaline phosphatase, gamma glutamyl transpeptidase and conjugated bilirubin. In acute obstruction the transaminase levels may be briefly very high.

If the stones obstruct the main pancreatic duct, the serum amylase concentration may rise sharply and there may be clinical pancreatitis.

Haematological changes. The polymorph leucocyte count may be raised; the level depends on the acuteness and severity of the cholangitis.

Blood culture should be performed repeatedly during the febrile period and the antibiotic sensitivity of any organism determined. Although the usual organisms encountered are the colonic ones, such as *E. coli* and anaerobic streptococci, other unusual ones such as

Pseudomonas must be sought. Bile should be taken at ERCP for culture.

X-rays of the abdomen may show calculi in the gallbladder, or more medially and posteriorly in the common bile duct.

Ultrasound may show dilated intra-hepatic ducts although more often these are undilated. Stones in the lower end of the common bile duct are often missed by ultrasound.

Cholangiography, preferably by the endoscopic route, confirms the presence of stones.

Diagnosis

This is not difficult if jaundice follows biliary colic and febrile episodes. Too often, however, there is only vague indigestion, no fever, no gallbladder tenderness and an unhelpful white blood count. Alternatively, the patient may present with painless jaundice and sometimes itching. The condition must then be differentiated from other forms of cholestasis, including neoplastic, and acute virus hepatitis (table 12.2). The bile in total biliary obstruction due to carcinoma is rarely infected and cholangitis is unusual unless there has been previous endoscopic cholangiography or stenting.

Residual common duct stones

Between 5 and 10% of patients having a cholecystectomy with exploration of the common bile duct will have retained stones. Calculi in the intra-hepatic ducts are especially liable to be overlooked. Residual bile duct calculi may be suspected if the patient experiences pain when the T-tube draining the bile duct is temporarily clamped. Cholangiography reveals filling defects. Sepsis and cholangitis occur post-operatively. In many instances, however, the residual bile duct calculi remain silent for many years.

Management of common duct stones

This depends on the clinical situation — emergency or elective—on the age and general condition of the patient and on the facilities and clinical expertise available. Antibiotics will be given for their systemic effect to treat or prevent septicaemia, and this is probably more relevant than their entry into bile. They are only temporarily effective in controlling the septicaemia if the bile duct is completely obstructed. Drainage is needed. Other measures include control of fluid and electrolyte balance and intramuscular vitamin K, if the patient is jaundiced.

Acute obstructive suppurative cholangitis

Clinical features that identify this syndrome are fever,

jaundice, pain, confusion and hypotension (*Reynold's pentad*) [145]. Renal failure and thrombocytopenia, as part of a disseminated intravascular coagulopathy, develop later. This situation is an emergency.

Laboratory tests should include blood cultures, as well as white cell and platelet count and, prothrombin time renal function tests. *Ultrasound* should show a dilated biliary system with or without stones. Even if negative, *endoscopic cholangiography* should be done if the clinical features suggest bile duct disease.

Treatment is by intensive broad spectrum antibiotics and emergency decompression of the biliary tract, as well as resuscitation with intravenous fluids. Antibiotics should cover Gram-negative colonic bacteria [185]. The combination of an aminoglycoside (gentamicin or netilmicin), ureidopenicillin (piperacillin or azlocillin) and metronidazole (for anaerobes) is a good choice. Most cases are caused by common duct stones. ERCP is done with sphincterotomy and stone removal, if coagulation and anatomy permit. If not, then a nasobiliary tube is inserted.

The aim of any procedure is to *guarantee decompression of the biliary system*. The endoscopic approach is now accepted as the first choice, although there is still a mortality of around 5–10% [90, 94]. If this method fails, percutaneous trans-hepatic external bile drainage is the second choice. Surgical operation carries a greater mortality than non-surgical techniques being between 16 and 40% [94]. After decompression there is usually rapid resolution of septicaemia and toxaemia. If not, drainage of the biliary system should be checked, or another source of sepsis sought, such as empyema of the gallbladder or liver abscess.

Antibiotics should be continued for one week, particularly if there are gallbladder stones, since empyema can be a complication of cholangitis.

Such severe cholangitis may also complicate malignant strictures after there has been previous intervention, for example cholangiography without drainage, or alternatively endoprosthesis insertion. The management is the same: antibiotics and biliary decompression.

Acute cholangitis

The same principles govern the treatment of cholangitis of a lesser degree, but endoscopic therapy can be done electively if the patient's condition allows.

Malaise and fever are followed by shivering and sweating (*Charcot's intermittent biliary fever*). Not all features of Charcot's triad (fever, pain, jaundice) may be present. Laboratory tests include white cell count, renal and liver function tests and blood cultures. Ultrasound may show biliary tract disease.

The choice of antibiotic depends upon the state of the patient and local policy. Ampicillin, ciprofloxacin [56] or

a cephalosporin usually suffices. Cholangiography is timed according to the state of the patient and the response to antibiotics. Stones are removed after endoscopic sphincterotomy. If the stones cannot be extracted, bile drainage is provided by insertion of a naso-biliary tube or endoprosthesis (fig. 31.13). This management is necessary independent of whether the gallbladder is *in situ* or not. Subsequent decisions on cholecystectomy are discussed below.

Multivariate analysis has identified seven features associated with a poor outcome in a mixed group of patients with cholangitis treated surgically and by non-surgical techniques. These were acute renal failure, cholangitis associated with liver abscess or liver cirrhosis, cholangitis secondary to high malignant biliary strictures or after percutaneous trans-hepatic cholangiography, female gender and age over 50 years [49].

Common duct stones without cholangitis

These are treated by elective endoscopic cholangiography, sphincterotomy and stone removal. Antibiotics are given to cover the procedure. Stone removal without sphincterotomy is possible, in most cases after balloon dilatation of the sphincter [106, 113]. Pancreatitis occurs

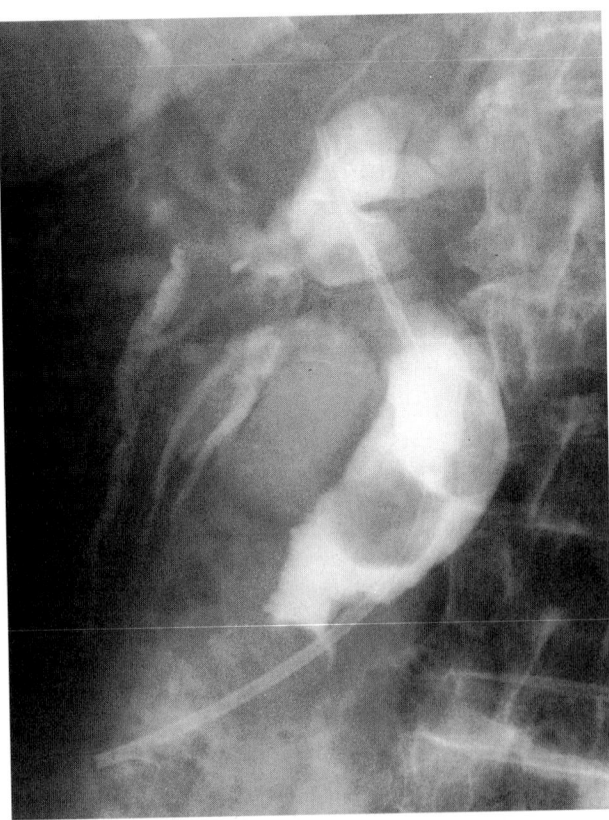

Fig. 31.13. ERCP in a patient with acute cholangitis. The common bile duct contains a large stone which could not be removed. Stent inserted to provide drainage.

in 4–10%. Randomized studies against sphincterotomy are awaited.

Patients with gallbladder *in situ*

Endoscopic sphincterotomy is definitive for residual post-cholecystectomy stones with only 10% having further biliary problems [61], a similar outcome to surgical treatment.

If the gallbladder is still *in situ* and contains stones, subsequent management depends upon the age and clinical state of the patient. In the elderly, several studies have shown that, after endoscopic sphincterotomy, only 5–10% need cholecystectomy for gallbladder disease during 1–9 year follow-up [39, 75]. In this group it is reasonable to leave the gallbladder *in situ* unless problems arise. In younger patients — the age point is as yet undefined — cholecystectomy is generally recommended because of the concern that complications will occur in the long term.

Acute gallstone pancreatitis

Gallstones travelling down the bile duct may produce acute pancreatitis as they pass through the ampulla. The stones are usually small and pass into the faeces. The inflammation then subsides. Sometimes the stone does not pass out of the ampulla and pancreatitis persists and may be severe. Abnormal liver function tests, particularly transaminases, and ultrasound are the most useful tests to identify the patient with pancreatitis due to gallstones [35]. Early ERCP and sphincterotomy to remove the stone(s) has been shown to reduce complications and cholangitis in patients with severe, but not mild, pancreatitis [45, 123]. The optimal timing and selection of patients awaits further study.

Biliary sludge may also cause attacks of acute pancreatitis [92].

Large common duct stones

Stones greater than 15 mm in diameter are difficult or impossible to remove with a standard basket or balloon after sphincterotomy. Some may pass spontaneously. There are several options (table 31.4), which will depend upon local expertise and enthusiasm.

Mechanical lithotripsy may crush the stone but is limited by basket design and stone shape and size. 90% success is possible with the latest baskets [164].

The easiest method particularly in the poor risk patient is the insertion of an *endoprosthesis* (fig. 31.13), which may be long term, or temporary before surgical or endoscopic duct clearance. Early complications are seen in 12%, with a mortality of 4% [122]. Biliary colic, cholangitis and cholecystitis are late complications [136].

Table 31.4. Non-surgical treatment options for large common duct stones

Mechanical lithotripsy ('crushing basket')
Endoprosthesis
Extracorporeal shock-wave lithotripsy
Contact dissolution therapy
Electrohydraulic lithotripsy
Laser lithotripsy

Extracorporeal shock-wave lithotripsy can fragment 70–90% of large common duct stones with subsequent clearance of fragments through the sphincterotomy in the majority of patients, with less than a 1% 30-day mortality [158, 186].

Dissolution therapy with methyl tert-butyl ether instilled via a nasobiliary tube may clear stones but there are practical problems in administration [84].

Endoscopic electrohydraulic and laser lithotripsy remain experimental [125].

Trans T-tube tract removal of stones

Retained stones can be removed percutaneously along the T-tube tract in 77–96% of patients [127] with a complication rate of 2–4% (cholangitis, pancreatitis, tract perforation). The T-tube should have been in place for 4–5 weeks before stone removal to allow a fibrous tract to form. This method is complementary to endoscopic sphincterotomy, which with a T-tube in place is successful in about 75% [127]. The endoscopic approach may be favoured in the older patient, or when there is patient intolerance of the T-tube, or the size or path of the T-tube is not optimal.

Intra-hepatic gallstones

Stones in the intra-hepatic ducts are particularly common in certain parts of the world such as the Far East and Brazil where they are associated with parasitic infestation. Gallstones form in chronically obstructed bile ducts due to such conditions as anastomotic biliary-enteric stricture, primary sclerosing cholangitis, or Caroli's disease. They are usually of brown pigment type. Secondary hepatic infection results in multiple abscesses.

Percutaneous techniques using large bore transhepatic catheters, combined with surgery if necessary, can clear stones in over 90% of patients, leaving the majority symptom-free [137]. The percutaneous transhepatic cholangioscopic approach can clear intra-hepatic stones in over 80% [78]. There is stone recurrence in 50% of patients with duct strictures.

Mirizzi's syndrome

Impaction of a gallstone in the cystic duct or neck of the gallbladder can cause partial common hepatic duct obstruction [118]. Recurrent cholangitis follows and the stone may erode into the common hepatic duct creating a single cavity [29].

Diagnosis is by endoscopic or percutaneous cholangiography (fig. 31.14). Ultrasound shows gallstones lying outside the hepatic duct. Surgery consists of removing the cystic duct, the diseased gallbladder and the impacted stone.

Biliary fistulae

External

These follow procedures such as cholecystotomy, transhepatic biliary drainage or T-tube choledochotomy. Very rarely they follow gallstones, carcinoma of the gallbladder or trauma.

Because of the sodium and bicarbonate content of bile, patients with external biliary fistulae run a risk of severe hyponatraemic acidosis and rise in blood urea levels.

Distal biliary obstruction contributes to the failure of the fistula to heal and the placement of an endoscopic or percutaneous biliary stent is followed by healing without the need for further difficult re-operations.

Internal

In 80% these are due to long-standing calculous cholecystitis. The inflamed gallbladder, containing stones, adheres and ruptures into a segment of the intestine, usually the duodenum and less often the colon (fig. 31.15). The ejected gallstones may be passed or cause intestinal obstruction (*gallstone ileus*), usually in the terminal ileum.

Post-operative biliary strictures, especially after multiple efforts at repair, may be complicated by fistula formation, usually hepatico-duodenal or hepatico-gastric. The fistulae are short, narrow and liable to block.

Biliary fistulae may also follow rupture of a chronic duodenal ulcer into the gallbladder or common bile duct. Fistulae may also develop between the colon and biliary tract in ulcerative colitis or Crohn's disease, especially if the patient is receiving corticosteroid therapy.

Rarely, in a patient with duct stones, a fistula can develop between the hepatic duct and portal vein with massive bilaemia, shock and death [6].

Clinical features

There is a long history of biliary disease. The fistula may

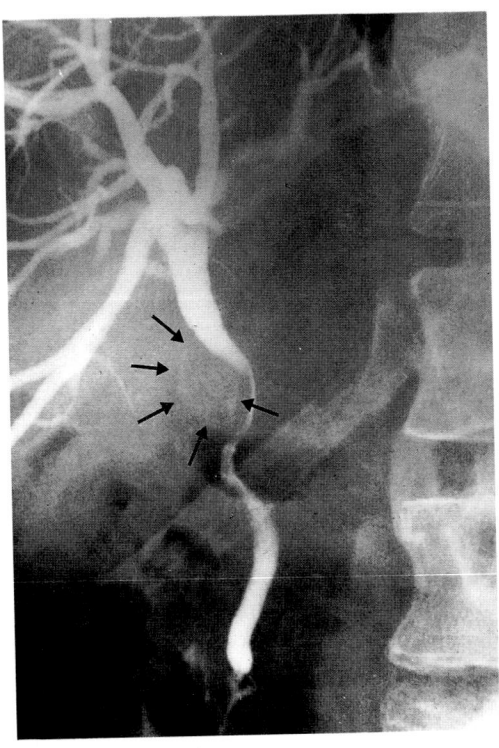

Fig. 31.14. Percutaneous cholangiography in Mirizzi's syndrome shows a large gallstone impacted in the cystic duct (arrowed) which has caused partial obstruction to the common hepatic duct.

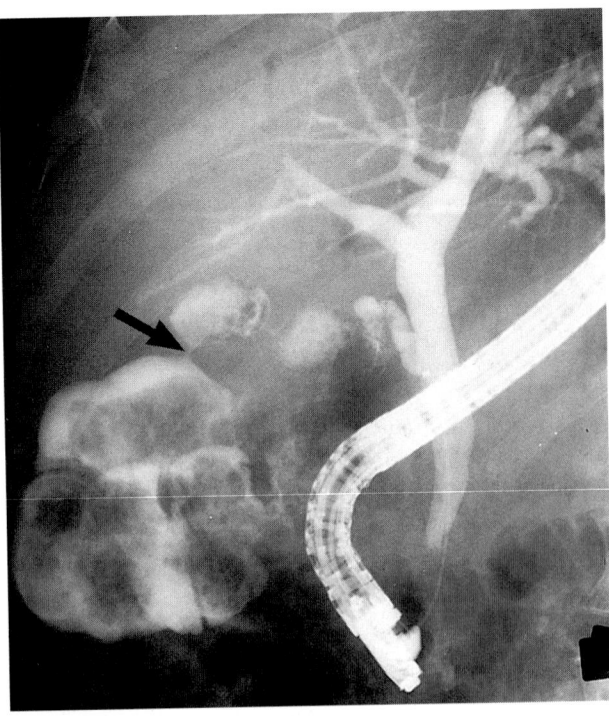

Fig. 31.15. ERCP showing a fistula between the gallbladder and colon (large arrow).

be symptomless and, when the gallstones have discharged into the intestine successfully, the fistula closes. Such instances are often diagnosed only at the time of a later cholecystectomy.

About one-third give a history of jaundice or are jaundiced on admission [155]. Pain may be absent or as severe as biliary colic. The features of cholangitis may be present. In cholecystocolic fistula the common bile duct may be filled with calculi, putrefying matter and faeces, which cause the severe cholangitis. Bile salts entering the colon produce severe diarrhoea. Weight loss is profound.

Radiological features

These include gas in the biliary tract and the presence of a gallstone in an unusual position. A barium meal, in the case of a cholecysto-duodenal fistula, or a barium enema, in the case of a cholecystocolic fistula, may fill the biliary tree. Small bowel distension may be noted.

ERCP should be diagnostic (fig. 31.15).

Treatment

Fistulae due to gallbladder disease are treated surgically. Adherent viscera are separated and closed and cholecystectomy and drainage of the common bile duct performed. The operative mortality is high, being about 13% [155].

Endoscopic treatment of common duct stones can result in closure of cholecystocolic and bronchobiliary fistulae [20, 112].

Gallstone ileus

A gallstone over 2.5 cm in diameter entering the intestine causes obstruction, usually of the ileum, less often of the duodeno-jejunal junction, duodenal bulb, pylorus or even colon [23]. The impacted gallstone may excite an inflammatory reaction in the intestinal wall, or cause intussusception.

Gallstone ileus is very rare but is the cause of a quarter of all cases of non-strangulated intestinal obstruction in patients over 65 [89].

The patient is usually an elderly, afebrile female possibly with a preceding history suggestive of chronic cholecystitis. The onset is insidious, with nausea, occasional vomiting, colicky abdominal pain and a somewhat distended but flaccid abdomen. Complete intestinal obstruction leads to rapid physical deterioration.

A plain X-ray of the abdomen may reveal loops of distended bowel with fluid levels and possibly the obstructing stone. Gas may be seen in the biliary tract and gallbladder, indicating a biliary fistula.

The plain film on admission is diagnostic in about 50%

of patients. Ultrasound, barium studies, and CT provide diagnostic information in a further 25%. Leucocytosis is not usual unless there is associated cholangitis with pyrexia.

Pre-operative diagnosis is made in about 70% of cases [23].

The prognosis is poor and worsens with age.

Treatment

After the patient's general condition has been restored by intravenous fluids and electrolytes, the intestinal obstruction should be relieved surgically. This may be done by manual propulsion of the stone or by enterotomy. Whether fistula repair and cholecystectomy are also done at the time of the first operation to relieve intestinal obstruction depends upon the operative feasibility and the clinical state of the patient [23]. Mortality is about 20%.

Haemobilia [196]

Haemorrhage into the biliary tract may follow trauma including surgical and needle liver biopsy, aneurysms of the hepatic artery or one of its branches, extra- or intrahepatic tumours of the biliary tract, gallstone disease, inflammation of the liver especially helminthic or pyogenic, rarely varicose veins related to portal hypertension and sometimes in association with primary liver cancer. Iatrogenic disease such as liver biopsy and percutaneous trans-hepatic cholangiography and bile drainage now accounts for 40% [196].

Clinical features are pain related to the passage of clots, jaundice and haematemesis and melaena. Minor episodes may be shown only by positive occult blood tests in faeces.

Diagnosis is suspected whenever upper gastrointestinal bleeding is associated with biliary colic, jaundice or a right upper quadrant mass or tenderness.

ERCP or percutaneous cholangiography may show the clot in the ducts (fig. 31.16).

Treatment

Many clear spontaneously. Otherwise the treatment consists of angiographic embolization [32]. Surgical exploration and drainage of the common bile duct may be indicated if bleeding and colic do not subside.

Bile peritonitis

Aetiology

Post-cholecystectomy. Bile may leak from small bile channels between the gallbladder and liver or from an im-

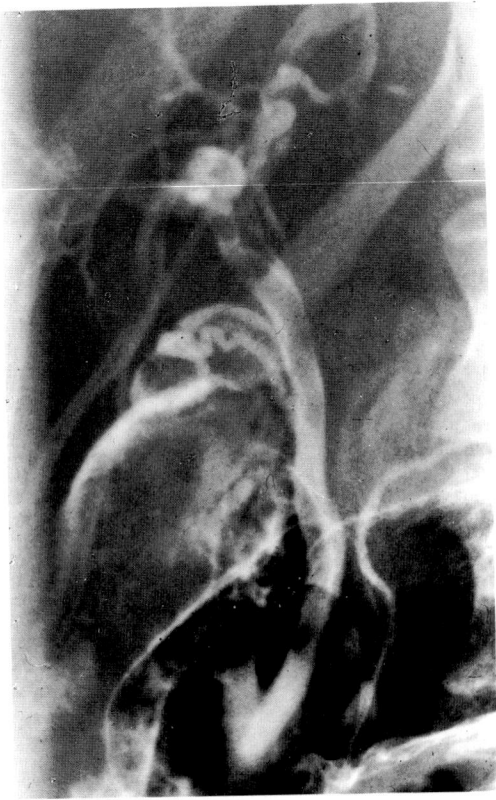

Fig. 31.16. ERCP in haemobilia shows filling defects, representing blood clot in the bile ducts.

perfectly ligated cystic duct. If the biliary pressure is raised, perhaps by a residual common duct stone, leakage is facilitated and the subsequent paraductal bile accumulation favours the development of biliary stricture.

Post-transplantation. Leakage of bile from the bile duct anastomosis is a recognized complication of liver transplantation.

Rupture of the gallbladder. Empyema or gangrene of the gallbladder may lead to rupture and the formation of an abscess; this is localized by previous inflammatory adhesions.

Trauma. Crushing or gunshot wounds may involve the biliary tree. Needle biopsy of the liver or percutaneous cholangiography may rarely be complicated by puncture of the gallbladder or of a dilated intra-hepatic bile duct in a patient with deep cholestasis. Oozing of bile rarely follows operative liver biopsy.

Spontaneous. Biliary peritonitis may develop in patients with prolonged, deep obstructive jaundice without demonstrable breach of the biliary tree. This is presumably due to bursting of minute intra-hepatic bile ducts.

Common bile duct perforation is exceedingly rare. The factors concerned are similar to those for perforated gallbladder. They include increases of intra-ductal pressure, calculous erosion and necrosis of the duct wall secondary to thrombosis [85].

Spontaneous perforation of the extra-hepatic bile ducts is a rare cause of jaundice in infancy, the most common site being at the confluence of the cystic and common hepatic duct [98]. Pathogenesis is unknown.

Clinical picture

This depends on whether the bile is localized or free in the peritoneal cavity, sterile or infected. Free rupture of bile into the peritoneal cavity causes severe shock. Due to the irritant effect of bile salts, large quantities of plasma are poured into the ascitic fluid. The onset is with excruciating, generalized, abdominal pain. Examination shows a shocked, pale, motionless patient, with low blood pressure and persistent tachycardia. There is board-like rigidity of the diffusely tender abdomen. Paralytic ileus is a frequent complication. Bile peritonitis should always be considered in any patient with unexplained intestinal obstruction. In a matter of hours secondary infection follows and the temperature rises while abdominal pain and tenderness persist.

Laboratory findings are non-contributory. There may be haemoconcentration. Abdominal paracentesis reveals bile, usually infected. Serum bilirubin rises and this is followed by increase in alkaline phosphatase levels. Cholescintigraphy or cholangiography will show the leakage of bile. Bile drainage by the endoscopic or percutaneous route has improved the prognosis.

Treatment

Fluid replacement is imperative. Paralytic ileus may demand intestinal intubation. Antibiotics are given to prevent secondary infection.

Rupture of the gallbladder is treated by cholecystectomy. Biliary leakage from the common bile duct can be treated by endoscopic stenting (with or without sphincterotomy) or naso-biliary drainage. If the leak does not seal over in 7–10 days, surgery may be necessary.

Association of gallstones with other diseases

Colorectal and other cancers

Population surveys show that gallstone sufferers do not seem at increased risk from other malignancies except perhaps that of the gallbladder [111] and extra-hepatic bile ducts [42].

Faecal bile acids and cholesterol metabolites may promote colorectal oncogenesis [160]. Cholecystectomy may allow greater exposure of conjugated primary bile acids to anaerobic intestinal bacteria and so the increased production of carcinogens. Cholecystectomy and gallstones and colorectal cancer have been linked, although the association was not confirmed in recent studies [3, 47]. The association may be related to increased diagnostic efforts in symptomatic post-cholecystectomy patients incidentally detecting early colorectal cancers.

Diabetes mellitus

About 30% of all diabetics over 20 years old have gallstones, compared with 11.6% of the general population of the same age. The older diabetic tends to be obese, and this may be the important factor in gallstone formation. Chronic pancreatitis and gallstones are associated and chronic pancreatitis can produce mild diabetes.

Patients with diabetes may have large, poorly contracting and poorly filling gallbladders [86]. A 'diabetic neurogenic gallbladder' syndrome has been postulated.

Patients with diabetes mellitus undergoing cholecystectomy, whether emergency or elective, have increased complications. These are probably related to associated cardiovascular or renal disease and to more advanced age [134].

References

1 Aaron JS, Wynter CD, Kirton OC *et al.* Cytomegalovirus associated with acalculous cholecystitis in a patient with acquired immune deficiency syndrome. *Am. J. Gastroenterol.* 1988; **83**: 879.

2 Abei M, Nuutinen H, Kawczak P *et al.* Identification of human biliary alpha$_1$-acid glycoprotein as a cholesterol crystallization promoter. *Gastroenterology* 1994; **106**: 231.

3 Adami HO, Meirik O, Gustavsson S *et al.* Colorectal cancer after cholecystectomy: absence of risk increase within 11–14 years. *Gastroenterology* 1983; **85**: 859.

4 Afdhal NH, Smith BF. Cholesterol crystal nucleation: a decade-long search for the missing link in gallstone pathogenesis. *J. Hepatol.* 1990; **11**: 699.

5 Amaral JF, Thompson WR. Gallbladder disease in the morbidly obese. *Am. J. Surg.* 1985; **149**: 551.

6 Antebi E, Adar R, Zweig A *et al.* Bilemia: an unusual complication of bile duct stones. *Ann. Surg.* 1973; **177**: 274.

7 Barkun JS, Barkun AN, Sampalis JS *et al.* Randomised controlled trial of laparoscopic versus mini cholecystectomy. *Lancet* 1992; **340**: 1116.

8 Barkun JS, Fried GM, Barkun AN *et al.* Cholecystectomy without operative cholangiography: implications for common bile duct injury and retained common bile duct stones. *Ann. Surg.* 1993; **218**: 371.

9 Barton JR, Russell RCG, Hatfield ARW. Management of bile leaks after laparoscopic cholecystectomy. *Br. J. Surg.* 1995; **82**: 980.

10 Bateson MC. Gallstone epidemiology. *Curr. Gastroenterol.* 1986; **5**: 120.

11 Bateson MC, Bouchier IAD, Maudgal DP *et al.* Calcification of radiolucent gallstones during treatment with ursodeoxycholic acid. *Br. Med. J.* 1981; **283**: 645.

12 Behar J, Lee KY, Thompson WR *et al.* Gallbladder contrac-

13 Bennion LJ, Ginsberg RL, Garnick MB *et al.* Effects of oral contraceptives on the gallbladder bile of normal women. *N. Engl. J. Med.* 1976; **294**: 189.

14 Berci G. Cholangiography and choledochoscopy during laparoscopic cholecystectomy, its place and value. *Digest. Surg.* 1991; **8**: 92.

15 Bergman JJGHM, van den Brink JR, Rauws EAJ *et al.* Treatment of bile duct lesions after laparoscopic cholecystectomy. *Gut* 1996; **38**: 141.

16 Berr F, Mayer M, Sackmann MF *et al.* Pathogenic factors in early recurrence of cholesterol gallstones. *Gastroenterology* 1994; **106**: 215.

17 Boston Collaborative Drug Surveillance Program. Oral contraceptives and venous thromboembolic disease: surgically confirmed gall-bladder disease and breast tumours. *Lancet* 1973; **i**: 1399.

18 Boston Collaborative Drug Surveillance Program. Gallbladder disease, venous disorders, breast tumours: relation to estrogens. *N. Engl. J. Med.* 1974; **290**: 15.

19 Bouchier IAD. Postmortem study of the frequency of gallstones in patients with cirrhosis of the liver. *Gut* 1969; **10**: 705.

20 Brem H, Gibbons GD, Cobb G *et al.* The use of endoscopy to treat bronchobiliary fistula caused by choledocholithiasis. *Gastroenterology* 1990; **98**: 490.

21 Carey MC, Small DM. The physical chemistry of cholesterol solubility in bile: relationship to gallstone formation and dissolution in man. *J. Clin. Invest.* 1978; **61**: 998.

22 Cheslyn-Curtis S, Gillams AR, Russell RCG *et al.* Selection, management, and early outcome of 113 patients with symptomatic gall stones treated by percutaneous cholecystolithotomy. *Gut* 1992; **33**: 1253.

23 Clavien P-A, Richon J, Burgan S *et al.* Gallstone ileus. *Br. J. Surg.* 1990; **77**: 737.

24 Cobden I, Lendrum R, Venables CLO *et al.* Gallstones presenting as mental and physical debility in the elderly. *Lancet* 1984; **i**: 1062.

25 Corazziari E, Jensen PF, Hogan WJ *et al.* Functional disorders of the biliary tract. *Gastroenterol. Int.* 1993; **6**: 129.

26 Cornwell EE, Rodriguez A, Mirvis SE *et al.* Acute acalculous cholecystitis in critically injured patients. *Ann. Surg.* 1989; **210**: 52.

27 Cox MR, Wilson TG, Luck AJ *et al.* Laparoscopic cholecystectomy for acute inflammation of the gall bladder. *Ann. Surg.* 1993; **218**: 630.

28 Crumplin MKH, Jenkinson LR, Kassab JY *et al.* Management of gallstones in a district general hospital. *Br. J. Surg.* 1985; **72**: 428.

29 Csendes A, Carlos Diaz J, Burdiles P *et al.* Mirizzi syndrome and cholecystobiliary fistula: a unifying classification. *Br. J. Surg.* 1989; **76**: 1139.

30 Cucchiaro G, Watters CR, Rossitch J *et al.* Deaths from gallstones: incidence and associated clinical factors. *Ann. Surg.* 1989; **209**: 149.

31 Cuschieri A, Berci G. *Laparoscopic Biliary Surgery.* Blackwell Scientific Publications, Oxford, 1990.

32 Czerniak A, Thompson JN, Hemingway AP *et al.* Hemobilia: a disease in evolution. *Arch. Surg.* 1988; **123**: 718.

33 Davids PHP, Ringers J, Rauws EAJ *et al.* Bile duct injury after laparoscopic cholecystectomy: the value of endoscopic retrograde cholangiopancreatography. *Gut* 1993; **34**:

1250.

34 Davidson BR, Neoptolemos JP, Carr-Locke DL. Endoscopic sphincterotomy for common bile duct calculi in patients with gallbladder *in situ* considered unfit for surgery. *Gut* 1988; **29**: 114.

35 Davidson BR, Neoptolemos JP, Leese T *et al.* Biochemical prediction of gallstones in acute pancreatitis: a prospective study of three systems. *Br. J. Surg.* 1988; **75**: 213.

36 Diehl AK, Beral V. Cholecystectomy and changing mortality from gallbladder cancer. *Lancet* 1981; **i**: 187.

37 Donald JJ, Cheslyn-Curtis S, Gillams AR *et al.* Percutaneous cholecystolithotomy: is gall stone recurrence inevitable? *Gut* 1994; **35**: 692.

38 Dowling RH. The enterohepatic circulation. *Gastroenterology* 1972; **62**: 122.

39 Dowsett JF, Vaira D, Polydorou A *et al.* Interventional endoscopy in the pancreaticobiliary tree. *Am. J. Gastroenterol.* 1988; **83**: 1328.

40 Dunn D, Fowler S, Nair R *et al.* Laparoscopic cholecystectomy in England and Wales: results of an audit by the Royal College of Surgeons of England. *Ann. R. Coll. Surg. Engl.* 1994; **76**: 269.

41 Editorial. Empyema of the gallbladder — a forgotten disease. *Lancet* 1984; **i**: 606.

42 Ekborn A, Hsieh C, Yuen J *et al.* Risk of extrahepatic bile duct cancer after cholecystectomy. *Lancet* 1993; **342**: 1262.

43 Erlinger S, Go AL, Husson J-M *et al.* Franco-Belgian Cooperative Study of ursodeoxycholic acid in the medical dissolution of gallstones: a double-blind, randomized, dose-response study, and comparison with chenodeoxycholic acid. *Hepatology* 1984; **4**: 308.

44 Ewins DL, Javaid A, Coskeran PB *et al.* Assessment of gall bladder dynamics, cholecystokinin release and the development of gallstones during octreotide therapy for acromegaly. *Q. J. Med.* 1992; **83**: 295.

45 Fan S-T, Lai ECS, Mok FPT *et al.* Early treatment of acute biliary pancreatitis by endoscopic papillotomy. *N. Engl. J. Med.* 1993; **328**: 228.

46 Fornari F, Imberti D, Squillante MM *et al.* Incidence of gallstones in a population of patients with cirrhosis. *J. Hepatol.* 1994; **20**: 797.

47 Friedman GD, Goldhaber MK, Queensbury CP Jr. Cholecystectomy and large bowel cancer. *Lancet* 1987; **i**: 906.

48 Geenen JE, Hogan WJ, Dodds WJ *et al.* The efficacy of endoscopic sphincterotomy after cholecystectomy in patients with sphincter of Oddi dysfunction. *N. Engl. J. Med.* 1989; **320**: 82.

49 Gigot JF, Leese T, Dereme T *et al.* Acute cholangitis: multivariate analysis of risk factors. *Ann. Surg.* 1989; **209**: 435.

50 Gilat T, Feldman C, Halpern Z *et al.* An increased familial frequency of gallstones. *Gastroenterology* 1983; **84**: 242.

51 Gleeson D, Ruppin DC, Saunders A *et al.* Final outcome of ursodeoxycholic acid treatment in 126 patients with radiolucent gallstones. *Q. J. Med.* 1990; **279**: 711.

52 Glenn F, Becker CG. Acute acalculous cholecystitis. *Ann. Surg.* 1982; **195**: 131.

53 Goldstein F, Thornton JJ, Szydlowski T. Biliary tract dysfunction in giardiasis. *Am. J. Dig. Dis.* 1978; **23**: 559.

54 Gomez NA, Gutierrez J, Leon CJ. Acute acalculous cholecystitis due to *Vibrio cholerae*. *Lancet* 1994; **343**: 1156.

55 Greiner L, Munks C, Wolfgang H *et al.* Gallbladder stone fragments in feces after biliary extracorporeal shock-wave lithotripsy. *Gastroenterology* 1990; **98**: 1620.

56 Gumaste VV. Selected summary: antibiotics and cholangitis. *Gastroenterology* 1995; **109**: 323.

57 Halevy A, Gold-Deutch R, Negri M *et al.* Are elevated liver enzymes and bilirubin levels significant after laparoscopic cholecystectomy in the absence of bile duct injury? *Ann. Surg.* 1994; **219**: 362.

58 Halpern Z, Dudley MA, Kibe A *et al.* Rapid vesicle formation and aggregation in abnormal human biles. A time-lapse video-enhanced contrast microscopy study. *Gastroenterology* 1986; **90**: 875.

59 Hauer-Jensen M, Karesen R, Nygaard K *et al.* Predictive ability of choledocholithiasis indicators. A prospective evaluation. *Ann. Surg.* 1985; **202**: 64.

60 Hawass ND. False negative sonographic finding in emphysematous cholecystitis. *Acta Radiol.* 1988; **29**: 137.

61 Hawes RH, Cotton PB, Vallon AG. Follow-up 6 to 11 years after duodenoscopic sphincterotomy for stones in patients with prior cholecystectomy. *Gastroenterology* 1990; **98**: 1008.

62 Health and Policy Committee, American College of Physicians. How to study the gallbladder. *Ann. Intern. Med.* 1988; **109**: 752.

63 Heaton KW, Emmett PM, Symes CL *et al.* An explanation for gallstones in normal-weight women: slow intestinal transit. *Lancet* 1993; **341**: 8.

64 Henriksson P, Einarsson K, Eriksson A *et al.* Estrogen-induced gallstone formation in males. *J. Clin. Invest.* 1989; **84**: 811.

65 Hernandez CA, Lerch MM. Sphincter stenosis and gallstone migration through the biliary tract. *Lancet* 1993; **341**: 1371.

66 Hickman MS, Schwesinger WH, Page CP. Acute cholecystitis in the diabetic. A case control study of outcome. *Arch. Surg.* 1988; **123**: 409.

67 Hobbs KEF. Laparoscopic cholecystectomy. *Gut* 1995; **36**: 161.

68 Hofmann AF. Medical dissolution of gallstones by oral bile acid therapy. *Am. J. Surg.* 1989; **158**: 198.

69 Holan KR, Holzbach RT, Hermann RE *et al.* Nucleation time: a key factor in the pathogenesis of cholesterol gallstone disease. *Gastroenterology* 1979; **77**: 611.

70 Holzbach RT, Marsh M, Olszewski M *et al.* Cholesterol solubility in bile: evidence that supersaturated bile is frequent in healthy man. *J. Clin. Invest.* 1973; **52**: 1467.

71 Hood K, Gleeson D, Ruppin DC *et al.* Prevention of gallstone recurrence by non-steroidal anti-inflammatory drugs. *Lancet* 1988; **ii**: 1223.

72 Hood KA, Gleeson D, Ruppin DC *et al.* Gall stone recurrence and its prevention: the British/Belgian gall stone study group's post-dissolution trial. *Gut* 1993; **34**: 1277.

73 Hopman WPM, Jansen JBMJ, Rosenbusch G *et al.* Role of cholecystokinin and the cholinergic system in intestinal stimulation of gallbladder contraction in man. *J. Hepatol.* 1990; **11**: 261.

74 Hussaini SH, Pereira SP, Murphy GM *et al.* Composition of gall bladder stones associated with octreotide: response to oral ursodeoxycholic acid. *Gut* 1995; **36**: 126.

75 Ingoldby CJH, El-Saadi J, Hall RI *et al.* Late results of endoscopic sphincterotomy for bile duct stones in elderly patients with gallbladder *in situ*. *Gut* 1989; **30**: 1129.

76 Inoue K, Fuchigami A, Higashide S *et al.* Gallbladder sludge and stone formation in relation to contractile function after gastrectomy. *Ann. Surg.* 1992; **215**: 19.

77 Jacyna MR, Bouchier IAD. Cholesterolosis: a physical

cause of 'functional' disorder. *Br. Med. J.* 1987; **295**: 619.

78 Jan Y-Y, Chen M-F. Percutaneous trans-hepatic cholangioscopic lithotomy for hepatolithiasis: long-term results. *Gastrointest. Endosc.* 1995; **42**: 1.

79 Janowitz J, Kratzer W, Zemmler T *et al.* Gallbladder sludge: spontaneous course and incidence of complications in patients without stones. *Hepatology* 1994; **20**: 291.

80 Jazrawi RP, Pazzi P, Petroni ML *et al.* Postprandial gallbladder motor function: refilling and turnover of bile in health and cholelithiasis. *Gastroenterology* 1995; **109**: 582.

81 Johnston DE, Kaplan MM. Pathogenesis and treatment of gallstones. *N. Engl. J. Med.* 1993; **328**: 412.

82 Jüngst D, Brenner G, Pratschke E *et al.* Low-dose ursodeoxycholic acid prolongs cholesterol nucleation time in gallbladder bile of patients with cholesterol gallstones. *J. Hepatol.* 1989; **8**: 1.

83 Jüngst D, Lang T, von Ritter C *et al.* Cholesterol nucleation time in gallbladder bile of patients with solitary or multiple cholesterol gallstones. *Hepatology* 1992; **15**: 804.

84 Kaye GL, Summerfield JA, McIntyre N *et al.* Methyl-*tert*-butyl ether dissolution therapy for common bile duct stones. *J. Hepatol.* 1990; **10**: 337.

85 Kerstein MD, McSwain NE. Spontaneous rupture of the common bile duct. *Am. J. Gastroenterol.* 1985; **80**: 469.

86 Keshavarzian A, Dunne M, Iber FL. Gallbladder volume and emptying in insulin requiring male diabetics. *Dig. Dis. Sci.* 1987; **32**: 824.

87 Kibe A, Holzbach RT, LaRusso NF *et al.* Inhibition of cholesterol crystal formation by apolipoproteins in supersaturated model bile. *Science* 1984; **225**: 514.

88 Kirtley JA Jr, Holcomb GW Jr. Surgical management of diseases of the gallbladder and common bile duct in children and adolescents. *Am. J. Surg.* 1966; **111**: 39.

89 Kurtz RJ, Heimann TM, Kurtz AB. Gallstone ileus: a diagnostic problem. *Am. J. Surg.* 1983; **146**: 314.

90 Lai ECS, Mok FPT, Tan ESY *et al.* Endoscopic biliary drainage for severe acute cholangitis. *N. Engl. J. Med.* 1992; **326**: 1582.

91 Lee SP, Hayashi A, Kim YS. Biliary sludge: curiosity or culprit? *Hepatology* 1994; **20**: 523.

92 Lee SP, Nicholls JF, Park HZ. Biliary sludge as a cause of acute pancreatitis. *N. Engl. J. Med.* 1992; **326**: 589.

93 Lennard TWJ, Farndon JR, Taylor RMR. Acalculous biliary pain: diagnosis and selection for cholecystectomy using the cholecystokinin test for pain reproduction. *Br. J. Surg.* 1984; **71**: 868.

94 Leung JWC, Sung JY, Chung SCS *et al.* Urgent endoscopic drainage for acute suppurative cholangitis. *Lancet* 1989; **i**: 1307.

95 Leung JWC, Sung JY, Costerton JW. Bacteriological and electron microscopy examination of brown pigment stones. *J. Clin. Microbiol.* 1989; **27**: 915.

96 Leuschner U, Güldütuna S, Hellstern A. Pathogenesis of pigment stones and medical treatment. *J. Gastroenterol. Hepatol.* 1994; **9**: 87.

97 Liddle RA, Goldstein RB, Saxton J. Gallstone formation during weight-reduction dieting. *Arch. Intern. Med.* 1989; **149**: 1750.

98 Lilly JR, Weintraub WH, Altman RP. Spontaneous perforation of the extrahepatic bile ducts and bile peritonitis in infancy. *Surgery* 1974; **75**: 664.

99 Lindberg EF, Grinnan GLB, Smith L. Acalculous cholecystitis in Viet Nam casualties. *Ann. Surg.* 1970; **171**: 152.

100 Lundgren O, Svanvik J, Jivegard L. Enteric nervous system ii. Physiology and pathophysiology of the gallbladder. *Dig. Dis. Sci.* 1989; **34**: 284.

101 McClure J, Banerjee SS, Schofield PS. Crohn's disease of the gallbladder. *J. Clin. Pathol.* 1984; **37**: 516.

102 Macintyre IMc, Wilson RG. Laparoscopic cholecystectomy. *Br. J. Surg.* 1993; **80**: 552.

103 Maclure KM, Hayes KC, Colditz GA *et al.* Weight, diet and the risk of symptomatic gallstones in middle-aged women. *N. Engl. J. Med.* 1989; **321**: 563.

104 McMahon AJ, Fullarton G, Baxter JN *et al.* Bile duct injury and bile leakage in laparoscopic cholecystectomy. *Br. J. Surg.* 1995; **82**: 307.

105 McMahon AJ, Russell IT, Baxter JN *et al.* Laparoscopic versus minilaparotomy cholecystectomy: a randomised trial. *Lancet* 1994; **343**: 135.

106 Macmathuna P, White P, Lennon J *et al.* Endoscopic sphincteroplasty: a novel and safe alternative to papillotomy in the management of bile duct stones. *Gut* 1994; **35**: 127.

107 McSherry CK, Ferstenberg H, Calhoun WF *et al.* The natural history of diagnosed gallstone disease in symptomatic and asymptomatic patients. *Ann. Surg.* 1985; **202**: 59.

108 Majeed AW, Troy G, Nicholl JP *et al.* A randomized, prospective, single-blind comparison of laparoscopic versus small-incision cholecystectomy. *Lancet* 1996; **347**: 989.

109 Makino I, Chijiiwa K, Higashijima H *et al.* Rapid cholesterol nucleation time and cholesterol gall stone formation after subtotal or total colectomy in humans. *Gut* 1994; **35**: 1760.

110 Maringhini A, Ciambra M, Baccelliere P *et al.* Biliary sludge and gallstones in pregnancy: incidence, risk factors, and natural history. *Ann. Intern. Med.* 1993; **119**: 116.

111 Maringhini A, Moreau J, Melton J III *et al.* Gallstones, gallbladder cancer, and other gastrointestinal malignancies. An epidemiologic study in Rochester, Minnesota. *Ann. Intern. Med.* 1987; **107**: 30.

112 Marshall T, Kamalvand K, Cairns SR. Endoscopic treatment of biliary enteric fistula. *Br. Med. J.* 1990; **300**: 1176.

113 May GR, Cotton PB, Edmunds SEJ *et al.* Removal of stones from the bile duct at ERCP without sphincterotomy. *Gastrointest. Endosc.* 1993; **39**: 749.

114 May GR, Sutherland LR, Shaffer EA. Efficacy of bile acid therapy for gallstone dissolution: a meta-analysis of randomised trials. *Aliment. Pharmacol. Ther.* 1993; **7**: 139.

115 May RE, Strong R. Acute emphysematous cholecystitis. *Br. J. Surg.* 1971; **58**: 453.

116 Meguid MM, Aun F, Bradford ML. Adenomyomatosis of the gallbladder. *Am. J. Surg.* 1984; **147**: 260.

117 Millat B, Fingerhut A, Deleuze A *et al.* Prospective evaluation in 121 consecutive unselected patients undergoing laparoscopic treatment of choledocholithiasis. *Br. J. Surg.* 1995; **82**: 1266.

118 Mirizzi PL. Sindrome del conducto hepatico. *J. Int. Chir.* 1948; **8**: 731.

119 Mok HYI, Druffel ERM, Rampone WH. Chronology of cholelithiasis. Dating gallstones from atmospheric radiocarbon produced by nuclear bomb explosions. *N. Engl. J. Med.* 1986; **314**: 1075.

120 Nagase M, Hikasa Y, Soloway RD *et al.* Gallstones in western Japan: factors affecting the prevalence of intrahepatic gallstones. *Gastroenterology* 1980; **78**: 684.

121 National Institutes of Health Consensus Development

Conference. Statement on gall stones and laparoscopic cholecystectomy. *Am. J. Surg.* 1993; **165**: 390.

122 Navicharen P, Rhodes M, Flook D *et al*. Endoscopic retrograde cholangiopancreatography (ERCP) and stent placement in the management of large common bile duct stones. *Aust. N.Z. J. Surg.* 1994; **64**: 840.

123 Neoptolemos JP, Carr-Locke DL, London NJ *et al*. Controlled trial of urgent endoscopic retrograde cholangiopancreatography and endoscopic sphincterotomy versus conservative treatment for acute pancreatitis due to gallstones. *Lancet* 1988; **2**: 979.

124 Neoptolemos JP, Hofmann AF, Moossa AR. Chemical treatment of stones in the biliary tree. *Br. J. Surg.* 1986; **73**: 515.

125 Neuhaus H, Hoffmann W, Zillinger C *et al*. Laser lithotripsy of difficult bile duct stones under direct visual control. *Gut* 1993; **34**: 415.

126 Núñez L, Amigo L, Mingrone G *et al*. Biliary aminopeptidase-*N* and the cholesterol crystallisation defect in cholelithiasis. *Gut* 1995; **37**: 422.

127 Nussinson E, Cairns SR, Vaira D *et al*. A 10 year single centre experience of percutaneous and endoscopic extraction of bile duct stones with T tube *in situ*. *Gut* 1991; **32**: 1040.

128 Offner GD, Gong D, Afdhal NH. Identification of a 130-kilodalton human biliary concanavalin A binding protein as aminopeptidase N. *Gastroenterology* 1994; **106**: 755.

129 Ohya T, Schwarzendrube J, Busch N *et al*. Isolation of a human biliary glycoprotein inhibitor of cholesterol crystallization. *Gastroenterology* 1993; **104**: 527.

130 O'Leary DP. Biliary cholesterol transport and the nucleation defect in cholesterol gallstone formation. *J. Hepatol.* 1995; **22**: 239.

131 Parangi S, Oz MC, Blume RS *et al*. Hepatobiliary complications of polyarteritis nodosa. *Arch. Surg.* 1991; **126**: 909.

132 Pattinson NR, Chapman BA. Distribution of biliary cholesterol between mixed micelles and non-micelles in relation to fasting and feeding in humans. *Gastroenterology* 1986; **91**: 697.

133 Pauletzki J, Sailer C, Kluppelberg U *et al*. Gallbladder emptying determines early gallstone clearance after shock-wave lithotripsy. *Gastroenterology* 1994; **107**: 1496.

134 Pellegrini CA. Asymptomatic gallstones. Does diabetes mellitus make a difference? *Gastroenterology* 1986; **91**: 245.

135 Pelletier G, Delmont J, Capdeville R *et al*. Treatment of gallstones with piezoelectric lithotripsy and oral bile acids. *J. Hepatol.* 1991; **12**: 327.

136 Peters R, Macmathuna P, Lombard M *et al*. Management of common bile duct stones with a biliary endoprosthesis. Report on 40 cases. *Gut* 1992; **33**: 1412.

137 Pitt HA, Venbrux AC, Coleman J *et al*. Intrahepatic stones: the transhepatic team approach. *Ann. Surg.* 1994; **219**: 527.

138 Pixley F, Wilson D, McPherson K *et al*. Effect of vegetarianism on development of gallstones in women. *Br. Med. J.* 1985; **291**: 11.

139 Plevris JN, Bouchier IAD. Defective acid base regulation by the gall bladder epithelium and its significance for gall stone formation. *Gut* 1995; **37**: 127.

140 Podda M, Zuin P, Battezzati PM *et al*. Efficacy and safety of a combination of chenodeoxycholic acid and ursodeoxycholic acid for gallstone dissolution: a comparison with ursodeoxycholic acid alone. *Gastroenterology* 1989; **96**: 222.

141 Portincasa P, Di Ciaula A, Baldassarre G *et al*. Gallbladder motor function in gallstone patients: sonographic and *in vitro* studies on the role of gallstones, smooth muscle function and gallbladder wall inflammation. *J. Hepatol.* 1994; **21**: 430.

142 Raja LA, Rothenberg RE, Odom JW *et al*. The incidence of intra-abdominal surgery in acquired immunodeficiency syndrome: a statistical review of 904 patients. *Surgery* 1989; **105**: 175.

143 Ransohoff DF, Gracie WA. Treatment of gallstones. *Ann. Intern. Med.* 1993; **119**: 606.

144 Ransohoff DF, Gracie WA, Wolfenson LB *et al*. Prophylactic cholecystectomy or expectant management for silent gallstones. *Ann. Intern. Med.* 1983; **99**: 199.

145 Reynolds BM, Dargan FL. Acute obstructive cholangitis: a distinct clinical syndrome. *Ann. Surg.* 1959; **150**: 299.

146 Rhodes M, Allen A, Dowling RH *et al*. Inhibition of human gall bladder mucus synthesis in patients undergoing cholecystectomy. *Gut* 1992; **33**: 1113.

147 Roberts KM, Parsons MA. Xanthogranulomatous cholecystitis: clinico-pathological study of 13 cases. *J. Clin. Pathol.* 1987; **40**: 412.

148 Ros E, Zambon D. Post cholecystectomy symptoms. A prospective study of gallstone patients before and two years after surgery. *Gut* 1987; **28**: 1500.

149 Roslyn JJ, Binns GS, Hughes EFX *et al*. Open cholecystectomy: a contemporary analysis of 42 474 patients. *Ann. Surg.* 1993; **218**: 129.

150 Roslyn JJ, Pitt HA, Mann LL *et al*. Gallbladder disease in patients on long-term parenteral nutrition. *Gastroenterology* 1983; **84**: 148.

151 Roslyn JJ, Thompson JE, Darvin H *et al*. Risk factors for gallbladder perforation. *Am. J. Gastroenterol.* 1987; **82**: 636.

152 Sackmann M, Niller H, Klueppelberg U *et al*. Gallstone recurrence after shock-wave therapy. *Gastroenterology* 1994; **106**: 225.

153 Sackmann M, Pauletzki J, Delius M *et al*. Noninvasive therapy of gallbladder calculi with a radiopaque rim. *Gastroenterology* 1992; **102**: 988

154 Sackmann M, Pauletzki J, Sauerbruch T *et al*. The Munich gallbladder lithotripsy study: results of the first five years with 711 patients. *Ann. Intern. Med.* 1991; **114**: 290.

155 Safaie-Shirazi S, Zike WL, Printen KJ. Spontaneous enterobiliary fistulas. *Surg. Gynecol. Obstet.* 1973; **137**: 769.

156 Sandstad O, Osnes T, Skar V *et al*. Common bile duct stones are mainly brown and associated with duodenal diverticula. *Gut* 1994; **35**: 1464.

157 Sarin SK, Negi VS, Dewan R *et al*. High familial prevalence of gallstones in the first-degree relatives of gallstone patients. *Hepatology* 1995; **22**: 138.

158 Sauerbruch T, Holl J, Sackmann M *et al*. Fragmentation of bile duct stones by extracorporeal shock-wave lithotripsy: a five-year experience. *Hepatology* 1992; **15**: 208.

159 Schoenfield LJ, Berci G, Carnovale RL *et al*. The effect of ursodiol on the efficacy and safety of extracorporeal shock wave lithotripsy of gallstones. *N. Engl. J. Med.* 1990; **323**: 1239.

160 Schottenfeld D, Winiwar SJ. Cholecystectomy and colorectal cancer. *Gastroenterology* 1983; **85**: 966.

161 Schriever CE, Jungst D. Association between cholesterol phospholipid vesicles and cholesterol crystals in human gallbladder bile. *J. Hepatol.* 1989; **9**: 541.

162 Shaffer E, Small DM, Biliary lipid secretion in cholesterol gallstone disease. *J. Clin. Invest.* 1977; **59**: 828.

163 Sharpstone D, Colin-Jones DG. Chronic, non-visceral

abdominal pain. *Gut* 1994; **35**: 833.

164 Shaw MJ, Mackie RD, Moore JP *et al*. Result of a multicentre trial using a mechanical lithotripter for the treatment of large bile duct stones. *Am. J. Gastroenterol.* 1993; **88**: 730.

165 Shea WJ, Demas BE, Goldberg HI *et al*. Sclerosing cholangitis associated with hepatic arterial FUDR chemotherapy: radiographic-histologic correlation. *Am. J. Roentgenol.* 1986; **146**: 717.

166 Shiffman ML, Sugerman HJ, Kellum J *et al*. Changes in gallbladder bile composition following gallstone formation and weight reduction. *Gastroenterology* 1992; **103**: 214.

167 Shiffman ML, Sugerman HJ, Moore EW. Human gallbladder mucosal function. *Gastroenterology* 1990; **99**: 1452.

168 Shimizu M, Miura J, Tanaka T *et al*. Porcelain gallbladder: relation between its type by ultrasound and incidence of cancer. *J. Clin. Gastroenterol.* 1989; **11**: 471.

169 Stewart L, Way LW. Bile duct injuries during laparoscopic cholecystectomy: factors that influence the results of treatment. *Arch. Surg.* 1995; **130**: 1123.

170 Stolzel U, Koszka C, Wolfer B *et al*. Relief of heterogeneous symptoms after successful gall bladder stone lithotripsy and complete stone disappearance. *Gut* 1994; **35**: 819.

171 Strasberg SM, Soper NJ. Management of choledocholithiasis in the laparoscopic era. *Gastroenterology* 1995; **109**: 320.

172 Strasberg SM, Toth JL, Gallinger S *et al*. High protein and total lipid concentration are associated with reduced metastability of bile in an early stage of cholesterol gallstone formation. *Gastroenterology* 1990; **98**: 739.

173 Sugerman HJ, Brewer WH, Schiffman ML *et al*. A multicenter, placebo-controlled, randomised, double-blind, prospective trial of prophylactic ursodiol for the prevention of gallstone formation following gastric-bypass-induced rapid weight loss. *Am. J. Surg.* 1995; **169**: 91.

174 Swidsinski A, Ludwig W, Pahlig H *et al*. Molecular genetic evidence of bacterial colonization of cholesterol gallstones. *Gastroenterology* 1995; **108**: 860.

175 The ACG Committee on FDA-Related Matters. GI drug column. *Am. J. Gastroenterol.* 1990; **85**: 497.

176 Thijs C, Knipschild P, Brombacher P. Serum lipids and gallstones: a case–control study. *Gastroenterology* 1990; **99**: 843.

177 Thistle JL, Cleary PA, Lachin JM *et al*. The natural history of untreated cholelithiasis during the National Cooperative Gallstone Study (NCGS). *Gastroenterology* 1982; **82**: 1197.

178 Thistle JL, May GR, Bender CE *et al*. Dissolution of cholesterol gallbladder stones by methyl *tert*-butyl ether administered by percutaneous transhepatic catheter. *N. Engl. J. Med.* 1989; **320**: 633.

179 Thornton J, Symes C, Heaton K. Moderate alcohol reduces bile cholesterol saturation and raises HDL cholesterol. *Lancet* 1983; **ii**: 819.

180 Thornton JR, Heaton KW, Espiner HJ *et al*. Empyema of the gallbladder—reappraisal of a neglected disease. *Gut* 1983; **24**: 1183.

181 Thomas WEG, Thornton JR, Thompson MH. Staphylococ-

cal acalculous cholecystitis. *Br. J. Surg.* 1981; **68**: 136.

182 Ulloa N, Garrido J, Nervi F. Ultracentrifugal isolation of vesicular carriers of biliary cholesterol in native human and rat bile. *Hepatology* 1987; **7**: 235.

183 Valdiviesco V, Covarrubias C, Siegel F *et al*. Pregnancy and cholelithiasis: pathogenesis and natural course of gallstones diagnosed in early puerperium. *Hepatology* 1993; **17**: 1.

184 van Campenhout I, Prosmanne O, Gagner M *et al*. Routine operative cholangiography during laparoscopic cholecystectomy: feasibility and value in 107 patients. *Am. J. Roentgenol.* 1993; **160**: 1209.

185 van den Hazel SJ, Speelman P, Tytgat GNJ *et al*. Role of antibiotics in the treatment and prevention of acute and recurrent cholangitis. *Clin. Infect. Dis.* 1994; **19**: 279.

186 Van der Hul RL, Plaisier PW, Van Blankenstein M *et al*. Extracorporeal shock wave lithotripsy of common bile duct stones in patients with increased operative risk. *Eur. J. Surg.* 1994; **160**: 31.

187 Vander Velpen GC, Shimi SM, Cuschieri A. Outcome after cholecystectomy for symptomatic gall stone disease and effect of surgical access: laparoscopic versus open approach. *Gut* 1993; **34**: 1448.

188 Van Steenbergen W, Ponette E, Marchal G *et al*. Percutaneous transhepatic cholecystostomy for acute complicated cholecystitis in elderly patients. *Am. J. Gastroenterol.* 1990; **85**: 1363.

189 Verbanck JJ, Demol JW, Ghillebert GL *et al*. Ultrasound-guided puncture of the gallbladder for acute cholecystitis. *Lancet* 1993; **341**: 1132.

190 Vlahcevic ZR, Bell CC Jr, Buhac I *et al*. Diminished bile acid pool size in patients with gallstones. *Gastroenterology* 1970; **59**: 165.

191 Vlahcevic ZR, Bell CC Jr, Gregory DH *et al*. Relationship of bile acid pool size to the formation of lithogenic bile in female Indians of the southwest. *Gastroenterology* 1972; **62**: 73.

192 Walters JRF, Hood KA, Gleeson D *et al*. Combination therapy with oral ursodeoxycholic and chenodeoxycholic acids: pretreatment computed tomography of the gall bladder improves gall stone dissolution efficacy. *Gut* 1992; **33**: 375.

193 Welbourne CRB, Mehta D, Armstrong CP *et al*. Selective preoperative endoscopic retrograde cholangiography with sphincterotomy avoids bile duct exploration during laparoscopic cholecystectomy. *Gut* 1993; **37**: 576.

194 Williamson RCN. Acalculous disease of the gallbladder. *Gut* 1988; **29**: 860.

195 Yap L, Wycherley AG, Morphett AD *et al*. Acalculous biliary pain: cholecystectomy alleviates symptoms in patients with abnormal cholescintigraphy. *Gastroenterology* 1991; **101**: 786.

196 Yoshida J, Donahue PE, Nyhus LM. Hemobilia: review of recent experience with a worldwide problem. *Am. J. Gastroenterol.* 1987; **82**: 448.

Chapter 32
Benign Stricture of the Bile Ducts

Benign strictures of the biliary system are uncommon and usually follow surgery, in particular cholecystectomy, laparoscopic or open (table 32.1). They may also complicate liver transplantation. Other causes are primary sclerosing cholangitis (Chapter 15), chronic pancreatitis and abdominal trauma.

Clinical features are cholestasis with or without sepsis and pain. Diagnosis is by cholangiography. In most cases the underlying cause is clear from the clinical data.

Post-cholecystectomy

Pathogenesis

The bile duct may be ligated, sectioned, perforated by suture material, or damaged by cautery or laser. Several

Table 32.1. Causes of benign bile duct stricture

Post-surgical
    cholecystectomy
    recurrence at bile duct/bowel anastomosis
    extensive hepatic resection
    liver transplantation

Inflammatory
    primary sclerosing cholangitis
    chronic pancreatitis
    radiotherapy

Trauma

Idiopathic

factors contribute to duct injury. There may be mistaken interpretation of the anatomy due to oedema or haemorrhage around an inflamed gallbladder, anomalies of the cystic duct or right hepatic duct (fig. 32.1), or lack of operator experience. Some surgeons advocate careful dissection of the neck of the bladder before dividing either cystic duct or artery. Meticulous dissection of the cystic duct at the infundibulum of the gallbladder is crucial to avoid bile duct injury.

Risk factors for *laparoscopic bile duct injury* include obesity, bleeding, acute cholecystitis and scarring in Calot's triangle (the area between the cystic duct and common hepatic duct). Uncertain anatomy, inexperience and a long procedure are also associated with damage [25, 26]. The threshold at which the decision is made to convert from laparoscopic to open surgery is also important.

A bile duct stricture may also follow prolonged T-tube drainage, cholecystotomy, rough probing of the duct for calculi and attempts at operative cholangiography especially with a normal sized duct. A calculus in the common bile duct is an insufficient cause. Bile leakage after surgery may form peri-ductal abscesses with constriction of the adjoining duct.

Pathological changes

Complete ligation, clipping or transection will become clear clinically in the immediate peri-operative period. With partial injury, the occlusion develops slowly. The

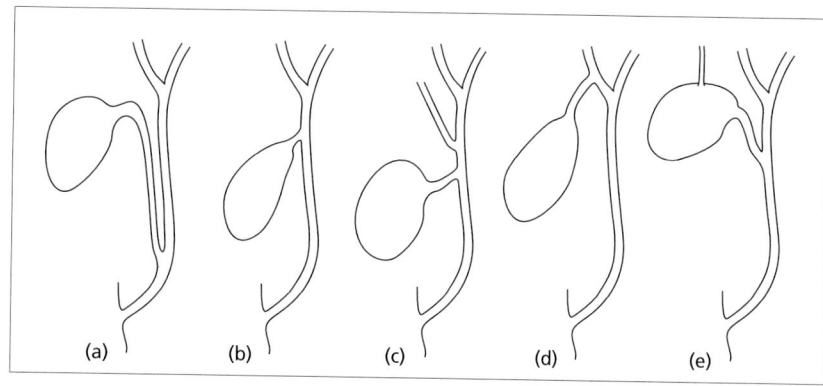

Fig. 32.1. Bile duct anatomy and anomalies associated with problems at cholecystectomy: (a) long cystic duct running adjacent to common duct; (b) short cystic duct; (c) anomalous right hepatic duct joins common duct outside liver; (d) cystic duct originates from right hepatic duct; (e) persistent duct between gallbladder and liver.

(a)   (b)   (c)   (d)   (e)

stricture is usually found in the common hepatic duct, or right hepatic duct particularly when the anatomy is anomalous. Less frequently there is damage to the common bile duct.

The bile duct above the stricture is dilated and thickened, and below is replaced over a variable length by a fibrous cord difficult to identify at operation. The intra-hepatic ducts may be dilated depending on the completeness of the obstruction.

The obstructed bile is viscid and usually infected, with debris or biliary mud. Small calculi may form above the stricture and in the intra-hepatic ducts.

The liver shows cholestasis. Biliary cirrhosis with portal hypertension and splenomegaly will develop with time if the obstruction is not recognized and relieved.

Clinical features

Post-cholecystectomy strictures are more common in females because they have more biliary surgery. Seventy per cent are less than 50 years old.

Bile duct damage occurs in approximately 1 in 400 open cholecystectomies [16]. The incidence is similar for laparoscopic cholecystectomy (1 in 200–400) [6, 15] although it is higher during the initial 'learning curve'. Since strictures can present many years after cholecystectomy, this rate is at present based on a relatively short follow-up experience.

If unrecognized at the time of cholecystectomy, presentation depends upon the degree of damage. Post-operative anorexia, nausea, vomiting, pain, abdominal distension, ileus and delayed recovery should raise the possibility of damage [25], although the presentation is usually more obvious. Complete transection of the main bile duct usually gives pain (bile peritonitis), fever and cholestatic jaundice 3–7 days post-operatively. Alternatively, an external biliary fistula develops. Such a fistula, even for a few days, suggests that biliary damage has occurred and that there is a bile leak. A stricture may follow. The fistula may drain intermittently with episodes of jaundice when it is closed. Sub-hepatic abscesses may develop.

Ligation or clipping the main duct gives escalating cholestatic jaundice with or without cholangitis.

If the bile duct injury is partial, there may be cholestasis early after operation, but it may be several months before obvious jaundice is apparent. This is the period of slow, constrictive fibrosis. Intermittent attacks of cholangitis with or without jaundice usually accompany all grades of biliary stricture. The cholangitis is marked by fever, sometimes very high, with a rigor, sweating and epigastric pain followed by dark urine and pale stools (*Charcot's intermittent biliary fever*). Itching may develop. Milder episodes are also seen which may be anicteric.

The patient may think that they have caught a chill, or had a short-lived viral infection.

With current awareness of the complications of laparoscopic cholecystectomy, and the availability of ERCP and other imaging, patients should not develop the chronic complications of biliary obstruction. The exception is the rare patient in whom multiple surgical attempts have been unsuccessful in providing unimpeded bile flow. Non-surgical methods should not be persisted with at the expense of long-term biliary cirrhosis, except after all attempts in a specialist tertiary referral centre to correct the stricture surgically.

With chronic cholestasis, secondary sclerosing cholangitis and then biliary cirrhosis follow particularly when there is recurrent sepsis. The patient becomes pigmented with clubbing of the fingers. Skin xanthomas are a very late feature. The liver is enlarged and firm. The spleen becomes palpable. Gastrointestinal bleeding due to portal hypertension is a late event; liver failure is terminal. In this now rare circumstance, transplantation has to be considered although the multiple previous operations and biliary sepsis are relative contraindications.

Patients unfortunate enough to suffer bile duct damage at cholecystectomy may become increasingly introspective as the months pass. They keep the most detailed notes of their symptoms and, understandably, become querulous and suspicious of their medical advisers. They need considerable support.

Investigations

Serum biochemistry is of increasing or intermittent cholestasis. The alkaline phosphatase, gamma-glutamyl transpeptidase and bile acid levels may be raised even if the serum bilirubin, which is usually rising, is normal.

Haematological findings include a mild, normochromic, normocytic anaemia. A moderate leucocytosis accompanies the febrile episodes.

Blood cultures may show enteric organisms, in particular *Escherichia coli*, during attacks of cholangitis.

Radiology. Ultrasound will usually show dilated ducts, but normal size ducts do not rule out duct injury with bile leak or intermittent obstruction. Radionuclide biliary imaging may show a leak (see fig. 29.8c). ERCP is the choice for cholangiography (fig. 32.2). When there is complete obstruction or transection of the duct, percutaneous cholangiography and bile duct catheterization are part of the pre-operative work-up and management.

Diagnosis

The history of recent cholecystectomy, the post-

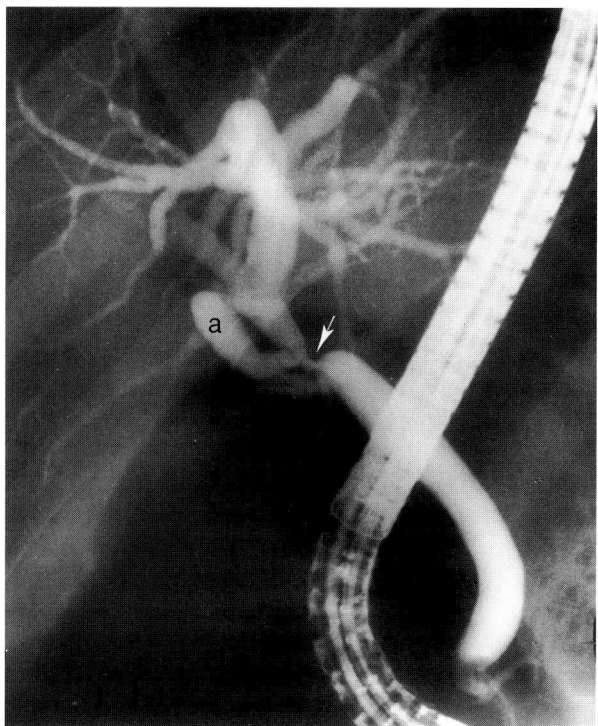

Fig. 32.2. Benign bile duct stricture following laparoscopic cholecystectomy (arrow). Note anomalous right-sided bile duct (a).

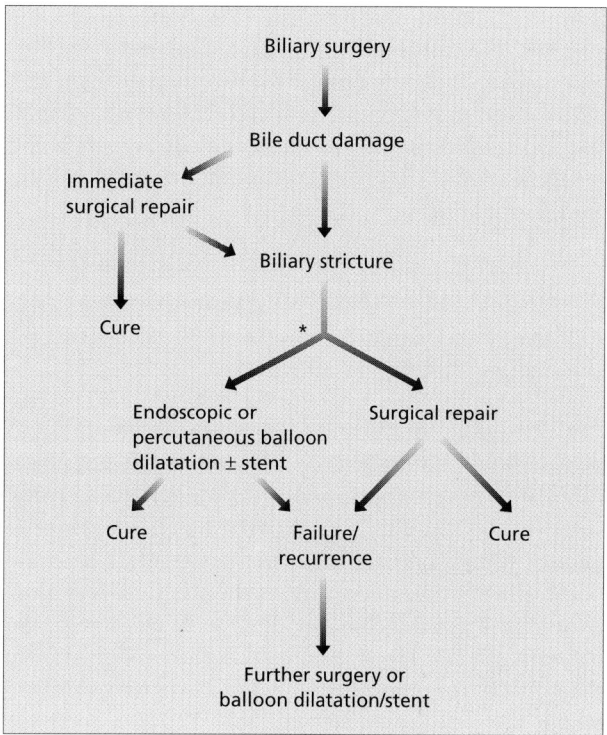

Fig. 32.3. The management of benign biliary stricture. *Choice depends on anatomy, clinical data and expertise available.

operative features and the biochemical and imaging data should lead to cholangiography and the correct diagnosis.

Treatment (fig. 32.3)

Prevention

The majority of strictures would be prevented if (i) cholecystectomy was only performed by experienced surgeons; (ii) the top down approach were used with thorough dissection at the junction of gallbladder infundibulum and cystic duct; and (iii) there were an appropriate threshold for conversion from laparoscopic to open surgery. This is particular so in the presence of acute cholecystitis.

No structure must be clamped or divided until the anatomy has been defined. Important technical points include good exposure, a dry operative field and adequate assistance [18]. The cystic artery must be ligated *before* the cystic duct is tied. Traction on the gallbladder should be avoided.

The place of routine intra-operative cholangiography during laparoscopic cholecystectomy is controversial [4]. If a selective cholangiography policy is followed, the rate of residual stones is low. Some emphasize the importance of showing duct anatomy to reduce duct

damage, but duct damage may still occur despite cholangiography.

Medical

Fluid and electrolyte balance must be maintained particularly in the jaundiced patient and those with a biliary fistula. Antibiotic therapy, based if possible on blood and bile culture, will improve septicaemia but if there is bile duct obstruction, bile duct catheterization and drainage by the endoscopic or percutaneous route is essential to treat sepsis. Bile collections may need percutaneous drainage.

Surgical versus non-surgical intervention [1, 28]

The overriding principle is the importance of referral to a specialist hepato-biliary centre where there will be a joint approach by surgeon, radiologist and endoscopist. For the completely obstructed bile duct (or completely transected duct) surgery is necessary after investigation and preparatory percutaneous bile drainage as appropriate to the individual patient. Bile leakage from cystic duct stump or tiny ducts in the gallbladder bed can usually be managed endoscopically by stent insertion [1]. For the incomplete stricture, although some may be treated non-surgically, for example by endoscopic balloon dilatation and stenting, long-term results are awaited. Overall data from patients having operative treatment in a specialist centre show a good result in 75% with a mean follow-up of 7 years [2]. Thus although non-surgical treatment may be successful in the short and medium term [1], the surgical option has to be considered throughout.

Balloon dilatation and stenting

A dilating balloon may be introduced by the endoscopic or percutaneous trans-hepatic route.

The *endoscopic route* is preferred if the papilla is accessible (Chapter 29). A large channel endoscope is used to allow passage of the balloon catheter. After diagnostic cholangiography a guide wire is placed through the stricture (fig. 29.18). Over this the balloon catheter is passed. Metal markers on the catheter allow accurate positioning of the balloon across the stricture. A sphincterotomy is usually done to allow easy passage of the balloon catheter. The size of balloon chosen depends on the tightness of the stricture, but the eventual aim is to inflate a 6–8 mm diameter balloon. The time that the balloon is kept inflated is not standardized and depends upon the firmness of the stricture and how easily it dilates. In some percutaneous series 15–20 min inflation is used but this depends upon the sedation and analgesia. Dilatation may be very painful. Long inflation times are not as practical with the endoscopic route.

After endoscopic balloon dilatation, one or more endoprostheses may be inserted to splint the stricture for a year (a period chosen empirically) to reduce the risk of re-stenosis [9].

There is greater experience with the *percutaneous trans-hepatic approach* for balloon dilatation. This method has been available for longer and many biliary strictures, particularly those after surgical repair, can only be reached from above, trans-hepatically.

The bile duct is catheterized percutaneously in the usual way (see Chapter 29). A guide-wire, usually a steerable variety, is negotiated through the stricture, the balloon catheter passed across the stricture and the balloon inflated (fig. 32.4). Again, dilatation to 6–8 mm is usual. Smaller diameter balloons are available for the tighter stricture. After dilatation, an internal–external catheter with numerous side holes sitting above and below the dilated area is left in place. Dilatation can be repeated as often as necessary. The length of time that the balloon is left inflated varies from centre to centre, being 5 to 20 min [27, 31]. Similarly, there are wide differences in the time for which an internal–external drain is left in place after dilatation. Some centres do this only for a few days while others leave the tube in for 6–9 months. How these variables affect outcome is not known [19].

Normally several sessions of dilatation are performed

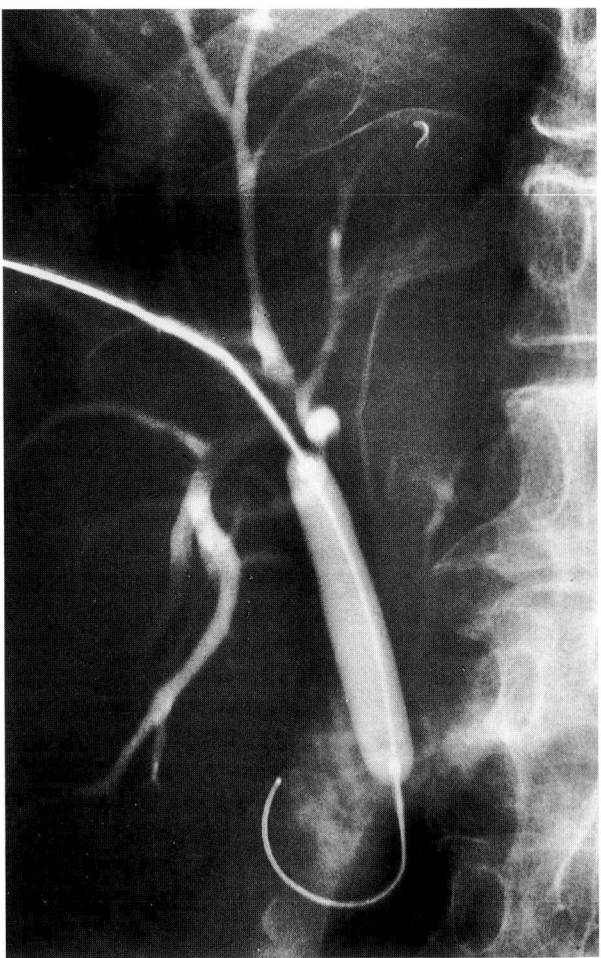

Fig. 32.4. A balloon, introduced trans-hepatically, has been inflated to dilate a benign biliary stricture.

under local anaesthesia and/or intravenous sedation/analgesia. To reduce hospital stay and improve results, a study has been done of balloon dilatation under general anaesthesia at a single session. Results using this approach are as good as with intravenous sedation and multiple procedures [12].

Success rates vary considerably, some reporting 90% patency with a mean follow-up of 3 years [12]. Differences in outcome reflect several factors including the definition of failure, the duration of follow-up and the features of the stricture.

Percutaneous balloon dilatation is usually used initially without endoprosthesis insertion, to avoid leaving a foreign body in the biliary system. In those patients where strictures recur after balloon dilatation, and surgery is not considered appropriate (by a specialist biliary surgeon), a stent may be inserted. With anastomotic strictures, the problem of this approach is the inaccessibility of the stent if it needs to be removed.

Many types of stent are available and there are insufficient data to recommend one over another. Metal stents

(Gianturco and Wallstent) have been used, and one series showed 55% success with a follow-up of 3 years [14].

The percutaneous trans-hepatic approach carries the risks of all other trans-hepatic procedures. Major complications include *sepsis*. 20% may have *haemobilia* [22] for which hepatic arterial embolization may be necessary. Dilatation may produce *bile duct perforation* [7].

No trials compare surgery with balloon dilatation. A retrospective comparison has shown better results with surgical repair than with percutaneous balloon dilatation (88 versus 55%) with a lower rate of bleeding complications [22]. There remains little doubt that surgical repair is the first choice in most cases. Percutaneous, and where possible endoscopic, balloon dilatation has a role in selected patients, particularly those with many previous operations and portal hypertension.

Operative [2, 28]

Operations should be undertaken under antibiotic cover as soon as possible after the original bile duct injury, before obliterative cholangitis, adhesion formation and secondary changes in the liver have added to the risk and technical difficulties. The surgeon attempting the first repair carries a great responsibility because failure reduces the chance of subsequent cure. The best surgeon should therefore be the first to re-operate rather than each intervention being undertaken by one of greater skill and reputation than his predecessor.

The operation chosen will depend mainly on two factors — the site and length of the stricture and the amount of duct available for repair. Any operation must provide excision of the stricture with mucosal apposition between the duct lining and the intestinal mucosa. The anastomosis must be as large as possible and not under tension.

Even if sufficient duct is available proximally, excision of the stricture and end-to-end anastomosis of the duct is rarely performed. Differences between the calibre of the duct above and below the stricture are too great for a satisfactory anastomosis. Recurrent stricture occurs in 58% of cases.

End-to-end anastomosis should not be performed if: (i) the ends are greater than 2 cm apart; (ii) the injury is not recognized at the time of surgery; (iii) the duct diameter is less than 4 mm [5].

The usual operation is anastomosis of the proximal bile duct to the intestine. An entero-anastomosis is added to minimize reflux from the intestines which would lead to cholangitis. The usual operation is therefore between proximal duct and a Roux-en-Y segment of jejunum (*choledochojejunostomy*). In the case of high stricture, the hepatic duct is used (*hepatico-jejunostomy*) (fig. 32.5).

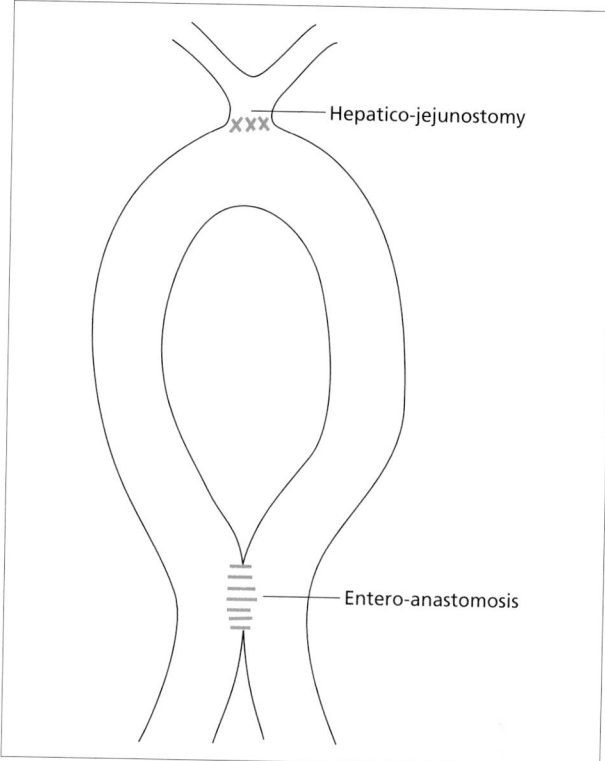

Fig. 32.5. Repair of a high biliary stricture by hepaticojejunostomy and entero-anastomosis.

The need for and duration of splinting of the anastomosis with silastic or other tubing is controversial. Some have recommended 6–12 months of splinting [23], but the impact of trans-anastomotic tubes on the long-term outcome of the repair is questionable [2].

Long-term percutaneous access to the stricture is made possible by the subcutaneous fixation of an extension of the Roux-en-Y loop beyond the biliary anastomosis. The position of the end of the bowel loop under the skin is marked by metal clips so that it can be found by X-ray fluoroscopy. Percutaneous entry into the loop allows cholangiography and, if necessary, further stricture dilatation [10].

Portal hypertension may be controlled by repairing the stricture, otherwise a porta-caval shunt may be necessary. This may be exceedingly difficult due to the adhesions from previous operations and a spleno-renal or meso-caval anastomosis may be the only shunt possible.

Outcome

Following surgical correction of a bile duct stricture in a specialist hepato-biliary unit, a good result, defined as loss of biliary symptoms and no further intervention necessary during a follow-up of 7.2 years, was achieved in 76% of 110 patients [2]. The operative mortality was low (1.8%). These results parallel reports from other specialist centres [22]. Factors associated with a poor outcome are discontinuity of right and left intra-hepatic ducts at the time of stricture repair, three or more attempts at operative repair before referral, hypoalbuminaemia, high serum bilirubin, the presence of liver disease and portal hypertension [2].

Bile duct/bowel anastomotic stricture

Choledocho-jejunostomies and hepatico-jejunostomies may stricture. About 20–25% of patients with such anastomoses will need a further procedure—surgical or radiological. Of the recurrent strictures, two-thirds occur within 2 years and 90% by 5 years [21]. If the patient remains symptom-free for 4 years post-operatively, there is a 90% chance of complete cure. This happy result reduces with the number of operations, but *can* follow many attempts at repair.

Clinical features

Restricturing presents as fever, rigors and jaundice. There may be pain. Previous episodes of mild flu-like symptoms may precede the major attack. Cholangitis does not necessarily indicate re-stenosis, but can be due to intra-hepatic strictures or stones, or improperly constructed enteric loops up to the anastomosis [17].

Investigations

Investigations in the acute phase show leucocytosis and abnormal liver function tests, often with a transient rise in transaminase (due to short-term acute obstruction) with later elevation of alkaline phosphatase and gamma glutamyl transpeptidase.

Radiology

A plain film of the abdomen may show air in the biliary tree (fig. 29.1) and the site of the stricture. Air in the ducts does not necessarily imply a fully patent anastomosis. Ultrasound may show dilated ducts but often does not because of the intermittent nature of the obstruction. Cholangiography by the percutaneous trans-hepatic route shows whether the anastomosis is strictured (fig. 32.6); careful observation of the rate of flow of contrast across the anastomosis is more important than the X-ray film images examined later. If there has been prolonged partial obstruction with recurrent cholangitis, the changes of secondary sclerosing cholangitis may be seen (fig. 32.7).

ERCP can be used for investigation of choledocho-duodenostomies. Entry via a subcutaneous access loop of intestine is an alternative approach for the hilar anastomosis [8].

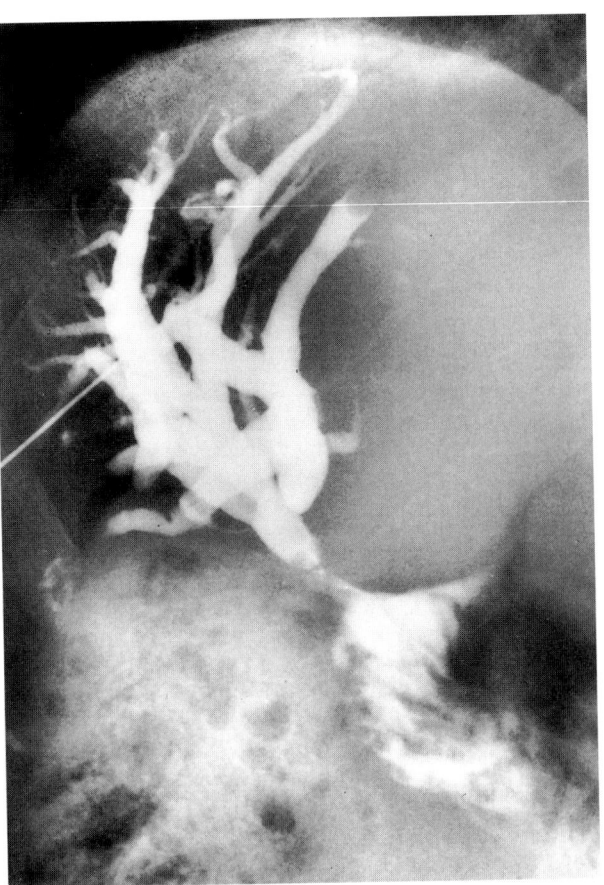

Fig. 32.6. Percutaneous trans-hepatic cholangiogram in a patient with hepatico-jejunostomy following post-cholecystectomy stricture. There is re-stenosis at the anastomosis with dilatation of the ducts in the right lobe.

Investigation of the patient with cholangitis but an apparently patent anastomosis is a challenge, since no one imaging technique can be relied upon to demonstrate the cause [17].

Treatment

This is based on the surgical and non-surgical methods discussed above. Usually access to the biliary system is only possible percutaneously. The importance of a specialist team of surgeon and radiologist is paramount [2].

For the patient with chronic cholestasis, fat-soluble vitamins supplements may be necessary (Chapter 13).

Post liver transplantation

Pathogenesis

Biliary complications follow in 10–20% of patients and include stricture, bile leak, fistulae and cholangitis. Strictures may be *anastomotic* due to technical factors, inflammation after a leak, and fibrosis, or *non-anastomotic*,

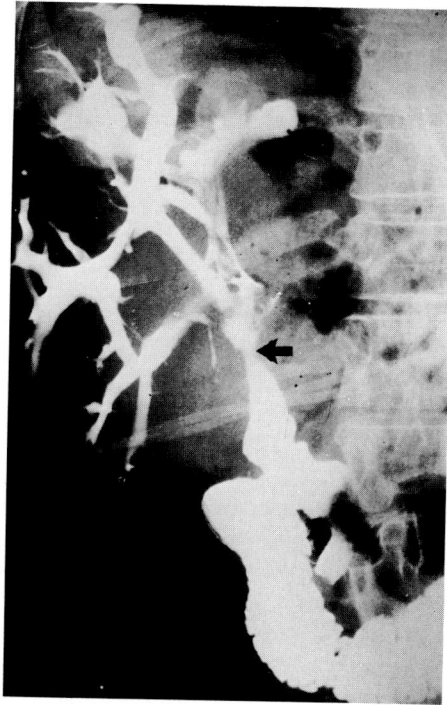

Fig. 32.7. Biliary stricture with patent choledocho-jejunostomy (arrow). Repeated attacks of cholangitis have led to secondary sclerosing cholangitis shown by irregular stenosis and dilatation of the intra-hepatic bile ducts.

forming above the anastomosis towards the hilum of the liver. The latter are sometimes due to duct ischaemia.

The blood supply to the distal (recipient) duct is rich due to collateral flow. That of the proximal (donor) duct is more tenuous [30], relying on the peri-biliary plexus derived from the reconstructed hepatic artery. Non-anastomotic leakage of bile with necrosis is seen after hepatic artery thrombosis [33]. Development of non-anastomotic strictures seems to be independent of the method of bile duct reconstruction whether choledocho-choledochostomy or Roux-en-Y anastomosis. The majority of hilar strictures occur by 3 months after transplantation [32].

Apart from ischaemia, suggested mechanisms of non-anastomotic stricturing are decreased healing due to high dose steroids, infection and chronic ductopenic arteriopathic rejection.

Biliary leaks are associated with T tubes, either due to dislodgement, or occurring at the time of removal. T-tube splinting of the anastomosis has been used to reduce biliary problems, but if this is omitted the complication rate is no higher [24].

Clinical features

Liver function tests deteriorate with or without sepsis. Other causes of altered liver function tests will be consid-ered and excluded by liver biopsy and viral serology. The differential diagnosis includes rejection, sepsis else-where, cytomegalovirus infection, recurrence of under-lying disease and drug toxicity.

Investigations

Intermittent rises and falls in serum bilirubin and/or wide fluctuations in the serum transaminase level, unre-sponsive to changes in immunosuppressive therapy, may indicate biliary tract pathology [29].

Ultrasound may show duct dilatation or a collection. Doppler ultrasound is done to check hepatic arterial flow. If ultrasound is normal a clinical decision is taken between liver biopsy or cholangiography. ERCP will show a biliary leak or stricture.

Treatment

Although surgical revision or conversion of the anasto-mosis is often needed, balloon dilatation and stent inser-tion has been used for post-transplantation stricture, both anastomotic and non-anastomotic [20, 32] with variable success. Features correlating with the success of non-surgical approaches await analysis.

Primary sclerosing cholangitis
(Chapter 15)

Extra- and intra-hepatic bile ducts are diffusely involved in approximately 80% of patients. If the patient develops persistent jaundice or recurrent sepsis, investigations are necessary to show whether there is a dominant stricture, that is one which appears to be causing significant obstruction compared with the diffuse changes else-where. Ultrasound may show duct dilatation; ERCP will show a dominant stricture if present. Brush cytology is necessary. Differentiation of benign stricturing from cholangiocarcinoma is difficult and often impossible.

Balloon dilatation with or without stenting can produce clinical improvement [11]. The differentiation between clinical deterioration caused by intra-hepatic disease and liver cell failure, and that due to remediable duct stricturing is often difficult but important so as not to delay transplantation inappropriately.

Other causes

Chronic pancreatitis may cause low bile duct obstruction (see Chapter 33), as may radiotherapy [3], a penetrating or sclerosed [13] duodenal ulcer, and trauma. The stric-ture occurring after resection of the head of the pan-creas is likely to be caused by recurrence of tumour, but benign strictures due to vascular insufficiency are also possible. This is related to the balance of blood supply to the bile duct proximally and distally. When necessary the bile duct should be divided as near to the ampulla as possible where the blood supply is better.

Summary

In all benign strictures of the bile duct, the outcome depends on the experience and judgement of the team of surgeon, endoscopist and radiologist, in selecting and performing the most suitable corrective procedure tailored to the individual patient.

References

1 Bergman JJGHM, van der Brink GR, Rauws EAJ *et al*. Treatment of bile duct lesions after laparoscopic cholecystectomy. *Gut* 1996; **38**: 141.

2 Chapman WC, Halevy A, Blumgart LH *et al*. Postcholecystectomy bile duct strictures: management and outcome in 130 patients. *Arch. Surg.* 1995; **130**: 597.

3 Cherqui D, Palazzo L, Piedbois P *et al*. Common bile duct stricture as a late complication of upper abdominal radiotherapy. *J. Hepatol.* 1994; **20**: 693.

4 Clair DG, Carr-Locke DL, Becker JM *et al*. Routine cholangiography is not warranted during laparoscopic cholecystectomy. *Arch. Surg.* 1993; **128**: 551.

5 Csendes A, Diaz JC, Burdiles P *et al*. Late results of immediate primary end to end repair in accidental section of the common bile duct. *Surg. Gynecol. Obstet.* 1989; **168**: 125.

6 Dunn D, Fowler S, Nair R *et al*. Laparoscopic cholecystectomy in England and Wales: results of an audit by the Royal College of Surgeons of England. *Ann. R. Coll. Surg. Engl.* 1994; **76**: 269.

7 Foutch PG, Sivak MV Jr. Therapeutic endoscopic balloon dilatation of the extrahepatic biliary ducts. *Am. J. Gastroenterol.* 1985; **80**: 575.

8 Hatfield ARW, Craig PI, Lanzon-Miller S *et al*. Percutaneous choledochoscopy in the management of benign biliary disease. *Gut* 1992; **33**: S34.

9 Huibregtse K. Endoscopic treatment of postoperative biliary strictures. In: *Endoscopic Biliary and Pancreatic Drainage*, p. 59. Georg Thieme Verlag, Stuttgart, 1988.

10 Hutson DG, Russell E, Schiff E *et al*. Balloon dilatation of biliary strictures through a choledochojejuno-cutaneous fistula. *Ann. Surg.* 1984; **199**: 637.

11 Johnson GK, Geenen JE, Vennu RP. Endoscopic treatment of biliary duct strictures in sclerosing cholangitis: follow-up assessment of a new therapeutic approach. *Gastrointest. Endosc.* 1987; **33**: 9.

12 Lee MJ, Mueller PR, Saini S *et al*. Percutaneous dilatation of benign biliary strictures: single-session therapy with general anesthesia. *Am. J. Roentgenol.* 1991; **157**: 1263.

13 Luman W, Hudson N, Choudari CP *et al*. Distal biliary stricture as a complication of sclerosant injection for bleeding duodenal ulcer. *Gut* 1994; **35**: 1665.

14 Maccioni F, Rossi M, Salvatori FM *et al*. Metallic stents in benign biliary strictures: 3-year follow-up. *Cardiovasc. Intervent. Radiol.* 1992; **15**: 360.

15 McMahon AJ, Fullarton G, Baxter JN *et al*. Bile duct injury and bile leakage in laparoscopic cholecystectomy. *Br. J. Surg.* 1995; **82**: 307.

16 McSherry CK. Cholecystectomy: the gold standard. *Am. J. Surg.* 1989; **158**: 174.

17 Matthews JB, Baer HU, Schweizer WP *et al*. Recurrent cholangitis with and without anastomotic stricture after biliary-enteric bypass. *Arch. Surg.* 1993; **128**: 269.

18 Moossa AR, Mayer AD, Stabile B. Iatrogenic injury to the bile duct: who, how, where? *Arch. Surg.* 1990; **125**: 1028.

19 Morrison MC, Lee MJ, Saini S *et al*. Percutaneous balloon dilatation of benign biliary strictures. *Radiol. Clin. North Am.* 1990; **28**: 1191.

20 O'Connor TP, Lewis WD, Jenkins RL. Biliary tract complications after liver transplantation. *Arch. Surg.* 1995; **130**: 312.

21 Pellegrini CA, Thomas MJ, Way LW. Recurrent biliary stricture. Patterns of recurrence and outcome of surgical therapy. *Am. J. Surg.* 1984; **147**: 175.

22 Pitt HA, Kaufman SL, Coleman J *et al*. Biliary stricture: is dilatation an acceptable alternative to operation? *Ann. Surg.* 1989; **210**: 417.

23 Pitt HA, Miyamoto T, Parapatis SK *et al*. Factors influencing outcome in patients with postoperative biliary strictures. *Am. J. Surg.* 1982; **144**: 14.

24 Rolles K, Dawson K, Novell R *et al*. Biliary anastomosis after liver transplantation does not benefit from T tube splintage. *Transplantation* 1994; **57**: 402.

25 Rossi RL, Schirmer WJ, Braasch JW *et al*. Laparoscopic bile duct injuries: risk factors, recognition, and repair. *Arch. Surg.* 1992; **127**: 596.

26 Schol FPG, Go PMNYH, Gouma DJ. Risk factors for bile duct injury in laparoscopic cholecystectomy: analysis of 49 cases. *Br. J. Surg.* 1994; **81**: 1786.

27 Skolkin MD, Alspaugh JP, Casarella WJ *et al*. Sclerosing cholangitis: palliation with percutaneous cholangioplasty. *Radiology* 1989; **170**: 199.

28 Stewart L, Way LW. Bile duct injuries during laparoscopic cholecystectomy: factors that influence the results of treatment. *Arch. Surg.* 1995; **130**: 1123.

29 Stratta RJ, Wood P, Langnas AN *et al*. Diagnosis and treatment of biliary tract complications after orthotopic liver transplantation. *Surgery* 1989; **106**: 675.

30 Terblanche J, Allison HF, Northover JMA. An ischemic basis for biliary strictures. *Surgery* 1983; **94**: 52.

31 Trambert JJ, Bron KM, Zajko AB. Percutaneous transhepatic balloon dilatation of benign biliary strictures. *Am. J. Roentgenol.* 1987; **149**: 945.

32 Ward EM, Kiely MJ, Maus TP *et al*. Hilar biliary strictures after liver transplantation: cholangiography and percutaneous treatment. *Radiology* 1990; **177**: 259.

33 Zajko AB, Campbell WL, Logsdon GA *et al*. Cholangiographic findings in hepatic artery occlusion after liver transplantation. *Am. J. Roentgenol.* 1987; **149**: 485.

Chapter 33
Diseases of the Ampulla of Vater and Pancreas

Peri-ampullary carcinoma

The region of the head of the pancreas is a common site for carcinoma [44]. The tumour may arise in the head of the pancreas itself, more often from ductular epithelium than acinar cells, the lining of the low bile duct, the ampulla (papilla) or rarely the duodenum. Tumours arising from any of these sites have the same overall effect (fig. 33.1), and will be considered as a group. They are often termed 'cancer of the head of the pancreas'. However, the prognosis is very different. 87% of patients with carcinoma of the ampulla and 47% of those with malignancy of the duodenum have a potentially operable tumour compared with only 22% of those arising in the head of the pancreas [28].

Aetiological factors include cigarette smoking, diet, previous partial gastrectomy and diabetes mellitus [44]. In some patients there is a strong family history, suggesting genetic predisposition [26]. There is no consistent relationship to coffee drinking or alcohol intake.

Molecular changes

K-*ras* gene mutation, particularly at codon 12, is found in the majority of pancreatic carcinomas and more frequently than in other tumours [18]. Mutations can be detected by polymerase chain reaction on formalin-fixed paraffin embedded tissue, or needle biopsy or aspirated material. Abnormally high p53 gene expression is found in 60% of pancreatic carcinoma, predominantly in ductal tumours [31]. These changes are common in other tumours, adding little to the understanding specifically of pancreatic carcinogenesis. Detection of K-*ras* mutations in pancreatic duct brushings [43] may aid diagnosis, but is presently a research tool.

Pathology

Histologically, the tumour is an adenocarcinoma, whether arising from pancreatic duct, acinus or bile duct. The ampullary tumours have a papillary arrangement and are often of low-grade malignancy; fibrosis is prominent. They tend to be polypoid and soft, whereas the acinar tumours are infiltrative, large and firm.

Obstruction of common bile duct

This results from direct invasion causing a scirrhous reaction, from annular stenosis, and from tumour tissue filling the lumen. The duct may also be compressed by the tumour mass.

The bile ducts dilate and the gallbladder enlarges. An

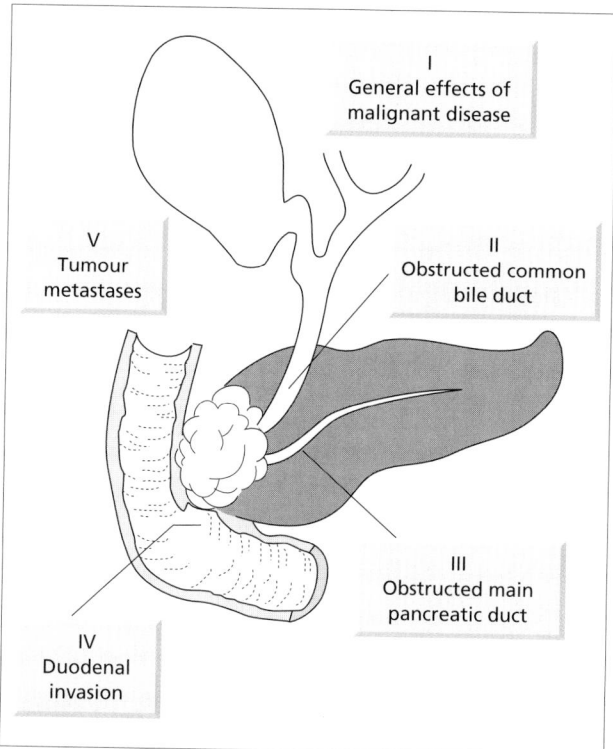

Fig. 33.1. The effects of carcinoma in the ampullary region. I, General effects of malignant disease—weakness and weight loss. II, Obstructed common bile duct. Dilated gallbladder and bile ducts—jaundice, hepatomegaly and pruritus. III, Obstructed main pancreatic duct—fibrous atrophy of pancreas, steatorrhoea and occasional glycosuria. IV, Duodenal invasion —occasional duodenal obstruction, positive stool occult blood and occasional melaena. V, Tumour metastases. Nerves—back and epigastric pain; regional glands, liver, lungs and peritoneum.

633

ascending cholangitis in the obstructed duct is rare. The liver shows the changes of cholestasis.

Pancreatic changes

The main pancreatic duct may be obstructed as it enters the ampulla. The ducts and acini distal to the obstruction dilate and later rupture, causing focal areas of pancreatitis and fat necrosis. Later all the acinar tissue is replaced by fibrous tissue. Occasionally, particularly in the acinar type, fat necrosis and suppuration may occur in and around the pancreas.

Diabetes mellitus or impaired glucose tolerance is frequent. Apart from destruction of insulin-producing cells by the tumour, this may be due to production of islet amyloid polypeptide (IAPP) by islet cells adjacent to the tumour [32].

Spread of the tumour

Direct extension in the wall of the bile duct and infiltration through the head of the pancreas is common with the acinar although not with the ampullary type. The second part of the duodenum may be invaded, with ulceration of the mucosa and secondary haemorrhage. The splenic and portal veins may be invaded and may thrombose with resultant splenomegaly.

Involvement of regional nodes is found in approximately a third of operated cases. Perineural lymphatic spread is common. Blood-borne metastases, with secondaries in liver and lungs, follow invasion of the splenic or portal veins. There may also be peritoneal and omental metastases.

Clinical features

Both sexes are affected, but males more frequently than females in a ratio of 2 : 1. The sufferer is usually between 50 and 69 years old.

The clinical picture is a composite one of cholestasis with pancreatic insufficiency, and the general and local effects of a malignant tumour (fig. 33.1).

Jaundice is of gradual onset, progressively deepening, but ampullary neoplasms can cause mild and intermittent jaundice. *Itching* is a common but not invariable feature, and when present comes after jaundice. Cholangitis is unusual.

Cancer of the head of the pancreas is not always painless. Pain may be experienced in the back, the epigastrium and right upper quadrant, usually as a continuous distress worse at night and sometimes ameliorated by crouching. It may be aggravated by eating.

Weakness and weight loss are progressive and have usually continued for at least 3 months before jaundice develops.

Although frank steatorrhoea is rare, the patient often complains of a change in bowel habit, usually diarrhoea.

Vomiting and intestinal obstruction may follow invasion of the second part of the duodenum. Ulceration of the duodenum can erode a vessel with haematemesis or, more commonly, occult bleeding.

Difficulty in making a diagnosis may make the patient depressed. It then becomes easy to believe mistakenly, that the patient is psychoneurotic.

Examination. The patient is jaundiced and shows evidence of recent weight loss. Theoretically, the gallbladder should be enlarged and palpable (*Courvoisier's law*). In practice, the gallbladder is only felt in about half the patients, although at subseqeunt laparotomy a dilated gallbladder is found in three-quarters. The liver is enlarged with a sharp, smooth, firm edge. Hepatic metastases are rarely detected. The pancreatic tumour is usually impalpable.

The spleen is palpable if involvement of the splenic vein has caused thrombosis. Peritoneal invasion is followed by ascites.

Lymphatic metastases are more usual with cancer of the body rather than head of the pancreas [46]. Occasionally, however, axillary, cervical and inguinal glands may be enlarged and Virchow's gland in the left supraclavicular fossa may be palpable.

Occasionally, widespread venous thromboses simulate thrombophlebitis migrans.

Investigations

Glycosuria occurs in 15–20% and with it there is an impaired oral glucose tolerance test.

Blood biochemistry. The serum alkaline phosphatase level is greatly raised. The serum amylase and lipase concentrations are sometimes persistently elevated in carcinoma of the ampullary region. Hypoproteinaemia with, later, peripheral oedema may be found.

There are no reliable serum tumour markers with sufficient specificity or sensitivity for clinical purposes [44]. CA242 shows slightly better sensitivity than CA19/9 but is still only positive in about half of early stage tumours. [19].

Haematology. Anaemia is mild or absent. The leucocyte count may be normal or raised, with a relative increase in polymorphonuclear leucocytes. The erythrocyte sedimentation rate is usually raised.

Differential diagnosis

The diagnosis must be considered in any patient over 40 years with progressive or even intermittent cholestasis. The suspicion would be strengthened by persistent or unexplained abdominal pain, weakness and weight loss, diarrhoea, glycosuria, positive faecal occult blood, hepatomegaly, a palpable spleen or thrombophlebitis migrans.

Radiology

Ultrasound and *CT scanning* can detect pancreatic masses as small as 2 cm in diameter. They will also show dilatation of the bile ducts and pancreatic duct, hepatic metastases and extra-hepatic spread of the primary lesion. Although ultrasound is more readily available and less expensive, it may be made difficult by intestinal gas. CT is often preferred (fig. 29.5) and the newer methods such as spiral (helical) and high resolution dynamic CT allow a diagnostic accuracy rate of greater than 95% [14]. MRI at present has no advantages.

Percutaneous ultrasound or CT-guided *fine needle aspiration* of the pancreatic mass is safe and has a sensitivity of 57–96% [30, 44]. There is a small risk of seeding of tumour cells along the needle track [33].

ERCP can usually demonstrate the pancreatic and bile ducts, allow biopsy of any ampullary lesion (fig. 33.2), and provide bile or pancreatic juice or brushings from the stricture for cytological examination (fig. 33.3) [20]. The appearance of the bile duct and/or pancreatic duct stricture gives a good indication of the underlying malignant cause of the stricture (fig. 29.11a) but occasionally appearances are deceptive and tissue diagnosis should still be sought. Unusual tumours such as lymphoma need to be identified since they may respond to conventional therapy.

In the patient with vomiting, *barium meal* will show the extent of duodenal invasion and obstruction.

Tumour staging

This gives an indication of whether the tumour is resectable or not. Clinical evidence, chest radiograph,

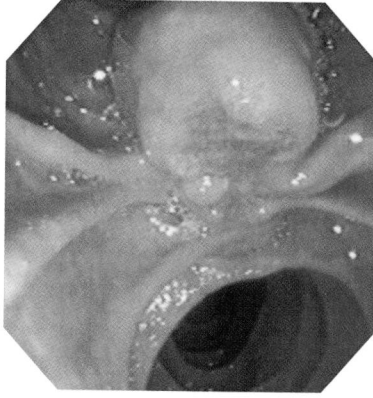

Fig. 33.2. Abnormal ampulla at ERCP. Note irregular surface with nodularity. Biopsy showed adenocarcinoma.

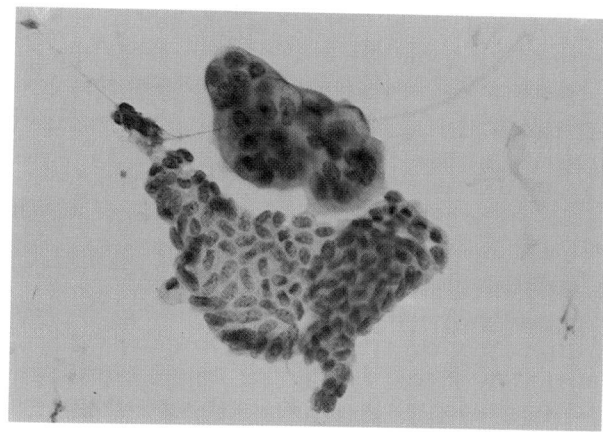

Fig. 33.3. Brush cytology taken from a low common bile duct stricture. There is a sheet of benign biliary epithelial cells and above this a small group of large polymorphic cells characteristic of adenocarcinoma.

CT or ultrasound will show obvious metastatic disease. Dynamic (contrast-enhanced) CT is highly accurate in predicting irresectability but less accurate in predicting resectability [14, 15]. Thus it can detect vascular invasion, but is less reliable in showing adjacent tissue invasion or local or distant metastases. Angiography shows comparable results in assessing resectability, with major vessel occlusion precluding resection and encasement making it unlikely [13]. Although advances in CT obviate the need for angiography to assess resectability in some centres, angiography is still appropriate before surgery in many cases to delineate the vascular anatomy, which can be atypical in up to one-third of patients.

Laparoscopy is valuable to show and biopsy minute hepatic metastases and peritoneal and omental seedings. Negative results from laparoscopy, CT and angiography correspond to a 78% resectability rate [46].

CT portography is useful to detect liver metastases, but adds little to the local staging of the pancreatic lesion.

Endoscopic ultrasonography is a new technique in which a high-frequency transducer at the tip of an endoscope is used to visualize the pancreatic and peripancreatic tissue through stomach and duodenal wall. In expert hands it is highly accurate for primary tumour (T) staging (85%) and showing vascular invasion (87%), but less so for regional lymph node (N) staging (74%) [35]. However, experience is limited, it is operator dependent and time-consuming, and is not routinely available.

Prognosis

The prognosis of pancreatic carcinoma is grave. After biliary bypass surgery the mean survival is about 6 months. The acinar type carries a worse prognosis than the ductal type, because regional lymph glands are involved earlier. Only the minority, between 5 and 20%, have resectable tumours.

Resection has had an operative mortality of approximately 15–20% [17], but recent reports have shown this to fall to 5% and less in specialist centres with a few expert surgeons performing more operations [44]. A recent report from a superspecialist unit of zero mortality after 145 consecutive pancreatico-duodenal resections is exceptional [8].

Coincident with reduced operative mortality has been a rise in reported 5-year survival to around 20% [6]. This may reflect earlier detection of disease through the newer scanning techniques, or selection of patients with less extensive spread of disease. Disease recurrence, however, remains a problem. Total pancreatectomy does not lead to longer survival than the less extensive Whipple's procedure and produces exocrine insufficiency and brittle diabetes [4].

The overall outlook for carcinoma of the pancreas however is grim with only 23 of 912 patients with carcinoma of the pancreas in one series surviving 3 years and only two of these being considered cures [10].

Prognosis for carcinoma of the ampulla is better, with 85% surviving 5 years after resection if the tumour has not spread beyond the margins of the sphincter of Oddi, and 11–25% if extension is greater [47]. Pancreatico-duodenectomy is the treatment of choice. Local resection can be done as an alternative to extensive surgery in selected patients [3].

Treatment

Resection

A decision to attempt resection depends on the clinical state of the patient and the staging of the tumour derived from radiological imaging. Difficulties in removal arise because of the inaccessibility of the pancreas on the posterior wall of the abdomen in the vicinity of vital structures. The operability rate is therefore very low.

The classical procedure is *pancreatico-duodenectomy* (*Whipple's operation*) which is performed in one stage with removal of related regional lymph nodes, the entire duodenum and the distal third of stomach. This operation was modified in 1978 [42] to preserve antral and pyloric function (pylorus-preserving pancreatico-duodenectomy). This reduces post-gastrectomy symptoms and marginal ulceration, and improves nutrition [23]. Survival is the same as those having the classical procedure. The continuity of the biliary passages is restored by anastomosis of the common bile duct with the jejunum. Pancreatico-jejunostomy drains the duct of the remaining pancreas. The continuity of the intestinal tract is restored by duodeno-jejunostomy.

Frozen section examination of the resection margins is mandatory.

Prognostic factors are tumour size, histological blood vessel invasion and lymph node status. The best indicator is lymph node histology. If negative at resection, 5-year survival is 40–50%, compared with 8% in those with nodes positive for metastasis [7]. Prognosis is also related to whether or not there is histological evidence of vascular invasion (median survival 11 versus 39 months).

Carcinoma of the ampulla is also usually treated by pancreatico-duodenectomy. Local resection (ampullectomy) is an alternative in selected patients with pre-malignant or malignant ampullary tumours [3]. Endoscopic photodynamic therapy has produced remission or reduced tumour bulk of ampullary carcinoma in a series of patients unsuitable for surgery [1]. This technique uses endoscopic delivery of red light (630 nm) to tumour sensitized with haematoporphyrin given intravenously.

Palliative procedures

The choice lies between surgical bypass and endoscopic or percutaneous transhepatic insertion of an endoprosthesis (stent).

For the jaundiced patient with vomiting due to duodenal obstruction, choledochojejunostomy and gastroenterostomy is necessary. For the patient with bile duct obstruction alone, some argue for prophylactic gastric bypass surgery at the time of biliary bypass but most would make this decision at the time of operation, according to the size of the tumour.

The choice between surgical and non-surgical relief of biliary obstruction depends upon the expertise available and the clinical status of the patient.

Endoscopic stent insertion (fig. 33.4) is successful in up to 95% of patients (60% after the first session) and has a lower 30-day mortality than surgical bypass [38]. When the endoscopic approach fails, the percutaneous, or combined percutaneous/endoscopic approach [34] can be used (see Chapter 29).

Percutaneous stent insertion (fig. 29.20) has a similar mortality, early morbidity and mean survival time (19 versus 15 weeks) to palliative surgery partly due to the complications of the trans-hepatic approach (haemorrhage, bile leakage) [5]. Endoscopic stent insertion has a lower complication rate and mortality than the percutaneous route [40].

Within 3 months of insertion 20–30% of plastic stents need to be replaced because of obstruction by biliary sludge [39]. *Metal mesh expandable stents* can be inserted endoscopically or percutaneously (fig. 29.16). They remain patent significantly longer than plastic stents (mean 273 versus 126 days) [11]. However, because of

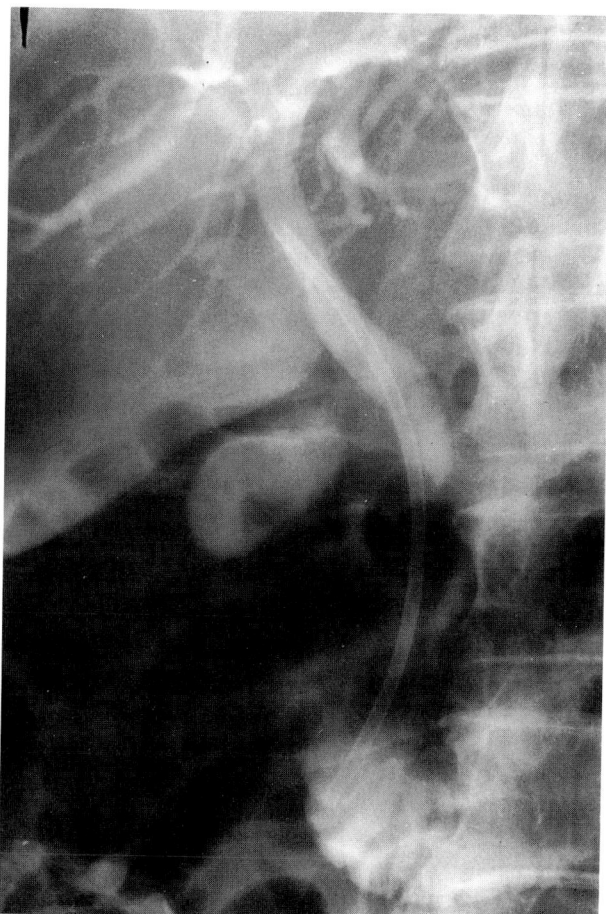

Fig. 33.4. Polyethylene 10 French endoprosthesis inserted across low common bile duct stricture by the endoscopic route. Note good flow of contrast into duodenum and decompressed biliary system.

their cost, they are best restricted to those patients with irresectable periampullary carcinoma who at the time of first stent change for obstruction are judged likely to have slower progression and a longer survival [29].

The non-surgical insertion of a stent is particularly applicable to old, poor-risk patients especially when a large, clearly inoperable pancreatic mass has been imaged or where there is extensive metastatic disease. For the younger patient with irresectable disease, surgical bypass should still be considered if longer than average survival is expected.

With all the approaches now available, no patient with carcinoma of the pancreas should die jaundiced or with intolerable itching.

Adjuvant treatment

Pre-operative adjuvant chemotherapy and radiotherapy have produced disappointing results. Selected patients may benefit from adjuvant combined radiotherapy and

chemotherapy after radical resection [16]. In irresectable patients, no chemotherapeutic or irradiation protocol has given definitive benefit.

Coeliac plexus block (percutaneously under X-ray screening, or at operation), may reduce pain for a few months, but in over half of patients pain returns [24].

Benign villous adenoma of the ampulla of Vater [36]

This leads to biliary colic and obstructive jaundice. The ampullary tumour is seen and biopsied at ERCP.

Dysplasia may be present on biopsy. CEA and CA19/9 are found on immunohistochemistry [48]. These lesions should be regarded as potentially premalignant. Local resection or pancreatico-duodenectomy is indicated [3]. In patients unfit for surgery stenting is palliative. Endoscopic photodynamic therapy is valuable but at present experimental [1].

Cystic tumours of the pancreas [45]

These may be benign or malignant and include cystic adenocarcinoma, cystic adenoma (serous and mucinous) and papillary cystic tumours. They may be misdiagnosed as pseudocysts. 40% of patients are asymptomatic. Work-up is by CT, angiography and ERCP. Cyst fluid analysis (cytology, tumour markers) may be valuable in differentiating the type of tumour [22]. 44% of lesions are malignant. In general, resection should be attempted. Frozen and even routine histology may be misleading. Mucinous cystic neoplasm should be considered potentially malignant.

Endocrine tumours of the pancreas [37]

These include insulinoma, carcinoid tumour, gastrinoma, VIPoma, PPoma and somatostatinoma. They present with either the systemic effects of the hormone released or a mass effect with pain or jaundice. A variable proportion are malignant, depending on the endocrine type. Treatment is by surgical resection or debulking, and medical measures to counter the effect of any hormone released. Overall 5-year survival is 40–60%.

Chronic pancreatitis

Pancreatitis, usually of alcoholic aetiology, can cause narrowing of the intra-pancreatic portion of the common bile duct [2]. The resultant cholestasis may be transient during exacerbations of acute pancreatitis. It is presumably related to oedema and swelling of the pancreas. More persistent cholestasis follows encasement of the intra- and peri-pancreatic bile duct in a progressively fibrotic pancreatitis. Pseudocysts of the head of the pancreas and abscesses can also cause biliary obstruction and persistent cholestasis.

Bile duct stenosis affects about 8% of patients with chronic alcoholic pancreatitis and this figure would be higher if more cholangiograms were done. It should be suspected if the serum alkaline phosphatase is more than twice elevated for longer than 1 month. ERCP shows a smooth narrowing of the lower end of the common bile duct, sometimes adopting a 'rat tail' configuration (fig. 33.5). The main pancreatic duct may be tortuous, irregular and dilated. Pancreatic calcification may be present.

Liver biopsy shows portal fibrosis [27], features of biliary obstruction, and sometimes biliary cirrhosis. Features of alcoholic liver disease are unusual.

Splenic vein thrombosis is a complication of chronic pancreatitis.

Management

Early diagnosis of a biliary stricture due to pancreatitis is essential as biliary cirrhosis and acute cholangitis can develop in the absence of clinical jaundice.

The patient must abstain completely from alcohol.

The place of surgery is controversial. Clinical, laboratory and imaging data do not necessarily distinguish those patients with significant bile duct obstruction from those with alcoholic liver disease or normal liver histology [21]. Liver biopsy is valuable in deciding whether surgical decompression of the bile duct is necessary. Plastic and metal mesh stents successfully relieve bile

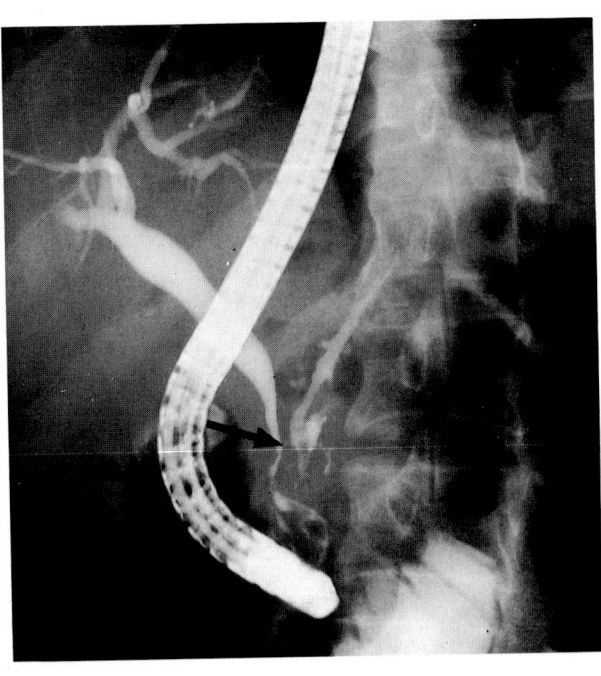

Fig. 33.5. Endoscopic retrograde cholangio-pancreatography in a patient with alcoholic chronic pancreatitis. Note the 'rat tail' narrowing of the distal common bile duct (arrow).

duct obstruction due to chronic pancreatitis [12], but long-term data are needed to judge whether this is an appropriate method of treatment. Acute cholangitis, biliary cirrhosis and protracted jaundice are absolute indications for surgery [41]. Choledocho-enterostomy is the usual procedure [9].

Obstruction of the common bile duct by enlarged lymph glands

This is extremely rare. The enlarged glands are nearly always metastatic, frequently from a primary in the alimentary tract, lung or breast, or from a hepato-cellular carcinoma.

Malignant glands in the porta hepatis are associated with deep jaundice, the main bile ducts usually being invaded rather than compressed. Secondary deposits in the hepatic parenchyma may also invade the bile ducts, causing obstruction.

Glands along the common duct may be enlarged in non-malignant conditions, but the bile duct usually escapes compression. Jaundice in infections such as tuberculosis, sarcoidosis or infectious mononucleosis is not obstructive but due to direct hepatic involvement or haemolysis.

Glandular enlargement in the reticuloses does, very rarely, cause obstruction to the common bile duct, but jaundice complicating these diseases is more often due to hepatic parenchymal involvement, to increased haemolysis or is of an obscure cholestatic type (see Chapter 4).

Other causes of extrinsic pressure on the common bile duct

Duodenal ulceration

This is an extremely rare cause of obstructive jaundice. Perforation, so that the ulcer impinges against the bile duct or causes adhesive peritonitis, may rarely result in biliary obstruction. This can also follow scarring as the ulcer heals or endoscopic sclerosis for bleeding [25].

Duodenal diverticulum

Diverticula of the duodenum are often found near the ampulla of Vater, but rarely cause obstruction of the bile duct. When they do so, obstruction is partial and jaundice intermittent.

References

1 Abulafi AM, Allardice JT, Williams NS *et al*. Photodynamic therapy for malignant tumours of the ampulla of Vater. *Gut* 1995; **36**: 853.

2 Aranha GV, Prinz RA, Freeark RJ *et al*. The spectrum of

biliary tract obstruction from chronic pancreatitis. *Arch. Surg.* 1984; **119**: 595.

3 Asbun HJ, Rossi RL, Munson JL. Local resection for ampullary tumours: is there a place for it? *Arch. Surg.* 1993; **128**: 515.

4 Baumel H, Hugier M, Manderscheid JC *et al.* Results of resection for cancer of the exocrine pancreas: a study from the French Association of Surgery. *Br. J. Surg.* 1994; **81**: 102.

5 Bornman PC, Harries-Jones EP, Tobias R *et al.* Prospective controlled trial of transhepatic biliary endoprosthesis versus bypass surgery for incurable carcinoma of head of pancreas. *Lancet* 1986; **i**: 61.

6 Cameron JL. The current management of carcinoma of the head of the pancreas. *Annu. Rev. Med.* 1995; **46**: 361.

7 Cameron JL, Crist DW, Sitzman JV *et al.* Factors influencing survival following pancreaticoduodenectomy for pancreatic cancer. *Am. J. Surg.* 1991; **161**: 120.

8 Cameron JL, Pitt HA, Yeo CJ *et al.* One hundred and forty-five consecutive pancreatico-duodenectomies without mortality. *Ann. Surg.* 1993; **217**: 430.

9 Carter DC. Pancreatitis and the biliary tree: the continuing problem. *Am. J. Surg.* 1988; **155**: 10.

10 Connolly MM, Dawson PJ, Michelassi F *et al.* Survival in 1001 patients with carcinoma of the pancreas. *Ann. Surg.* 1987; **206**: 366.

11 Davids PHP, Groen AK, Rauws EAJ *et al.* Randomized trial of self-expanding metal stents versus polyethylene stents for distal malignant biliary obstruction. *Lancet* 1992; **340**: 1488.

12 Deviere J, Cremer M, Baize M *et al.* Management of common bile duct stricture caused by chronic pancreatitis with metal mesh self expandable stents. *Gut* 1994; **35**: 122.

13 Dooley WC, Cameron JL, Pitt HA *et al.* Is preoperative angiography useful in patients with periampullary tumors? *Ann. Surg.* 1990; **211**: 649.

14 Freeny PC, Traverso WL, Ryan JA. Diagnosis and staging of pancreatic adenocarcinoma with dynamic computed tomography. *Am. J. Surg.* 1993; **165**: 600.

15 Fuhrman GM, Charnsangavej C, Abbruzzese JL *et al.* Thin section, contrast enhanced computed tomography accurately predicts the resectability of malignant pancreatic neoplasms. *Am. J. Surg.* 1994; **167**: 104.

16 Gastrointestinal Tumor Study Group, Kalser MH, Ellenberg SS. Further evidence of effective adjuvant combined radiation and chemotherapy following curative resection of the pancreatic head. *Cancer* 1987; **59**: 2006.

17 Gudjonsson B. Cancer of the pancreas: 50 years of surgery. *Cancer* 1987; **60**: 2284.

18 Hruban RH, van Mansfield ADM, Offerhaus GJA *et al.* K-*ras* oncogene activation in adenocarcinoma of the human pancreas. *Am. J. Pathol.* 1993; **143**: 545.

19 Kawa S, Tokoo M, Hasebe O *et al.* Comparative study of CA 242 and CA 19-9 for the diagnosis of pancreatic cancer. *Br. J. Cancer* 1994; **70**: 481.

20 Kurazawinski TR, Deery A, Dooley JS *et al.* A prospective study of biliary cytology in 100 patients with bile duct strictures. *Hepatology* 1993; **18**: 1399.

21 Lesur G, Levy P, Flejou J-F *et al.* Factors predictive of liver histopathological appearance in chronic alcoholic pancreatitis with common bile duct stenosis and increased serum alkaline phosphatase. *Hepatology* 1993; **18**: 1078.

22 Lewandrowski K, Lee J, Southern J *et al.* Cyst fluid analysis in the differential diagnosis of pancreatic cysts: a new approach to the preoperative assessment of pancreatic cystic lesions. *Am. J. Roentgenol.* 1995; **164**: 815.

23 Lillemoe KD. Current management of pancreatic carcinoma. *Ann. Surg.* 1995; **221**: 133.

24 Lillemoe KD, Cameron JL, Kaufman HS *et al.* Chemical splanchnicectomy in patients with unresectable pancreatic cancer: a prospective randomized trial. *Ann. Surg.* 1993; **217**: 447.

25 Luman W, Hudson N, Choudari CP *et al.* Distal biliary stricture as a complication of sclerosant injection for bleeding duodenal ulcer. *Gut* 1994; **35**: 1665.

26 Lynch HT. Genetics and pancreatic cancer. *Arch. Surg.* 1994; **129**: 266.

27 Morgan MY, Sherlock S, Scheuer PJ. Portal fibrosis in the livers of alcoholic patients. *Gut* 1978; **19**: 1015.

28 Nix GAJJ, Van Overbeeke IC, Wilson JHP *et al.* ERCP diagnosis of tumors in the region of the head of the pancreas. Analysis of criteria and computer-aided diagnosis. *Dig. Dis. Sci.* 1988; **33**: 577.

29 O'Brien S, Hatfield ARW, Craig PI *et al.* A three-year follow-up of self expanding metal stents in the endoscopic palliation of longterm survivors with malignant biliary obstruction. *Gut* 1995; **36**: 618.

30 Parsons L, Palmer CH. How accurate is fine-needle biopsy in malignant neoplasia of the pancreas? *Arch. Surg.* 1989; **124**: 681.

31 Pellegata NS, Sessa F, Renault B *et al.* K-*ras* and *p53* gene mutations in pancreatic cancer: ductal and nonductal tumors progress through different genetic lesions. *Cancer Res.* 1994; **54**: 1566.

32 Pemert J, Marsson J, Westermark GT *et al.* Islet amyloid polypeptide in patients with pancreatic cancer and diabetes. *N. Engl. J. Med.* 1994; **330**: 313.

33 Rashleigh-Belcher HJC, Russell RCG, Lees WR. Cutaneous seeding of pancreatic carcinoma by fine-needle aspiration biopsy. *Br. J. Radiol.* 1986; **59**: 182.

34 Robertson DAF, Ayres R, Hacking CN *et al.* Experience with a combined percutaneous and endoscopic approach to stent insertion in malignant obstructive jaundice. *Lancet* 1987; **ii**: 1449.

35 Rosch T. Endoscopic ultrasonography in pancreatic cancer. *Endoscopy* 1994; **26**: 806.

36 Rosenberg J, Welch JP, Pyrtek LJ *et al.* Benign villous adenomas of the ampulla of Vater. *Cancer* 1986; **58**; 1563.

37 Rothmund M, Stinner B, Arnold R. Endocrine pancreatic carcinoma. *Eur. J. Surg. Oncol.* 1991; **17**: 191.

38 Smith AC, Dowsett JF, Russell RCG *et al.* Randomised trial of endoscopic stenting versus surgical bypass in malignant low bileduct obstruction. *Lancet* 1994; **344**: 1655.

39 Speer AG, Cotton PB, Rode J *et al.* Biliary stent blockage with bacterial biofilm. A light and electron microscopy study. *Ann. Intern. Med.* 1988; **108**: 546.

40 Speer AG, Cotton PB, Russell RCG *et al.* Randomized trial of endoscopic versus percutaneous stent insertion in malignant obstructive jaundice. *Lancet* 1987; **ii**: 57.

41 Stahl TJ, Allen MO'C, Ansel HJ *et al.* Partial biliary obstruction caused by chronic pancreatitis: an appraisal of indications for surgical biliary drainage. *Ann. Surg.* 1988; **207**: 26.

42 Traverso LW, Longmire WP Jr. Preservation of the pylorus in pancreaticoduodenectomy. *Surg. Gynecol. Obstet.* 1978; **146**; 959.

43 Van Laethem J-L, Vertongen P, Deviere J *et al.* Detection of c-K-*ras* gene codon 12 mutations from pancreatic duct brush-

ings in the diagnosis of pancreatic tumours. *Gut* 1995; **36**: 781.

44 Warshaw AL, Fernandez-Del-Castillo C. Pancreatic carcinoma. *N. Engl. J. Med.* 1992; **326**: 455.

45 Warshaw AL, Compton CC, Lewandrowski K *et al.* Cystic tumors of the pancreas: new clinical, radiologic, and pathologic observations in 67 patients. *Ann. Surg.* 1990; **212**: 432.

46 Warshaw AL, Zhuo-yun G, Wittenberg J *et al.* Preoperative staging and assessment of resectability of pancreatic cancer. *Arch. Surg.* 1990; **125**: 230.

47 Yamaguchi K, Enjoji M. Carcinoma of the ampulla of Vater. A clinico-pathologic study and pathologic staging of 109 cases of carcinoma and five cases of adenoma. *Cancer* 1987; **59**; 506.

48 Yamaguchi K, Enjoji M. Adenoma of the ampulla of Vater: putative precancerous lesion. *Gut* 1991; **32**: 1558.

Chapter 34
Tumours of the Gallbladder and Bile Ducts

Benign tumours of the gallbladder

Papilloma

Multiple, small, papillomatous tumours, consisting of hypertrophied villi laden with cholesterol esters, may be found in as many as 80% of surgically removed gallbladders. They are often associated with cholesterosis.

Papillomas are seen in about 0.3% of cholecystograms. In a functioning gallbladder they appear as concave filling defects, pointing towards the centre on the lateral wall. They are about 5–10 mm in diameter and may be multiple. They are differentiated from gallstones by their fixed position.

Adenoma

These very rare, small, single tumours are usually fundal, where they form a semi-solid or cystic papillary mass. Adenoma is usually a symptom-free, incidental finding although detached tumour particles may cause biliary colic.

These tumours are found incidentally at surgery, or during ultrasound being performed for gallstones although stones may obscure the adenoma [17]. In cholecystograms, an adenoma is usually seen at the fundus as a small circular or semicircular translucent filling defect. Adenomas greater than 1 cm in diameter have a higher risk of malignant change and should be removed [17].

Carcinoma of the gallbladder

This is an uncommon neoplasm. Gallstones coexist in about 75% of cases and chronic cholecystitis is a frequent association. There is no definite evidence of a causal relationship. Whatever causes gallstones predisposes to cancer.

The calcified (porcelain) gallbladder is particularly likely to become cancerous [38]. The common gallbladder papillomas are not pre-cancerous. It may complicate ulcerative colitis. An anomalous pancreatico-biliary ductal union, greater than 15 mm from the papilla of Vater, is associated with congenital cystic dilatation of the common bile duct and with gallbladder carcinoma [29]. Regurgitation of pancreatic juice may be tumorigenic.

Chronic typhoid infection of the gallbladder increases the risk of gallbladder carcinoma by 167-fold [6] emphasizing the need for antibiotic treatment to eradicate the chronic typhoid and paratyphoid carrier state, or for elective cholecystectomy.

Papillary adenocarcinoma starts as a wart-like excrescence. It grows slowly into, rather than through, the wall until a fungating mass fills the gallbladder. Mucoid change is associated with more rapid growth, early metastasis and gelatinous peritoneal carcinomatosis. *Squamous cell carcinoma* and *scirrhous* forms are recognized. The *anaplastic type* is particularly malignant. The most common tumour is a differentiated adenocarcinoma [7, 15] which may be papillary.

The tumour usually arises in the fundus or neck, but rapid spread may make the original site difficult to locate. The rich lymphatic and venous drainage of the gallbladder leads to early spread to related lymph nodes, causing cholestatic jaundice and widespread dissemination. The liver bed is invaded and there may also be local spread to the duodenum, stomach and colon resulting in fistulae or external compression.

Clinical. The patient is usually an elderly, white female, complaining of pain in the right upper quadrant, nausea, vomiting, weight loss and jaundice [15]. Sometimes an unsuspected carcinoma is found in a cholecystectomy specimen at histology. These small lesions may not even be recognized at the time of operation [12].

Examination may reveal a hard and sometimes tender mass in the gallbladder area.

Serum, urine and *faeces* show the changes of cholestatic jaundice if the bile duct is compressed.

Liver biopsy shows the histological picture of biliary obstruction but does not indicate the cause, because hepatic metastases are uncommon.

Ultrasound scanning shows a mass in the gallbladder lumen or totally replacing the gallbladder. With early lesions the differentiation between gallbladder carcinoma and a thickened wall due to acute or chronic cholecystitis is difficult.

CT may also show a mass in the area of the gallbladder. Ultrasound and CT detect carcinoma of the gallbladder in 60–70% of cases [34].

By the time an abnormality is shown by ultrasound or CT, extension is likely and the chance of total removal low. MRI scanning can help to show the extent of disease and contribute to staging [42].

ERCP shows external compression of the bile duct in the jaundiced patient. *Angiography* shows displacement of hepatic and portal blood vessels by the mass.

In only 50% of patients is a correct pre-operative diagnosis made [10].

Prognosis

This is generally hopeless because the majority are inoperable at the time of diagnosis. Distant metastases are already present in 50% of cases [15]. The only long-term survivors are those in whom the tumour was found incidentally at the time of cholecystectomy for gallstones (carcinoma *in situ*).

Median survival from diagnosis is 3 months, with only 14% alive at 1 year [10]. Papillary and well-differentiated adenocarcinomas have longer survival than tubular and undifferentiated types [21]. The results of radical resection including partial hepatectomy and radical lymphadenectomy are conflicting [8, 15] with some series showing no survival benefit and others claiming increased survival.

Treatment

Cholecystectomy has been recommended for all patients with gallstones in an effort to prevent the development of carcinoma in the gallbladder. This seems drastic for a common condition, and would lead to a large number of unnecessary cholecystectomies.

The pre-operative diagnosis of carcinoma of the gallbladder should not preclude laparotomy although the results of surgical treatment are disappointing. Radical resection including partial hepatectomy has been attempted but with unsatisfactory results and no convincing evidence of improved survival [15]. The same applies to irradiation therapy [22].

Endoscopically or percutaneously placed biliary prostheses relieve bile duct obstruction.

Other tumours

Rarely leiomyosarcoma, rhabdomyosarcoma [2], oat cell carcinoma [23] and carcinoid tumours develop in the gallbladder.

Benign tumours of the extra-hepatic bile duct

These extremely rare tumours usually remain undetected until there is evidence of biliary obstruction and cholangitis. They are rarely diagnosed pre-operatively.

Recognition is important as resection is curative.

Papilloma is a polypoid tumour which projects into the lumen of the common bile duct. It is a small, soft, vascular tumour, which may be sessile or pedunculated. These tumours may be single or multiple; they may be cystic. Occasionally they undergo malignant change [32]. Cholangiography may show a smooth mass projecting into the bile duct. Mucus secretion from the tumour can cause obstructive cholangitis.

Adenomyoma can be found anywhere in the biliary tract. It is firm and well circumscribed and varies in size up to 15 cm in diameter. It is cured by resection [9].

Fibroma is small and firm and causes early bile duct obstruction.

Granular cell tumour is of mesenchymal origin. It affects young women, usually black, causing cholestasis [5]. It must be distinguished from cholangiocarcinoma or localized sclerosing cholangitis. Tumours are uniformly resectable and curable.

Carcinoma of the bile duct (cholangiocarcinoma)

Carcinoma of the bile duct seems to be increasing. This must in part reflect wider application of newer diagnostic imaging and cholangiographic techniques. Diagnosis of site of origin and spread are more exact.

Carcinoma may arise at any point in the biliary tree from small intra-hepatic bile ducts to the common bile duct (fig. 34.1). The clinical picture and treatment differ according to the site. Surgery has made few advances largely because of the inaccessibility of hilar tumours but there is wider awareness of the need to identify those patients where resection might be possible since even if not curative, surgical treatment may prolong survival with good quality of life. In those who are inoperable, the enthusiastic invasive radiologist and endoscopist make sure that no patient dies with jaundice and/or pruritus.

Associations

Bile duct cancer is associated with ulcerative colitis with or without sclerosing cholangitis (Chapter 15). The majority of patients with primary sclerosing cholangitis who develop cholangiocarcinoma have ulcerative colitis. Patients with primary sclerosing cholangitis and ulcerative colitis who also have colorectal neoplasia

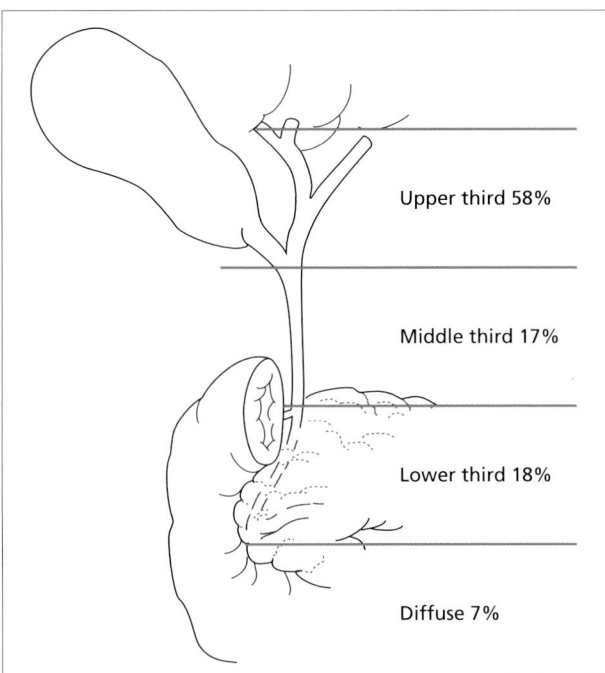

Fig. 34.1. Site of cholangiocarcinoma. The majority occur in the upper third of the bile duct [46].

(dysplasia/carcinoma) are at greater risk of cholangiocarcinoma than those without colonic neoplasia [4].

In a group of 70 patients with primary sclerosing cholangitis followed prospectively for a mean of 30 months, 15 patients died of liver failure. Five of 12 patients (40%) having an autopsy had cholangiocarcinoma—7% of the total group [41].

All members of the congenital fibropolycystic family may be complicated by adenocarcinoma (Chapter 30). These include congenital hepatic fibrosis, cystic dilatation (Caroli's syndrome), choledochal cyst, polycystic liver and von Meyenburg complexes. Cholangiocarcinoma may be associated with biliary cirrhosis due to biliary atresia.

The liver fluke infestations of the Orient may be complicated by intra-hepatic (cholangiocellular) cholangiocarcinoma. In the Far East (China, Hong Kong, Korea, Japan), where *Clonorchis sinensis* is prevalent, cholangiocarcinoma accounts for 20% of primary liver tumours. These arise in the heavily parasitized bile ducts near the hilum.

Opisthorchis viverrini infestation is important in Thailand, Laos, and western Malaysia [26]. These parasites induce DNA changes and mutations through the production of carcinogens and free radicals, and the stimulation of cellular proliferation of intra-hepatic bile duct epithelium [35].

The risk of extra-hepatic bile duct carcinoma is significantly lower 10 years or more after cholecystectomy, suggesting a link with gallstones [16].

Bile duct cancers are not closely associated with cirrhosis unless it is of the biliary type.

Pathology

The confluence of cystic duct with main hepatic duct or the right and left main hepatic ducts at the porta hepatis are common sites of origin (fig. 34.1) and the tumour extends into the liver. It causes complete obstruction of the extra-hepatic bile ducts with intra-hepatic biliary dilatation and enlargement of the liver. The gallbladder is collapsed and flaccid. If the tumour is restricted to one hepatic duct, biliary obstruction is incomplete and jaundice absent. The lobe of the liver drained by this duct atrophies and the other hypertrophies.

In the common bile duct the tumour presents as a firm nodule or plaque which causes an annular stricture which may ulcerate. It spreads along the bile duct and through its wall.

Local and distant metastases, even at autopsy, are found in only about half of the patients. They involve peritoneum, abdominal lymph nodes, diaphragm, liver or gallbladder. Blood vessel invasion is rare and extra-abdominal spread is unusual.

Histologically the tumour is usually a mucin-secreting adenocarcinoma with cuboidal or columnar epithelium (fig. 34.2). Spread along neural sheaths may be noted. Tumours around the hilum are sclerosing with an abundant fibrous stroma. More distal ones are nodular or papillary.

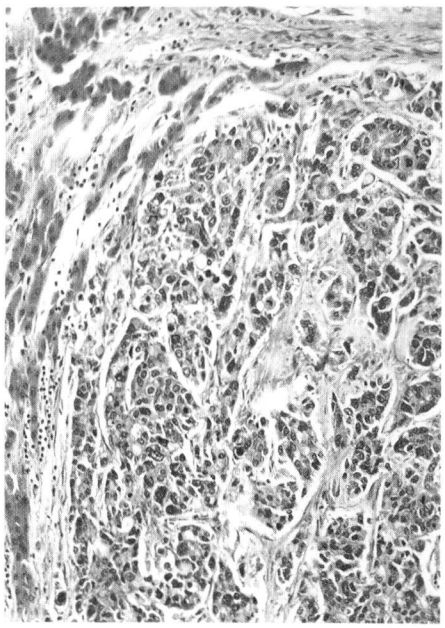

Fig. 34.2. Bile duct carcinoma: a papillary fibrous stroma is seen. (Stained H & E, ×40.)

Molecular changes

Point mutations in codon 12 of the *K-ras oncogene* are found in cholangiocarcinoma [50]. *p53 protein* is expressed particularly in high grade mid and distal duct cholangiocarcinomas [14]. *Aneuploidy* (divergence from the normal chromosome content) is found in hilar cholangiocarcinoma [43] and is associated with neural invasion and shorter survival.

Cholangiocarcinoma cells contain *somatostatin receptor* RNA and cell lines have specific receptors. Cell growth is inhibited by somatostatin analogues. Radionuclide scanning with a labelled somatostatin analogue has detected a cholangiocarcinoma [45].

Clinical features [46]

This tumour tends to occur in the older age group, patients being about 60 years old. Slightly more males than females are affected.

Jaundice is the usual presenting feature, followed by pruritus—a point of distinction from primary biliary cirrhosis. Jaundice may be delayed if only one main hepatic duct is involved. The trend of the serum bilirubin level is always upward, but periods of clearing of jaundice are found in up to 50% [24].

Pain, usually epigastric and mild, is present in about one-third of patients. Diarrhoea may be related to steatorrhoea. Weakness and weight loss are marked.

The condition may be associated with chronic ulcerative colitis, often following long-standing cholestasis due to sclerosing cholangitis.

Examination. Jaundice is deep. The patient is usually afebrile until the terminal stage. Cholangitis is unusual unless the bile ducts have been interfered with surgically, endoscopically or percutaneously.

The liver is large and smooth, extending 5–12 cm below the costal margin. The spleen is not felt. Ascites is unusual.

Investigations

Serum biochemical findings are those of cholestatic jaundice. The serum bilirubin, alkaline phosphatase and γ-glutamyl transpeptidase levels may be very high. Fluctuations may reflect incomplete obstruction or primary involvement of one hepatic duct.

The serum mitochondrial antibody test is negative and α-fetoprotein is not increased.

The *faeces* are pale and fatty and occult blood is often present. *Glycosuria* is absent.

Anaemia may be greater than that seen with ampullary carcinoma; the explanation is unknown—it is not due to blood loss. The leucocyte count is high normal with increased polymorphs.

Hepatic biopsy shows the features of large bile duct obstruction. Tumour tissue is not obtained. It may be extremely difficult to get histological proof of malignancy.

It is important to obtain *cytology* from the area of the bile duct stricture. This is best done on brushings taken from the stricture at the time of endoscopic or percutaneous procedures, or on fine needle aspirates done under ultrasound or fluoroscopy. Malignant cells are detected in 60–70% of patients [13, 27]. Analysis of bile simply aspirated at cholangiography is much less helpful.

The tumour marker CA19/9 increases in some cholangiocarcinoma but high levels have also been reported in benign disease, making it less helpful in screening. Use of CA19/9 and CEA together may give a higher accuracy [40].

Scanning

Ultrasound is particularly helpful showing dilated intrahepatic ducts. A tumour mass may be shown in 40% of cases. Ultrasound (real time together with Doppler) accurately detects neoplastic involvement of the portal vein, both occlusion and wall infiltration, but is less good in showing hepatic arterial involvement [31]. Intraduct ultrasound is still experimental but can provide important information on tumour extension in and around the bile duct [44].

CT scan shows intra-hepatic bile duct dilatation, but the tumour is difficult to demonstrate as it is isodense with the rest of the liver. CT will show lobar atrophy and the relationship of the caudate lobe to the hilar tumour. Spiral CT with computerized reconstruction is a new technique which should allow accurate analysis of the relationship between vascular and bile duct anatomy at the hilum.

MRI imaging detects the larger intra-hepatic (cholangiocellular) carcinoma but adds little to ultrasound and CT for the extra-hepatic type. MRI cholangiography, in which imaging data are used to give a reconstruction of the biliary (and pancreatic) tree, is available in some centres (see fig. 29.7), and may be valuable.

Cholangiography

Endoscopic or percutaneous cholangiography, or both, is essential, and should be performed in all patients with the picture of cholestasis and dilated intra-hepatic ducts shown by ultrasound or CT.

Cytology or transpapillary forceps biopsy at the time of ERCP may reveal tumour.

Endoscopic retrograde. The normal common bile duct and gallbladder are visualized and the obstruction at the hilum identified (fig. 34.3).

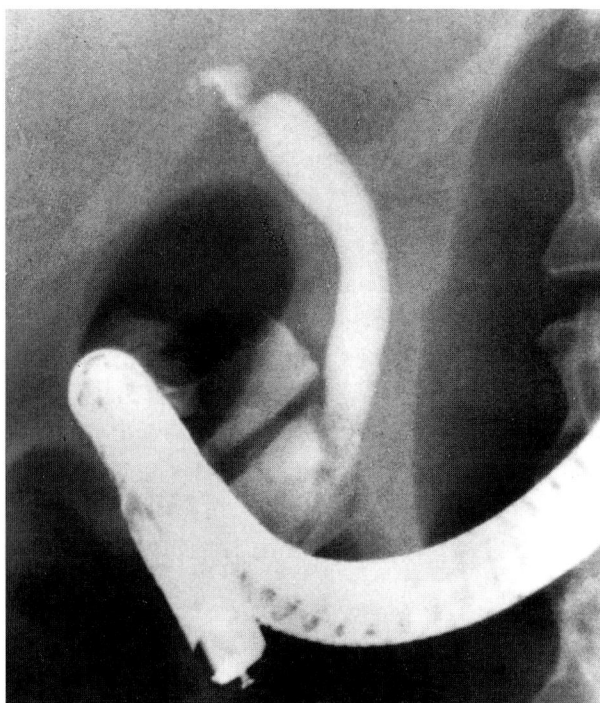

Fig. 34.3. Carcinoma of bile ducts at the hilum of the liver. ERCP shows a common bile duct of normal calibre terminating in an irregular obstruction.

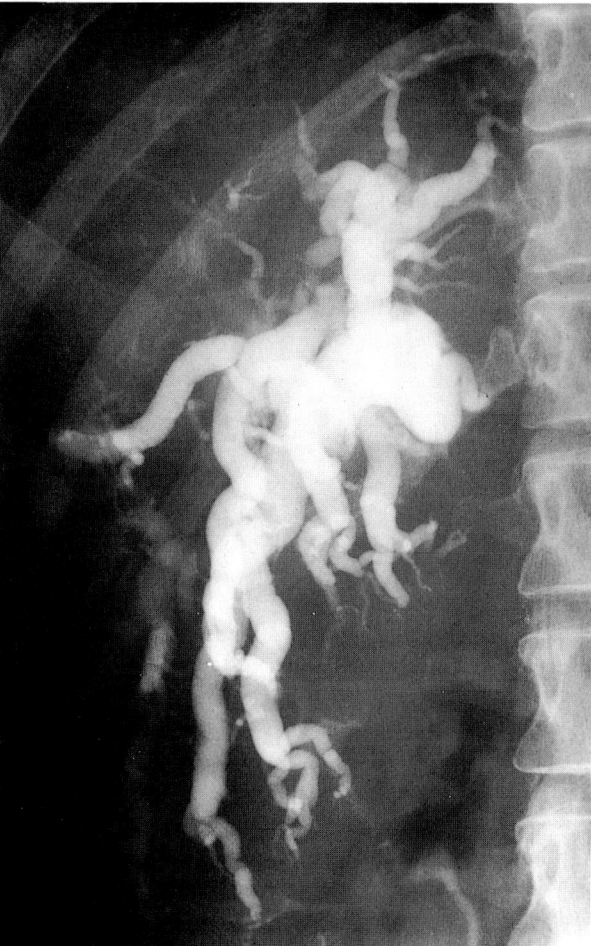

Fig. 34.4. Same patient as in fig. 34.3. Percutaneous trans-hepatic cholangiography shows gross dilatation of intra-hepatic bile ducts and no contrast material enters the common bile duct.

Percutaneous. The obstruction is blunt or nipple-like (fig. 34.4). Intra-hepatic bile ducts are always dilated. When right and left hepatic ducts are individually obstructed, puncture of both systems may be necessary to outline the obstruction accurately.

Angiography

Digital subtraction angiography (DSA) shows hepatic artery and portal vein and their intra-hepatic branches. It remains an essential part of the pre-operative assessment of irresectability.

Diagnosis

In the patient with deepening cholestatic jaundice the clinical diagnosis is likely to be carcinoma of the peri-ampullary region. Other possibilities are drug jaundice, primary sclerosing cholangitis (Chapter 15) and primary biliary cirrhosis (Chapter 14). Cholangiocarcinoma is an unusual cause but it should be detected if an orderly work-up is used (see fig. 13.20). History and examination are usually unhelpful.

The first step in the cholestatic patient is ultrasound scanning. Intra-hepatic bile ducts will be dilated in cholangiocarcinoma. The common duct is normal, equivocal or may be dilated down to an extra-hepatic

tumour. Cholangiography—endoscopic or percutaneous — is done to show the level and characteristics of the stricture. Cytology and biopsy are performed.

Sometimes cholestatic patients reach surgery without cholangiography because on the basis of scanning the cause of obstruction is assumed to be carcinoma of the pancreas or stones. When the common duct is found to be normal, palpation of the hilum is negative, and operation cholangiography (without intra-hepatic bile duct filling) is 'clear', the diagnosis may still be in doubt. The hilar mass is too high and too small to be detected. The significance of a large green liver with a collapsed gall-bladder may not be realized.

If ultrasound does not show dilated bile ducts in the cholestatic patient, other causes (Chapter 13) need to be considered including drug jaundice (history) and primary biliary cirrhosis (antimitochondrial antibody). Liver histology will help. If primary sclerosing cholangitis is possible, cholangiography is diagnostic. ERCP should be done in any cholestatic patient with non-dilated bile ducts where the diagnosis remains in question.

With scanning and cholangiography it should be possible to diagnose the bile duct stricture due to cholangiocarcinoma. At the hilum, the differential diagnosis is metastatic gland, in the mid-duct carcinoma of the gallbladder, and in the periampullary region carcinoma of the pancreas. Differentiation will depend upon history and other imaging techniques.

Prognosis

Prognosis depends on the site of the tumour. Those distally placed are more likely to be resectable than those at the hilum. The histologically differentiated do better than the undifferentiated. Polypoid cancers have the best prognosis.

If unresected, the 1-year survival is 50%, with 20% surviving at 2 years and 10% at 3 years [18]. This reflects that some tumours are slow growing and metastasize late. Jaundice can be relieved surgically or by endoscopic or percutaneous stenting. The tumour kills by its site making it inoperable, rather than by its malignancy. Average survival after resection is longer, making proper assessment in patients fit for surgery essential.

Staging

If the clinical state of the patient does not rule out surgery the resectability and extent of tumour is assessed. Metastases, usually late, should be sought.

Low and mid common bile duct lesions are usually resectable although angiography and venography are needed to exclude vascular invasion.

The more frequent hilar cholangiocarcinoma is more problematic (table 34.1). If cholangiography shows involvement of the secondary hepatic ducts in both hepatic lobes (fig. 34.5, type IV) or angiography shows encasement of the main portal vein or hepatic

Table 34.1. Criteria of irresectability for hilar cholangiocarcinoma

---

Bilateral bile duct involvement or multifocal disease on
  cholangiography
Main trunk of portal vein encased/occluded
Bilateral involvement of hepatic arterial or portal vein branches or
  both
Unilateral hepatic artery involvement and extensive contralateral
  bile duct involvement

---

artery, the lesion is irresectable. A palliative procedure is needed.

If the tumour is limited to the hepatic duct bifurcation, affects one lobe of the liver only, or only obstructs the portal vein or hepatic artery on the same side, the lesion may be resectable. Pre-operative imaging is aimed at establishing whether after surgical removal a viable unit of liver remains [47]. This must contain a biliary radicle large enough to anastomose to bowel, and a normal portal vein and hepatic arterial branch. At surgery, further assessment is done with intra-operative ultrasound and a search for lymph node involvement.

Treatment

Surgery

Tumours of the lower bile duct may be resected with a 1-year survival of about 70% [30]. More proximal tumours may be resected by local or major liver surgery including excision of the whole bifurcation of the common hepatic duct, lobectomy if necessary and bilateral hepatico-jejunostomy.

Some advocate caudate lobectomy, based on the observation that two to three bile ducts from this lobe drain directly into the main bile ducts adjacent to the confluence of the hepatic ducts and thus are likely to be involved by tumour.

The   proportion   of   cholangiocarcinomas   being

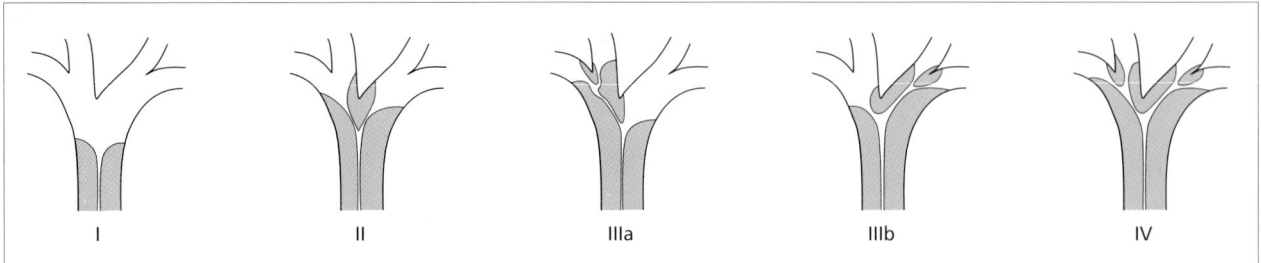

Fig. 34.5. Classification of hilar cholangiocarcinoma according to involvement of bile ducts. Resectability of type I to III depends on angiographic findings. Type IV (bilateral involvement of secondary hepatic ducts) indicates incurable disease. In inoperable patients median survival after stent insertion depends upon the extent of tumour [39].

resected has increased from 5–20% of patients in the 1970s to 40% or more in specialist centres in the 1990s [3, 47]. This relates to earlier diagnosis and referral to a tertiary centre, more accurate and complete pre-operative assessment, and a more aggressive surgical approach. The problem is to achieve a resection with tumour negative margins. Mean survival after aggressive resection of hilar cholangiocarcinoma is 2–3 years with good palliation for most of this time [3, 30, 49]. Local resection of Bismuth type I and II tumours (fig. 34.5) carries a perioperative mortality of 5% or less. Liver resection is needed for type III lesions, and carries a greater morbidity and mortality.

Liver transplantation is not appropriate for cholangiocarcinoma because of early recurrence in the majority [49].

Surgical palliative procedures include anastomosis of jejunum to the segment III duct in the left lobe which is usually accessible despite the hilar tumour (fig. 34.6). Jaundice is relieved for at least 3 months in 75% of patients [20]. If segment III bypass is not possible (atrophy, metastases), a right-sided intra-hepatic anastomosis to the segment V duct can be done [47].

Non-surgical palliation

In those patients unfit for surgery or with irresectable tumours, jaundice and itching may be relieved by placing an endoprosthesis across the stricture either by the endoscopic or percutaneous route.

By the endoscopic route, stents can be inserted successfully in about 90% of patients if a combined endoscopic/percutaneous procedure is included after a failed endoscopic attempt. The major early complication is cholangitis (7%). 30-day mortality is between 10 and 28% depending upon the extent of the tumour at the hilum and the mean survival is 20 weeks [39].

Percutaneous trans-hepatic endoprosthesis insertion is also successful but carries with it a higher risk of complications such as bleeding and bile leakage (Chapter 29). Metal mesh endoprostheses, which expand to 1 cm diameter in the stricture after insertion on a 5 or 7 French catheter, are more expensive than plastic types, but have longer patency for peri-ampullary strictures [11, 25]. They may be used for hilar strictures. Early studies suggest a similar advantage over plastic endoprostheses [48] but their insertion requires an experienced operator.

There are no trials comparing surgical versus non-surgical palliation. There are benefits and disadvantages of both approaches [33]. Generally, non-operative techniques are appropriate for high-risk patients expected to have a shorter survival [28].

Internal radiotherapy using [192]iridium wire or radium needles may be combined with biliary drainage [19]. The value of this technique is unproven. Cytotoxic drugs are ineffective. External radiotherapy has appeared to show some benefit in retrospective studies but in a randomized trial showed no benefit [37]. Symptomatic treatment is that of chronic cholestasis (Chapter 13).

Cholangiocellular carcinoma

This intra-hepatic bile duct derived tumour is classified as a primary hepatic carcinoma. It becomes symptomatic as it enlarges producing abdominal pain rather than jaundice. It grows rapidly with early metastasis and a particularly poor prognosis. There is an association with Thorotrast (thorium dioxide), an intravenous contrast medium used many years ago. Scanning shows an intra-hepatic mass [1]. Distinction from hepato-cellular carcinoma may be difficult. Hepatic venous and portal vein involvement are rare. Surgery is the only chance for effective treatment. Liver resection has given a median survival of 13 months; patients having transplantation for irresectable tumours survive a median of 5 months [36].

Metastases at the hilum

Cholestatic jaundice developing following the diagnosis of carcinoma elsewhere (in particular the colon) may be due to diffuse metastases within the liver or duct obstruction by nodes at the hilum. Differentiation between the two is by ultrasound. If dilated bile ducts are shown and the patient is symptomatic with itching, biliary obstruction can be relieved by insertion of an

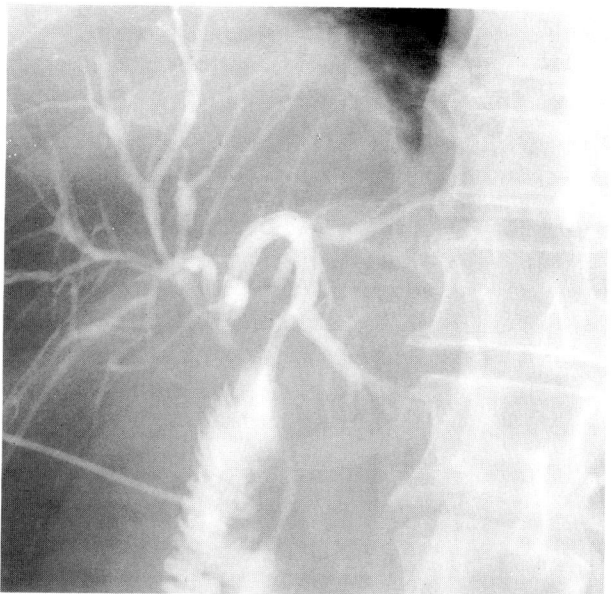

Fig. 34.6. Check cholangiogram after surgical bypass for hilar cholangiocarcinoma. The anastomosis is between the jejunum and the third segment duct of the left lobe.

endoprosthesis by the endoscopic or percutaneous approach. Palliation is achieved depending upon the extent of tumour but the 30-day mortality is greater and the survival significantly shorter compared with endoprosthesis insertion for primary bile duct malignancy [39].

References

1 Adjei ON, Tamura S, Sugimura H *et al.* Contrast-enhanced MR imaging of intrahepatic cholangiocarcinoma. *Clin. Radiol.* 1995; **50**: 6.

2 Al-Jaberi TM, Al-Masri N, Tbukhi A. Adult rhabdomyosarcoma of the gall bladder: case report and review of published works. *Gut* 1994; **35**: 854.

3 Baer HU, Stain SC, Dennison AR *et al.* Improvements in survival by aggressive resections of hilar cholangiocarcinoma. *Ann. Surg.* 1993; **217**: 20.

4 Broomé U, Löfberg R, Veress B *et al.* Primary sclerosing cholangitis and ulcerative colitis: evidence for increased neoplastic potential. *Hepatology* 1995; **22**: 1404.

5 Butterly LF, Schapiro RH, LaMuraglia GM *et al.* Biliary granular cell tumor: a little-known curable bile duct neoplasm of young people. *Surgery* 1988; **103**: 328.

6 Caygill CPJ, Hill MJ, Braddick M *et al.* Cancer mortality in chronic typhoid and paratyphoid carriers. *Lancet* 1994; **343**: 83.

7 Chao T-C, Greager JA. Primary carcinoma of the gallbladder. *J. Surg. Oncol.* 1991; **46**: 215.

8 Chijiiwa K, Tanaka M. Carcinoma of the gallbladder: an appraisal of surgical resection. *Surgery* 1994; **115**: 751.

9 Cook DJ, Salena BJ, Vincic LM. Adenomyoma of the common bile duct. *Am. J. Gastroenterol.* 1988; **83**: 432.

10 Cubertafond P, Gainant A, Cucchiaro G. Surgical treatment of 724 carcinomas of the gallbladder. Results of the French Surgical Association Survey. *Ann. Surg.* 1994; **219**: 275.

11 Davids PHP, Groen AK, Rauws EAJ *et al.* Randomized trial of self-expanding metal stents versus polyethylene stents for distal malignant biliary obstruction. *Lancet* 1992; **340**: 1488.

12 de Aretxabala X, Roa I, Brugos L *et al.* Gallbladder cancer in Chile: a report on 54 potentially resectable tumors. *Cancer* 1992; **69**: 60.

13 Desa LA, Akosa AB, Lazzara S *et al.* Cytodiagnosis in the management of extrahepatic biliary stricture. *Gut* 1991; **32**: 1188.

14 Diamantis I, Karamitopoulou E, Perentes E *et al.* p53 protein immunoreactivity in extrahepatic bile duct and gallbladder cancer: correlation with tumour grade and survival. *Hepatology* 1995; **22**: 774.

15 Donohue JH, Nagorney DM, Grant CS *et al.* Carcinoma of the gallbladder: does radical resection improve outcome? *Arch. Surg.* 1990; **125**: 237.

16 Ekbom A, Hsieh C, Yuen J *et al.* Risk of extra hepatic bile duct cancer after cholecystectomy. *Lancet* 1993; **342**: 1262.

17 Farinon AM, Pacella A, Cetta F *et al.* Adenomatous polyps of the gallbladder. Adenomas of the gallbladder. *HPB Surgery* 1991; **3**: 251.

18 Farley DR, Weaver AL, Nagorney DM. 'Natural history' of unresected cholangiocarcinoma: patient outcome after non-curative intervention. *Mayo Clin. Proc.* 1995; **70**: 425.

19 Fletcher MS, Brinkley D, Dawson JL *et al.* Treatment of hilar carcinoma by bile drainage combined with internal radiotherapy using 192-iridium wire. *Br. J. Surg.* 1983; **70**: 733.

20 Guthrie CM, Banting SW, Garden OJ *et al.* Segment III cholangiojejunostomy for palliation of malignant hilar obstruction. *Br. J. Surg.* 1994; **81**: 1639.

21 Hisatomi K, Haratake J, Horie A *et al.* Relation of histopathological features to prognosis of gallbladder cancer. *Am. J. Gastroenterol.* 1990; **85**: 567.

22 Houry S, Schlienger M, Huguier M *et al.* Gallbladder carcinoma: role of radiation therapy. *Br. J. Surg.* 1989; **76**: 448.

23 Johnstone AK, Zuch RH, Anders KH. Oat cell carcinoma of the gallbladder: a rare and highly lethal neoplasm. *Arch. Pathol. Lab. Med.* 1993; **117**: 1009.

24 Klatskin G. Adenocarcinoma of the hepatic duct at its bifurcation within the porta hepatis. An unusual tumour with distinctive clinical and pathological features. *Am. J. Med.* 1965; **38**: 24.

25 Knyrim K, Wagner HJ, Pausch J *et al.* A prospective, randomized, controlled trial of metal stents for malignant obstruction of the common bile duct. *Endoscopy* 1993; **25**: 207.

26 Kurathong S, Lerdverasirikul P, Wongpaitoon V *et al.* *Opisthorchis viverrini* infection and cholangiocarcinoma. A prospective, case-controlled study. *Gastroenterology* 1985; **89**: 151.

27 Kurzawinski TR, Deery A, Dooley JS *et al.* A prospective study of biliary cytology in 100 patients with bile duct strictures. *Hepatology* 1993; **18**: 1399.

28 Lai ECS, Chu KM, Lo C-Y *et al.* Choice of palliation for malignant hilar biliary obstruction. *Am. J. Surg.* 1992; **163**: 208.

29 Misra SP, Dwivedi M. Pancreaticobiliary ductal union. *Gut* 1990; **31**: 1144.

30 Nagorney DM, Donohue JH, Farnell JH *et al.* Outcomes after curative resections of cholangiocarcinoma. *Arch. Surg.* 1993; **128**: 871.

31 Neumaier CE, Bertolotto M, Perrone R *et al.* Staging of hilar cholangiocarcinoma with ultrasound. *J. Clin. Ultrasound* 1995; **23**: 173.

32 Neumann RD, Livolsi VA, Rosenthal NS *et al.* Adenocarcinoma in biliary papillomatosis. *Gastroenterology* 1976; **70**: 779.

33 Nordback IH, Pitt HA, Coleman J *et al.* Unresectable hilar cholangiocarcinoma: percutaneous versus operative palliation. *Surgery* 1994; **115**: 597.

34 Oikarinen H, Paivansalo M, Lahde S *et al.* Radiological findings in cases of gallbladder carcinoma. *Eur. J. Radiol.* 1993; **17**: 179.

35 Parkin DM, Ohshima H, Srivatanakul P *et al.* Cholangiocarcinoma: epidemiology, mechanisms of carcinogenesis and prevention. *Cancer Epidemiol. Biomarkers Prevention* 1993; **2**: 537.

36 Pichlmayr R, Lamesch P, Weimann A *et al.* Surgical treatment of cholangiocellular carcinoma. *World J. Surg.* 1995; **19**: 83.

37 Pitt HA, Nakeeb A, Abrams RA *et al.* Perihilar cholangiocarcinoma. Postoperative radiotherapy does not improve survival. *Ann. Surg.* 1995; **221**: 788.

38 Polk HC. Carcinoma and calcified gallbladder. *Gastroenterology* 1966; **50**: 582.

39 Polydorou AA, Cairns SR, Dowsett JF *et al.* Palliation of proximal malignant biliary obstruction by endoscopic endoprosthesis insertion. *Gut* 1991; **32**: 685.

40 Ramage JK, Donaghy A, Farrant JM *et al.* Serum tumor

markers for the diagnosis of cholangiocarcinoma in primary sclerosing cholangitis. *Gastroenterology* 1995; **108**: 865.

41 Rosen CB, Nagorney DM, Wiesner RH *et al.* Cholangiocarcinoma complicating primary sclerosing cholangitis. *Ann. Surg.* 1991; **213**: 21.

42 Sagoh T, Itoh K, Togashi K *et al.* Gallbladder carcinoma: evaluation with MR imaging. *Radiology* 1990; **174**: 131.

43 Sato Y, van Gulik TM, Bosma A *et al.* Prognostic significance of tumour DNA content in carcinoma of the hepatic duct confluence. *Surgery* 1994; **115**: 488.

44 Tamada K, Ido K, Ueno N *et al.* Preoperative staging of extrahepatic bile duct cancer with intraductal ultrasonography. *Am. J. Gastroenterol.* 1995; **90**: 239.

45 Tan CK, Podila PV, Taylor JE *et al.* Human cholangiocarcinomas express somatostatin receptors and respond to somatostatin with growth inhibition. *Gastroenterology* 1995; **108**: 1908.

46 Tompkins RK, Saunders KD, Roslyn JJ *et al.* Changing patterns in diagnosis and management of bile duct cancer. *Ann. Surg.* 1990; **211**: 614.

47 Vauthey J-N, Blumgart LH. Recent advances in the management of cholangiocarcinomas. *Semin. Liver Dis.* 1994; **14**: 109.

48 Wagner H-J, Knyrim K, Vakil N *et al.* Plastic endoprostheses versus metal stents in the palliative treatment of malignant hilar biliary obstruction: a prospective randomized trial. *Endoscopy* 1993; **25**: 213.

49 Washburn WK, Lewis WD, Jenkins RL. Aggressive surgical resection for cholangiocarcinoma. *Arch. Surg.* 1995; **130**: 270.

50 Watanabe M, Asaka M, Tanaka J *et al.* Point mutation of K-*ras* gene codon 12 in biliary tract tumors. *Gastroenterology* 1994; **107**: 1147.

Chapter 35
Hepatic Transplantation

In 1955, Welch performed the first transplantation of the liver in dogs [149]. In 1963, Starzl and his group carried out the first successful hepatic transplant in man [129].

The number of transplants is escalating and, in 1994, 3450 patients were transplanted in the USA. Elective liver transplantation in low risk patients has a 90% 1-year survival [12, 127]. Improved results can be related to more careful patient selection, to better surgical techniques and post-operative care, and to greater willingness to retransplant after rejection [82]. Better immunosuppression has contributed.

Selection of patients

The patient selected for transplant should suffer from irreversible, progressive disease for which there is no acceptable, alternative therapy. The patient and his family must understand the magnitude of the undertaking and be prepared to face the difficult early postoperative period and life-long immunosuppression.

Shortage of donors makes selection particularly difficult. It is usually done by a transplantation selection committee. Candidates are divided into the chances of dying—low risk, moderate risk and high risk. Unfortunately, the category may deteriorate while the patient is waiting. Results (and costs) are much better if the patient is low risk (ambulatory) compared with high risk (intensive care).

In the USA, demand for liver transplants is increasing but with little change in the numbers of donors. The size of the waiting list now exceeds the number of transplants performed in 1 year (fig. 35.1). Thus, the low risk patient may have to wait 6–12 months for an organ. A patient with fulminant liver failure will only wait 4 days. Those with rare blood groups B and AB wait longest. Donor livers suitable for children are particularly rare and this has led to the 'split liver' technique (see fig. 35.6).

Candidates (tables 35.1, 35.2, fig. 35.2)

In Europe, the pattern of primary indication for liver transplantation is changing (fig. 35.2). The main indication is cirrhosis, including primary biliary cirrhosis. More patients with acute and subacute hepatic failure and with biliary atresia are being included and fewer with cancer.

Cirrhosis

All patients with end-stage cirrhosis should be considered for liver transplantation. Selection of the right time

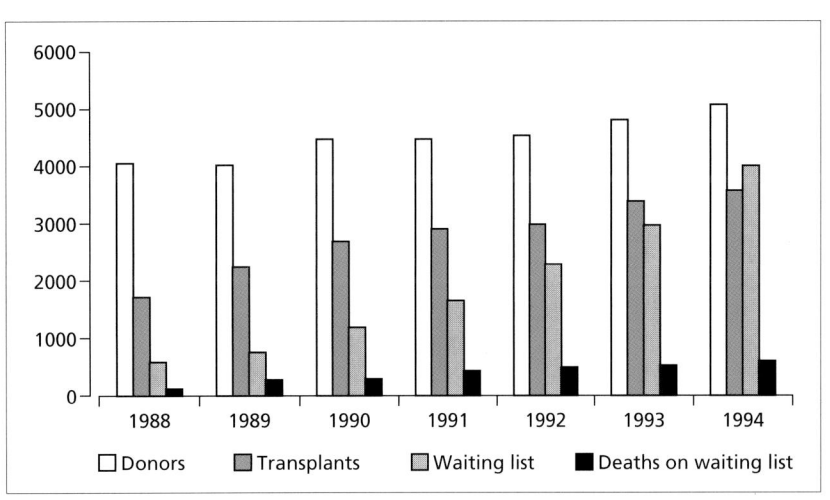

Fig. 35.1. Cadaveric donor organ utilization 1986–93 (data from the United Network for Organ Sharing (UNOS) Scientific Registry, August 1995).

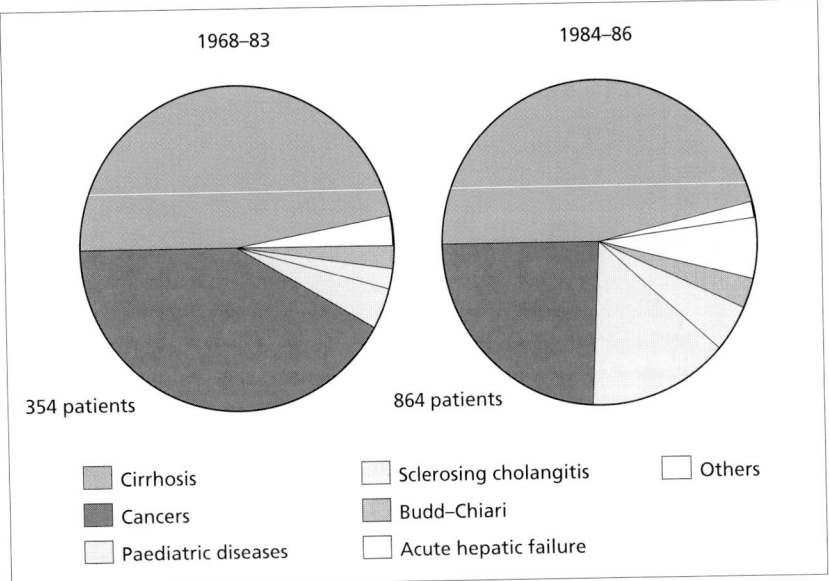

1968–83

1984–86

354 patients

864 patients

☐ Cirrhosis

☐ Sclerosing cholangitis

☐ Others

☐ Cancers

☐ Budd–Chiari

☐ Paediatric diseases

☐ Acute hepatic failure

Fig. 35.2. Changing patterns of primary indications for liver transplantation [13].

Table 35.1. Percentage survival of 9966 patients according to diagnosis of cirrhosis, acute liver failure and cancer (data from European Liver Transplant Registry, 1993)

Diagnosis	% 1-year survival	% 2-year survival	% 3-year survival
Cirrhosis	80	73	71
Acute liver failure	60	56	54
Cancer	64	42	36

is difficult. The patient must not be moribund, so that the transplant will fail, or be capable of leading a relatively normal life for a long period so that transplant is unnecessary. Indications include a prothrombin time more than 5 seconds prolonged, serum albumin concentration less than 30 g/litre, and intractable ascites. Bleeding oesophageal varices (see Chapter 10), after failure of medical treatment and sclerotherapy, is a good indication. The cost of transplant is little different from that of long-term medical and surgical management of complications such as bleeding, coma and ascites.

The patients are poor operative risks because of impaired blood coagulation and portal hypertension, so that blood loss is great. The technical difficulties are greater when cirrhosis is present, particularly when the liver is small and difficult to remove. Survival is much the same for all forms of cirrhosis.

Autoimmune chronic hepatitis

Transplantation is being performed at the stage of cirrhosis, and also for the major side-effects of corticosteroid therapy such as bone thinning and recurrent infections. The liver disease does not seem to recur post-transplant (Chapter 17).

Table 35.2. Possible candidates for hepatic transplantation

Cirrhosis
Cryptogenic
Autoimmune
Virus B (HBV DNA negative)
Virus D
Virus C
Alcoholic (Chapter 20)

Cholestatic liver disease
Primary biliary cirrhosis
Biliary atresia
Primary sclerosing cholangitis
Secondary sclerosing cholangitis
Graft-versus-host disease
Chronic hepatic rejection
Cholestatic sarcoidosis (Chapter 26)
Chronic drug reactions (rare)

Primary metabolic disease (see table 35.3)

Fulminant liver failure (Chapter 8)

Malignant disease (Chapter 28)
Hepato-cellular carcinoma
Epithelioid haemangio-endothelioma
Hepatoblastoma

Miscellaneous
Budd–Chiari syndrome (Chapter 11)
Short-bowel syndrome

Transplantation for chronic viral hepatitis

Hepatic transplantation performed for *acute* fulminant viral hepatitis (A, B, D and E) is not followed by graft reinfection as the viral levels are very low (Chapter 16).

In the chronic situation, however, graft reinfection is very common.

Hepatitis B

Results in patients with chronic hepatitis B are disappointing, probably owing to extra-hepatic viral replication, particularly in monocytes [71]. The 1-year survival is 80%, but the 2-year survival is only 50–60%. Transplantation should only be considered if the patient is serum HBV-DNA and HBeAg negative [71]. In HBV-positive patients, the post-transplant course is usually severe with an escalated course, with cirrhosis or cirrhosis and liver cancer in 2–3 years. Re-transplant results in even shorter time before recurrence and liver failure [138].

Post-transplant, a severe *fibrosing cholestatic hepatitis* may develop with ballooning of hepatocytes and ground-glass change. This may be related to high cytoplasmic expression of viral antigens in the presence of immunosuppression [10, 32]. HBV may sometimes be cytopathic. Attempts to prevent reinfection of the graft by interferon have largely failed [73]. Long-term use of hepatitis B immunoglobulin reduces recurrent infection if given to HBV-DNA-positive patients in the anhepatic stage, then daily for 1 week, then monthly for 1 year, and probably longer [115]. It is very costly. Lamivudine given before and after transplant may control reinfection. Ganciclovir may reduce HBV replication [48]. Hepato-cellular carcinoma can develop in the transplanted liver [78].

Hepatitis delta

Transplantation is almost always followed by infection of the graft. HDV RNA and HDAg can be detected in the new liver and HDV RNA in the serum [159]. Hepatitis only develops if there is concomitant or super infection with hepatitis B virus.

Hepatitis B infection is inhibited by delta infection and hepatitis B recurrence may be reduced by delta infection. In general, survival is good after transplant for delta infected patients with a 1-year survival of 76% and a 2-year survival of 71% [30].

Hepatitis C

End-stage HCV disease is an increasing indication for liver transplantation accounting for about one-third of patients (see below).

In virtually all patients, the transplant will be followed by reinfection of the graft [35, 102]. This is usually from the host as the genotype before and after transplant is similar. Factors influencing recurrence include genotype 1b [43]. The disease can be transmitted from a donor who is anti-HCV positive (fig. 35.3). This is becoming rare

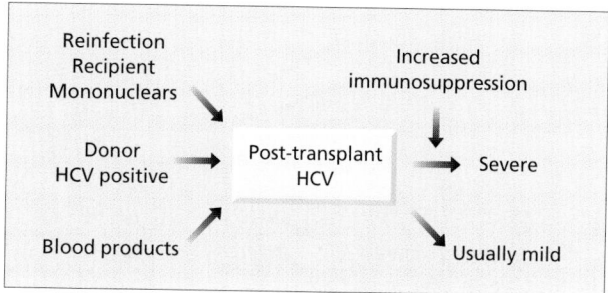

Fig. 35.3. Mechanisms for recurrent HCV hepatitis after liver transplantation.

now that donors are screened for HCV. Similarly in spite of large amounts of blood transfused, the chances of receiving HCV-positive blood and of developing of hepatitis C are low.

Patient and graft survival are excellent with a 1-, 2- and 3-year survival of 94, 89 and 87%, respectively, in cirrhotic patients [7].

After transplant there is a 10-fold increase in the level of serum HCV RNA [51, 114], found even in the absence of histological hepatitis. More usually, activity is related to the amount of corticosteroid and other chemotherapy being used [123].

Reinfection is more frequent after multiple episodes of rejection [123].

The recurrent hepatitis is of varying severity. It is usually mild, compatible with a normal life expectancy and an excellent survival rate [87]. However, longer follow-up is showing an increasing number of patients developing chronic hepatitis and cirrhosis [42]. Persistent HCV can cause severe graft damage especially with HCV genome type 1b [47].

Interferon therapy is only transiently effective [156] and may increase hepatic rejection. Combination of interferon with ribavirin seems more successful; hepatic histology is improved and graft rejection reduced [15].

Neonatal hepatitis

This disease of unknown aetiology is associated with jaundice, giant cell hepatitis and rarely liver failure necessitating liver transplant which is curative [24].

Alcoholic liver disease

In the West, these patients are likely to provide the largest number of candidates for transplant. The selection and the results obtained are discussed in Chapter 20.

Cholestatic liver disease

End-stage biliary disease, usually involving the small intra-hepatic bile ducts, is an excellent indication for

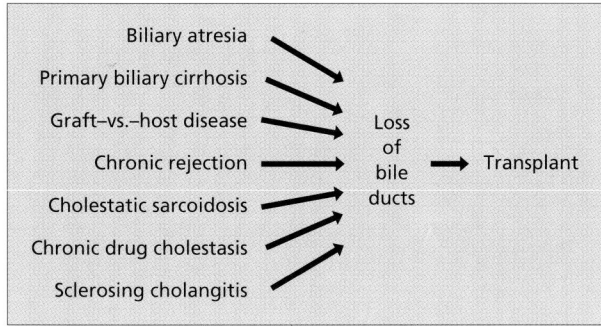

Fig. 35.4. Diseases with disappearing bile ducts treated by liver transplantation.

hepatic transplantation (fig. 35.4). Hepato-cellular function is usually preserved until late and the timing of the transplant is easy. In every case the liver shows an advanced biliary cirrhosis, often combined with loss of bile ducts (*'disappearing bile duct syndrome'*).

Primary biliary cirrhosis (Chapter 14)

One-year survival after transplantation is over 75% [40]. A patient with primary biliary cirrhosis and primary pulmonary hypertension had a triple-transplant of liver, lung and heart and was well 7 years later [147].

Extra-hepatic biliary atresia (Chapter 24)

This indication comprises 35–67% of paediatric liver transplants. Results are excellent and long-term survivors have good physical and mental development [99, 113].

The Pittsburgh Group report 12 of 20 children surviving between 1 and 56 months, although 19% needed a second transplant and post-transplant surgery was necessary in 37% [39]. In another series of 36 patients, operated at an average age of 30 months, the calculated 3-year survival was 75% [151].

A previous Kasai procedure increases the operative difficulty and morbidity.

Alagille's syndrome

Transplant is required only in the very severe sufferers [25]. Associated cardiopulmonary disease may be fatal and careful pre-operative assessment is necessary [140].

Primary sclerosing cholangitis

Sepsis and previous biliary surgery provide technical problems. Nevertheless, the results for transplantation are good, 1-year survival being 70% and 5-year survival 57% (see Chapter 15). Cholangiocarcinoma is a com-

plication that greatly reduces long-term survival. Colon cancer is the most frequent cause of death [92].

Langerhans' cell histiocytosis accounts for 15–39% of sclerosing cholangitis. It has been successfully treated by liver transplant [158].

Other end-stage cholestatic diseases

Hepatic transplantation has been performed for graft-versus-host cirrhosis in a bone marrow recipient [109]. Other rare indications include cholestatic sarcoidosis (Chapter 26) and chronic drug reactions (for instance, to chlorpromazine).

Primary metabolic disease

Liver homografts retain their original metabolic specificity. Consequently, liver transplantation is used for patients with inborn errors of metabolism that result from defects in hepatic function. Patients suffering from these conditions are good candidates. Selection depends on the prognosis and the likelihood of the later complication of primary liver tumours.

Liver transplantation for metabolic disorders is divided into those performed for *end-stage liver disease* or pre-malignant change and those performed for major *extra-hepatic features* (table 35.3). Overall survival is 85.9% over 5.5 years follow-up [99].

Table 35.3. Liver transplantation for metabolic disorders

End-stage disease or premalignant change
α_1-antitrypsin deficiency
Wilson's disease
Tyrosinaemia
Galactosaemia
Glycogen storage diseases
Protoporphyria
Neonatal haemochromatosis
β-thalassaemia
Cystic fibrosis
Byler's disease

Major extra-hepatic features
Primary oxaluria type 1
Homozygous hypercholesterolaemia
Crigler–Najjar syndrome
Primary coagulation disorders
   (factor VIII, IX, protein C)
Urea cycle defects
Mitochondrial respiratory chain defects
Primary familial amyloidosis

End-stage liver disease

α_1-antitrypsin deficiency

This is the most common metabolic disease leading to liver transplantation. Only a few sufferers will have significant liver disease, but macronodular cirrhosis will develop in about 15% before the age of 20 years. Hepatocellular carcinoma is a complication. The plasma α_1-antitrypsin deficiency is corrected and the lung disease stabilizes after the transplant. Advanced pulmonary disease is a contraindication unless both lungs and liver are transplanted.

Wilson's disease

Liver transplants have to be considered in patients presenting with the clinical picture of fulminant hepatitis, in young cirrhotic patients with severe hepatic decompensation who have failed to improve after 3 months' adequate D-penicillamine treatment, and in effectively treated patients who have developed severe hepatic decompensation following discontinuance of penicillamine [132]. The 1-year survival after transplant is about 68%. Copper metabolism returns to normal.

Neurological manifestations reverse at varying rates [104].

Glycogen storage diseases

Liver transplantation has been successfully performed for types I and IV [84], with survival and continued growth into adult life [66].

Galactosaemia

A few patients diagnosed late developed advanced cirrhosis in childhood and early adult life and are candidates for transplantation [99].

Protoporphyria

This can lead to end-stage cirrhosis and so be an indication for liver transplantation [17, 55, 116]. Post-operatively, the high level of protoporphyrin in erythrocytes and faeces persists and the disease is not cured.

Tyrosinaemia

Hepatic transplantation is curative and should be considered early before the development of hepato-cellular carcinoma [88].

Neonatal haemochromatosis

This can be rapidly fatal. It may represent a number of disorders. Transplantation gives variable results.

β-thalassaemia

Combined heart and liver transplantation has been reported for end-stage, iron-induced organ failure in an adult with homozygous β-thalassaemia [95].

Cystic fibrosis

Hepatic transplantation is indicated for predominant liver involvement [88]. *Pseudomonas* and *Aspergillus* infection may be complications. Pulmonary function may improve after the transplant.

Byler's disease

This familial, intra-hepatic cholestasis results in death from cirrhosis or heart failure. The low serum apolipoprotein A1 concentration is corrected by transplant performed for cirrhosis [21].

Major extra-hepatic features

Oxaluria

Primary oxaluria type I, due to deficiency of hepatic peroxismal alanine-glyoxylate aminotransferase, is corrected by simultaneous hepatic and renal transplantation [148]. Cardiac dysfunction reverses [112]. Perhaps the hepatic transplantation should be done before renal damage has developed [29].

Homozygous hypercholesterolaemia

Liver transplant produces an 80% decrease in serum lipids. Cardiac transplant or coronary bypass are also usually necessary [11, 108, 142].

Crigler–Najjar syndrome

Liver transplant is indicated to prevent neurological sequelae when the serum bilirubin level is very high and cannot be controlled by phototherapy [64].

Primary coagulation disorders

The transplant is performed for end-stage cirrhosis due to hepatitis B or C. Factor VIII and IX production is maintained post-transplant and haemophilia and haemophilia A are cured [75]. Protein C deficiency is corrected.

Urea cycle enzyme deficiencies

Transplantation has been performed for ornithine trans-carbamylase deficiency as urea cycle enzymes are predominantly located in the liver [72, 139]. The decision concerning the need for transplantation is difficult as some urea cycle disorders allow a normal life style.

Mitochondrial respiratory chain defects

These may cause liver disease in neonates associated with hypoglycaemia and post-prandial hyperlacticacidaemia. They have been treated by liver transplant [49].

Primary familial amyloidosis

Transplant is performed for the intractable polyneuropathy. Neurological improvement is variable [135].

Fulminant liver failure (Chapter 8)

Indications include fulminant viral hepatitis, Wilson's disease, acute fatty liver of pregnancy, drug overdose (for instance, paracetamol), and drug-related hepatitis such as that due to isoniazid-rifampicin [14].

Malignant disease (Chapter 28)

Hepatic transplantation has been disappointing in patients with liver tumours despite pre-operative attempts at identifying extra-hepatic spread. Patients with cancer have a low operative mortality, but the worst long-term survival. Carcinomatosis is the usual cause of death. Tumour recurs in 60%, perhaps because of the immunosuppressants necessary to prevent rejection.

The peri-operative survival is 76%, but the 1-year survival only 50% and the 2-year survival 31% [13]. For all tumours transplanted, the overall actual 5-year survival is 20.4%. These results are believed to justify transplantation [110].

Hepatocellular carcinoma (Chapter 28)

The tumour must be 5 cm or less. If multifocal, only three tumours less than 3 cm each should be considered. Staging laparoscopy is important at the time of transplant [118]. Vascular invasion, even microscopic, increases the recurrence rate and mortality [81]. Pre-operative chemotherapy or chemoembolization may delay recurrence [145].

The 2-year survival is 50 versus 83% for non-malignant conditions. This raises the question of whether donor livers are being wisely used to treat malignant disease [135].

Transplantation may be preferable to resection for small tumours discovered incidentally in a patient with compensated cirrhosis.

Fibrolamellar carcinoma

The tumour is localized to the liver and cirrhosis is absent. This may be the best tumour candidate for transplantation.

Epithelioid haemangio-endothelioma

This presents as multiple focal lesions in both lobes of an otherwise normal liver. The course is unpredictable and recurrence is likely in 50%. Metastatic spread does not contraindicate surgery and this does not correlate with survival [65]. It can be successfully treated by liver transplantation.

Hepatoblastoma

Transplantation results in a 50% survival at 24–70 months [68]. Microscopic vascular invasion and anaplastic epithelium with extra-hepatic spread are bad signs.

Hepatic apudomas

Transplantation is occasionally used for palliation, even if secondaries are present [6, 83].

Abdominal cluster operations for right upper quadrant malignancy

Most of the organs derived from the embryonic foregut are removed including liver, duodenum, pancreas, stomach and intestine. With powerful immunosuppressants, donor lympho-reticular cells circulate without causing clinical graft-versus-host disease and become those of the recipient without causing rejection [118, 131]. The procedure is clearly very radical and patients usually die from recurrent tumour.

Cholangiocarcinoma

This is an unsatisfactory indication as tumour recurrence is usual and 1-year survival is 0% [103].

Miscellaneous

Budd–Chiari syndrome (Chapter 11)

Although liver transplants have been performed with success, recurrence of thrombosis is likely especially if there is underlying myeloproliferative disease.

Short bowel syndrome

Small bowel plus liver transplantation has been performed for short bowel syndrome with secondary liver failure [50].

Transplantation also has to be considered for *cystic fibrosis* with accompanying cirrhosis, and for adult *Niemann–Pick disease*.

Absolute and relative contraindications
(table 35.4)

Absolute

These include uncorrectable cardiopulmonary disease, ongoing infection, metastatic malignancy, AIDS and severe brain damage.

Transplant should not be done if the patient cannot comprehend the magnitude of the undertaking and the exceptional physical and psychological commitment required [82].

Relative (higher risk)

Patients are at higher risk if they have advanced liver disease and are being treated in an intensive care unit and particularly if they are ventilation-dependent.

Children do particularly well but technical difficulties increase below the age of 2 years. There is no absolute contraindication on account of advanced age and biological age is more important than chronological; general and nutritional state must be considered. Nevertheless, age does not usually exceed 60 years.

Table 35.4. Absolute and relative contraindication to liver transplantation

Absolute
Psychological, physical and social inability to tolerate the procedure
Active sepsis
Metastatic malignancy
Cholangiocarcinoma
AIDS
Advanced cardiopulmonary disease

Higher risk
Age more than 60 or less than 2 years
Prior porta-caval shunt
Prior complex hepato-biliary surgery
Portal vein thrombosis
Re-transplant
Multiorgan transplants
Obesity
Serum creatinine more than 2 mg/dl
Cytomegalovirus mismatch
Advanced liver disease

In a small series, transplant of female donor livers into male recipients was associated with a poorer outcome [61], but this must be confirmed with larger numbers.

Risk increases with body weight more than 100 kg.

Retransplantation, or multi-organ transplant clearly add to the risk.

A pre-transplant serum creatinine level exceeding 2.0 mg/dl is the most accurate predictor of post-transplant death [31].

CMV mismatch (R – D+) adds to the risk.

Portal vein thrombosis makes the transplant more difficult and survival is reduced. However, the operation is usually possible [133]. An anastomosis is made between the donor portal vein and the recipient confluence of superior mesenteric vein and splenic vein, or a venous graft from the donor is used.

Previous porta-caval shunts make the operation more difficult and a distal spleno-renal shunt can be used. Transjugular intra-hepatic portal-systemic stent shunt (TIPS) for variceal bleeding is the most satisfactory preliminary to transplantation [2]. It offers no technical problems.

Retransplantation is associated with increased technical problems. Previous complex surgery in the upper abdomen may also make the transplant technically impossible.

General preparation of the patient

A standard protocol is used. The procedure is discussed fully with patient and relatives and consent given.

The usual clinical, biochemical and serological investigation of any patient with liver disease is detailed.

Blood group, HLA and DR antigens are recorded. Antibodies to cytomegalovirus and hepatitis C are measured and markers of hepatitis B infection noted.

In patients with malignant disease, metastases must be sought by all possible techniques.

The hepatic arterial tree must be visualized and any anatomical abnormality, including an aberrant origin of the hepatic artery and a pre-duodenal portal vein, noted. The portal vein and the inferior vena cava must be seen. A selective right renal arteriogram is also performed as failure to recognize a high right kidney may result in unavoidable right nephrectomy. Demonstration of the bile ducts pre-operatively is performed by cholangiography, usually endoscopic. Ultrasound and CT scanning are routine. A careful cardio-pulmonary assessment should include measurement of pulmonary venous pressure.

The pre-transplant medical 'work-up' takes about 10 days. It includes psychiatric counselling and confirmation of the diagnosis. The patient may wait many months for a suitable donor liver and, during this period, intensive psychosocial support is necessary.

The patient should receive hepatitis B, pneumococcal and influenza vaccination.

Donor selection and operation

Selection is standardized [106]. There is however, variability between centres in defining 'good' or 'bad' livers. Increasing demand has led to use of a liver previously regarded as less satisfactory but with no significant increase in graft loss.

Informed consent is given by the relatives. The donor is aged between 2 months and 55 years of age, a victim of brain injury that has resulted in brain death. Cardiovascular and respiratory functions are sustained by mechanical ventilation. The recovery of livers and other vital organs from heart-beating cadavers minimizes the ischaemia that occurs at normal body temperatures and is a major contribution to graft success.

A donor should suffer from no other disease including diabetes and should not be obese; fatty change should be excluded by liver histology [134]. The donor should not have had periods of prolonged hypotension or anoxia or have suffered from cardiac arrest.

Transplant across A, B and O blood groups may be followed by severe rejection. It should be avoided unless necessitated by an emergency situation [52].

HLA matching is more difficult and indeed there is some evidence that selected HLA class II mismatches may be advantageous, particularly in preventing the vanishing bile duct syndrome [93].

Hepatitis B and C viral markers, CMV antibodies and HIV testing should be done.

The operative details of the donor and recipient operation are discussed elsewhere [22, 82, 120]. The hepatic structures are dissected and the liver is pre-cooled through the splenic vein with Ringer's lactate and 1000 ml of the University of Wisconsin (UW) solution perfused through the aorta and portal vein [63]. A cannula in the distal inferior vena cava provides a vent for venous outflow. After removal, the cold liver is further flushed with an additional 1000 ml UW solution through the hepatic artery and portal vein and stored in this solution in a plastic bag on ice in a portable cooler. This routine has extended the preservation time to 11–20 hours so that the recipient operation may be semi-elective and not performed at unsocial hours. The same surgeon can perform both donor and recipient procedures. Further advances in organ preservation [16] include use of a perfusion machine once the liver arrives at the transplant centre. Graft viability may be assessed by nuclear magnetic resonance.

If possible, and particularly for elective procedures, the size and shape of the donor liver should be matched to that of the recipient. It must certainly not be larger, and if possible should be smaller. Occasionally a small-sized liver is transplanted into a larger patient. The donor liver increases in size at the rate of about 70 ml per day until it achieves the volume expected for the recipient's size, age and sex [144].

The recipient operation (fig. 35.5)

The average operative time is 7.6 (4–15) hours. An average of 17 (2–220) packed cells are transfused. A cell-saver is useful, saving approximately a third of the blood lost into the abdominal cavity. This is aspirated, repeatedly washed and the red cells resuspended and infused.

The hilar structures and the vena cava above and below the liver are dissected, cross-clamping and dividing the various vessels just as the liver is removed.

During the implantation of the new liver, it is necessary to occlude the splenic and vena cava circulations. During this anhepatic phase, the use of a pump-driven veno–venous bypass prevents pooling in the lower part of the body and thus splanchnic congestion. The cannulas are placed in the inferior vena cava (via the femoral vein) and the portal vein, and run to the subclavian vein [122].

The veno–venous bypass allows increased operative time, less bleeding, and an easier technique.

All vascular anastomoses are completed before opening the blood supply to the liver. Portal vein thrombosis must be excluded. Hepatic arterial anomalies are

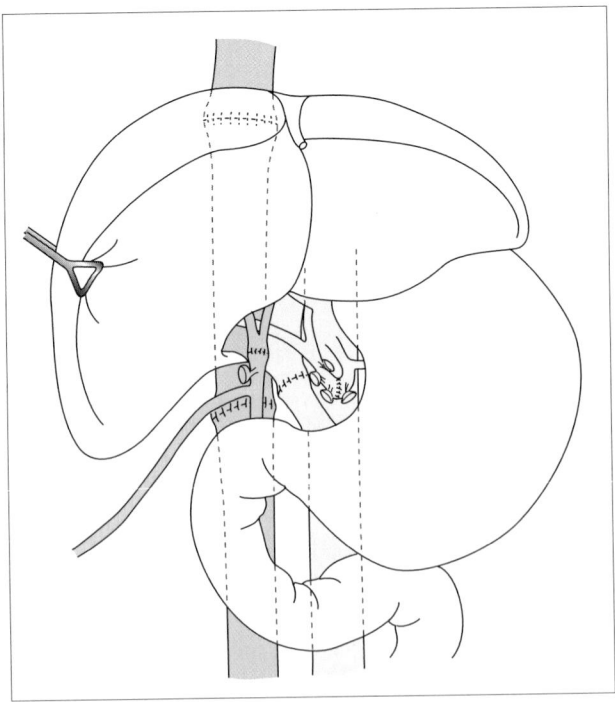

Fig. 35.5. Completed orthotopic liver transplantation. Biliary tract reconstruction is by duct-to-duct anastomosis.

frequent, and vessel grafts from the donor should be available for arterial reconstructions.

The usual order of anastomases is (i) supra-hepatic vena cava, (ii) intra-hepatic vena cava, (iii) portal vein, (iv) hepatic artery and (v) biliary system. The bile duct is usually reconstructed by direct anastomosis with a T-tube stent. If the recipient bile duct is diseased or absent, end-to-side Roux-en-Y choledocho-jejunostomy is chosen. Before closing the abdomen, the surgeon usually waits a period of about one hour so that any remaining bleeding points may be identified and closed.

Reduced size segmental (split liver) transplantation

Because of the difficulty in obtaining small donor livers for young children, segments of adult livers have been used [12] (fig. 35.6). This provides two viable grafts from a single donor liver, although usually only the left lobe or left lateral segment is used [38, 98]. The weight ratio of recipient to donor should be about 3 : 4. 75% of paediatric patients now receive reduced size liver transplants.

Results are not quite as satisfactory as with full liver grafts (75 versus 85% survival at 1 year [18]). There are more complications including increased intra-operative blood loss and inadequate allograft perfusion due to portal vein hypoplasia [8]. Graft loss and biliary complications are increased over adult transplants [14, 38].

Living-related liver transplantation

In special circumstances, usually in children, a liver graft, usually the left lateral segment may be used from a living-related donor [38, 60]. Donation is restricted to relatives who must give free and informed consent. This provides a readily available graft of excellent quality when there are no cadaveric livers available. The recipient should have terminal disease or reside in a country where cadaveric transplantation is not permitted. With advanced surgical experience and anaesthesiology and critical care, the risk to the donor is less than 1% [157]. The operative stay averages 11 days and the blood loss is only about 200–300 ml. Rarely, the donor may have operative and post-operative complications such as injuries to bile duct and spleen or abscesses.

The procedure is largely used in paediatrics [19]. It has been used in primary biliary cirrhosis [58]. It has also been used in fulminant hepatic failure where a cadaveric donor is not available at short notice. This has the disad-

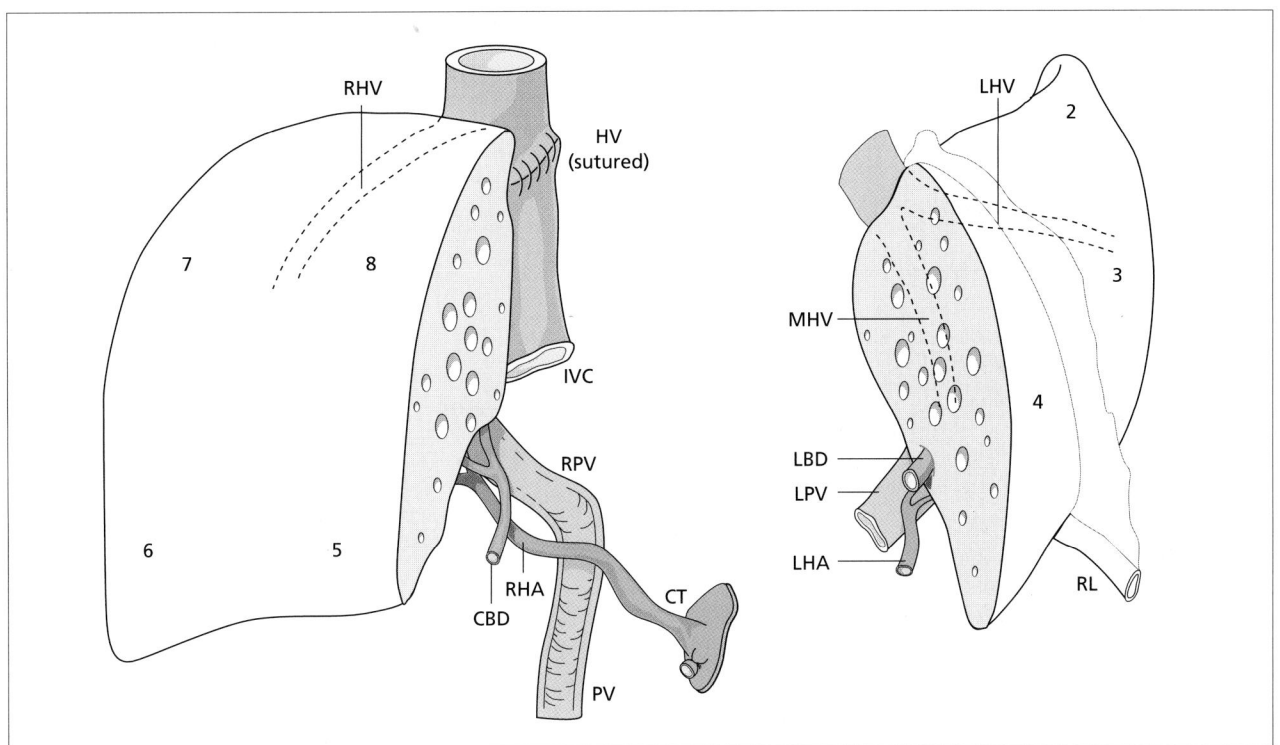

Fig. 35.6. Diagram of the two grafts after preparation from one donor liver. Note that all the main vascular and biliary structures remain attached to the right lobe and that the left lobe is supplied by lobar pedicles (IVC = inferior vena cava; PV = portal vein; CT = coeliac trunk; CBD = common bile duct; HV = hepatic vein; RPV = right portal branch; RHA = right branch of hepatic artery; RHV = right hepatic vein; LHA = left branch of hepatic artery; LPV = left portal branch; LBD = left bile duct; LHV = left hepatic vein; MHV = middle hepatic vein). Numbers indicate hepatic segments [38].

vantage of inadequate time to prepare the donor both psychologically and pre-operatively, including the collection of his or her autologous blood.

Auxiliary heterotropic liver transplantation

Healthy liver tissue is introduced somewhere in the body leaving the native liver *in situ* [90]. It may be indicated in fulminant hepatic failure where there is a chance that the patient's own liver will regenerate. It may also be used in the treatment of some metabolic defects.

A reduced size graft is usually used. The left lobe of the donor liver is excised and the right lobe anastomosed to the portal vein and aorta of the recipient. The donor liver hypertrophies and the recipient's own liver atrophies.

Immunosuppression is discontinued when the host liver has recovered. At this time the auxiliary is likely to atrophy and may be removed.

Xeno-transplantation

A patient with end-stage cirrhosis who was HBV-positive and HIV-positive, received a baboon liver. The early result was good, but the patient succumbed at 70 days to bacterial, viral and fungal infection [128]. This experience has not been repeated and there are ethical concerns and animal rights questions.

Liver transplantation in paediatrics

The mean age is about 3 years, but successful transplant has been performed at less than 1 year old [9]. A major problem is scarcity of paediatric donors which may necessitate adult reduced-liver or split-liver donations.

Post-transplant, growth is good and the quality of life excellent [151].

The small size of the vessels and bile ducts poses technical problems. Pre-transplant anatomy should be identified by CT or, preferably, MRI. Hepatic artery thrombosis occurs in at least 17% [136]. Re-transplants are frequent. Biliary complications are also common.

One-year survival is 75.5% for children who are less than 3 years old [97]. Renal function may deteriorate post-transplant and this is not solely due to cyclosporine A. Infections are frequent, particularly varicella, Epstein–Barr [86], mycobacteria [79], *Candida* [67] and CMV.

Immunosuppression

Multiple therapy is usually given which varies between centres. Most centres use a combination of cyclosporine and corticosteroids.

Cyclosporine may be given pre-transplant orally, or

intravenously if oral intake is not possible. It is combined with methylprednisolone intravenously.

After transplant, the patients receive cyclosporine intravenously in divided doses, until oral intake is adequate when it is continued in divided doses, together with intravenous methylprednisolone, tapering to 0.3 mg/kg per day by the end of the first week. When oral intake is possible, it is continued by mouth. Other centres do not use cyclosporine pre-transplant, but prescribe azathioprine together with methylprednisolone, starting cyclosporine only when renal function is adequate. Long-term maintenance is usually with 5–10 mg cyclosporine kg/day.

Cyclosporine side-effects include nephrotoxicity but the glomerular filtration usually stabilizes after a few months. Nephrotoxicity is enhanced by drugs such as the amino glycosides. Electrolyte disturbances include hyperkalaemia, uricacidaemia and a fall in serum magnesium. Other complications include hypertension, weight gain, hirsuties, gingival hypertrophy and diabetes mellitus. Lymphoproliferative diseases can be seen long term. Cholestasis can develop. Neurotoxicity is shown by mood alterations, seizures, tremor and headaches.

Cyclosporine and tacrolimus can interact with other drugs so changing blood levels (table 35.5).

Cyclosporine is costly, has a narrow therapeutic index and its use has to be monitored carefully. Trough blood levels have to be taken, initially frequently, and then at regular intervals. The dose is based on the nephrotoxicity of the drug. Side-effects may necessitate reducing the dose, and indeed replacing cyclosporine with azathioprine.

Tacrolimus (FK506) is a macrolide antibiotic somewhat similar to erythromycin. It is more poweful than cyclosporine in inhibiting interleukin-2 (IL2) synthesis

Table 35.5. Interactions between cyclosporine (and tacrolimus) and other drugs

Increase cyclosporine levels
Erythromycins
Ketoconazole
Corticosteroids
Metoclopromide
Verapamil
Diltiazem
Tacrolimus

Decrease cyclosporine levels
Octreotide
Phenobarbitone
Phenytoin
Rifampicin
Septrin (Bactrim)
Omeprazole

and expression of IL2 receptors. It has been used to salvage patients with repeated liver rejection [130]. It is comparable to cyclosporine in terms of patient and graft survival [141]. There are, however, fewer episodes of acute and refractory rejection and less concurrent need for corticosteroid immunosuppression. There are more adverse effects necessitating discontinuation. These include nephrotoxicity, diabetes, diarrhoea, nausea and vomiting. Neurological complications (tremors and headache) are more common with tacrolimus than cyclosporine [41]. The main indication for tacrolimus continues to be refractory rejection.

Azathioprine side-effects include myelosuppression, cholestasis, peliosis hepatitis, peri-sinusoidal fibrosis and veno-occlusive disease.

Cell migration and chimerism

Donor cells have been identified in recipients of liver transplantation. This chimerism could influence the host immune system with development of tolerance to donor tissues. After 5 years immunosuppression might be stopped without allograft rejection [126]. Unfortunately, complete withdrawal is possible in only about 20% and significant reduction in 55% [155]. Patients transplanted for autoimmune hepatitis may suffer a recurrence when immunosuppression is reduced.

Post-operative course

This is not easy, particularly in the adult. Further surgery such as draining abscesses, biliary reconstruction or control of bleeding may be necessary.

Re-transplantation is required in 20–25% of patients [121]. The main indications are primary graft failure, hepatic arterial thrombosis and chronic rejection, often with cytomegalovirus infection. Renal dialysis may be required. Results are not so satisfactory as for the first transplant.

Factors determining an adverse result include poor pre-transplant nutrition, Child's grade C, a raised serum creatinine level and severe coagulation abnormalities. Poor results are related also to the amount of blood products required during surgery, the need for renal dialysis post-transplant and severe rejection. The operation is easier in those without cirrhosis and portal hypertension, and the peri-operative mortality is considerably less.

The causes of death are surgical—technical complications (either immediate or late), biliary leaks, and hepatic rejection, with or without infections often related to large doses of immunosuppressants.

The patient usually spends about 10 days in intensive care, 2 months in hospital or attending outpatients and is fully rehabilitated in 6 months. The patients' quality of life and well being is greatly improved but follow-up of 9-month survivors showed that only 43% were working [5]. The patients age, duration of disability before transplant and type of job significantly affected the post-transplant employment status.

More than 87% of paediatric survivors are fully rehabilitated with normal growth, both physical and psychosocial.

Post-transplantation complications

(table 35.6)

The three major problems are:
1 primary graft non-function (days 1–2);
2 infections (days 3–14 and on); and
3 rejection (from 5–10 days).

The presenting features of all three are very similar, namely large, firm, tender liver, increasing jaundice, fever and leucocytosis. Specialist investigations must be available [57]. These include CT [37], ultrasound and Doppler imaging, HIDA scanning, angiography, and percutaneous and endoscopic cholangiography.

Protocol liver biopsies are taken of the donor liver pre-transplant and 5 days, 3 weeks and 1 year after transplantation. No particular feature in the donor liver biopsy predicts function after transplantation. However,

Table 35.6. Complications of liver transplantation

Weeks	Complications
1	Primary graft non-function
	Bile leaks
	Renal
	Pulmonary
	CNS
1–4	Cellular rejection
	Cholestasis
	Hepatic artery thrombosis
5–12	CMV hepatitis
	Cellular rejection
	Biliary complications
	Hepatic artery thrombosis
	Hepatitis C
12–26	Cellular rejection
	Biliary complications
	Hepatitis B
	EBV hepatitis
	Drug-related hepatitis
>26	Ductopenic rejection (rare)
	CMV hepatitis
	EBV hepatitis
	Portal vein thrombosis
	Disease recurrence
	(HBV, HCV, tumours)

zonal or severe focal necrosis and neutrophil infiltration predicts a poor early course [62].

Primary graft non-function

This affects less than 5% of patients between the first 24 and 48 hours. It is related to inadequate preservation of the donor liver, particularly a long (more than 30 hours) cold preservation time and especially warm ischaemia time [134], to hypoacute rejection or shock in the recipient. It is marked by worsening state, hyperdynamic instability, renal dysfunction, lacticacidosis with increases in prothrombin time, bilirubin, transaminases and potassium (fig. 35.7). Blood glucose falls.

Re-transplantation is the only treatment and should not be delayed in the hope of spontaneous improvement.

Technical complications

Surgical complications will develop in about a half and will greatly increase the 6 months' mortality rate (32% versus 11%) [74]. They are most frequent in children with small vessels and bile ducts.

Doppler ultrasonography or, if necessary, arteriography is used for detection of hepatic arterial, hepatic venous, portal venous or inferior vena caval stenosis or thrombosis [96].

Routine ultrasound or CT is used to evaluate hepatic parenchymal abnormalities, peri-hepatic collections and biliary dilatation.

Cholangiography through the T-tube is used to define biliary abnormalities. HIDA scanning may be used to show biliary leaks.

Guided biopsy allows aspiration of fluid collections.

Sub-capsular hepatic necrosis. This is related to disproportionate size between donor and recipient. It can be visualized by CT scanning and usually resolves spontaneously [1].

Bleeding. This is more likely if removal of a diseased liver has left a raw area on the diaphragm or if there have been adhesions from previous surgery or infection. Treatment is by transfusion and reoperation if necessary.

Vascular complications

Hepatic artery thrombosis is most frequent in children. It may be related to the hypercoagulable state developing in the first few days after transplant. It may be acute, marked by clinical deterioration, fever and bacteraemia. The thrombosis may be silent, presenting days to weeks later as a bile leak. Loss of the hepatic artery supply may result in necrosis of the complete donor bile duct. Hepatic infarction, abscess formation and intra-hepatic biloma can follow (fig. 35.8). Doppler ultrasound is diagnostic and the findings are confirmed by angiography. Re-transplantation is usually the only treatment although stenoses of vascular anastomoses have been treated with balloon angioplasty [108].

Portal vein thrombosis is often silent, presenting with variceal bleeding weeks to months after transplant. A spleno-renal shunt is occasionally effective treatment and balloon angioplasty has been done. Re-transplant is often necessary.

Hepatic vein occlusion is common in patients who have had liver transplantation for the Budd–Chiari syndrome.

Occasionally there is stricture of the supra hepatic vena caval anastomosis and this can be treated by balloon dilatation.

Biliary tract complications

Bile secretion recovers spontaneously over a 10–12-day

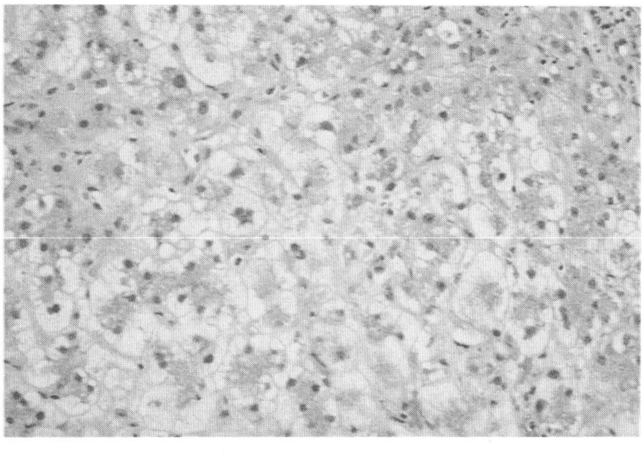

Fig. 35.7. Graft ischaemia 2 days after liver transplantation. Hepatocytes are swollen with loss of cytoplasm. (Stained H & E, ×350.)

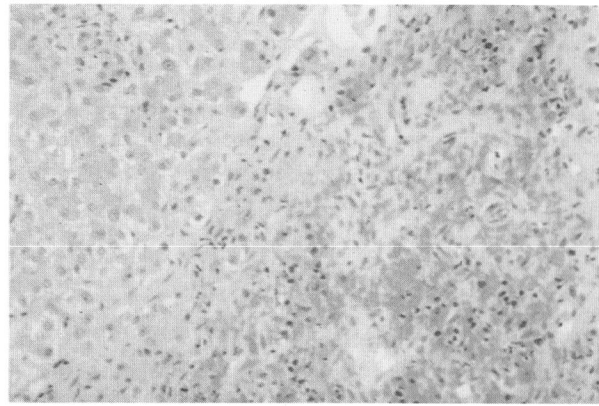

Fig. 35.8. Hepatic infarction, 3 days post-transplant, due to hepatic artery thrombosis. An area of necrotic, infarcted hepatocytes with haemorrhage adjoins normal liver tissue. (Stained H & E, ×150.)

Table 35.7. Biliary complications of liver transplantation

Leaks
Early (3–4 weeks)
    Anastomotic
    T-tube
Late (4 months) after T-tube removal

Strictures
Anastomotic (6–12 months)
Intra-hepatic (3 months)

period and is strongly dependent upon bile salt secretion [125]. Complications include bile leaks, malposition of T-tubes and bile duct obstruction, usually stricture [76, 147] (table 35.7).

Bile leaks may be early (first 30 days) related to the bile duct anastomosis or late (about 4 months) after T-tube removal [105]. Abdominal pain and peritoneal signs may be masked by immunosuppression.

Early leaks are diagnosed by routine T-tube cholangiography on the third day or, after T-tube removal, by ERCP [124]. HIDA scanning may be useful.

Bile leaks are usually treated by insertion of a naso-biliary catheter with or without a stent. Anastomotic leaks, especially from Roux-en-Y choledocho-jejunostomy, usually require surgery.

Extra-hepatic anastomotic strictures. These present after about 5 months with intermittent fever and fluctuating serum biochemical abnormalities. They are treated by percutaneous cholangiography or ERCP, dilatation and stenting.

Non-anastomotic or 'ischaemic-type' biliary strictures develop in 2–19% [44]. They are associated with multi-factorial damage to the hepatic arterial plexus around bile ducts. Factors include prolonged cold ischaemia time, hepatic arterial thrombosis, ABO blood group incompatibility, rejection, foam-cell arteriopathy and a positive lymphocytotoxic cross-match. Peri-biliary arteriolar endothelial damage contributes to segmental microvascular thrombosis and hence to multiple segmental biliary ischaemic strictures.

Ischaemic strictures usually develop after several months. They are treated by balloon dilatation and stenting. Re-transplant may be necessary if conservative methods have failed. Early strictures usually require retransplant for their correction.

Renal failure

Oliguria is virtually constant post-transplant, but in some renal failure is more serious. The causes include pre-existing kidney disease, hypotension and shock, sepsis, nephrotoxic antibiotics and cyclosporine or tacrolimus. They accompany severe graft rejection or overwhelming infection. Dialysis does not improve survival.

Pulmonary complications

Mechanical factors contribute. Air passing through an abnormal pulmonary vasculature can cause cerebral air emboli.

In infants, death *during* liver transplantation may be related to platelet aggregates in small lung vessels [49]. Intravascular catheters, platelet infusions and cell debris from the liver may contribute.

The right diaphragm is paralysed and right lower lobe atelectasis is common. In one series, 20% of patients underwent bronchoscopy [70]. Adult respiratory distress syndrome with thrombocytopenia can be related to endotoxaemia. It requires intubation [89].

Pleural effusion is virtually constant and in about 18% aspiration is necessary. About 20% have pulmonary infections, including pneumonia, empyema, and lung abscesses. The causes are frequently opportunist.

A post-transplant hyperdynamic syndrome tends to normalize with time [46].

The hepato-pulmonary syndrome (Chapter 6) is usually corrected by liver transplant but only after a stormy post-transplant course with prolonged hypox-aemia, mechanical ventilation and long intensive care [69].

During and after the operation, circulatory overload may lead to pulmonary oedema, especially in those with pre-existing pulmonary hypertension.

Non-specific cholestasis

This is frequently seen in the first few days, serum bilirubin peaking at 14–21 days. Liver biopsy suggests extra-hepatic biliary obstruction but cholangiography is normal. Factors concerned include mild preservation injury, sepsis, haemorrhage and renal failure. If infection is controlled, liver and kidney function usually recover but a prolonged stay in the intensive care unit is usually necessary.

Rejection

Immunologically, the liver is a privileged organ with regard to transplantation, having a higher resistance to immunological attack than other organs. The liver cell probably carries fewer surface antigens. Nevertheless, episodes of rejection of varying severity, are virtually constant.

Cellular rejection is initiated through the presentation of donor HLA antigens by antigen-presenting cells to host-helper T cells in the graft. These helper T cells secrete IL2 which activates other T cells. The accumulation of activated T cells in the graft leads to T-cell mediated cytotoxicity and a generalized inflammatory response [3].

Hyper-acute rejection is rare and is due to presensitization to donor antigens. Acute (cellular) rejection is fully reversible, but chronic (ductopenic) is not. The two may merge into one another [45]. The diagnosis of rejection from opportunistic infections is difficult and protocol liver biopsies are essential. Increased immunosuppression to combat rejection favours infection.

Acute cellular rejection

This is seen between 5 and 30 days post-transplant. The patient feels ill, there is mild pyrexia and tachycardia. The liver is enlarged and tender. Serum bilirubin, transaminases and prothrombin time increase. The liver enzyme changes lack specificity and a liver biopsy is essential.

Primary targets for the infiltrating immunocytes are epithelial cells of the bile ducts and endothelium of hepatic arteries and veins. Rejection is shown by the classical triad of portal inflammation, bile duct damage (fig. 35.9) and sub-endothelial inflammation of portal and terminal hepatic veins (endothelialitis) (fig. 35.10). Eosinophils may be conspicuous [53], and hepatocellular necrosis may be seen.

Rejection may be graded into mild, moderate and severe [34, 59] (table 35.8). Follow-up biopsies may show eosinophils, resembling a drug reaction, and infarct-like areas of necrosis, perhaps secondary to portal venous obstruction by lymphocytes. Hepatic arteriography shows separation and narrowing of hepatic arteries (fig. 35.11). Very rarely, the acute rejection may continue as graft-versus-host disease [111]. Low hepatic tissue con-

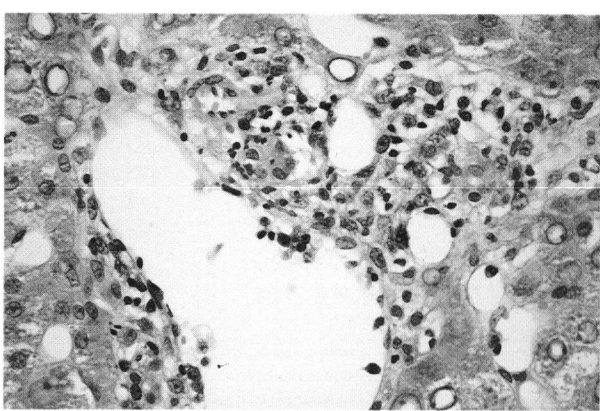

Fig. 35.10. Acute cellular rejection 8 days post-transplant. Liver biopsy shows portal zone infiltration with mononuclear cells and endothelialitis of cells lining the portal vein. (Stained H & E, ×100.)

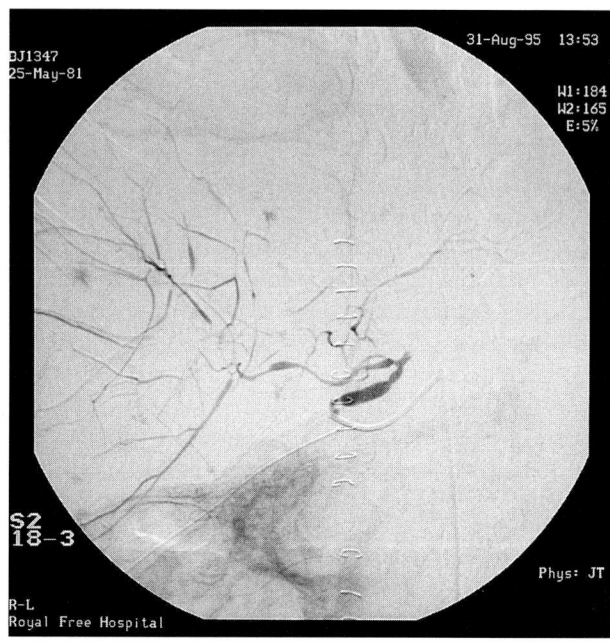

Fig. 35.11. Hepatic arteriogram in acute cellular rejection shows separation of intra-hepatic arterial tree with marked narrowing.

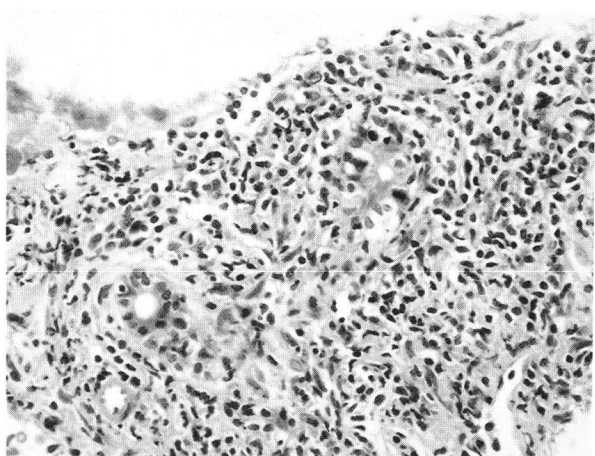

Fig. 35.9. Acute rejection: a damaged bile duct infiltrated with lymphocytes is seen in a densely cellular portal tract. (Stained H & E, ×100.)

centrations of cyclosporine or tacrolimus are associated with cellular rejection [117]. In 85%, treatment is successful by increasing immunosuppression. Boluses of methylprednisolone (3000 mg) are given on alternate days. Those who are steroid-resistant receive OKT3 murine monoclonal antibody for 10–14 days. Tacrolimus rescue may also be tried. Those failing to respond to these measures proceed to ductopenic rejection. Retransplant may be needed if the rejection continues.

Table 35.8. NIDDK-LTD nomenclature and grading of liver allograft rejection [34]

Acute rejection*		Chronic (ductopenic) rejection†	
Grade	Histopathological findings	Grade	Histopathological findings
A0 (none)	No rejection		
A1 (mild)	Rejection infiltrate in some, but not most, of the triads, confined with the portal spaces	B1 (early or mild)	Bile duct loss, without centrilobular cholestasis, perivenular sclerosis, or hepato-cellular ballooning or necrosis and dropout
A2 (moderate)	Rejection infiltrate involving most or all of the triads, with or without spillover into lobule. No evidence of centrilobular hepatocyte necrosis, or dropout	B2 (intermediate/moderate)	Bile duct loss, with one of the following four findings: centrilobular cholestasis, perivenular sclerosis, hepato-cellular ballooning, necrosis and dropout
A3 (severe)	Infiltrate in some or all of the triads, with or without spillover into the lobule, with or without inflammatory cell linkage of the triads, associated with moderate–severe lobular inflammation and lobular necrosis and dropout	B3 (late or severe)	Bile duct loss, with at least two of the following four findings: centrilobular cholestasis, perivenular sclerosis, hepato-cellular ballooning, or centrilobular necrosis and dropout

* The diagnosis of acute rejection is based on the presence of at least two of the following three findings: (1) predominantly mononuclear but mixed portal inflammation; (2) bile duct inflammation/damage; and (3) subendothelial localization of mononuclear cells in the portal and central veins. Thereafter, the severity of rejection is graded on the above findings.
† Bile duct loss in >50% of triads must be present for the diagnosis.

Chronic ductopenic rejection

Bile ducts are progressively damaged and ultimately disappear [152]. The mechanism seems to be immuno-logical with aberrant expression of HLA class II antigens on bile ducts. Donor–recipient HLA class I mismatch with class I antigen expression on bile ducts is contributory.

Ductopenic rejection is defined as loss of interlobular and septal bile ducts in 50% of portal tracts. Duct loss is calculated by the ratio of hepatic artery and numbers of bile ducts within a portal tract (normal greater than 0.7). Preferably 20 portal tracts should be studied [59]. Foam-cell obliterative arteriopathy increases the bile duct damage. Ductopenic rejection may be graded histologically into mild, moderate and severe (table 35.8) [34].

Bile duct epithelium is penetrated by mononuclear cells resulting in focal necrosis and rupture of the epithelium. Eventually bile ducts disappear and portal inflammation subsides (fig. 35.12). Larger arteries (not seen in a needle biopsy) show sub-intimal foam cells, intimal sclerosis and hyperplasia. Centrizonal necrosis and cholestasis develop and eventually biliary cirrhosis.

Ductopenic rejection usually follows early cellular rejection (at about 8 days) with bile duct degeneration (at about 10 days) and ductopenia (at about 60 days) [143]. The onset is usually within the first 3 months but can be sooner. Cholestasis is progressive.

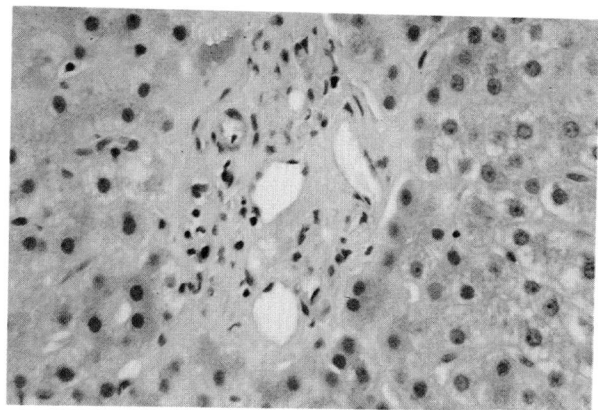

Fig. 35.12. Chronic ductopenic rejection. Bile ducts have disappeared from the portal tract which contains only a hepatic arterial branch, a portal vein and no inflammation. (Stained H & E, ×350.)

Hepatic angiography shows markedly narrowed hepatic arteries with no peripheral filling and often with branch vessel occlusions (fig. 35.13) [150]. Major hepatic arterial occlusions lead to bile duct stricturing shown by cholangiography (fig. 35.14). CMV cholangitis can also lead to the sclerosing cholangitis picture.

Ductopenic rejection is not usually reversed by increasing the immunosuppression although some patients, seen early, respond to tacrolimus and steroids.

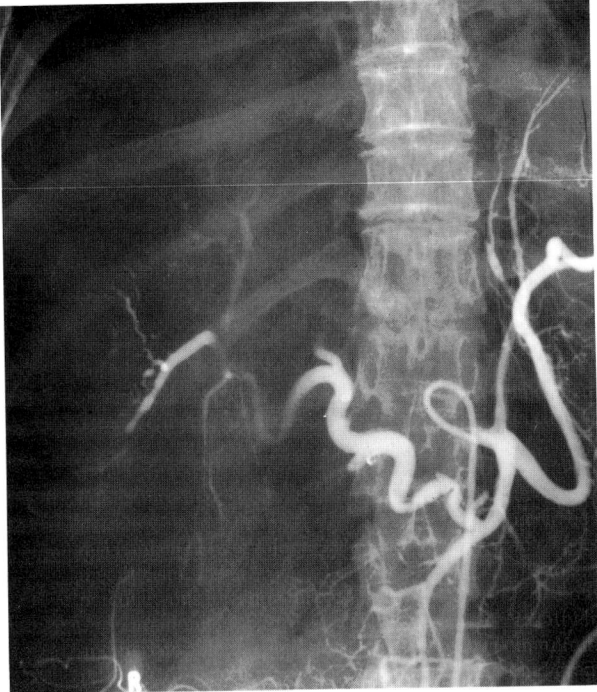

Fig. 35.13. Chronic rejection: coeliac angiogram shows pruning of intra-hepatic arterial tree. Filling did not improve later in the series.

Usually re-transplant is the only effective treatment. Irreversible ductopenic rejection is decreasing with better immunosuppression.

Infections

Over 50% will experience an infection in the post-transplant period [36, 54]. This may be primary, reactivation or related to opportunistic organisms (fig. 35.15). It is important to note the degree of immunosuppression and history of any previous infection [146].

Bacterial

These are seen during the first 2 weeks post-transplant and are usually related to technical complications. They include pneumonia, wound sepsis, liver abscess and biliary sepsis. They may be related to invasive procedures and vascular lines. They are usually of endogenous origin and selective bile decontamination is used prophylactically by some centres.

CMV

This infection is a virtually constant complication of liver transplantation and is symptomatic and serious in 30%. It may be primary (infection coming from the transfused blood or donor liver), or may be a secondary reactiva-

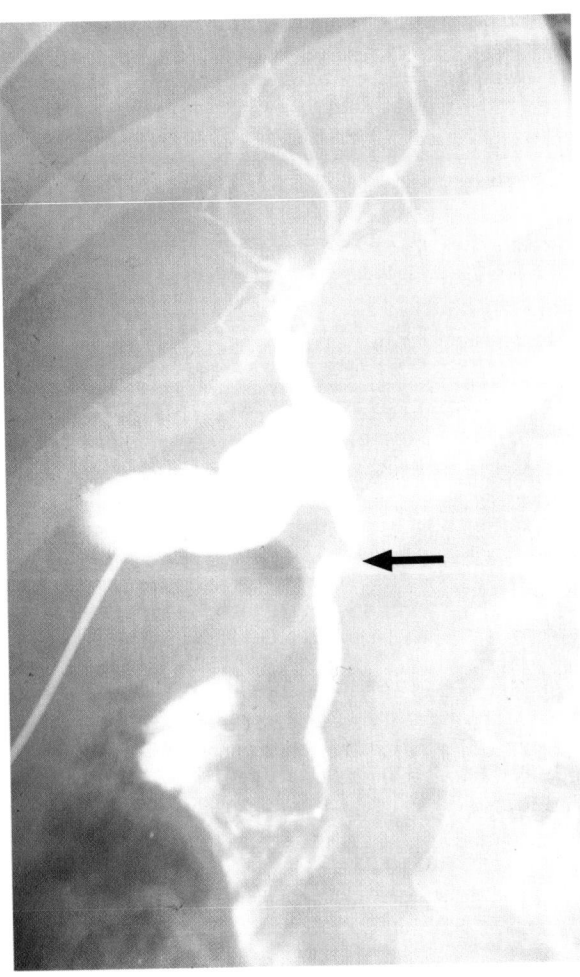

Fig. 35.14. A T-tube cholangiogram at 1 year post-transplant shows a stricture (arrowed) at the site of the original bile duct anastomosis.

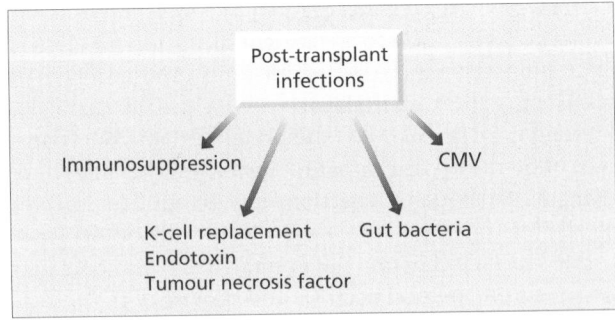

Fig. 35.15. Mechanisms of infection in liver transplant recipients.

tion. The single, most important risk factor is a positive donor with CMV antibodies [48]. It could be largely prevented by using sero-negative donors.

Infection is increased in those receiving antilymphocyte therapy, having a retransplant or with hepatic artery thrombosis.

Infection presents within 90 days post-transplant, the peak at 28–38 days. It continues for months or even years in those with poor graft function who require heavy immunosuppression. CMV is the most common cause of hepatitis in the liver allograft patient [100].

The picture is of a mononucleosis-like syndrome with fever and increased transaminases. The lungs are particularly involved in the severely affected. Chronic infection is associated with cholestatic hepatitis and the vanishing bile duct syndrome.

'Pizza-pie' retinitis and gastroenteritis are other features.

Liver biopsy shows clusters of polymorphs and lymphocytes with CMV intra-nuclear inclusions (fig. 35.16). Bile duct atypia and endothelialitis are absent. Immuno-staining, using a monoclonal antibody against an early CMV antigen, allows early diagnosis (fig. 35.17) [101]. The shell-vial cell culture technique is positive within 16 hours.

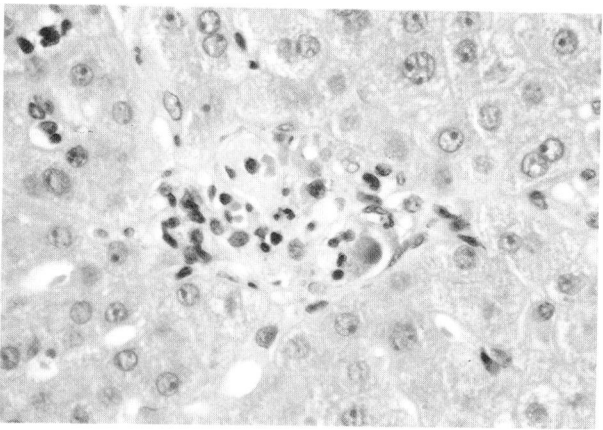

Fig. 35.16. Cytomegalovirus hepatitis 4 weeks post-transplant. A focus of inflammation shows hepatocytes containing inclusion bodies. (Stained H & E, ×160.)

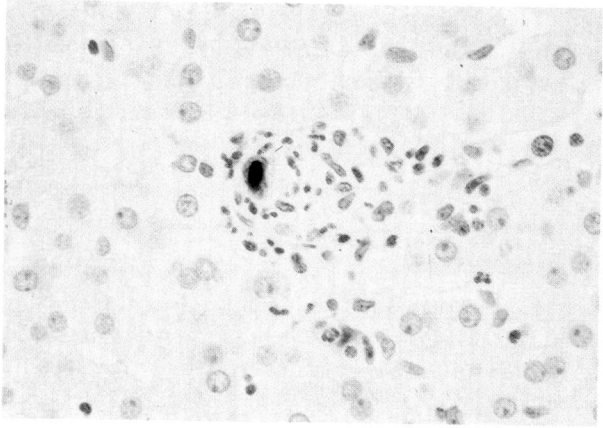

Fig. 35.17. Immunoperoxidase staining (×160) confirms the presence of CMV as a brown intra-nuclear deposit.

Gancyclovir long-term from the first post-operative day to day 100 almost completely eliminates CMV infection [154]. Unfortunately, it is expensive and the drug must be given intravenously.

If possible, immunosuppression must be reduced. Chronic CMV is an indication for re-transplant.

Herpes simplex virus

This infection is usually related to immunosuppression-induced reactivation. Liver biopsy shows confluent areas of necrosis with surrounding viral inclusions. This infection has virtually disappeared with prophylactic acyclovir.

Epstein–Barr virus

This is most frequent in children as a primary infection. It causes a mononucleosis–hepatitis picture [85] (fig. 35.18). It is often asymptomatic. The diagnosis is made serologically (see Chapter 16). A *lymphoproliferative syndrome* is a complication, shown as a diffuse lymphadenopathy or widespread polyclonal lympho-proliferation in internal organs. Treatment is by lowering immunosuppression and giving high-dose acyclovir. A monoclonal B-cell lymphoma can develop and this has a poor prognosis.

Adenovirus

These infections are seen in children. They are usually mild, but fatal hepatitis can develop. There is no recognized treatment.

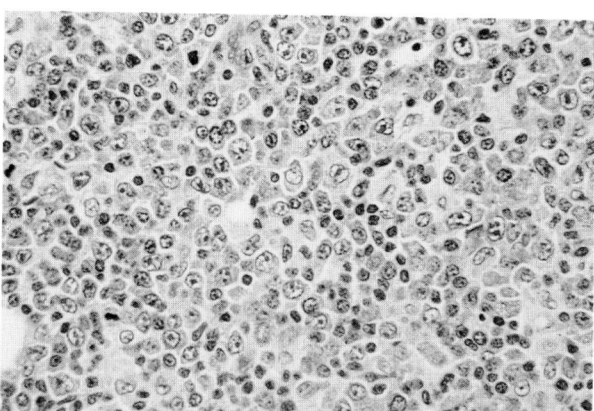

Fig. 35.18. Epstein–Barr-associated lymphoproliferative syndrome in a child aged 3 years, 6 months post-transplant. A lymph node from the porta hepatis shows sheets of lymphocytes replacing the normal lymph gland architecture. (Stained H & E, ×300.)

Varicella

This can complicate transplants in children. It is treated with intravenous gancyclovir [80].

Nocardia

This infection usually affects the chest but skin and cerebral lesions may also occur [107].

Fungal infections

Candida is the most usual, seen at 16 days and usually within the first 2 months [146]. It is treated with amphotericin B but survival is reduced.

Pneumocystis pneumonia

This presents in the first 6 months. It is diagnosed by bronchoscopy and broncho-alveolar lavage. It is prevented by bactrim (septrin) prophylaxis one tablet daily for the first 6 months post-transplant.

Malignancies

Six per cent of organ transplant recipients will develop cancer, usually within 5 years of the transplant [137]. Many are related to immunosuppression. Malignancies include lymphoproliferative diseases, skin cancers and Kaposi's sarcoma [56, 137]. Yearly cancer surveillance is essential for all patients post-transplant.

Drug-related toxicity

This must always be considered in any reaction whether hepatitic or cholestatic. Causative drugs include azathioprine, cyclosporine, tacrolimus, antibiotics, antihypertensives and antidepressants.

Disease recurrence

Hepatitis B appears at 2–12 months and may lead to cirrhosis and liver failure within 1–3 years. Hepatitis C is seen at any time after the first 4 weeks. Hepato-cellular malignancies recur in the graft or as metastases, usually within the first 2 years.

The possible recurrence of primary biliary cirrhosis is discussed in Chapter 14. Budd–Chiari syndrome may reappear quite soon after transplantation when anticoagulation is stopped [119].

Central nervous system toxicity

Severe central nervous changes can follow liver transplantation [4, 20, 33]. Half the patients show fits, children being more susceptible than adults [4, 28]. Cyclosporine-associated fits are controlled by phenytoin but this induces (accelerates) cyclosporine metabolism.

Central pontine myelinolysis is related to sudden alterations in serum electrolytes, perhaps in combination with cyclosporine. CT scan shows white-matter lucencies.

Cyclosporine is bound to lipoprotein fractions in the blood. Patients with low serum cholesterol values are at particular risk of central nervous system toxicity after the transplant [4].

Cerebral infarction is related to peri-operative hypotension, or air/microthrombus embolism.

Psychosis may complicate high-dose steroid treatment for rejection.

Cerebral abscess is part of the general infection.

Headaches in the first few weeks can persist. Cyclosporine has been incriminated but in most instances the cause is obscure [20].

Tremor is a common side-effect of immunosuppressants including corticosteroids, tacrolimus, cyclosporin and OKT3. It is usually mild, but occasionally requires reduction or cessation of medication.

A second transplant is associated with more and greater mental abnormalities, seizures and focal motor defects [77].

Bone disease

Patients having liver transplants usually have some previous degree of hepatic osteodystrophy. The bones deteriorate post-transplant with vertebral collapse in 38% during the second 3 months. The cause is multifactorial and includes cholestasis, corticosteroid therapy and bed rest. Recovery takes place with time.

Ectopic soft tissue calcification [91]

This can develop diffusely and is associated with respiratory insufficiency and bone fractures. It is secondary to hypocalcaemia due to citrate infused in fresh frozen plasma, and in addition renal failure and secondary hyperparathyroidism. Tissue injury and administration of exogenous calcium lead to the soft tissue calcium deposition.

Conclusion

Hepatic transplantation is a tremendous undertaking that does not begin or end with the surgery. It can only be performed in special centres, prepared and able to provide facilities.

The patient and his family need psychiatric and social support. There must be a back-up programme to procure organs. The survivor requires life-long medical and surgical supervision, together with costly drugs, both immunosuppressive and antibiotic.

Attending physicians must keep in touch with the transplant centre. They should be aware of possible late complications, particularly infections, chronic rejection, biliary complications, lymphoproliferative and other malignancies.

It is not surprising that the cost is high. Technical advances, the training of more transplant teams and less costly immunosuppression will lower the cost. It must be compared with hospital costs of the last year of life of patients with liver disease who would have been candidates for transplantation had circumstances permitted [153].

References

1 Abecassis J-P, Pariente D, Hazebroucq V *et al.* Subcapsular hepatic necrosis in liver transplantation: CT appearance. *Am. J. Roentgenol.* 1991; **156**: 981.

2 Abouljoud MS, Levy MF, Rees CR *et al.* Comparison of treatment with transjugular intra-hepatic portosystemic shunt or distal splenorenal shunt in the management of variceal bleeding prior to liver transplantation. *Transplantation* 1995; **59**: 226.

3 Adams D. Mechanisms of liver allograft rejection in man. *Clin. Sci.* 1990; **78**: 343.

4 Adams DH, Ponsford S, Gunson B *et al.* Neurological complications following liver transplantation. *Lancet* 1987; **i**: 949.

5 Adams PC, Ghent CN, Grant DR *et al.* Employment after liver transplantation. *Hepatology* 1995; **21**: 140.

6 Arnold JC, O'Grady JG, Bird GL *et al.* Liver transplantation for primary and secondary hepatic apudomas. *Br. J. Surg.* 1989; **76**: 248.

7 Ascher N, Lake JR, Emond J *et al.* Liver transplantation for hepatitis C virus-related cirrhosis. *Hepatology* 1994; **20**: 24S.

8 Badger IL, Czerniak A, Beath S *et al.* Hepatic transplantation in children using reduced size allografts. *Br. J. Surg.* 1992; **79**: 47.

9 Beath SV, Brook GD, Kelly DA *et al.* Successful liver transplantation in babies under 1 year. *Br. Med. J.* 1993; **307**: 825.

10 Benner KG, Lee RG, Keeffe EB *et al.* Fibrosing cytolytic liver failure secondary to recurrent hepatitis B after liver transplantation. *Gastroenterology* 1992; **103**: 1307.

11 Bilheimer DW, Goldstein JL, Grundy SM *et al.* Liver transplantation to provide low-density-lipoprotein receptors and lower plasma cholesterol in a child with homozygous familial hypercholesterolemia. *N. Eng. J. Med.* 1984; **311**: 1638.

12 Bismuth H, Houssin D. Reduced sized orthotopic liver grafts in hepatic transplantation in children. *Surgery* 1984; **95**: 367.

13 Bismuth H, Castaing D, Ericzon BG *et al.* Hepatic transplantation in Europe. First report of the European liver transplant registry. *Lancet* 1987; **ii**: 674.

14 Bismuth H, Samuel D, Castaing D *et al.* Orthotopic liver transplantation in fulminant and subfulminant hepatitis—the Paul Brousse experience. *Ann. Surg.* 1995; **222**: 109.

15 Bizollon T, Ducerf C, Trepo C. New approaches to treatment of hepatitis C virus infection after liver transplantation using ribavirin. *J. Hepatol.* 1995; **22** (Suppl. 2).

16 Blankenstejn JD, Terpstra OT. Liver preservation: the past and the future. *Hepatology* 1991; **13**: 1235.

17 Bloomer JR, Weimer MK, Bossenmaier IC *et al.* Liver transplantation in a patient with protoporphyria. *Gastroenterology* 1989; **97**: 188.

18 Broelsch CE, Whitington PF, Emond JC *et al.* Liver transplantation in children from living related donors. Surgical techniques and results. *Ann. Surg.* 1991; **214**: 428.

19 Broelsch CE, Burdelski M, Rogiers X *et al.* Living donor for liver transplantation. *Hepatology* 1994; **20**: 49S.

20 Bronster DJ, Emre S, Mor E *et al.* Neurologic complications of orthotopic liver transplantation. *Mt. Sinai J. Med.* 1994; **61**: 63.

21 Burdelski M, Rodeck B, Latta A *et al.* Treatment of inherited metabolic diseases by liver transplantation. *J. Inherit. Metab. Dis.* 1991; **14**: 604.

22 Busuttil RW, Shaked A, Millis JM *et al.* One thousand liver transplants. The lessons learned. *Ann. Surg.* 1994; **219**: 490.

23 Cames B, Rahier J, Burtomboy G *et al.* Acute adenovirus hepatitis in liver transplant recipients. *J. Pediatr.* 1992; **120**: 33.

24 Casavilla FA, Reyes J, Tzakis A *et al.* Liver transplantation for neonatal hepatitis as compared to the other two leading indications for liver transplantation in children. *J. Hepatol.* 1994; **21**: 1035.

25 Cardona J, Houssin D, Gauthier F *et al.* Liver transplantation in children with Alagille syndrome—a study of twelve cases. *Transplantation* 1995; **60**: 339.

26 Chardot C, Candinas D, Mirza D *et al.* Biliary complications after paediatric liver transplantation: Birmingham's experience. *Transplant. Int.* 1995; **8**: 133.

27 Chazouilleres O, Kim M, Combs C *et al.* Quantitation of hepatitis C virus RNA in liver transplant recipients. *Gastroenterology* 1994; **106**: 994.

28 Cilio MR, Danhaive O, Gadisseux JF *et al.* Unusual cyclosporin related neurological complications in recipients of liver transplants. *Arch. Dis. Child.* 1993; **68**: 405.

29 Cochat P, Faure JL, Divry P *et al.* Liver transplantation in primary hyperoxaluria type 1. *Lancet* 1989; **i**: 1142.

30 Colledan M, Grendele M, Gridelli B *et al.* Long-term results after liver transplantation in B and delta hepatitis. *Transplant. Proc.* 1989; **21**: 2421.

31 Cuervas-Mas V, Millan J, Gavaler JJ *et al.* Prognostic value of preoperatively obtained clinical and laboratory data in predicting survival following liver transplantation. *Hepatology* 1986; **6**: 922.

32 Davies SE, Portmann BC, O'Grady JG *et al.* Hepatic histological findings after transplantation for chronic hepatitis B virus infection, including a unique pattern of fibrosing cholestatic hepatitis. *Hepatology* 1991; **13**: 150.

33 De Groen PC, Aksamit MD, Rahela J *et al.* Central nervous system toxicity after liver transplantation. *N. Engl. J. Med.* 1987; **317**: 861.

34 Demetris AJ, Seaberg EC, Batts KP *et al.* Reliability and predictive value of the National Institute of Diabetes and Digestive and Kidney Diseases liver transplantation database. Nomenclature and grading system for cellular rejection of liver allografts. *Hepatology* 1995; **21**: 408.

35 DiBisceglie AM. Liver transplantation for hepatitis C: the promise and the challenge. *Hepatology* 1995; **22**: 660.

36 Dominguez EA. Long-term infectious complications of liver transplantation. *Semin. Liver Dis.* 1995; **15**: 133.

37 Dupuy D, Costello P, Lewis D *et al*. Abdominal CT findings after liver transplantation in 66 patients. *Am. J. Roentgenol.* 1991; **156**: 1167.

38 Emond JC, Whitington PF, Thistlethwaite JR *et al*. Transplantation of two patients with one liver: analysis of a preliminary experience with 'split-liver' grafting. *Ann. Surg.* 1990; **212**: 14.

39 Esquivel CO, Iwatsuki S, Gordon RD *et al*. Indications for pediatric liver transplantation. *J. Pediatr.* 1987; **111**: 1039.

40 Esquivel CO, Van Thiel DH, Demetris AJ *et al*. Transplantation for primary biliary cirrhosis. *Gastroenterology* 1988; **94**: 1207.

41 European FK 506 Multicentre Liver Study Group. Randomized trial comparing tacrolimus (FK 506) and cyclosporin in prevention of liver allograft rejection. *Lancet* 1994; **344**: 423.

42 Feray C, Gigou M, Samuel D *et al*. The course of hepatitis C virus infection after liver transplantation. *Hepatology* 1994; **20**: 1137.

43 Feray C, Gigou M, Samuel D *et al*. Influence of the genotypes of hepatitis C virus on the severity of recurrent liver disease after liver transplantation. *Gastroenterology* 1995; **108**: 1088.

44 Fisher A, Miller CM. Ischemic-type biliary structures in liver allografts — the Achilles heel revisited. *Hepatology* 1995; **21**: 589.

45 Freese DK, Snover DC, Sharp HL *et al*. Chronic rejection after liver transplantation: a study of clinical, histopathological and immunological features. *Hepatology* 1991; **13**: 882.

46 Gadano A, Hadengue A, Widmann JJ *et al*. Hemodynamics after orthotopic liver transplantation: study of associated factors and long-term effects. *Hepatology* 1995; **22**: 458.

47 Gane EJ, Portmann BC, Naoumov NV *et al*. Long-term outcome of hepatitis C infection after liver transplantation. *N. Engl. J. Med.* 1996; **334**: 815.

48 Gish RG, Lau JYN, Brooks L *et al*. Ganciclovir treatment of hepatitis B virus infection in liver transplant recipients. *Hepatology* 1996; **23**: 1.

49 Goncalves I, Hermans D, Chretian D *et al*. Mitochondrial respiratory chain defect: a new etiology for neonatal cholestasis and early liver insufficiency. *J. Hepatol.* 1995; **23**: 290.

50 Grant D, Wall W, Mimeault R *et al*. Successful small-bowel/liver transplantation. *Lancet* 1990; **335**: 181.

51 Gretch DR, Bacchi CE, Gorey L *et al*. Persistent hepatitis C virus infection after liver transplantation: clinical and virological features. *Hepatology* 1995; **22**: 1.

52 Gugenheim J, Samuel D, Reynes M *et al*. Liver transplantation across ABO blood group barriers. *Lancet* 1990; **336**: 519.

53 Gupta SD, Hudson M, Burroughs AK *et al*. Grading of cellular rejection after orthotopic liver transplantation. *Hepatology* 1995; **21**: 46.

54 Hadley S, Samore MH, Lewis WD *et al*. Major infectious complications after orthotopic liver transplantation and comparison of outcomes in patients receiving cyclosporin or FK 506 as primary immunosuppression. *Transplantation* 1995; **59**: 851.

55 Herbert A, Corbin D, Williams A *et al*. Erythropoietic protoporphyria: unusual skin and neurological problems after liver transplantation. *Gastroenterology* 1991; **100**: 1753.

56 Hertzler G, Gordon SM, Piratzky J *et al*. Case report: fulminant Kaposi's sarcoma after orthotopic liver transplantation. *Am. J. Med. Sci.* 1995; **309**: 278.

57 Holbert BL, Campbell WL, Skolnick ML. Evaluation of transplanted liver and postoperative complications. *Radiol. Clin. North Am.* 1995; **33**: 521.

58 Ichida T, Matsunami H, Kawasaki S *et al*. Living related-donor liver transplantation from adult to adult for primary biliary cirrhosis. *Ann. Intern. Med.* 1995; **122**: 275.

59 International Working Party. Terminology of hepatic allograft rejection. *Hepatology* 1995; **22**: 648.

60 Jurim O, Shackleton CR, Mc Diarmid SV *et al*. Living-donor liver transplantation at UCLA. *Am. J. Surg.* 1995; **169**: 529.

61 Kahn D, Govaler JS, Makowka L *et al*. Gender of donor influences outcome after orthotopic liver transplantation in adults. *Dig. Dis. Sci.* 1993; **38**: 1485.

62 Kakizoe S, Yanaga K, Starzl TE *et al*. Evaluation of protocol before transplantation and after reperfusion biopsies from human orthotopic liver allografts: considerations of preservation and early immunological injury. *Hepatology* 1990; **11**: 932.

63 Kalayoglu M, Sollinger HW, Stratta RJ *et al*. Extended preservation of the liver for clinical transplantation. *Lancet* 1988; **i**: 617.

64 Kaufman SS, Wood RP, Shaw BW Jr *et al*. Orthotopic liver transplantation for type I Crigler–Najjar syndrome. *Hepatology* 1986; **6**: 1259.

65 Kelleher MB, Iwatsuki S, Sheahan DG. Epithelioid hemangioendothelioma of liver: Clinicopathological correlation of 10 cases treated by orthotopic liver transplantation. *Am. J. Surg. Pathol.* 1989; **13**: 999.

66 Kirschner BS, Baker AL, Thorp FK. Growth in adulthood after liver transplantation for glycogen storage disease type I. *Gastroenterology* 1991; **101**: 238.

67 Klingspor L, Stintzing G, Tollemar J. Deep *Candida* infection in child liver transplant recipients: serological diagnosis and incidence. *Acta. Paediatr.* 1995; **84**: 424.

68 Koneru B, Flye MW, Busuttil RW *et al*. Liver transplantation for hepatoblastoma: the American experience. *Ann. Surg.* 1991; **213**: 118.

69 Krowka MJ. Hepatopulmonary syndrome: what are we learning from interventional radiology, liver transplantation and other disorders? *Gastroenterology* 1995; **109**: 1009.

70 Krowka MF, Cortese DA. Pulmonary aspects of chronic liver disease and liver transplantation. *Mayo Clin. Proc.* 1985; **60**: 407.

71 Lake JR, Wright TL. Liver transplantation for patients with hepatitis B: what have we learned from our results. *Hepatology* 1991; **13**: 796.

72 Largilliere C, Houssin D, Gottrand F *et al*. Liver transplantation for ornithine transcarbamylase deficiency in a girl. *J. Pediatr.* 1989; **115**: 415.

73 Lavine JE, Lake JR, Ascher NL *et al*. Persistent hepatitis B virus following interferon alfa therapy and liver transplantation. *Gastroenterology* 1991; **100**: 263.

74 Lebeau G, Yanaga K, Marsh JW *et al*. Analysis of surgical complications after 397 hepatic transplantations. *Surg. Gynecol. Obstet.* 1990; **170**: 317.

75 Lerut JP, Laterre PF, Lavenne-Pardonge E *et al*. Liver transplantation and haemophilia A. *J. Hepatol.* 1995; **22**: 583.

76 Letourneau JG, Hunter DW, Payne WD *et al.* Imaging of and intervention for biliary complications after hepatic transplantation. *Am. J. Roentgenol.* 1990; **154**: 729.

77 Lopez OL, Estol C, Colina I *et al.* Neurological complications after liver transplantation. *Hepatology* 1992; **16**: 162.

78 Luketic VA, Shiffman ML, McCall JB *et al.* Primary hepatocellular carcinoma after orthotopic liver transplantation for chronic hepatitis B infection. *Ann. Intern. Med.* 1991; **114**: 212.

79 McDiarmid SV, Blumberg DA, Remotti H *et al.* Mycobacterial infections after pediatric liver transplantation: a report of three cases and review of the literature. *J. Pediatr. Gastroenterol.* 1995; **20**: 425.

80 McGregor RS, Zitelli BJ, Urbach AH *et al.* Varicella in pediatric orthotopic liver transplant recipients. *Pediatrics* 1989; **83**: 256.

81 McPeake J, Williams R. Liver transplantation for hepatocellular carcinoma. *Gut* 1995; **36**: 644.

82 Maddrey WC (ed.) *Transplantation of the Liver* (2nd edn). Norwalk: Appleton & Lange 1994.

83 Makowka L, Tzakis AG, Mazzaferro V *et al.* Transplantation of the liver for metastatic endocrine tumors of the intestine and pancreas. *Surg. Gynecol. Obstet.* 1989; **168**: 107.

84 Malatack JJ, Finegold DN, Iwatsuki S *et al.* Liver transplantation for type 1 glycogen storage disease. *Lancet* 1983; **i**: 1073.

85 Malatack JJ, Gartner JC Jr, Urbach AH *et al.* Orthotopic liver transplantation, Epstein–Barr virus, cyclosporine and lymphoproliferative disease: a growing concern. *J. Pediatr.* 1991; **118**: 667.

86 Martinez OM, Villanueva JC, Lawrence-Miyasuki L *et al.* Viral and immunological aspects of Epstein–Barr virus infection in pediatric liver transplant recipients. *Transplantation* 1995; **59**: 519.

87 Marzano A, Smedile A, Abate M *et al.* Hepatitis type C after orthotopic liver transplantation: reinfection and disease recurrence. *J. Hepatol.* 1994; **21**: 961.

88 Mieles LA, Esquivel CO, Van Thiel DH *et al.* Liver transplantation for tyrosinemia: a review of 10 cases from the University of Pittsburgh. *Dig. Dis. Sci.* 1990; **35**: 153.

89 Miyata T, Yokoyama I, Todo S *et al.* Endotoxaemia, pulmonary complications and thrombocytopenia in liver transplantation. *Lancet* 1989; **ii**: 189.

90 Moritz MJ, Jarrell BE, Munoz SJ *et al.* Regeneration of the native liver after heterotopic liver transplantation for fulminant hepatic failure. *Transplantation* 1993; **55**: 952.

91 Munoz SJ, Nagelberg SB, Green PJ *et al.* Ectopic soft tissue calcium deposition following liver transplantation. *Hepatology* 1988; **8**: 476.

92 Narumi S, Roberts JP, Emond JC *et al.* Liver transplantation for sclerosing cholangitis. *Hepatology* 1995; **22**: 451.

93 Neuberger JM, Adams DH. Is HLA matching important for liver transplantation? *J. Hepatol.* 1990; **11**: 1.

94 Notten A, Sproat IA. Hepatic artery thrombosis after liver transplantation: temporal accuracy of diagnosis with Duplex US and the syndrome of impending thrombosis. *Radiology* 1996; **198**: 553.

95 Olivieri NF, Liu PP, Sher GD *et al.* Brief report: combined liver and heart transplantation for end-stage iron-induced organ failure in an adult with homozygous beta-thalassaemia. *N. Engl. J. Med.* 1994; **330**: 1125.

96 Orons PD, Zajko AB. Angiography and interventional procedures in liver transplantation. *Radiol. Clin. North Am.* 1995; **33**: 541.

97 Otte JB. Recent developments in liver transplantation: lessons from a 5-year experience. *J. Hepatol.* 1991; **12**: 386.

98 Otte JB, De Ville de Goyet J, Sokal E *et al.* Size reduction of the donor liver is a safe way to alleviate the shortage of size-matched organs in pediatric liver transplantation. *Ann. Surg.* 1990; **211**: 146.

99 Otte G, Herfarth C, Senninger N *et al.* Hepatic transplantation in galactosaemia. *Transplantation* 1989; **47**: 902.

100 Paya CV, Hermans PE, Wiesner RH *et al.* Cytomegalovirus hepatitis in liver transplantations. *J. Infect. Dis.* 1989; **160**: 752.

101 Paya CV, Holley KE, Wiesner RH *et al.* Early diagnosis of cytomegalovirus hepatitis in liver transplant recipients: role of immunostaining, DNA hybridization and culture of hepatic tissue. *Hepatology* 1990; **12**: 119.

102 Pereira BJG, Milford EL, Kirkman RL *et al.* Transmission of hepatitis C virus by organ transplantation. *N. Engl. J. Med.* 1991; **325**: 454.

103 Pichlmayr R, Weimann A, Ringe B. Indications for liver transplantation in hepatobiliary malignancy. *Hepatology* 1994; **20**: 335.

104 Polson RJ, Rolles K, Calne RY *et al.* Reversal of severe neurological manifestations of Wilson's disease following orthotopic liver transplantation. *Q. J. Med.* 1987; **64**: 685.

105 Popescu I, Sheiner P, Mor E *et al.* Biliary complications in 400 cases of liver transplantation. Prospective analysis of 93 conservative orthotopic liver transplantations. *Mt. Sinai J. Med.* 1994; **61**: 57.

106 Pruim J, Klompmaker IJ, Haagsma EB *et al.* Selection criteria for liver donation: a review. *Transplant. Int.* 1993; **6**: 226.

107 Raby N, Forbes G, Williams R. *Nocardia* infection in patients with liver transplants or chronic liver disease: radiologic findings. *Radiology* 1990; **174**: 713.

108 Revell SP, Noble-Jamieson G, Johnston P *et al.* Liver transplantation for homozygous familial hypercholesterolaemia. *Arch. Dis. Child.* 1995; **73**: 456.

109 Rhodes DF, Lee WM, Wingard JR *et al.* Orthotopic liver transplantation for graft-versus-host disease following bone marrow transplantation. *Gastroenterology* 1990; **99**: 536.

110 Ringe B, Wittekind C, Bechstein WO. The role of liver transplantation in hepatobiliary malignancy: a retrospective analysis of 95 patients with particular regard to tumor stage and recurrence. *Ann. Surg.* 1989; **209**: 88.

111 Roberts JP, Ascher NL, Lake J *et al.* Graft-versus-host disease after liver transplantation in humans: a report of four cases. *Hepatology* 1991; **14**: 274.

112 Rodby RA, Tyszka TS, Williams JW. Reversal of cardiac dysfunction secondary to type 1 primary hyperoxaluria after combined liver-kidney transplantation. *Am. J. Med.* 1991; **90**: 498.

113 Ryckman FR, Fisher RA, Pederson SH *et al.* Liver transplantation in children. *Semin. Pediatr. Surg.* 1992; **1**: 162.

114 Sallie R, Cohen AT, Tibbs CJ *et al.* Recurrence of hepatitis C following orthotopic liver transplantation: a polymerase chain reaction and histological study. *J. Hepatol.* 1994; **21**: 536.

115 Samuel D, Bismuth A, Mathieu D *et al.* Passive immunoprophylaxis after liver transplantation in HBsAg-positive patients. *Lancet* 1991; **337**: 813.

116 Samuel D, Boboc B, Bernuau J *et al*. Liver transplantation for protoporphyria: evidence for the predominant role of the erythropoietic tissue in protoporphyrin overproduction. *Gastroenterology* 1988; **95**: 816.

117 Sandborn WJ, Lawson GM, Cody TJ *et al*. Early cellular rejection after orthotopic liver transplantation correlates with low concentrations of FK 506 in hepatic tissue. *Hepatology* 1995; **21**: 70.

118 Selby R, Kadry Z, Carr B *et al*. Liver transplantation for hepatocellular carcinoma. *World J. Surg*. 1995; **19**: 53.

119 Seltman HJ, Dekker A, Van Thiel DH *et al*. Budd–Chiari syndrome recurring in a transplanted liver. *Gastroenterology* 1983; **84**: 640.

120 Shaw BW Jr, Wood RP. The operative procedures. In W.C. Maddrey, ed. *Transplantation of the Liver*. Elsevier, New York, 1988, p. 87.

121 Shaw BW, Gordon RD, Iwatsuki S. Retransplantation of the liver. *Semin. Liver Dis*. 1985; **5**: 394.

122 Shaw BW Jr, Martin DJ, Marquez JM *et al*. Venous bypass in clinical liver transplantation. *Ann. Surg*. 1984; **200**: 524.

123 Sheiner PA, Schwartz ME, Mor E *et al*. Severe or multiple rejection episodes are associated with early recurrence of hepatitis C after orthotopic liver transplantation. *Hepatology* 1995; **21**: 30.

124 Sheng R, Sammon JK, Zajko AB *et al*. Bile leak after hepatic transplantation: cholangiographic features, prevalence, and clinical outcome. *Radiology* 1994; **192**: 413.

125 Shiffman ML, Carithers RL Jr, Posner MP *et al*. Recovery of bile secretion following orthotopic liver transplantation. *J. Hepatol*. 1991; **12**: 351.

126 Starzl TE, Demetris AJ, Trucco M *et al*. Cell migration and chimerism after whole-organ transplantation: the basis of graft acceptance. *Hepatology* 1993; **17**: 1127.

127 Starzl TE, Demetris AJ, Van Thiel D. Liver transplantation. *N. Engl. J. Med*. 1989; **321**: 1014, 1092.

128 Starzl TE, Fung J, Tzakis A *et al*. Baboon to human liver transplantation. *Lancet* 1993; **341**: 65.

129 Starzl TE, Marchioro TL, von Kaulla KN *et al*. Homotransplantation of the liver in humans. *Surg. Gynecol. Obstet*. 1963; **117**: 659.

130 Starzl TE, Todo S, Fung J *et al*. FK 506 for liver, kidney and pancreas transplantation. *Lancet* 1989; **ii**: 1000.

131 Starzl TE, Todo S, Tzakis A *et al*. The many faces of multivisceral transplantation. *Surg. Gynecol. Obstet*. 1991; **172**: 335.

132 Sternlieb I. Wilson's disease: indications for liver transplants. *Hepatology* 1984; **4**: 15S.

133 Stieber AC, Zetti G, Todo S *et al*. The spectrum of portal vein thrombosis in liver transplantation. *Ann. Surg*. 1991; **213**: 199.

134 Strasberg SM, Howard TK, Molmenti EP *et al*. Selecting the donor liver: risk factors for poor function after orthotopic liver transplantation. *Hepatology* 1994; **20**: 829.

135 Suhr OB, Holmgren G, Steen L *et al*. Liver transplantation in familial amyloidotic polyneuropathy. *Transplantation* 1995; **60**: 933.

136 Tan KC, Yandza T, de Hemptinne B *et al*. Hepatic artery thrombosis in pediatric liver transplantation. *J. Pediatr. Surg*. 1988; **23**: 927.

137 Tan-Shalaby J, Tempero M. Malignancies after liver transplantation: a comparative review. *Semin. Liver Dis*. 1995; **15**: 156.

138 Todo S, Demetris AJ, Van Thiel D *et al*. Orthotopic liver transplantation for patients with hepatitis B virus-related liver disease. *Hepatology* 1991; **13**: 619.

139 Todo S, Starzl ET, Tzakis A *et al*. Orthotopic liver transplantation for urea cycle enzyme deficiency. *Hepatology* 1992; **15**: 419.

140 Tzakis AG, Reyes J, Tepetes K *et al*. Liver transplantation for Alagille's syndrome. *Arch. Surg*. 1993; **128**: 337.

141 U.S. Multicenter FK 506 Liver Study Group. A comparison of tacrolimus (FK 506) and cyclosporin for immunosuppression in liver transplantation. *N. Engl. J. Med*. 1994; **331**: 1110.

142 Valdivielso P, Escolar JL, Cuervas–Mons V *et al*. Heart and liver transplantation in a patient with familial hypercholesterolemia. *Ann. Intern. Med*. 1988; **108**: 204.

143 Van Hoek B, Ringers J, Kroes ACM *et al*. Temporary heterotopic auxiliary liver transplantation for fulminant hepatitis B. *J. Hepatol*. 1995; **23**: 109.

144 Van Thiel DH, Gavaler JS, Kam I *et al*. Rapid growth of an intact human liver transplanted into a recipient larger than the donor. *Gastroenterology* 1987; **93**: 1414.

145 Venook AP, Fenel LD, Roberts JP *et al*. Liver transplantation for hepatocellular carcinoma: results with preoperative chemoembolization. *Transplant. Surg*. 1995; **i**: 242.

146 Wade JJ, Rolando N, Hayllar K *et al*. Bacterial and fungal infections after liver transplantation: an analysis of 284 patients. *Hepatology* 1995; **21**: 1328.

147 Wallwork J, Williams R, Calne RY. Transplantation of liver, heart and lungs for primary biliary cirrhosis and primary pulmonary hypertension. *Lancet* 1987; **ii**: 182.

148 Watts RWE, Morgan SH, Danpure CJ *et al*. Combined hepatic and renal transplantation in primary hyperoxaluria type I: clinical report of nine cases. *Am. J. Med*. 1991; **90**: 179.

149 Welch CS. A note on transplantation of the whole liver in dogs. *Transplant. Bull*. 1955; **2**: 54.

150 White RM, Zajko AB, Demetris AJ *et al*. Liver transplant rejection. Angiographic findings in 35 patients. *Am. J. Roentgenol*. 1987; **148**: 1095.

151 Whitington PF, Balistreri WF. Liver transplantation in pediatrics: indications, contraindications, and pretransplant management. *J. Pediatr*. 1991; **118**: 169.

152 Wiesner RH, Ludwig J, Vanhoek B *et al*. Current concepts in cell-mediated hepatic allograft rejection leading to ductopenia and liver failure. *Hepatology* 1991; **14**: 721.

153 Williams JW, Vera S, Evans LS. Socioeconomic aspects of hepatic transplantation. *Am. J. Gastroenterol*. 1987; **82**: 1115.

154 Winston DJ, Wirin D, Shaked A *et al*. Randomized comparison of gancyclovir and high-dose acyclovir for long-term cytomegalovirus prophylaxis in liver transplant recipients. *Lancet* 1995; **346**: 69.

155 Williams R. Liver transplantation: effects of withdrawing long-term immunosuppression (in preparation; 1995).

156 Wright TL, Combs C, Kim M *et al*. Interferon-α therapy for hepatitis C virus infection after liver transplantation. *Hepatology* 1994; **20**: 773.

157 Yamaoka Y, Morimoto T, Inamoto J *et al*. Safety of the donor in living-related liver transplantation — an analysis of 100 parental donors. *Transplantation* 1995; **59**: 224.

158 Zandi P, Panis Y, Debray D *et al*. Pediatric liver transplantation for Langerhans' cell histiocytosis. *Hepatology* 1995; **21**: 129.

159 Zignego AL, Dubois F, Samuel D *et al*. Serum hepatitis delta virus RNA in patients with delta hepatitis and in liver graft recipients. *J. Hepatol* 1990; **11**: 102.

Index